OXFORD MEDICAL PUBLICATIONS

THE THEORY AND PRACTICE
OF PUBLIC HEALTH

THE THEORY AND PRACTICE
OF PUBLIC HEALTH

Edited by

W. HOBSON
B.Sc., M.D., D.P.H.

Consultant in Medical Education to the
World Health Organization; Formerly Professor of Social
and Industrial Medicine, University of Sheffield;
World Health Organization Visiting Professor,
Government of India; Adviser in Medical Education,
European Office, World Health Organization,
Copenhagen, and Chief of Staff Training,
World Health Organization, Geneva

FOURTH EDITION

LONDON
OXFORD UNIVERSITY PRESS
NEW YORK   TORONTO
1975

Oxford University Press, Ely House, London W.1

GLASGOW NEW YORK TORONTO MELBOURNE WELLINGTON
CAPE TOWN IBADAN NAIROBI DAR ES SALAAM LUSAKA ADDIS ABABA
DELHI BOMBAY CALCUTTA MADRAS KARACHI LAHORE DACCA
KUALA LUMPUR SINGAPORE HONG KONG TOKYO

ISBN 0 19 264222 7

© Oxford University Press 1961, 1965, 1969, 1975

First Edition 1961
Fourth Edition 1975

PRINTED IN GREAT BRITAIN
BY RICHARD CLAY (THE CHAUCER PRESS) LTD
BUNGAY, SUFFOLK

CONTENTS

CONTRIBUTORS

MICHAEL ROWLAND ALDERSON, M.D., D.P.H., D.C.H., D.Obst.R.C.O.G. *Professor of Medical Information Science, University of Southampton.*

WILLIAM FERGUSON ANDERSON, O.B.E., C.St.J., F.R.C.P. (Glas.), F.R.C.P. (Lond.), F.R.C.P. (Ed.). *David Cargill Professor of Geriatric Medicine, University of Glasgow.*

JOHN SELWYN ALFORD ASHLEY, M.B., Ch.B., M.F.C.M. *Senior Research Fellow in Medical Care, London School of Hygiene and Tropical Medicine.*

LEO BARIĆ, Ph.D., D.H.E., D.S.W. *Senior Lecturer, Department of Community Medecine, University of Manchester.*

LUIZ MARINO BECHELLI, M.D. *Professor and Head of Department of Dermatology, Faculdade de Medicina de Ribeirão Preto, University of São Paulo, Brazil.*

THOMAS HENRY BEWLEY, M.A., M.D., F.R.C.Psych., F.R.C.P.I. *Consultant Psychiatrist, St. Thomas's and Tooting Bec Hospitals, London.*

ROBERT FREDERIC BRIDGMAN, M.D. *Formerly Chief Medical Officer, Organization of Medical Care, World Health Organization, Geneva.*

COLIN FRASER BROCKINGTON, M.A., M.D., M.Sc., D.P.H., M.R.C.P. Barrister-at-Law. *Professor Emeritus of Social and Preventive Medicine, University of Manchester.*

SIR JOHN BROTHERSTON, M.A., M.D., F.R.C.P. (Ed.), F.R.C.P. (Glas.), D.P.H., Dr.P.H., F.R.S. (Ed.). *Chief Medical Officer, Scottish Home and Health Department, Edinburgh.*

FRANK EDWARD BRUCE, M.Sc.(Eng.), S.M., F.I.C.E., F.I.P.H.E., F.R.S.H. *Reader in Public Health Engineering, Imperial College of Science and Technology, University of London.*

JOHN PRINCE BULL, C.B.E., M.A., M.D., F.R.C.P. *Director, Medical Research Council Industrial Injuries and Burns Unit, Birmingham Accident Hospital.*

LUCAS JOHN HARMSWORTH BURTON, M.A., M.R.C.S., L.R.C.P., D.P.H., F.R.S.H. *Division of Health Manpower Development, World Health Organization, Geneva.*

JAMES RONALD BUSVINE, Ph.D., D.Sc., F.I.Biol. *Professor of Entomology as Applied to Hygiene, London School of Hygiene and Tropical Medicine.*

JOCELYN CHAMBERLAIN, M.B., B.S., D.C.H., M.F.C.M. *Senior Lecturer in Community Medicine, University College Hospital Medical School and the Royal Free Hospital School of Medicine.*

ANDREW BARNETT CHRISTIE, M.A., M.D., F.R.C.P., F.F.C.M., D.P.H., D.C.H. *Physician Superintendent, Fazakerley Hospital, Liverpool; Head of Department of Infectious Diseases, University of Liverpool.*

JOHN C. COLLINS, B.Sc., M.S.E., M.I.C.E., F.R.S.H. *Radiological Protection Officer, The University of Manchester.*

BRANKO CVJETANOVIĆ, M.D. *Chief Medical Officer, Bacterial Diseases, Division of Communicable Diseases, World Health Organization, Geneva.*

CHARLES D. FLAGLE, M.Sc., Dr.Eng. *Professor of Operations Research, and Professor of Public Health Administration, The Johns Hopkins University, Baltimore.*

GEORGE DICK FORWELL, M.B., Ch.B., Ph.D., F.R.C.P. (Ed.), D.P.H., D.I.H. *Principal Medical Officer, Scottish Home and Health Department, Edinburgh.*

HERBERT MICHAEL GILLES, K.O.S.J., B.Sc., M.D., F.R.C.P., F.F.C.M., D.T.M. and H. *Professor of Tropical Medicine, University of Liverpool.*

E. VAN GUNST, *Head of the Indoor Climate Division, Research Institute for Public Health Engineering, T.N.O., Delft.*

SVEN RICHARD SIXTEN HARALDSON, Dr. Med., D.H.E., C.F.P. *Scandinavian School of Public Health, Göteborg. Formerly Adviser on National Health Planning, World Health Organization.*

PETER HENDERSON, C.B., M.D., D.P.H. *Late Senior Principal Medical Officer, Department of Education and Science, London.*

YNGVE HOFVANDER, M.D. *Associate Professor, Pediatric Clinic, University Hospital, Uppsala; Consultant to the Swedish International Development Authority (SIDA) in Tropical Nutrition and Pediatrics.*

GROUP CAPTAIN PETER HOWARD, O.B.E., M.B., B.S., Ph.D., M.R.C.P., F.R.Ae.S. *Consultant Adviser in Aviation Physiology to the Royal Air Force Medical Branch.*

JAN VAN IERLAND, *Research Officer, Sound and Light Division, Research Institute for Public Health Engineering, T.N.O., Delft.*

DERRICK BRIAN JELLIFFE, M.D., F.R.C.P., F.A.P.H.A., F.A.A.P. *Head, Population, Family and International Health Division, School of Public Health, and Professor of Public Health and of Pediatrics, School of Medicine, University of California at Los Angeles.*

LEO A. KAPRIO, M.D., M.P.H., Dr.P.H. *Regional Director for Europe of the World Health Organization, Copenhagen.*

GEORGE STEWART KILPATRICK, M.D., F.R.C.P. (Ed.), M.R.C.P. *Dean of Clinical Studies, The Welsh National School of Medicine, and Senior Lecturer, Department of Tuberculosis and Chest Diseases, The Welsh National School of Medicine, University of Wales.*

PETER MICHAEL LAMBERT, M.B., Ch.B., D.P.H., M.F.C.M. *Senior Medical Statistician, Office of Population Censuses and Surveys, London.*

PATRICK JOSEPH LAWTHER, M.B., D.Sc., F.R.C.P. *Professor of Environmental Medicine in the University of London at St. Bartholomew's Hospital Medical College; Director, Medical Research Council Air Pollution Unit.*

JOHN ALEXANDER HUGH LEE, *Professor of Preventive Medicine, University of Washington, Seattle.*

ROBERT FRANCIS LESLIE LOGAN, M.D., F.R.C.P., D.I.H. *Professor of Organization of Medical Care, London School of Hygiene and Tropical Medicine.*

WILLIAM PHILIP DOWIE LOGAN, M.D., Ph.D., D.P.H., F.R.C.P. *Director, Division of Health Statistics, World Health Organization, Geneva.*

JEREMY NOAH MORRIS, D.Sc., F.R.C.P., D.P.H., D.C.H. *Professor of Public Health, University of London at the London School of Hygiene and Tropical Medicine.*

BRANKO NIŽETIĆ, M.D., D.Oph.(Parma), M.P.H. *Reader in Ophthalmology, University of Rome, Regional Officer for Public Health Ophthalmology, World Health Organization, Copenhagen.*

H. Ph. L. DEN OUDEN, *Staff Member, Research Institute for Public Health Engineering, T.N.O., Delft.*

The late MORLEY PARRY. *Sometime Food Hygiene Advisory Officer, Department of Health and Social Security, London.*

DONALD DARNLEY REID, M.D., D.Sc., F.R.C.P. *Professor of Epidemiology and Director, Department of Statistics and Epidemiology, London School of Hygiene and Tropical Medicine.*

JOHN ALEXANDER FRASER ROBERTS, C.B.E., F.R.S., M.A., M.D., D.Sc., F.R.C.P. *Geneticist, Paediatric Research Unit, Guy's Hospital Medical School, London. Formerly Director, Clinical Genetics Research Unit, Medical Research Council.*

THOMAS FERGUSON RODGER, C.B.E., B.Sc., M.B., F.R.C.P. (Ed.), F.R.C.P. (Glas.), D.P.M. *Professor of Psychological Medicine, University of Glasgow.*

FRANZ W. ROSA, M.D., M.P.H., *Team Leader, Intercountry Family Health Advisory Services, World Health Organization, Western Pacific Region, Manila.*

ARMAND PETER RUDERMAN, Ph.D. *Professor of Health Administration, School of Hygiene, University of Toronto.*

GOVINDAN SAMBASIVAN, M.B.B.S., D.T.M. *Formerly Director, Division of Malaria Eradication, World Health Organization, Geneva.*

RICHARD SELWYN FRANCIS SCHILLING, M.D., F.R.C.P., M.F.C.M., D.Sc., D.P.H., D.I.H. *Professor of Occupational Health and Director of the T.U.C. Centenary Institute of Occupational Health, London School of Hygiene and Tropical Medicine.*

DUCO ANTON SCHREUDER, Dr.Techn. *Institute for Road Safety Research SWOV, Voorburg, The Netherlands.*

ANDREW BEST SEMPLE, C.B.E., V.R.D., M.D., D.P.H., F.F.C.M. *Professor of Community and Environmental Health, University of Liverpool.*

CHARLES L. SENN, P.E., M.S.P.A. *Lecturer in Public Health, University of California at Los Angeles. Professor of Health Sciences, San Fernando Valley State College.*

KENNETH SODDY, M.D., F.R.C.Psych. *Physician in charge, Children's and Adolescents' Psychiatric Department, University College Hospital, London.*

JAMES HARLAN STEELE, D.V.M., M.P.H. *Professor of Environmental Health, School of Public Health, University of Texas.*

ALAN STOLLER, M.R.C.S., L.R.C.P., D.P.M., F.A.N.Z.P., F.R.C.Psych., F.A.C.M.A. *Chairman, Mental Health Authority, Melbourne, Victoria, Australia.*

MERVYN SUSSER, M.B., M.R.C.P. (Ed.), D.P.H. *Professor and Head, Division of Epidemiology, School of Public Health and Administrative Medicine, Columbia University, New York.*

GEORGE REGINALD WADSWORTH, M.D. *Late Professor of Physiology, University of Singapore.*

MICHAEL DONALD WARREN, M.D., M.R.C.P., F.F.C.M. *Professor of Health Services Administration and Director of the Health Services Research Unit, University of Kent at Canterbury.*

WILLIAM HARDY WICKWAR, M.A.(Lond). *Professor Emeritus of Political Science, University of South Carolina; Director of Planning, Richland Memorial Hospital, Columbia, South Carolina.*

RICHARD ROBERT WILLCOX, M.D., M.R.C.P. *Consultant Venereologist, St. Mary's Hospital, London, and King Edward VII Hospital, Windsor.*

THOMAS WILSON, C.B.E., M.D., D.P.H., D.T.M., D.T.H. *Emeritus Professor of Tropical Hygiene, University of Liverpool.*

PREFACE TO THE FOURTH EDITION

The fourth edition follows the third edition after an interval of five years. The book has catered for the needs not only of post-graduate students but there have also been considerable demands by undergraduate students in the newly developing countries and especially in certain parts of Africa. This is under-standable because more of the doctors' work there is concerned with public health than it is in highly developed countries. The front line doctor has also to be something of an administrator since it is expected that he will be the manager and co-ordinator of a team of auxiliaries and many of the clerical tasks will be delegated to them.

Since the last edition it has become the practice in the United States to use the term Community Medicine for departments of preventive medicine or public health; it is felt, however, that the book is now so well known by its familiar title that it would be a mistake to change it.

The term community medicine emphasizes the importance of the provision of comprehensive medical care services as well as preventive services. Socialist countries have always used the term public health because it is understood to include the provision of comprehensive care services (including hospital services) and thus there is no problem in continuing to use this term provided this is understood.

The changing fashion in names is well illustrated by the University of Sheffield; just after the war the term 'social medicine' was popularized by the influence of John Ryle, the new Department at Sheffield was called 'Social and Industrial Medicine'; in 1960 it was changed to 'Preventive Medicine and Public Health' and in 1972 was changed to 'Community Medicine'.

In this new edition continuing emphasis has been given to the use of managerial sciences in public health and the use of computers which has made possible the development of models, for example of epidemics; this use of simulation is a valuable new tool in planning the control of communicable disease and the organization and evaluation of health services [see especially CHAPTER 16, Typhoid Fever; CHAPTER 25, Tuberculosis; CHAPTER 29, Public Health Ophthalmology; and CHAPTERS 3, 41, 42, 45 and 46 on the planning and organization of health services].

It is sometimes thought that the managerial sciences are of value only in highly developed countries; on the contrary there are many simple techniques which can assist in helping the administrator with very limited resources.

In the programme guide for the World Health Organization Regional Office for Africa, the regional director has made this point, I quote, 'In Africa this means utilizing effective manage-ment techniques in order to obtain maximum yield from team work and local resources'.

Since the last edition there has been a complete reorganiza-tion of the N.H.S. in Britain with a great deal of emphasis placed on the use of managerial sciences in health management and planning, including the use of medical information systems. This has been covered in a new chapter entitled Statistics as a Basis for Health Management and Planning as well as in additions to the chapter on Systems of Medical Care.

In the last five years several new developments and changes have taken place which has necessitated a number of other new chapters. In the first edition I said that the complete eradica-tion of malaria might be achieved within 10–15 years. Un-happily the earlier promise has not yielded the results expected and the problem is so complex and difficult that a separate new chapter has been added on this topic. Family planning has also required a separate chapter in view of the importance given to it in recent times. Perhaps mention should be made of a new chapter on public health ophthalmology; this is a fresh ap-proach which tackles the problem of eye diseases as a whole, and has been reflected in the recent appointment of a medical officer for this purpose in the World Health Organization Regional Office for Europe, Copenhagen.

Clinicians are becoming more interested in the public health aspects of their work because of their participation in meetings of groups of experts to discuss control programmes; three new chapters have been added of special interest to clinicians: The Public Health Aspects of Certain Skin Diseases; Public Health Ophthalmology; The Venereal Diseases and Treponematoses, of interest not only to the venereologist and public health specialist but to all clinicians, in view of the recent resurgence of these diseases; The Control of Infection in Hospital; and The Evaluation of Screening Procedures. New chapters have also been added on rabies, the health problems of nomad peoples, and dependence as a public health problem. Several chapters have been completely rewritten, for example, air-borne infections, water and food-borne infections, administra-tive aspects of communicable disease control, health of mother and infant, occupation and health, the social services and health of the community. The pollution of the environment has again received special attention.

I wish to express my deep regret at the death of Dr. L. G. Norman, Chief Medical Officer, London Transport, and also of Mr. Morley Parry, formerly Food Hygiene Advisory Officer, Department of Health and Social Security, London. In addition a number of authors have retired from writing chapters. I wish to thank them for their valuable contributions in the past. They include: K. G. Bergin, Christine Cockburn, Robert Cruickshank, A. W. Schoen, Ian Taylor, B. B. Waddy, and T. B. Weber.

I also wish to welcome the following newcomers: M. R. Alderson, L. Barić, L. M. Bechelli, T. H. Bewley, A. B. Christie, B. Cvjetanović, S. R. Sixten Haraldson, P. Howard, D. B. Jelliffe, P. M. Lambert, B. Nižetić, F. W. Rosa, G. Sambasivan, R. S. F. Schilling, A. B. Semple, R. R. Willcox, W. H. Wickwar, and Jocelyn Chamberlain.

I wish to draw the reader's attention to a policy which is being developed of joint authorship for a number of chapters in which a senior and experienced contributor has been assisted by a colleague especially interested in research in the field.

As in previous editions efforts have been made to ensure that contributions reflect developments in public health in all parts of the world. Contributors have been recruited not only from Europe but also from North and South America, India and Australia.

It is unfortunate that with the increasing size of the book coupled with the high costs of publishing, the price has had to be raised, this is particularly unfortunate in the case of those undergraduate students who may wish to buy the book.

Myrtleville, Co. Cork,   W. HOBSON
   July 1974

PREFACE TO THE FIRST EDITION

Doctors and others concerned with the everyday problems of health and sickness approach their problems from varying points of view, depending on the way they have been trained and upon the particular kind of work they are engaged in. There are two important and essentially different lines of approach; the first is that concerned with the problem of health and sickness in the individual, and the second, the problem of health and disease in the community as a whole. Let us consider the first.

For at least 5,000 years the practising physician has been chiefly concerned with the cure of the sick individual, taking payment for services rendered and making a living from so doing; one can say therefore that in one respect he has had a vested interest in disease. The growth of knowledge in many fields has brought with it an increasing amount of specialization; this came to its height before the Second World War when clinical medicine had become highly 'departmentalized'. After the end of the war, however, there came an increasing awareness of the need to consider the person from what Smuts has called the holistic point of view, to look on the 'person' as a whole, as a part of his family and as a part of the community in which he lives. It has become increasingly apparent that both in diagnosis and treatment it is important for the physician to take into account the social and emotional aspects of illness. Many physicians in treating their patients are also concerned with the preventive aspects of illness and with the promotion of health in their patients. The family doctor, paediatrician, geriatrician, obstetrician, industrial physician, and even the general physician and surgeon, all in their special fields, are becoming more and more aware of the importance of considering the physical and emotional environment in relation to sickness, not only in practising their art but also in teaching and research. I believe that these topics should be included in textbooks of clinical medicine because they are part of the knowledge which the doctor needs for the handling of his patient in a full and comprehensive manner. This does not, of course, preclude the fact that there is a place for specialized textbooks on the social aspects of disease.

This new concept was emphasized by Ryle (1948) when he became the first Professor of Social Medicine at Oxford University just after the Second World War. He referred to this branch of medicine as 'Social Medicine'; whereas public health places the emphasis on the environment and deals with communities, social medicine derives its inspiration from the field of clinical experience and deals with individuals. Social medicine is really concerned with *the social aspects of disease in the sick person*. As far as hospital practice is concerned, it includes the whole of the work of the almoner's department. This includes social diagnosis and therapeutics and the organization of after-care, rehabilitation, and resettlement.

The second line of approach to sickness became important when it was realized that in order to combat epidemic disease it was necessary to consider a disease from a totally different aspect. Men began to ask, 'How can we prevent this disease from entering our country?' and when it had entered, 'How can we get rid of it?' From this developed the concept that the State had a responsibility for the health of the community as a whole, and there came into being public health organizations in which were employed administrators, doctors, nurses, engineers, and chemists to deal with the many problems.

The attack first of all was on the purely physical environment and on the communicable diseases, later on the organization and development of medical and social services became important as public health measures. Today there are new problems connected with non-communicable diseases such as accidents, radiation hazards, mental ill health, peptic ulcer, cancer, heart disease, the chronic rheumatic diseases, and the problems of old age; these can be tackled by such methods as health education, early detection of disease, and the provision of the necessary special services to deal with the problems. This pattern of development, which began in the economically highly-developed countries, is now being followed in the newly-developing countries. During recent years a totally new concept has emerged, namely the possibility of eradication of disease in the world as a whole. This can only be achieved by a 'wholly holistic' approach, i.e. by considering the whole community of man as the unit with which we deal; this has been made possible by the formation of the World Health Organization. Malaria is the first disease in history to be attacked simultaneously all over the world with the aim of complete eradication within a given period of time. It is expected that this will be achieved within 10–15 years; consideration is now being given to the eradication also of smallpox, diphtheria, and tuberculosis. This is truly a long way from the concept of the sick patient who comes to the doctor complaining of illness which the doctor diagnoses and treats. The efforts to control common diseases are not always popular with the practising physician, however. I am reminded at this point of the doctor I met in an Indian village who was complaining that since the teams of DDT sprayers had been to the village there had been no more malaria and he had as a result lost his livelihood. There are also other problems created by the large-scale control of killing diseases, i.e. over-population and the danger of malnutrition. It is probable that we could reduce the prevalence of 'chronic bronchitis' and lung cancer considerably in Western Europe if we were able to eliminate atmospheric pollution and cigarette smoking. Unfortunately we do not have the 'know how' with regard to these problems, and attempts to change old-established habits, such as smoking, by propaganda have so far failed.

The control or eradication of disease requires the participation and co-operation of large numbers of people of widely different interests, including politicians, administrators, doctors, teachers, and especially the people themselves. Certainly the doctor must play a large part in this work: it is important to realize that the function of a doctor now and in the future is not merely to treat the sick or even to promote health in the patient, he has a fuller and larger role, he must also play his part as an important member of a team concerned with disease control and eradication. If he is a public health officer or a medical administrator he will have to play a much greater part than, say, a physician in a hospital or a teacher of physiology in a medical school. There is clearly a great deal which the family doctor will have to know and which he will have to consider if he is to practise 'comprehensive medicine', i.e. to take into account the preventive and social aspects of illness when dealing with patients, and to play his part fully in community schemes for the control of disease and the promotion of health. The great majority of doctors and even teachers of medicine do not think on these lines, while the teaching curricula of many medical schools are still based on the anatomo-pathological concepts of the nineteenth century. Can we do anything to alter this state of affairs? Certainly many medical schools are making valiant efforts to effect changes. As far as textbooks are concerned there are plenty which give details of the work of the public health officer and the laws which govern his work in any one particular country. The majority of these books have been written by single authors, usually medical officers of health, and are intended for undergraduate and graduate students of the country of origin. They contain much detail of history, law, and administration for the examination requirements of the country concerned. These textbooks are usually unsuitable for students, whether undergraduate or postgraduate, from other countries or for administrators who wish to acquire some ideas on the best way to organize health services. It is true that customs and practices vary in different countries, and they will affect the way in which he will cope with problems within the family or the way in which health services are administered, nevertheless there is a great deal of basic knowledge and many fundamental principles relating to family care and health administration which are common to people everywhere; moreover, comparison of the relative advantages and disadvantages of different systems can be of great value in deciding what are the best ways of providing new services or of changing old ones. I have tried to fill this gap and to provide a textbook covering the community aspects of medicine which will give basic information of value to those engaged in health work in different parts of the world. The book has been planned also to provide for the requirements of postgraduate students in public health. It covers, for example, all the areas outlined by the National Board for Specialists in Public Health in the United States, and for the M.P.H. of North America and the D.P.H. (England), with the sole exception of biometrics; this is so specialized that it requires a textbook of its own. It is hoped also that undergraduate students will find it useful as a book of reference, particularly where 'public health' forms an important part of the undergraduate curriculum, for example, in Africa, South-East Asia, and South America where many doctors have to combine the functions of a public health doctor with those of treating the sick in a setting where prevention of disease is of enormous importance. For the postgraduate public health student reading an elective or special subject the book will need to be supplemented by further reading. A number of key references have been carefully selected from this point of view and these are listed under various headings at the end of each chapter.

A great deal of thought has been given to the title of the book. The word hygiene indicates to many those topics concerned with sanitation or with personal habits and cleanliness. The term 'social hygiene' has been used to describe services provided for diseases of special social importance, such as venereal disease, juvenile delinquency, problem families, etc. Some consider social medicine to be synonymous with schemes for social security or so-called socialized medicine, while Ryle's concept, as stated previously, is a wider one and embraces the social aspects of disease affecting the sick individual.

The term preventive medicine indicates that prevention is something which the doctor practises apart from cure; this separation is artificial; in dealing with a patient there should only be comprehensive medicine. Fifty years ago, the term preventive medicine meant little more than the use of immunizing procedures. In the United States preventive medicine has now a much wider meaning and is used to describe different levels of prevention, from prevention of illness to the prevention of disability or progression of disease! The term 'preventive medicine' is therefore capable of a wide variety of definitions depending upon individual concepts and, indeed, this idea has only to be extended a short stage farther, i.e. to the prevention of pain or of death, and the whole of medicine becomes preventive. In any case, not all aspects of preventive medicine can be covered by the work of the public health doctor, some form part of the work of the doctor treating individual patients, e.g. health education of patients, after care and rehabilitation. There is also some confusion of thinking when one refers to the work of assistant medical officers of health working in local authority clinics, most of this is not public health at all, immunization of persons, routine examinations are part of clinical medicine although the *organization* of clinics and services of this nature is public health.

We must not ignore the importance of the idea of the promotion of health; this is particularly stressed in the Constitution of the World Health Organization. The term 'positive health', however, now seems to have fallen into disfavour.

It seems to me that the best term to use to describe the community approach is one which has withstood the test of time, namely, 'public health'. A comprehensive definition has been given by Winslow (1951); it reads as follows:

'Public Health is the science and the art of preventing disease, prolonging life and promoting physical health and efficiency *through organized community efforts* for the sanitation of environment, the control of community infections, the education of the individual in principles of personal hygiene, the organization of medical and nursing service for the early diagnosis and preventive treatment of disease, and the development of the social machinery which will ensure to every individual in the community a standard of living adequate for the maintenance of health.'

It emphasizes the fact that no sound distinction, therefore, can be drawn between sanitation, preventive medicine, curative medicine, health promotion, and improvements of standards of living. All are parts of a comprehensive public health programme in the modern sense. The prime purpose of Public Health is to modify man's environment and his own behaviour in order to promote health and change the natural history of disease. The practice of public health is based on a number of scientific disciplines such as physics, chemistry, physiology, microbiology, parasitology, pathology, engineering, sociology, psychology, and statistics, but has one which belongs essentially to itself, namely, epidemiology. We can define epidemiology quite simply as the study of causes of morbidity and mortality within groups of people as distinct from their study within the individual person. Its methods of study are essentially statistical in nature.

Throughout this work the importance of the 'epidemiological approach' has always been kept in mind, not only in solving the problems of controlling disease but also in finding the most efficient ways of organizing health services, so-called 'operational research'. It is in this last respect that we can see the emergence of a new scientific discipline in the practice of public health, namely, public health administration. This is a subject which has now found acceptance in many universities as a subject worthy of academic study basing its work on studies in operational research and using techniques such as 'the case study method' developed by schools of business administration. It is sometimes said that administrators are born, not made; this is untrue, they are made by experience and training, and just as some men are more fitted to become surgeons so others are more fitted for the difficult task of administration. If we compare public health with clinical medicine then we can say that epidemiology is the diagnostic tool of public health and public health administration its therapeutic armamentarium.

W. HOBSON

Copenhagen,
February 1961

General Works on Public Health
and Related Subjects

Anderson, C. L. (1970) *Health Principles and Practice*, 6th ed., St. Louis.

Anderson, C. L. (1973) *Community Health*, 2nd ed., London.

Bhargava, G. S., ed. (1971) *War Against Disease; On the Health Front in South East Asia*, New Delhi.

Blum, H. L. (1969) *Health Planning 1969*, American Public Health Association Western Regional Office, San Francisco.

Boyer, J. L. (1967) *Précis d'Hygiène et de Médecine Preventive*, 4e éd., Paris.

Brockington, C. F. (1968) *World Health*, 2nd ed., London.

Brockington, C. F. (1965) *The Health of the Community*, 3rd ed., London.

Bryant, J. (1969) *Health and the Developing World*, Ithaca.

Burton, L. E., and Smith, H. H. (1970) *Public Health and Community Medicine for the Allied Professions*, Baltimore.

Clark, D. W., and MacMahon, B., eds (1967) *Preventive Medicine*, Boston.

Confrey, E. A., ed. (1961) *Administration of Community Health Services*, Chicago.

Cottrell, J. D. L. (1969) The teaching of public health in Europe, *Wld Hlth Org. Monogr. Ser.*, No. 58; also in French.

Davey, T. H., and Wilson, T. (1965) *Davey and Lightbody's Control of Disease in the Tropics*, 3rd. ed., London.

Davies, M. J. B. (1971) *Preventive Medicine, Community Health and Social Services*, 2nd ed. London.

Douglas-Wilson, I., and McLachlan, G., eds. (1974) *Health Service Prospects*, London.

Ehrlick, P. R., and Ehrlick, Anne H. (1970) *Population, Resources Environment. Issues in Human Ecology*, San Francisco.

Forsyth, Gordon (1973) *Doctors and State Medicine*, 2nd ed., London.

Gernez-Rieux, Ch., et Gervois, M. (1971) *Eléments de Médecine Préventive, Hygiène et Médecine Sociale*, 3e éd., Paris.

Godber, G. E. (1970) *Medical Care. The Changing Needs and Pattern*, London.

Goodman, N. M. (1971) *International Health Organizations and their work*, 2nd ed., London.

Greenwood, M. (1935) *Epidemic and Crowd Diseases*, London.

Grundy, F. (1964) *Preventive Medicine and Public Health*, 5th ed., London.

Hanlon, J. J. (1969) *Principles of Public Health Administration*, 5th ed., St. Louis.

Hilleboe, H. E., and Schaefer, M. (1967) *Papers and Bibliography on Community Health Planning*, Albany.

Hilleboe, H. E., and Larimore, G. W., eds (1965) *Preventive Medicine*, 2nd ed., Philadelphia.

Hobson, W. (1963) *World Health and History*, Bristol.

Hughes, C. C. (1969) *Disease and 'Development' in Africa*, Michigan.

Karb, S. L., and Steuart, G. W., eds (1963) *A Practice of Social Medicine*, Edinburgh.

Katz, A. M., and Felton, J. S. (1965) *Health of the Community*, New York.

King, M. (1966) *Medical Care in Developing Countries*, Nairobi.

Lathem, W., and Newbery, A. (1970) *Community Medicine, Teaching, Research and Health Care*, New York.

Lapeyssonie, L. (1970) *Eléments d'hygiène et de santé publique sous les tropiques*, 2e éd., Paris.

Leavell, H. R., and Clarke, E. G. (1965) *Preventive Medicine for the Doctor in his Community; an Epidemiological Approach*, 3rd ed., New York.

Mackintosh, J. M. (1965) *Topics in Public Health*, Edinburgh.

Maegraith, B. (1973) *One World. Heath Clark Lectures for 1970*, London.

McKeown, T., and Lowe, C. R. (1966) *An Introduction to Social Medicine*, Oxford.

Maxcy, K. F., ed. (1965) *Rosenau's Preventive Medicine and Public Health*, 9th ed., New York.

Omran, A. R. ed. (1974) *Community Medicine in Developing Countries*, New York.

Paul, H. (1964) *The Control of Diseases*, 2nd ed., Edinburgh.

Prywes, M., and Davies, A. M. (1968) *Health Problems in Developing States*, New York.

Roberts, L., and Shaw, K. M. (1966) *A Synopsis of Hygiene (Jameson and Parkinson)*, 12th ed., London.

Smillie, W. G. (1963) *Preventive Medicine and Public Health*, 3rd ed., New York.

Smolensky, J., and Haar F. B. (1972) *Principles of Community Health*, 3rd ed., Philadelphia.

Suchman, E. A. (1963) *Sociology and the Field of Public Health*, New York.

Susser, M., and Watson, W. (1971) *Sociology in Medicine*, 2nd ed., London.

Wegman, M. E. *et al.*, eds. (1973) *Public Health in the Republic of China*, New York.

World Health Organization. *Int. Dig. Hlth Leg. Cum. Indexes* 1948–54; 1955–59: 1960–64:; and Vol. 14 (1963) through to Vol. 24 (1973).

World Health Organization Regional Office for Africa (1970) *An Integrated Concept of the Public Health Services in Africa*, Brazzaville; also in French.

World Health Organization (1971) *Fourth Report on the World Health Situation (1965–1968)*, Geneva.

World Health Organization (1972) *Health Hazards of the Human Environment*, Geneva.

World Health Organization (1972) *World Directory of Schools of Public Health*, 2nd ed., Geneva. (French edition published 1973).

World Health Organization (1974) The work of WHO in 1973, *Off. Rec. Wld Hlth Org.*, **213**.

World Health Organization Statistics Annual for 1970, Geneva.
    (1973) Volume 1. *Vital Statistics and Causes of Death.*
    (1974) Volume 2. *Infectious Diseases: Cases, Deaths and Vaccinations.*
    (1974) *Health Personnel and Hospital Establishments.*

I

THE HISTORY OF PUBLIC HEALTH

C. FRASER BROCKINGTON

PUBLIC HEALTH FROM THE DAYS OF THE ANCIENTS UNTIL THE RENAISSANCE OF LEARNING

'On the State of Public Health', the phrase coined by John Simon, we can hardly speak with accuracy before the nineteenth century; for diseases continued to be largely undifferentiated and unclassified, and records of birth and deaths were not kept. All the evidence suggests that, with few exceptions of time and place, it was bad. Human life was short and hazardous and human communities died, like creatures of the wild, from a multitude of accidental causes. Against a host of invaders, noxious agents, and brutal assaults, the human race survived; but there was such fearful mortality that the population of the world advanced only slowly, and at different times and places it is known to have declined. The importance of each cause of death throughout the world will often have varied. Deliberate destruction of young life at various times may have played an important role; to this many earlier civilizations, Egyptian, Hebrew, Hindu, Chinese, Greek, Roman, and Teutonic, resorted, although such practices were strongly countered by religious sanctions, which have had their roots in the urge for survival. The killing of female infants has been a deeply rooted custom among nomads and hunters in Africa, south-west Asia, and India; it was practised in England before and after the Black Death; it caused the cessation of population growth in Japan between 1750 and 1850 during the Tokugawa era. Abortion, by artificial interference and by medicines, has also been widely practised; sometimes, as on the Pacific atoll of Yap today, it has caused a heavy decline in population. Yet such man-made hazards, including deaths in war and famine, have generally been of less importance than disease as a cause of death. In particular, infant and child mortality throughout many thousands of years continued grievously heavy. In enlightened Rome, famous for her aqueducts, public baths, thermae, and *Cloaca Maxima*—symbolizing a preoccupation with sanitation hardly less marked than that of Chadwick nearly 2,000 years later—and in Greece, it was customary to wait a week before naming the babies, for so few survived. Plague, smallpox, typhus, and other of the major killing epidemic diseases made periodic invasions, while chronic endemic infections, such as tuberculosis and malaria, reduced vitality and shortened life. In 400 B.C. the life expectancy of Grecian city dwellers, calculated from burial inscriptions, was about thirty years; and this may well be the general picture covering five thousand years of civilization. Some diseases, as still today, long remained localized, so that parts of the world were free while others suffered; but, in general, all diseases since differentiated seem to have affected man since earliest time. Indeed, a catalogue of conditions identified in Egyptian mummies, and in the writings of the Ancients, is almost as imposing as the latest nosology in the eighth revision of the *International Statistical Classification of Diseases, Injuries, and Causes of Death*.

Thus, there is nothing new in public health as a human need. Every community has in some measure felt the need for it. Disease and the impairment of vitality must always have been a disadvantage, however much the value system of a group made it possible to ignore the effects. The same sorts of hazards to health—epidemic spread, nutritional disorders, occupational risks, the perils of child bearing, the inadequacies of child care—have long prevailed.

From earliest civilizations some form of public health has existed—as a conscious effort by authority to apply social, scientific, and medical knowledge to the protection of the health of the community. Crete, Egypt, Greece, and Rome, all, at some time, built model towns and had finely developed sanitary systems. In Rome public baths were available to everyone; here the workers went in the evening 'to wash and to undo the fatigues of the day'. Inoculation against smallpox was practised in India and China before the Christian era. Rome built leprosaria and, like Greece, sought to regulate prostitution. The latrine and the flush closet were invented not as some have said during the European Renaissance, but in Crete 3,000 years before, or earlier. The Arabic civilization carried on where Rome and Greece left off; Cordoba and other Arabian cities had health departments with sanitary inspectors. The Arabs built the first hospitals with differentiation between patients (Khairallah, 1946). Europe in the Middle Ages continued to isolate leprosy and almost eliminated it. It also evolved, with hesitation and many second thoughts, primitive measures of limiting epidemic spread by the *cordon sanitaire*.

The cult of personal health is as old as medicine itself; at least as regards the foundation of maxims for healthy living. Indeed, the Ancients prided themselves upon their ability to dispense wisdom about how to live; although much of it was speculative and coloured by the hot and cold theory of disease. Some of the teaching in the major religions can also be regarded as a form of public health—aiming at sobriety, cleanliness, the avoidance of excretal pollution, the maintenance of family life, isolation of sufferers from infectious maladies, and the ritual abstention from food likely to convey parasites.

Barriers to the Development of Public Health

If public health has been an ever-present need there have been many forces acting against it. That which most readily springs to mind is ignorance of the scientific bases of health.

Environmental hygiene, as conducted by the Ancients and developed by the Arabs and in China, had little scientific background, except in the practice of inoculation against smallpox. Avicenna, in his *Qanun*, is said to have recogized the spread of disease by water; but it is more likely that the sanitary systems of ancient times depended upon aesthetic rather than scientific considerations. Contagion was recognized; indeed, Galen knew that phthisis was contagious; but the Greek theory of miasma, basically a belief in the odours of putrefaction as a cause of epidemics, had little, if any, relationship to the modern concept of the biology of infection. This miasmic theory, which gave little opportunity for specific public health action in the field of infectious disease, although it may have encouraged general sanitary measures, was stubbornly held for over two thousand years. Alongside this, the Hippocratic concept of disease—in its simplest form postulating the existence of a balance of four cardinal humours, blood, phlegm, black and yellow bile, themselves endowed with elementary qualities—hot, moist, dry, and cold—was equally unhelpful; for it denied the specificity of disease, which, with few exceptions, long continued unrecognized.

Nevertheless, although in comparison with modern times, ignorance of the scientific basis of health has been immense, it has never been such that effective public health could not have been developed. Social barriers have been of far greater importance in retarding progress in public health than has mere ignorance. Many scientific discoveries, which could have been so applied to public health, have passed unnoticed for want of a champion; much as did Hero's steam engine in Alexandria (A.D. 135) for lack of the values upon which an industrial society is built. The connexion between marshy terrain and malaria had been noted in Roman times and certainly by the eighteenth century drainage had proved itself to be an effective preventive. Quinine, in malaria, was being used prophylactically from the middle of the eighteenth century. We have had the technical knowledge for malaria eradication for a long time; but lacked the organization, the driving force, and, perhaps most of all, the sense of urgency necessary for its effective use. Why, we might equally well ask, did the Roman Empire not develop a service for maternity and child welfare, based upon the teaching of mothercraft in Galen's first volume of hygiene? Why did Rome not have an industrial health service? Many of the ill effects of industrial processes were already known; the 'trembling' due to inhalation of mercury vapour and lead paralysis were described by writers in Rome and Greece; and many early writers referred to the short-lived fate of those condemned to work in mines. Galen wrote that 'the life of many men is involved in the business of their occupation and it is inevitable that they should be harmed by what they do'. He added 'and it is impossible to change it'—symbolizing in his scepticism the long centuries when public health remained in the wilderness.

As the centuries passed the opportunities for effective action increased; but with little response. The Arabs described smallpox, anthrax, measles, and scabies as specific diseases, but with little change in public health practice, except perhaps to enhance the growing belief in contagion and the possibilities of preventing epidemic spread. The cure and prevention of scurvy was known to the Renaissance explorers—certainly by Jacques Cartier (1535), to whom the natives of the New World demonstrated the virtues of stewed pine cones in the treatment of his scorbutic sailors. But scurvy continued to lower the stamina of the northern hemisphere for many centuries—even after the final scientific proof of the effectiveness of oranges and lemons which James Lind was to provide on H.M.S. *Salisbury* (1748).

Likewise, the value of mercury for the treatment of syphilis was known at the beginning of the sixteenth century, within a few years of the epidemic spread of the disease. Benvenuto Cellini records in his autobiography that he himself drank the milk of a goat inuncted with mercury. Here was the basis of a system of clinics for the treatment of venereal disease; but none was adopted, save in France (1770) and Denmark (1790), until modern time. Such examples of knowledge slowly accumulating to little purpose, its benefits long denied to societies by social barriers of one sort or another, might be multiplied many times.

Such social forces have been many and varied. Public health could mean little to peoples whose food supplies were precarious and when a lack of general education made communication difficult. The value system, upon which the western world now leans heavily in its development of new health measures, has too often itself served as a deterrent, since health is not an absolute quality, but has the value which the culture of society accords it. In at least one major religion, health of the body was long thought to be of little account, and disease was a grace to purify the soul. Such an attitude continues to be common in many parts of the world today. The fact that none knew the size of the problem—at least till John Graunt analysed the *Bills of Mortality*—was a more serious handicap than we, in the age of statistics, can easily appreciate. And above all else, lack of organization, of responsible people, and of trained staff have been stubborn deterrents—themselves dependent upon a general failure to regard health and disease as proper subjects for public action.

Indeed, the most important social barrier has undoubtedly been the absence of recognition by authority of any precise obligation to develop public health services. Thus, the Ancients who wrote profusely about hygiene did not seem to consider public health in its widest sense. Galen's *Hygiene* was written for the intelligent few. The thoughts which came to him in Pergamos (A.D. 175), when, as physician to the School of Gladiators, he walked the wards of the Aesculapian hospital in sight of the Acropolis, were directed to the privileged. Barbarians and slaves were disregarded when he began to develop 'a certain art of hygiene'. So, too, in the cities of Rome and Greece, the aqueducts, fountains, and sewers still left masses of the people living in squalor in overcrowded tenement blocks. In the form we know it today—the highest measure of health for all—public health has never, until recently, been a national objective; for Galen was no exception in writing for the civilized citizens of the city states of Greece and Rome, and not for the barbarian hordes. This was the outlook of most people until the Renaissance, and, even after that, of all except the enlightened few. Nor is this surprising, since the struggle for freedom from ill health for all had necessarily to follow upon the other great battles for universal privileges which now began to be waged—to be free from tyranny, to be equal before the law, to vote; these were necessarily the first objectives, and upon their achievement, in the normal course of history, public health has depended.

The climate of opinion favourable to public health, when it did come, depended more upon enlightened self-interest than on a visionary dedication; the development of a social conscience often followed when diseases of squalor were seen to endanger the lives and health of the rich and poor alike; and when the health of industrial workers became an important consideration in improving output. There was little evidence until then that the authorities recognized any direct and continuing responsibility for the health of the people. Thus we approach the Renaissance of Learning with little, if anything, accomplished more than in the days of Rome and Greece. In terms of world population, which must reflect public health, numbers remained almost static; a probable 275 millions in A.D. 1000 had become about 400 millions by the time of the Renaissance of Learning.

PUBLIC HEALTH AFTER THE RENAISSANCE OF LEARNING

From about 1500 in Europe there began a growth of ideas about public health which, with the passage of time, led to action. The great minds of many countries began to evolve schemes for the improvement of the human race. The earliest of these was named by its author, Thomas More, *Utopia* (1516), and it was to this fictitious dreamland that many followed—the land where hygiene protected health and medicine restored it; where all that was needed was to hand, from hospitals to pure water, insurance against sickness and unemployment, health examinations before marriage. . . . English, French, Dutch, Italians, all had their pipe dreams. Daniel Defoe wrote *Essay on Projects* (1697); Ludovico Muratori, *Della Publica Felicita* (1749); Joseph Benoît-Fodéré (1798), *Les Lois éclairées*. . . . But all these ideas, and many others, were little more than ferments, each leavening a little the societies in which they appeared—none of which were ready yet to be organized, or organized yet to be ready, for any of the social services which we, today, find commonplace. Ramazzini's great work on occupational disease (1700) must have set people thinking; but the immediate effect upon the world's workers cannot have been very great. Progress in the understanding of disease processes, coupled with a growth of social conscience, led in various if limited ways, to public health action. Workers began to be protected against the worst risks of the most obvious poisonings; ingenious devices, including masks to put over the mouth and nose, and extraction conduits for sucking out the foul vapours of the workshops, were early inventions. Mercurial poisoning among the gilders caused a distinguished merchant of gilded bronzes in France to finance research through the Royal Academy of Sciences resulting in a reasonably effective suction device, the *'fourneau d'appel'*.

At the beginning of the sixteenth century in European countries compulsory parish registration began and when, a century later, the slow process of classifying disease was started, the study of vital and health statistics was the natural result. John Graunt (1662) analysed the London *Bills of Mortality*, the weekly compilations of deaths obtained by house-to-house visiting, from the sixteenth century; so began a process without which all public health must remain in the dark. 'Vague conjecture,' as William Farr was to remark two centuries later, 'began to be replaced by numerical expression.' In the middle of the eighteenth century (1758) Sweden created an official statistical commission charged with the tabulation of vital records received from the clergy. Civil registration of births and deaths followed—pioneered in the British colony of Massachusetts Bay (1639), it was extended by the *Napoleonic Code* (1792) to the whole of France, and thus influenced vital registration throughout western Europe, Latin America, and parts of the Middle East. Registration of births and deaths in England and Wales (1836) had the same, and perhaps even more, influence—largely because of the appointment of William Farr to the office of the Registrar General in Somerset House, London; it was to influence the course of events throughout the English-speaking world, including the Dominions and the United States.

Attempts were made from about 1600 onwards to establish services to meet one need or another, as these appealed to men of action; of these, many and varied, the following are but examples. Thus it was that St. Vincent de Paul (1576–1660), the parish priest of Châtillon-les-Dombes, began home nursing through his Sisters of Charity (1617). 'Before your establishment,' he said in one of his Conferences, 'there was never a community destined to serve the sick in their homes.' Robert Owen (1800) showed that care for the worker, besides immensely benefiting health, increased rather than diminished output. Of equal, if not greater, significance, national and local health organizations also began to appear; municipal doctors of many European states, and particularly the *Kreisphysikus* in Prussia, became effective agents for arousing public interest. *Bureaux de Santé*, with limited objectives to combat the plague, were established as early as the sixteenth century in the big towns of southern France. But none of these were effective by modern standards; all failed for one reason or another—including the Voluntary Board of Health at Manchester (1795), the *Comité de Salubrité publique* in Paris (1802), the *Collegium Medicum* in Denmark (1740)—either on account of lack of authority, or money, or of personnel.

The possibilities of public health action began to benefit from additions to scientific knowledge about the causation of disease; notably James Lind's experiment on board H.M.S. *Salisbury* (1748), which finally proved that oranges and lemons could prevent and cure the scourge of scurvy; and that of Edward Jenner (1796), which demonstrated the prevention of smallpox by vaccination. Jenner's work followed upon a century during which the age-old practice of inoculation had been popularized by the indefatigable Lady Mary Wortley Montague (1689–1762). From the beginning of the nineteenth century vaccination began to be practised as a public health measure, with and without compulsion. Lind's work on scurvy had less immediate effect, except that it led after half a century to preventive action in the British Navy. Of much more importance was the establishment of a preventive service in general for naval seamen, which followed Lind's *An Essay on the Most Effectual Means of Preserving the Health of Seamen* (1757). Pringle (1752) and Colombier (1775) wrote on the subject of army health. Such preventive services were the prototypes of those for infant hygiene, maternal and child health, and school health, which were to be developed a century and a half later. Thus the growth of public health presents itself as a multitude of small changes not always easy to distinguish, rather than as a few spectacular events.

After 1650 industrialization began to have an effect upon living standards; this was particularly so in England, where the Industrial Revolution started. Mechanical aids to living were now to influence health in a thousand new ways. In the next 150 years world population advanced sharply, and by the date when Malthus wrote (1798), it had already doubled to reach some 920 millions, suggesting that the state of public health had begun to improve, if not spectacularly, in all parts of the world, except perhaps in Africa. In particular, infant mortality and child mortality had begun to lessen and life to lengthen out. In this setting the movement to towns, in that part of the world where the Industrial Revolution had begun, which resulted in the industrial slums, provided an even greater contrast with the improving standard of living. The time for action had come.

PUBLIC HEALTH IN THE NINETEENTH CENTURY

Modern public health was the result of a growth of understanding and sense of responsibility among peoples in Europe, who, although they had a common cultural setting, were living in very different conditions and under different forms of government. Naturally therefore, this new social service had many points of origin. Two of these are of particular importance, that of Johann Peter Frank (1745–1821), who wrote about public health, mainly as social medicine, and as a police measure; and that of Edwin Chadwick (1800–90), whose main concern was with sanitation and with local government. Frank's *System einer Vollständigen Medicinischen Polizey*, an expression of the autocracy under which he and his forbears had lived, grew naturally out of *cameralism*. The benevolent dictator, or enlightened ruler, sitting with his advisers *in camera*, sought ways and means to raise his country's wealth; conceiving the idea of people themselves as the natural wealth of his country, he began to take steps to preserve their life and health and so to increase his estate.

Frank's system concerned itself with almost every aspect of public health, with the exception of industrial hygiene, and the emphasis was upon hospitals and medical care. Frank saw illhealth as an expression of poverty, a philosophy which he boldly stated in his oration as Dean of the Medical School in Austrian Lombardy (1790). Chadwick's public health was, to some extent, an expression of the political philosophy of his country, a distrust of autocratic rule; but it was also a child of the Industrial Revolution, which by the second quarter of the nineteenth century had given rise to remarkable changes in both the environment and the demography of a small island. Chadwick, influenced by his earlier association with Jeremy Bentham, began, like Frank, to see in poverty the main cause of ill health; and his first, and to many most striking, achievement was the reform of English Poor Law, with a uniform locally elected administration which gave, among other things, free medical care to the poor. Practical experience of the new industrial slums, however, soon convinced him that the most important forces were acting in the opposite direction; he came to see disease as a cause of poverty, 'the pecuniary cost of noxious agencies' as he described it. A nation-wide survey, using the Poor Law medical officers as the surveyors, resulted in *The Sanitary Condition of the Labouring Population* (1842), a powerful indictment of insanitary living, mirrored against rising standards.

Chadwick and, to a less extent, the public health pioneers on the Continent were aided by the arrival of cholera. In the first quarter of the nineteenth century this disease, with all the dramatic urgency of the plague, had spread from India relentlessly across the Continent; its course was watched everywhere with apprehension. It provided the final irresistible challenge to the complacent acceptance of slum living. It focused the attention of government and people on the need for sanitation. Doctors began to connect ill health more specifically with pollution of the environment; local citizens of initiative and public spirit began to see the need for public measures of control. Chadwick was able to marshal these forces and to bring them to a successful conclusion. His Public Health Act (1848), must for ever be a landmark in the history of world public health. He will always be famed for hammering home relentlessly his conviction that health depends upon sanitation. Chadwick's empirical system of sanitation, dependent upon an inviolable circuit of incoming and outgoing fluids, as an essential of urban life, has been as momentous for man's progress as Harvey's scientific discovery of the circulation of the blood. If Chadwick were alive today he would find nine-tenths of the world still suffering the torment of intestinal infections from which most of Europe and the New World, in following his teachings, has escaped. But Chadwick should be remembered even more for his less-considered teachings; the use of local government in public health administration, and of the medical officer of health as a specialist adviser. It was his evangelism which began the participation of the people in protecting their own health, by franchise from among themselves for voluntary service on local Boards of Health and through giving the means to finance the services needed out of their own pockets. It was his idea that doctors should discharge a function towards society as a whole, as well as towards the treatment of sick individuals.

Chadwick's public health, emphasizing the environmental rather than the personal aspects of hygiene, with the hospital little considered, influenced developments in North America and in the British dominions and colonies. The influence on America was striking; Shattuck's monumental report on health conditions in Massachusetts (1850) followed Chadwick's main lines of thought; America looked across the Atlantic to a country that 'had far outstripped any country in the world in the direction of state medicine' (Hanlon, 1969). American public health was based on local government with 'the role of national government confined primarily to providing plans, financial aid, advice and supervision' (Wyatt, 1951). Such differences as have developed in the American scene are derived from two contingencies; the fact that she did not follow Chadwick's new Poor Law with all that this entailed in social thinking; and the influence of federalism, which has led the States to develop along their own lines.

Public health on the continent of Europe followed a very different course. The administration, although widely different in detail, tended towards centralization, to state control and state officials; of this, France is the greatest exponent, with its public health services based on the *département* under the supreme authority of the prefect and with a medical director on the staff of the central organization. France has dealt with preventive work essentially by means of national circulars, with all the advantages of central stimulation and the disadvantages of a lack of local autonomy. Continental countries have also developed public health with emphasis upon personal rather than environmental hygiene. French Utopians in the nineteenth century dwelt upon the need for organized medical care. Condorcet (1793), in *L'Esquisse d'un Tableau historique des Progrès de l'Esprit humain*, wanted a system of insurance to do away with poverty; Jules Guérin (1848), editor of the Parisian journal *Gazette Médicale* asked that medicine should be dedicated to society; Philippe Buchez (1839), asked for a national health service in France with 16,000 district doctors, each giving free treatment to approximately 2,000 persons.

The French prefects received their first national circular about hospitals in 1840. European countries began to build state hospitals at an early date and, as Newsholme recorded of Denmark, they established 'an admirable system of municipal and county hospitals . . . supported out of taxes, which removed hospital treatment from the category of problems still to be solved' (Newsholme, 1931). European countries also tended to develop insurance against sickness. This continental pattern of public health spread in its turn to colonial territories dependent upon it; and, by the chance of association with Germany, to Japan.

Public health began with little scientific basis for action. At the time of Chadwick's Act (1848), and the first International Health Congress in Paris (1851), diseases were still largely undifferentiated and there was no absolute proof of the bacterial origins of much of it. The six months spent in Paris during 1851 by delegates from twelve nations was mainly a debate between contagionists and miasmatists, as it might have been in Sydenham's day. Yet evidence for the germ theory was piling up. Oliver Wendell Holmes in America and Semmelweiss in Vienna in the early nineteenth century added puerperal fever to the lengthening list of diseases known to be conveyed by human contact. John Snow, practising medicine in Soho, London, published his 'slender pamphlet' on cholera (1849); and in 1854, through further research, gave convincing evidence of its water-borne spread. William Budd did the same for typhoid (1856). The specificity of disease was becoming plain, and infectious disease, under the generic term 'fever', began to be sorted out into its component parts. Burdon Sanderson's study of tuberculous material (1867–68) made it almost certain that infection was a biological process. The second half of the nineteenth century was heralded by Pasteur's identification of bacteria, with the final rout of the theory of spontaneous generation. Koch isolated the tubercle bacillus in 1882, and, in rapid succession, scientists in different parts of the globe did the same for many other common maladies. Public health began now to look like an exercise in practical bacteriology; a realization particularly favourable to countries that had adopted the Chadwick pattern, but of importance to all through the development of artificial immunization and the tracing of carriers. Thus we entered the golden age of environmental hygiene, particularly in Great Britain, where public health laws followed one another in bewildering succession and where local government grew in importance, with medical officers of health and sanitarians employed in increasing numbers. In the United States the first State Board of Health was set up in Louisiana in 1855 following the great epidemic of yellow fever in 1853, and Massachusetts followed 14 years later in 1869 in order to protect and promote the public health (Freedman, 1969).

The bacteriological concept of disease processes, interpreted by Joseph Lister (1827–1912), together with the evolution of professional nursing following the teaching of Florence Nightingale (1820–1910), also gave birth to the modern hospital. In earlier civilizations the hospital had been little more than a place of refuge; a grave misfortune for whomsoever entered its portals. Infection, the spread of pathogenic organisms from patient to patient and ward to ward, had been a constant nightmare. The growth of the modern hospital, beginning with the simple laws of antisepsis and of aseptic rituals, quite transformed the public health scene, gradually shifting the balance of emphasis, already precarious, from prevention to cure.

For a time also the science of bacteriology obscured other equally significant aspects of public health. Bacteria occupied the forefront of the stage. But public health was soon falling back again on social issues. Miss Nightingale began to preach household hygiene (1858) as the answer to Britain's excessive infant mortality. John Simon (1816–1904) began his famous survey—or series of surveys—to determine the chief causes of excess mortality in 1858; and by 1871, when his period as Chief Medical Officer to the Privy Council in London came to an end, he had quite transformed the general understanding of public health problems. This episode in public health history, in which nation-wide studies were conducted by doctors of distinction in a wide range of important health problems—diet, infantile mortality, dust as a cause of pulmonary disease, worm infestations, lead, arsenic, and mercury poisoning in industry, housing, etc.—has probably no equal in world public health history.

In consequence of this, and of pioneer work in the rest of Europe and the United States, public health broadened its front with new services and fresh developments in professional work. The public health nurse appeared on the scene in Britain and the United States at about the same time (1872); Pierre Budin, Variot, and others in Paris, and Ballantyne in England, sought practical answers to antenatal and neonatal disorders. Nurses going into the homes, together with clinics at which mothers and babies might attend for advice, shifted the emphasis of public health work once again to a consideration of habits of living. The discovery of the tubercle bacillus, it was now realized, had done little to solve the problem of the white scourge; Philip and others began to study the social aspects of this disease and to find at least the beginning of a means to remedy them. Thus, personal hygiene, in its many forms, came now to fill an increasing part of the public health picture, developing many new aspects to meet the risks of the vulnerable classes. *Social hygiene*, one of its offspring, evolved services to protect mother and young child, school child, homeless children, industrial workers; schemes for tuberculosis and venereal disease; and, as ideas further developed during the century, for problem families, the handicapped, the aged, and the mentally ill. Two other offspring of personal hygiene, children of earlier years, began to grow in strength and quality: *preventive medicine* extended its techniques in immunization, in health education, and in preventive examinations; *social medicine* extended the participation of curative medicine in public health through organized medical services. *Social insurance* began to combat poverty in various countries of Europe and the Commonwealth.

The origins of social medicine are not easy to define. They might be found in Galen's *Hygiene*, or, perhaps more realistically, in Frank's omnibus of social medicine. But the term itself was first used by Grotjahn (1869–1931). Most of the pioneers of personal hygiene were exponents of social medicine, which is essentially the approach of the clinician to the problems of community health. However, the world waited until 1943 for the first Chair to be created with social medicine in its title, when John Ryle (1889–1950) went from the Regius Professorship of Physic at Cambridge to the Chair of Social Medicine at Oxford. No more moving statement of the ideals to which John Ryle subscribed can be imagined than that which he propounded on his American lecture tour. In *Changing Disciplines* (1948) he wrote:

'Thirty years of my life have been spent as a student and teacher of clinical medicine. In these thirty years I have watched disease in the ward being studied more and more thoroughly—if not always more thoughtfully—through the high power of the microscope; disease in man being investigated by more and more elaborate techniques and, on the whole, more and more mechanically. Man, as a person and as a member of a family and of much larger social groups, with his health and sickness intimately bound up with the conditions of his life and work—in the home, the mine, the factory, the shop, at sea, or on the land—and with his economic opportunity, has been inadequately considered in this period by the clinical teacher and hospital research worker. The medicine of the teaching schools has, as I have suggested, undergone a gradual conversion to a highly technical exercise in bedside pathology and therapeutic method. The morbid "material" of the hospital ward consists very largely—if we exclude the emergencies—of end-result conditions for which, as a rule, only a limited amount of relief repays the long stay, the patient investigation, and the anxious expectancy of the sick man or woman. With aetiology—the first essential for prevention—and with prevention itself the majority of physicians and surgeons have curiously little concern. Nor have they at present the opportunity, nor yet the appropriate types of training or assistance, requisite for the study of aetiology or prevention. Their material is mainly selected by four factors: the gravity, the difficulty or the rarity of their cases, or their suitability otherwise for admission to a hospital. Some of the most common diseases, the less lethal diseases, and the beginnings of disease are even considered as providing "poor teaching material". Health and sickness in the population and their possible correlations with significant and measurable social or occupational influences are outside their province.'

Public health has been developed in the countries of the western world in widely different ways; measures have been evolved, generally, only when pressing needs have come to be felt. Denmark began a system of gratuitous treatment for venereal disease, irrespective of social and financial station, as early as 1790; Britain followed 150 years later (1916), and Switzerland, for indigents only, even later (1931). Smallpox vaccination was made compulsory in Germany over a century before this step was taken in France. Sweden established a statistical commission in 1758, whereas Britain began official analysis of vital statistics only in 1837. Holland and Scandinavia developed the midwife to a high professional standing shortly after the turn of the century while Britain lagged behind some twenty-five years; the United States has not thought it necessary to have midwives. Sanitary hygiene began through national legislation in 1848 in England and not until fifty years later (1902) in France. Instances of wide differences in timing and emphasis could be multiplied many times. The philosophy of public health has been given many interpretations; and the human being, subjected broadly to the same occupational, ecological, nutritional, psychological, and other hazards, has nowhere been given any uniform protection. Recent develop-

ments in comprehensive medical care have tended to hasten the development of a common pattern. Britain, Australia, New Zealand, the United States, and Canada are now engaged, more deeply even than the Scandinavian countries where such developments were pioneered, in operating schemes of medical care, financed by the State or by insurance, according to taste. The final phase of public health in the western world is witnessing an increasing centring of interest upon the hospital; as specialist medicine and surgery develop their technical skills the future in Europe and the New World may well be a fight to prevent the hospital from taking control.

PUBLIC HEALTH AFTER THE FIRST AND SECOND WORLD WARS

The rest of the world awaited the influence of world wars before embarking upon public health practice in any real sense —apart from the initiation which colonial territories experienced from their parent bodies. After the First World War, Turkey, Russia, and Yugoslavia, at once engaged upon gigantic efforts to 'develop', began their own schemes of public health with little if any reference to the European pattern. Russia and Yugoslavia adopted a scheme based upon principles which had been long discussed in Europe, but never practised: complete integration of curative and preventive services; medicine as a social service; the predominance of preventive medicine; community participation, largely by means of Soviets; and health centres as the basis of day-to-day work. Yugoslavia, with Andrija Stampar as its adviser, also introduced the Institute of Hygiene, combining administrative work with research, an ingenious device to ensure that practical schemes for applying epidemiology, industrial hygiene, bacteriology and parasitology, food hygiene, maternal and child health, nutrition, etc., will be kept in touch with scientific developments. The distinctive new feature in this east European scene has been the subordination of medicine to the needs of the community. Thus enlightened authority has been able to impose upon the medical profession that which deliberate democratic choice has found difficulty in doing. The fifty years which have elapsed since these three exciting adventures in large-scale public health schemes organized on a national basis were begun, have provided dramatic proof of the possibilities of public health even in under-developed countries, if backed with sufficient authority and direction; success has been most marked in Russia, where the health picture is now, in its main aspects, that of a developed country.

After the Second World War the movement for public health became general, aided by the World Health Organization, which began to function in late 1948. Many new countries, Indonesia, Burma, Thailand, India, Pakistan, and some South American States, have taken part in a general awakening, urgent and impulsive. For these countries health problems of even greater magnitude than those of Russia, Turkey, and Yugoslavia in the 1920's, or of Europe in the early nineteenth century, had to be faced. Communicable diseases have been even more widespread; and these have been exacerbated by nutritional disorders almost unknown to Europe. Intestinal infections and infestations of many kinds, and many special diseases, such as yaws, leprosy, and filariasis, have for long prevailed. Widespread lack of sanitation has caused untold illness. Childbirth remains in the hands of the village handywomen;

doctors, nurses, sanitarians, and other auxiliaries hardly exist. In Indonesia, where there is one doctor to 57,000 people, it is said that a woman dies in childbirth every quarter of an hour and a baby every minute.

Moreover, the social framework upon which health services depend for their support has in most cases hardly begun to develop; there is an absence of scientific background, and the existence of deeply rooted customs and beliefs which make progress in public health more difficult. It is inevitable that success in these circumstances, and in the short period of time which has elapsed, has been limited. Centralized schemes for the eradication of special diseases, undertaken with the help of international bodies or financed by interested nations, have been the most distinctive development. The provision of a basic public health system has, for the most part, yet to be devised; but in many areas model health units have been set up in which personnel can be trained and schemes suitable to the country tried out. Within such limits, as in Russia, Turkey, and Yugoslavia, the health centre has become the necessary component in day-to-day working. If there is little sign yet of the development of strong public health schemes such as those seen in the western world, the first step at least has been taken.

This last stage in public health is too young for critical analysis. Certainly much has been accomplished in little time. The World Health Organization is determined upon world eradication of malaria; this scourge and other crippling diseases are being energetically attacked. But permanent improvement in health, for the vast regions of the world where development is still in its early stages, must await strong national public health systems [see CHAPTER 51].

Public health has moved far since Galen dreamed of hygiene on the Acropolis at Pergamos. Disease and ill health, with the marshalling of so many forces against them, have given ground, and particularly rapidly during the past half century. Ultimate success in the conquest of many diseases can now be seen; and a final goal in which infectious and nutritional disorders have been overcome throughout the world is no idle dream. But it would be wrong to leave this short account without a note of warning for the many new problems that present themselves as others recede. Not for nothing has man escaped

from the immediate hazards of an ecological struggle in which survival is bought at a fearful cost in life. In this struggle at least his numbers were slow to advance and his maximum birth rate did little more than compensate, as an average of many years, for his high mortality. Already the success of public health in reducing mortality, more rapidly than changing customs can permit of corresponding reductions in the birth rate, is introducing a serious problem of over-population. In countries where public health has been longest in effective operation, and where natality has responded to the new pattern of living, the demographic structure has undergone profound change, with a shift of population to older groups. Thus, over-population and ageing are new challenges no less demanding than some of the infectious diseases which are passing. Moreover, where public health has succeeded emphasis has shifted from infectious to degenerative disease, now equally prevalent; some due to real increase, but mostly a manifestation of demographic changes resulting in a higher proportion of old people. New hazards also have arisen as the pattern of life changes with 'development'; carcinoma of the lung can be related to excessive smoking and smoke-laden atmospheres; suicide, alcoholism, and supposedly stress diseases are directly or indirectly nervous phenomena, the response of the human to the strains of a highly organized society. There is much still barring the way to Utopia.

Finally, history records a growth of understanding of the nature of health and of the value which society places upon it. For Galen and the aristocracy of ancient Greece, health was a state of reasonable activity and freedom from pain; in Elizabethan England scurvy and the ague, just as today pinta in South America and perhaps chronic bronchitis in England, have been accepted as normal. Society has been prepared to overlook disease when inevitable, widespread, and not wholly incapacitating and to accept as healthy a large measure of impaired functioning. But this rationalization has receded as the western world has steadily set its sights higher. Much, today, that we see as abnormal in the physical, mental, and social field was in comparatively recent times regarded as normal. Mere absence of disease is no longer enough. Utopians must be positively healthy.

REFERENCES AND FURTHER READING

Brockington, C. F. (1965) *Public Health in the Nineteenth Century*, Edinburgh.
Brockington, C. F. (1966) *A Short History of Public Health*, 2nd ed., London.
Carr-Saunders, A. M. (1965) *World Population: Past Growth and Present Trend*, London.
Frank, J. P. (1941) The people's misery: mother of diseases, *Bull. Hist. Med.*, **9**, 81.
Frazer, W. M. (1950) *A History of English Public Health, 1834–1939*, London.
Freedman, B. (1969) Letter, *J. Amer. med. Ass.*, **210**, 1104.
Goodman, N. M. (1969) International health, *Lancet*, i, 45.
Hanlon, J. J. (1969) *Principles of Public Health Administration*, 5th ed., St. Louis.
Hobson, W. (1963) *World Health and History*, Bristol.
Howard-Jones N. (1974) The scientific background of the International Sanitary Conferences, *Wld Hlth Org. Chron.*, **28**, 4–9.
Khairallah, A. A. (1946) *Outline of Arabic Contributions to Medicine*, Beirut.

Lambert, R. (1963) *Sir John Simon and English Sanitary Administration (1816–1904)*, London.
Newsholme, A. (1931) *International Studies on the Relation between the Private and Official Practice of Medicine with special reference to the Prevention of Disease*, conducted for the Milbank Memorial Fund, London.
Rosen, J. (1953) Cameralism and the concept of medical police, *Bull. Hist. Med.*, **27**, 21.
Ryle, J. A. (1948) *Changing Disciplines*, London.
Sand, R. (1952) *The Advance to Social Medicine*, London.
Shattuck, L. (1948) *Report of the Sanitary Commission of Massachusetts, 1850*, Cambridge, Mass.
Sigerist, H. E. (1951) *A History of Medicine*, New York.
Simon, Sir J. (1890) *English Sanitary Institutions*, London.
Trevelyan, G. M. (1944) *English Social History*, London.
World Health Organization (1958) *The First Ten Years of WHO*, Geneva.
World Health Organization (1968) *The Second Ten Years of WHO*, Geneva.
Wyatt, L. R. (1951) *Intergovernmental Relations in Public Health*, Minneapolis.

2

VITAL STATISTICS

W. P. D. LOGAN and P. M. LAMBERT

HISTORICAL

Vital statistics are the maps and milestones of public health. The principal subdivisions of vital statistics are:

1. Demographic statistics (population, marriages, and fertility).
2. Mortality statistics (numbers and causes of death).
3. Morbidity statistics (illnesses and injuries, incapacity, hospitalizations, etc.).

In the history of vital statistics two names qualify for special mention. John Graunt, haberdasher and train-band captain of the City of London, and Fellow of the Royal Society, published in 1662 his *Natural and political observations mentioned in a following index, and made upon the Bills of Mortality*. The London Bills of Mortality were commenced during the previous century and were weekly compilations of the burials, baptisms, and marriages recorded in each parish. Graunt described the mechanism of collection of the data in the following words:

'When any one dies, then, either by tolling or ringing of a bell, or by bespeaking of a grave of the *sexton*, the same is known to the *searchers*, corresponding with the said *sexton*:

'The *searchers* hereupon (who are ancient matrons sworn to their office) repair to the place where the dead corpse lies, and *by view of the same*, and by other enquiries, they examine by what *disease* or *casualty* the corpse died. Hereupon they make their report to the *parish clerk*, and he, every *Tuesday* night, carries in an accompt of all the *burials* and christenings happening that week to the Clerk of the Hall. On Wednesday the general accompt is made up and printed, and on Thursday published and dispersed to the several families who will pay four shillings *per annum* for it.'

In his *Observations* Graunt noted the excess of male over female births, the excess of the death rate of the city over that of the country, and the very high mortality of young children. The parish clerks of London deserve our gratitude for their perseverance in publishing the bills which the citizens took in weekly for no other reason that Graunt could discover than curiosity about increase and decrease of burials and rare casualties 'so as they might take the same as a text to talk upon in the next company'; and in the plague time, 'that so the rich might judge of the necessity of their removal, and that tradesmen might conjecture what doings they were like to have in their respective dealings'. Similar bills were commenced in some other English and continental cities, but they were allowed to lapse, leaving the series incomplete.

It is of interest that an echo of those weekly tables of London deaths, started in the sixteenth century, is heard still today in the General Register Office of England and Wales where the staff refer colloquially to the London table in the Weekly Return as 'the London Bill'.

The other great name in the history of vital statistics is that of Dr. William Farr (1807–83), who became 'Compiler of Abstracts' to the General Register Office on 10 July 1839, two years after the establishment of that Office, and continued there until his retirement on 1 February 1880. For almost the whole of Farr's forty years at the General Register Office the Registrar General was Major Graham, and the combination of the outstanding statistical capacity of the one with the administrative capacity of the other rendered it a period in which were established practically all the foundations of the vital statistics of the present day. The First Annual Report of the Registrar General contains the first of a long series of 'letters' by Farr, addressed to the Registrar General, on the causes of death in England and on a variety of related matters. Of this series of letters it has been said that they were from first to last marked by a lucid marshalling of the facts, a masterly command of all the resources of method and numerical investigation, and an unaffected and vigorous English, breaking out every now and again, when stimulated by a clear view of some wide generalization, into passages of great eloquence and pure philosophy.

Farr's writings were marked by two great features, an inherent scientific accuracy, and a reverberant prose style, that invites quotation. A typical sample, written in 1864, is the following:

'To what then is the high mortality of London men in the working ages of life due? It is not want of work. Their hands and heads are sufficiently employed to insure exercise. The drainage of their dwellings, and their water supply, is in many districts scanty; habits of ablution are not cultivated; and their skin is often unclean. They live too frequently in crowded rooms, from which fresher air than they breathe is excluded. It is the same in the workshops, where the air is in many trades loaded with dust, which induces bronchitis. Workshops are sometimes ill constructed for the supply of air for breathing, and the men themselves throw obstacles in the way of ventilation. Spirits and other stimulants are by certain numbers—such as the publicans—taken to a fatal excess. These latter causes to some extent account for the excess in the mortality of men over the mortality of women.

'The whole subject of the mortality of men in towns requires careful investigation. It is of national importance; for the workmen in all large towns suffer as much and often more than the workmen of London.'

Some of the important events and dates in the development of vital statistics are listed in TABLE 1.

TABLE 1

*Chronology of Important Events in the Development of
Civil Registration and Vital Statistics*

YEAR	AREA	REMARKS
Circa 1250 B.C.	Egypt	Early in the reign of Egyptian King Rameses II, there appears to have been in force a somewhat elaborate registration system. Whether at that remote time it applied equally to all classes of the population would seem doubtful, but where the system did apply it could scarcely have excluded records of births and deaths.
578–534 B.C.	Rome	Citizens were required to give account of newly born children within 30 days of birth, while officials were appointed throughout the provinces for the purpose of recording the relevant facts relating to births, adolescents, and deaths.
A.D. 720	Japan	Registration of live births, deaths, and marriages compulsory in some parts of Japan.
1532	England	Ordinance required Bills of Mortality which were weekly records of burials issued by the clergy of the Established Church containing data relating to the number of deaths, and deaths from plague, in the various parishes of London.
1538	England	Every priest of the Established Church of England was required to keep a book or register in which should be recorded 'every Sunday in the presence of the Wardens or of one of them, every wedding, baptism, or burial occurring in the parish during the previous week'.
1597	England	Convocation of Canterbury required inscription of parish registers on parchment, the preparation of duplicate copies of all entries, weekly entries to be read aloud by parish priest each week at conclusion of one of the Sunday services when the names of the clergyman and church-wardens were to be inscribed at the foot of each completed page of the register and a copy of each register to be forwarded at the end of each year within one month after Easter to the Bishop of the diocese for preservation among the episcopal archives.
1617	Ireland	Appointment of first known Registrar General of Births, Marriages, and Burials—Sir George Keare. Continued only three years, and no records are extant.
1620	Canada	Ecclesiastical registration of baptisms, burials, and marriages instituted.
1628	Finland	Compulsory civil registration of live birth, death, stillbirth, and marriage established.
1639	United States of America	Civil registration of birth, death, and marriage required in Massachusetts Bay colony.
1662	England	John Graunt published results of his studies under title *Natural and Political Observations . . . made upon the Bills of Mortality*—the first real study in vital statistics.
1681	Ireland	Sir William Petty's 'Observations upon the Dublin Bills of Mortality' appeared.
1693	England	Edmund Halley read before the Royal Society his paper, *An Estimate of the Degrees of the Mortality of Mankind Drawn from Curious Tables of the Births and Funerals in the City of Breslau; with an attempt to ascertain the Price of Annuities upon Lives.*
1795	Canada	System of registration by Roman Catholic clergy extended to Protestant congregations by the Act of 1795.
1837	England	Births, Marriages and Deaths Registration Act, which became effective 1 July 1837, provided for voluntary registration of live births, deaths, and marriages.
1839	England	Dr. William Farr appointed to the General Register Office as Compiler of Abstracts.
1845	Northern Ireland	Compulsory civil registration of non-Catholic marriages established.
1855	New Zealand	Compulsory civil registration of live birth, death, and marriage established.
1855	Scotland	Compulsory civil registration of live birth, death, and marriage established.
1864	Northern Ireland	Compulsory civil registration of live birth, death, and Roman Catholic marriage established.
1864	Ireland	Compulsory civil registration of live birth, death, and marriage established.
1875	England and Wales	Compulsory civil registration of live birth, death, and marriage established.
1886	Burma, India and Pakistan	Births, Deaths and Marriages Registration Act provided for voluntary, not compulsory, civil registration.
1893	International	Establishment of the International List of Causes of Death.
1897	Ceylon	Compulsory civil registration of live birth, death, and stillbirth established.
1913	New Zealand	Compulsory civil registration of stillbirth established.
1927	England and Wales	Compulsory civil registration of stillbirth established.
1939	Scotland	Compulsory civil registration of stillbirth established.
1965	International	Eighth Revision of the International Classification of Diseases.
1967	International	Adoption of World Health Organization Nomenclature Regulations, 1967.

(Source: *Handbook of Vital Statistics Methods* (1955) United Nations, New York.)

METHODS OF COLLECTION

Vital statistics can be obtained systematically in three ways:

1. By registration, which may be defined as the continuous and permanent recording of the occurrence and the characteristics of vital events (births, marriages, deaths) primarily for their value as legal documents and secondarily for their usefulness as a source of statistics.

2. By enumeration, represented by the census of population and by sickness surveys.

3. By special returns—notifications of infectious disease, certificates of incapacity for work, abstracts of hospital case records, and the like.

In England and Wales—and, with only slight differences in detail, in the other countries of the British Isles—the central government department responsible for the collection and compilation of vital statistics is the Office of Population Censuses and Surveys (formerly the General Register Office). The director of this office is the Registrar General, a permanent civil servant. This department supervises the registration of births, marriages, and deaths in the many hundreds of local registration offices throughout the country and in addition compiles vital statistics for the country as a whole and for its constituent administrative and other areas. The vital statistics division of the Office operates in two principal sections, one concerned with census, population, and fertility, and the other concerned with medical, i.e. mortality and morbidity, statistics.

The arrangements for central and local registration and the compilation of national vital statistics in a number of countries are shown in TABLE 2.

The first census of modern times appears to have been in Canada in the Colony of New France in 1666. The first complete census of a European country was in Iceland in 1703, followed by Sweden in 1749. In England and Wales the first census took place in 1801 and has been repeated at regular ten-year intervals with the single exception of 1941.

The census contributes two essential pieces of information to public health workers:

1. A numerical description of the population and its social, environmental, economic, and other characteristics, necessary for a proper comprehension of the human community that constitutes the field of application of public health.

2. The statistical denominators that are required for the calculation of mortality and morbidity rates, so that numbers of deaths or of illnesses can be measured in relation to the number of persons at risk.

In Great Britain in 1753 a Bill was introduced in Parliament

TABLE 2

Administration of Civil Registration and Compilation of National Vital Statistics

Country	Registration		Vital statistics
	Local	National	
South Africa	District Registrar	Registrar General's Office	Bureau of Census and Statistics
Canada	Provincial Department of Public Health	—	Dominion Bureau of Statistics
U.S.A.	State Department of Health	—	Public Health Service
Ceylon	Divisional Registrar	Registrar General's Department	Registrar General's Department
India	Health Department or Land Revenue Department	—	Directorate General of Health Services
Pakistan	Municipal Health Department	—	Director General of Health
Ireland	District Registrar's Office	General Register Office	Central Statistical Office
United Kingdom:			
England and Wales . . .	Local Registration Office	Office of Population Censuses and Surveys	Office of Population Censuses and Surveys
Northern Ireland . . .	Local Registration Office	General Register Office	General Register Office
Scotland . . .	Local Registrar's Office	General Register Office	General Register Office
Australia	District Registry Office	—	Commonwealth Bureau of Census and Statistics
New Zealand	District Registrar's Office	Registrar General	Census and Statistics Department —Department of Health

(Source: *Handbook of Vital Statistics Methods* (1955).)

At the international level the principal agencies concerned with vital statistics are: 1. the Statistical Office of the United Nations which compiles vital statistics from the member states and publishes them in its *Demographic Yearbook*; and 2. the World Health Organization, which compiles vital statistics relating to the health of its member states and publishes them in its *World Health Statistics Annual*. The existence of these organizations and their publication of carefully compiled comparative tables of vital statistics for the majority of the countries of the world has in recent years opened up a new field in the development and utilization of vital statistics.

DEMOGRAPHIC STATISTICS
THE CENSUS OF POPULATION

The numbering of the people is recorded on various occasions in Biblical history from the time of Moses. King David had an unfortunate experience in 1017 B.C. when his census provoked Divine wrath and drew on Israel a three-day pestilence in which 'there died of the people from Dan even to Beer-sheba seventy thousand men' (2 Samuel xxiv, 15).

for taking and registering an annual account of the total number of the people, but was rejected, one of the opposing Members of Parliament declaring that he did not believe 'that there was any set of men . . . so presumptuous and so abandoned as to make the proposal . . . I hold this project to be totally subversive of the last remains of English liberty'. But by 1801 circumstances had changed, and on Monday, 10 March a census was held. For a detailed account of the censuses from 1801 to 1931 the reader is referred to a report by the Interdepartmental Committee on Social and Economic Research which describes the various items the successive censuses have included.

An account of the census of 1961 is contained in the *General Report* for that census, and describes the planning and organization and the subsequent production of a series of reports covering special aspects. The legal authority for the 1961 census was the Census Act 1920, which is a permanent Act applicable to censuses generally, the Census Order, 1960, which was an Order in Council, and the Census Regulations 1960, wherein the detailed machinery and the precise forms to be used were prescribed. The census was taken on Sunday, 23 April 1961. The method was that 69,000 enumerators (for

England and Wales), employed to take the census under the supervision of Census Officers (the local Registrars of Births and Deaths), left a schedule at each household within his assigned district some days before the census day, for compulsory completion by the head of the household, and collected it shortly after the census day.

The full list of questions for 1961 is somewhat larger than in the 1951 census, but owing to the introduction of sampling methods at the enumeration stage, nine people out of ten were asked for less information than at any previous census this century. The questions asked on the schedule, for each person in the household as far as appropriate, were:

> Name and Surname
> Relationship to Head of Household
> Usual Residence
> Sex
> Age
> Single, Married, Widowed
> Date of Marriage and end of first marriage
> Children born in marriage
> Birthplace
> Nationality

In addition, there was a question about household arrangements (piped water supply, cooking-stove, kitchen sink, water-closet, bath), and a record was made on the schedule of ownership, renting, the total number of persons and the number of rooms. Questions asked from a 10 per cent. sample of the population were those relating to personal occupation, employment, place of work, status in employment, education, scientific and technological qualifications, change of usual residence or duration of stay at present usual residence, and persons usually resident in private households who were absent on census night.

The latest census took place on the night of 25/26 April 1971. The *General Report* has not yet been issued.

Population

The census provides two estimates of the population of the country as a whole and of local areas:

TABLE 3
Population and Decennial Rates of Change England and Wales 1871–1971

	Population	Decennial increase per cent. of population	Increase due to births	Decrease due to deaths	Natural increase	Inward (+) or outward (−) balance of migration
1871	22,712,266	—	—	—	—	—
1881	25,974,439	14·4	37·9	22·8	15·1	−0·7
1891	29,002,525	11·7	34·3	20·3	14·0	−2·3
1901	32,527,843	12·2	31·6	19·2	12·4	−0·2
1911	36,070,492	10·9	28·6	16·1	12·4	−1·5
1921	37,886,699	4·9	23·0	12·4	8·2	−3·2
1931	39,952,377	5·5	18·3	12·6	6·0	−0·5
1951	43,757,888	4·7	16·6	11·9	4·0	+0·6
1961	46,104,548	5·4	16·3	11·8	4·5	+0·8
1971	48,749,575	5·7	18·1	12·1	5·9	−0·2

(Source: *Registrar General.*)

1. *De facto* population, which is the number of persons enumerated in the area at the census. This is also called the enumerated population.

2. *De jure* population, which is the number of persons ordinarily resident in each area, regardless of where they happen to have been enumerated at the census. This may also be called the resident population.

The trend of population in England and Wales since 1871 is shown in TABLE 3.

Intercensal Movements of Population

Between one census and the next it is necessary to adjust the census figures annually to allow for population changes that have taken place. For the country as a whole this is not an unduly difficult matter, and is done simply by deducting the number of deaths and of emigrants and by adding the number of births and of immigrants. In this connexion two terms are often used:

1. Natural increase—the excess of births over deaths during a given period.

2. Net inward or outward balance of migration—the difference between the natural increase and the actual increase of the population.

Sex–Age Structure of the Population

One of the notable features of population change during this century is the diminishing proportion of young people and the

TABLE 4
Population Age Distribution (Persons) (England and Wales)

	1881	1970	2001
All ages	100	100	100
0–	36	24	23
15–	45	39	42
45–	14	24	21
65–	5	13	13

(Source: *1972 Population Projections.*)

increasing proportion of the elderly, i.e. 'ageing of the population'.

For England and Wales TABLE 4 shows the age distribution of the population in 1881, 1970, and 2001, and indicates that the ageing tendency is not expected to continue.

World Population

The world population picture in 1965 and a projection to the year 1985 are shown in TABLE 5. The 50 per cent. increase in

TABLE 5
World Population (in millions)

	1965	1985 ('medium' projection)	Annual increase (%)
Total . . .	3,289	4,934	2·5
East Asia . .	852	1,182	1·9
South Asia . .	981	1,694	3·6
Europe . .	445	515	0·8
U.S.S.R. . .	231	287	1·2
Africa . .	303	530	3·7
Northern America .	214	280	1·5
Latin America .	246	435	3·8
Oceania . . .	17·5	26·8	2·7

(Source: *U.N. Population Division.*)

the world's population during these 20 years will produce many problems in the field of international public health.

Fertility Statistics

The sources of fertility statistics are: 1. the census; 2. registration of births; 3. special surveys.

Questions on fertility in marriage have been asked at the 1951 and subsequent censuses. Prior to 1951, the last such questions were asked in 1911. The only comprehensive inquiry on the subject during the intervening years was the sample Family Census taken in 1946 by the Royal Commission on Population. Detailed current information has, however, been collected at the registration of births since 1938 under the Population (Statistics) Act of that year.

The data obtained at the 1961 census were published in a Census Fertility Report. The Census tables contain figures about the total number of children born to a woman (family size), including details of women who had not yet had a child (infertility) and about women who had a child in the year ending on census date (current fertility). These data are presented for women classified by age either at marriage or at census date, by duration of marriage, by how many times married, the difference of age between husband and wife, geographical, occupational, and educational details.

The percentage of married women who had children was as follows:

	All married women under 50 (i.e. including incomplete families)	Married women aged 45–49 (completed families)
No child . . .	19	15
1 child	27	26
2 children . . .	29	29
3 children . . .	14	15
4+ children . . .	11	14
Mean family size . .	1·78 children	2·02 children

Classified by social class of husband, women aged 45–49 married only once showed the following gradient of fertility:

Social class	Mean family size
I. Professional, etc. . .	1·78
II. Intermediate . . .	1·70
III. Skilled . . .	2·18
IV. Partly skilled . . .	2·15
V. Unskilled . . .	2·43

POPULATION REPLACEMENT AND FERTILITY TRENDS

The *Net Reproduction Rate* is a conventionally used index of population replacement that is now tending to go out of fashion, since, though it provides a convenient summary of the events of a year, it is an unsatisfactory guide to long-term prospects.

In algebraic form it may be expressed thus:

$$\text{Net Reproduction Rate (female) for a given year} = \sum_{x=15}^{x=45} \frac{\text{No. of live births (female) to women aged } x}{\text{No. of women aged } x} \times f_x$$

where f is a factor introduced to allow for the proportion of newborn girls who will not survive to the age of their mother.

Analysis of the births of any one period, such as a year, can give misleading results when either the family size or the timing of births is changing. What is necessary is to take a group of people, such as those born or married in a particular period, and to follow them through their reproductive lives. Such a group is called a cohort and the study of fertility records in this form cohort analysis. An analysis of this kind based on census and registration data provides a striking demonstration of the changes which have occurred in family size during the last three generations, from an average of six children per completed family in the middle of the nineteenth century to little more than two children per family by about 1920, since when there has been little change.

ANNUAL BIRTH RATES AND FERTILITY STATISTICS

These are derived from registration of births. In England and Wales the information recorded at birth registration under the Births and Deaths Registration Act, 1953, includes date and place of birth, name and sex of child, name and birthplace of each parent, and occupation of father. Legitimacy or illegitimacy is not recorded as such, but if the parents are not married the father's name is not entered in the register unless he attends the registration.

The Birth Rate (live births) is ordinarily calculated as follows:

$$\text{Live Birth Rate per thousand population} = \frac{\text{No. of live births}}{\text{No. of population}} \times 1{,}000$$

For *stillbirths* the rate is sometimes calculated in the same way, but more usually a different denominator is used, viz.

$$\text{Stillbirth Rate per thousand total births} = \frac{\text{No. of stillbirths}}{\text{No. of births, live and still}} \times 1{,}000$$

Birth rates for local areas are calculated not on the basis of the births actually occurring in a given area but after 'transfer' of the births to the area of usual residence of the mother. A birth rate can then be calculated in the way described. Since the sex–age composition of the population of a local area will influence its birth rate, the rate can be further adjusted, 'standardized', by the application of an *Area Comparability Factor (Births)* which will compensate for local differences in population sex–age structure. This is done routinely by the Registrar General for England and Wales (see page 144 of the *1965 Statistical Review*, Part III, Commentary).

Under the Population Statistics Act, 1938, as amended by the Population (Statistics) Act, 1960, additional information of a confidential character, used only for statistical purposes, is also elicited at birth registration. This additional information is used as the basis for a series of annual fertility tables in which births are tabulated in relation to age of each parent, region, parity, geographical region, and duration of marriage.

The distinction should be noted between registration of a birth, which is a civil act performed usually by a parent attending the local Register Office of Births and Deaths, and notification of birth, which is done by the doctor or midwife who attends a woman in childbirth and which is made to the local Medical Officer for Environmental Health to enable him to carry out his statutory duties in relation to maternity and child welfare. Local arrangements usually exist, however, whereby the Registrar of Births and Deaths and the Medical Officer of Health exchange information periodically so that each may know of births coming to the notice of the other.

MORTALITY STATISTICS

The basis of mortality statistics is the information recorded at registration of death. This information includes the date and place of death, the name and usual place of residence of the decedent, his sex, age, and occupation (in the case of married women, occupation of husband), and the cause of death.

The cause of death is reported to the Registrar of Births and Deaths on a medical certificate of cause of death. In England and Wales the certificate in use corresponds closely with that recommended by the World Health Organization for international use. In this certificate [see FIG. 1] the medical practitioner in attendance upon the decedent records, in Part I, the immediate cause of death together with any underlying disease that directly gave rise to it, and in Part II any significant associated diseases that contributed to the death but did not directly lead to it. In coroners' cases—mainly deaths from violent or unknown causes—when an autopsy takes place the pathologist reports the cause of death on a form similar to the international pattern. As a further, and indispensable, step towards international comparability, causes of death are classified in accordance with the *International Statistical Classification of Diseases, Injuries, and Causes of Death* (ICD), the eighth revision of which was made in 1965 and came into operation in 1968. The ninth revision, which is in the course of preparation, will be published in Spanish as well as in English and French. The *International Classification of Diseases*, which originated in 1893 as the *International List of Causes of Death*, was greatly modified at its sixth revision in 1948 so as to be used for morbidity statistics as well as for causes of death, and it is now generally used for both purposes as well as providing for the indexing of hospital diagnostic records.

Cause of Death		Approximate interval between onset and death
I		
*Disease or condition directly leading to death**	(*a*) . . . . due to (or as a consequence of)	. . . .
Antecedent causes Morbid conditions, if any, giving rise to the above cause, stating the underlying condition last	(*b*) . . . . due to (or as a consequence of) (*c*)	. . . .
II		
Other significant conditions contributing to the death, but not related to the disease or condition causing it	. . . .	. . . .

* This does not mean the mode of dying, e.g., heart failure, asthenia, etc. It means the disese, injury, or complication which caused death.

FIG. 1. International form of medical certificate of cause of death.

It comprises a three-digit list of categories starting at No. 000 and going on to 999, with a large number of fourth-digit subdivisions for optional use. In accordance with the World Health Organization Nomenclature Regulations, member states publishing mortality or morbidity statistics must do so by the three- or four-digit list, or by one of the approved condensed lists: List A of 150 categories, List B of 50 categories (for mortality), List C of 70 categories (for morbidity), List D of 300 categories for hospital morbidity, and List P of 100 categories for perinatal morbidity and mortality.

In England and Wales deaths registered as having occurred in a local area other than that in which the decedent normally resides are 'transferred' to the area of normal residence. There are arrangements whereby the local Medical Officer of Health may be supplied by the Registrar of Births and Deaths with registration particulars of all deaths occurring in his area. The Medical Officer of Health is also informed, in due course, of deaths transferred into his area.

In England and Wales provisional mortality statistics are published weekly and quarterly in the *Registrar General's Weekly and Quarterly Returns*. Final figures for each year are published in the *Registrar General's Annual Statistical Review*, Part I (Medical Tables), and further statistics are contained in the volume entitled Part III (Commentary), the successor to what was published for many years as the *Text*. In the neighbourhood of each census, the Registrar General also publishes a number of *Decennial Supplements*, such as Life Tables, an Occupational Mortality Supplement, and an Area Mortality Supplement.

DEATH RATES

What is usually described as a *Crude Death Rate* is calculated by relating the total number of deaths registered in a given period to the estimated number of the total population at risk. The denominator is usually taken for convenience as the estimated population at the mid-point of the period. The period will often be a year. If it is not, the rate should be adjusted to make it the equivalent of an annual rate. For example:

(1) Crude Death Rate for 1972 per 1,000 $= \dfrac{\text{Total deaths, all ages, 1972}}{\text{Estimated population at 30 June 1972}} \times 1{,}000$

(2) Mean Annual Crude Death Rate for 1968–72 per 1,000 $= \dfrac{\text{Total deaths, all ages, 1968–72}}{\text{Sum of estimated population at 30 June each year 1968–72}} \times 1{,}000$

Alternatively, this could be calculated as follows:

$$\text{Mean Annual Crude Death Rate 1968–72 per 1,000} = \frac{\text{Total deaths, all ages, 1968–72}}{\text{Estimated population 30 June 1970}} \times \frac{1,000}{5}$$

$$(3) \text{ Crude Death Rate 2nd quarter 1972 per 1,000} = \frac{\text{Total deaths, all ages, 2nd quarter 1972}}{\text{Estimated population 30 June 1972}} \times 4,000$$

Sex–Age Death Rates

Death rates for specific sex–age groups of the population are calculated in a similar way, but it is important to note that in the denominator as well as the numerator only the specific sex–age group should be included. For example, death rate in 1972, of females aged 15–44:

$$\text{Death Rate 1972 per 1,000 females aged 15–44} = \frac{\text{Deaths of females aged 15–44 in 1972}}{\text{Estimated female population aged 15–44 at 30 June 1972}} \times 1,000$$

Crude Death Rates and Sex–Age Rates for Specified Causes

For death rates for specified causes the only change to be made in the above formulae is that the numerator should include only deaths from the specified cause. The denominator remains unchanged.

Thus,

$$\text{Death Rate, 1972, from bronchitis per 1,000 men aged 45–64} = \frac{\text{Deaths from bronchitis in men aged 45–64, 1972}}{\text{Estimated male population aged 45–64 at 30 June 1972}} \times 1,000$$

TRENDS AND COMPARISONS OF DEATH RATES—STANDARDIZATION

A death rate has little meaning on its own. It is only when comparisons are made that death rates assume meaning. The comparisons that are made with death rates are of several types. The principal are:

1. Comparison of one sex–age group with another, i.e. the study of sex–age differences.
2. Comparison of one year with another, i.e. the study of time trends.
3. Comparison of one local area with another, i.e. the study of area differences.
4. Comparison of one occupational group with another, i.e. the study of occupational differences.

For all comparisons in which specific rates by sex and age are not used, i.e. when death rates of all ages, or over a wide range of ages, are being compared, it is advisable to *standardize* the rates. This is done in order to eliminate the misleading effects that might be caused by differences in the sex–age composition of the populations whose mortality is being compared.

There are two basic methods for the standardization of death rates (and incidentally also of morbidity rates) by sex and age, a *direct* method and an *indirect* method. In many circumstances the two methods will yield practically the same answer. The choice of the method to be used is sometimes no more than a matter of taste. In other circumstances there is sometimes felt to be a real advantage in using one rather than the other; and sometimes the form in which the data are available allows no choice, precluding the use of one and requiring the use of the other method.

Direct Standardization

Suppose we wish to compare the death rates (all ages) in a series of local areas A, B, . . . etc. In order to apply direct standardization we require to know:

TABLE 6

Standardization of Death Rates
Direct Standardization (Hypothetical Data)

Age in years	Standard population		Local death rates per 1,000		No. of deaths in standard thousand	
	Actual, millions	Reduced to 1,000 total	Area A	Area B	Area A	Area B
			Male			
0–	5·2	115	2·0	2·5	0·2	0·3
15–	9·0	200	1·6	1·8	0·3	0·4
45–	5·4	120	12·0	14·0	1·4	1·7
65+	2·1	47	80·0	85·5	3·8	4·0
			Female			
0–	5·0	111	1·7	2·0	0·2	0·2
15–	9·0	200	1·0	1·4	0·2	0·3
45–	6·1	136	7·4	8·0	1·0	1·1
65+	3·2	71	54·2	63·0	3·8	4·5
Total	45·0	1,000	18·4	6·5	10·9	12·5

Standardized Death Rate   10·9   12·5

Comparative Mortality Factor (C.M.F.) $= \dfrac{10·9}{11·8\star} \times 1,000$ $= \dfrac{12·5}{11·8\star} \times 1,000$

$= 924$ $= 1,059$

---

* 11·8 is the Crude Death Rate in the Standard Population [see TABLE 7].

1. The death rates for specific sex–age groups in A, B, etc.

2. The distribution by the same sex and age groups of a 'standard population', usually the population of the country as a whole. For convenience this standard population may be reduced in total size to a million, 'the standard million' or a thousand, depending upon whether rates per million or per thousand are wanted.

In essence the method of direct standardization shows what the all ages death rate would be in a standard population if each of its sex–age groups experienced the death rates recorded in the various local populations [TABLE 6].

Indirect Standardization

Again comparing the death rates in a series of local areas A, B, etc., for the method of indirect standardization we have to know:

1. The death rates for specific sex–age groups in the standard population;

2. The distribution by the same sex–age groups of the population of the local areas, A, B, ... etc.

This yields a correcting factor which is then applied to the crude local rate to produce a local standardized rate [TABLE 7].

The additional steps required in this indirect method compared with the direct method do not make it arithmetically any more troublesome, but make it a little more difficult to describe and to understand.

Expressed in algebraic symbols, where for each sex–age group:

P = Standard population,
M = Standard death rate,
p = Local population,
m = Local death rate, and
Σ = Summation of all sex–age groups.

1. The local standardized death rate (direct method) $= \dfrac{\Sigma mP}{P}$

2. The local standardized death rate (indirect method) $= \dfrac{\Sigma mp}{\Sigma p} \times f$

where $f = \dfrac{\Sigma MP}{\Sigma P} \div \dfrac{\Sigma Mp}{\Sigma p}$

TABLE 7
Standardization of Death Rates
Indirect Standardization (Hypothetical Data)

Age in years	Standard rates per 1,000	Population (thousands)		Expected deaths at standard rates	
		Area A	Area B	Area A	Area B
		Male			
0–	2·4	2	12	4·8	28·8
15–	1·6	5	28	8·0	44·8
45–	13·5	11	6	148·5	81·0
65+	82·9	5	2	414·5	165·8
		Female			
0–	1·8	3	14	5·4	25·2
15–	1·1	6	28	6·6	30·8
45–	7·6	13	7	98·8	53·2
65+	60·5	5	3	302·5	181·5
Total	11·8	50	100	989	611

Index rates 989 ÷ 50   611 ÷ 100
= 19·8   = 6·1
Correcting factors 11·8 ÷ 19·8   11·8 ÷ 6·1
= 0·60   = 1·93
Standardized rates 18·4 × 0·60   6·5 × 1·93
= 11·0   = 12·5

Standardized Mortality Ratio (S.M.R.) $= \dfrac{\text{Actual deaths}}{\text{Expected deaths}} \times 100$

$= \dfrac{922 \times 100}{989}$ $= \dfrac{647 \times 100}{611}$
= 93   = 106

The next step is to calculate the number of deaths that would occur at each age in the local population at standard rates, and thence to estimate what the standard all ages rate would have been with the local population sex–age distribution. Comparing this rate with the actual standard rate indicates whether the local population distribution tends to put the standard rate up or down, i.e. whether it favours high or low mortality.

Standardized Mortality Ratio

Instead of expressing mortality as a standardized death rate in the form of so many deaths per 1,000 population, the mortality comparison may be put in the form of a ratio between the number of deaths registered in the local area and the number that would have been registered in the same area if standard death rates for each sex–age group had occurred. The comparison is usually expressed as a percentage [TABLE 7].

The *Standardized Mortality Ratio* (S.M.R.) is therefore

$$\frac{\text{Actual deaths}}{\text{Expected deaths}} \times 100$$

or, in algebraic form, S.M.R. $= \dfrac{\Sigma\, mp}{\Sigma\, Mp} \times 100$

Since this method of standardization involves multiplication of standard death rates by local population, i.e. $\Sigma\, Mp$, it is a process of indirect standardization; this can also be seen by noting the complete similarity between the items of information used in the calculation in TABLE 7. However, by not requiring the calculation of an *index rate* or a *correcting factor* the S.M.R. is probably easier to understand in principle than an indirectly standardized *rate*, though the amount of calculation needed is little less.

Corresponding with the S.M.R., a standardized form of mortality ratio can also be calculated by direct standardization [TABLE 6], yielding what was called, when it was formerly used in connexion with occupational mortality, a *Comparative Mortality Factor* (C.M.F.) expressible in algebraic notation as

$$\frac{\Sigma\, mP}{\Sigma\, MP} \times 1,000$$

STANDARDIZED RATES, RATIOS, AND INDICES USED IN OFFICIAL STATISTICS

Although all of them are based either on direct or indirect standardization, the standardized rates, etc., used by the Registrar General for various purposes are sometimes calculated in special ways and presented in special forms.

The standardized rates, ratios, and indices principally used in recent years have been:

1. FOR ANNUAL TRENDS

(i) Up to 1941: Directly standardized death rates based upon a standard million population corresponding in its sex–age constitution with that of England and Wales in 1901.

(ii) From 1942 to 1957: A *Comparative Mortality Index* (C.M.I.), in which death rates in the given year were compared with that of 1938 taken as unity, the rates for both years being standardized on the basis of a population sex–age distribution that was the average of the two years. For a full explanation see the *Registrar General's Statistical Review*, Part I, 1941, page 320.

(iii) Since 1958: A *Standardized Mortality Ratio* (S.M.R.) comparing the death rate each year with the mean annual rate for 1950–52, and more recently for 1968, taken as 100.

2. AREA MORTALITY

(i) For annual comparisons, the crude rate for each local area is multiplied by an Area Comparability Factor (A.C.F.), and the rate so adjusted is then related to the rate for the country as a whole, taken as unity, a special adjustment also being made to allow for patients in chronic sick and psychiatric hospitals. This is a process of indirect standardization in which the A.C.F. is the correcting factor, and may be used unchanged for several years, so long as the sex–age distribution of the local population does not change much.

(ii) In the decennial supplement for 1951 and 1961 area comparisons were made by Standardized Mortality Ratios whereby the mortality for each area was compared with that of the country as a whole taken as 100. Recently S.M.R.s have been used also for annual area comparisons.

3. OCCUPATIONAL MORTALITY

(i) In the Decennial Occupational Mortality analyses from 1881 to 1921 comparisons were made by means of a Comparative Mortality Factor (C.M.F.) in which the deaths of men aged 20–64 in separate occupational groups were compared with that of all men of that age-range in the country, the mortality of the latter taken as 1,000. As already mentioned, this was a method of direct standardization, the standard population being adjusted in size so as to yield exactly 1,000 deaths.

(ii) In the Decennial Supplements from 1931 onwards use was made of a Standardized Mortality Ratio (S.M.R.) expressing the mortality at ages 20–64 (15–64 in 1961) in separate occupational groups as a percentage of that for all men of corresponding age [see also CHAPTER 38].

4. EQUIVALENT AVERAGE DEATH RATE (E.A.D.R.)

This is a special, and very simple form of standardization occasionally used for miscellaneous purposes. The E.A.D.R. for a given age-range is expressed as the average of the death rates of the separate age-groups composing the total age-range covered. For example, an E.A.D.R. at ages 0–64 would be the average of the death rates of the fourteen quinary age-groups 0–4, 5–9, 10–14, . . . 60–64. This is tantamount to direct standardization on the basis of a hypothetical standard population in which the numbers of the population are equal in each of the separate age–groups.

OTHER METHODS OF PRESENTATION OF MORTALITY STATISTICS

1. LIFE TABLES AND EXPECTATION OF LIFE

The life table is a special way of presenting the mortality experience of a given population for a particular period of time. It is not, as is sometimes supposed, a method of forecasting future mortality, but is a method of describing past mortality. What the life table shows is how a hypothetical cohort of individuals would die off, from birth onwards, if the cohort were subject to the mortality rates of a specified year or years. The average length of life experienced by this cohort, from the time they started until all are dead, is the expectation of life.

Though extensively used in life-assurance practice, the life table method of displaying mortality is of less interest for public health purposes, and a Medical Officer of Health will seldom want, other than for his own personal satisfaction, to work out a life table for his own area. However, the *expectation of life* which is derived from the life table, is a very well known mortality function; but, since it measures past not future mortality experience, it has no real prognostic significance and is not quite the simple statistic it is popularly thought to be.

A National Life Table is calculated in England and Wales at the period around each census. Life Table No. 11 was calculated on the mortality of 1950–52 and Life Table No. 12 was calculated for years 1960–62. In addition to these periodic life tables, which are prepared with great precision and present the data by single years of age, abridged life tables

TABLE 8

Extract from English Life Table No. 12, 1960–62

Age x	Males					Females				
	l_x	d_x	p_x	q_x	$\overset{\circ}{e}_x$	l_x	d_x	p_x	q_x	$\overset{\circ}{e}_x$
0	100,000	2,449	0·97551	0·02449	68·09	100,000	1,896	0·98104	0·01896	74·00
1	97,551	153	0·99843	0·00157	68·80	98,104	124	0·99874	0·00126	74·43
25	95,753	95	0·99901	0·00099	45·84	97,105	52	0·99946	0·00054	51·08
45	92,433	369	0·99601	0·00399	27·05	94,685	269	0·99716	0·00284	32·06
65	68,490	2,499	0·96352	0·03648	11·95	81,286	1,470	0·98192	0·01808	15·26
85	10,169	1,897	0·81341	0·18659	3·90	23,115	3,405	0·85271	0·14729	4·58
106	3	1	0·57391	0·42609	—	—	—	—	—	—
107	2	1	0·56825	0·43175	—	—	—	—	—	—
108	—	—	—	—	—	3	1	0·54097	0·45903	—
109	—	—	—	—	—	2	1	0·53421	0·46579	—

(Source: *Registrar General's Decennial Supplement 1961*, Life Tables.)

are published annually and triennially which present the data by 5-year age intervals.

An extract from English Life Table No. 12 is given in TABLES 8 and 9. The meaning of the various column headings is as follows:

Age x—successive exact ages, 0, 1, 2, etc.

l_x—the number of persons surviving to age x

d_x—the number of persons dying between age x and age $x + 1$ (i.e. between one age and the next)

p_x—the probability of surviving from age x to age $x + 1$

q_x—the probability of dying between age x and age $x + 1$

$\overset{\circ}{e}_x$—expectation of life at age x, i.e. the average length of life to be lived beyond exact age x.

TABLE 9

*Expectation of Life at Birth and at Age 1 year
English Life Tables Nos. 1 to 12*

English life table	Years	Expectation of life at			
		Birth		Age 1 year	
		Male	Female	Male	Female
No. 1	1841	40	42	47	48
2	1838–44	40	42	47	47
3	1838–54	40	42	47	47
4	1871–80	41	45	48	50
5	1881–90	44	47	51	53
6	1891–1900	44	48	52	55
7	1901–10	49	52	56	58
8	1910–12	52	55	58	60
9	1920–22	56	60	60	63
10	1930–32	59	63	62	65
11	1950–52	66	72	68	72
12	1960–62	68	74	69	74
	1968–70	69	75	69	75

(Source: Registrar General. The last line is from *Abridged Life Table 1968–70*.)

The extract from Life Table No. 12 shows that, under conditions of mortality experienced in England and Wales in 1960–62, out of 100,000 boys born, 97,551 would survive to age 1, 95,753 to age 25, and so on; that is to say, at these levels

of mortality less than 5 per cent. of males would die before age 25. By age 65, more than two-thirds (68,490) of the original group would still be alive, decreasing rapidly to little more than 10 per cent. (10,169) at age 85; and the male life table comes to an end with the last two survivors aged 107. Throughout their life females fare better than males; 98,104 would survive to age 1, 97,105 to age 25, 81,286 to age 65 and 23,115 to age 85. The cohort is reduced to its final 2 by age 109.

Expectation of life at birth ($\overset{\circ}{e}_x$) was 68·09 for boys and 74·00 for girls; at 1 year, however, expectation of life was slightly higher, since the relatively high mortality of the first year of life was now past. At age 65 the expectation of life of men was 11·95 years and of women 15·26 years, not much more than they were 50 years ago. Improvements in mortality during this century, though touching all ages, have inevitably been much greater among the young than the old.

2. LOSS OF EXPECTED YEARS OF LIFE

The death of a child aged 1 year represents a much greater loss of potential lifetime than that caused by the death of a man aged 80, who could not reasonably be expected to have lived much longer anyway. Accordingly, a cause of death operating mainly among young children might be responsible for a greater loss of expected years of life than that occasioned by another cause, possibly giving rise to many more deaths, but operating mainly among elderly persons. Similarly, looked at from the point of view of capacity for work, and taking the working years as 15 to 64, the death of a child under the age of 15 entails the loss of a full working lifetime of 50 years, whereas the death of a man aged exactly 60 involves the loss only of 5 years of working life.

In order to measure the effects of mortality from a small number of causes in terms of this concept of loss of expected years of life and loss of expected years of working life the Registrar General for England and Wales annually publishes a small table, an example of which appears in TABLE 10.

3. COHORT ANALYSIS

The conventional approach to a set of death rates, either from all causes or from a particular disease, is to study: 1. the

TABLE 10

Years of Life Lost due to Mortality from Certain Causes: Numbers of Deaths from Certain Causes, Death Rates per 10,000 Population, Mean Ages at Death, Years of 'Working Life' Lost, and Years of 'Total Life' Lost per 10,000 Population, 1970
(England and Wales)

The last two columns present figures for years of 'working life' lost (taken at ages 15–64) and for years of 'total life' lost (to age 85); The method of calculation has been: (*a*) to calculate the mean age at death from all causes for each of the age groups 0–, 5–, 15–, 25–, 45–, 65 and over; (*b*) to deduct each mean age from 85; alternatively, for the 'working life' comparison, to deduct each mean age or 15, whichever is the greater, from 65; (*c*) to multiply each difference so obtained by the number of deaths from the particular disease in the respective age group; (*d*) to total the products, and (*e*) to divide by the population at all ages to produce the rates shown.

ICD No.	Cause of death	Total deaths		Mean age at death	Years of life lost per 10,000 population	
		Number	Rate per 10,000 population		Ages 15–64	Total to age 85
	All causes:					
	Male	293,093	123	66·6	641	2,270
	Female	282,141	112	72·8	383	1,374
010–012, 019·0	Tuberculosis of respiratory system inc. late effects:					
	Male	1,025	0	64·8	2	8
	Female	372	0	61·9	1	3
140–209	Cancer (all sites):					
	Male	62,550	26	66·5	105	456
	Female	53,179	21	67·3	89	324
162	Cancer of trachea, bronchus and lung:					
	Male	24,913	10	66·1	36	179
174	Cancer of breast:					
	Female	10,677	4	64·1	23	78
410–414	Ischaemic heart disease:					
	Male	80,844	34	68·4	105	542
	Female	58,473	23	76·1	24	191
Rem. 393–429	Other heart disease, hypertension:					
	Male	18,622	8	71·8	21	113
	Female	28,111	11	77·0	16	97
480–493	Pneumonia, bronchitis (chronic and unspecified), emphysema and asthma:					
	Male	41,275	17	70·7	56	259
	Female	31,584	13	75·2	33	131
531–533	Peptic ulcer:					
	Male	2,309	1	69·4	3	15
	Female	1,456	1	75·2	1	5
E800–E949	Accidents:					
	Male	9,583	4	44·1	88	161
	Female	7,691	3	65·2	27	61

(Source: *Registrar General's Quarterly Return for England and Wales*, No. 490, Second Quarter, 1971, H.M.S.O., London.)

trend of the rates for given sex–age groups at successive periods of time, to see whether the disease seems to be increasing or decreasing; and 2. the sex–age distribution of the death rates for selected periods of time to see what kind of sex–age mortality pattern the disease presents.

To take a particular example, TABLE 11 gives death rates of men from cancer of tongue by 5-year age-groups and 5-year

TABLE 11

Cancer of Tongue
(Death rates per million men)

Age	1921–25	1926–30	1931–35	1936–40	1941–45	1946–50	1951–55
45–	**62**	40	24	13	10	5	5
50–	142	**105**	62	40	22	13	7
55–	244	205	**151**	88	50	34	26
60–	345	333	269	**198**	119	64	42
65–	420	422	399	297	**229**	134	85
70–	449	445	448	403	337	**238**	155
75–79	485	485	487	500	393	333	**287**

(Source: *General Register Office Study No. 13.*)

periods of time. The conventional way of studying these data would be to note: 1. that at each age-group there has been a progressive and substantial decline in mortality, the decline at ages 50–54 being from 142 to 7, i.e. by 95 per cent., and at ages 75–79 from 485 to 287, i.e. by 40 per cent.; and 2. that at each period of time there was a steep rise in mortality from the youngest to the oldest age-group shown; in 1921–25 the rate increased from 62 at 45–49 to 485 at 75–79, and in 1951–55 it increased from 5 to 287.

Whether, however, we follow a row of figures horizontally—an age-group at successive time-periods—or vertically—the age distribution of the rates in a given time-period—we are looking at successive rates in different groups of people; men aged 45–49 in 1921–25 are not the same men as those aged 45–49 in 1926–30, and the rates in 1951–55 at ages 45–49 refer to a different group of men from those for 50–54, and so on.

If, however, we move diagonally across the table from top left to bottom right we are then able to follow the death rates for the same cohort of men as they grow older at successive intervals of time. For example, the cohort who were aged 45–49 in 1921–25, with a rate of 62, had a rate of 105 at ages 50–54,

151 at ages 55–59, and so on up to 287 at ages 75–79. This is the only cohort that can be followed in the table through all seven age-periods; but the cohort who were aged 45–49 in 1926–30 (with a rate then of 40) and the cohort aged 50–54 in 1921–25 (rate 142) can each be followed diagonally through six age-periods; and other cohorts similarly but for diminishing durations.

Cohort analysis is not used routinely in vital statistics, since the more conventional methods are ordinarily sufficient. But it is a useful auxiliary way of studying mortality data and, if used circumspectly, can sometimes draw attention to trends that might otherwise be overlooked.

SOME SPECIAL ASPECTS OF MORTALITY STATISTICS

The Interpretation of Trends in Time

One of the most useful contributions of mortality statistics is the information they provide about trends of death rates, either from all causes or from selected causes.

In studying a series of death rates, annual, quinquennial, etc., the following sources of error or difficulty must be kept in mind and allowance made for their possible effects.

1. SEX AND AGE CHANGES IN THE POPULATION

This difficulty has already been mentioned above in the section on methods of standardization. Except over comparatively short periods of time, as from one year to the next, during which the population sex–age structure cannot have altered significantly, it is always advisable, by one method or another, to standardize the rates and so minimize the influence of sex–age changes. Changes in the relative numbers in the two sexes need be considered only when rates for *persons* (males and females) are under consideration. For rates for the sexes separately, an adjustment only for age change is necessary.

TABLE 12

Death Rates and Standard Mortality Ratio
All Causes (England and Wales)

	Crude death rate per 1,000 persons	S.M.R.
1909	14·6	219
1925	12·1	153
1938	11·6	119
1957	11·5	91
1970	11·7	87
Reduction (per cent.) 1909 to 1970 . . .	19·9 per cent.	60 per cent.

(Source: Registrar General.)

TABLE 12 shows that the crude death rate declined from 14·6 to 11·7 per thousand between 1909 and 1970, a decline of 19·9 per cent. But if standardization is performed, so as to make allowance for sex–age changes in the population during that period, the reduction in mortality can be shown to have been by 60 per cent.

2. CHANGES IN DISEASE CLASSIFICATION AND IN METHODS OF STATISTICAL ASSIGNMENT

The International List of Causes of Death came into use in England and Wales in 1911, following its second revision. The List has been revised at approximately 10-year intervals since then, the eighth (1965) revision coming into operation in 1968. Changes in classification can have considerable effect upon the recorded trends of some causes. This was particularly so when the sixth revision came into operation in 1950. A still greater upset to annual comparability took place in England and Wales in 1940, when the system of selecting cause of death for statistical assignment was altered. Previously when more than one cause was certified selection was made on the basis of arbitrary rules of priority. Since 1940 the cause selected has been the 'underlying cause' as indicated by the way the certifier has filled in the death certificate.

Ordinarily in publishing serial death rates covering a number of years the Registrar General adjusts the earlier figures, so far as it is practicable to do so, to make them comparable with the later ones; and following each Revision he publishes tables showing for the same period, e.g. one year, deaths classified by both revisions. This dual tabulation provides a bridge from one revision to the next, and facilitates the calculation of conversion factors for adjusting the earlier figures.

The effects of successive changes of classification upon four important causes of death are shown in TABLE 13, the years for which dual tabulations were made being 1939, 1949, 1957, and 1967.

3. CHANGES IN FASHIONS OF DIAGNOSIS

Throughout the years new medical discoveries are constantly being made, new ideas of aetiology and of the relationships between different diseases are developed, new diseases are identified and labelled, new disease descriptions come into fashion to displace the terminology favoured by an earlier generation, and means of diagnosis are constantly being improved. With the language and the practice of medicine constantly changing, it is inevitable that the way death certificates are filled in, the arrangement of the diseases reported, and the terms used to describe them will also change; and such changes in terminology, in fashions of certification, in diagnostic precision will in turn lead to distortions in the resultant mortality statistics. Sometimes, as when a new disease is described, there may follow a rapid increase in the number of reported deaths as doctors quickly get to know about it. But the disease may not have been becoming more lethal or more prevalent; it may simply have become more widely recognized.

TABLE 13

Death Rates per Million Persons, All Ages, in Accordance with Successive Revisions of the International Classification
(England and Wales)

Revision of International Classification	Coronary disease	Hyper-tension	Bronchitis	Nephritis
4th, 1929 . .	121	3	843	392
4th ⌠ 1939 . .	473	32	375	317
5th ⌡ 1939 . .	433	42	762	358
5th ⌠ 1949 . .	996	144	706	259
6th ⌡ 1949 . .	1,093	389	672	156
6th ⌠ 1957 . .	1,700	434	600	97
7th ⌡ 1957 . .	1,719	436	603	93
7th, 1967 . .	2,383	232	575	55
8th, 1967 . .	2,675	231	538	46

(Source: Registrar General.)

Sometimes evidence of a direct transfer from one disease label to another can be established by adding the two together and showing that the gains in one are balanced by the losses in the other, a technique that has been repeatedly applied since the time of John Graunt.

On occasion, however, the influence of changing fashion in nomenclature or of improvements in diagnosis cannot be estimated with any degree of precision, though they may be suspected, or even assumed, to have been playing a big part in producing an apparent trend. Two outstanding examples at the present time are deaths from coronary disease [TABLE 13] and deaths from cancer of lung, both of which have recorded enormous increases in recent decades, particularly in men. It is beyond all reasonable doubt that a new fashion in terminology has contributed to the apparent increase in coronary disease, and, similarly, modern methods of diagnosis have contributed to the apparent increase in cancer of lung. How much of the increase in each instance is to be accounted for in this way, and how much of the increase is due to the real rise in the prevalence of the two diseases is difficult to assess.

Infant Mortality

Infant mortality comprises deaths of children under 1 year of age. It is usually expressed as a rate per 1,000 live births, during the same period, thus:

$$\text{Infant Mortality Rate in 1972 per 1,000 live births} = \frac{\text{Deaths under 1 year of age in 1972}}{\text{Live births in 1972}} \times 1,000$$

Some of the children dying under age 1 in a given year would, however, be born not in that year but in the previous year, so the numerator and denominator do not quite correspond. Ordinarily the error introduced is quite trivial, but during periods when the birth rate is fluctuating violently it may become significant. Because of the fluctuations in the

of life but also because of its close correlation with social conditions.

The following definitions are used in connexion with the separate periods of the first year:

Neonatal mortality = deaths under 4 weeks
Early neonatal mortality = deaths under 1 week
Late neonatal mortality = deaths between 1 and 4 weeks
Postneonatal mortality = deaths over 4 weeks and under 1 year
Perinatal mortality = stillbirths and deaths under 1 week. (A stillbirth is a foetal death after the 28th week of pregnancy.)

Neonatal and postneonatal rates are expressed per thousand *live* births, as for infant mortality rates; but the perinatal rate

TABLE 15
Neonatal and Postneonatal Mortality Rates per 1,000 Live Births (England and Wales, 1969)

	Neonatal		Postneonatal	
	Male	Female	Male	Female
Birth injury and difficult labour	2·80	1·71	0·01	0·01
Anoxic and hypoxic conditions	4·01	2·66	0·02	0·01
Immaturity unqualified	1·98	1·71	0·01	0·01
Congenital malformations	2·57	2·29	1·17	1·24
Pneumonia and bronchitis	0·68	0·46	2·88	2·20
Intestinal infectious disease	0·11	0·06	0·47	0·42
Accidental suffocation	0·06	0·04	0·58	0·37
All causes (including causes not listed above)	13·72	10·25	6·60	5·39

(Source: Registrar General.)

is expressed per thousand *total* births, live and still, as is also the stillbirth rate.

TABLE 14
Infant Mortality Rate, its Principal Subdivisions, and Stillbirth Rate (England and Wales)

	Rates per 1,000 live births					Rates per 1,000 total births	
	Infant mortality rate (under 1 year)	Neonatal mortality rate (under 4 weeks)	Early neonatal mortality rate (under 1 week)	Late neonatal mortality rate (1 week and under 4 weeks)	Postneonatal mortality rate (4 weeks and under 1 year)	Perinatal mortality rate (stillbirths + early neonatal)	Stillbirth rate
1928	65·3	31·1	21·6	9·5	34·2	60·8	40·1
1938	52·8	28·3	21·1	7·1	24·5	58·6	38·3
1948	33·9	19·7	15·6	4·1	14·2	38·5	23·2
1958	22·5	16·2	13·8	2·4	6·4	35·0	21·5
1970	18·2	12·3	10·6	1·7	5·9	23·5	13·0

(Source: Registrar General.)

birth rate associated with the First and Second World Wars, the Registrar General on each occasion introduced temporarily a correction to the simple infant mortality rate. Thus for the period 1940–57 the rate was expressed per thousand *related* live births to take account of births in the previous year. This correction has since been abandoned as being no longer required.

The infant mortality rate occupies a special position in vital statistics, not only because of its value as an indicator of loss

The trend of the above rates in recent decades, and the contrast between the causes of neonatal and postneonatal mortality, are shown in TABLES 14 and 15 [see also CHAPTER 34].

Maternal Mortality

Maternal mortality comprises deaths due to maternal causes (ICD Eighth Revision, Nos. 630–678), viz. complications of pregnancy; abortion; complications of delivery; and of the puerperium.

The *Maternal Mortality Rate* is expressed as deaths from maternal causes per thousand *total* births, live and still, during the same year. The numerator and denominator do not completely match since: 1. some deaths result from births occurring in the previous year; 2. some deaths, e.g. those from abortion, are not associated with any birth; 3. a proportion of maternities give rise to multiple births. These are minor sources of inaccuracy and do not affect the usefulness of the rate. Prior to 1958 there was no time limit beyond which a death resulting from some maternal complication could not be assigned to

TABLE 16

Trend of Maternal Mortality and of Associated Maternal Mortality
(*Death Rates per 1,000 Total Births, England and Wales*)

	Maternal causes except abortion	Abortion	Total maternal mortality	Associated maternal mortality
1931	3·43	0·68	4·11	1·38
1938	2·70	0·55	3·24	0·82
1948	0·86	0·16	1·02	0·31
1955	0·50	0·10	0·59	0·17
1970	0·14	0·04	0·18	0·07

(Source: Registrar General.)

maternal causes. As a result, a small proportion of maternal deaths were recorded among women of very advanced ages, attributed to childbearing many years before. This misleading situation was corrected at the Seventh Revision of the International Classification, with the result that from 1958 onwards deaths have been assigned to maternal causes only when they occur within *one year* of the maternal complication.

In England and Wales, in addition to deaths assigned to maternal causes, a further group of deaths are classified as deaths 'not due to, but associated with maternal causes'. These are deaths assigned to some other cause indicated by the certifier as being responsible, but with a maternal complication mentioned on the death certificate as an associated condition. They are not included in the maternal mortality rate.

The trend of maternal mortality in England and Wales in recent years is shown in TABLE 16.

Occupational Mortality

In the years around each census the Registrar General carries out an analysis of occupational mortality. At death registration the occupation of the deceased person is recorded, or, if a married woman, the occupation of her husband. Similar information about occupation in respect of the population in general is obtained at the census. On the basis of the two pieces of information, occupational death rates can be calculated.

There are a number of limitations and difficulties to be kept in mind. In the first instance, the occupational descriptions given at the census and at death registration are given in different circumstances and very often by different people (at the census by the head of the household, at death registration by an informant, usually a near relative), so that they are liable to disagree, sometimes to a considerable degree. Secondly, it is the last occupation that is recorded, and this may not have been the usual occupation. Thirdly, when the data are broken down to small occupational groups for separate

causes of death, numbers become small and chance fluctuations in the figures become a source of difficulty. And finally there is considerable selection by people of jobs on the basis of their physical fitness, so that the mortality recorded for a particular occupation may be low because that occupation selects only fit people for entry into it (or only fit people would seek to enter it, which comes to the same thing) or, on the other hand, be high because it is regarded as a light job suitable for people in poor health.

In the Classification of Occupations of 1960 there were 27 occupational orders divided into just over 200 unit groups and the mortality of these during the period 1959–63 was tabulated and published in a Decennial Supplement on Occupational Mortality. Such analyses have been made decennially since 1851 (except 1941), the two previous ones being for 1930–32 and 1949–53 [Table 17]. The number of unit groups was much smaller than in 1951 in order to conform as far as possible with the International Standard Classification of Occupation recommended by the International Labour Office, and also because the previous classification had been found to be too elaborate.

TABLE 17

Standardized Mortality Ratios—Men Aged 15–64
(*England and Wales, 1959–63*)
(*Selected Occupations*)

Coal mine faceworkers . . .	180
Publicans	147
Fishermen	144
Telephone operators . . .	129
Bakers	118
Butchers	105
Postmen, mail sorters . .	95
Medical practitioners . .	89
Draughtsmen	79
Clergy	62
Teachers	60

(Source: *Registrar General's Decennial Supplement 1961*, Occupational Mortality.)

In addition to tabulating mortality by individual occupational groups, extensive use is also made of a classification of occupations into five Social Classes, depending upon the *general standing within the community* of the occupations concerned. It is not a classification of individuals but of the occupational group to which they belong. The five Social Classes are:

I. Professional, etc., occupations (e.g. law, medicine, the Church)
II. Intermediate occupations (e.g. employers, managers, farmers)
III. Skilled occupations (e.g. fitters, clerks, engine drivers)
IV. Partly skilled occupations (e.g. machine minders)
V. Unskilled occupations (e.g. labourers, kitchen hands)

The tabulation of the mortality of married women by husband's occupation provides a useful check upon the occupational mortality distributions of men. If the mortality of the men and of their wives is similar, it may be assumed—provided wives do not work in the same occupation—that no specific occupational factor is at work, since that would affect the men only; on the other hand, if the mortality of men and married women for a given occupational group differs substantially, the presumption is that an occupational factor is present.

In calculating mortality for occupations and social classes, the principal measurement used is a Standardized Mortality Ratio (S.M.R.) at ages 15–64, the standard being all men (or all married women, or single women) at those ages. At ages 65 and over the discrepancies between occupational statements at census and death registration become too large to relate the two directly, and mortality from separate causes is measured by a Proportionate Mortality Ratio (P.M.R.) in which for a given occupation the proportion of deaths assigned to a particular cause is compared, per cent., with the corresponding proportion for all men (or women). This is calculated for ages 65–74 only.

TABLE 18, which shows the social class distribution of mortality of men aged 15–64, indicates that for some causes of death,

TABLE 18
Standardized Mortality Ratios—Men Aged 15–64
(England and Wales)

	Social class				
	I	II	III	IV	V
All causes:					
1921–23 . . .	82	94	95	101	125
1930–32 . . .	90	94	97	102	111
1949–53 . . .	98	86	101	94	118
1959–63 . . .	76	81	100	103	143
Selected causes 1959–63					
Tuberculosis .	40	54	96	108	185
Malignant neoplasm of					
stomach . .	49	63	101	114	163
Leukaemia . .	106	100	103	97	108
Coronary disease,					
angina . .	98	95	106	96	112
Bronchitis . .	28	50	97	116	194
Ulcer of stomach .	46	58	94	106	199

(Source: *Registrar General's Decennial Supplement 1961,*
Occupational Mortality.)

such as respiratory tuberculosis and bronchitis, there is a gradient of increasing mortality from Social Class I to Social Class V, while for other causes such as leukaemia or coronary disease no obvious gradient in either direction can be discerned. As regards all causes changes in social class assignments of occupations in 1959–63 has led to a more pronounced rising gradient from Social Class I to V than was apparent on previous occasions.

In addition to the deaths of adults these occupational mortality analyses concern themselves also with deaths of infants. Here the denominator is obtained, not from the census, but from the statements of father's occupation given at birth registration. Infant mortality by social class has always shown

TABLE 19
Infant Mortality by Social Class
Rates per 1,000 Live Births (Legitimate Only)

	All classes	Social class				
		I	II	III	IV	V
1921	79·1	38·4	55·5	76·8	89·4	97·0
1930–32	61·6	32·7	45·0	57·6	66·8	77·1
1949–53	29·5	18·7	21·6	28·6	33·8	40·8
1964–65*	17·5	12·7		17·2		20·8

(Source: Registrar General; and Spicer and Lipworth (1966).)

a steep rising gradient from Social Class I to Social Class V [TABLE 19] [see also CHAPTER 38].

Area Mortality

An Area Mortality report is a further part of the *Registrar General's Decennial Supplements* [see also CHAPTER 39].

For a very long time this was an analysis of deaths, in local areas, registered during the 10 years from one census to the next. In the 1951 Supplement a departure was made from tradition, and deaths were analysed for the period 1950–53 and related to the local area populations determined at the 1951 census. Death rates by sex and age from a number of causes were tabulated individually for the City of London and the Metropolitan Boroughs, for each of the County Boroughs, and for each Administrative County. Rates at all ages were standardized and expressed as Standardized Mortality Ratios, with England and Wales taken as 100.

TABLE 20
Standardized Mortality Ratios
Regions of England and Wales
(1959–1963)
(England and Wales = 100)

	Breast (female)	Cervix (female)
London and South-East . .	107	87
Midlands	104	97
Eastern	103	87
South Western . . .	101	94
North Midland . . .	99	103
Southern	98	93
North Western . . .	95	113
East and West Ridings . .	95	118
Wales	94	107
Northern	86	119

(Source: *Registrar General's Decennial Supplement 1961,*
Area mortality.)

In addition to the individual local areas, death rates and S.M.R.s were calculated for the ten Standard Regions, the six conurbations, and the five urban/rural aggregates. A similar study was carried out for the 5 years 1959–63 [TABLE 20].

International Mortality Statistics

The existence of the International Statistical Classification of Diseases, Injuries, and Causes of Death, and the World Health Organization's recommendations regarding its use, go a long way towards making possible the comparison of death rates for different countries, and such rates are now accessible in regular international publications. But the international comparison of death rates still remains an uncertain business even for those experienced in such matters. The principal causes of incomparability are the following:

1. International differences in the form of death certificate used, and in the way the causes of death are tabulated in different statistical offices.

2. International differences in the proportions of deaths certified by qualified medical practitioners.

3. International differences in the amount of specialized diagnostic facilities available to medical practitioners.

4. International differences in the ideas and preferences of

medical practitioners regarding the certifying of various causes of death, in the terminology used, and in their views upon the interrelationships of one disease with another.

The possible existence of causes of incomparability such as these renders it difficult to know what to make of the very large differences in rates, for example from ischaemic heart disease, and from bronchitis [TABLE 21]. The death rate from heart disease in the United States and the United Kingdom was approximately four times higher than in France, where there is no shortage of doctors or of facilities for diagnosis, and over eight times higher than in Japan; and the death rate from bronchitis in England and Wales was four times that of the United States. Recent investigations lead to the conclusion that

TABLE 21
Death Rates, All Ages per 100,000 Persons (1968)
(ICD 8th Revision 1965)

	Ischaemic Heart Disease (A83)	Bronchitis Emphysema and Asthma (A93)
United States . .	338	17
Japan . . .	35	15
France . . .	77	12
Ireland . . .	250	67
England and Wales .	285	67
Northern Ireland .	282	57
Scotland . . .	332	54
Yugoslavia . . .	46	17
Australia . . .	278	30
New Zealand . .	252	33

(Source: *World Health Statistics Annual, 1968.*)

these differences are not entirely artificial but derive at least to some degree from differences between countries in environment, diet, habits, and ways of life.

MORBIDITY STATISTICS

Attempts at the systematic statistical measurement of sickness were made from time to time during the eighteenth and nineteenth centuries in connexion with the experience of the early friendly societies (sick funds), the Army and Navy, major epidemics, and admissions to hospital. An account of these early efforts was given by Farr in a chapter on Vital Statistics that he contributed, in 1837, to McCulloch's *A Statistical Account of the British Empire*. Developments in the hospital field during the nineteenth century have been sketched in *Hospital Morbidity Statistics* (General Register Office Study No. 4, 1951).

Morbidity statistics provide a picture of the amount of illness, disability, and injury within a population. The public health administrator, at first primarily concerned with the prevention of infectious diseases, soon came to realize that there were many other conditions about which information was required in order that he might implement the work in the community for which he was responsible. To the hospital administrator a knowledge of the amount and nature of the diseases prevailing in his area is of paramount importance if he is to provide adequate facilities for dealing with them. Morbidity data are needed for the planning, development, and management of programmes concerned with all aspects of social security in its widest sense. Industrial undertakings and other organizations engaged in production or concerned with the national economy need morbidity statistics in order to assess and to reduce the effects of sickness upon the availability of man-power. Persons engaged in medical research utilize morbidity statistics in studying the aetiology and pathogenesis of sickness, and in seeking methods of prevention or cure. Finally, social research workers need morbidity statistics in order to correlate sickness of varying severity and duration with the social and economic factors that are themselves inextricably bound up with how patients react to their sickness.

In summary, the uses of morbidity statistics are:

1. Control of infectious diseases.
2. Planning for development of preventive services.
3. Ascertainment of relationship to social factors.
4. Planning for provision of adequate treatment services.
5. Estimation of economic importance of sickness.
6. Research into aetiology and pathogenesis.
7. Research on efficacy of preventive and therapeutic measures.
8. National and international study of distribution of diseases and impairments.

The following list indicates the very wide range of types and sources of morbidity statistics that are available:

Sickness surveys.
Mass diagnostic and screening surveys (e.g. tuberculosis).
Census enumeration of sick persons or of certain defects.
Notifications of infectious disease.
Registration of certain diseases (e.g. cancer).
Certification of certain conditions for special benefits or allowances (e.g. maternity benefits).
Records of road accidents.
Industrial accidents and diseases.
Hospital in-patient and out-patient records.
Home-visiting and nursing services.
Special clinics (e.g. tuberculosis, venereal disease).
General practitioners' clinical records.
Social security schemes and voluntary health plans and funds.
Pensioners' and veterans' medical records.
Life and sickness insurance records.
Records of health welfare centres (e.g. antenatal and child welfare).
School medical records (routine examinations and sickness absenteeism).
Records of physical examinations and sickness absenteeism in industry, civil service, etc.
Sickness and recruitment records of Armed Forces.

THE MEASUREMENT OF MORBIDITY

Morbidity statistics must take account of several factors which do not affect mortality statistics, in that, as distinct from death, illness may occur many times in the same person, have a duration ranging from hours to years, vary in severity from the most trivial to the most serious, and lead to varying degrees of disturbance to the patient's ordinary mode of life from minimum disability to lengthy hospitalization.

Morbidity can be measured in terms of three units:

1. *persons* who are ill;
2. the *spells* of illness that are experienced;
3. the *duration* of these illnesses.

Morbidity can also be measured in terms of:

1. Spells of illness *commencing*, or persons becoming ill, during a defined period. This is called *incidence*.

2. Spells of illness *current*, or persons ill, during a defined period. This is called *period prevalence*.

3. Spells of illness *current*, or persons ill at a particular point of time within the period or at an average point of time within the period. This is called *point prevalence*.

4. The duration of these illnesses, expressed either as *average duration* or as frequency distributions of durations either in relation to spells or to ill persons.

NATIONAL MORBIDITY STATISTICS IN ENGLAND AND WALES

Morbidity Statistics Compiled by the Office of Population Censuses and Surveys (formerly the General Register Office [TABLE 22]

1. NOTIFIABLE INFECTIOUS DISEASES

A regular series of the number of cases of notifiable infectious diseases has been published in the Registrar General's

TABLE 22
Miscellaneous Representative Morbidity Statistics in England and Wales

Notifiable Infectious Diseases
(Final numbers after correction)

	1950	1960	1970
Meningococcal infection*	1,149	630	525
Scarlet fever .	65,878	32,166	13,138
Whooping cough .	157,752	58,030	16,597
Diphtheria .	959	49	22
Acute poliomyelitis .	7,752	378	7

* From 1st October 1968 a sub-category of Acute meningitis.

Survey of Sickness
Bronchitis: Mean monthly prevalence rates per 10,000 persons, 1950

	\multicolumn{3}{c}{Age}	All ages
	16–44	45–64	65+	16+
Males .	193	650	892	426
Females	236	406	852	383

Hospital In-patient Inquiry
Discharge rates per 10,000 population by principal diagnosis at ages 45–64, 1968

Male		Female	
Hernia with or without obstruction . . .	65·7	Benign neoplasm of uterus	36·6
Acute myocardial infarction	51·4	Utero-vaginal prolapse .	35·3
Peptic ulcer . . .	34·3	Cholelithiasis and cholecystitis . .	22·5
Malignant neoplasm of bronchus, trachea and lung . . .	32·6	Arthritis and spondylitis .	22·4
		Varicose veins of lower extremities . .	21·1
Bronchitis . .	31·4		

General Practitioners' Records
Ulcer of stomach. Patient consulting rate per 1,000 males, all ages. May 1955–April 1956

	Urban	Semi-urban	Rural
North . .	19	10	11
Midlands and Wales .	16	13	9
South . .	14	13	9

Cancer Registration
Percentage of patients registered in 1961 surviving 5 years*

Site	Male	Female
Stomach	5	5
Rectum	21	23
Bronchus, trachea and lung . .	5	4
Breast	—	44
Cervix uteri (excluding *in situ*) . .	—	44
Prostate	17	—

* Crude minimum survival rates uncorrected.

Mass Miniature Radiography
Tuberculosis rates, all ages per 1,000 examinations (1967)

Examinee group	Male	Female
Hospital in- and out-patients . .	5·0	4·3
General practitioner referrals . .	9·1	6·2
Contacts . . .	3·0	2·7
General public volunteers . .	2·2	1·6
All groups, including groups not mentioned above	2·6	1·9

Legally Induced Abortions in 1970
By age and main operation

	Under 19	20–24	25–34	35 and over	Not stated
Dilatation . .	7,775	10,921	10,969	4,720	642
Vacuum aspiration	6,931	9,480	11,325	5,208	732
Hysterotomy .	1,228	1,607	5,714	4,280	279
Hysterectomy .	4	33	343	649	22
Other and not stated .	1,092	1,153	1,040	334	84

Congenital Malformations
Rates per 10,000 births by sex and type of birth
(England and Wales, 1970)

Site	Total	\multicolumn{2}{c}{Live}	\multicolumn{2}{c}{Still}
		Male	Female	Male	Female
All babies . .	176	167	144	1,220	2,110
Limbs . .	67	64	66	144	180
Central nervous system .	40	20	25	883	1,815
Cleft lip/palate .	14	15	11	53	48
External genitalia .	12	21	2	28	4
Cardiovascular system .	9	10	8	25	22

TABLE 22 (contd.)
Mental Health Statistics
First admission rates to mental illness hospitals
per million, all ages

	1969	
	Males	Females
All diagnoses	1,554	2,114
Depressive psychoses, involutional melancholia	492	840
Psychoneuroses	219	372
Schizophrenia, schizo-affective disorders, paranoia	239	261
Psychoses of the senium . . .	132	241

National Insurance Statistics
Numbers of insured persons (1,000s) absent from work
on specified dates (1970)

	3 March	2 June	1 Sept	1 Dec.
Sickness .	969	826	789	880
Injury .	61	59	55	58

(Source: *Registrar General's Quarterly Return*,
3rd Quarter 1971, No. 491, H.M.S.O., London.)

Weekly Return since 1895, starting first with certain London fever hospitals and attaining nation-wide coverage in 1922 when the present series of statistics based on returns made weekly by Medical Officers of Health to the Registrar General first began. The statistics published weekly show the number of cases of each disease notified in every local-authority area in England and Wales. They are followed every quarter by figures corrected for diagnosis and analysed by sex and age, and published in the Registrar General's Quarterly Return, and consolidated for the whole year in the Annual Statistical Review.

2. SURVEY OF SICKNESS

In 1944 a continuous sample survey of the nation's health was begun and continued until the beginning of 1952. The data were derived from the people themselves, not from clinical records or medical notifications, and one aim was to assess the quantity of minor illnesses that do not lead to medical care as well as those that do. Each month a different sample of about 4,000 people, selected as a representation of the population of England and Wales aged 16 and over, was interviewed by field workers of the Social Survey Unit of the Central Office of Information. The results were published in various reports, notably Nos. 2 and 12 of the General Register Office Special Studies. Recently a health section of the General Household Survey has been introduced but no data had been published at the time of writing.

3. HOSPITAL IN-PATIENT INQUIRY

Starting in 1949 a programme has been developed for the compilation of hospital morbidity statistics. This programme covers all the National Health Service hospitals of England and Wales except hospitals (and departments in general hospitals) for psychiatric diseases and for mental subnormality. It is based on individual case summary forms completed on discharge and a 10 per cent. sample of all patients discharged is used for analysis. Statistics are compiled by sex and age, diagnosis, duration of stay, and area of residence, as well as by hospital

region, length of time on waiting list, and department of hospital in which treated. A special type of return is made for maternity cases.

4. GENERAL PRACTITIONERS' RECORDS

During the three years 1951–54 ten medical practitioners kept records in a form suitable for analysis by the General Register Office. Each consultation between doctor and patient was recorded, showing date and place of consultation, the number and type of medical certificates issued, any referral to hospital, and the diagnosis (or other reason for consultation) (General Register Office Studies Nos. 7 and 9).

A much larger inquiry covering some 100 practices in different parts of the country was held in the twelve months May 1955 to April 1956. This was in collaboration with the College of General Practitioners, and the 170 doctors taking part were members of the College interested in general practitioner research. The records were analysed in relation to sex, age, diagnosis, area, and occupation (General Register Office Study No. 14). A fresh inquiry on a similar large scale was held in the 12 months from November 1970 but the results are not yet available.

5. NATIONAL CANCER REGISTRATION

Since 1945 there has been a national scheme for the registration of cancer patients. The information is obtained only in respect of hospital patients (in-patients and out-patients). On provisional diagnosis, a registration card is sent to the General Register Office and this is followed by an abstract card confirming the diagnosis, and giving fuller details about the patient and the clinical, histological, and treatment data. The abstract cards are passed back and forward between the registering hospital and the General Register Office at intervals so that each case can be followed up year after year until death. The objectives of the national cancer registration scheme are two-fold (i) to obtain data on the incidence of cancer, by site, sex, age, and stage of disease, and (ii) to calculate survival rates for 1, 2, 3, . . . years. Particular attention is given to the five-year survival rate, either expressed as a crude rate or corrected to allow for mortality from other causes.

6. MASS MINIATURE RADIOGRAPHY

Since 1954 there has been national compilation of statistics from returns made by Mass Miniature Radiography Units in England and Wales. Units submit each month a 10 per cent. sample of examinee record cards. These are analysed by sex, age, previous history, type of examinee, and previous X-ray. Details of all significant abnormal findings are analysed and related to the 10 per cent. sample of all examinations. Results are published in Part 3 Commentary of the Registrar General's Statistical Review (until 1968 they also appeared in the Annual Reports of the Chief Medical Officer of the Department of Health and Social Security). A General Register Office Study for the period 1955–57 has also been published.

7. ABORTION STATISTICS

Medical practitioners who terminate a pregnancy under the regulations of the Abortion Act 1967 are required to notify the circumstances on a prescribed form to the Chief Medical Officer of the Department of Health and Social Security. From these forms statistics are compiled by a special unit of the Office of Population Censuses and Surveys. Marital status, age, parity, area of residence, type of operation and reasons for termination are among the variables analysed in these statistics which appear in the Registrar General's Weekly and Quarterly Returns and in a Supplement to the Statistical Review.

8. CONGENITAL MALFORMATIONS

Following the discovery that the drug *Thalidomide* was capable of producing a particular type of congenital abnormality when taken during pregnancy, arrangements were made to monitor the occurrence of congenital abnormalities that are easily recognized at birth. This information is collected by Medical Officers for Environmental Health and relayed at monthly intervals to the Office of Population Censuses and Surveys.

The information is normally collected in conjunction with Birth Notification whereby Medical Officers for Environmental Health are advised of all births in their district. Among the variables included in the statistics which appear in the Registrar General's Return for the September Quarter are sex, area, type of birth, and type of malformation

Morbidity Statistics Compiled by the Department of Health and Social Security

MENTAL HEALTH INQUIRY

Since 1949 statistics have been compiled from individual summary records of all patients in all National Health Service hospitals for mental illness and the mentally handicapped. Cards relating to patients admitted, discharged, transferred, or died are sent monthly to the Department of Health and Social Security and annual statistics are compiled giving sex, age, diagnosis, area, social class, duration of stay. Information on the number of patients in these hospitals at the end of each year is based on censuses which were carried out at the end of 1954 and 1963 and the records of admissions, discharges, and deaths over the period.

Of particular interest has been the establishment of a follow-up index. Cards of patients admitted to a mental hospital for the first time during 1954–56 are filed in an alphabetical index, and subsequent admissions and discharges of these patients are entered in the index so as to build up a longitudinal history of periods spent in hospital by each patient.

STATISTICS ANALYSING CERTIFICATES OF INCAPACITY FOR WORK

Since 1949 the Ministry of Pensions and National Insurance (now incorporated in the Department of Health and Social Security) has analysed the medical certificates submitted to it in respect of insured persons incapacitated from work and claiming either sickness benefit or injury benefit.

Broadly the whole of the civilian *working* population aged 15 and over can qualify under the National Insurance Act for sickness benefit without limit of income, including not only those employed under contract of service but also the self-employed. Only comparatively small sections of the working population are excluded, the most numerous being those employed married women who elect not to be insured in their own right. The National Insurance (Industrial Injuries) Act applies, broadly speaking, to all civilians working for an employer under contract of service or apprenticeship, corresponding closely with the class of 'employed persons' under the main scheme.

Weekly numbers of new claims for sickness and for injury benefit, classified by regions of the country, are published in the Registrar General's Weekly Return, and the estimated number of insured persons absent from work on a selected day each month owing to certified sickness or industrial injury (or prescribed disease) is published in the Registrar General's Quarterly Return.

Annual analyses are carried out for each twelve-month period from June to June. Though this may cause inconvenience in comparing the figures with calendar-year statistics derived from other sources, it eases problems of administration in periods of winter epidemics and also has the advantage of including the figures for each winter in a single set of annual tables.

The total number of claims received each year run into many millions, and the analysis is based upon a 5 per cent. sample. The statistics are not published, but an annual 'Digest' is issued to Medical Officers for Environmental Health and other interested persons on request This digest tabulates the claims by sex, age, region, diagnosis, number of persons claiming, number of claims, days of incapacity, and other related items.

STATISTICS OF THE ACTIVITIES OF HEALTH SERVICES

Alongside mortality and morbidity statistics there has been developing in recent years an interest in statistics that describe

TABLE 23

Miscellaneous Health Service Statistics

Number of population per physician (1966–67)

Israel	420
U.S.S.R.	450
U.S.A.	650
Australia	850
England and Wales	860
Canada	880
India	4,830
Ethiopia	65,380

Hospital Beds and their Utilization 1967

	Beds	Admissions
	(per 10,000 population)	
U.S.S.R.	102	2,063
Italy	101	1,342
Mongolia	100	1,562
England and Wales	97	1,036
United States	84	1,475
Israel	82	1,266

Hospital Beds by Specialty (1967)
Percentage distribution

	England and Wales	U.S.A.	U.S.S.R.
Total	100	100	100
General Medicine and Surgery	42	55	69
Maternity	2	0·1	3
Paediatric	1	1	4
Mental	28	32	10
Tuberculosis	2	1	8
Others	25	11	6

not the levels of health of the community but the health services available to the community and the way these services are used. Such statistics are needed for the organization both of curative and preventive services, for national health planning, and for the evaluation of health programmes.

The variety of services provided makes it difficult to present a complete description of the statistics used, but the following is a general outline of statistics relating to hospital services (World Health Organization Technical Report Series No. 261).

A. Statistics relating to the hospital

1. Resources of the hospital

   (a) Beds by specialty
   (b) Special departments, services, and facilities
   (c) Personnel—medical, nursing, other professional and technical, other including administrative and general service staff
   (d) Educational facilities

2. Utilization of hospital resources

   (a) Statistics of patient movement
   (b) Statistics of days of care
   (c) Statistics of other professional services

3. Financial data

   (a) Total annual current income of hospital
   (b) Total annual capital expenditure
   (c) Total annual current operating expenditure

B. Statistics relating to the patient

   (a) Numbers of patients discharged by sex, age, diagnosis, and days of hospitalization
   (b) In addition for long-stay institutions, number of patients resident on a given day (e.g. first day of year)
   (c) Area of residence of patient

PRINCIPAL SOURCES OF OFFICIAL VITAL STATISTICS OF ENGLAND AND WALES

1. REGISTRAR GENERAL'S WEEKLY RETURN

2. REGISTRAR GENERAL'S QUARTERLY RETURN

3. REGISTRAR GENERAL'S ANNUAL STATISTICAL REVIEW
   Part I Tables Medical
   Part II Tables Population
   Part III Commentary
   Supplements on Cancer and Abortion.

4. REGISTRAR GENERAL'S DECENNIAL SUPPLEMENT
   Life Tables
   Occupational Mortality
   Area Mortality

5. CENSUS REPORTS
   Preliminary Report
   General Report

6. GENERAL REGISTER OFFICE STUDIES ON MEDICAL AND POPULATION SUBJECTS

7. REPORT ON HOSPITAL IN-PATIENT ENQUIRY (Department of Health and Social Security/Office of Population Censuses and Surveys)

8. STATISTICAL REPORT SERIES (Department of Health and Social Security)

9. ANNUAL DIGEST OF HEALTH STATISTICS FOR ENGLAND AND WALES (Department of Health and Social Security)

10. ANNUAL DIGEST OF STATISTICS ANALYSING CERTIFICATES OF INCAPACITY (Department of Health and Social Security)

11. ANNUAL ABSTRACT OF STATISTICS (Central Statistical Office)

SELECTED REFERENCES

(Additional to the Official Sources listed above)

General

Benjamin, B. (1959) Elements of Vital Statistics, London.

Case, R. A. M. (1956) Cohort analysis of mortality rates as an historical or narrative technique, Brit. J. prev. soc. Med., 10, 159.

Greenwood, Major (1948) Medical Statistics from Graunt to Farr, London.

Hill, A. Bradford (1971) Principles of Medical Statistics, 9th ed., London.

Humphreys, Noel A., ed. (1885) Vital Statistics: a Memorial Volume of Selections from the Reports and Writings of William Farr, London.

Moriyama, I. M. (1964) Uses of vital records for epidemiological research, J. Chron. Dis., 17, 889.

Puffer, R. R., and Wynne Griffith, G. (1967) Patterns of urban mortality, Pan American Health Organization, Scientific Publ. No. 151, Washington, D.C.

Puffer, R. R., and Serrano, C. V. (1973) Patterns of mortality in childhood, Pan American Health Organization Scientific Publ. No 262, Washington D.C.

Spicer, C. C. and Lipworth, L. (1966) General Register Office Studies on Medical and Population Subjects, No 19.

Swaroop, S. (1960) Introduction to Health Statistics, Edinburgh.

World Health Organization Regional Office for Europe (1961) Report of a European Technical Conference on Mortality Statistics, Copenhagen.

World Health Organization Regional Office for Europe (1964) Report on the Application of Automatic Data Processing Systems in Health Administration, Copenhagen.

World Health Organization Regional Office for Europe (1965) European Conference on Health Statistics, Copenhagen.

World Health Organization Regional Office for Europe (1967) Symposium on the Use of Electronic Computers in Health Statistics and Medical Research, Stockholm, Sweden, 6-10 June 1966. Mimeo. Euro-341, Copenhagen.

Hospital Morbidity Statistics

Committee on the Danish National Morbidity Survey (1959) The Hospital Survey of Denmark, The Morbidity Survey of 1950, Copenhagen.

Fraenkel, M., and Erhardt, C. L. (1955) Morbidity in the Municipal Hospitals of the City of New York, New York.

Norris, V. (1959) *Mental Illness in London*, Institute of Psychiatry, Maudsley Monograph No. 6, London.

Cancer

Dorn, H. F., and Cutler, S. J. (1959) *Morbidity from Cancer in the United States*, Public Health Monograph 56, Public Health Service Publication No. 590. Vol. II (1970)

International Union Against Cancer (1966) *Cancer Incidence in Five Continents*, Berlin, Vol. II (1970).

National Cancer Institute (1964) *International Symposium on End Results of Cancer Therapy*, Monograph 15, Washington.

Stocks, P. (1959) Cancer registration and studies of incidence by survey, *Bull. Wld Hlth Org.*, **20**, 697.

Sickness Surveys

CANADA. Dominion Bureau of Statistics (1953–57) *Canadian Sickness Survey 1950–51*, Special Compilation, Nos. 1–11, Ottawa.

DENMARK. The Committee on the Danish National Morbidity Survey; Lindhardt, Marie (1960) *Sygdomsundersøgelsen I Danmark 1951–1954*, Copenhagen. English version, 1961.

JAPAN. Ministry of Health and Welfare (1956) Division of Statistics, *The National Health Survey in Japan* (roneoed).

NETHERLANDS. Oliemans, A. P. (1969) Morbiditeit in de huisart spraktijk (Report on the National Morbidity Survey carried out by the Netherlands College of General Practitioners, Leiden).

UNITED STATES. United States Department of Health, Education and Welfare, National Center for Health Statistics, Vital and Health Statistics Publication Series Nos. 1–22 (formerly Public Health Service Publication No. 1000.

International Vital and Health Statistics

World Health Organization, *World Health Statistics Annual*, formerly *Annual Epidemiological and Vital Statistics*, Geneva (annual). It consists of three volumes: Vol. 1. Vital Statistics and Causes of Death; Vol. 2. Infectious Diseases: Cases, Deaths and Vaccinations; Vol. 3. Health Personnel and Hospital Establishments. The current edition published in 1974 relates to statistics for 1970.

World Health Organization Expert Committee on Health Statistics, Various Reports, *Wld Hlth Org. techn. Rep. Ser.*, Nos. 5, 25, 53, 133, 164, 218, 261, 336, 364, 389, 429, 472.

United Nations Statistical Office, *Demographic Yearbook*, New York (annual).

United Nations (1968) *Compendium of Social Statistics 1967*, New York.

3
STATISTICS AS A BASIS FOR HEALTH MANAGEMENT AND PLANNING

M. R. ALDERSON

INTRODUCTION

This chapter discusses the use of routine statistics as a basis for health management and planning. In order to put current developments into perspective there is a fairly lengthy prologue giving: the history of the development of the hospital statistics; a discussion of the use of routine data; and the contribution that routine data can make to the genesis of ideas. The chapter then goes on to describe the data that is currently available, and how this is used in managing the health service. A distinction is drawn between the management needs for information on a day-to-day basis, and periodic review of the functioning of the total health care system. The information needs of planners are discussed separately, as their requirements are rather different; it is suggested that their needs can be met by the basic management information system, providing there is the facility to mount special studies on a once-off basis.

History

It is appropriate to consider the history of this subject for three reasons: the major determinant of the future is the past; it is salutory to observe how few 'current' ideas are really new; and it is important to observe how many years pass before sound ideas are implemented. This latter observation may temper the enthusiasm to implement new approaches with the patience that is so often required.

Logan and Lambert [p. 8] have discussed the historical development of vital registration. One rather different scheme warrants mention; the first major collection of data in England occurred in the eleventh century AD, shortly after the Battle of Hastings. For the purpose of ascertaining and recording the special dues owing to the Crown, William sent into each county commissioners whose inquiries are preserved in the Domesday Book. It is interesting to note that in the collection of this 'management data', which he required for his new kingdom, William took the trouble of having the whole inventory checked by a team of assessors independently of those who collected the basic data.

A leading article in *The Lancet* (1835–36) drew attention to the failure of London hospitals and public medical charities to publish statistics about the patients treated in these institutions. This was contrasted with the production of such information by hospitals abroad. A few years later, *The Lancet* (1840–41) returned to the same theme; by that time a committee of the Council of the Statistical Society of London had made steps for the provision of data relating to hospital statistics. The first report of this committee appeared in the *Journal of the Statis-*

tical Society (1842) and contained data for six general hospitals in London. The tabulations showed the number of persons in the hospitals, the number of each sex suffered from different diseases by age, the month in which patients were admitted, and the time that they remained under treatment. The report discussed the possibility of collecting information about the mortality and duration of diseases left to nature, and stated that no such thing could ever be contemplated as it would entail depriving patients of treatment. However, it was pointed out that without some standard of comparison, medical science could make very little further progress. Two years later, the second report of the Committee appeared (*Journal of the Statistical Society*, 1844). Further data appeared in an article in the *Journal of the Statistical Society* (1862); fourteen general hospitals provided information for 1861, but in subsequent reports the number of London hospitals participating dropped year by year until 1865 when only ten hospitals furnished returns. In the report for 1865 (*Journal of the Statistical Society*, 1866), it was pointed out that some alternative system might have to be established due go the failing response from the hospitals. In the following year an analysis was presented by Guy (1867), giving five-year figures for thirteen London hospitals. He suggested that the mortality of different hospitals was mainly due to the causes which determined the nature and severity of the cases they treated. Following this report there were no further regular publications of hospital morbidity data by the Royal Statistical Society.

A very careful discussion of the problems of collecting and interpreting hospital statistics was presented by Bristowe and Holmes (1863) in the sixth report of Sir John Simon, the Medical Officer of the Privy Council. They discussed the problems of using case fatality rates and also the use of an index of 'unsuccess in medical treatment'. Somewhat more optimistic proposals were made by Florence Nightingale (1863), who advocated the regular collection of a wide range of standard items to ascertain the results of particular treatments and special operations. She suggested that the whole question of hospital economics, as influenced by diets, medicines, and comforts, should be examined and that data on out-patients be collected. Farr (1875) advocated an even greater extension; he suggested a return should be made of the cases of sickness in the civil population.

It is interesting to recollect that about this period, equipment for mechanically processing data was being developed by Charles Babbage (Morrison and Morrison, 1961). Babbage never produced a working machine, but working from his papers, Scheutz developed a somewhat simpler calculating machine. A replica of this was used for the calculations required for the production of the English Life Tables in 1863; this work was carried out under the supervision of Farr at the General Register Office.

Despite all this enthusiasm, the advance from then onwards was slow; it was not until the local health authorities took over the management of hospitals in 1929 that interest reawakened, and large-scale recording and analysis of hospital statistics began (Spears and Gould, 1936–37). With the advent of the Second World War and the organization of the emergency medical service a system for collecting records was instituted; every fifth record for patients admitted to their hospitals during 1940–46 was examined and its salient features coded for statistical analysis. About this time the Nuffield Provincial Hospitals Trust set up Bureau of Health and Sickness Records at Oxford and Glasgow. The work of the Glasgow unit was described in the report *Hospital and Community* (1948); this gave details of a one-year pilot inquiry to find out what facts of value could be gained from an intelligent and systematic study of hospital records about sickness in the community, and to discover the difficulties and shortcomings inherent in such a study. This was thought to be the first study that gave a complete picture of all types of hospital-treated sickness for a defined population. Ryle (1948) discussed the concept of the Oxford Bureau, and showed how the collection of morbidity data stretching beyond hospital admission was a logical extension of the collection of analyses of mortality data. Some preliminary results from the work of the Oxford Bureau were described by Cotton (1958).

The introduction of the National Health Service in 1948 provided the opportunity for the commencement of a national scheme for collecting hospital morbidity statistics. MacKay (1951) described the scheme and suggested that the data would be valuable for management purposes. We are thus, after a lengthy description of the history and development of data collection systems, approaching the theme of this chapter. Thus far there has been a marked absence of comment about data relating to community health problems. Logan and Lambert [p. 10] have already dealt with mortality data, which was the cornerstone of public health information systems in the nineteenth century. He has also mentioned the sources of morbidity data that reflect community health. The relative paucity of routine data on the incidence and prevalence of disease in the community, and of patient care delivered by the family doctor is discussed in a later section of this chapter.

The Use of Routine Data

Before elaborating on the use of management information in the health service, it is important to reflect that such systems rely on routine data. It has already been pointed out that a number of early pioneers had great faith in the use of routine data; but before rushing on fired by the enthusiasm of these individuals, it is appropriate to consider the problems of using such data. Claude Bernard (1948) suggested that, in the nineteenth century, a physician observing a disease in different circumstances, reasoning about the influences of these circumstances, and deducing consequences which are controlled by other observations, was a person who reasoned experimentally even though he made no experiments. Yule (1924) pointed out that the student of social facts could not experiment, but had to deal with circumstances operating beyond his control;

such a person must take the records as they occur and endeavour, as best as he can, to interpret the observed variation. Topley (1940) pointed out that it was wrong to force experiment and observation into sharply separated categories; he suggested that this was almost as dangerous a heresy as the antithesis between science and art. Hill (1962) acknowledged his preference for the experimental approach, but at the same time stated that it did not lead him to repudiate or even to underrate the claims of accurate and designed observations. Dudley (1970) agreed that when gathering data and drawing conclusions the doctor was inevitably a scientist, although the controlled rigour of the internal scientific programme may not be wholly possible in the complex clinical situation. He suggested that as uncertainty and complexity increased there was a move away from the identifiable components of scientific method, but this did not mean that a scientific attitude need be abandoned.

The opposite point of view was put by Platt (1952), who observed that major advances in knowledge were the fruit of careful experiments planned in advance to test specific hypotheses, and that data recorded other than as part of a specific research project would yield little of value. Acheson (1967) has suggested that the two extreme propositions—that all routinely recorded data are of potential value to research, and that no routinely recorded data are of value to research—are equally absurd.

The Genesis of Ideas

Shegog (1971) commented that currently there was no developed science of medical information. If, therefore, we are to develop a science of medical information, it is important to consider the way in which new ideas are conceived and developed. It is imperative that thought should be given to the mode by which knowledge is first acquired in relation to the use of routine data; how does one progress from a position of ignorance, through a hunch, to a tentative but testable hypothesis, which can then be explored by preliminary and detailed studies? The most difficult stage in this recursive cycle of investigation is the identification of hunches that warrant further study; can the examination of routine data facilitate the identification of such hunches? Published work describing advances in knowledge often fail to reveal the source of the basic hunch, and even in one's own research work it is not always easy to identify the genesis of an idea and trace its origin. Pearson (1892), in his book *The Grammar of Science*, discussed the scope of science and laid stress on the method by which facts are handled; he suggested that it is the method by which they are dealt that forms 'a science'. Hogben (1940) observed that the Hindu and the Arabs had a need for constant reckoning in commercial undertakings, and this was associated with a high development of arithmetic; he suggested that the need to progress with practical applications was a powerful stimulus to advance in knowledge. Jay (1970) in an article entitled 'Creative Intercourse', commented that the concept of a single creative person was incorrect, and in fact two interacting minds were needed. In support of this he mentioned that before Michelangelo started work on the Medici Chapel he engaged in a prolonged discussion with his patron the Pope and they exchanged some fifty letters. Medawar (1969) pointed out that good scientists study the most important problems that they think they can solve; it is after all their professional business to solve problems, not merely to grapple with them. He agreed that devising an hypothesis was a 'creative act' in the sense that it was the invention of a possible world, or a possible fragment of the world; experiments were then performed to find out whether or not that imagined world was, to an adequate approximation, the real one. Medawar (1969) also suggested that what scientists do has never been the subject of a scientific inquiry, and pointed out that it is no use looking to scientific papers, for they not merely conceal but actively misrepresent the reasoning that went into the work they describe.

A leading article in the *British Medical Journal* (1971) stated that it is a truism that great scientific discoveries are not suddenly snatched out of the sky. Sherrington (1922) quoted Pasteur: 'To have the fruits there must have been cultivation of the tree'; he then qualified this by pointing out that although there is merit in appreciating the possibilities of earlier work, that is only a preliminary to the main achievement. Spence (1953) suggested that the recognition of new phenomena took shape in the mind endowed with imagination and insight, but he also stressed the need for skill in collecting and systematizing knowledge. He felt that the analysis of routine records was spurred on by the hope that this enabled one to proceed from ignorance to testable hypotheses in a surer fashion than relying on the casual acquisition of knowledge.

The above argument suggests that the careful application of scientific method tailored to particular needs, and introduced *pari passu* with a careful consideration of progress in parallel fields, may result in the development of a science of medical information. This chapter now turns to an appraisal of the current attitudes to, and use of management information in, the health field. Progress has been slow, and some of the ideas of pioneers such as Farr and Nightingale have still not been implemented. This lengthy prologue has been provided as a guide to the future direction and rate of progress of the subject.

HEALTH INFORMATION SYSTEMS

Logan and Lambert [p. 14] have discussed the routine mortality and morbidity statistics that are available. One item that is worth special comment is the scheme developed in England and Wales entitled Hospital Activity Analysis (H.A.A.). This system was first described by Benjamin (1965) as an attempt to develop a basic information system for hospital departments. He stated that the object of such a system would be to provide the hospital consultant with feedback of information about the operation of his own department, quickly, and in sufficient detail to enable him to review his own experience continuously within his own environment.

Benjamin (1971) described an information system as a centralized collection of information or reference to information which:

1. Is intended to be used for certain very specific purposes (e.g. to serve the needs of a particular service in a local authority).

2. Is very highly organized with respect to storage, updating, editing, retrieval, and manipulation.

3. May contain material which is either numerical, literary, or geographical and which in its primary state may exist in a wide variety of formats (documents, punch cards, magnetic tapes, etc.).

4. Will provide both routine periodical reports and answers to most *ad hoc* inquiries.

A recent Civil Service Department report (1971) reviewed the use of management information systems, and suggested that, although a vast amount has been and is being written about 'Integrated Management Information Systems', in the main these publications scratch superficially across the surface of a complex subject. A search of literature relating to the development of management information systems identifies many articles, but not one that makes one dissent from this suggestion. Cross and Roberts (1970), in an interesting discussion of management controls in medical care, point out that over the past twenty-one years in which the National Health Service has been developing, the national plans for information accession, retrieval, and processing are largely irrelevant to the management problems that confront the managers. Examination of the literature certainly does not suggest that there is any readily transplantable system functioning in either America or Scandinavia or the Continent that could be grafted on to the health service in this country. The next section therefore deals with the climate of opinion in respect of the introduction and use of information in the management of the health service. This is a necessary prelude to the discussion of a model information system.

Current Attitudes to Management in the National Health Service

The Salmon Report on 'Senior Nursing Staff Structure' (Ministry of Health, 1966) emphasized that the Chief Nursing Officer would have to develop effective channels of communication between nurses and other hospital officers and within the nursing service itself. It was felt that this was an important feature of the Chief Nursing Officer's job and necessary in order to obtain due consideration of proposals for better organization of the service.

The Department of Health and Social Security (1967) in the first report of the Joint Working Party on the Organization of Medical Work in Hospitals—the 'Cogwheel Report'—discussed how medical staff could become more involved in organizational problems. This report suggested that specialties should be grouped into divisions with the aim of reviewing hospital bed usage against the background of community needs, organization of out-patient and in-patient services, and review of clinical practice. It was suggested that this would require a study of data on waiting lists, out-patient waiting time, and time spent in hospital by patients awaiting operation or investigation; the use of resources in terms of man-power and equipment should also be considered by divisions. It was pointed out that a system would be required for supplying relevant data in order for the divisions to achieve their function. The *British Medical Journal* (1968) discussed the causes of long waiting lists for admission to hospital and of delays in out-patients; they suggested that a senior member of the staff should have the special obligation of periodically reviewing the matter in his own hospital.

The Department of Health and Social Security (1969) report on the functions of the district general hospital stressed that the best use would be made of specialized and expensive hospital facilities only if the community based services were seen to be capable of providing effective community care where hospital care is not really required. The report pointed out that it is easier to plan these services together, not separately.

The Department of Health and Social Security (1970) produced a second Green Paper on the future structure of the National Health Service. Unification of the health services was recommended with the formation of Area Health Authorities; it was proposed that there should be a Medical Officer at Area Health Board level, who would be responsible for helping his colleagues monitor the need for, and outcome from, all clinical services. One of the main tasks of this 'Community Physician' would be to develop the quantity and quality of information about health needs and the working of Area Health Services. It was hoped that the Community Physician would be able to take advantage of the new opportunities of collaboration through the system recommended in the Cogwheel Report. About this time a leading article in the *British Medical Journal* (1970) suggested that the result of putting the Salmon and Cogwheel proposals into practice so far had been an improvement in the effectiveness of hospital management. Not everyone, however, felt that this introduction of Salmon and Cogwheel had been an advantage; Paulley (1971) suggested that under the Cogwheel system patients and hospital departments would not have a fair deal. Similar views were echoed by Morley (1971). The Department of Health and Social Security (1971) issued a consultative document on National Health Service reorganization; this stressed the need to measure progress against clear objectives. The document suggested that the central department should have the ultimate responsibility for monitoring the performance of the health service.

The effective management of health was discussed by Logan, Klein, and Ashley (1971), who suggested that there was need for the continuing capacity to monitor the results of decisions taken, and that up till then the National Health Service had been largely run on the basis of a well-meaning stewardship.

Dollery (1971), in an article on the quality of health care and and its attainment, suggested that there was need for a continuing external but professional evaluation of the performance of health services. He advocated providing this initially on a pilot and voluntary scale as an Audit of Health Care (A.H.C.) that would review the work of the N.H.S. He suggested that this A.H.C. should be mainly concerned with studying staffing, organization, and facilities; he believed that it could do much useful work without the necessity of attempting a detailed definition of what constitutes good quality care. Ultimately, he felt that the remit of the A.H.C. could cover all aspects of health services, but that in the first few years it would be wise to restrict it to well-defined and substantial problems that were widely admitted to be unsatisfactory at present. Smith (1971) suggested that if doctors were to serve their patients as well in the future as they have in the past, then they should accept A.H.C.s as a necessary, even if distasteful, arrangement. Ashford (1971) stated that intelligence and evaluation must play a central role in an efficient health care system, and that the intelligence function involved the monitoring of current performance of the system, with a view to the application of controlled measures where necessary. He said that this was one of the major tasks of management within the health service and

particularly so at the national level. A similar point has been made by Warren (1971).

Another voice of warning was raised by Seddon (1971), who quoted Pickering's phrase, 'the extraordinary proliferation of non-producers'; he suggested that Hospital Activity Analysis might merely aggravate this problem, and at the same time irritate the producers in the health service. Forsyth and Sheik (1971), reviewing the mechanics of medical management in Cogwheel systems, reported that many committees found the available data misleading; apart from the usefulness of the material, the accuracy and validity of the data were often questioned. They pointed out that there was considerable difficulty in the use of information in the Cogwheel system. Cumming and Goldsmith (1971) suggested that there was great need for someone with experience, skill, and time to work closely with divisions and the Medical Executive Committee to clarify and define those management problems that should be tackled.

Current Use of Routine Data

Heasman (1964) presented data, derived from the 10 per cent. sample processed centrally for the 'Hospital In-Patient Inquiry', on the variation and duration of stay for two common surgical conditions. He showed considerable variation in the lengths of stay between individual hospital groups, and between regions. He suggested that statistically controlled studies were needed to show objectively the effect of different lengths of stay in hospital for uncomplicated cases. In a series of papers (Heasman, 1968, 1970; Heasman and Carstairs 1971), the system used in Scotland for presenting in-patient statistics to consultants has been described. The earlier paper discusses the derivation of the data, and the latter papers present some of the results and the problems posed by circulating such material to consultants.

Wall and Cross (1968) discussed the use of Hospital Activity Analysis data in the Birmingham Region; they gave examples of how the data can be analysed to assist regional planning and to provide a basis for examining the work of hospitals. McNay (1969) reported experience in the use of H.A.A. in the Newcastle area; he emphasized that, partly due to the lack of computer time, the data were used primarily to investigate specific problems rather than produce routine output for transmission to all consultants in the Region. *Ad hoc* analysis in response to specific management or planning problems had been used in the following three functions:

1. To assist long-term planning.
2. To assist in the evaluation of proposals for major changes in hospital provision.
3. To assist in the evaluation of minor changes in the provision of services within the hospitals and within departments.

Wall and Wharton (1970) have shown how H.A.A. data can be used to illustrate the hospital in-patient work-load created by the care of persons aged 65 and over. Kemp, Damblen, and Lindsay (1971) have described how the basic Scottish system can be adapted to the local collection and use of extended clinical particulars for an orthopaedic hospital. Ferguson and Murray (1970) have shown how the standard Scottish form for maternity data can be adapted for use as a normal delivery discharge letter to the family doctor. Rowe (1971) predicted that by the end of 1971, 76 per cent. of all discharges and deaths for general in-patients in England and Wales would be covered by H.A.A.; Wales and Scotland already had 100 per cent. coverage. He considered that the three following analyses were of most use in looking at the management of the service:

1. Time on waiting list, by age and sex, by specialty or diagnosis, and by consultant or firm.
2. Average duration of stay by specialty and diagnosis for each hospital, by sex and age of patient.
3. Number of days from admission until first operation.

He went on to say, however, that the real benefits from H.A.A. had been obtained from using the bank of data to supply information on particular problems as and when they had arisen.

Problems Inherent in Using Routine Data

Any routine data collection system is open to the accusations that: the data is erroneous; there is considerable delay in production of the material; the material when produced is inappropriate to the uses for which the scheme was designed or to which people endeavour to put it; the total system is so inflexible that it is unable to respond to the specific requirements of individuals contributing data to the system; the output is unacceptable to the potential users. It is important to discuss each of these separate issues in turn, and indicate some of the remedies that are required.

1. ERRORS IN THE BASIC DATA

Many studies have shown that there are problems with the accuracy of routine data. Heasman and Lipworth (1966) have commented upon the accuracy of certification of death, while Lockwood (1971) reported the accuracy of Scottish hospital morbidity data. In a series of publications, Alderson has discussed the problems with regard to mortality data (1965), sickness absence data (1968), occupational mortality data (1972a), cancer registration data (1972b), and hospital discharge data (Alderson and Meade, 1967; Alderson, 1972c). A number of other authors have commented on the issues involved in the error rate of basic data. The answer to the problem is not simple, but one important point is that it is necessary to have a clear idea about the overall accuracy of routine data. Only when one has a clear idea of the error rate for each specific item is it possible to interpret the basic data with due caution. Sometimes, by having a clear-cut idea of the error rate material, one can in fact reinforce faith in the data by showing that the accuracy is better than had been imagined. Another reason for carrying out such studies is that by doing so one will often identify loopholes in the system which can be adjusted to improve the accuracy of specific items. Study can, in fact, separate the items into three rather different classes; in the first category, the error rate is so trivial that no special steps need be taken, and the material can be interpreted as though it was completely accurate; secondly, some items have an error rate that creates difficulty with interpretation, and examination of the cause of this may suggest minor alterations in the system that can be implemented and thereby improve the error rate; thirdly, some items may be so inaccurate that effort is not justified in trying to improve their accuracy. These items have therefore to be handled as they are, or removed entirely from the data collection system. One major cause of dropping an item from the routine system is not solely the error rate, but the fact that it is an item that is very frequently recorded as 'not known'. Careful examination of the error rate of the basic data can also provide guidance in the preparation of edit programmes to be used on input of the data into the computer system; these may be so adjusted that unlikely and impossible answers are identified before the master file is created.

2. DELAY IN THE PRODUCTION OF MATERIAL

Often, the staff involved in collecting the basic data are doing this as one of many duties; in such circumstances pressure of other work can easily cause the routine data collection to be put last in a series of jobs that have to be done. Where staff are specifically set aside for data collection they will often work on their own, with no arrangement for relief for holidays and sickness; this again creates delay. Where the material passes through many hands (from the basic collection of data, abstraction from patient's notes, coding, and then data preparation), each of these links in the chain can create an added delay. In busy hospitals there is often difficulty in obtaining the case records, or discussing a specific problem with the medical staff where there is difficulty about abstracting some of the items. Some of this delay can be overcome by more generous allocation of staff for the specific data collection system, and also by periodic examination of the system to identify simpler ways of capturing the data. For a number of statistical systems, data collection is a quite separate exercise grafted on to the functioning of an organization; where the data is captured as a by-product of some operational procedure, there is a greater chance of collecting this without undue delay. This point will be examined in the next main section, 'Towards an Ideal Management Information System'.

3. INFLEXIBILITY OF THE BASIC SYSTEM

Often data collection systems have been devised and controlled from central government. Where the system is a national one, there is often great difficulty in devising an agreed national form; once this has been drawn up and arrangements made for collecting the basic data, there is reluctance to permit variants on the basic form. However, it is imperative that any data collection system for use in management of the health service should be of value at local level, and the system must be sufficiently flexible so that it can be moulded to meet local needs. Unless this happens, all enthusiasm for the basic system will wither away. Therefore, there is need to cater for local interest; this may be the collection of additional clinical particulars or the insertion of additional administrative and patient items for management purposes. The simplest variant to permit is the extension of the number of items that are collected; this is easily arranged if the number of additional items are few, and the basic system provides for additions on the statistical form and in the computer file. More difficult to allow for is a collection of extended additional particulars. In such a case the fresh material may be considered as a sub-file providing there is adequate linkage so that the common particulars do not have to be recorded and processed twice over.

Difficulty can be experienced from local pressures for variations in standard codes. This can be dealt with most satis-factorily by using additional digits to extend the standard codes. This may provide the extra specificity required but still ensure comparability of the basic information with that coded elsewhere.

4. INAPPROPRIATENESS OF ITEMS

The main source of data in England (H.A.A.) allows a very incomplete examination of the functioning of the hospital service. The data provides some information about work-load, but this is unrelated to information about the staffing situation in the hospital, or the other resources required in caring for in-patients. One needs to examine the information on work-load in relation to staffing, data about the facilities available in terms of buildings and equipment, and the internal organiza-tion of the hospital. This material must be so moulded into the system that at the same time one can examine the cost in relation to the through-put of patients. The H.A.A. data is event-type material relating to isolated episodes of in-patient care; Acheson (1967) who set up the Oxford Record Linkage Study in 1961, has demonstrated how linkage of routinely available data for births, marriages, deaths, and hospital dis-charges can be achieved. He has shown how the provision of person-based, rather than event-based, statistics adds an extra dimension in the analysis of routine data. More information about the care of out-patients is desirable, and the relationship between out-patient attendances and admission to hospital: subsequently, patients on discharge should be followed through, to relate an episode of hospital admission to atten-dances at out-patients and readmission should this occur. Only when such a linked file is built up will there accumulate in-formation on outcome of care. Case fatality rate (which is available from the simple event-type data) provides very limited hard information about outcome; nothing is currently available in the way of the soft but highly relevant information such as patient satisfaction.

Some of the problems mentioned under this section can be dealt with by improved handling of the routinely available data, in particular the institution of linked files, which bring together subsequent events occurring to any given individual. However, some of the other problems can only be dealt with by collating series of sets of data that are currently discreet within the health service (such as the information on work-load, staffing, and on costs).

5. UNACCEPTABILITY OF THE ANALYSES

Within the health service there is a fairly healthy scepticism about the acceptance and use of routine data. Often, routine data will provide little that is not already known to individuals dealing with day-to-day problems; when they try and use the system they run up against the other four problems mentioned above. Until something is done about the accuracy, the delay, the inappropriateness, and the inflexibility of the system, it will be difficult to get ready acceptance of management data. There has to be a subtle re-education of the potential users of the system. Great care should be taken to see that the informa-tion is presented in a sensible and intelligible way; this can often only be done by patient trial and error, with discussion among individuals and gradual improvement in the feedback. Of course, where the output is part of an *ad hoc* analysis, or a

planned collection of extended data, there is a far greater chance of the information being used. Only by successful use will there gradually be a change in the attitude and climate leading to greater acceptance of such material. Wofinden (1971) in an article on the planning of health centres pointed out that in a democratically operated National Health Service strongly influenced by the doctors it was almost impossible to put logical plans into practice. This is a further comment emphasizing the point made earlier that, however accurate and carefully presented is data for management or planning pur-poses, there is still the problem of translating information into action.

Alderson (1971) suggested that the basic system should be restricted in nature; he pointed out that the enthusiasm of a few had to be balanced against the inertia of the lowest com-mon denominator in the data collection system. A similar point was made by Weir (1970) who commented that although com-puters were of considerable benefit in handling management information they should only be used to do now what was considered necessary but had previously been impracticable. He emphasized that they should be used to analyse information rapidly, but that this should only be information that was known to be both accurate and useful. A number of papers have been written on the ways of improving capture of the basic data; Ellis-Martin (1971) suggested how the basic patient and administrative data could be obtained by the use of a multipart pre-registration form. Riddle (1971) has examined alternative ways of capturing H.A.A. data; he has been looking at the possibility of using bar-marked sheets, or forms suitable for optical character reading. He suggested that document reading methods should be given serious consideration if the collection of patient data was extended from in-patients to out-patients. He felt that it would not be possible to find the punch operators and accommodation for their machines within the health service for conventional input on punch cards or paper tape.

Grogono and Woodgate (1971) have discussed the develop-ment of an index for measuring health. They suggested that the index could be used to allot priorities in treatment and to apply cost benefit techniques to health; they stated that the develop-ment of their index was stimulated by the current statistics used to represent efficiency in the hospital; they were highly critical of the use of mean bed occupancy, and suggested that their index might be of greater use to measure priorities and progress with the application of treatment.

Towards an Ideal Management Information System

The preceding sections have touched on the currently available data, the way these are handled, and the problems that occur. Reference has been made to actual use of informa-tion in the health service, but the literature does not identify any currently operating information system that is ideal. It is therefore necessary to consider what are the basic steps in setting up a model intelligence system in the health service. Four steps are required:

1. Examination of the resources for the intelligence system, both resources of information and of staff and equipment for handling this information.

2. Separately one requires to examine the problems faced

by all levels of management in the National Health Service; including study of the problems facing those responsible for administering the hospitals, local health authorities, and family practice services, at national and local level.

3. Having identified the problems that management faces, one wants to identify how information is currently used and whether a decision on current problems is reached without need for or use of information.

4. One then requires to sit and quietly think how the current resources of information can be brought together and used for a more profitable examination of the problems faced by management.

Providing there is acceptance of the basic solution derived under step (4), one then requires to introduce an innovation in provision of information; if possible, this introduction should be monitored so that the outcome of the provision of information is observed. Unless this is carefully done it will be impossible to determine whether the provision of information has aided management and justified the cost of the system.

Ockenden and Bodenham (1970) reported on a study undertaken in Scotland in which they examined the place of computers in the health service. They emphasize the application of computers in information handling and suggest that as part of the improvement in information handling there should be a chief officer appointed at Regional level, of equal status to the Senior Administrative Medical Officer, the Board Secretary, and the Treasurer. They refer to this new post as that of Senior Information Processing Officer and in their report discuss the functions of such an individual. Heasman (1971), in an article on computers in a central health organization, states that one of their main uses is in the accumulation of data banks. He suggests that there are three main applications of the data: first, administrative functions such as the carrying out of population surveillance; secondly, statistical analyses such as the examination of trends of mortality and morbidity, statistics for the management, organization, and planning of the service, and statistics as a basis for epidemiological studies; thirdly, he suggests that data banks should be assembled which can be used to answer *ad hoc* management, clinical, or research inquiries. He is thus distinguishing between the routine production of statistical analyses, the use of the basic data as a sampling frame for specific studies, and the answering of *ad hoc* queries by a specific interrogation of the data held in the bank. He then goes on to describe how the basic data could be fed into this system; he suggests that the foundation is data relating to spells of hospital admission, with a different approach being required for obstetrics, neonatal paediatrics, and psychiatry. He states that there is a major need for a wide-scale study of data concerning out-patients but that he feels that in the foreseeable future regular collection of data from general practice will not be feasible. McKeown and Lowe (1968) have, however, pointed out the value of a measurement of ill health in the community such as was obtained in England and Wales from 1942 to 1952 from the survey of sickness. They suggest that there is need to regularly carry out such a survey to check on the running of the health service. Bodenham and Wellman (1972) have carried out a further examination of the needs of the health service authorities for information for managerial and administrative purposes. In their recent report they have

discussed how the information system might be organized in Scotland. Heasman (1972) made some specific comments about the proposals for Scotland with regard to the Unification of the Health Service and the information needs of this service. Bispham, Thorne, and Holland (1971), in an article on the information requirements for planning, provide a clear discussion of the basic data that should be provided. Beginning with population and demographic data they then comment on the need for mortality data and a range of morbidity data to be included. This article concentrates, however, on the types of information required rather than the specific mechanisms for collecting and collating this data. Ashford (1971) has also discussed the way the current information system in England and Wales could be amended.

Moser (1970) has discussed the current changes in the social statistics that are collated in England and Wales. He pointed out that nothing more effectively aids improvement in the statistics than an attempt to integrate them into a single framework. He referred to a long-term project aimed at producing an integrated system of social statistics for the country which would provide information on social conditions, social resources, and the flow of people through various activities and institutions; ultimately, the analyses of this material might be linked with analyses of financial and man-power resources.

All these authors seem to be agreed on the need to collate and study population, demographic, mortality, and morbidity data. In order to manage the health service there must be available precise information about the health problems of the community and how these are currently being dealt with, the resources required to deal with these problems, and some indication of outcome of medical care. Although at the present time many of the routinely available statistics are collected from separate systems set up solely for the purpose of capturing and processing statistics, the advent of computers offers the possibility of linking the capture and processing of information more closely to the operation of the health care system. An examination has therefore been carried out of the way in which a computer operating in a batch-processing mode might assist with the operation of some aspects of the health service and at the same time capture information. The more a computer is involved in operational activities within the health service, the greater the possibility of capturing comprehensive data. If this can be operated through a batch-processing system it may be possible to use computer personnel and other trained staff with the minimum of interference to the medical and paramedical staff in their day-to-day work. The system should be so devised that it co-ordinates the flow of information to give maximum use of any captured item and removes any unnecessary duplication of data recording and, wherever possible, removes need for clerical work or a repetitive nature. Although it has been suggested that the system should be expanded to cover as much of the total health care system as possible (in order to give a flow of information about total health care), every item collected and stored on the system should be carefully scrutinized to see that only data that is of sufficient accuracy, and of proven value, is stored.

Knox (1968) has described the introduction of batch processing into a hospital environment, while Cross, Droar, and Roberts (1968) discuss the methods used for identification of in-patients. Such a scheme can be extended to provide standard identification particulars for those patients for whom an out-patient appointment is requested. The system could be used to schedule the out-patient attendances and from first attendance at out-patients co-ordinate requests for investigation, reattendances at out-patients, or placement on the waiting list. The system should handle the waiting list and call-up patients for admission; as in the system described by Cross and his colleagues a file should be kept of current in-patients; if the system was associated with a request and reporting system for biochemical and other investigations, it would be possible to accumulate such data into an historical file. On discharge the system should be responsible for initiating a simple standardized discharge summary and appropriate follow-up of the patient. If the initial booking for out-patients was carried out as in some hospitals, with screening of the family doctor's letter, there might be recording even at this stage of provisional diagnosis or reason of attendance. In order to handle the waiting list effectively, the system should know the provisional diagnosis from out-patients, and the clinician's opinion of resources required on admission (such as complex investigation or planned surgery). All hospitals will have some manual system for booking theatre time for cold surgery, and it should be possible to link the data on theatre use into the basic patient file.

Such a system would provide for the collection of considerable data about the work-load carried by hospitals, including out-patient work-load. It might be possible to associate the use of service departments with specific medical problems (as distinct from the current system which tends to count the work-load in service departments without relating this to the medical problems for which the investigations are performed). Extended particulars are available in other systems for recording particulars about staffing and costs in the health service. Careful examination should be made of the way in which this data is currently collected and attempts must be made to relate staffing and costs to the work-load data. If the computer system were responsible for scheduling follow-up of patients discharged from the wards it should be possible to accumulate some index of outcome; it would certainly be possible to relate a spell of in-patient care to subsequent attendances at out-patients, to transfer to other hospitals, or to readmission. Although these items would not directly provide a measure of outcome they would certainly be an indication of progress and an advance on the simple analysis of case fatality rate.

Though the hospital service is an expensive segment of the total health service, the majority of contacts that individual people make with the various branches of the health service are to a great extent concerned with medical care outside hospital. A number of studies have shown that there is wide variation in the way in which family doctors handle their work-load, with a fifty-fold variation in referral rate to hospital. Most general medical problems, such as the care of expectant mothers, the care of young children, the care of young chronic sick, and the care of the mentally ill, are not dealt with solely by facilities for care in the community or care in hospital. It is important to have for management purposes (and, as will be discussed in the next section, for planning purposes) basic data about the health problem of a defined population and information that identifies the total resources by which this health problem is being handled. For instance, with the care of the expectant mother it is important to know what proportion of high-risk mothers are cared for in the community, and what proportion reach hospital. Studies such as the national birthday trust survey (Butler and Bonham, 1963) have shown that allocation of resources is not directly related to risk. It is therefore necessary to collect information about the health problems of the community and contacts with general practitioners and other community health staff.

Some practitioners are now trying to use a computer to assist with the screening of young children, the middle-aged, or the elderly; such work has been described by Hodes (1969). Such work can be readily mounted from a computer-held file of patients in the practice; once this is available one gets as an immediate by-product the age and sex register of the practice (though the use of this is more for research than actual practice administration or patient care). A rather different class of scheme is one where the doctor collects particulars of the work-load that he is carrying; this may be done for the purpose of studying practice administration, or for general interest, and has been described by Dinwoodie (1969). If the diagnostic particulars are recorded they may be used to initiate follow-up of the chronic sick and 'at-risk' groups in the practice; this approach has been discussed by Dinwoodie and Grene (1971).

Alderson (1972d) has suggested there is need to establish, at least for a sample of family practitioners, a computer-based practice list. This list could then be used to initiate scheduling of special groups cared for by the family doctor, such as young children, screening for cervical cancer, screening of middle-aged males for cardiovascular or respiratory disease, and surveillance of the elderly. Mention of these functions is not meant to imply that such screening is of proven value, but that if practitioners wish to carry out periodic surveillance of these groups in their practice an automated practice list should facilitate call-up of the patients. For specific conditions where continued surveillance is required the system could be used to schedule long-term follow-up, as for instance with patients who have had a gastrectomy, or patients who have had radio-active iodine treatment for thyrotoxicosis. Where the family doctor is able to spell out, perhaps in conjunction with his hospital colleagues, a specific programme of supervision for those suffering from chronic disease, the system again should be able to assist with scheduling reattendance. Extension of the practice-based system to each of these applications would mean that some basic data about the work-load carried in the practice was being collected; this should provide a foundation for the *ad hoc* collection of extended particulars of morbidity treated in family practice. To date, the health service has provided for the collection of information from the hospital service but has made no routine provision for collection of data from family practice. It is suggested that it is necessary, at least on a sample basis, to have the facility to continually collect material about morbidity in the population and work-load in family practice.

It is not suggested that the systems outlined above for collecting data from family practice and hospital care would provide a bank of data that could answer all the queries being raised in the day-to-day management of the health service. It is suggested, however, that the system should produce timely, accurate and more appropriate data than is currently available. With careful planning, the system should be more flexible than has been the case in the past with national data collection systems. Providing the contributors to the system can be sufficiently motivated, the output from the data may gradually become more acceptable to the clinicians and managers in the health service. Florence Nightingale and Farr were suggesting data collection systems of the order of complexity of that outlined above; computers have altered the situation in that ease of storage and transmission of data had radically altered. Feasibility and evaluation studies are currently required to quantify the cost of a system such as that outlined above, and to demonstrate the uses to which data can be put, and the impact on medical care that might ensue.

INFORMATION SYSTEMS AND PLANNING

This section considers planning carried out in the health service at national, regional, or area level. The term 'planning' is used by different people to mean very different things; it can be defined as the process culminating in decisions regarding the future provision of the correct balance of domiciliary, out-patient, and in-patient facilities for the investigation, treatment, and care of all 'perceived health needs' of the community. The planning process involves a lengthy time scale and is particularly concerned with planning for the health needs of the next generation. Excluded from this definition is the examination of current resources and current demands resulting in the short-term real location of these resources in order to more effectively meet these demands 'tomorrow'. This latter process is part of the day-to-day functions of management and has been covered in the previous section. This is in contrast to the definition used by McSwiney (1970) who included the production of day-to-day services as one of the four major areas in the operation of a hospital which required planning. Bispham, Holland, and Stringer (1971) have pointed out that planning involves different activities at the national, regional, and area levels. They suggest that at the national level there is concern with the overall administrative structure of the services and with the general framework of policy; at regional level there is need for co-ordination of area services and planning of the provision for super-specialties (such as neurosurgery or radiotherapy) which require a population greater than that of a single area); while at area level the main concerns are the detailed allocation of resources and provision for the more common acute and chronic conditions.

A recent World Health Organization report (1971) pointed out that there were currently four broad approaches to planning which were described as follows:

1. DEDUCTIVE PLANNING

This is where broad policies and objectives are established at the highest level of the organization, and detailed proposals for implementation flow downwards to those who provide services. Standards tend to be 'normative' in the sense that they are developed by experts or derived from current experiences and activity.

2. INDUCTIVE PLANNING

In this, local experiences, services, and practices are identified and efforts made to co-ordinate and consolidate them so that greater benefits can be made more widely available. The objective is to improve what is already available in the expec-

tation that the overall services to the entire population will thereby be improved.

3. IMPRESSIONISTIC PLANNING

This is the type of *ad hoc* professional and institutional decision-making to which most clinicians and administrators have been accustomed in the past. Decisions and choices are made on the basis of experience, pressures, minimal information, and rough estimates of needs and possibilities. The process is more intuitive and political in character than rational or scientific and can scarcely be regarded as planning in the strict sense of the term.

4. IDEALISTIC PLANNING

The aims of the plan are stated only in the form of unobtainable ideas. Action is encouraged by exhortation, but precise objectives or methods of achieving them are not specified.

The simplest way to plan is to identify the current work-load, quantify the resources used to meet this work-load, and relate this to the population in the catchment area; in this way 'norms for provision of care' can be derived. These norms can then be applied to the projected population figures in order to obtain anticipated requirements. Such an approach is likely to perpetuate the fault in the current system. Bispham, Holland, and Stringer (1971) have pointed out that the studies of Barrow-in-Furness and Teesside were not able to establish objective criteria of need for medical care; the ten-year hospital plan for England and Wales used the findings from these studies, and thus the recommended bed ratios are based on current demand. They point out that this is an inadequate measure of need. Planning has been done by applying a 'norm' for requirements to population projections. In order to produce a more precise approach one requires detailed information about the diseases currently affecting the population, and on to this one needs to build estimates of: trends in the incidence of disease; possible changes in the attitudes of the population to health and health care; future variations in delivery of care; impending changes in therapy; and the affect that any new therapy is likely to have on the prognosis of disease.

The routine data, especially the data that have been discussed in the previous section of this paper, are somewhat limited. If the data can provide clear-cut guidance about the major (i.e. costly) segment of the health service this is of some help. It is, however, a rather limited picture upon which to base long-term planning. Two rather different types of change can occur in the delivery of medical care; first are minor alterations and innovations, second are major changes resulting from advances in knowledge or technology. At any one point in time evidence can usually be produced to show that the complete health needs of a population are not being met; there is obviously, therefore, evidence that immediate changes might be instituted. Some of the unmet demand can be catered for by minor adjustment in the delivery of health care. The reason why all these changes are not implemented is usually that there is a shortage of total funds, and the capital and staff available cannot be stretched to meet all the demands upon the health service. It is here, however, that the techniques of operational research can come into play; providing one knows the current demand and the way in which this is being met, one can build a model of the health care system, simulate change in the system, and observe in the model the repercussions that alteration in the development of resources has on workload.

There are at least five steps that may be recognized in such a planning process; these are first a situational analysis, then formulation of alternative tactical approaches, a decision phase, discussion and implementation, and finally evaluation. The World Health Organization (1971) pointed out that these steps probably form part of all methods and systems of health planning whatever their political and cultural background, whether or not the overall process is explicitly divided up into these steps. Statistics are relevant to at least three of these steps. The information system should obviously play a part in the situation analysis; and this phase involves the collection, presentation, and examination of factual data. Navarro and Parker (1970) in their article 'Models in Health Services Planning', discuss three alternative approaches to the handling of basic data in planning. They cover prediction (i.e. ordinary statistical forecasting); simulation, with the observation of possible changes in the health services system, and the repercussions that these changes have on the present and future utilization and resources; their third model involves goal-seeking, a technique which determines that alternative which minimizes cost or changes in resources that are required to achieve in a given time period specified utilization patterns. Another World Health Organization report (1970a) discussed the use of computers and multivariate regression methods in the study of the determinants of mortality. They advocate this approach with the use of sophisticated methods to analyse mortality data, in order to improve the prediction of future trends. Evaluation is linked to the continued collection of data in the information system, but this subject is dealt with by Warren [CHAPTER 46].

It is of little use just studying data (even if it is accurate data) which demonstrates the current demand for health services; of even less use is the examination of data that solely refers to demand for a particular segment of the health services. In order to build up a conceptual model of the functioning of the health service, one really requires to know how many people are out and about in the community suffering from incipient or overt disease and who have not contacted the National Health Service. One then requires to know what proportion of patients contact their family doctor, and for all those who do contact the family doctor how he deals with their particular problem. Does he rely on his clinical judgement or does he use direct access investigations; does he prescribe treatment; does he continue to see the patient at intervals; or does he refer the patient to the hospital services? For those patients referred to out-patients, one wants to know at first attendance in what proportion a clinical diagnosis is made, what proportion have investigations, what proportion are asked to reattend out-patients, and how many times are they brought back to out-patients, and what proportion are put on the waiting list for admission. For those patients admitted to hospital, one wants to know what investigations and what operative procedures are carried out, and what is the total length of stay. For all these alternative forms of care, one requires information about outcome; both hard data on mortality, recurrence or complications, and soft data about return to active life, and

satisfaction of both the patient and his family with the care provided. It should then be possible to look at the total resources currently involved in providing health care; and the costs entailed in the provision of such care. It is impossible to conceive of a routine information system that could collect precise and accurate particulars about the total uses of the health service. It is even more unlikely that the system could actually tell why some patients with raised blood pressure go to their doctor, and why others do not. No information system could tell why some family doctors treat the patient without investigation, why some carry out investigations themselves or make use of direct access information, and why some refer their patients to out-patients. However, unless we know the answer to these questions we cannot confidently comment on the potential for change in the health care system.

Matthews (1971) has discussed the problem of extrapolating local findings to a wider population. He points out that it is unlikely that studies of samples of the population in every district of the country, and on a wide range of conditions, will ever be practicable. This is, of course, almost self-evident; he then points out the question of whether the prevalence of disease in one population may be deduced from that in another. He suggests that further research is needed to check on this, and to determine what other characteristics should be recorded in an attempt to make such extrapolation possible. Many health planners now dream of having a single index of the health status of the community that would serve as a guide to the requirements for a range of health problems. It is extremely unlikely that in fact a single index can be derived, as it can in the economic field, where a monetary unit can be derived from a number of highly diverse components. To be satisfactory an index of health would have to have the following requirements: availability; completeness of coverage; quality (i.e. not varying with time and place); universality; ease of calculation; acceptance; reproducibility; specificity; sensitivity; and validity. Coming down to the needs for area planning, Gatherer (1971) has pointed out that the community health specialist must be aware of factors in his own area which are likely to affect the health of people living there, and that he will need to use all available techniques to give him the information that he requires, and supplement the data that is routinely available.

FIGURE 2 shows actual and projected livebirths for the United Kingdom over the past thirty-five years, with projections for the next forty years. This shows how the 1955 projection was quite inaccurate due to a sudden rise in the annual number of births. Five years later the next projection assumed that the climb in births was of a temporary nature. This appeared to be wrong and five years later the demographer then assumed that the rise in the number of births was going to be steady; no sooner has this decision been made than in fact the annual number of births dropped. It will be interesting to examine this chart in years to come to see whether the 1970 projection is any more accurate; this has suggested that the decline in births over the past five years is a temporary feature. It is worth noting that in 1965, ten years after the 1955 projection, the actual number of births was some 31 per cent higher than had been projected ten years earlier. A moment's reflection shows what an impact this variation can have on planning of maternity services, and facilities for the care of young children.

Smith (1968) points out that planning involves prediction and that prediction is always subject to the possibility of error. He emphasizes this with a specific example regarding the introduction of new drugs for the treatment of mental illness; these have been associated with a reduction in the average duration of hospital stay. He points out that this is not immediately translatable into planning, as it may reduce the total demand for hospital admission, by shortening the average duration of mental illness; on the other hand, the improved efficiency of treatment may result in the increased popularization of hospital treatment of illnesses that currently are left untreated or are treated in the community because of the lack of suitable or useful hospital treatment. One could also mention in this context the importance of resolving a difference between the effect

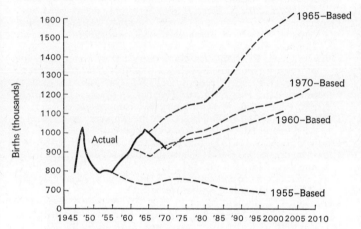

Fig. 2. Actual and projected live births—United Kingdom.

of treatment upon the length of stay, and the relapse rate of patients so treated. Many authors, such as Williams and Bray (1971), make passing reference to the value of routine statistics in relation to planning; often such reference is made without any clear indication of how the statistics actually assist in the planning process. A recent World Health Organization report (1970b) has pointed out that the various roles in planning must be subjected to a systematic analysis, in order to delineate more sharply the functions for which training is required. Experience has shown that health statisticians all too often find difficulty in providing health planners with statistical information that is relevant to their needs. The converse of this is that health planners frequently fail to determine precisely what were their needs. There are a number of problems in this exchange of information between the health planner and the statistician; particularly, there is a need to define the types of statistics required, and to demonstrate how the data can be used to provide health indicators.

One problem to be guarded against in the use of routine statistics is the derivation of judgements about the efficacy of different forms of treatment. The examination of the routine data should only be used to identify variation in delivery of health care, and variation in outcome. Hill (1963) has discussed the gradual development of the method of clinical trials, in order to provide specific guidance about the efficacy of treat-

ment. Cochrane (1972) has demonstrated how this technique may be extended from the use of basic trials for treatments into control trials which throw light upon the value of different ways of delivering health care.

Problems in the Use of Data in Relation to Planning

Townsend (1962) pointed out, after a survey of the residential facilities provided for the elderly, that we would look back in horror at some of the cruelties perpetrated in the 1860s, just as our descendants a hundred years hence will look back in horror at some of the cruelties that we perpetrate today. Forsyth and Logan (1960) discussed the relationship between beds used, the size of the waiting list, and actual need. They were aware that the waiting list might have a stifling effect on referral for admission, and that admission could occur for social reasons as well as for medical care. Forsyth and Logan (1968), after discussing a mass of data relating to use of out-patient clinics, pointed out that there was a great need for meaningful statistical information to serve as a basis for planning. They commented that official statistics were few, and in some respects misleading; they acknowledged that the Ministry of Health, Regional Hospital Boards, and Hospital Management Committees were understaffed both qualitatively and quantitatively in relation to problems involved in collecting and analysing the kind of information that was required for planning. Meredith and his colleagues (1968) emphasized the need for specific studies to illuminate general problems; they pointed out nine reasons why a patient's transfer to 'second-line beds' might be delayed, and acute beds become blocked. Such information, of course, is not available from the routine statistics, which can, however, comment upon variation in length of stay in acute beds.

Forsyth, Thomas, and Jones (1970) present data about a planning exercise in the Liverpool Region. They discuss the problem of translating findings of any study into action, and point out that this is by no means a simple matter. They refer to problems of parochialism, powerful personalities, political pressure, emotion, and prejudice which constantly act against the unbiased planning of hospital services.

It has already been pointed out that there is need to take into account the attitudes of the general population to seeking health care; in this context it is interesting to note that even in Russia, with its excellent provision of doctors and other staff, hospitals, out-patient establishments, and polyclinics, Popov (1971) has demonstrated an iceberg of morbidity in an urban population. He showed that there were persons in the community with disease which required medical care, for which they had not contacted the health services.

A recent article by Pendreigh and his colleagues (1972) has discussed the problem of determining the requirements for treatment of renal failure. It has been pointed out that in order to plan for the treatment and management of end-stage renal failure it is important to determine the number of patients likely to benefit from maintenance haemodialysis or renal transplantation. They review the findings of nine surveys carried out in different countries and then describe a detailed survey carried out in Scotland. It is interesting to note that in order to carry out this survey they have relied primarily upon hospital consultants to notify patients with chronic renal failure; a second and very important source of notification was family doctors. The routine data on hospital in-patients and death registration were only used to supplement the other sources of information. Although the routine sources of data could have identified the patients suffering from renal disease, inquiries would still have had to be made to individual con-sultants in order to identify the severity of renal disease and the suitability of individual patients for haemodialysis or renal transplantation. Only this special inquiry has been able to provide the data required for planning.

REFERENCES

Acheson, E. D. (1967) *Medical Record Linkage*, London.

Alderson, M. R. (1965) M.D. Thesis, London University.

Alderson, M. R. (1968) Data on sickness absence in some recent publications of the Ministry of Pensions and National Insurance, *Brit. J. prev. soc. Med.*, **21**, 1.

Alderson, M. R. (1971) Selection of data from patients records, in *Computers in Radiotherapy* (*Proceedings of the Fourth International Conference on Computers in Radiotherapy*), eds. Glicksman, A. S., Cohen, M., and Cunningham, J. R., Special Report No. 5 British Institute of Radiology.

Alderson, M. R. (1972*a*) Some sources of error in British occupational mortality data, *Brit. J. industr. Med.* **29**, 245.

Alderson, M. R. (1972*b*) Cancer registration, in *Cancer Priorities*, ed. Bennett, G., British Cancer Council.

Alderson, M. R. (1972*c*). Unpublished report, Medical Information Unit, Wessex Regional Hospital Board. *Spectrum 1971*, ed. Abrams, M. E., London.

Alderson, M. R. (1972*d*) The Wessex Plan for computing, in

Alderson, M. R. (1974) Health information systems, *WHO Chronicle*, **28**, 52.

Alderson, M. R. and Meade, T. W. M. (1967) Accuracy of diagnosis on death certificates compared with that in hospital records, *Brit. J. prev. soc. Med.*, **21**, 22.

Ashford, J. R. (1971) The uses of information within the health services; the challenges of technical change, in *Challenges for Change, Essays on the Next Decade in the National Health Service*, ed. McLachlan, G., London.

Benjamin, B. (1965) Hospital activity analysis, *Hospital*, **61**, 221.

Benjamin, B. (1971) The use of statistics in the management of health and welfare services, in *Management of Health Services*, eds. Gatherer, A., and Warren, M. D., Oxford.

Bernard, C. (1948) *An Introduction to the Study of Experimental Medicine*, quoted by Ryle, J. D. (1948).

Bispham, K., Holland, W. W., and Stringer, J. (1971) Planning for health, *Hospital*, **67**, 82.

Bispham, K., Thorne, S., and Holland, W. W. (1971) Information for area health planning, in *Challenges for Change*, ed. McLachlan, G., London.

Bodenham, K. E., and Wellman, F. (1972) *Foundations for Health Service Management,* a Scicon Report for the Scottish Home and Health Department on the requirements for a Health Service Information System, London.

Bristowe, and Holmes, (1863) in *Sixth Report of Medical Officer to Privy Council*, London.

British Medical Journal (1968) Leading Aritcle, *Brit. Med. J.* **3**, 448.

British Medical Journal (1970) Leading Article, *Brit. Med. J.*, **4**, 635.

British Medical Journal (1971) Leading Article, *Brit. Med. J.*, **2**, 120.

Butler, N. R., and Bonham, D. G. (1963) *Perinatal Mortality*, London.

Civil Service Department (1971) Management Studies No. 2; *Computers in Central Government Ten Years Ahead*, London, H.M.S.O.

Cochrane, A. L. (1972) *Effectiveness and Efficiency, Random Reflections on Health Services*, Rock Carling Monograph, London.

Cotton, H. (1948) The collection of morbidity data from hospitals, *J. roy. statist. Soc.*, **3**, 14.

Cross, K. W., Droar, J., and Roberts, J. L. (1968) Electronic processing of hospital records, in *Computers in the Service of Medicine*, Vol. I, eds. McLachlan, G., and Shegog, R. A., London

Cross, K. W., and Roberts, J. L. (1970) Management controls in medical care, *Hospital*, **66**, 45, 81 and 121.

Cumming, G., and Goldsmith, O. (1971) Inclined planes or cogwheels?, in *In Low Gear?, An Examination of Cogwheels*, ed. McLachlan, G., London.

Department of Health and Social Security (1967) *First Report of the Joint Working Party on the Organisation of Medical Work in Hospitals*, London, H.M.S.O.

Department of Health and Social Security (1969) *The Functions of a District General Hospital*, Report of the Committee of the Central Health Services Council, London, H.M.S.O.

Department of Health and Social Security (1970) *The Future Structure of the National Health Service*, London, H.M.S.O.

Department of Health and Social Security (1971) *National Health Service Re-organisation—Consultative Document*, London, H.M.S.O.

Dinwoodie, H. P. (1969) An elementary use of a computer for morbidity recording in general practice, *Hlth Bull.*, **27**, 6.

Dinwoodie, H. P., and Grene, J. D. (1971) Computers in general practice, in *Principles and Practice of Medical Computing*, eds. Whitby, L. G., and Lutz, W., Edinburgh.

Dollery, C. T. (1971) The quality of health care, in *Challenges for Change*, ed. McLachlan, G., London.

Dudley, H. A. S. (1970) The clinical task, *Lancet*, **ii**, 1352.

Ellis-Martin, K. G. (1971) Capturing data for hospital activity analysis, *Med. Record*, **12**, 35.

Farr, W. (1875) *Supplement to 35th Annual Report of the Registrar General*, London, H.M.S.O.

Ferguson, J. B. P., and Murray, A. (1970) Survey of the use of Form S.M.R.M. (Scottish Medical Record—Maternity) as a normal delivery discharge letter, *Hlth Bull.*, **28**, 30.

Forsyth, G., and Sheikh, J. M. (1971) The mechanics of medical management, in *In Low Gear?, An Examination of Cogwheels*, ed. McLachlan, G., London.

Forsyth, G., and Logan, R. F. L. (1960) *The Demand for Medical Care*, London.

Forsyth, G., and Logan, R. F. L. (1968) *Gateway or Dividing Line?, A Study of Hospital Outpatients in the 1960s*, London.

Forsyth, G., Thomas, R. G., and Jones, S. P. (1970) Planning in practice, a half term report, in *Problems and Progress in Medical Care*, 4th Series, London.

Gatherer, A. (1971) Planning services, in *Management and the Health Services*, eds. Gatherer, A., and Warren, M. D., Oxford.

Goodwin, C. S. (1972) Medical information systems, *Lancet*, **ii**, 871.

Grogono, A. W., and Woodgate, D. J. (1971) Index for measuring health, *Lancet*, **ii**, 1024.

Guy, W. A. (1867) On the Mortality of London Hospitals, *J. statist. Soc.*, **30**, 392.

Heasman, M. A. (1964) How long in hospital?, *Lancet*, **ii**, 539.

Heasman, M. A. (1968) Scottish hospital in-patient statistics—sources and uses, *Hlth Bull.*, **26**, 10.

Heasman, M. A. (1970) Scottish consultant review of in-patient statistics (SCRIPS), *Scot. med. J.*, **15**, 386.

Heasman, M. A. (1971) The use of computers in a central organisation and record linkage, in *Principles and Practice of Medical Computing*, eds. Whitby, L. G., and Lutz, W., Edinburgh.

Heasman, M. A. (1972) The information system in an integrated health service, in *Spectrum 1971*, ed. Abrams, M. E., London.

Heasman, M. A., and Carstairs, V. (1971) In-patient management: variations in some aspects of practice in Scotland, *Brit. med. J.*, **1**, 495.

Heasman, M. A., and Lipworth, L. (1966) *Accuracy of Certification of Cause of Death*, Studies on Medical and Population Subjects No. 20, General Register Office, London, H.M.S.O.

Hill, A. B. (1962) Observation and experiment, in *Statistical Methods in Clinical and Preventive Medicine*, Edinburgh.

Hodes, C. (1969) The computer and screening techniques in general practice, *J. roy. Coll. gen. Practit.*, **18**, 330.

Hogben, L. (1940) *Mathematics for the Million*, London.

Hospital and Community (1948) *Hospital Treated Sickness Amongst the People of Stirlingshire*, a report of the Glasgow Health and Sickness Records Bureau, London.

Jay, A. (1970) Creative intercourse, in *Management and Machiavelli*, p. 93, Harmondsworth.

Journal of the Statistical Society (1842) Report of the Committee on Hospital Statistics, *J. statist. Soc.*, **5**, 168.

Journal of the Statistical Society (1844) Second Report of the Committee of the Statistical Society of London on Hospital Statistics, *J. statist. Soc.*, **7**, 14.

Journal of the Statistical Society (1862) Statistics of the General Hospitals of London, 1861, *J. statist. Soc.*, **25**, 384.

Journal of the Statistical Society (1866) Statistics of Metropolitan and Provisional General Hospitals for 1865, *J. statist. Soc.*, **29**, 596.

Kemp, I. W., Damblen, D. L., and Lindsay, E. D. (1971) A system for collection of orthopaedic clinical data, *Hlth Bull.*, **29**, 88.

Knox, E. G. (1968) Introducing a computer to a hospital, experiences of the experiment at Birmingham, in *Computers in the Service of Medicine*, eds. McLachlan, G., and Shegog, R. A., London.

Lancet (1835–36) Leading Article, *Lancet*, 55.

Lancet (1840–41) Leading Article, *Lancet*, 649.

Lockwood, E. (1971) Accuracy of Scottish hospital morbidity data, *Brit. J. prev. soc. Med.*, **25**, 76.

Logan, R. F. L., Klein, R. E., and Ashley, J. S. A. (1971) Effective management of health, *Brit. med. J.*, **2**, 519.

Matthews, G. K. (1971) Measuring need and evaluating services, in *Portfolio for Health, the Role and Programme of the D.H.S.S. in Health Services Research*, ed. McLachlan, G., London.

MacKay, D. (1951) *Hospital Morbidity Statistics*, Studies on Medical and Population Subjects No. 4, General Register Office, London, H.M.S.O.

McKeown, T., and Lowe, C. R .(1968) *An Introduction to Social Medicine*, Oxford.

McNay, R. A. (1969) Hospital activity analysis, experience in the area of the Newcastle Regional Hospital Board, *Hospital*, **65**, 308.

McSwiney, B. A. (1970) Planning: priorities and objectives, in *Resources in Medicine—A Collection of Papers on Management in Medicine Based on a Seminar Held at St Thomas's Hospital*, London.

Medawar, P. B. (1969) Hypothesis and imagination, in *The Art of the Soluble*, Harmondsworth.

Meredith, J. S., Anderson, M. A., Price, A. C., and Leithead, J. (1968) *'Hostels' in Hospitals? The Analysis of Beds in Hospitals by Patient Dependency*, London.

Ministry of Health (1966) *Report of the Committee on Senior Nursing Staff Structure*, London, H.M.S.O.

Morley, E. P. (1971) Cogwheel, *Brit. med. J.*, **1**, 292.

Morrison, P., and Morrison, E. (1971) *Charles Babbage and His Calculating Engines*, New York.

Moser, C. A. (1970) Some general developments in social statistics, *Social Trends*, **1**, 7.

Navarro, V., and Parker, E. D. (1970) Models in health services planning, in *Data Handling in Epidemiology*, ed. Holland, W. W., London.

Nightingale, F. (1863) *Notes on Hospitals*, 3rd ed., London.

Ockenden, J. M., and Bodenham, K. E. (1970) *Focus on Medical Computer Development, a Study of the British Scene by Scientific Control Systems Ltd.*, London.

Paulley, J. W. (1971) Salmon and Cogwheel, *Brit. med. J.*, **1**, 113.

Pearson, K. (1892) *The Grammar of Science*, London

Pendreigh, D. M., Howitt, L. F., MacDougall, A. J., Robson, J. S., Heasman, M. A., Kennedy, A. C., MacLeod, M., and Stewart, W. K. (1972) Survey of chronic renal failure in Scotland, *Lancet*, **i**, 304.

Platt, R. (1952) Wisdom is not enough: reflections on the science and art of medicine, *Lancet*, **ii**, 977.

Popov, G. A. (1971) Principles of health planning in the U.S.S.R., *Wld Hlth Org. Publ. Hlth Pap.* No. 43.

Riddle, J. W. (1971) A new approach to the capture of H.A.A. data, *Med. Record*, **12**, 6.

Rowe, R. G. (1971) History and present use of H.A.A., in *Proceedings, Journées Banques De Données*, Paper 1, Afcet-IRIA.

Ryle, J. A. (1948) *Changing Disciplines: Lectures on the History, Methods and Motives of Social Pathology*, London.

Seddon, H. (1971) Some reflections on medical records, *Brit. med. J.*, **4**, 103.

Shegog, R. (1971) Personal communication.

Sherrington, J. (1922) *Brit. med. J.*, **2**, 1139.

Smith, A. (1968) *The Science of Social Medicine*, London.

Smith, G. (1971) Case for a medical ombudsman, *The Times*, 4th November.

Spears, N. E., and Gould, C. A. (1936–37) Mechanical tabulation of hospital records, *Proc. roy. Soc. Med.*, **30**, 633.

Spence, J. (1953) The methodology of clinical science, *Lancet*, **i**, 629.

Topley, W. W. C. (1940) *Authority, Observation and Experiment in Medicine*, London.

Townsend, P. (1962) *The Family Life of Old People*, London.

Wall, M., and Cross, K. W. (1968) Recording and analysis of in-patient data on a regional basis, *Hospital*, **64**, 354.

Wall, M., and Wharton, D. A. (1970) The elderly in hospital, *Hospital*, **66**, 414.

Warren, M. D. (1971) Evaluation of services, in *Management and the Health Services*, eds. Gatherer, A., and Warren, M. D., Oxford.

Wier, R. D. (1970) Committees or computers, *Scot. med. J.*, **15**, 416.

Williams, L. M., and Bray, J. C. (1971) The use of computers for administrative purposes in the National Health Service, in *Principles and Practice of Medical Computing*, eds. Whitby, L. G., and Lutz, W., Edinburgh.

Wofinden, R. C. (1971) Health centres: problems and possibilities, *Community Medicine*, **125**, 175.

World Health Organization (1970a) Programmes for analysis of mortality trends and levels, *Wld Hlth Org. techn. Rep. Ser.*, No. 440.

World Health Organization (1970b) Training in national health planning, *Wld Hlth Org. techn. Rep. Ser.*, No. 456.

World Health Organization (1971) Statistical indicators for the planning and evaluation of public health programmes, *Wld Hlth Org. techn. Rep. Ser.*, No. 472

Yule, G. (1924) *Report of the Industrial Health Research Board (No. 28)*, London.

FURTHER READING

International Epidemiological Association (1973) Uses of epidemiology in planning health services, *Proc. Sixth Internat. Sc. meeting, Belgrade*, Belgrade.

Gatherer, A., and Warren, M. D., eds. (1971) *Management and the Health Services*, Oxford.

McLachlan, G., ed. (1971) *Challenges for Change, Essays on the Next Decade in the National Health Service*, London.

McLachlan, G., ed. (1971) *In Low Gear?, An Examination of Cogwheels*, London.

Seder, Richard H. (1973) Planning and politics in the allocation of health resources, *Amer. J. Pub. Hlth*, **63**, 774.
World Health Organization (1974) Modern management methods and the organization of health services, *Publ. Hlth. Pap.*, No. 55.

ADDENDUM; RECENT CHANGES IN RELATION TO USE OF INFORMATION FOR HEALTH MANAGEMENT AND PLANNING

Since the chapter was submitted in early 1972 there have been a number of changes in relation to the use of information in health service management which require brief mention. This is a field that is currently changing rather rapidly, particularly in relation to the reorganization of the health service. The consultative document already mentioned was followed by a White Paper (DHSS, 1972a) which again referred to the use of information. Further detail was provided in two other reports from the DHSS, the Report of the Working Party on Medical Administrators (DHSS, 1972b) and that on Management Arrangements for the Reorganized National Health Service (DHSS, 1972c). Alderson (1973a) has reviewed the comments in these reports on the use of management information, and related these to a system for handling information. Since that date there has been the appointment of specialists in community medicine at regional level with specific responsibility for information and research, whilst the job descriptions for the area medical officer and the district community physician also emphasize their roles in the establishment of information systems. Powles and his colleagues (1972) have reviewed the information requirements for planning, whilst Fox (1973) has commented that though there is plenty of information available for comprehensive planning there is lack of a structured system for handling this. It has been accepted that a planning and monitoring system should be introduced in the reorganized health service, and HRC(73)8 (DHSS, 1973) discussed the development of the planning system. This has now been tested in a few pilot areas, and further official guidance is awaited. The basic data required is comparable to that already collected by each of the liaison committees preparing area profiles; the draft forms however suggest that consolidating the material for the different functions of the district and area based services into an overall picture will be difficult. Tagg (1973) has emphasized that budgetary control must include study of the efficient use of resources in relation to results achieved. There is no agreed system for quantifying need or efficient use of resources that can be immediately applied in every district.

Reference has already been made to the work of Acheson (1967); a different aspect of record linkage is the proposal for a national cohort study, which has been published by the Office of Population Censuses and Surveys (OPCS 1973a). This report discusses 'proposals to link birth registration, internal migration, overseas migration, census of population, notification of cancer, and death registration for a one per cent sample of the population. This study started with a sample generated from the 1971 Census and has been updated by the addition of the above particulars. The cohort study will be a statistical exercise, providing tabular data for management, medical studies, and fertility studies.

World Health Organization Regional Office for Europe (1974) Report of a Conference on Health Information Systems, Copenhagen 1973 (Euro 4914), Copenhagen.

Reference is made in the main chapter to the need for information about the workload carried in primary medical care. A major advance was the first national study of morbidity in general practice conducted in England and Wales in 1955/56; a second survey was launched in 1970 and a paper on the method has now been published by the OPCS (1973b). The second survey aims to provide information about morbidity seen in general practice, the extent to which family doctors make use of facilities outside their practices, patients' consulting patterns, including the use of home visits and attendances at practice premises. The study has been extended for a second year and will perhaps lead to a system of continuous morbidity information from general practice on a larger scale than hitherto. Another approach to the collection of data on the illness in the community was touched upon by the Working Party on Collaboration Report (1973); this includes a discussion on the use of registers of the population in defined areas and associated files of contacts with the health and personal social services. The report recommended a systematic programme of studies on the organization and use of such registers. A major advance in the collection of information about the health status of the general population has now been made with the establishment of a General Household Survey; an introductory report on this survey has now been published by the OPCS (1973c). This is a continuing household sample survey organized throughout Great Britain, which has the central objective of making available a substantially improved flow of social statistics. One aspect that is covered in the survey is health data, and the preliminary report provides material about the chronic sickness in the community, incapacity from short-term sickness, contact with the family practitioners, use of outpatient facilities in hospital, and inpatient spells. This material is available by age, sex, locality, occupational group, and reported diagnostic categories.

Knox, Morris and Holland (1972) reviewed the information requirements in the unified health service and made proposals about the planning of such systems. Ashford, Ferster, and Pethybridge (1973) have commented upon the information requirements for management at the district level in the reorganized NHS. The chapter touches upon the requirements for comprehensive information systems which illuminate the actual functioning of the complete services provided for a community. Alderson (1973b) has further described one way in which a comprehensive information system might develop in this country. In two recent papers Yates (1973a and 1973b) has reported upon actual uses of information for management at hospital level, indicating how routinely available data has to be complemented by that provided from special studies.

REFERENCES

Alderson, M. R. (1973a) Information systems in the unified health service, in *The Future—and Present Indicatives*, ed. McLachlan, G., London.

Alderson, M. R. (1973*b*) Towards a health information system, *Hlth Soc. Serv. J.*, **83**, 1524.

Ashford, J. R., Ferster, J., and Pethybridge, R. J. (1973) Information requirements for district management in the reorganised NHS, in *The Future—and Present Indicatives*, ed. McLachlan, G., London.

Department of Health and Social Security (1972*a*) *National Health Service Reorganisation; England.*, Cmnd 5055, London, H.M.S.O.

Department of Health and Social Security (1972*b*) *Report of the Working Party on Medical Administrators* (Hunter Report), London, H.M.S.O.

Department of Health and Social Security (1972*c*) *Management Arrangements for the Reorganised N.H.S.*, London, H.M.S.O.

Department of Health and Social Security (1973) Development of planning in the reorganised N.H.S., HRC (73)8, London.

Knox, E. G., Morris, J. N., and Holland, W. W. (1972) Planning medical information systems in a unified health service, *Lancet*, **ii**, 696.

Office of Population Censuses and Surveys (1973*a*) *Cohort Studies; New Developments.* Studies on medical and population subjects No. 25, London, H.M.S.O.

Office of Population Censuses and Surveys (1973*b*) Morbidity statistics from general practice, *Second National Study Preliminary Report, Method*, London, O.P.C.S.

Fox, J. (1973) Technological components of health planning: Part 2, Information, *Community Med.*, **129**, 356.

Office of Population Censuses and Surveys (1973*c*) *The General Household Survey Introductory Report*, London, H.M.S.O.

Powles, J. ed. (1972) *The Organisation of Information Services: Final Report of the Workshop*, Area 44 Health Services Project.

Tagg, T. A. J. (1973) National Health Service reorganisation: specific financial aspects, *Hosp. Serv. Fin.*, **21**, (6), 12.

Working Party on Collaboration between the N.H.S. and Local Government (1973) *Report on its activities from June to July 1973*, London, H.M.S.O.

Yates, J. M. (1973*a*) Information for the management of clinical work in hospitals, in *The Future—and Present Indicatives*, ed. McLachlan, G., London.

Yates, J. M. (1973*b*) Monitoring in the hospital service, *Hosp. Hlth Serv. Rev.*, **69**, 322.

FURTHER READING

Brooke, Eileen M. (1974) The current and future use of registers in health information systems, *Wld Hlth Org. Offset publ. Ser.*, No. 7.

The Statistician, Vol. 21, No. 4, December 1972. This issue contained invited papers all dealing with medical information systems.

4

EPIDEMIOLOGICAL METHODS IN THE STUDY OF DISEASE

D. D. REID

The *Oxford English Dictionary* definition of epidemiology as 'that branch of medical science which treats of epidemics' is not very informative. Nor, if Tyndall's dictum that 'reproductive parasitic life is at the root of epidemic disease' which the *Dictionary* cites is definitive, is it in tune with modern usage. In the investigative medicine of today epidemiological methods, although largely developed to study disease due to parasitic organisms in human populations, are now quite generally applied to all illnesses of obscure origin. This extension of the field of epidemiological inquiries is discussed in more detail in CHAPTER 27. The general principles of the methods concerned are, however, most readily set out in terms of their traditional use in the study of acute and chronic infectious disease.

Epidemics are, in Greenwood's term, 'crowd diseases' affecting groups of people; and epidemiology thus deals with the characteristic behaviour of such diseases within the complex matrix of human populations. As a science of groups rather than of individuals it is, inevitably and essentially, statistical in nature; and it uses simple numerical techniques to achieve its aim of so clarifying the pattern of disease behaviour that the discovery of its origin and mode of spread will give the key to its control. The basic methods involve the collection and arrangement of observations on the occurrence of disease. Their purpose is to relate disease incidence to three main axes of classification—personal, temporal, and spatial. This entails a close study of:

1. The personal characteristics, e.g. diet, social class, occupation, or habits of life, common to all those affected by a specific disease.
2. The time of disease onset in relation to contemporary changes, e.g. in environment or habit, and the appearance of patterns in the timing of onset of cases within an outbreak.
3. The geographic or spatial distribution of disease, e.g. in relation to the physical environment.

These simple basic methods do not, of course, cover the whole field of epidemiological technique. The epidemiologist may be concerned in such disparate problems as the ascertainment of disease prevalence in communities by sampling inquiries, the testing of prophylactic measures by controlled field trials, or the mathematical basis of the theory of epidemic behaviour. But in the primary task of disease investigation these simple systematic arrangements of field observations form a useful guide to action. This chapter is, therefore, largely confined to a discussion of their application in the epidemiological approach to the study of disease incidence—the discovery of its nature and cause, its mode of spread, its natural history in individual or community, and the modifying effects of environment.

THE DISCOVERY OF NATURE AND CAUSE

In the probing observational stage of epidemiological inquiry about the nature and cause of disease, three basic associations are taken to indicate a likely cause and effect relationship between a disease 'D' and a factor 'A'. These are: that the incidence of 'D' varies in time with fluctuations in the force of the factor 'A'; that 'D' is found only in the presence of 'A'; and, conversely, that it is never observed in its absence. In practice, particularly in the more complex chronic disease of later life, such a simple set of rules may not be very appropriate; but they apply quite closely to the identification of causes in the acute disorders.

The example traditionally used to display the epidemiological approach is the work of Snow on cholera. Certainly, in the Broad Street epidemic of 1854 he illustrated the crucial value of classification of his observations by timing, location, and personal characteristics. The time distribution of the date of onset in the patients affected showed the quick upsurge in the first few days of the epidemic which we now recognize as typical of the explosive character of an outbreak following the simultaneous exposure of a large number of people to a common source of infection. Again, the geographical distribution of cases of cholera in the district of Soho at the time clearly showed a concentration centred on the area served by the Broad Street pump. But complete conviction of the water supply from that pump as the source of the epidemic came from Snow's demonstration that the persons affected had all drunk water from the particular pump, while those living in the district who escaped had drawn their water supply from a different source. Thus, by splitting up the Soho population in various ways according to their place of residence and their drinking habits, Snow was able to produce circumstantial, but convincing, evidence about the origin of cholera in some living organism passed from person to person through the medium of an infected water supply.

Perhaps a less-well-known example of the application of essentially the same principle of analysis is the earlier study of an 'epidemic' of non-infectious disease a century before. John Huxham, who practised in Plymouth, published an account of 'a disorder exceedingly epidemical', marked by severe colic culminating in palsy or epilepsy, which ravaged the west of England in 1724. He noted its seasonal incidence with a rapid rise in the autumn, the association of severity with bountiful apple harvests, its appearance in the cider-drinking county of Devon, and its concentration among the 'lowest Sort of People' for whom apples were a staple of diet, and cider, 'being cheaper than the smallest beer', the drink 'the joyful populace drank abundantly'. Huxham thus rightly associated the disease with apples, but wrongly concluded that the drinking of cider itself was the cause of the disease. He went on to suggest that the 'crude, gross, tartar' thus drawn into the blood affected the secretion of the humours—an early example of the danger of decisions about causation based on the circumstantial evidence of association which may be all that preliminary epidemiological surveys can give. On the other hand, fresh evidence of the same kind served to put Sir George Baker on to the true cause of the disease, for, some years later, he pointed out that the disease was not found in the cider-producing counties of Hereford, Worcester, and Gloucester, but that a disorder which was clinically similar had been common in Poitou in France, where the vintners had made sour wines more palatable by mixing them with litharge. Then, in a way which is typical of modern epidemiological research, he went from the field back to the laboratory for confirmatory evidence of his proposition that lead was, in fact, the agent of disease and that Huxham's theory that the tartar in the apples had corrupted the bile was untenable. Final proof came from the demonstration in the cider of lead which came from the apparatus in which Devon cider was then stored. These methods, involving the division of the population into groups which are homogeneous in respect of age or habit, and the comparison of the incidence of disease among them, still form the basis of epidemiological investigation. Associations observed, e.g. between habits and disease, then give clues about causation which can be followed up by more detailed clinical inquiries and perhaps confirmed by laboratory experiment.

UNCOVERING THE MODE OF SPREAD

Prevention of infectious disease usually demands the interruption of the chain of transmission from person to person. In the practice of preventive medicine, therefore, it is obviously essential to know not only the nature of the causative agent of

Time Charts

A time chart of an outbreak of measles affecting a family group is illustrated in FIGURE 3. To a family of two parents and four children the oldest child returns from school in the acute infectious stage of the disease. The day of onset in this, the *Index* or *Primary Case*, is plotted as day 1 on the time chart. The interval between the day of sickening in this introducing

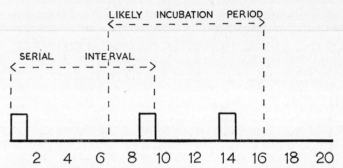

FIG. 3. Time chart of an outbreak of measles illustrating changes from the day of onset in number of days.

case and the onset of measles in the next child affected is plotted on the chart as the *Serial Interval*. This is not the same as the incubation period which intervenes between contact and sickening; but it is the most practical index of the transfer of infection from person to person. During the likely incubation period of this disease (7–16 days) two of the three remaining children sickened on the ninth and fourteenth days; and these are termed the *Secondary Cases*.

The simplest and best measure of the communication of infection among a group susceptible to it is the *Secondary Attack Rate*. This may be defined as the attack rate of a specific disease among the remaining susceptible members (of a closed group) within a stated period of time after its introduction into that group by an index or primary case. In the present example the

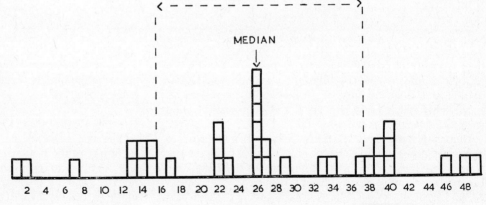

FIG. 4. Time chart showing the number of cases of measles in an epidemic from the first recorded case to the last.

disease but also the foci from which it is disseminated through the community and the manner and route of such spread. To do this, quite simple techniques are required—the drawing of time charts or maps and the calculation and tabulation of comparative rates either of the risk of transfer or of attack in different groups of the population.

parents had been rendered immune by previous infection, but the three remaining children were susceptible; and if two contracted measles within the likely incubation period of the disease the secondary attack rate would have been $\frac{2}{3} \times 100$ or $66\frac{2}{3}$ per cent. This secondary attack rate is one of the most useful measures of the risk of the transfer of infection in different diseases or of the same disease in different circumstances. But it can be effective only when, as in a disease like measles, all the susceptibles affected exhibit a definite clinical response to adequate doses of the infecting organism. Where immunity cannot be determined from the previous history, the denominator can be taken as the number of individuals in contact with the index case.

Time charts of outbreaks in larger communities can give vital clues about the nature of the epidemic source. The quick explosive course of the outbreak that follows the simultaneous exposure of susceptibles to a common source of infected food or water was early noted by Snow. In general, the pattern of the

Epidemic Maps

'Spot maps' are usually intended to illustrate the distribution in space of the patients affected in any outbreak of disease so that any associations, whether with food or water supplies, can be readily appreciated. They may be modified, as in FIGURE 5, to describe the route and rate of the spread of measles through an urban community. The day of the peak of the epidemic, as defined by the onset of the median case, in each sector of the district is charted and the route of the spread of the wave of infection from school to school is readily followed along the main routes of communication in the area. Some indication of the

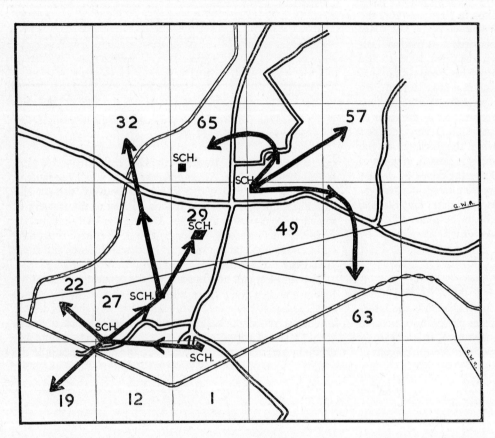

FIG. 5. Spot map to illustrate the distribution in space of patients affected in an outbreak of disease.

time sequence of cases in epidemics depends on the mode of transfer of infection varying from the slow, sporadic appearance of contact-spread illnesses like scabies or venereal disease to the fairly steady rapid rise and fall of air-borne infections such as influenza or measles.

FIGURE 4 shows how the time chart of the outbreaks of measles in schools or in different parts of a town can be most simply described and classified. The 'peak' of these epidemics can be most simply defined by the median day of the outbreak, i.e. the day of onset of the central case or the mid-point of the interval between the two central cases. In the illustration it is the twenty-sixth day. The rate of the epidemic spread within the area can also be defined in terms of the interquartile range, i.e. the interval between the dates enclosing the middle 50 per cent. of the cases. In the example in FIGURE 4 it is the interval between the fifteenth and the thirty-eighth day.

speed of movement of the epidemic wave through the area is given by the time between the peaks of the epidemics in each half-mile-square sector of the map.

Disease Incidence in Population Groups

The analysis of the distribution of disease in a community according to the personal characteristics of all exposed to the risk of attack consists simply of a comparison of the incidence rates in various sub-groups of the population. As pointed out in the preceding chapter, these rates are expressed in terms of the number of fresh instances of the specified disease per 1,000 persons exposed to risk over a stated period of time. In other words, the 'exposure to risk' is measured by the total person-time periods over which the population in question was exposed to the risk of attack. In the analysis of such observations the population is progressively split first, in the conventional way, into age and sex groups; and then, according to the preliminary results thus obtained, by such characteristics as occupation, diet, or water supply. In the investigation of an outbreak of paratyphoid fever, for example, a high attack rate among children would suggest a further subdivision of the whole population according to their milk, ice-cream, or confectionery supply to seek possible indications of excessive incidence in a group exposed to the risk of infection from some dietetic source they have in common. The results may be made more readily intelligible by diagrams or graphs, but the points of excessive risk of attack are usually obvious enough.

In such field investigations it may be helpful to have some systematic approach to the uncovering of sources and likely mode of spread in an outbreak of infectious illness. TABLE 24 gives an outline of the characteristic patterns of epidemic behaviour according to the mode of transfer of infection. In prolonged outbreaks one type of pattern may merge into another, as when the first wave of water-borne epidemic is succeeded by a secondary wave of case-to-case spread within affected households. Nevertheless, this broad scheme may serve to indicate the first steps in the solution of an epidemiological problem.

through a district such as is seen in infectious illness; and the groups of the population particularly vulnerable to the disease were those, like women of child-bearing age in poor families, who were likely to be most adversely affected by poor feeding.

The same process of investigation can be usefully extended to isolate and define different disease entities which, although not differing very much clinically, may have a distinctly different pattern of epidemic behaviour. Cruickshank (1953) has illustrated this point by contrasting the epidemiological characteristics of two clinically similar but not identical types of impetiginous lesion of the face. The first, characterized clinically by encrusted lesions with erythema and some local adenitis, has a seasonal distribution reminiscent of scarlet fever. It affects young schoolchildren, and spreads rapidly within closed communities. The other is a more strictly localized bullous lesion commonly seen in men in the Armed Forces serving in hotter climates; and it spreads less easily in barracks and similar environments. In this particular context it is possible to use laboratory methods to confirm that the first type of lesion shares the epidemic distribution of scarlet fever because of a common association with streptococcal infection, while the

TABLE 24

Epidemic Patterns According to Mode of Spread

AXIS OF CLASSIFICATION	MODE OF SPREAD			
	Contact		Ingestion	Vector
	Direct	Air-borne	Food, milk, or water	
Time				
Epidemic curve	Sporadic	Rapid	Explosive	Slow
Seasonal maximum	None	Winter	Summer	Depends on vector
Places	Closed communities, e.g. institutions	Universal	Confined to district of supply	Confined to vector area
Persons	Members of closed groups	Younger of all classes	Common diet or source of water supply	Exposed by occupation or habitation

EPIDEMIOLOGICAL DIFFERENTIAL DIAGNOSIS

Progress in the understanding of the causes of specific diseases has come from the recognition of clinical entities within some hitherto undifferentiated mass of clinical phenomena. Such differentiation, which allows greater precision in the ascertainment of cause, has usually been effected by detailed clinical description and a classification of syndromes by a grouping of the signs and symptoms most commonly found in association with each other. The identification of disease entities may also be furthered, however, by a study of the epidemic behaviour of the various syndromes concerned. In pellagra, for example, Goldberger (1916) used epidemiological methods to discover that it was more likely to be due to dietetic deficiency than to infection by a neurotropic virus. It was true that the disease affected some families more than others, but its seasonal distribution, unlike the major forms of infectious illness, showed a peak in incidence just before the harvest was gathered in. Further, the time sequence of dates of onset of cases in families or communities gave no hint of the regularity in incubation period which a parasitic infection might be expected to produce. In the same way, there was no geographic spread

second type is more usually the result of staphylococcal infection. In the acute respiratory infections, where laboratory aid may not be so immediately helpful, the same approach—a form of epidemiological diagnosis—may, as in the distinction of serum hepatitis or infectious jaundice, be of considerable practical importance.

STUDYING THE NATURAL HISTORY OF DISEASE

The natural history or the course of development of a disease can be related, particularly in chronic or recurrent illness, to the characteristics of the individual and, more especially perhaps in the acute infections, to the changing circumstances of large populations. Methods of measuring individual susceptibility or community resistance are thus of practical importance.

The Susceptibility of Individuals

In the commoner infectious diseases, such as measles or whooping cough, obvious clinical infection is usually followed by prolonged immunity, and a simple clinical history thus suffices to establish the individual's susceptibility. In the streptococcal diseases infection by one strain may not produce immunity to another; and repeated attacks of clinically similar illness may result. In these circumstances a more detailed history of illness and exposure to diffcrent sources may be required to elucidate problems of infection and cross-immunity. Pickles (1939) gives a fascinating account of the way in which, in the special circumstances of a rural general practice, careful tabulation of times of onset in relation to exposures to other cases gave vital information about the duration of infectiousness and the specificity of the immunity which followed illness of various types.

The problem of repeated attacks of the same type of illness is, however, particularly acute in both apparently infectious illnesses like the non-specific respiratory infections and in neurotic illnesses or other constitutional disorders. The early studies of personal susceptibility to repeated attacks of disability were directed to the problem of accidents affecting factory workers observed over a period of time. The numbers of individuals sustaining 0, 1, 2, 3, etc., accidents were tabulated, and it was noted that a small proportion of those thus observed accounted for a high percentage of the total number of such injuries. A more sophisticated mathematical analysis showed, however, that although such a result was not unlike the distribution which might have occurred purely by chance, the chance hypothesis, which postulated that all those observed were equally 'susceptible' to accidents, did not fit the data very adequately. On the other hand, a theoretical distribution based on an unequal personal liability to accident did give a reasonably close description of the observed distribution of the various number of accidents sustained per person. Although the same general method has been effectively applied to sickness data, there are both theoretical and practical objections to its use as a sole indication of 'prone-ness' or susceptibility to disease. Not only may other theoretical models based on different premises give an equally good fit between observation and expectation, but the equality in exposure over the whole period of observation which is an important basic assumption may be difficult to ensure in practice.

In the study of the susceptibility of children to repeated upper respiratory infections, for example, it is thus often simpler to see whether there is a correlation between the number of such illnesses suffered by the individuals in a group in one year with the number suffered in the next. Such a consistency is made explicit in the correlation coefficient which measures the closeness of the association between an individual's experience relative to other members of his class from year to year; and the size of the coefficient indicates the relative importance of such differences in individual susceptibility in the total variation in incidence of the specific disease in these particular circumstances. In school classes, for example, a correlation analysis of this type suggested that in these conditions consistent individual differences in susceptibility were numerically important in respiratory affections (Reid, 1958).

Long-term histories of the sickness experience of individuals may be available in the health records of occupational groups or sickness insurance agencies. By the analysis of such records, it may be possible to demonstrate the influence of personal susceptibility or habits on the evolution of chronic disease. A comparison of the frequency of absence because of illness in bronchitic workers with that in their unaffected colleagues showed that permanent disability is preceded by unduly frequent attacks of less serious respiratory infections in earlier life.

In the same way, some indication of an excessive incidence of different types of illness—peptic ulcer, lung cancer, or coronary thrombosis—in these same bronchitic individuals may point to a common origin in heavy cigarette smoking (Reid and Fairbairn, 1958).

Data Linkage

The linking of two or more medical records relating to the same individual is being increasingly used to determine, for example, the long-term consequences for health of a particular experience or exposure in foetal or early life. A recent example concerns the linking of notifications of infectious disease such as chickenpox in a pregnant woman to the death certificate for the child resulting from that pregnancy. In this way, an excess risk of death from leukaemia among children was attributed to maternal infection during pregnancy (Adelstein and Donovan, 1972).

Data linkage may have other epidemiological applications (Heasman, 1970). The value of hospital admission data as an index of the incidence of a chronic relapsing disease can be enhanced by linking repeated admissions for the same individual. Duplication of cases is thus avoided and a better estimate of the frequency of new cases, for example of ulcerative colitis, can be made. Again, the natural history of malignant disease in its later stages can be defined by linking records of hospital care to death certificates. This is of special importance in relation to disease registers where all the cases, perhaps of cancer or cardiovascular disease, occurring in a defined area are recorded at the time and followed up until death.

Retrospective and Prospective Inquiries

Unfortunately, sufficiently detailed personal histories are seldom available, and the relevance of personal characteristics or habits to disease experience is most frequently assessed by comparing the distribution of such features in the personal histories, elicited by interrogation, of sick patients with that in a suitable group of individuals not suffering from the illness in question. This 'control' group is usually drawn from the same population and matched in respect of some major characteristics, e.g. age and sex, with the sick individuals. Comparisons between 'sick' and 'control' groups will then reveal major differences, e.g. in dietary habit, between patients with coronary thrombosis and their unaffected controls which may have aetiological significance.

Such comparisons of past history (i.e. retrospective studies) are useful pointers to personal qualities or habits which distinguish the sick from the well. But the interpretation of their results is open to the objection that the answers given by a patient suffering from cancer of the lung, e.g. about smoking habits or family history of malignant disease, are likely to be coloured by his present symptoms and anxieties or that the investigator may be prejudiced in his interpretation of these answers by his knowledge of the patient's condition.

Some of these objections may be met by the prospective type of inquiry where a large sample of the apparently well population is interrogated about their personal habits, e.g. in diet or smoking, and then followed up over a long period of time. Observations on the occurrence of diseases such as lung cancer or coronary thrombosis among this population will then allow the calculation of incidence rates, in groups with contrasting smoking or dietetic habits, which are unaffected by the personal bias in response associated with the retrospective type of inquiry. As the studies on the role of smoking in cancer of the lung have shown, both types of inquiry can be used in turn to give confirmatory evidence of an aetiological association between habit and disease (Hammond and Horn, 1958; Doll and Hill, 1956).

Disease Evolution in the Community

The study of the evolution of disease in the community largely depends on the analysis of vital statistical information on sickness or death due to the specific infectious or other type of illness. The rates concerned have been defined in the previous chapter, but some examples may be given here of their application in epidemiology.

Standardized death rates are useful as summary measures of the mortality experience of populations of widely different age or sex structure; and they are particularly useful in the broad comparisons of mortality in different countries and in the study of the long-term trends of disease. In a country like Britain with a steadily increasing proportion of older people, crude death rates are liable to give false impressions of the changing importance of a specific disease in a community. On the other hand, such summary measures may obscure important features of disease experience in the changing circumstances of different sections of the community. It is thus essential to look at the time trends in disease within specific age and sex groups. In pulmonary tuberculosis in recent years, for example, the death rate has certainly been falling. But this decline has not been shared equally by all groups, for a marked decline among young women has to be contrasted with a much smaller fall among middle-aged males.

Such trends may often be more readily interpreted by setting out the experience of 'cohorts' of individuals who have been born in a specified decade and whose death rate at each succeeding stage of the life of their generation is compared with that of people born in other decades and followed through in the same way. Springett (1952) has given a useful account of the development of such methods in the field of pulmonary tuberculosis, where they have explained how the contemporary shift in the peak of mortality towards middle and later life is a reflection of declining infection rates in childhood and a relative deterioration in the experience of the survivors of earlier generations or 'cohorts' born in the past century in this country. The use of such methods can be readily extended to other diseases, e.g. in the study of the epidemic of lung cancer affecting the generation who began to smoke cigarettes during or after the First World War and who are now past middle age.

THE MEASUREMENT OF ENVIRONMENTAL INFLUENCES ON DISEASE

There are three basic elements in the balance of natural forces determining the incidence of human disease—the pathogenic agent, the susceptible host, and the physical environment which may affect either. In the respiratory infections, for example, a lowering change in atmospheric temperature may reduce the resistance of the host and, by increasing crowding in poorly ventilated buildings, enhance the rate of transfer of the infective agent. Since the immediate environment of house or work place can often be readily altered, some measure of its influence on disease incidence is essential if the likely preventive effect of such a change is to be assessed.

The Use of Statistical Analysis

The traditional approach to this problem is through the analysis of vital statistical data on the mortality experience of populations in relation to different indices of environmental conditions. Statistical techniques such as the calculation of coefficients of correlation are often used to explore the relative closeness of the association between disease incidence and various indices of environmental conditions. The statistical correlation between disease rates from bronchitis in different areas and the local air pollution level, for example, is greater than its correlation with indices of domestic overcrowding. Although the apparent effects of various factors can be sorted out in this way, the problem is to decide whether these interrelated factors have independent effects. More sophisticated statistical methods such as partial regression analysis are usually needed, in order to assess the residual relationship between disease incidence and either of these factors after the effects of the other has been taken into account (Fairbairn and Reid, 1958). Similarly, in dealing with correlations over a period of time between the simultaneous variations in, e.g. humidity and air-borne respiratory infections, rather complex methods of smoothing out the general seasonal trends are required in order to distinguish the presumptive effects of humidity on the spread of disease from the possible effects of contemporary fluctuations in temperature, e.g. on the susceptibility of the hosts. By such methods, Holland et al. (1961), showed that the rate of admission to London hospitals for respiratory conditions was related to the prevailing levels of air pollution and, quite independently, to changes in temperature. Useful as such methods are in exploring possible aetiological relationships, cause and effect should not be too readily assumed and the possible role of some other factor not included in the preliminary analysis, such as regional differences in smoking habits, should always be kept in mind.

Field Observations

In environmental studies some of the simple measures of epidemic behaviour already described can be readily applied; and the interpretation of the results obtained can be furthered by the use of ancillary bacteriological and other methods of investigation. The secondary attack rate within a small closed community, such as the family or classroom, can be used as a measure of the rate of transfer of infection to determine the effect on such risks of differing conditions of ventilation or overcrowding. In a study of the effects of domestic crowding on acute minor respiratory illness the secondary attack rate was compared among members of families of five living in three grades of domestic conditions. TABLE 25 shows that there is a small but statistically significant rise in the secondary attack rate with each increase in the crowding of the home (Brimblecombe et al., 1958). Differences in the completeness of disease reporting by the various families might explain such results, and bacteriological measures of the person-to-person spread of organisms in these circumstances were used to amplify the clinical data. As TABLE 25 shows, a similar rate based on the frequency of transfer of a type-specific organism from the throat of its introducer into the household to the throats of the others in the home confirmed the suggestion that overcrowding did result in an increased risk of the transfer of infection. By such studies, the influence of one of the environmental factors in respiratory disease can be isolated and its importance assessed.

TABLE 25

Clinical and Bacteriological Measures of Transfer of Infection in Different Housing Conditions

	Type of housing		
	Un-crowded	Crowded	Over-crowded
Clinical secondary attack rate (per cent.)	13·5	16·4	17·4
Bacterial-transfer rate (per cent.)	11·2	13·8	16·0

The same sort of combination of clinical and bacteriological measures may prove helpful in studies of cross-infection in schoolroom or barracks. The risk of transfer of measles in classrooms, for example, can be readily measured by the secondary attack rate among susceptible children exposed to a primary case. In one such study (Reid *et al.*, 1956), there was a significant association between these secondary attack rates in classrooms and the level of counts made by a slit sampling apparatus of *Streptococcus salivarius* coming from the mouths of children in these rooms. The implication of such a correlation would seem to be that conditions of ventilation and class behaviour which favoured the wide aerial dissemination of infected droplets from the nose and throat also allowed the ready transfer of measles virus. Such suggestions may be most satisfactorily confirmed by the controlled field trial of measures designed to so improve environmental conditions that the risk of transfer of infection is minimized. In this instance, air sterilization by ultra-violet irradiation of the upper air of schoolrooms produced a significant lowering in the measles secondary attack rate there compared with the rate in control classrooms not thus equipped (Medical Research Council, 1954).

Prevalence Survey Methods

In the wider field of factory or community there is also scope for the parallel use of vital statistical and clinical or bacteriological methods in the assessment of the different infective hazards of various environments. Population surveys either by mass miniature radiography in adults or of tuberculin skin test results in children in different parts of the country, may corroborate vital statistical evidence about the sources of infection in town and country. In cities, where contact with human infections is frequent, the high notification rates for pulmonary tuberculosis among young urban males are associated with both a high rate of prevalence of active lesions found by radiographic surveys and a high rate of tuberculin skin test conversion among adolescents. On the other hand, the bovine origin of the high death rates from non-pulmonary forms of the disease in the rural areas is suggested by the high proportion of tuberculin reactors among school entrants there (Medical Research Council, 1952). The proportion of tuberculin reactors at different ages can also be used to estimate the risk of infection in different time periods. This has recently been done on the

basis of a field survey in Uganda where bovine infection is uncommon and B.C.G. vaccination seldom carried out (Stott *et al.*, 1973).

The automation of laboratory techniques and the development of sensitive and precise serological tests has made large-scale surveys entirely practicable. These are now extensively used to describe the distribution in different communities, and in different age and sex groups within them, of immune responses to specific infections even in the absence of clinical manifestations or history. Thus a clear rise among older children in the titre for malaria antibodies with different antigens (*P. vivax* and *P. falciparum*) showed that, despite a widespread antimalarial campaign, transmission of the disease was still taking place although no parasites were found in films of peripheral blood (Draper, Voller, and Carpenter, 1972).

Increasingly, epidemiological studies on disease causation involve the clinical interrogation or examination of representative samples of contrasted populations. Mortality studies based on death certification are subject to possible bias associated with the diagnostic habits in doctors working in different areas. Moreover, the death certificate tends to concentrate on the terminal condition and gives less information on the earlier stages of the disease and the social circumstances or personal habits which may initiate or aggravate it. Yet detailed knowledge of these facts is essential for any intelligent attempt at disease control or prevention.

The usual approach is to draw, by some process of random selection, representative samples of populations whose reported mortality experience is markedly different. To this sample are then applied standard clinical questionnaires designed to elicit the essential clinical history in a uniform fashion, and then some physical test to assess the degree of any functional disability. In the study of chronic bronchitis, for example, a questionnaire on respiratory disease history and symptoms, current and past personal habits and circumstances and a simple test of lung function were used to examine randomly selected samples from doctors' practices in different parts of the country (College of General Practitioners, 1961). By such methods, the social class distribution of the disease was confirmed, and the effects of cigarette smoking and the urban environment were elucidated.

International and Migrant Studies

The use of standardized clinical techniques has made feasible the comparison of the results of prevalence surveys in different countries. This allows the confirmation of any major international differences in disease experience that were suggested by differences in reported death rates and which may be of aetiological importance. TABLE 26 shows, for example, how surveys of the prevalence of respiratory symptoms can support the suggestion in the death rate from chronic lung disease of a clear ranking from high rates in England to very low rates in Japan. The concurrent collection of data on personal characteristics such as smoking can also provide clues to possible causes for these international differences in the frequency of respiratory disease (Reid and Fletcher, 1971).

A special form of international study exploits the unique opportunity for making crucial observations afforded by the migration of people from country to country. Among immigrants to Israel, for example, the prevalence of multiple sclerosis is 29 per 100,000 for those born in Europe and 9 per 100,000 for those coming from either Africa or Asia (Alter, 1973). Similar observations have been made in other countries. Migrant studies need not be confined to international comparisons. Movement within a country where there are major

TABLE 26
Prevalence of Chronic Phlegm Production in London, Eastern Cities of the United States and Tokyo, and National Death-rates from Chronic Lung Disease in 1965–67

	Prevalence in men aged 40–59 in the population (per cent.)	National death-rate/100,000 men aged 45–54
London	33	41
Eastern cities of the United States	24	18
Tokyo	4	4

environmental differences may be equally informative. TABLE 27 shows, for example, how both life-time residence and movement from a place of birth to region of death may affect the risk of dying from multiple sclerosis (Kurtzke *et al.*, 1971). The effect seems to depend in part on age at migration. Observations such as these have led to speculation about the role of exposure to infection in early childhood and the development of relative immunity to the disease (Dean, 1970).

TABLE 27
Multiple Sclerosis Mortality per 100,000 Population in United States by Region of Birth and Region of Death (Kurtzke, 1971)

Region of Birth	Region of Death	
	North	South
North	1·00	0·87
South	0·68	0·46

Twin Studies in Epidemiology

The separation of the genetic from the environmental elements in the individual disposition to disease has been attempted by the technique of twin studies. The basic concept is simple. Uniovular or monozygotic pairs of twins are identical in their genetic endowment while binovular or dizygotic pairs are no more genetically alike than ordinary brothers or sisters. Generally speaking, twins are reared in the same family environment. If genetic factors are of special importance in a particular disease, the genetically identical or monozygotic twins are more likely to be similarly affected by that disease than dizygotic pairs would be. The degree of this similarity in disease experience is usually measured by a concordance rate which indicates the risk, when one of a pair is affected, of his co-twin being similarly diseased. Thus, if in a series of 6 sets of twins both were affected in 4 sets and only one in each of the remaining 2 pairs, the probability of any one of the 10 affected probands having an affected co-twin would be 8 out of 10, i.e. a concordance rate of 80 per cent. In recent years, national twin registries have been established, e.g. in Sweden and

Denmark, by listing all live twin births occurring in a defined period and following them through to either death or survival into adult life. In this way an unbiased sample of twins is obtained and the difficulties of interpreting results based on pairs of twins seen in hospital practice avoided. Typical of the results now accruing are those from the Danish Twin Registry given in TABLE 28 (Hauge *et al.*, 1968). The concordance rates for both infectious and non-infectious disease vary widely. For rheumatic fever, the concordance rate is much higher in monozygotic than in dizygotic twins and the inference is that genetic factors are relatively important in this disease. For deaths from acute infections on the other hand, the difference is much less, so that the environmental circumstances such as chance exposure to infection are presumably dominant.

Twin studies may also be used to detect the effect of differing environmental agents on each of a set of genetically identical twins who have been reared separately or who have been exposed to a different degree to some external pathogen. Among sets of male monozygotic or identical twins, for

TABLE 28
Occurrence of Selected Somatic Diseases in the Danish Twin Register Based on a Survey of 4,368 Same-Sexed Pairs

Disease	Proband–Concordance Rates per cent.	
	Monozygotic	Dizygotic
Cerebral apoplexy	36	19
Coronary occlusion	33	27
Tuberculosis	54	27
Rheumatic fever	33	10
Rheumatoid arthritis	50	5
Death from acute infection	14	11
Bronchial asthma	63	38
Epilepsy	54	24

example, the prevalence of chronic cough is 15 per cent. among smokers and 8 per cent. among non-smokers (Cederlöf *et al.*, 1966). Since the twins are constitutionally matched, this natural experiment allows the unequivocal assessment of the effect of smoking on respiratory symptoms.

The Use of the Computer

The development of the electronic computer has had important consequences for epidemiological research. As already noted, it can be used to simulate epidemic behaviour in different populations. It can also allow the practical application of more refined methods for the statistical analysis of large amounts of data. Multivariate analysis, involving the interrelations of many variables can now be planned without undue regard to the amount of arithmetical manipulation which previously often prohibited its use. In large studies, particularly where a follow-up is included, the computer can perform clerical duties such as reproducing addresses or updating records with efficiency and accuracy. Galloway (1966) has illustrated this by using the computer to produce, for every birth in an area, letters to parents arranging a series of visits, at appropriate intervals, to an immunization clinic.

Of increasing importance is the facility that the computer

has in linking the records of the same individual held no different files. Data linkage can, of course, be done by hand, but the speed of search by the computer through files held on magnetic tape or disc makes large-scale studies practicable.

OTHER EPIDEMIOLOGICAL METHODS
Theoretical Epidemiology

The rise and fall of the incidence rate of an infectious disease in a community depends on the proportion of the population who are susceptible, the number of infective cases, and the range of effective contacts which they make during their period of infectiousness. The introduction of a large number of children in the infectious stage of measles into a residential school where contact is prolonged and intimate enough to allow the effective transfer of infection is bound to lead to a sharp epidemic. Conversely, when the wave of infection has affected nearly all the susceptible children this 'exhaustion of susceptibles' inevitably leads to the decline and end of the epidemic. The number of fresh cases produced in each successive generation of the epidemic can be estimated by mathematical formulae which take all three of these basic factors into account. Where transmission is through an intermediate insect or other vectors, the formulae have to allow for the duration of life and biting habits of these vectors as well as the length of time during which they carry infection.

Increasingly sophisticated methods of mathematical model building have been developed (Dietz, 1967); and these are useful in the planning of disease control or in comparing the results of the application of alternative theories of epidemic behaviour with the observed rise and fall of the epidemic curve. Such methods have been used, for example, in estimating the epidemiological consequences of alterations in the duration of infectivity of the mosquito vector in malaria (Macdonald, 1953) or in the proportion of children susceptible to measles in the population (Abbey, 1952). Stochastic models, where the element of chance contact is more precisely taken into account, have given good fits to field data on the spread of infection in families and similar communities. Again, the introduction of the electronic computer has made feasible the repeated simulation of epidemic behaviour to provide models of what might happen in certain conditions of contact, infectivity or immunity in a population (Bailey, 1967). A set of random numbers generated in the computer is used to introduce the element of chance, e.g. in contact with an infectious case. One such computer simulation was designed to predict the likely effect of the use of live poliomyelitis virus vaccine on the spread of another virus infection through a suburban population (Elveback *et al.*, 1968).

WHO has developed models for the evaluation of disease control programmes e.g. in the case of trachoma (see Sundaresan and Asaad, 1973) and also in typhoid fever [see CHAPTER 16].

Screening Procedures

One approach to disease control of infectious and non-infectious disease is the detection and protection of susceptible individuals. In the control of tuberculosis, for example, tuberculin skin test surveys are used to pick out those whose negative reaction implies that they have not yet been exposed to the immunizing effect of infection. In these subjects vaccination can confer a worthwhile degree of protection against the larger infective doses experienced in adult life.

The same principles are being increasingly applied in attempts to control the non-infectious diseases. Here, there is seldom a clear-cut distinction between the susceptible and the immune. Indeed, it is useful to consider susceptibility, e.g. to ischaemic heart disease, as a normally distributed characteristic like height or blood pressure. The identification of individuals at the extreme of this distribution may be regarded as those most at risk of serious disease on whom preventive measures should be concentrated. The school child with a family or personal history of respiratory illness and poor lung function on testing for ventilatory ability, for example, might well be the subject of intensive health education, e.g. on the hazard of smoking.

Field Trials

The practice of epidemiology clearly requires a catholic choice of technical methods. More often than not, the inferences about disease causation that come from epidemiological studies are circumstantial in that they are based on observed associations rather than on planned experiments. Corroborative evidence may be derived from the results, e.g. of bacteriological techniques, and confidence in the conclusions from field studies thus increased. The ultimate proof of cause and effect can usually come only from the field trial of methods of disease prevention or control based on the aetiological theories which these field inquiries suggest. In such trials the methods involved (Hill, 1958) are simply those which govern experimentation in other branches of science.

The procedure is simple in concept if difficult to execute in practice. Volunteers are usually arranged into classes according to age and sex, and then each class is divided by some process of random allocation into two groups. To one is given the new prophylactic under test while the other group, receiving some other preparation, serves as a control. The subsequent disease experience of both groups in similar conditions is then followed up. The relative frequency of disease, as defined in some standard terms, is then taken as the criterion by which preventive efficacy is judged. Field trials of vaccines against influenza, for example, followed these principles to demonstrate the degree of superiority of the Asian type over polyvalent Virus A and a Virus B vaccine (Medical Research Council, 1958). The same methods have been applied in a wider context where community groups rather than individuals are the unit of observation. Field trials of the value of fluoridation of water supplies in the prevention of dental caries illustrate the general principle that successful prevention is the ultimate test of success in investigating the causes and method of spread of disease (Ast *et al.*, 1956).

Epidemiological methods are thus at the core of the practice of preventive medicine. Their increasing application in the field of chronic or degenerative diseases is emphasized in CHAPTER 27. But whatever their field of application, they must be used with rigour in the discovery of causes and in the assessment of the methods of control to which these discoveries may lead.

REFERENCES

Abbey, Helen (1952) An examination of the Reed–Frost theory of epidemics, *Hum. Biol.*, **24**, 201.

Adelstein, A. M., and Donovan, J. W. (1972) Malignant disease in children whose mothers had chickenpox, mumps, or rubella in pregnancy, *Brit. med. J.*, **4**, 629.

Alter, M. (1973) Multiple sclerosis in migrant populations, *Triangle*, **12**, 1, 25.

Ast, D. B., Smith, D. J., Wachs, B., and Cantwell, K. T. (1956) Newburgh–Kingston caries fluorine study, XIV. Combined clinical and roentgenographic dental findings after ten years of fluoride experience, *J. Amer. dent. Ass.*, **85**, 314.

Bailey, N. T. J. (1967) The simulation of stochastic epidemics in two dimensions, *Proc. 5th Berkeley Symp. Math. Statist. Probab.*, **4**, 237.

Brimblecombe, F. S. W., Cruickshank, R., Masters, P. L., Reid, D. D., and Stewart, G. T. (1958) Family studies of respiratory infections, *Brit. med. J.*, **1**, 119.

Cederlöf, R., Friberg, L., Jonsson, E., and Kaij, L. (1966) Respiratory symptoms and angina pectoris in twins with reference to smoking habits. An epidemiological study with mailed questionnaire, *Arch. environm. Hlth*, **13**, 726.

College of General Practitioners (1961) Chronic bronchitis in Great Britain, *Brit. med. J.*, **2**, 973.

Cruickshank, R. (1953) Epidemiology of some skin infections, *Brit. med. J.*, **1**, 55.

Dean, G. (1970) The multiple sclerosis problem, *Scien. Amer.*, **223**, 1, 40.

Dietz, K., (1967) Epidemics and rumours: A survey, *J. roy. Statist. Soc.*, A. **130**, 505.

Doll, R., and Hill, A. B. (1956) Lung cancer and other causes of death in relation to smoking, a second report on the mortality of British doctors, *Brit. med. J.*, **2**, 1071.

Draper, C. C., Voller, A., and Carpenter, R. G. (1972) The epidemiologic interpretation of serologic data in malaria, *Amer. J. trop. Med. Hyg.*, **21**, 696.

Elveback, L. R., Ackerman, E., and Young, G. (1968) A stochastic model for competition between viral agents in the presence of interference, *Amer. J. Epidem.*, **87**, 373.

Fairbairn, A. S., and Reid, D. D. (1958) Air pollution and other local factors in respiratory disease, *Brit. J. prev. soc. Med.*, **12**, 94.

Galloway, T. McL. (1966) Computers. Their use in local health administration, *Roy. Soc. Hlth J.*, **86**, 213.

Goldberger, J. (1916) Pellagra: causation and method of prevention, *J. Amer. med. Ass.*, **66**, 471.

Hammond, E. C., and Horn, D. (1958) Smoking and death rates: report on 44 months of follow-up of 187,783 men, *J. Amer. med. Ass.*, **166**, 1159, 1294.

Hauge, M., Harvald, B., Fischer, M., *et al.* (1968) The Danish Twin Register, *Acta Genet. med. (Roma)*, **17**, 315.

Heasman, M. A. (1970) Uses of record linkage in epidemiology, in *Data Handling in Epidemiology*, ed. Holland, W. W., p. 83, London.

Hill, A. B. (1958) The experimental approach in preventive medicine, Harben Lectures 1957, *J. roy. Inst. publ. Hlth*, **21**, 177, 209.

Holland, W. W., Spicer, C. C., and Wilson, J. M. G. (1961) Influence of the weather on respiratory and heart disease, *Lancet*, ii, 338.

Kurtzke, J. F., Kurland, L. T., and Goldberg, I. D. (1971) Mortality and migration in multiple sclerosis, *Neurology (Minneap.)*, **21**, 1186.

Macdonald, G. (1953) The analysis of malaria epidemics, *Trop. Dis. Bull.*, **50**, 871.

Medical Research Council (1952) National tuberculin survey, 1949–50, *Lancet*, **i**, 775.

Medical Research Council (1954) *Air Disinfection with Ultra-violet Irradiation. Its Effects on Illness among Schoolchildren*, Special Report Series No. 283, London, H.M.S.O.

Medical Research Council (1958) Trial of an Asian influenza vaccine. 4th Progress Report to the M. R. C. by its Committee on Influenza and other Respiratory Virus Vaccines, *Brit. med. J.*, **1**, 415.

Newell, K .W. (1968) Some World Health Organization Multi-disciplinary Studies. Paper read at the Fifth Scientific Meeting of the International Epidemiological Association. 24–31 August 1968.

Pickles, W. N. (1939) *Epidemiology in Country Practice*, Bristol.

Reid, D. D. (1958) Environmental factors in respiratory disease, Milroy Lectures, *Lancet*, **i**, 1237, 1289.

Reid, D. D., and Fairbairn, A. S. (1958) The natural history of chronic bronchitis, *Lancet*, **i**, 1147.

Reid, D. D., and Fletcher, C. M. (1971) International studies in chronic respiratory disease, *Brit. med. Bull.*, **27**, 59.

Reid, D. D., Lidwell, O. M., and Williams, R. E. O. (1956) Counts of air-borne bacteria as indices of air hygiene, *J. Hyg. (Lond.)*, **54**, 524.

Springett, V. H. (1952) An interpretation of statistical trends in tuberculosis, Milroy Lectures, *Lancet*, **i**, 521, 575.

Stott, H., Anil Patel, Sutherland, I., Thorup, I., Smith, P. G., Kent, P. W., and Rykushin, Y. P. (1973) The risk of tuberculous infection in Uganda. Derived from the Findings of National Tuberculin Surveys in 1958 and 1970, *Tubercle (Edinb.)*, **54**, 1.

Sundaresan, T. K., and Asaad, F. A. (1973) The use of simple epidemiological models in the evaluation of disease control programmes: A case study of trachoma, *Bull. Wld Hlth Org.*, **48**, 709.

FURTHER READING

For general texts on epidemiology with particular emphasis on the infectious fevers see *Principles of Epidemiology* by I. Taylor and J. Knowelden (1964), 2nd ed., London, and *Epidemiology: Man and Disease* by J. P. Fox, C. E. Hall and L. R. Elveback (1970), London. *The Uses of Epidemiology* by J. N. Morris (1970), 2nd ed. reprint, Edinburgh, gives an interesting introduction to the applications of epidemiology in the study of chronic disease. *Epidemiology: Principles and Methods* by B. MacMahon and T. F. Pugh (1971) gives a useful account of the principles of aetiological inquiry. *Statistical Methods in Clinical and Preventive Medicine* (1962) by Professor Sir Austin Bradford Hill is an excellent review of the use of statistical methods in the solution of clinical and epidemiological problems. Some of the technical issues in the conduct of field studies are discussed in *Medical Surveys and Clinical Trials* edited by L. J. Witts (1964), 2nd ed., London, while an introduction to their appli-cation in psychiatry is given in *Epidemiological Methods in the Study of Mental Disorders* by D. D. Reid (1960), World Health Organization, Geneva, and its sequel *The Scope of Epidemiology in Psychiatry* by Tsung-yi Lin and C. C. Standley (1962), World Health Organization, Geneva. A World Health Organization monograph by G. A. Rose and H. Blackburn (1968) describes *Cardiovascular Survey Methods. Cancer Epidemiology: Methods of Study* by A. M. Lilienfeld, E. Pedersen and J. E. Dowd (1967), Baltimore, serves the same purpose in respect of malignant disease. The report of a World Health Organization Committee on Twin Studies is given in *Acta Genetica et Gemellologia* (1966), **15**, 2, 109, and a symposium on migrant studies in chronic disease covered examples in many countries (*Israel Journal of Medical Sciences* (1971), **7**, 12, 1333–1596). Theoretical epidemiology is discussed in *The Mathematical Theory of Epidemics* (1957) by N. T. J. Bailey. The collected papers of the late George Macdonald on this subject have been published under the title of *Dynamics of Tropical Disease* edited by L. J. Bruce-Chwatt and V. J. Glanville (1973), London. The practical aspects of the use of computers in epidemiology are discussed in *Principles and Practice of Medical Computing* by L. G. Whitby and W. Lutz (1971), Edinburgh, and in *Data Handling in Epidemiology* (1970) edited by W. W. Holland, London. Record linkage is discussed from both the theoretical and practical point of view in *Medical Record Linkage* by E. D. Acheson (1967), London. Another useful work is I.E.A. (1973) Uses of epidemiology in planning health services. *Proc. Sixth Internat. Sc. Meeting, Belgrade.* The teaching of epidemiology is covered in *Epidemiology: A Guide to Teaching Methods,* edited by C. R. Lowe and J. Kostrzewski, 1973, London.

5

HEALTH ASPECTS OF COMMUNITY DEVELOPMENT AND HOUSING

C. L. SENN

Urbanization and Population Explosion

One of the most striking phenomena of our times is the rate at which people are moving from rural areas to large and capital cities. The influx of persons and families who have little funds, training and formal education has created major urban social, economic, and health problems. Many of those concerns were discussed at the World Health Assembly in Geneva, in 1967. The topic for these 'Technical Discussions', chosen by the Executive Board, was 'The Challenge to Public Health of Urbanization'. The author served as principal consultant.

Participants emphasized the essentiality of health administration co-operation and leadership in securing adequate attention to health factors in physical, social, and economic planning at the top administrative and political levels of national, regional,

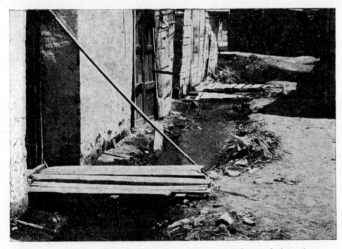

FIG. 6. Squatter housing borders open sewer in an Asian city.

and municipal government. Plans must include those of short range which aim at mitigating against the most serious, immediate consequences of the sudden change from life in rural areas and small communities to living conditions in crowded squatter settlements or overcrowded living units in the oldest and most densely developed areas of the inner city. Problems range from malnutrition to drug dependence, from increased rates of communicable disease to prostitution and venereal disease. High on the list of priorities is suitable shelter in a satisfactory environment. In fact, these are also important health factors for the total population.

Man's housing and the community in which he lives significantly affect many of life's necessities, such as: adequate quantities of nutritious, safe, and healthful food; a plentiful and safe water supply; unpolluted air; suitable and comfortable shelter; effective systems of waste disposal; convenient and efficient transportation and communication; education, cultural, social, and health facilities and opportunities; various personal and community services and conveniences; and employment in a healthful environment to enable man to properly support his family. The goals of physical, economic, and social community and regional planning are those prescribed in our definition of 'health'—'physical, mental, and social well-being'.

Participants in the World Health Assembly Discussions noted that cities, when properly planned and of the optimum size, can best provide those facilities, services, and environmental health conditions essential for modern, healthful living. However, when cities are not properly planned and regulated urbanization results in serious health and social problems. To achieve maximum health benefits, environmental health planning should be an integral part of community development. In many countries the rate of population increase of urban centres and capital cities is exceeding the ability of the people and their governments to plan and build required housing and facilities. In developing countries the in-migration from rural areas and villages, coupled with a high birth rate and reduced death rate, has resulted in huge 'squatter settlements' of makeshift habitations, ringing cities or crowding nearby hill-sides. Many such areas are without community water supplies, sewers, or refuse collection. Some are without roads, so access is only by paths up steep hill-sides. Housing is usually crowded on land, crowded with occupants, and built of cast-off or rudely erected native materials; floors are dirt, and toilet and drainage facilities do not exist or are grossly unsanitary, primitive units shared by many families. Coping with such existing health and sanitation problems and planning programmes to halt such unregulated community development is a problem which requires the concerted effort of many governmental agencies, and especially the leadership of the health and environmental control administrations.

In older cities of Europe and the United States the Industrial Revolution produced huge blocks of tenement and multiple-family buildings crowded together along narrow streets. Little open space was provided to admit light and ventilation or permit outdoor recreation and relaxation; living units lacked sufficient space, adequate windows, efficient heating, suitable plumbing, proper food storage and preparation equipment, and other facilities requisite for healthful housing. Burning of soft coal on fireplace grates and in stoves, furnaces, and steam generating boilers produced smoke, soot, and sulphur, which caused, together with smoke, fume, and odour-liberating industries, serious air-pollution problems.

More recently, the air-pollution problem has been aggravated by a phenomenal increase in automotive vehicles in many cities and by emissions by refineries and new chemical industries. The resulting smoke, sulphur, hydrocarbons, lead, fumes, photochemicals, dust, and soot are leading to statistically demonstratable higher bronchitis, emphysema, and similar respiratory diseases and excess death rates among the elderly in air-polluted sections of some cities. Heavy traffic on narrow streets and crowded express highways produces noise, congestion, and tension, and is producing new accident hazards. Many urban areas which were not designed for today's traffic and parking needs cannot be adequately corrected without major demolitions, replanning, and reconstruction [see also CHAPTER 14].

Large families from rural areas, many being minority groups, some from other countries, and most with low incomes and no experience in urban living, crowd into the oldest and most deteriorated neighbourhoods of urban centres. When large numbers of persons with inadequate education and training and neither decent housing nor permanent employment opportunities move into cities, serious social problems commonly result, including prostitution and venereal disease, dependence upon alcohol and drugs, malnutrition, increased tuberculosis rates, and sometimes increased crime and violence. Massive community and government action is necessary to solve such problems. An important goal is to enable the people to obtain a residential environment suitable for family living, relaxation, recreation, and wholesome social contacts.

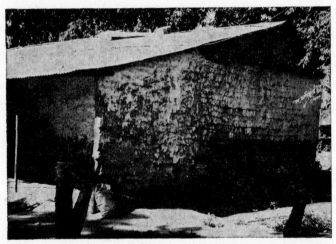

FIG. 7. Chagas' disease-transmitting triatomine bugs breed in this type of housing in Venezuela.

When regional planning and regulation is ineffective, developments which spring up beyond the central city's control and services are without proper public water supplies, sewerage, drainage, refuse collection, building and health regulations, transportation to jobs in the city, and other services and facilities. Solutions are dependent upon development of co-ordinated regional, economic, social, physical, and health planning, controls, and services. In such programmes the health and environmental control administrations should be full partners, represented by personnel qualified in environmental health planning and engineering, as well as in other health disciplines [see CHAPTERS 6, 7, 8 and 9].

The steps being taken to cope with the current urbanization phenomenon include:

Arresting migration to major cities by: improving economic, educational, and living conditions of farm workers and village residents; establishing new industries in existing small towns or in new towns.

Checking the growth of large cities by: moving industries, businesses, and government offices to cities of declining populations or to new settlements; building new housing in well-planned satellite communities; prohibition or restraints against expansion of existing industries in the largest cities.

Village and town improvement involves providing community water and sewerage systems, and solid-waste collection and disposal. Successful programmes also include improving health services, schools, and other community services. In some countries newly planned villages are built for families, and nearby land is provided for them to farm. They are taught new techniques and co-operatively use equipment which increases farm production and produces a suitable income. The objective is to enable agricultural workers to enjoy many of the city's benefits, and thereby reduce the urge to move to the city. An example of this type of programme exists in Venezuela, where the health administration develops and guides such villages, which are governed by committees composed of local residents. The families pay for their own piped water supply, and build their own schools, clinics, etc. They have easy access to markets, health and hospital services, secondary schools, and other services and facilities in large communities around which the planned villages are built.

The maximum size a major city should attain and whether there should be any artificial restraint on size is not universally accepted, and depends upon many factors. Planners of the U.S.S.R. are attempting to limit the population of Moscow to its present size by moving industry and people to new towns. London planners are seriously trying to curtail its population growth by building new towns and moving certain government operations and industries to regions and cities where growth has stopped or populations are declining. Brazil utilized a new concept in establishing a new inland national capital, Brasilia, to slow the trend of population concentration along the coast. Stockholm planners developed new, nearly self-sustaining satellites, connected to the central city by express highways and subways. These consist of groups of nearly self-sufficient neighbourhoods built around a central core of business, industry, and transportation. Most cities are developing concentrated programmes for urban renewal, are modernizing their mass transportation and express highway systems, and are concentrating on control of air, water, and land pollution, and noise abatement [see CHAPTER 8].

Health Administration Participation

Improvements in housing and communities are dependent upon many agencies and individuals. The first essential is a national policy which enunciates goals and objectives. This should be based upon data on existing conditions in order to form the basis for setting priorities. One source of data is the national census of housing. The methods available for implementing plans, goals, and priorities vary according to the political, economic, and social policies of each country. Ideally, at the top level of government, official procedures are established to bring together the total concept of physical, social, and economic planning, with active participation of health and environmental authorities.

Economic policies are directed towards determining what part of the country's, region's, or city's resources will be devoted to community development and housing. Social and economic planning considers the question of how much will be financed by the Government, and in other than socialistic economies, how much will be the responsibility of the private sector. There are major factors in developing plans for improved housing and community facilities for the low-income groups.

Physical planners suggest the form and design of communities and their facilities, utilities, and related services.

There is considerable variation in the opinion of experts concerning the 'ideal' size for cities and new towns. Most experts believe a population of over 20,000 is necessary to support desirable cultural, educational, medical, and community services. British new towns were planned for populations ranging from 20,000 to probably 100,000. The U.S.S.R. and Czechoslovakian planners favour upper limits of 300,000. Other urbanization experts now believe a planned population for new cities of 1,000,000 or more is not too high. A committee of governmental officials, including members of Congress, mayors and others from the United States, after studying European new-town developments, in a report entitled *The New City* (1969), recommended that the national government support the building of a hundred new towns of 100,000 persons and ten of one million each.

Relationships of the Residential Environment to Health

There is an abundance of evidence that the provision of an approved community water supply piped to the dwelling unit or its premises is an essential element for preventing enteric diseases and for maintenance of personal and household cleanliness. Similarly, lack of approved toilet facilities, private for each family, produces significant outbreaks of enteric disease and leads to problems of irregularity. Lack of acceptable excreta disposal facilities in urbanizing areas of developing countries results in widespread illness and death from Ascaris, hookworm, and other helminth infestations. Lack of sewers and resultant accumulations of highly polluted water in ditches and privy vaults is producing extensive outbreaks of urban filariasis in places like Rangoon, Burma, and Georgetown, Guiana. Studies in the United States and Africa have shown that diarrhoeal disease rates are relatively high where flies are numerous and have access to human waste and subsequently to human food. A 1971 publication of the Pan American Health Organization estimated there are 250 million cases of urban filariasis in the world.

Research to establish cause-and-effect relationships between housing and health among slum residents of cities which have a safe piped water system and community sewers has not produced conclusive data linking environmental conditions with an above-normal incidence of communicable disease. Certain specific environmental defects, however, are significant. In some cities a high incidence of rat-bites, rat-bite fever, and rodent-borne murine typhus are correlated with high rodent populations. Plague is a constant threat in some areas of the world, unless rats are effectively controlled. Huge numbers of cases of helminth infestations and enteric disease are occurring among children exposed to the grossly unsanitary conditions usually found in toilet rooms shared by more than one family.

For decades it has been known that small children develop severe and sometimes permanent mental impairment when they have access to and chew on peeling layers of lead paint. The problem is being given increased attention today. Hall (1972) estimated that as many as 50,000 cases of lead poisoning now exist in children in the United States.

Carbon monoxide produces death and physical impairment when fuel-burning heaters are not properly vented to the out-of-doors.

An analysis of the data tends to indicate that variables like nutrition, employment, age, and other factors, make it difficult to verify the assumption that housing is a major contributor to the higher-than-community-average disease rate among slum dwellers. In a position paper for the First Invitational Conference on Health Research in Housing and Its Environment (1970), Professor Ido de Groot and his colleagues presented data to indicate that inadequate space (crowding) within dwelling units is not a primary cause for transmission of respiratory disease. They argued that 'personal space' (the distance between individuals in normal household contacts) is far more significant than room space ('or the distance from room occupants to walls and ceilings').

Studies in Baltimore, in the United States, by Wilner and Walkley and their colleagues (1962) compared health and social conditions, and accident rates of families in the slum housing with those of families of similar economic and ethnic characteristics who had moved to new, acceptable, government-financed housing projects. The study showed that while some demonstrably higher rates on intestinal and respiratory illness were found among young slum dwellers, investigation of 'social well-being' produced the most significant data. Only 14 per cent. of the slum dwellers were 'satisfied with their living and storage space' compared with 85 per cent. of the housing-project occupants; 30 per cent. of slum dwellers 'invited friends to come to their living quarters', while this figure for good housing occupants was 75 per cent.; 18 per cent. of the slum dwellers considered the neighbourhood 'a good place to raise their children' compared with 59 per cent. of the occupants of housing projects who answered that question.

Martin (1967) reviewed the literature and summarized statistical analyses in Britain concerning the relationships between overcrowding of living quarters and other related environmental factors, to selected indices of health. He noted that advances in medicine, such as antibiotics and chemotherapy, and more readily available medical care for the poor, have drastically reduced the incidence and severity of many ill-health conditions formerly associated with 'slums' and 'overcrowding'. He noted that 'with the decline in infant mortality rates the importance of socio-economic factors, including domestic overcrowding, has diminished but not to the point of disappearance'.

In his summary, Martin noted that the effects of environmental defects on certain groups in a community 'may be more serious than they may appear from community health indices'. He further stated: 'The evidence shows the clear association of health with socio-economic conditions, overcrowding, and air pollution. When these are eliminated, the influence of other factors is slight.'

The Residential Environment and Injury Prevention

A WHO working document prepared by MacQueen (1964; see also Neutra and McFarland, 1970), quoted in WHO's Public Health Paper No. 25, analyses 1,223 home accidents per year per 100,000 population in Aberdeen, Scotland [see also CHAPTER 28]. Among the housing features which were found to be requisite to reducing home accidents were:

1. Good lighting of stairways, and readily accessible light switches at entrances to and exits from rooms and hallways.
2. Stairs with treads somewhat wider than the rise, and with surfaces in good repair, and handrails which provide suitable support, but not a temptation for children to slide.
3. Sufficient conveniently located electric outlets to minimize long and numerous cords.
4. Electric outlets and switches located so they cannot be reached from the bathtub, cabinets for medicines and potential poisons located beyond the reach of small children.
5. Heaters guarded and located to minimize burns and fires.

Neutra and McFarland (1970) stated that in the United States, 'in 1968, 20 million persons were injured in home accidents of whom 110,000 were permanently disabled and 28,500 were killed'. Their analysis of the major causes listed: 'falls, fires, pedestrian accidents, bicycle accidents, and poisonings'.

Wilner's and his colleagues' (1962) Baltimore studies showed that the rate of accidents was one-third higher in 'slum housing' areas than in an acceptable residential environment. Health and environmental administrations are gradually accepting a more significant role in programmes to reduce the toll from such accidents, which are producing more disability, damage to health and mortality than communicable diseases.

WHO's Public Health Paper No. 26 (1965) on 'Domestic Accidents' gives a more comprehensive account of the relationship between the residential environment and accidents.

Planners are giving special attention to designing new developments so that small children may walk from their living unit to their play areas without crossing a street or driveway. In planning new, and replanning old, neighbourhoods, heavy traffic is routed around, rather than through, residential neighbourhoods. Adequate street lighting and good design, construction, and maintenance of walks aid in reducing night accidents, as well as being a deterrent to crime and violence [see CHAPTER 7].

Mental Health Implications

Lemkau (1970) reviewed the literature and drew upon his long experience as a Professor of Mental Health to assess the currently accepted relationships between mental health and the residential environment. As in every element in the study of the effect of housing and health, he concluded that there is a relationship between good housing and good mental health. However, the magnitude or significance of this relationship is difficult to measure because of the many other related variables.

Lemkau further stated: 'Crowding makes irritations and interruptions inevitable, causing personal clashes which can grow into the deep seated repressed bitternesses that are conceded to be of importance in some mental diseases'. He is convinced that crowding and its associated effects are allied with mental well-being, and cites many illustrations which prove the point.

For instance, Martin (1967) notes that while rehousing of individuals and families may improve their physical environments, mental stress may result from being moved away from familiar surroundings and friends.

Social Factors

Controlled experiments with rats, such as those of Calhoun (1962), and observations of the behaviour of rats and other animals in nature, as discussed by Carstairs (1969), show that dramatic adverse sociological effects result from severe overcrowding. Calhoun's rats were allowed to multiply in what was arranged to be comparable to relatively dense residential

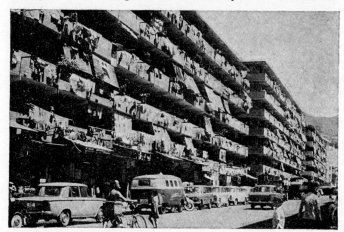

FIG. 8. Resettlement housing in Hong Kong.

environment. As they became more and more crowded together they developed strong tendencies to be socially disorganized, and lost their normal tendencies towards cooperative living. They even ignored normal responsibilities of raising their young. These series of experiments, coupled with other studies and observations, are commonly cited as probable indicators of the effects of crowding and congestion on man. On the other hand, Mitchell's (1970) five-year sociological study of high-density housing in Hong Kong, and elsewhere, included large numbers of interviews of conditions in which more than one family, and many children, shared a small, one-room living unit. A surprising result of that study was the conclusion that 'densities do not affect deeper and more basic levels of emotional strain and hostility'. He further said, 'Although high densities and other physical features of housing do not effect deeper levels of strain, the social features of housing have an important impact on these strains'. Among the most significant adverse conditions is the doubling-up of basic families in a single unit, especially those not related to each other. The strain of crowding in a small unit is eased if individuals can escape from the living unit, a factor which indicates that the surrounding environment may be important as a substitute for a more spacious indoor environment. This tendency to 'escape' was also cited by Mitchell as a factor in reducing parental control over children who must 'escape'. As in the Baltimore studies, it was noted that 'high-density housing also discourages interaction and friendship practices among neighbours and friends'.

Wilner and Baer (1970) note that, unlike other animals, man possesses the ability to alter his physical environment (adjustment) and to 'change his evaluation of the environment thereby "redefining" what constitutes beneficial surroundings (adaptation)'.

Adjustment, adaptation, and group activities are surprisingly strong factors in producing social satisfaction among residents of some of the most crude and substandard squatter settlements. These factors include a sense of pride in those who built and now own 'their own home'. This is an important factor, which is often completely lacking in governmentally operated housing 'projects'. In the squatter settlements there is usually an informal but surprisingly effective system of 'self-government' while in most governmentally operated housing there is a tendency towards a degree of regulation which the occupants consider to be an objectionable form of regimentation.

Parisot (1961), Lemkau (1970), Martin (1967), Chave (1967), and others, have noted and recognized that the provision of trained and competent social-worker type personnel can play an important role in producing a suitable social environment in housing project areas, new towns and complexes of huge high-rise apartment buildings. Bazell, in *Science* (1971), noted that public housing projects, urban renewal and enforcement of housing codes have failed to overcome the problems associated with living in the congested areas of the Harlem district of New York City. However, a programme which focuses upon working with the people to educate them and change their attitudes is a promising element of a comprehensive programme which is proving effective in improving what they call 'preventive maintenance'. An associate in environmental medicine of that project is quoted as saying, 'Large-scale preventive maintenance of tenement housing could do more for the health of East Harlem residents than the services of a thousand doctors'.

The United Nations Department of Economic and Social Affairs has issued many publications and reports on the economic and social implications of urbanization, community development and housing. For instance, the trend of population shift to urban areas and large cities is projected to 1980, when in the more developed regions of the world over 60 per cent. of the population will live in 'big cities' and only 10 per cent. in rural areas and small towns (United Nations Department of Economics and Social Affairs, 1968).

The United Nations' publication, *Improvement of Slums and Uncontrolled Settlements* (1971a) provides a rather comprehensive and somewhat quantitative analysis of the problem. It is stated that 'a thousand million people are living in substandard housing'. By the year 2,000 the urban population is likely to be twenty times what it was in 1920.

Another publication of that agency, *Social Aspects of Housing and Urban Development* (United Nations Department of Economic and Social Affairs, 1970a) discusses the dwelling as a means of strengthening family life. The publication states:

The critieria used in evaluating the elements are these— which is not to say they are either the best or the only criteria that should be applied:

(*a*) Does it enable the family to achieve or sustain feelings of personal, or human dignity?
(*b*) Does it permit the family to stay together, or does it force separations before the family wishes them?
(*c*) Does it permit the family to eat, sleep and perform all daily functions in accordance with the family's standards of decency and its requirements for privacy?
(*d*) Does it stimulate and assist in the expression of the family's rise in aspirations?
(*e*) Does the family feel the dwelling to be so much theirs (regardless of the method of tenure) that they adorn it, making it the outward visible symbol of an inner spiritual grace?

Broad Assessment of Health Effects

The difficulty of separately assessing the effects on health of each contributing factor has precluded the achievement of convincing, scientific proof of specific causal relationships of housing to health. This does not mean that such relationships do not exist. The difficult problem is to separate the stresses, and separately or additively evaluate their effects on various individuals. Too much of the past research in this area has been to assess effects on the health of young, normal, healthy students, members of the Armed Forces, and others who would normally be least affected. Other comparative analyses were concerned with communicable disease rates, without having the methodology to link cause and effect accurately.

Many of the current dramatic changes resulting from urbanization, industrialization, the population explosion, modern transportation and man's ability to drastically modify the environment, are creating new health problems. In developing regions these include major threats from communicable diseases, especially when developments spring up without adequate control and consideration of the health consequences of the new environment. Such problems include the traditional ones of enteric disease from contaminated water and food, the extremely high incidence of infestation with *Ascaris* and other parasites, and insect- and rodent-borne disease.

In addition, other major disease threats result when communities develop without adequate consideration of the potential health problems which are associated with certain environmental conditions. For instance, dependence upon vaccination, in place of control of the *Aëdes aegypti* mosquito, has been a causative factor in serious outbreaks of haemorrhagic fever in urban-type regions which are developed without public water supplies and where the mosquito develops in stored water. Another all-too-common disease of epidemic proprotions results from the installation of public water supplies in developments where adequate sewerage and drainage are not available. The resulting accumulations of polluted water are a favourite breeding site for the mosquito *Culex fatigans* which transmits urban filariasis. The result is infection of as many as 25 per cent. of the population and, as mentioned above, an estimated current global infection of 250 million persons with this dread disease.

Building of dams, and the resultant stored water, has provided an environment which is ecologically favourable for developing the snail which serves as the intermediate host for the cercaria which produces schistosomiasis. In addition, storage and distribution of irrigation water completely change the economy and living habits of the region, while reservoirs force relocation of persons who had lived on what becomes flooded land.

Within and surrounding large and capital cities, there is a constantly mounting real and potential impairment of the health of a large segment of the population by increasing levels of air pollution, noise and congestion. These effects are far more difficult to assess than diseases which established epidemiological procedures can trace to a single micro-organism or parasite. As mentioned above, not enough is known about the additive and synergistic effects of various stresses to scientifically and positively quantify cause-and-effect relationships. Participants in the Health Research Conference on Housing and Its Environment (1970) had reluctantly to conclude that not enough is now known to establish 'limits of human tolerance to crowding, congestion, and noise in the residential environment'. Participants concluded that we must find better ways to learn what levels of environmental and housing quality are most desired, and which of these can be provided with the available resources and technology. Economists at the conference cautioned that imposition of unrealistically high standards for housing and the residential environment may divert resources from other necessities and thereby unduly restrict the ability to acquire or provide other of life's necessities and amenities, some of which may be more important.

Assessment of health effects, then, includes but goes far beyond analysis of morbidity and mortality, traditional epidemiology and the direct identification of clinical symptoms with specific causes. Among the suggested guidelines are:

1. In planning and evaluating the residential environment, utilize as a guide the WHO definition of 'health'.
2. Expanded research to enable better separation and independent evaluation of the many factors which may, collectively, produce adverse health effects, including 'physical, mental and social well-being.
3. Development of a better methodology for assessing and evaluating the resident's likes and dislikes, satisfactions and irritations, and values as contrasted with unimportant elements.
4. Acceptance of the great variations in desires of individuals, depending on their age, family composition, economic status, likes and dislikes, whether employed or retired, etc.
5. Understanding of the necessity of fully taking into account the effects of climate and social customs when designing or improving housing and communities.

OBJECTIVES OF HOUSING AND COMMUNITY DEVELOPMENT PROGRAMMES

Guidelines, criteria, and principles or standards are usually desirable to assist in achieving the maximum in quality, including health effects. While professionals, other than health specialists, are usually more directly in charge of planning and designing communities and housing, environmental health expertise can contribute much if officially involved in the early stages of the planning and decision-making processes at all levels of government. This participation and action is essential in each phase of the programmes. These include:

1. Planning of new towns, regions, developments, and areas.
2. Developing programmes for urban renewal or other major improvements of existing residential areas.

3. Conducting routine and continuous housing and environment maintenance and operational programmes.

An excellent statement of the health objectives of programmes is contained in the WHO report of the Expert Committee on the *Public Health Aspects of Housing* (1961). That report summarizes the human wants and needs which the housing and community should satisfy.

More recently, a committee of the American Public Health Association, with participation by representatives of WHO, developed a new and somewhat comprehensive report *Basic Health Principles of Housing and Its Environment* (1971). This publication includes those elements of housing and neighbourhood design, occupancy and maintenance which a multidisciplinary committee of experts considered to be important to health. The following is the list of principles, criteria or goals which are explained and 'justified' in the publication.

Living Unit and Structure
HUMAN FACTORS

1. Shelter against the elements.
2. Maintenance of a thermal environment that will avoid undue heat loss but permit adequate heat dissipation from the human body.
3. Indoor air of acceptable quality.
4. Daylight, sunlight, and artificial illumination:

   (a) Admittance of sunlight.
   (b) Avoidance of daylight and sun obstruction.
   (c) Provisions for regulation and controlling daylight and sunlight.
   (d) Provision of suitable and adequate artificial illumination.

5. In family units, facilities for sanitary storage, refrigeration, preparation and service of nourishing and satisfactory foods and meals.
6. Adequate space, privacy and facilities for the individual and arrangement and separation for normal family life.
7. Opportunities and facilities for home recreation and social life.
8. Protection from noise from without, from other units and from certain other rooms, and control of reverberation.
9. Design, materials and equipment which facilitate performance of household tasks and functions without undue physical and mental fatigue.
10. Design, facilities, surroundings, and maintenance to produce a sense of mental well-being.
11. Control of the health aspects of materials.

SANITATION AND MAINTENANCE

1. Design, materials, and equipment to facilitate clean, orderly, and sanitary maintenance of the dwelling and personal hygiene of the occupants.
2. Water piping of approved, safe materials installed and supplied to fixtures within each living unit which avoids introducing contamination.
3. Adequate, private, sanitary, water-flushed toilet facilities within family units.
4. Plumbing and drainage system designed, installed and

maintained, so as to protect against leakage, stoppage, over-flow and escape of odours.

5. Facilities for sanitary disposal of food, waste, storage of refuse, and sanitary maintenance of premises to reduce the hazard of vermin and nuisances.

6. Design and arrangements for proper drainage of roofs, yards, and premises, and for conducting such drainage from the buildings and premises.

7. Design and maintenance to exclude and facilitate control of rodents and insects.

8. Facilities for the suitable storage of belongings.

9. Programme to assure maintenance of the structure, facilities, and premises in good repair and in a safe and sanitary condition.

SAFETY AND INJURY PREVENTION

1. Construction, design, and materials of a quality necessary to withstand all anticipated forces which affect structural stability.

2. Construction, installation, materials, arrangement, facilities, and maintenance to minimize danger of explosions and fires and their spread.

3. Design, arrangement, and maintenance to facilitate ready escape in case of fire or other emergency.

4. Protection against all electrical hazards including shocks and burns.

5. Design, installation, and maintenance of fuel-burning and heating equipment to minimize exposure to hazardous or undesirable products of combustion, prevent fires or explosions, and protect persons against related hazards.

6. Design, maintenance and arrangement of facilities, including lighting, to minimize hazards of falls, slipping, or tripping.

7. Facilities for safe and proper storage of drugs, insecticides, poisons, detergents, and deleterious substances.

8. Facilities and arrangements to promote security of the persons and belongings.

Residential Environment

COMMUNITY OR INDIVIDUAL FACILITIES

1. An approved community water supply, or where not possible, an approved individual water supply system.

2. An approved sanitary sewerage system or, where not possible, an approved individual sewage disposal system.

3. An approved community refuse collection and disposal system or, where not possible, arrangements for sanitary storage and disposal.

4. Avoidance of building on land subject to periodic flooding, and adequate provision of surface drainage to protect against flooding and to prevent mosquito breeding.

5. Provision of vehicular and pedestrian circulation to provide for freedom of movement and contact with community residents while adequately separating pedestrian from vehicular traffic.

6. Street and through-highway location, and traffic arrangements to minimize accidents, noise, and air pollution.

7. Provision of such other services and facilities as may be applicable to the particular area, including public transportation, schools, police and fire protection, electric power, health, community, and emergency services.

8. Community housekeeping and maintenance services, e.g. street cleaning, tree and parkway maintenance, weed and rubbish control, and other services requisite to a clean and aesthetically satisfactory environment.

QUALITY OF THE ENVIRONMENT

1. Development controls and incentives to protect and enhance the residential environment.

2. Arrangement, orientation, and spacing of buildings to provide for adequate light, ventilation, and admission of sunlight.

3. Provision of conveniently located space and facilities for off-street storage of vehicles.

4. Provision of useful, well-designed, properly located space for play, relaxation and community activities for daytime and evening use in all seasons.

5. Landscaping, plantings, trees, and green areas properly arranged and maintained.

6. In communities, improved streets, gutters, walks, cross-walks, and access ways.

7. Suitable lighting facilities for streets, walks, and public areas.

ENVIRONMENT CONTROL PROGRAMMES

1. Control sources of air and water pollution and local sources of ionizing radiation.

2. Control of rodent and insect propagation, pests, domestic animals, and livestock.

3. Inspection, education, and enforcement programmes so that premises and structures are maintained in such condition and appearance as not to exert a blighting influence on the neighbourhood.

4. Community noise control and abatement.

5. Building and development regulations.

Few countries or communities could achieve conformance with all of the listed elements of a healthful residential environment. The principles are, therefore, intended to be used to evaluate existing standards and practices; and only those principles which are deemed to be particularly significant and applicable, and which are economically attainable, would be included in the establishing priorities and standards. Also, it is recognized that many features which could be included in the design of a new development or in new housing would be difficult, if not impossible, to achieve without major re-building of existing developments and buildings.

Environmental Planning

The United Nations' publication, *Human Settlements* (1971*b*), states that environmental planning seeks to 'direct the forces that shape human settlements to bring the man-made elements of the environment into greater harmony with the natural elements, to improve the quality of human life and prevent its further deterioration and impairment'. The paper's list of objectives of planning begins with 'a healthy environment with adequate and safe housing, clean air and pure water, parks and open spaces, agreeable streets and minimal noise and other disturbing elements'. Among the other listed goals are opportunities for social and cultural activities in an identifiable community, provision for human needs, cultural enrichment and creative use of leisure time, and access to natural beauty and wilderness.

Team Approach to Planning

Before new communities are built a site-selection study should evaluate topography, soil, drainage, climate, prevailing winds, sources of water of suitable quality and sufficient quantity, locations for disposal of liquid and solid wastes, and all factors which may affect health. In this effort the environmental and sanitarian engineer play an important role. Potentially air-polluting industries and operations are to be located where prevailing winds normally convey pollutants away from the community. Housing is oriented to maximize benefits of sun exposure (where desired) and to maximize or minimize, as the case may be, effects of prevailing winds. Building, plumbing, heating, and ventilating, electrical and other codes, standards, and policies are reviewed by health specialists to assure that new and remodelled housing provides attainable features necessary for health. In drafting those codes care should be taken to not restrict or prevent use of new materials or new methods. These include use of plastic water pipe and drainage systems, prefabrication and other innovations. Housing codes and standards or requirements are adopted to provide authority for health and housing inspectors to require that units be properly maintained, are not overcrowded, and are periodically rehabilitated to meet modern standards. The latter is important, so that as standards for new housing improve, existing older housing is periodically rehabilitated to reasonably conform to these new standards.

Economic and social planning and administrative officials and agencies should participate in the physical planning process because satisfactory modern housing cannot usually be provided and maintained for the lowest income families without some form of governmental assistance. This is the basis for 'housing estates' in Britain, 'public housing' in the United States, and various forms of public housing or rent subsidies in many other countries. Under some housing estate plans, the amount paid for rent includes the fee for electricity, gas, and water. In the United States each unit in public housing is equipped with a refrigerator and a cooking range.

Financial assistance to low-income families is sometimes provided in the form of government grants and low-interest loans to improve and modernize their housing. In Britain the Public Health Inspectors play an important role in determining which buildings qualify for such assistance, and in certifying that improvements can reasonably bring the unit into compliance with their basic housing standards. Under one plan property owners pay one-half of the cost of improvement and the government the other half, within certain limits. Final government payments are not made to owners until the Public Health Inspector certifies compliance with established minimum requirements. In some Scandinavian countries the government closely regulates housing. Stockholm has acquired most vacant land in and surrounding the city, and housing is built by co-operative societies. The rents they charge are regulated so that they not only cover all normal costs but also provide funds for periodic rehabilitation, and to enable replacing the buildings after sixty years of use should such

replacement be necessary or desirable. The design is carefully regulated and reviewed by experts who issue instructions intended to assure maximum conformance with good health and social practices. Their codes also provide for sanitary regulation by the health department.

In socialistic economies much of the housing is the property of the state; rents represent but a fraction of the cost, and housing managers supervise maintenance and occupancy. The health ministry maintains overall sanitary control to assure that health standards are met in design, construction, operation, and maintenance.

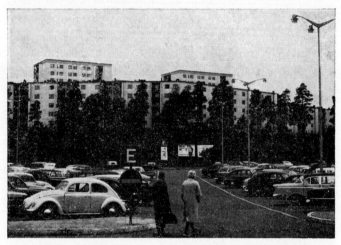

FIG. 9. Swedish new towns preserve natural landscape.

In some developing countries families are encouraged and helped in programmes of 'aided self help' housing. An example is Cuidad Kennedy in Bogota, Colombia, where thousands of families have utilized government facilities and technical help to make concrete blocks and beams and fabricate their own housing. Health factors are important elements of urban renewal conducted programmes to improve and rebuild substandard neighbourhoods. Studies by health administrations aid in setting priorities, and in deciding which areas should be rehabilitated and which should be cleared. In some countries, like the United States, federal funds are provided to assist cities in making comprehensive surveys and scientific evaluations of existing housing and environmental conditions of the whole community. Data from such studies are analysed to determine what corrective action is needed and to develop master plans which schedule various urban renewal projects and programmes. The type of corrective action required may range from minor repairs to major rehabilitation and slum clearance. Short- and long-range plans are scheduled, so noted substandard conditions are brought up to desired and attainable standards within a specified number of years. Success is dependent upon firm government policies and laws, financial assistance where needed, and a well-organized public education programme to secure co-operation of property owners, managers, and occupants. Among the factors considered in deciding whether to rehabilitate or clear and rebuild are historic, cultural, and touristic value of buildings and areas which should be preserved and the adverse psychological effect of uprooting people and families from familiar homes and neighbourhoods.

Housing Standards and Codes

The regulation and planning of housing and community development, whether by codes and laws or by government policy, usually involve several somewhat important steps. New developments and major urban renewal programmes are generally subject to conformance with a regional or community master plan. This establishes policy concerning such essentials as the physical relationship of residential areas to commercial and service centres, industries and places of employment, major transportation systems and elements (such as airports) and various community services such as schools, health care facilities, public service organizations like police and fire protection, cultural, recreational, and open space and various utilities.

At the micro-scale of development there are usually controls on such elements as density in terms of number of living units per unit area of land, building height, open space and various other 'development controls'. This phase of control considers the question of public water and sewerage systems, drainage, utilities, streets, walks, exterior lighting, spacing of buildings, parking for automotive vehicles and transportation.

Another element in the control programme is the standards for buildings and living units. In developing these, it is desirable to consider the above 'Basic Health Principles', and to include those which are most applicable and attainable. This is another element of planning in which there is need to officially provide for review of the basic plans and standards by authorities with expertise and competence in the health and social fields.

The acceptability of the residential environment is dependent upon maintenance, occupancy and use of existing housing and its environment. Some countries adopt 'minimum housing codes' which set basic requirements that are applicable to all existing housing. In addition, community environmental control programmes are directly related to quality of the residential environment. These include measures to control rodents and vectors, air pollution and noise control, and good solid waste management and 'community housekeeping'.

A significant development is the trend towards factory or industrialized housing construction. To produce the best housing at the lowest cost usually involves research and development at the national level. To enable use of new materials and innovative methods, the designers must not be restricted by detailed specifications which describe how to build, but rather, should simply meet essential performance characteristics which describe such elements as structural and fire safety, thermal and noise insulation, etc. In setting standards, a most difficult question to answer includes the minimum amount of space for various family compositions; the degree of separation of space into separate rooms for sleeping, living, etc.; minimum ceiling heights; window placement; required noise attenuation characteristics of walls, doors, ceiling–floor combinations and other elements which separate one room or living unit from the other, and exclusion of exterior noise from public corridors; minimum provisions for heating; design and equipment for avoiding excessively hot and humid indoor environment; the arrangement of living units and their environment to produce optimum conditions for social contacts, relaxation, and recreation.

Building and housing codes or practices represent a compromise between the desirable and the attainable. For this reason the specific requirements should be flexible and capable of adjustment not only to permit use of proven new methods and materials but to increase in quality as the country's economic and social standards rise. On the other hand, if codes are too far advanced for a country's or region's social and economic status they are not enforceable, and the result is worse than if a realistic standard was adopted. Some codes which have been adopted in the United States and elsewhere specifically provide that certain standards now applicable to new housing shall not apply to buildings erected before the new, higher standards were adopted. For instance, older buildings need not be provided with running hot water or private toilets and bath for each family. Some codes of Britain and elsewhere in Europe specifically apply only to buildings which are officially determined to be unfit for habitation. Other requirements apply only to housing for the working class or to multiple-family housing. Such codes should not be amended to require that all housing shall meet specified minimum requirements deemed necessary for health, comfort, and safety, regardless of when they were built. Naturally, some compromises and exceptions must be made for less-essential features when full compliance with these items would present unusual problems. For instance, modern building codes should require sound-proofing of walls and of the floor–ceiling separation between living units to reduce noise transmission by a specified amount, usually ranging from 40 to 52 decibels. It would usually be impractical to require that an existing building be constructed to fully meet such requirements. Similarly, reconstruction of existing buildings to reduce the indoor effects of outdoor noises may not be practical. For instance, studies in Britain indicate that the noise from certain busy streets can only be satisfactorily controlled by sound insulating windows which would be kept locked. This might necessitate complete air conditioning. Studies in the United States show that it is possible to suitably insulate living units from noise of departing jet aircraft by installing similar windows, sound deadening roofs and walls, and otherwise modifying building construction. The cost for sound-proofing an existing building, of several thousand dollars per living unit, would normally be prohibitive.

Current codes require housing design, insulation, construction, and heating facilities capable of maintaining the indoor temperatures above 21° C. in the coldest weather. For hot desert regions and warm, humid climates future codes may properly require insulation, design, and construction to minimize indoor heat and air-conditioning units which cool and dehumidify. Health administrations should review building, plumbing, heating and ventilating, electrical, housing, and related codes and standards to assure that health factors are covered as well as is practical within existing national, regional, or local economic and social conditions.

Since many present housing standards are not based upon scientific study, physiologists, psychiatrists, epidemiologists, sociologists, environmental specialists, and health scientists should conduct much more research to determine what specific features of housing and its environment are most desirable and necessary, and thereby assist governments in establishing scientifically proven levels and conditions for incorporation in codes and standards. In Great Britain housing standards are covered by Building Regulations (1972).

New Materials and Methods

New building materials and methods are constantly being tested to ensure that they will perform their intended functions, will endure exposure to anticipated adverse conditions and will not create conditions hazardous to health or safety. For example, among these newer materials is plastic pipe for water and drainage. This is light, relatively inexpensive, can be installed with a minimum of tools, and is especially desirable for use by individuals or groups who do their own work to build, improve, and maintain their housing. Other examples are plastic-covered electrical wiring conduit, various forms of plastic, asbestos-cement, epoxies, air-pressure blown cement, fibre glass, insulation, and factory-formed building components. Among the characteristics being evaluated are availability, cost, ease of installation and public acceptance. These factors are all relevant to the objective of providing the best-quality housing for the largest number of persons within the limitations of available finances and resources.

Goromosov, in a WHO Public Health Paper (1968), lists a considerable number of possible adverse effects for which new materials should be evaluated. These include toxicity and odour when testing new water pipe; tendency to produce static electricity when evaluating floor surfaces and covering; liberation of toxic fumes, gases, and smokes in case of fire; release of ionizing radiation from building components which contain radioactive materials, etc. High among the safety factors is the relative flammability of the materials. Another factor is the tendency of floor and stair surfaces to become slippery.

A number of national building research centres have comprehensive facilities for evaluating materials and construction methods. An example is the British Building Research Station where various 'factory-built' houses and modular units for housing are exposed to the weather (or a simulated adverse weather condition). Multistorey buildings constructed by assembling factory-built apartments are tested for structural strength; walls are subjected to acoustical tests to evaluate their noise attenuating qualities; various building components are evaluated for their insulating and thermal properties. In the United States, the Bureau of Standards is comprehensively evaluating a wide variety of new housing units built with innovative use of materials and methods.

Design of the Residential Environment

The amount and arrangement of open space, planning for traffic and circulation within the neighbourhood, and choice between detached single-family dwellings; dwellings with walls in common, referred to as terrace housing, row-housing and town houses; and multi-unit, multistorey apartment houses, are all factors which affect both the life style and the cost and amount of land utilized for housing. These are among the elements of urban planning. The WHO Expert Committee report on the 'Public Health Aspects of Metropolitan Planning and Development' (1965) outlined three goals of urban planning:

1. Improvement of existing conditions in the core area (urban renewal).

2. Orderly growth at the periphery.

3. The creation, if necessary, of satellite or independent new towns.

That Committee advocated comprehensive, integrated, overall regional economic, physical, and social planning; area-wide comprehensive planning of social services and systems especially significant to health, such as water supplies, sewerage and liquid-waste disposal, drainage, and solid-waste collection and disposal or utilization, air-pollution control, control of ionizing radiation, provision of well-designed housing and open space, including recreational facilities, health administration planning for public-health establishments, including hospitals, clinics, and facilities for care of children and the aged; drainage and sanitation to facilitate vector control; design, location, and control of industry and transportation systems to reduce air pollution, noise, and vibration in the residential environment. The Expert Committee advocated utilization of health expertise in all planning or programming related to health objectives.

Chave (1967) said that nine out of ten British families would prefer a single-family, detached home with its own yard. He said the terrace housing of new towns, which provides a small yard for each family, is a 'second choice'. In a number of countries, families living in apartment houses are assigned and may utilize an 'allotment garden' which is located within convenient walking distance. This enables the family to raise garden crops, maintain a small building in which they can sleep during the seasons when they are caring for their gardens, and satisfy a basic urge to be close to nature.

There is a growing tendency to minimize the amount of land area utilized for housing each family. This is especially important in countries where the most productive, limited agricultural land is being converted to residential use. Planners recognize that a policy of providing large plots of land for each family also increases the cost, necessitates more expenditure per family for streets, walks, water and sewer lines, electric and gas lines, street lighting and other necessities. Such developments also increase 'urban sprawl', increase the time required to get from home to work, and make it difficult to build and operate efficient public transport systems.

Routing of traffic around residential areas is an effective means of reducing hazards to the residents and minimizing the effect of traffic noise and air pollution.

More efficient use of land can be achieved by designs which provide for common use of land for play and open space in place of providing separate, private open spaces for each family. Such design patterns also significantly reduce costs of utilities and essential services.

At a housing seminar in Africa, held in 1962, participants from Kenya described a housing development of single-family homes with small, individual, wall-enclosed yards. At the juncture of the walls for each four yards, each family had an aqua-privy and sink or basin. The yard walls served as two of the walls for the toilet facility. A single, relatively small plastic drain line, and a single plastic water line served four families. A small public sewer line conveyed the sewage to an inexpensive and efficient stabilization pond. Participants in the seminar agreed that the project provided an excellent example of utilizing good planning to ensure provision of an essential water supply and sewerage system at a minimum cost.

A study by our students, in the United States, showed that similar savings are achieved by use of *cul-de-sac* streets. Traffic is so light that streets substitute for sidewalks. Small water and sewer lines suffice. In addition, that design pattern produced a desirable social environment because it promoted contact between children and adults and seemed to instill a sense of 'togetherness'.

This concept is becoming popular in designs which minimize the total area per dwelling unit, thereby enabling use of larger segments of open space by neighbourhood groups. In the United States these are called planned unit developments and include either groups of single-family or various types of multi-family housing arrangements. The land provided for use in common as recreation and open space is maintained by a 'Housing Association' co-operative, financed by nominal fees paid by residents of the development.

Density

Density is usually defined as the number of persons, or of dwelling units, per acre or hectare. Stevens (1964), who studied

regularly occurring consequences of severe overcrowding in man'.

The concept of considering an entire neighbourhood in a single, unified plan is practised by the U.S.S.R. health officials (WHO, 1964), who have adopted the 'microrayon' (neighbourhood) as their planning unit. Such neighbourhoods are 'divided from each other by green belts free of all buildings', and official policies require 'preservation of green, open spaces and the setting aside of green spaces between blocks of flats and in microrayons for recreation and children's games'. They further emphasize 'siting buildings in the area correctly, giving houses the best exposure to the sun and the most convenient orientation, insulating them from noise and other unfavourable effects of urban transport'. 'To establish favourable microclimate conditions in the microrayons and blocks of flats, there is a system of open planning and building; open spaces are planted with greenery, parks provided for recreation of the people, playgrounds for the children.' It should be noted that their design is largely for a pedestrian population. The bold assertions of their Ministry of Health—that designs for space,

TABLE 29
Gross Land Area Requirements

TYPE OF BUILDING	LAND FOR RESIDENTIAL USE		STREETS FOR RESIDENTIAL USE		COMMUNITY FACILITIES		STREETS FOR COMMUNITY FACILITIES		TOTAL AREA PER FAMILY
	Area	Per cent.	Area	Per cent.	Area	Per cent.	Area	Per cent.	
Single-family detached .	6,000	71	1,800	22	530	6	110	1	8,440
2-storey . . .	1,485	53	600	21	610	22	120	4	2,795
3-storey . . .	985	45	480	21	610	28	120	6	2,195
9-storey . . .	515	35	220	15	610	42	120	8	1,485
13-storey . . .	450	32	220	15	610	44	120	9	1,440

high-density housing developments in various countries, noted that the amount of space in the living unit affects the density. For twelve-storey apartment buildings, for instance, with 80 square feet per person, the maximum density was 1,000 persons per acre, while with 200 square feet per person, the density was 300 persons per acre.

Using a number of references, the author has compiled TABLE 29 showing the amount of gross land area required for five types of residential buildings.

With 8,440 square feet per family, one acre for five families would be required, compared with one acre for thirty families in thirteen-storey buildings. This estimate agrees with that of British authorities, who say that, even with thirteen-storey buildings, they do not recommend more than thirty-one families per acre. In their new towns with considerable open space, they have a density of fourteen families per acre in two-storey units.

The housing development of Wah Fu on Hong Kong Island, described by Mitchell (1970), has 7,788 flats on 24 acres, which is a density of 324 families, or 2,260 persons, per acre. As indicated in his paper, people can live and be reasonably 'happy' under such a density when they are adjusted to those conditions. On the other hand, Carstairs (1969), in 'Overcrowding and Human Aggression', says, '. . . it is possible to learn from studies of animals, both in their natural environment and under experimental conditions, and to note certain

green belts, freedom from noise and air pollution, solarization, daylight, and view are all based on considerations of health—is a factor that has not been as clearly and emphatically stated by health authorities of other countries.

Visits to Stockholm satellite communities and to other new Scandinavian developments reveal a great amount of concern for space and play areas. The Stockholm programme is effective, partly because the community owns the land surrounding the city and exercises strict control based upon health and sociological factors, as well as other considerations. Sociologists and health officials work in close collaboration with planners in reviewing development plans to establish criteria, and they suggest optimum attainable conditions as determined by their studies of human needs and wants.

Housing for Special Groups

The number of persons over 65 years of age is rapidly increasing as a result of advances in public health. Similarly, the public and governments have become aware of the need to provide suitable housing and social conditions for these people. Most countries no longer accept the concept that old, poor persons must live in a 'poorhouse' or 'home for the aged'. The modern aim is to prolong the time such persons may independently and comfortably occupy their own households. There are various expert opinions on what constitutes ideal housing and environmental conditions for the elderly. This difference of opinion is due, in part, to the fact that the choice of all persons is not alike. Some authorities recognize that some elderly like to be near young people, and advocate living units for the aged in buildings or areas occupied by young persons. Some have assumed that elderly persons prefer living units at ground level, and locate housing for elderly on the first floor, while families with children occupy other floors. However, British sociologists have found that many elderly persons enjoy living on the higher floors of buildings with elevators, away from noise from streets and children's play, and where they can enjoy a view of the neighbourhood. This arrangement allows mothers to be on the first floor, where they can readily supervise the outdoor play of their small children. In some countries, like the United States, France, and elsewhere, there are 'retirement communities' of individual cottages and single-storey, multiple-family units. These are provided with comprehensive conveniences, services, and opportunities for relaxation and recreation. While many elderly persons favour this form of life, and enjoy being away from children, others are depressed by observing the disappearance of their peers because of death or infirmity, and miss the laughter and gaiety of children and young people.

Because of their relatively low cost, efficient design, complete plumbing and heating facilities, ease of maintenance, and the good social atmosphere of 'mobile home parks', there is a marked increase in the number of aged persons moving into mobile homes, especially in the United States. Some are located in 'condominium' arrangements, whereby either conventional housing or mobile-home occupants purchase the land on which their units are located and pay their share towards the maintenance of community facilities, which include recreation buildings, hobby and home workshop areas, swimming-pools, park-like space, and sometimes golf courses. Each mobile home is equipped with a full kitchen and bath, and units provide from 500 to 1,100 or more sq. ft. ($\simeq$46 to 102 m².) of floor space. They are provided with built-in equipment, modern 'space age' insulation, and new 'factory finished' interior and exterior walls. They are surrounded by grass and flowers. Their design is efficient so that maintenance labour is reduced to a minimum.

With the trend towards industrialized or factory housing construction, there is evidence in the United States that design patterns established by the mobile-home industry will be followed in building units to be placed on conventional foundations, rather than on wheels. This type of housing has not been subject to compliance with traditional building and zoning codes, and therefore represents the type of housing built without the usual restraints of such codes.

Studies by Walkley (1966), our students and others indicate that there is a wide variety of attitudes and desires concerning housing and environments for the elderly. While some prefer living in special communities for the elderly, many others prefer to be in a neighbourhood where there are also young couples and children. Walkley found that some elderly people like to live near their children and grandchildren. Our studies indicate that many like to live in the central city where they can enjoy the 'activity' and social and cultural elements. Our studies show that some elderly people prefer traffic noise and the occasional screech of brakes to the quiet of a more secluded environment.

Our studies also indicate that the elderly place high value on proximity of services (including those for health, as well as stores and shops). If these centres are not near their living units, they appreciate efficient public transportation systems.

Among the most frequently expressed desires and preferences are:

1. Ability to keep comfortably warm and to avoid excessively high heat and relative humidity.
2. Ease of operation and maintenance, such as:
   (a) Electric outlets, switches and controls which can be reached without too much stooping and effort.
   (b) Hand-holds at toilets and baths.
   (c) Eye-level, rather than near floor-level ovens.
3. Noise levels which do not seriously interfere with sleep, and hearing radio and other means of communication.
4. Materials, design and arrangement which minimize labour for maintenance and performance of household tasks.
5. In certain latitudes, especially, sunlight and a pleasant view.
6. Facilities and arrangements which promote and permit social contacts and activities.

One reason why elderly persons leave their family homes is that they no longer need the extra rooms and space required when their children were with them. The extra space in the home and yard, no longer needed, necessitates work and expense which can be avoided by moving to a smaller unit. The type of smaller quarters they move to depends upon their income and financial resources. In several European countries governments provide special subsidies, assisting such persons to find suitable housing within their means. When no such subsidy is provided persons and couples on minimum pensions are likely to occupy units which are substandard in quality, size, and maintenance.

Attention is being given to the importance of providing special services for elderly persons who live in their own households. For instance, labour unions in Israel have built housing projects in which a one-room sleeping–living-room, plus a kitchen and bath are built for the elderly, on the ground floor. Upper floors are occupied by younger families. Maid service is provided, and nursing service is readily available to assure that such persons will receive needed attention. In Rotterdam the second floor of a large apartment house is occupied by old persons who need some help and care. Occupants are no longer able to do all their own housekeeping and cooking, so meals can be eaten in the community dining-room or are delivered to the individual's living unit. Maid service is provided; nursing and medical care are provided in an infirmary. Baths are given, or available, under supervision, in specially designed facilities to minimize the hazard of broken bones from otherwise common falls in the bathtub.

The goal should be to assist the elderly to maintain their own households as long as possible in the environment of their choice; then to make available care and facilities which prolong a maximum practical degree of independence. Finally, there is need for another type of facility for bed-ridden, elderly persons so they may receive the kind and amount of care necessitated by various types and degrees of infirmity and senility.

Programme Administration

Since public health is founded on the principle of 'prevention', the most productive efforts to improve health features of community development and housing are those directed towards planning, building, regulating, and controlling new developments so that they provide the best environmental conditions attainable within available resources, and in conformance with established social goals. This necessitates assignment by the health administration of competent specialists to represent health interests at national, regional, and local planning council and committee deliberations. Similarly, regardless of what agencies are responsible for developing and adopting standards and requirements for new housing, the health administration should actively participate in their development, and provide data, advice, and guidance on each item which relates to health.

A second necessity for a successful programme is environmental health control programmes which minimize air pollution and noise from both stationary and moving sources; systems for community refuse and other solid-waste storage, collection, and disposal; inspection and provision of community sanitation services which minimize rodents, flies, and other vermin; inspection, regulation, and testing to assure adequate control of food and milk; health regulation of places of employment; and community cleansing and maintenance to assure a wholesome and attractive residential environment.

A third step in community improvement is comprehensive programmes to rehabilitate or eliminate obsolescent and substandard or slum housing. This programme should begin with comprehensive surveys and studies. In some countries the first step is to review data from the national census of housing to determine the extent of the housing deficiency and the extent of overcrowding of units. In addition, special surveys are necessary to obtain specific data on the quality and quantity of housing and the environment. A study of such data coupled with economic and social studies form the basis for housing and environmental improvement and renewal programmes and policies. The methods used and items evaluated are described in the WHO Report of the Expert Committee on 'Appraisal of the Hygienic Quality of Housing and Its Environment' (1967). The Netherlands conducts comprehensive programmes to systematically survey and analyse such data for every dwelling unit, and maintains comprehensive files which can be instantly retrieved by electronic data-processing methods. In the United States federally sponsored and locally conducted 'Community Renewal Programmes' include social and economic studies as well as surveys of physical conditions, and the resulting report is a plan and schedule for urban renewal programmes. Under the Economic Commission for Europe, a vast amount of data are being accumulated to assist countries in developing such urban renewal survey and planning programmes. As computers and electronic data-processing become more generally available, more communities will use such facilities to maintain a continuous inventory of housing and its environment. In Rotterdam such systems enable instant retrieval of data concerning any building, block, or region of the city, both for planning urban renewal and for use in administration of their rent-control programme.

Urban renewal action programmes are the fourth step and the most significant in improving the environment of an older city. Surveys, coupled with public policy decisions by government leaders, determine whether a substandard area will be demolished or rehabilitated. A factor taken into account in deciding whether to rehabilitate or clear—in addition to economics—is the adverse mental health effects on residents who are uprooted from familiar surroundings when whole neighbourhoods are cleared. The choice between rehabilitation and clearance depends upon whether existing housing, environmental conditions, and the neighbourhood are capable of being transformed into acceptable standards by rehabilitation.

In some countries the health administration acts in an advisory capacity. In others health personnel play a major role; for instance, British Public Health Inspectors play a major role in urban renewal programmes. Under local Councils they utilize established criteria to determine whether existing living units are so grossly substandard as to necessitate clearance, or on the contrary, they qualify for rehabilitation. In the latter case a determination is made as to whether the buildings qualify for governmental financial aid. Their determination also indicates whole areas which should be demolished, and recommend, based upon established criteria, whether building owners shall be paid for the estimated remaining useful life of their property. Rehabilitation of some older units necessitates considerable ingenuity and rearrangement to provide window area for living-rooms and kitchens, to allocate space within the unit for bath and toilet facilities, to modernize kitchen and heating systems, and overcome original construction defects like damp walls or poorly insulated ceilings. Similarly, the environment may need modification, such as to provide open space to expose windows to the sky and admit breezes, to provide off-street parking and space for play or recreation. In some old and historic areas narrow streets are converted to pedestrian malls. Planners, architects, and housing experts of many cities and countries, like Copenhagen, Stockholm, and many other European cities, are making detailed surveys, studies, and plans for the rehabilitation of old, congested areas which their governments wish to rehabilitate and preserve. New and more efficient ways are needed to rehabilitate old buildings with a minimum of dislocation of the occupants.

A fifth step, and one usually taken only with some reluctance, is clearance and redevelopment of 'slum' areas. Much of this type of programme is underway in Moscow, London, cities in the United States, and elsewhere. The most serious social aspect of this type of programme is due to confiscation of homes and small businesses, and uprooting persons from familiar surroundings. This is usually hardest on the elderly. It is essential that residents of such areas be assured of suitable housing, employment, and assistance in social adjustment. Somes persons and families are moved to new housing in the same neighbourhood; some are given assistance in acquiring different houses and business locations; and some are moved to new towns. In the United States the urban renewal law requires that such families be rehoused in units which are 'decent, safe and sanitary, and at a rent they can afford to pay'. When owner-occupied units are cleared assistance is given to owners so that they may acquire another unit, if so desired.

A vital step in urban renewal programmes is officially established close working relationships between social, welfare, and health agencies, and economic specialists, housing project administrators, and all who have responsibilities for pro-grammes relating to housing and its environment, and related social, economic, and health conditions.

Another factor usually necessary to secure maximum benefits necessary from community improvement programmes is com-munity education and participation by community leaders to assist in developing public understanding and support. This is enhanced by organizing committees of citizens and civic, busi-ness, religious, and other groups who participate in goal setting and programme planning. Special educational programmes should explain objectives and seek support of students, families, and property owners and managers.

The legal profession plays an important role in developing laws, contracts, and various procedures to enforce standards and regulate the various housing programmes, co-operatives, and administrative agencies. Penalties for violating housing and environmental health regulations are often established in the housing and health codes. Regulatory procedures include per-mits and licences, rent-withholding authority, rent increases or supplements for qualifying units, and government contri-bution to cost of bringing up to established standards. In large communities housing-programme administration is improved by effective use of electronic data-processing systems. Data from the census of housing, special housing surveys, and all inspection and improvement or demolition programmes are then automatically recorded, analysed, and retrieved to plan programmes and to keep data up to date. The most advanced systems 'print-out' letters to property managers, analyse the results of inspection programmes, and schedule visits of inspectors.

Participation in Setting Goals and Standards

Each country should establish a national and regional pro-gramme and procedures whereby health and other administra-tions participate in physical, economic, and social planning and programme development. The role of such committees or com-missions depends upon the form of government and its political policies. For instance, in a socialistic economy community development and housing are financed and built by the govern-ment, and the overall economic committee has very broad responsibilities for deciding what portion of the gross national product will be allocated to community development, housing, and urban renewal. Under other systems the role and responsi-bilities of such committees depend upon the relative import-ance of the role of government, private enterprise, co-operatives, and other groups. In capitalistic systems private enterprise is primarily responsible, but is subject to controls and regulations. Some programmes are neither socialistic nor capitalistic, but as in the Scandinavian countries, such as Sweden, local govern-ment may own the land and co-operative associations build and operate housing under broad government supervision and con-trol. In other countries, like Britain, development is both by private enterprise and by government, and in some cases is accomplished by a combination of both.

Physical, economic, and social planners develop programmes within the framework of established governmental policies. Decisions may be based upon many factors, such as govern-ment policy to promote development of certain regions and enterprises; decisions to limit the growth of major cities; pro-grammes to develop new towns or satellite communities;

policies to limit the amount of good agricultural land which will be utilized to build housing; questions of whether the government will own and operate any or most housing, and if so, what part of the cost will be recovered as rent; whether to build communities with single-family homes or predominantly multiple housing with high population density per unit of land area. Within the framework of such policy decisions, regional plans are developed, including regional plans for transportation and communication, adequate and satisfactory water supplies, sewerage, sewage treatment, and waste-water re-use pro-grammes developed for whole drainage basins, collection and disposal or processing of solid wastes, location and regulation of industry to minimize the effects on community air pollution, noise and vibration, and minimize travel to and from the place of employment, zoning or master planning, which prescribes what areas are to be used for various residential, commercial, industrial use, or 'performance standards' for zoning pre-scribing limits of adverse effects on neighbouring property occupants; locations of airports, highways, parks, schools, and public buildings, and practically all physical features of the region.

Citizen Involvement and Education

A most dominant feature of modern housing concepts is the principle that the occupants and users should be more active and involved in the whole planning process. Health, sociologi-cal, and planning specialists are among the most important members of the teams which stimulate community involve-ment in planning new developments, urban renewal projects, and housing and environmental improvement programmes. Properly conducted, such studies aid in setting priorities and tend to ensure that adequate consideration is given to the features and elements most desired by the people who are most affected.

The United Nations' publication, *Social Aspects and Management of Housing Projects* (1970b), describes manage-ment policies concerning public housing programmes of a number of countries. Most of these countries recognize the importance of tenant education. Some advocate tenant partici-pation in decision-making and policy development. The Indian authority has recognized that tenants become 'enraged' by management rules and regulations. The policy in England and Wales was said to be to avoid issuing long lists of rules and prohibitions.

The report of a conference of housing project managers in the United States entitled *Housing Crisis—1969* strongly recommended creation of committees to represent tenants. The group noted that active tenant participation in policy matters tended to minimize the feeling of 'tenant regimentation'.

In a number of countries the trend is towards employment of 'home-makers' who advise tenants on a wide variety of social, economic and physical maintenance subjects. This type of programme recognizes that large-scale expenditures for new and rehabilitated housing do not produce maximum benefits unless adequate attention is paid to securing tenant adjustment to the environment and especially tenant acceptance of responsibility.

Public participation tends to promote community support and a pride in contributing to a better community. This spirit is usually enhanced by encouraging the people to become physically involved in housing and community improvement. An example is the Venezuela rural housing programme, in which the people are encouraged to improve and beautify their premises. Community groups also construct and operate modest health clinics and community halls, and build or improve the school facilities. They operate and finance their water and community housekeeping services.

Migration to large cities is continuing, with resultant growth in squatter settlements. Governments are realizing that this movement cannot be forcefully stopped.

In some countries and cities, like Costa Rica and Bangkok, governments are participating in planning the squatter settlements so that they can eventually be provided with streets, water mains, sewers, electric and other services. Residents are aided in providing rudimentary sanitation and are encouraged to improve their housing as funds become available. This appears superior to the usual situation whereby groups of squatters build their crude housing without regard to basic community planning.

THE FUTURE OF CITIES

The 'Outline Document' (1967) which the author prepared for the World Health Assembly Technical Discussions on 'The Challenge to Public Health of Urbanization' was based upon reports by national health ministries and WHO study teams. One African Minister of Health said his capital city grew from 125,000 to 200,000 between 1960 and 1966. Only 6 per cent. of the dwelling units have indoor piped water; there are no public sewers; most people use crude privies, and many do not even have room for a privy. In Calcutta, 79 per cent. of the population live in a single room or less; in some districts 30 to 50 persons share a single latrine. The city's growth rate projects to a population of 30 million by the year 2000. The problems are compounded by an inadequate and pollution-threatened public water supply, a grossly inadequate transportation system and generally deteriorating conditions.

Participants in those World Health Assembly Discussions emphasized the importance of health administration involvement, and utilization of health and environmental expertise, to guide, control and regulate urban growth. Many expressed the conviction that limits of growth should be set to control the size of major cities. However, in spite of all the existing problems in community development, residential environment planning, and housing, the participants concluded that the outlook was 'on the whole optimistic. It was thought that cities, properly guided and controlled, can provide a healthy and happy environment.'

REFERENCES AND FURTHER READING

Abrams, C. (1965) *The City is the Frontier*, New York.

American Public Health Association (1960) *Planning the Neighbourhood*, New York.

American Public Health Association (1963) *Housing an Aging Population*, New York.

American Public Health Association (1967) *Housing Maintenance and Occupancy Ordinance*, New York.

American Public Health Association (1971) *Basic Health Principles of Housing and its Environment*, New York.

Ashworth, H. (1957) *Housing in Great Britain*, London. (A useful reference book of facts and figures.)

Bancroft, G. (1972) Housing the elderly, *Lancet*, **i**, 683.

Banks, R. (1972) Designing housing for the elderly, *R. Soc. Hlth J.*, **92**, 151.

Bayley, E. and Dockery, A. (1972) Traffic pollution of the urban environment, *R. Soc. Hlth J.*, **92**, 6.

Bazell, R. (1971) Urban health and environment: a new approach, *Science*, **174**, No. 4013.

Beyers, G. H. (1965) *Housing and Society*, London. (An analysis of housing statistics and trends.)

Building Research Station, Garston, Herts. (1960) *Densities in Housing Areas*, London, H.M.S.O.

Building Research Station, Garston, Herts. (1964) *A Survey of Housing for Old People*, London, H.M.S.O.

Building Research Station, Garston, Herts. (1964) *A Review of British Research Relevant to Urban Planning*, London, H.M.S.O.

Calhoun, J. B. (1962) Population density and social pathology, *Scient. Amer.*, **206**, 139.

Carstairs, G. M. (1969) Overcrowding and human aggression, in *Violence in America*, New York.

Centre for Urban Studies (1964) *Public Health and Urban Growth*, Report No. 4, London.

Chave, S. P. W. (1967) Social and mental health aspects of urbanization, in *Challenge to Public Health Aspects of Urbanization*, Proceedings of a Seminar of Medical Officers of Health, February/March 1967, London.

Dewhurst, A. (1973) Housing and area improvements (U.K.), *R. Soc. Hlth J.*, **93**, 69.

Dutt, A. K. (1970) A comparative study of regional planning in Britain and the Netherlands, *Ohio J. Sci.*, **70**, 321.

Hall, J. A. (1972) A critical look at housing (U.K.), *R. Soc. Hlth J.*, **92**, 255.

Hall, S. (1972) Lead pollution and poisoning, *Environm. Sci. Techn.*, **6**, No. 1.

Hazemann, R. H. (1973) Social aspects of housing, *R. Soc. Hlth J.*, **93**, 13.

Jacob, M. (1972) Slum clearance and housing improvement (U.K.), *R. Soc. Hlth J.*, **92**, 258.

Jensen, R. (1966) *High Density Living*, London.

Laurer, G. R. (1973) The distribution of lead paint in New York City tenement buildings, *Amer. J. publ. Hlth.* **63**, 163.

Lemkau, P. V. (1970) Mental health and housing, in *Proceedings of the First Invitational Conference on Health Research in Housing and its Environment*, United States Department of Health, Education and Welfare, Rockville, Md.

Mackintosh, J. M. (1965) *Topics in Public Health*, Edinburgh.

Martin, A. E. (1967) Environment, housing and health, *Urban Studies*, **4**, No. 1.

Martin, H. L. (1970) The contribution of housing conditions to burns and scalds in children, *Med. Offr*, **124**, 281.

Mitchell, R. E. (1970) Personal and social consequences arising from high-density housing in Hong Kong and other major cities in Southeast Asia, in *Proceedings of the First Invitational Conference on Health Research in Housing and its Environment*, United States Department of Health, Education and Welfare, Rockville, Md.

Mitchell, R. E. (1971) Some social implications of high-density housing, *Amer. sociol. Rev.*, **36**, 18.

Mollers, S. L. (1960) *Housing in Northern Countries*, Copenhagen.

National Swedish Institute for Building Research (1967) *Quality of Dwellings and Housing Areas*, Report No. 27. (Published in agreement with the United Nations.)

Neutra, R., and McFarland, A. R. (1970) Accidents and the residential environment, in *Proceedings of the First Invitational Conference on Health Research in Housing and its Environment*, United States Department of Health, Education and Welfare, Rockville, Md.

Neutra, R. (1972) Accident epidemiology and the design of the residential environment, *Hum. Factors*, **13**, 405.

The New City (1969), New York.

Osborn, F. J., and Whittick, A. (1963) *New Towns: The Answer to Megalopolis*, Cambridge, Mass.

Pan American Health Organization (1967) *Environmental Health in Urban Planning*, Washington, D.C.

Pan American Health Organization (1971) Managing water resources, *PAHO Gaz.*, **3**, No. 3.

Parisot, J. (1961) Working paper for WHO Expert Committee on Public Health Aspects of Housing, Geneva.

Power, J. G. P. (1960) Health aspects of vertical living in Hong Kong, *Commun. Hlth*, **1**, 316.

Stanbury, C. A. (1960) *Housing: Looking to the Future*, London.

Stevens, P. M. H. (1964) *Densities in Housing Areas*, Department of Scientific and Industrial Research, Building Research Station, London, H.M.S.O.

United Nations Department of Economic and Social Affairs, New York.
  (1962) *Report of an* ad hoc *Group of Experts on Housing and Urban Development*.
  (1968) *Urbanization: Development of Policies and Planning*.
  (1969) *Basics of Housing Management*.
  (1970a) *Social Aspects of Housing and Urban Development*.
  (1970b) *Social Aspects and Management of Housing Projects: Selected Case Studies*.
  (1970c) *Social Programming of Housing in Urban Areas*.
  (1971a) *Improvement of Slums and Uncontrolled Settlements*.
  (1971b) *Human Settlements*.
  (1971c) *Symposium on the Impact of Urbanization on Man's Environment*.

United Nations Economic Commission for Africa (1965) *Housing in Africa*, New York.

United States Public Health Service (1967) *Report of the Environmental Health Planning Committee*, Washington, D.C.

Walkley, R. P. (1966) *Retirement Housing in California*, Berkeley, Calif.

Werskow, H. J. (1971) Pathogenesis of urban slums, *J. Amer. med. Ass.*, **215**, 1959.

Whittle, J. (1971) Housing at Thamesmead, *Roy. Soc. Hlth J.*, **91**, 28.

Wilner, D. M., and Baer, W. C. (1970) Sociocultural factors in residential space, in *Proceedings of the First Invitational Conference on Health Research in Housing and its Environment*, United States Department of Health, Education and Welfare, Rockville, Md.

Wilner, D. M., and Walkley, R. P. *et al.* (1962) *The Housing Environment and Family Life*, American Public Health Association, Baltimore, Md.

World Health Organization (1964) Housing programmes: The role of the public health agencies, *Wld Hlth Org. Publ. Hlth Pap.*, No. 25.

World Health Organization (1965) Domestic accidents, *Wld Hlth Org. Publ. Hlth Pap.*, No. 26.

World Health Organization (1967) Suggested outline for use by countries in discussing the challenge to public health of urbanization, in *A 201 Technical Discussions*, Geneva.

World Health Organization (1968) Physiological basis of health standards for dwellings, ed. Goromosov, M. S., *Wld Hlth Org. Publ. Hlth Pap.*, No. 33.

World Health Organization Expert Committee Report (1961). Public health aspects of housing, *Wld Hlth Org. techn. Rep. Ser.*, No. 225.

World Health Organization Expert Committee Reports (1965) Public health aspects of metropolitan planning and development, *Wld Hlth Org. techn. Rep. Ser.*, No. 297.

World Health Organization Expert Committee Reports (1967) Appraisal of the hygienic quality of housing and its environment, *Wld Hlth Org. techn. Rep. Ser.*, No. 353.

World Health Organization (1972) Report of a WHO Scientific Group: Development of environment criteria for urban planning, *Wld Hlth Org. techn. Rep. Ser.*, No. 511.

World Health Organization (1974a) uses of epidemiology in housing programmes and in planning human settlements. Report of a WHO Expert Committee on Housing and Health, *Wld Hlth Org. techn. Rep. Ser.*, No. 544.

World Health Organization (1974b) Health Aspects of urban development. Report of a seminar convened by WHO Regional Office for Europe, *Wld Hlth Org. Chron.*, **28**, 249.

World Health Organization Regional Office for Europe (1974) Report of a seminar on Health Aspects of Urban Development, Stuttgart 1973 (Euro 4108), Copenhagen.

For a list of references on *Tropical Housing* see References at end of CHAPTER 6.

6

THE EFFECT OF HEAT AND VENTILATION ON HEALTH

E. van GUNST and H. Ph. L. den OUDEN

INTRODUCTION

A general physiological requirement which determines man's capacity for a 'free and independent life' as defined by Claude Bernard (1878) is the maintenance of a remarkable degree of stability, or constancy, in respect of certain physical and chemical factors, e.g. temperature, oxygen, sodium chloride, etc., in the internal environment—namely in the blood and tissue fluids which surround the actively functioning cells of the body, as distinct from the air and solid surroundings which constitute the external environment of the individual. When discussing this conception Haldane (1929) pointed out that the exposed parts of the body are more affected by, and adapted to, variations in the external environment than tissues and organs more deeply situated. Moreover, bearing in mind that different physiological functions demand different conditions for efficiency, he concluded that: 'The medium in every separate part of the body must be normal for that part; and the great outstanding fact is that this normality is maintained, the normality constituting what we call health.'

In health, we daily experience phases of activity, fatigue, viz. decreased capacity for activity, and recovery, the over-all physiological requirement being that the recovery phase, which includes recreation as well as rest and sleep, shall completely abolish the state of disturbed normality of general or local fatigue caused by our purposeful activities and the environment to which we were exposed. Many factors collectively determine whether the individual can achieve such a desirable balance, and failure to do so inevitably leads to cumulative fatigue, as shown by decreasing capacity for daily work, aggravated sensations of personal discomfort or stress, and, sooner or later, actual impairment of health.

When attempting to deal with problems of this nature it is not only necessary to detect the particular factors concerned but also to ascertain whether the adjustment and control of other factors would help towards a satisfactory solution. Thus, for example, while excessive environmental warmth may appear to be a primary cause, the adoption of suitable clothing at work may alleviate or prevent thermal discomfort and stress. In field investigations it is helpful to have in mind a list or schedule of factors which can affect comfort, health, and working capacity, because they influence physiological balance from day to day. Such a list is given in TABLE 30, which shows the various factors grouped under the general headings of Activity, Environment, Time, and Personal.

In the scientific sense it may be stated that throughout life the human body is the servant of energy, because all forms of activity, whether conscious or subconscious, involve the use of energy rendered available for vital processes by those chemical reactions in the tissues which are covered by the term metabolism. Again, energy in many forms and intensities is present

TABLE 30

Factors Affecting Comfort, Health, Working Capacity, and Balance in Daily Cycle of Activity–Fatigue–Recovery

GROUP I ACTIVITY	1. MENTAL WORK: nature, concentration, use of special senses: posture.
	2. MUSCULAR WORK: energy expenditure, static and dynamic components of muscular effort in light, moderately heavy, and heavy work; posture and postural change.
	3. RECREATION: mental and physical.
GROUP II ENVIRONMENT	1. PHYSICAL: air temperature and temperature gradient, humidity, air movement, air change, mean radiant temperature of surroundings; heat transference by emission, reflection and absorption of radiant heat, convection, conduction, evaporation, and condensation; heating, ventilating, and air-conditioning systems; increased and decreased atmospheric pressure; gravity variations; wind force; contact pressure with solid objects; vibration; restriction of movement by clothing; seating and machine design; daylight and artificial lighting, intensity and distribution, glare, flicker, colour of surroundings, moving machinery, field of vision; noise and ultrasonic vibrations; electrical hazards; shortwave radiation, radioactive materials; protective clothing.
	2. CHEMICAL: air purity, ionization, and percentage composition; atmospheric pollution by gases, dust, smoke, fumes, and vapours; wet processes; contact with solvents, oils, and materials used in occupations.
GROUP III TIME	Continuous or intermittent work, rate and rhythm of work; duration of work per spell, day, and week; timing and length of rest pauses; rate of change of environment and duration of exposure to environmental factors.
GROUP IV PERSONAL	Individual make-up; age, sex, physique; state of fitness; diet balance and energy intake; personal hygiene, clothing, habits; education; aptitude and training for occupation; acclimatization to environmental factors; economic circumstances, responsibilities; family and home environment; sleep.

in the external environment, and each exerts some effect on the body. Fortunately, as in the case of heat, light, or sound, each type of energy gives rise to sensations or evokes physiological reactions which may lead us, if we will, to control it to advantage or to devise and adopt appropriate measures to protect the body as a whole or the organs of special sense against discomfort or actual harm.

While heat, light, and sound may readily be studied and measured by scientific methods, the assessment of the physical characteristics of an environment which collectively influence personal warmth, or daylight, or artificial lighting in relation to vision, or sounds which we call noise are much more complicated problems owing to the capacity which the human body possesses for adaptation to environmental conditions, individual variation, and such personal factors as age, sex, occupation, clothing, or habits, local customs and superstitions.

Problems of discomfort, fatigue, or stress due sometimes to the combined effects of environmental heat, light, and sound arise in many situations in the crowded industrialized communities of towns and cities, but they may indeed arise in houses, hospitals, schools, offices, or industries wherever their location if we fail to detect and control or eliminate the cause.

In the last analysis, survival in the face of severe environmental conditions depends on our subconscious and conscious reactions to the type and intensity of the stimuli associated with them. We need to remind ourselves that our sensitiveness to conditions causing discomfort or stress or even pain is a desirable and indeed an essential attribute, because such sensations warn us that general or local normality of health is threatened and that action is needed to control the environmental factors concerned.

A first step towards the practical solution of such field problems is to examine them from the physiological point of view and attempt to understand how and why the human body reacts to these physical factors. Then it is essential to give measurable and, as far as present-day knowledge permits, precise meanings to such terms as 'suitable', 'sufficient', 'desirable', or 'optimum' in respect of environmental heat, light, or sound in relation to physiological requirements and limitations. This being the case, it is necessary, in the present context, to define human requirements in terms which the architect and the heating, ventilating, illuminating, or acoustic engineer can interpret in terms of design, construction, fittings, and appliances which will enable the factors concerned to be controlled and the required conditions to be produced and maintained. Having regard to variations between individuals in a community, it is desirable to define a range rather than a single measure or standard for any environmental factor, so that within the range specified the requirements for the maintenance of health, comfort, and working capacity of the vast majority of persons will be satisfied when one has to stay a long time in the environment.

BODY TEMPERATURE REGULATION

If we are *thermally comfortable* we are quite unaware that heat is continuously being transferred from our bodies to the environment. Such continuous transfer or loss of heat from the body is necessary for the maintenance of stability in respect of temperature in the internal environment which is an essential physiological requirement. Even when *sitting at rest* the body heat production of an average adult amounts to approximately 100 kilocalories[1] per hour.

This heat is liberated by the metabolic processes which furnish the energy required for the rhythmic action of the heart and the muscles of respiration and other internal activities. Taking the weight of an average man as 70 kilograms and the

specific heat of the body as 0·83 gram-calorie, it may readily be calculated that his temperature would rise by at least 1·7° C. in one hour if this quantity of heat (100 kcal.) were retained in his body. Not only so, but because a rise in temperature of as little as 0·56° C. increases metabolic heat production by approximately 7 per cent., his temperature would mount with increasing rapidity.

The subconscious or conscious physiological reaction and the instinctive actions of the individual in response to stimulation by environmental heat or cold are all calculated to maintain or restore local or general temperature normality. It is therefore relevant to consider the physiological mechanisms and physical processes involved in the regulation of body temperature and the factors which facilitate or hinder the remarkably efficient thermostatic control of its internal environment shown by the human body in health.

Perhaps the most widely recognized characteristic of health is what is termed a 'normal' oral temperature of 36·9° C., with a daily range of 0·53° C. between late afternoon and early morning. The power which the living body possesses of maintaining its internal temperature practically constant at 37·5° C., irrespective of wide variations in the temperature of the external environment, is an attribute of fundamental importance. At about this temperature the dissociation of oxygen from haemoglobin and the chemical reactions of metabolism liberate energy at optimum rates as required for conscious and subconscious bodily activities.

Through the temperature sense organs associated with the so-called 'hot and cold' spots on the skin we subconsciously react to and become consciously aware of conditions which we describe as hot or cold. It has been shown that if the temperature of the skin is approximately 29° C. as small a change in its temperature as 0·2° C. may be detected.

It would be outside the scope of this section to deal with the nervous control of body temperature in detail. We should, however, remind ourselves that experimental research and clinical observation have shown that the higher levels of the central nervous system, particularly certain parts of the hypothalamus, are involved in the operation and co-ordination of the mechanisms concerned with body temperature control and regulation. Thus, there is evidence that warmth applied to the anterior part of the hypothalamus is followed by dilatation of the cutaneous blood vessels and sweating, both of which reactions are calculated to increase heat loss to the environment. On the other hand, the posterior part of the hypothalamus is concerned with the response to cold, namely, vasoconstriction and shivering, the first reducing heat loss to the environment and the second increasing internal heat production, both mechanisms in fact making some contribution to the maintenance of thermal balance. Having regard to the complexity of its structure, the variety of its tissues, and the diversity of function of its components, it is truly astonishing that the human body can exercise such an efficient thermostatic control of its heat content that, even when measured in the mouth, the daily variation in temperature is as small as 0·56° C.

The temperature of an inanimate object changes with that of its environment, but the internal temperature of the human body is kept practically constant in health by the maintenance of a balance between metabolic heat production and heat loss to the environment. While the exposure of the living body to

---

[1] One kilocalorie (kcal.) is the amount of heat required to raise the temperature of 1 kilogram of water 1° C.

variations in environmental heat or cold may evoke physiological reactions, e.g. changes in muscle tone, adrenaline secretion, or shivering, which affect the rate of body heat production, the regulation of body temperature mainly depends on the efficiency of the 'vital mechanisms', to use the words of Claude Bernard, which enable the rate of heat loss to the environment to be adjusted to balance metabolic heat production.

Bearing in mind that actual measurement in the laboratory and in industry has shown that body heat production may range from 1·6 kcal. per minute when sitting at rest to eight or more times this rate according to the severity of the muscular work performed, it is evident that in health the human body can adjust and control its rate of heat loss over a wide range of heat production.

Exposure to environmental heat or cold evokes physiological reactions which are calculated to increase or reduce the rate of heat loss to the environment. Thus the first response to heat is a reduced tone in the peripheral blood vessels which leads to an increase in the flow of warm blood to the skin and an increase in the thermal conductivity of the underlying tissues. Both of these reactions are calculated to promote heat loss by radiation and convection. They constitute what may be termed the fine-adjustment mechanism for body-temperature regulation, but if needed, the coarse-adjustment mechanism—the secretion of sweat—is evoked and the very powerful cooling effect of the evaporation of water is made use of. In this connexion it is of interest to note that when 1 gram of water evaporates, approximately 585 gram-calories of heat are absorbed.

On exposure to environmental cold, the first response is an increase in the tone of the peripheral blood vessels and a reduction in blood flow to the skin and in the thermal conductivity of the tissues. These fine-adjustment reactions are calculated to reduce heat loss by radiation and convection because they reduce the rate of heat transfer to the skin from the deeper parts of the body. If, however, they fail to control heat loss, then the coarse-adjustment mechanism—shivering—may be called into play in an attempt to increase body heat production to balance the increased rate of heat loss caused by the coldness of the environment.

In general terms it may be said that if, when sitting at rest, we are conscious of sweating or shivering, then the mechanisms concerned with body-temperature regulation are under stress, and the acute thermal discomfort experienced usually stimulates us to take steps to control the environment or escape from it.

It follows from such considerations that, having regard to the habitability of buildings, it is necessary to define environmental conditions which satisfy requirements for health and thermal comfort, and to specify in practicably measurable terms standards for those physical characteristics of indoor climate which should be controllable by building design and construction coupled with provisions for heating, ventilation, or air conditioning as necessitated by climate, and the activities and number of occupants of the building.

HEAT TRANSFER TO THE ENVIRONMENT

The controlling factors which determine the rates of heat transfer between the body and the environment by these physical processes are as follows:

1. By CONVECTION: the *Dry Bulb Temperature* of the air and the *Rate* of air movement.
2. By RADIATION: the *Radiant Temperature* of the solid surroundings.
3. By EVAPORATION: the *Humidity and Temperature* of the air and the *Rate* of air movement.

SYMBOLS:

C: heat exchange between the human body and the surrounding air, in kcal./hour.

R: heat exchange between the human body and neighbouring objects and walls, in kcal./hour.

E: heat emission of the human body by evaporation of perspiration, in kcal./hour.

M: metabolism, heat quantity generated within the human body, in kcal./hour.

α_c: surface coefficient for convection in kcal./m.² ° C. hour.

t_h: surface temperature of the human body, ° C.

T_h: surface temperature of the human body, ° K. (273 + t_h ° C.).

t_a: temperature of the surrounding air, ° C.

v: velocity of surrounding air in cm./sec.

A_h: surface area of the human body m.².

—As an average for males 1·8 m.².
 for females 1·65 m.².

—Radiation upright 75 per cent.
 sitting 50 per cent.

—Convection upright 100 per cent.
 sitting 75 per cent.

f_{hs}: configuration factor, 0–1. A value of 1 is obtained for the human body with its entire environment.

ε: emission coefficient.

σ: Stefan–Boltzmann coefficient $4\cdot96 \times 10^{-8}$ kcal./m.² hour ° K⁴.

T_s: mean radiant temperature, ° K.

p_h: vapour pressure for saturated air at the temperature of the human skin (35° C.) in mm. Hg.

p_a: vapour pressure of the air at the actual temperature in mm. Hg.

1. By means of CONVECTION, heat at the surface of the human body is transferred to the surrounding air, since customarily this surface has a temperature higher than the air. Under normal conditions the skin temperature will range between 33° and 29° C.

The total quantity of heat transferred in this manner by a human being will be proportional to the area of his body, A_h, as well as to the temperature difference existing between this surface and the surrounding air. The constant in this relationship is known as the convective heat-transfer coefficient, and its value will depend on the nature of the particular surface and on the velocity of the air striking along the surface.

It is known that:

$$C = \alpha_c \cdot A_h \cdot (t_h - t_a) \text{ in kcal./hour.}$$

$$\alpha_c = 1\cdot1 \sqrt{v} \text{ . kcal./m.² ° C. hour when } v \text{ in cm./sec.}$$
(Pierce Laboratory).

Characteristic is that neither the air temperature nor the air velocity will have identical values at all points in a space. When these differences become too large in the vicinity of the human body they can be sensed as uncomfortable in view of appreciable quantitative differences in the heat transferred from different parts of the human body. In this connexion it will be known that not all parts of the human body are equally sensitive to heat changes.

It will be apparent that a proper distribution of air temperature and of air velocity is a very important aspect with regard to the comfort of the resulting climatic conditions.

When heating is introduced the air temperature within a space will generally be found to increase from the floor to the ceiling. A temperature increase larger than 1·5–2° C. per metre will generally be experienced as uncomfortable. When introducing systems in which air is blown into a room in order to attain the desired temperature level this air supply may either be at a higher or lower temperature than that of the room. In this case one must see to it that the air movements within the space are such that the sensation of draught is avoided. Draught may be defined as a local air motion at a velocity which is too high for the air temperature, or at an air temperature which is too low for the particular air velocity. It is not so simple to define allowable limits for these aspects, and furthermore, the view of individual authors and per country may vary.

2. Due to the temperature it possesses, each surface will emit RADIATION in the form of electromagnetic waves. The quantity that is radiated will depend not only on the temperature but also on the nature of the surface.

Surfaces which clearly tend to reflect incident radiation (such as bright metal surfaces) will also emit little radiation. When radiation is transmitted to a body the non-reflected part of the radiation will be absorbed and transformed into heat. The extent to which radiation penetrates the human surface will depend on the wavelength.

For this radiation, the following order of wavelengths are encountered:

Solar	. . . .	$0·3–2·3\ \mu$
Industrial processes	. .	$2·5\ \mu$ } infra-red
Indoor climate	. .	$8–10\ \mu$ }

Estimation of the percentage of radiation reacting one surface from another surface emitting it is a geometric problem, and it is given by the size relation between the two surfaces and by their relative positions (configuration factor).

Under normal indoor conditions the effect from all the enclosing walls can be considered as a single entity having a single mean temperature, which may be determined from the actual temperatures of the various surface sections, while the enclosing walls will completely encompass the human body. These particulars determine the geometric picture obtained for the human body in relation to all the enclosing walls.

The quantity of radiation emitted by a body will also depend on its temperature expressed in ° Kelvin, the thermodynamic temperature.

The radiation exchange between the human body and its environment can be expressed mathematically by:

$$R = (A_h \cdot f_{hs} \cdot)(\varepsilon_h \cdot \varepsilon_s)\ \sigma \left[\left(\frac{T_h}{100} \right)^4 - \left(\frac{T_s}{100} \right)^4 \right] \text{ in kcal./hour}$$

Depending on the values of the temperatures T_h and T_s, the human body will either lose heat by radiation ($Q_r > 0$ when

$T_h > T_s$) or receive heat from radiation ($Q_r < 0$ when $T_h < T_s$).

An environment is comprised of various components of which the temperature can be subject to appreciable variation. This may be illustrated by the fact that the inner surface of a single window-pane will be at about 5° C. for an outside temperature of 0° C., while the temperature of the radiator surface will then amount to about 50–55° C.

Similar to conditions characteristic for heat exchange by convection, not all parts of the human body will be subject to equal radiation conditions.

A rough impression of non-permissible differences will be quoted from an investigation by Chrenko (1956). When applying radiant heating incorporated in the ceiling he advises that: (1) at head level the increase in radiant temperature may not exceed 2° C.; (2) at head level the increase in radiation intensity may not exceed 10·8 kcal./m.² hour.

As an initial approximation, the entire surroundings can be considered to be a single entity, and it is convenient to introduce the so-called mean radiant temperature. It represents that particular and homogeneous surface temperature of the enclosing walls which would result in the actual radiation heat exchange experienced by the human body. This radiant temperature can be calculated for any spot within the space from equations in which the configuration factor for this spot and the enclosing walls is a major item. For simplification purposes radiant temperature is generally assumed to be equal to the average surface temperature of the various wall sections.

3. The possibilities of heat loss for the human body by convection and radiation become rather limited when the environmental temperature increases: in that case the terms expressing temperature in the equations for C and R become increasingly irrelevant.

Under these conditions the human body reverts to its means of 'coarse adjustment', i.e. the mechanism of sweating. The initial unnoticeable stage of sweating progresses to evaporation at the skin's surface, in which case the sweat glands can secrete so much fluid that certain body-surface parts become moist. The climatic conditions of the environment will determine the quantity of sweat that is evaporated. The human body is unable to control the intensity of this evaporation.

It is also possible to express evaporation mathematically in the form of an equation.

The maximum quantity of heat, removed by evaporation from a uniformly wetted surface to air, can be expressed by:

$$E_{\max} = 3·3 \cdot v^{0·4}\ (P_h - P_a) \text{ kcal./hour}$$

v in cm./sec.

P in mm./Hg

Whether in fact this maximum quantity will actually evaporate depends, for example, on whether the total surface of the human body has become moist and the extent to which clothing will oppose this evaporation.

4. The quantity of heat to be transferred from the human body will be determined by the particular activity that is undertaken. The indoor climate is characterized by a number of facets which allow this heat loss. Utilizing its mechanisms of control, the human body will attempt to maintain the proper

balance with its internal temperature. Under these conditions the following formula is applicable:

$$M = \pm C \pm R + E$$

The human being has at its disposal a certain adaptation mechanism; under specific conditions this accommodation feature may result in the required equilibrium only after some acclimatization.

When expressing these various aspects numerically it is very important to realize that each particular type of heat balance need not imply that comfort has been achieved. It has already been pointed out that the three means of bodily heat loss can cause marked irregularities for the body surface, and these must be maintained within specific limits in order to warrant comfort. In addition, each one of the three means of heat exchange, i.e. C, R, and E (convection, radiation, and evaporation) should be subjected to limits. This latter aspect is mainly of importance during extreme conditions.

For complaints regarding indoor climatic conditions, these

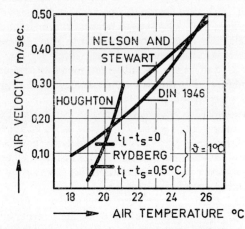

FIG. 10. Relation between allowable air velocity and air temperature.

facts deserve the necessary attention. In an appreciable number of complaints the criticizer is led astray from the correct conclusion.

First, it is necessary to investigate whether heat equilibrium can exist in a particular situation, after which it is advisable to determine the relation between the totals obtained for C, R, and E, and finally it is necessary to determine the differences in respectively C, R, and E which can occur over the various parts of the body.

Under normal conditions it is generally possible to review the heat balance from the total (combined) aspect; in the more extreme case any of the individual components C, R, or E may actually predominate. Customary complaints concern an air temperature which is too high (complaint: warm—too dry), as well as a radiant temperature that is too low (complaint: cold, draughty). High humidity impedes efficient evaporation of perspiration, and at the higher temperature levels this environmental type may be experienced as stuffy or close. When the humidity is too low (<30 per cent.) this can lead to throat complaints; for work that is not too severe this type of environment may induce excessive evaporation in workers who perspire and who may also complain of being cold.

Especially the complaint regarding draught is often caused

by excessive variation in one of the factors, such as excessive radiation to cold surfaces from one side of the body, excessive temperature differences between feet and head, and higher air velocities on certain body parts, such as neck or back [FIG. 10].

A thorough analysis of complaints is recommended; when complaints are received from groups of people inquiries often lead to locating the causes for discomfort and in addition show the correction that is necessary.

When it finally becomes impossible to maintain the required equilibrium in heat supply and demand between the human body and its environment an excess or shortage of heat supply will occur within the body. When the duration of this type of condition cannot be curtailed it will be necessary to introduce special technical measures. These measures, however, appear to fall outside the scope of this chapter, and one enters rather more into the specialized branch of industrial medicine, in which the term 'comfort' is often replaced by the keyword 'allowable'.

STANDARDS OF INDOOR WARMTH—COMFORT

1. In the first place it is only possible to refer to comfortable conditions when the heat supply and demand by the human body is in equilibrium with its environment. This fact alone does not suffice: it is, furthermore, essential that the three possible means of heat transfer are correlated and that in addition none of the alternatives for the heat transfer should be too irregular in its distribution over the surface of the human body.

To date, physiological research has not provided any precise delineation of the comfort zone in cases where the heat balance has firmly been established. The investigations are complicated, especially when analysed quantitatively, while differences mentioned in the introduction, such as age, sex, race, clothing, etc., introduce further complications.

Furthermore it is added that under comfortable climatic conditions the physiological reactions of the human being become notably feeble.

Limits of a zone within which the indoor climate can be assigned as comfortable has thus mainly been established from inquiries to groups of persons subjected to a test.

During the study of existing literature on this subject the following conclusions were derived: (1) An investigation of this type can result in reasonably reliable opinions provided the groups are not too small in numbers and, say, a few hundred people are consulted, while in addition the number of conditions to which the persons under test are exposed should not be too limited. (2) Any maximum in the number of votes received which denote a particular climatic condition as comfortable may be associated with the particular outdoor climate existing at the time. (3) It also appears that the time factor can be of influence on the voting and that opinions may be revised at a later date.

The above-mentioned conclusions are illustrated in FIGURE 11. It is customary that persons included in the inquiry are requested to stipulate their opinion regarding a particular environment by means of selected wording, which can vary from 'comfortable' to, for instance, 'much too hot' or in the case of the other extreme 'much too cold'.

2. In general, conditions of comfort are primarily expressed by means of the degree of comfort that is experienced for each

fundamental climatic factor. In order to allow proper design of the necessary provisions to offset discomfort, recommended values are denoted for: the air temperature, air humidity, air

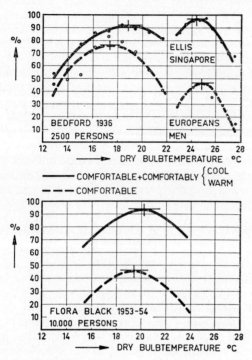

FIG. 11. Air temperature versus percentage observations indicating comfort.

velocity, and the radiant temperature. Handbooks concerning heating and ventilation from the various countries will generally quote recommended values.

TABLE 31
Thermal Comfort Sensations Scales

Heat scale		Moisture scale	
Sensation	Intensity index	Sensation	Intensity index
Unbearably hot .	+7	Unbearably moist .	+7
Much too hot .	+6	Much too moist .	+6
Too hot .	+5	Too moist .	+5
Hot .	+4	Moist .	+4
Too warm .	+3	Too humid .	+3
Warm .	+2	Humid .	+2
Comfortably warm .	+1	Comfortably humid .	+1
Neutral .	0	Neutral .	0
Comfortably cool .	−1	Comfortably dry .	−1
Cool .	−2	Dry .	−2
Too cool .	−3	Too dry .	−3
Cold .	−4	Parched .	−4
Too cold .	−5	Too parched .	−5
Much too cold .	−6	Much too parched .	−6
Unbearably cold .	−7	Unbearably parched .	−7

Freshness scale		Radiant heat scale	
Sensation	Intensity index	Sensation	Intensity index
Very stuffy .	+2	Heat . .	+ or ++
Stuffy .	+1	Neutral .	0
Comfortable .	0	Cold . .	− or −−
Fresh .	−1		
Very fresh .	−2		

Instruction

Decide which Intensity Indices ± correspond to the sensations you feel. Record them on the Thermal Survey Record Sheet, noting the time you have been in the environment, and your personal data.

The principal item which is generally quoted is the air temperature, which can differ somewhat for summer and winter conditions. An additional recommendation asserts that the sum of the air temperature and the mean radiant temperature should attain a specified value.

A fairly customary ruling is that a reduction in the radiant temperature by 1° C. can be compensated by raising the air temperature 1° C. For the conditions in Europe it is accepted that in the winter $t_1 + t_r = 40°$ C.

It has generally been accepted that the desirable humidity in the comfort zone is not particularly relevant as long as relative humidities between 30 and 70 per cent. are maintained. The presumption is reasonably applicable for persons at rest; when, however, bodily heat generation is increased due to moderate activity it is possible that some discomfort will be experienced at either extremity of this humidity range on account of excessive or insufficient evaporation.

Although it is possible to allow higher air velocities at the higher temperature levels, the rule of thumb that air velocities in excess of 25 cm./sec. involve certain risks is still more or less applicable. In this connexion it is pointed out that air velocities are much harder to control than temperature or humidity.

It will be clear that it is not practical to give recommendations here regarding desirable climatic levels for the various countries as well as for the different rooms of dwellings or public buildings. For this aspect, reference should be made to the books specified on pages 84–5.

From FIGURE 11 it is clear that not all persons will express satisfaction regarding a particular climate when an appreciable number of persons are consulted. When defining comfort zones a majority of satisfied persons suffices, for instance, when 70–80 per cent. consider the climate comfortable (comfortably warm —comfortable—comfortably cool).

3. Several methods have been developed to substitute the definition of comfort from the four basic components by utilizing a single integral characteristic. An initial attempt to this end was the combination of the temperature and air humidity. Climatic conditions having different values for the air temperature and the air humidity, but which did appear identical regarding the comfort experienced, were assigned with the same value of the *effective temperature*.

The *effective temperature* (E.T.) scale devised by Yaglou in the United States enables air temperature, humidity, and air movement to be expressed as the temperature of practically still saturated air which gives rise to an equivalent sensation of warmth as that experienced in the environment under examination. It should be noted, however, that there are two scales of effective temperature, the normal scale for persons wearing light indoor clothing, while the basic scale applies to persons stripped to the waist. Both scales were determined for persons doing sedentary or light muscular work. The effective temperature scales do not take into account radiant heat or cold, but the *corrected effective temperature* (C.E.T.) scale, as advocated by Bedford, overcomes this disadvantage by using the globe thermometer temperature instead of the dry bulb temperature of the air with the normal or basic scale nomograms. Reference to the normal scale nomogram [FIG. 12] shows that when radiant heat was present the E.T. was 21·2° C., but the C.E.T.(N) was 22·2° C.

The *equivalent temperature* scale, which was developed by

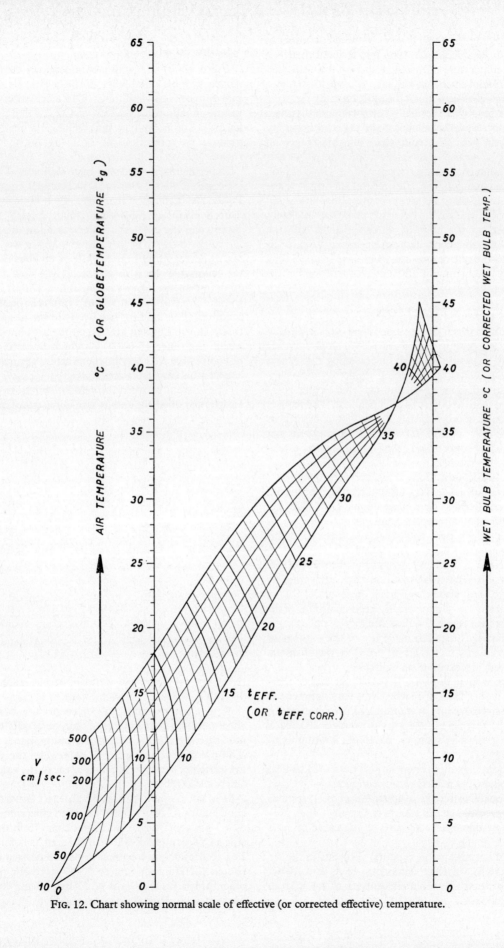

FIG. 12. Chart showing normal scale of effective (or corrected effective) temperature.

Dufton at the Building Research Station of the Department of Scientific and Industrial Research, takes into account the effect of the dry bulb temperature of the air, radiation from the surroundings and air movement on the rate of heat loss from a black body having a surface temperature substantially the same as that of the clothing of a thermally comfortable individual. This scale does not, however, allow for the effect of humidity on evaporative heat loss. The equivalent temperature of an environment may be measured directly by the EUPATHEOSCOPE or by taking simultaneous measurements of air temperature, globe thermometer temperature, and air velocity and determining their combined effect by means of a special nomogram. The equivalent temperature so determined is the dry bulb temperature of the air in a room in which the air is still, the temperature of the walls, floor, and ceiling being the same as that of the air, and the rate of heat loss from the eupatheoscope the same as that occurring in the environment under investigation.

VENTILATION

During breathing oxygen is consumed and carbon dioxide and water vapour are produced. For this reason alone some air renewal is already essential. An analysis regarding this aspect and other criteria provides the following result:

Oxygen Required. During breathing, the oxygen percentage is reduced from about 21 to 16·5 per cent. The oxygen consumption calculated on this basis (0·1 m.^{3}/hour oxygen or 0·5 m.^{3}/hour air per person for normal activity) is not decisive, since it is lower than the requirements established on alternative grounds.

Carbon Dioxide Production. This averages 0·020 m.^{3}/hour per person for normal activity, although more is produced during heavy work. Exhaled air contains 4 per cent. CO_2, i.e. 100 times the amount in atmospheric air.

The toxic limit is ±3 per cent. CO_2, the threshold limit value being 0·5 per cent.

Heat Production. A sedentary person generates about 100 kcal./hour of heat. Often other heat sources, such as machinery, solar radiation, etc., will also prevail in an enclosure.

Since the heat capacity of air is small, large quantities of air will be needed for heat removal unless cooling is applied.

Micro-organisms. Russia has made use of the number of various micro-organisms in the air in order to establish the ventilation required, for example on staircases.

Production of Water Vapour. Especially at higher temperatures and at higher rates of metabolism, very appreciable heat quantities are removed by evaporation of perspiration. In a temperate climate this for normal activity averages 40g./hour in winter and 50 g./hour in summer. At 26° C. it amounts to 65 g./hour.

Excessive humidity, resulting from various causes (industrial or domestic processes), is inducive to discomfort.

Other Products. During the evaporation of perspiration, for instance, disagreeable smells escape to the air. Other processes (industrial or domestic) may also be the cause of such smells.

The presence of harmful gases, vapours, or agents in the air can be more serious. Various countries have laid down MAC-values (*maximum allowable concentration*) for a large number of contaminants.

Ventilation Standards

From all of the aforementioned considerations, the CO_2 content is most suitable for calculating the desirable ventilation rate for average conditions. The calculation is based on the maximum allowable content of CO_2, which as such is neither harmful nor annoying, but which is a ready indication regarding the objectionable build-up of body odour in the room.

Experiments carried out by Lehmberg, Yaglou, and their colleagues (1935, 1936, 1937) at Harvard University School of Public Health showed that body odour intensities ranging from 'threshold' to 'overpowering' could be related to the fresh-air supply and the cubic space per person in the room. An odour intensity described as 'moderate' in that it was neither pleasant nor disagreeable and raised little or no objection was agreed as the 'allowable' limit in rooms. It was found that for seated adults when the air space available per individual was 11 m.^{3} a minimum fresh air supply of 17 m.^{3} per person per hour was required. This finding has been shown to apply in occupied rooms in the London area when the air temperature was kept within the range 15·6–20° C. which Bedford (1936) found to be compatible with warmth comfort for the majority of persons engaged on very light activities.

The relation between the ventilation required per person for a particular air space and its size is illustrated in FIGURE 13. The

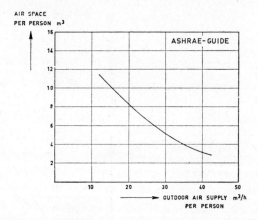

FIG. 13. Relation between air space and minimum outdoor air supply per person.

data concern American standards from Yaglou *et al.* (1936, 1937).

When, for example, school rooms are occupied only for short periods, after which they can be ventilated at an accelerated rate the normal ventilation can be based on this feature. The rise in CO_2 content will depend on the volume of space available per person and can increase to the value which is considered allowable.

It is not possible to specify an exact limit to the allowable concentration. A generally accepted maximum may be taken as 0·5 per cent. When entering a room from the fresh air outside a CO_2 content of 0·1–0·15 per cent. is definitely noticeable. For continuous indoor residence the desired ventilation rate should therefore amount to 30–17 m.^{3}/hour per person. The older American standards stipulated 17 m.^{3}/hour per person. More modern Russian recommendations quote higher figures.

In some cases it will not be the carbon dioxide but other contaminants which will be decisive. In kitchens and bathrooms of residences this will be the water vapour produced. Under industrial conditions toxic or explosive gases or vapours can be produced, and the ventilation required can be calculated from the quantities of gas or vapour that are released and the MAC-value which is desired.

Under domestic conditions contamination can result from the combustion products in the heating installations without a flue, especially when these contain the dangerous carbon monoxide (CO) if the combustion is incomplete. In addition, there is the danger of coal-gas, which also contains CO and which claims numerous victims during the winter months. Adequate ventilation would at any rate have prevented part of these accidents.

MEASUREMENTS OF INDOOR CLIMATE AND VENTILATION

The indoor climate governs the balance between internal heat generation and exterior heat loss for the human being.

This indoor climate is defined by four components: the air temperature, the humidity of the air, the air motion or air velocity, and the mean radiant temperature, while in addition some air renewal is called for.

The heat balance can be obtained at an appreciable number of combinations of these four components, but heat emission is experienced as comfortable only when this occurs within certain limiting values of these components.

In order to be able to classify whether an indoor climate falls within the comfort zone, it is necessary to determine the above-mentioned components *in situ* by means of measurements. It will also be necessary to know the air-renewal rate.

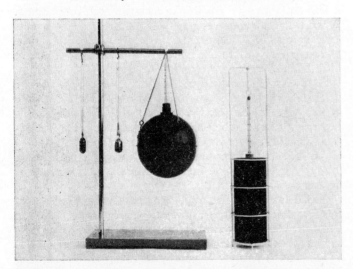

FIG. 14. Measurement of mean radiation temperature: two katathermo-meters—globe thermometer and resulting thermometer.

When reviewing the results of the measurements it is necessary to be aware of the fact that a comfort zone is not defined by fixed limits, but that these limits vary with the outdoor climate, the season of the year, the race, the individual, and the severity of the work performed (metabolism).

Regrettably no suitable instrument is as yet available which

indicates the degree of comfort by a single value, although in addition to instruments annotating values of individual components, a few instruments have been developed for recording the combined effect of two or more climatic components. The main disadvantage of these instruments is that they fail to react in similar manner to the human body, although that illusion might be obtained [FIG. 14].

When it is desired to change or improve environmental conditions it is essential that the values for individual components are known. Sometimes, however, instruments which record the influence of a combination of climatic components can prove useful in order to obtain a rapid and over-all impression.

A short summary of the most prominent instrument types will follow.

Instruments for Measuring the Air Temperature

The first instrument for establishing the temperature of the air is the mercury thermometer. It is cheap and accurate, the

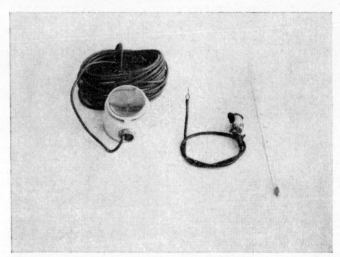

FIG. 15. Measurement of air temperature: resistance thermometer, thermocouple, ordinary thermometer.

simplest and most popular instrument. Since the heat equilibrium of the instrument is affected by the unwanted radiation heat exchange with the enclosing walls, the temperature read off on the thermometer in fact represents some intermediate point between the air temperature and the mean radiant temperature. In order to reduce the errors in air-temperature measurement, the thermometer bulb may be shielded against radiation. In addition, the bulb containing the mercury may be reduced in size, in this way both reducing the heat transfer by radiation and increasing the heat transfer by convection. Increasing the air velocity will considerably increase the convective transport.

When measurements are required at an appreciable number of places the electrical measuring technique is preferred. The principal instruments are:

1. Thermocouples, which consist of an electrical circuit comprising two wires of dissimilar metals. The difference in e.m.f. between the two junctions (of which one is maintained at constant temperature) is nearly proportional to the temperature difference. As the items utilized are only small, the radiant heat

exchange is negligible. Popular combinations of metals for these instruments are copper–constantan and iron–constantan.

2. Resistance thermometers, which depend on the change of electrical resistance of metals and semi-conductors with temperature change.

Although the design of the recording section for electrical instruments can generally be simple, bi-metal strips are often used for recording-type instruments at one point only. These strips consist of two metal layers having different coefficients of expansion, which deform in some specific manner at temperature changes [FIG. 15].

Instruments for Measuring the Mean Radiant Temperature

The mean radiant temperature can be accurately determined by averaging the surface temperatures established, for instance, by thermocouples.

It is also possible to utilize thermopiles, which consist of a number of thermocouples connected in series. The hot junctions are blackened in order to raise the absorption coefficient; an attempt is made to minimize variation in the temperature of the cold junctions [FIG. 16]. Depending on the distance away from the object, one obtains an average temperature of a section of the wall surface.

The globe thermometer of Vernon is an ordinary thermometer for which the sensitivity to radiation has been increased very materially by the addition of a black sphere made of thin metal having a diameter of about 15 cm. which encompasses the mercury bulb. Missenard's resultant thermometer is a similar instrument in which the sphere has been replaced by a black vertical cylinder.

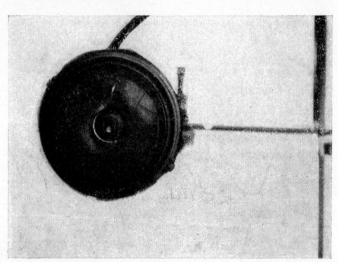

FIG. 16. Front view of a thermopile for measuring surface temperatures.

For determining the radiant temperature, Hill's katathermometer may also be used. This is a thermometer in which the glass reservoir, which is about 40 mm. long and 20 mm. in diameter, has been filled with alcohol or toluene. The instrument is heated and the time is recorded in which the instrument cools over the range of temperature, which is indicated

on the stem. This time interval is dependent upon the air temperature, the air velocity, the mean radiant temperature, and the calibration particulars of the instrument used. When using two instruments having different absorption coefficients the mean radiant temperature can be calculated. The method is tiresome, but cheap.

Instruments for Measuring the Humidity of the Air

Mankind is indifferent to a relatively large range of air humidities. Below a certain minimum difficulties may be

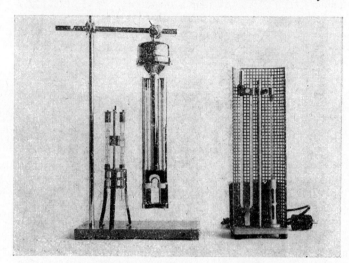

FIG. 17. Two types of psychrometers and electrolytic hygrometer.

caused by dehydration of mucous membranes in mouth and throat. The relative humidity of 30–40 per cent. can be considered a minimum, although in very dry and very cold climates it will not always be possible to maintain even these values. When the relative humidity is too high the heat emission by evaporation will be hampered; this aspect becomes important at higher temperature and during heavy work (high rate of metabolism).

Physically, humidity should preferably be assigned as the value of the vapour pressure of water expressed in millimetres of mercury. In practice, the use of the relative humidity is generally preferred, which denotes the percentage of the saturation pressure of water vapour at the existing temperature. It is also customary to define humidity by the weight relation water vapour/dry air expressed generally as grams of water vapour per kg. dry air.

A final indication of humidity can be obtained by stipulating the dewpoint of the air, i.e. the temperature to which air of the particular consistency must be cooled in order to become fully saturated without condensation.

The equation containing the various factors for denoting humidity requires a lot of calculation, and use of the psychrometric chart (or the Mollier diagram), in which the humidity is represented graphically, is generally preferred [TABLE 32].

The standard instrument for measuring humidity is the psychrometer [FIG. 17]. The instrument has two thermometers, one is plain (dry bulb) and the other has a wetted cloth at the bulb (wet bulb). The difference in the two thermometer readings is a measure of the humidity.

The relative humidity can be determined in three different

ways: (1) by calculation; (2) from a table; or (3) by the psychrometric chart. When calculating the relative humidity Sprung's equation is used:

$$p = p'\text{max.} - 0.5 \, (t_{db} - t_{wb})\frac{P_{\text{atm}}}{755}$$

in which $p'\text{max.}$ = saturation vapour pressure at the wet bulb temperature. (When ice is formed on the wet bulb the factor 0·5 should be replaced by 0·44.)

The value of $p'\text{max.}$ may be read off in the column '100 per cent. R.H.' and for the particular temperature from the left-hand side of TABLE 32. From the value calculated for p, the

TABLE 32
Vapour Pressure of Moist Air
(Barometric pressure 760 mm. Hg)

t_L °C.	Vapour pressure mm. Hg at a RH of . . . %										
	0	10	20	30	40	50	60	70	80	90	100
0	0	0·5	0·9	1·4	1·8	2·3	2·8	3·2	3·7	4·1	4·6
1	0	0·5	1·0	1·5	2·0	2·5	2·9	3·4	3·9	4·4	4·9
2	0	0·5	1·1	1·6	2·1	2·7	3·2	3·7	4·2	4·8	5·3
3	0	0·6	1·1	1·7	2·3	2·9	3·4	4·0	4·6	5·1	5·7
4	0	0·6	1·2	1·8	2·4	3·1	3·7	4·3	4·9	5·5	6·1
5	0	0·7	1·3	2·0	2·6	3·3	3·9	4·6	5·2	5·9	6·5
6	0	0·7	1·4	2·1	2·8	3·5	4·2	4·9	5·6	6·3	7·0
7	0	0·8	1·5	2·3	3·0	3·8	4·5	5·3	6·0	6·8	7·5
8	0	0·8	1·6	2·4	3·2	4·0	4·8	5·6	6·4	7·2	8·0
9	0	0·9	1·7	2·6	3·5	4·3	5·2	6·0	6·9	7·7	8·6
10	0	0·9	1·8	2·8	3·7	4·6	5·5	4·4	7·4	8·3	9·2
11	0	1·0	2·0	2·9	3·9	4·9	5·9	6·9	7·8	8·8	9·8
12	0	1·1	2·1	3·2	4·2	5·3	6·3	7·4	8·4	9·5	10·5
13	0	1·1	2·2	3·4	4·5	5·6	6·7	7·8	8·9	10·0	11·2
14	0	1·2	2·4	3·6	4·8	6·0	7·1	8·3	9·5	10·7	11·9
15	0	1·3	2·5	3·8	5·1	6·4	7·6	8·9	10·2	11·4	12·7
16	0	1·4	2·7	4·1	5·4	6·8	8·2	9·5	10·9	12·2	13·6
17	0	1·4	2·9	4·3	5·8	7·2	8·6	10·1	11·5	13·0	14·4
18	0	1·5	3·1	4·6	6·2	7·7	9·2	10·8	12·3	13·9	15·4
19	0	1·6	3·3	4·9	6·6	8·2	9·8	11·5	13·1	14·8	16·4
20	0	1·7	3·5	5·2	7·0	8·7	10·4	12·2	13·9	15·7	17·4
21	0	1·9	3·7	5·6	7·4	9·3	11·1	13·0	14·8	16·7	18·5
22	0	2·0	3·9	5·9	7·9	9·9	11·8	13·8	15·8	17·7	19·7
23	0	2·0	4·2	6·3	8·4	10·5	12·5	14·6	16·7	18·8	20·0
24	0	2·2	4·4	6·7	8·9	11·1	13·3	15·5	17·8	20·0	22·2
25	0	2·4	4·7	7·1	9·4	11·8	14·1	16·5	18·9	21·2	23·6
26	0	2·5	5·0	7·5	10·0	12·5	15·0	17·5	20·0	22·5	25·0
27	0	2·7	5·3	8·0	10·6	13·3	15·9	18·6	21·2	23·8	26·5
28	0	2·8	5·6	8·4	11·2	14·1	16·9	19·7	22·5	25·3	28·1
29	0	3·0	6·0	8·9	11·9	14·9	17·9	20·9	23·8	26·8	29·8
30	0	3·2	6·3	9·5	12·6	15·8	18·9	22·1	25·2	28·4	31·5
31	0	3·3	6·7	10·0	13·4	16·7	20·0	23·4	26·7	30·0	33·4
32	0	3·5	7·1	10·6	14·2	17·7	21·2	24·8	28·3	31·8	35·4
33	0	3·7	7·5	11·2	15·0	18·7	22·4	26·2	29·0	33·6	37·4
34	0	4·0	7·9	11·9	15·8	19·8	23·7	27·8	31·7	35·6	39·6
35	0	4·2	8·4	12·5	16·7	20·9	25·1	29·3	33·4	37·6	41·8
36	0	4·4	8·8	13·3	17·7	22·1	26·5	31·0	35·3	39·8	44·2
37	0	4·7	9·3	14·0	18·9	23·4	28·0	32·7	37·4	42·1	46·7
38	0	4·9	9·9	14·8	19·7	24·7	29·6	34·5	39·4	44·4	49·3
39	0	5·2	10·4	15·6	20·8	26·0	31·2	36·4	41·6	46·8	52·0
40	0	5·5	11·0	16·5	22·0	27·5	32·9	38·4	43·9	49·4	54·9
41	0	5·8	11·6	17·3	23·2	29·0	34·7	40·5	46·3	52·1	57·9
42	0	6·1	12·2	18·3	24·4	30·6	36·7	42·8	48·8	55·0	61·1
43	0	6·4	12·9	19·3	25·7	32·2	38·6	45·1	51·4	57·9	64·3
44	0	6·8	13·6	20·3	27·1	33·9	40·7	47·4	54·2	61·0	67·8
45	0	7·1	14·3	21·4	28·6	35·7	42·8	49·9	57·0	64·2	71·4
46	0	7·5	15·0	22·6	30·1	37·6	45·1	52·6	60·1	67·6	75·2
47	0	7·9	15·8	23·7	31·6	39·5	47·4	53·3	63·2	71·1	79·0
48	0	8·3	16·6	25·0	33·3	41·6	49·9	58·2	66·5	74·9	83·2
49	0	8·8	17·5	26·3	35·0	43·8	52·5	61·3	70·0	78·7	87·5
50	0	9·2	18·4	27·6	36·8	46·0	55·2	64·4	73·6	82·7	92·0

relative humidity (R.H.) may be established either from the table or it is calculated from:

$$\text{R.H.} = \frac{p}{p_{\text{max.}}} \cdot 100 \text{ per cent.}$$

R.H. may also be determined directly from the dry-bulb temperature and the psychrometric difference read off for $t_{db} - t_{wb}$ [FIG. 19].

A correct psychrometer reading can be obtained only when there is a minimum air velocity of *ca.* 2 m./sec. around the bulbs. This air velocity can be obtained by installing a small fan or by swirling the whole instrument around in the air. A fan driven by a spring is also used.

The *hair hygrometer* [FIG. 18] is based on the principle that human hair changes in length with variations in the relative

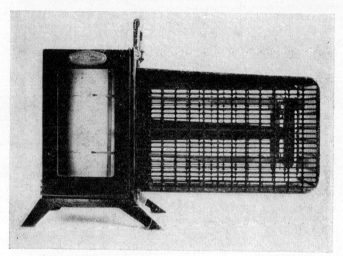

FIG. 18. Combined thermograph and hair hygrograph.

humidity. The actual connexion between hairlength and relative humidity is determined empirically, and when the meter is used correctly the results obtained from duplicate tests are practically identical. Recorder-type hygrometers are also popular, which may then be combined with a bimetal thermograph. The data obtained are recorded on a sheet of paper fixed around a vertical cylinder, which makes one complete revolution either per day or per week [FIG. 19].

More recently, lithium chloride cells have come into use. In these instruments the low saturation pressure resulting from a solution of lithium chloride in water is compared to the pressure of saturated water vapour at the same temperature. The cell is heated electrically until the saturation pressure of the LiCl$_{\text{aq.}}$ solution is just in equilibrium with the existing pressure of the water vapour in the air. By proper calibration of the instrument, it is possible to derive the dewpoint of the air from the temperature obtained from the cell. The advantages of this instrument are that it is relatively cheap and requires little maintenance. The more basic method of determining the dewpoint by cooling the moist air is applied only in the fairly expensive, recording-type instruments.

Instruments for Measuring the Air Velocity

For the measurements of indoor conditions only instruments denoting fairly low velocities are required. The lower limit can be considered to be 5–10 cm./sec.

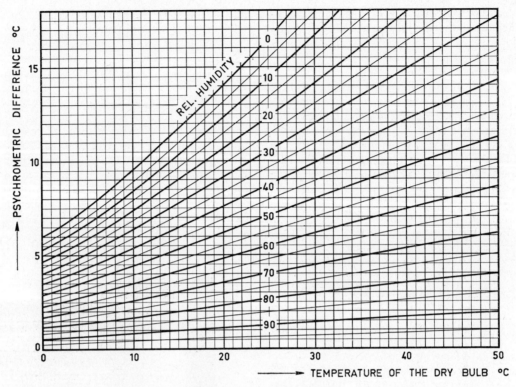

FIG. 19. Hygrometric chart.

In the group of mechanical instruments appreciable use is still made of the revolving-vane-type anemometer. This is a type of windmill very daintily constructed which is driven by

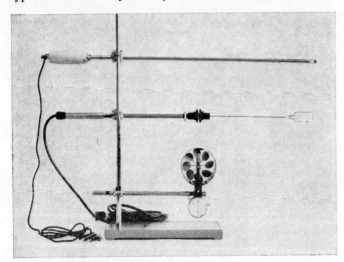

FIG. 20. Three types of anemometers: propeller vane, heated thermocouple, hot wire.

the wind force, while the velocity is determined by a counter. The counter generally registers the number of revolutions of the shaft; registration by electrical means is also feasible. Deviation of the wind direction up to 20 degrees from shaft axis is allowable. The delicate mechanism requires careful maintenance, and rapid fluctuations in the wind velocity cannot be recorded.

Another type of mechanical instrument is the deflecting-vane anemometer, which consists of a pivoted vane enclosed in a

case. Details of mechanism are shown in FIGURE 21. The air flowing through the instrument displaces a vane, which is coupled to an indicator, while indicator movement is resisted by a spring. The instrument is fairly large but robust, and can be used down to rather feeble wind speeds. Various attachments are available.

Measuring instruments which depend on cooling experienced by a heated object have the advantage that they are particularly sensitive at low velocities. The previously mentioned katathermometer operates by means of intermitted heating, but the time required for measuring is long.

A more recent type of instrument utilizes an electrically-heated wire or sphere, of which the temperature is determined.

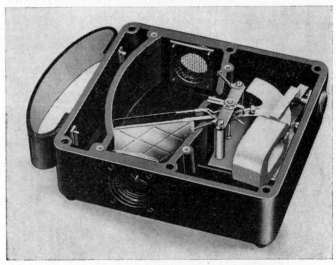

FIG. 21. Interior of a deflecting-vane anemometer.

It is sometimes necessary to correct for air-temperature variations. This is not the case for the instrument depicted in FIGURE 22, since the air velocity is related to the difference in temperature between the sphere and the air, which is determined thermo-electrically in this instance.

Some of the above-mentioned instruments are also suitable

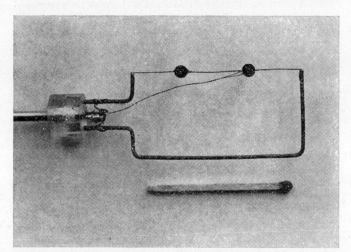

FIG. 22. Anemometer with heated and unheated junction of thermo-couple.

at the higher air velocities. A simple method of determining the air velocity in a duct consists of the Pitot tube, used in conjunction with a suitable manometer.

One of the instruments which is affected by various climatic factors is the katathermometer, which has already been mentioned. To this group also belong the globe thermometer and the Missenard resultant thermometer. All these three instruments are affected by three of the four climatic components; air temperature, radiant temperature, and air velocity. The instruments which are shaped as cylinders conform somewhat better to the human body than the spherical globe thermometer.

AIR RENEWAL

When air is supplied into and exhausted from an enclosure by means of special openings it is possible to calculate the rate of air change from the average velocity of the air through these openings. The measuring instrument should not, of course, cause any appreciable obstruction to the air flow. Away from the exhaust air opening the air velocity diminishes very rapidly. It is therefore preferable to measure the air supply at the inlet, although this quantity cannot be measured with high accuracy.

When the required ventilation results from cracks in windows and doors measurements cannot be made, and instead a tracer gas is used. The air-change rate can be established from the rate at which the concentration diminishes by means of the formula:

$$C_t = C_0 \, (e^{-at})$$

in which: C_t = concentration of tracer after t hours;

C_0 = initial tracer concentration;

$e = 2 \cdot 718$;

a = air change rate per hour.

Both physical and chemical methods can be used in the tracer technique. In a simple chemical method CO_2 is used as the tracer.

The physical methods involve, for instance, the addition of helium or hydrogen, which have a much higher heat conductivity than air, or using CO_2, which has a lower heat conductivity coefficient. In the Katharometer method the change in temperature is measured by an electrically-heated resistance held in the mixture of air and tracer.

Another alternative method involves the change in absorption of infra-red rays when, for example, CO_2 or N_2O are added.

REFERENCES AND FURTHER READING

General

The significance to health of stability in the internal environment of the body is examined and expounded in:

Bernard, C. (1878) *Les Phénomènes de la Vie*, Paris.
Cannon, W. B. (1939) *The Wisdom of the Body*, revised ed., London.
Haldane, J. S. (1929) *The Sciences and Philosophy*, London.

Body temperature regulation may be studied in:

Evans, C. Lovatt (1962) *Starling's Principles of Human Physiology*, 13th ed., London.

Adaptation to heat and cold, protective effect of clothing and health in relation to climate are reviewed and many references are given in:

Winslow, C. E. A., and Herrington, L. P. (1949) *Temperature and Human Life*, Princeton.

Body-heat production and muscular work grades; problems of heat, cold, and clothing are critically examined in:

Brown, J. R., and Crowden, G. P. (1963) Energy expenditure ranges and muscular work grades, *Brit. J. industr. Med.*, **20**, 277.

Burton, Allan C., and Edholm, Otto G. (1955) *Man in a Cold Environment*, London.
Liese, W. (1960) Neuere wärmephysiologische und hygienische Ergebnisse von klimatischer Bedeutung, *Ges. Ing.*, **81** (12), 363.

An authoritative and detailed examination of heating, ventilation, and air-conditioning requirements and methods; the use of effective, corrected effective, and equivalent temperature, scales of warmth with a good bibliography will be found in:

Bedford, T. (1964) *Basic Principles of Ventilation and Heating*, 2nd ed., London.

Recommendations for heating and ventilation in houses and other buildings are included in the following:

American Society of Heating, Refrigeration and Air-Conditioning (1965/1967) Fundamentals, systems, equipment.
British Standard Codes of Practice, *Heating and Thermal Insulation* (1949); *Ventilation* (1950) British Standards Institution, London.
Gagge, A. P., Burton, A. C., and Gazett, H. C. (1960) A practical system of units for the description of the heat exchange of man with his environment, *Science*, **94**, 428.
Institution of Heating and Ventilating Engineers (1965) *Guide*, London.

Nuffield Provincial Hospitals Trust (1955) *Studies in the Functions and Design of Hospitals*, London.

Royal College of Physicians, Report of Advisory Committee (1936) *Domestic Heating by Gas Considered from the Point of Health and Comfort*, London.

The use of instruments and nomograms for assessing the thermal environment are clearly described in:

Bedford, T. (1946) *Environmental Warmth and Its Measurement*, M.R.C. War Memorandum No. 17, London, H.M.S.O.

Thermal Comfort

Bedford, T. (1936) The warmth factor in comfort at work, *Rep. industr. Hlth Res. Bd (Lond.)*, No. 76, London, H.M.S.O.

Bedford, T. (1958) Research on heating and ventilation in relation to human comfort, *J. Heat. Pip. Air Condit.*, **30**, 127.

Benzinger, T. H. (1959) Physiologischer Mechanismus der physikalischen Wärmeregulation des Menschen, *Pflügers Arch. ges. Physiol.*, **270**, 72.

Black, Flora W. (1954) Desirable temperatures in offices. A study of occupant reaction to the heating provided, *J. Inst. vent. Engrs*, **22**, 319.

Brouha, L. (1961) Physiological reactions of men and women during muscular activity and recovery in various environments, *J. appl. Physiol.*, **16** (1), 133.

Chrenko, F. A. (1956) Heated floors and comfort, *J. Inst. heat. vent. Engrs*, **23**, 385.

Crowden, G. P. (1952) Optimum living conditions in temperate climates, *Practitioner*, **168**, 593.

Crowden, G. P. (1956) Environmental factors affecting comfort, health and working capacity, *J. roy. Inst. publ. Hlth*, **19**, 109.

Ellis, F. P. (1953) Thermal comfort in warm and humid atmospheres, *J. Hyg. (Lond.)*, **51**, 386.

European Community of Coal and Steel, High Authority (1961) *Arbeitsphysiologische und Arbeitspathologische Studies*, Ch. II.

Glickman, N. *et al.* (1950) Physiological examination of the effective temperature index, *J. Heat. Pip. Air. Condit.*, **22** (1), 157.

Grandjean, E., and Rhiner, A. (1963) Die Luftfeuchtigkeit und ihre Auswirkung auf die Behaglichkeit in Wohn- und Büroräumen, *Gesundheits-Ing.*, **84** (12), 362.

Hickish, D. E. (1955) Thermal sensations of workers in light industry in summer, *J. Hyg. (Lond.)*, **53**, 112.

Hickish, D. E. (1957) The thermal comfort of workers in light industries in summer in relation to environmental factors, Ph.D. Thesis, University of London.

Hill, L., Flack, M., McIntosh, J., Rowlands, R. A., and Walker, H. B. (1913) *The Influence of the Atmosphere on our Health and Comfort in Confined and Crowded Spaces*, Smithson, Misc. Coll. 60, No. 23, Pub. 2170.

Koch, W., Jennings, B. H., and Humphreys, C. M. (1960) Is humidity important? *ASHRAE Journal*, **2** (4), 63.

Krantz, P. (1964) Calculating human comfort, *ASHRAE Journal*, **6** (9), 68.

Newburgh, L. H. (1949) *Physiology of Heat Regulation*, Philadelphia.

Rydberg, J. (1962) Air introduction through perforated ceilings, *V.V.S. Tidskrift*, **33** (6), 227.

Taylor, P. F. (1952) Thermal comfort sensations and physiological reactions in relation to variations in indoor climate, Ph.D. Thesis, University of London.

Wenzel, H. G. (1961) Die Wirkung des Klimas auf den arbeitenden Menschen, in *Handbuch der gesamten Arbeitsmedizin*, Bd. I., ed. Baader, E. W. Berlin.

Wenzel, H. G. (1962) Die Einwirkung des Klimas auf den arbeitenden Menschen, *Heizung, Lüftung, Haustechnik*, **13**, 349.

Yaglou, C. P. (1947) A method for improving the effective temperature index, *Trans. Amer. Soc. heat. vent. Engrs*, **53**, 307.

Yaglou, C. P., and Miller, W. E. (1925) Effective temperature with clothing, *Trans. Amer. Soc. heat. vent. Engrs*, **31**, 89.

Heat Stress

Belding, H. S., and Hatch, T. F. (1955) Index for evaluating heat stress in terms of resulting physiological strains, *J. Heat. Pip. Air Condit.*, **27**, 129.

Bell, C. R., and Provins, K. A. (1962) Effects of high temperature environmental conditions on human performance, *J. occup. Med.*, **4** (4), 202.

Brouha, L. (1962) Physiological reactions to psychometric extremes, *ASHRAE Journal*, **4** (3), 83.

Brown, J. R., Crowden, G. P., and Taylor, P. F. (1959) Circulatory responses to change from recumbent to erect posture as an index of heat stress, *Ergonomics*, **2**, 262.

Brüner, H. (1959) Arbeitsmöglichkeiten unter Tage bei erschwerten klimatischen Bedingungen, *Int. Z. angew. Physiol.*, **18**, 31.

Crowden, G. P. (1949) A survey of physiological studies of mental and physical work in hot and humid environments, *Trans. roy. Soc. trop. Med. Hyg.*, **42**, 325.

Ellis, F. P. (1953) Symposium on Fatigue, *Tropical Fatigue*, Ergonomics Research Soc., London.

Fahnestock, M. K. (1963) Comfort and physiological responses to work, *ASHRAE Journal*, **5** (3), 25.

Inouye, T. *et al.* (1953) Effect of relative humidity in heat losses of men exposed to environments of 80, 76 and 72° F., *Trans. Amer. Soc. heat. vent. Engrs*, **59**, 329.

Ledent, P., and Bidlot, R. (1947) Que savons-nous des limites de températures humainement supportables?, Institut d'Hygiene des Mines-Hasselt, Communication 28.

Leithead, C. S., and Lind, A. R. (1964) *Heat Stress and Heat Disorders*, London.

Lind, A. R., Hellon, R. F., Weiner, J. S., and Jones, R. M. (1955) Tolerance of men to work in hot, saturated environments, *Brit. J. industr. Med.*, **12**, 296.

Lind, A. R., Hellon, R. F., Weiner, J. S., Jones, R. M., and Fraser, D. C. (1957) Reactions of mines-rescue personnel to work in hot environments, *Med. Res. Memor.*, No. 1, National Coal Board, London, H.M.S.O.

Mackworth, N. H. (1950) Researches on the measurement of human performance, *Spec. Rep. Ser. med. Res. Coun. (Lond.)*, No. 268, London, H.M.S.O.

MacPherson, R. K. (1949) *Tropical Fatigue*, Brisbane.

Pepler, R. D. (1958) Warmth and performance, *Ergonomics*, **2** (11), 63.

Smith, F. E. (1955) *Indices of Heat Stress*, M.R.C. Mem. No. 29, London, H.M.S.O.

Wenzel, H. G. (1961) Die Wirkung des Klimas auf den arbeitenden Menschen, in *Handbuch der gesamten Arbeitsmedizin*, Bd. I, ed. Baader, E. W. Berlin.

Wenzel, H. G. (1961) Messungen der körperlichen Leistungfähigkeit bei Hitzearbeit, *Zbl. Arb. wiss.*, **15**, 17.

World Health Organization Report of a WHO Scientific Group (1969) Health factors involved in working under conditions of heat stress, *Wld Hlth Org. techn. Rep. Ser.*, No. 412.

Wyndham, C. H. *et al.* (1953) Working efficiency of Africans in heat, *Arch. industr. Hyg.*, **7**, 234.

Heat Illness

Ellis, F. P. (1958) Heat illness, *J. roy. nav. med. Serv.*, **44**, 236.

Ladell, W. S. S., Waterlow, J. C., and Hudson, M. F. (1944) Desert climates: physiological and clinical observations, *Lancet*, ii, 491.

Leithead, C. S., Guthrie, J., De la Place, S., and Maegraith, B. (1958) Incidence, aetiology and prevention of heat illness on ships in the Persian Gulf, *Lancet*, ii, 109.

Minard, D., Belding, H. S., and Kingston, J. R. (1957) Prevention of heat casualties, *J. Amer. med. Ass.*, **165**, 1813.

Thomson, M. L. (1958) Heat exhaustion and allied disorders, *Med. Press*, **239**, 100.

Weiner, J. S., and Horne, G. O. (1958) A classification of heat illness, *Brit. med. J.*, **1**, 1533.

Acclimatization to Heat

Eichna, L. W., Ashe, W. F., Bean, W. B., and Shelley, W. B. (1945) The upper limits of environmental heat and humidity tolerated by acclimatised men working in hot environments, *J. industr. Hyg.*, **27**, 59.

Glickman, N. *et al.* (1947) Physiological adjustments of human beings to sudden change in environment, *Trans. Amer. Soc. heat. vent. Engrs*, **53**, 327.

Hellon, R. F., Jones, E. M., MacPherson, R. K., and Weiner, J. S. (1956) Natural and artificial acclimatisation to hot environments, *J. Physiol. (Lond.)*, **132**, 559.

Wyndham, C. H., Strydom, N. B., Cooke, H. M., and Maritz, J. S. (1960) The temperature responses of men after two methods of acclimatisation, *Arbeitsphysiologie*, **18** (2), 112

Wyndham, C. H., Strydom, N. B., Morrison, J. F., DuToit, F. D., and Kraan, J. G. (1954) A new method of acclimatisation to heat, *Arbeitsphysiologie*, **15**, 373.

Sweating and Salt Loss

Brebner, D. F., Kerslake, D. McK., and Waddell, J. L. (1958) The effect of atmospheric humidity on the skin temperatures and sweat rates of resting men at two ambient temperatures, *J. Physiol. (Lond.)*, **144**, 199.

Leithead, C. S., Leithead, L. A., and Lee, F. D. (1958) Salt deficiency heat exhaustion, *Ann. trop. Med. Parasit.*, **52**, 456.

Thomson, M. L., and Sutarman (1953) The identification and enumeration of active sweat glands in man from plastic impressions of the skin, *Trans. roy. Soc. trop. Med. Hyg.*, **47**, 412.

Houghten, F. C. *et al.* (1931) Heat and moisture losses from men at work and application to air conditioning problems, *Trans. Amer. Soc. heat. vent. Engrs*, **37**, 541.

Ladell, W. S. S. (1955) The effects of water and salt intake upon the performance of men working in hot and humid environments, *J. Physiol. (London)*, **127**, 11.

Lehmann, G. (1950) Schwitzen und Trinken bei Hitzearbeit, *Zbl. Arb. Wiss.*, **4**, 3.

Malhotra, M. S., Sharma, B. K., and Sivaraman, R. (1959) Requirements of sodium chloride during summer in the tropics, *J. appl. Physiol.*, **14** (5), 823.

Physiological Effects of Clothing

Brown, J. R., and Croton, L. M. (1957) An experimental method for the determination of the 'CLO' value of clothing, *J. Text. Inst.*, **48**, 10.

Chattopadhyay, S. K. (1958) Physiological effects of industrial protective clothing, Ph.D. Thesis, University of London.

Crockford, G. W., and Hellon, R. F. (1964) Design and evaluation of a ventilated garment for use in temperatures up to 200° C., *Brit. J. industr. Med.*, **21**, 187.

Hick, F. K. *et al.* (1952) Physiological adjustments of clothed human being to sudden changes in environment, *Trans. Amer. Soc. heat. vent. Engrs*, **58**, 189.

Inouye, T. *et al.* (1953) A comparison of physiological adjustments of clothed women and men to sudden changes in environment, *Trans. Amer. Soc. heat. vent. Engrs*, **59**, 35.

Yaglou, C. P., and Messer, A. (1941) The importance of clothing in air conditioning, *J. Amer. med. Ass.*, **117**, 1261.

Ventilation and Habitability of Dwellings

Bedford, T. (1960) Requirements for satisfactory heating and ventilation, *Ann. occup. Hyg.*, **2** (3), 167.

Brown, J. R. (1955) Physiological reactions of women to heat and humidity during work in the home, *Advanc. Sci. (Lond.)*, **11**, 415.

Crowden, G. P. (1951) The height of rooms in dwellings in relation to health and comfort, *J. roy. sanit. Inst.*, **71**, 108.

Crowden, G. P. (1955) The habitability of dwellings: heating and ventilation requirements, *Advanc. Sci. (Lond.)*, **11**, 411.

Davies, I. G. (1955) The improvement of back-to-back houses with special reference to ventilation, *Annual Report of the Medical Officer of Health of the City of Leeds for 1955*, p. 121.

De Heer, T., and Erkelens, H. J. (1963) Heat transmission by radiation: a new method of calculating the local and the total effects, *J. Inst. of heat. vent. Engrs*, **30** (1), 357.

Dick, J. B. (1955) Warmth and comfort in dwellings, *Advanc. Sci. (Lond.)* **11**, 422.

Houghten, F. C. *et al.* (1937) Cooling requirements for summer comfort air conditioning, *Trans. Amer. Soc. heat. vent. Engrs*, **43**, 145.

Lehmberg, W. H., Brandt, A. D., and Morse, K. (1935) A laboratory study of minimum ventilation requirements: ventilation box experiments, *J. Heat. Pip. Air Condit.*, **7**, 44.

Ministry of Labour and National Service (1953) *Heating and Ventilation in Factories*, 5th ed., London, H.M.S.O.

Olingsberg, R. (1967) Kaltlufteinblasung in belüfteten Räumen, *Gesundheits-Ing.*, **88**, 210.

Renbourne, E. T., Angus, T. C., Ellison, J. McK., Croton, L. M., and Jones, M. S. (1949) The measurement of domestic ventilation: an experimental and theoretical investigation with particular reference to the use of carbon dioxide as a tracer substance, *J. Hyg. (Lond.)*, **47**, 1.

Richards, S. J. (1957) Minimum ceiling heights in South Africa, Bulletin No. 15, National Building Research Inst., Pretoria.

Wenzel, H. G., and Müller, E. A. (1957) Untersuchungen der Behaglichkeit des Raumklimas bei 'Deckenheizung', *Int. Z. angew. Physiol.*, **16**, 335.

Yaglou, C. P., Riley, E. C., and Coggins, D. I. (1936) Ventilation requirements, Pt. 1, *J. Heat. Pip. Air Condit.*, **8**, 65.

Yaglou, C. P., and Witheridge, W. N. (1937) Ventilation requirements, Pt. 2, *J. Heat. Pip. Air Condit.*, **9**, 447.

Tropical Housing

Drew, J. B., Fry, M., Maxwell, E., and Frod, H. L. (1947) *Village Housing in the Tropics*, London.

Fry, M., and Drew, J. (1956) *Tropical Architecture in the Humid Zone*, London.

Rao, M. N. (1952) Comfort range in tropical Calcutta, *Indian J. Med. Res.*, **XL** (1), 45.

Raychaudbury, B. C. (1960) Thermal performance of light weight structures in tropics, *Proc. C.B.R.I.*, Second Research Workers Conf., Poorkee.

Report of Proceedings on Conference on Tropical Architecture (1953), London. Printed at University College (1954).

Richards, S. J., Van Straaten, J. F., and Van Deventer, E. N. (1960) Some ventilation and thermal considerations in building design to suit climate, *S. Afr. Architect. Rec.*, **45** (1).

Van Straaten, J. F., Richards, S. J., Lotz, F. J., and Van Deventer, E. N. (1965) Ventilation and thermal considerations in school building design, *C.S.I.R. Research Report*, No. 203, Pretoria.

Watford Building Research Station (1950) *Notes on Building, Housing and Planning in Tropical and Sub-Tropical Countries*.

Webb, C. G. (1952) Some observations of indoor climate in Malaya, *J. Inst. heat. vent. Engrs*, **19**, 187.

7

LIGHTING AND PUBLIC HEALTH

J. van IERLAND and D. A. SCHREUDER[1]

EFFECTS OF VISIBLE AND ULTRA-VIOLET RADIATION UPON MAN

NON-VISUAL EFFECTS

However important vision may be, visible and ultra-violet radiation have a still more vital function. The presence of such radiation—of a certain spectral composition, in a certain amount and in a certain rhythm—is a primary condition for many forms of life, including man and vegetation. Apart from affecting our bodies directly, this radiation affects our health by its influence upon the atmosphere, oxygen production by plants, and germicidal effects. The bactericidal effect is caused by ultra-violet radiation of 220–300 nm, with a maximum effectiveness at 265 nm. Ultra-violet radiation, especially in the region from 250 to 300 nm, is a factor in the production within the skin of pigments and vitamin D, necessary for the building up of our body and for our general resistance against harmful influences. Rickets in children is a well-known effect of vitamin D deficiency. Light is also applied in the prevention and cure of other diseases (Sausville et al., 1971).

As compared with data on the therapeutic application of ultra-violet radiation, convincing quantitative data as regards the required dose from the point of view of public health are scarce. In zones where health may be threatened by a shortage of ultra-violet radiation, somewhat arbitrarily the erythemal effect on white people has been introduced as a measure of its biological effect: the dose needed to cause just perceptible reddening of the untanned skin has been designated 1 mpe (*minimum perceptible erythema*). This erythemal threshold (1 mpe) has been found to be 4,000 ± 2,000 Fe sec., in which 1 Fe ('erythemal finsen') corresponds to 0.1 watt/m² at the wavelength of maximum erythemal efficiency (i.e. 297 nm). A person sunbathing at sea-level when the sun's altitude is 60 degrees would reach the lower boundary of this threshold within about 10 minutes; at the sun's altitude of 30 degrees it would take about half an hour. For people who are deprived of natural ultra-violet radiation, e.g. because of high latitudes, a daily dose of $\frac{1}{4}$ to $\frac{3}{4}$ mpe on face and hands has been proposed as a standard (Dantsig et al., 1967). Meanwhile the relevance of the spectral erythemal efficiency concept is questioned by some authors because of possible biological interaction of radiation of various wavelengths (Thorington and Parescandola, 1967).

Two criteria are used for the maximum permissible dose of ultra-violet radiation: erythema and conjunctivitis.

Usual lamps, including fluorescent, mercury, and iodine lamps, at usual values of illuminance,[3] produce only a negligible fraction of the value recommended for those who are deprived of natural ultra-violet radiation.

In fluorescent light, even with the largest fraction of ultra-violet radiation, there is no danger of overdose within 8 hours of exposure as long as levels are lower than 5,000 lux.[4] The risk of conjunctivitis would exist only from 150,000 lux onwards. With xenon lamps 500 lux from, without adequate shielding, erythema may occur within approximately one hour; conjunctivitis may occur within 20 minutes.

From everyday experience we know that a bright environment, especially if the light is white or of a bluish tint, is conducive to bodily and mental activity, expansive behaviour and cheerfulness. For many people only a small amount of light is sufficient to keep them from getting to sleep or even to wake them up. On the other hand, darkness or dim light, especially of a warmer reddish colour, fosters relaxation.

Such phenomena could be explained by the hypothesis that the state of our vegetative and hormonal system depends upon the amount and composition of light: a great amount of light, especially if it is white or bluish, might stimulate the function of the sympathetic system, causing an *ergotropic* condition (raised peripheral blood circulation, muscular tone, and adrenaline secretion, resulting in a readiness for bodily action). In dim light and light of a reddish tint the vagus functions would be dominant, resulting in a so-called *histotropic* condition for relaxation and digestion.

Support for the above hypothesis has been found in a direct connexion between special cells in the periphery of the retina and the hypophysis, the centre in the midbrain which regulates the vegetative system (Assenmacher, 1966; Wurtman, 1968; Goromosov, 1968). Further indications have been found in the changes of various involuntary functions (blood circulation and composition, function of the thyroid gland, etc.) in people who either had gone blind or who had recovered from blindness (in both cases as far as the blindness had a peripheral cause, so that primarily the amount of light on the retina was affected).

This field of study may be of growing importance for the design of lighting installations: it offers possibilities for the design of lighting for specific moods and attitudes.

VISION WITH RESPECT TO LIGHTING
General

The most obvious function of light is that of being a medium for vision. Man's appreciation of his environment and his ability for controlling it depend to a great extent on his sense of vision. Burner (1966) estimated that 40 per cent. of the sensory information reaching the cortex is of visual origin; in 80–90 per cent. of our manual activities vision plays a part.

---

[1] Dr Schreuder wrote the section on 'Public Lighting'.
[2] 1 nm. (nanometer) = 10^{-9} m. (metre) = $10^{-9} \times 3.28$ ft
[3] A short explanation of physical terms is given in an appendix on p. 104.

[4] $1 \text{ lux} = 1 \frac{\text{lumen}}{\text{m.}^2} = 0.093 \frac{\text{lumen}}{\text{sq. ft}}$

The structure of our visual sensory organ and its many ways of adaptation enable man to carry out a wide variety of visual tasks. Thus he can perceive the form, detail, and colour of near and distant objects in a bright light by *photopic* vision, for which the cones in the fovea are used, or merely become aware of objects in his visual field by *scotopic* vision, if the light is dim, by making use of the rods which predominate in the peripheral parts of the retina.

Possibilities for adjustment to various circumstances are: *fixation* by movements of head and eyes, including a change in the mutual position of the latter (*convergence*), and by changes in the convexity of the lens (*accommodation*), according to the distance of the object. *Adaptation* to the brightness of the visual field, results primarily from the fact that, according to the brightness, the cones are connected with the brain in larger or smaller units (the latter condition rendering the possibility of discrimination of smaller detail). To a lesser extent it results from the pupil reflex controlling the pupil size.

Peripheral vision is essential for the guidance of eye movements and other automatic responses to the environment. Logan (1967) illustrates its significance as follows: a man without foveal vision would not be able to perform regular duties in an office or workshop; he would hardly be handicapped, however, in, for example, agricultural activities, and anyhow he would be able to find his way. On the other hand, a man without peripheral vision, could perform, e.g. an office task, but, missing the possibilities for orientation and adequate reflexes, he would be seriously handicapped in everyday life.

Visual Performance. A great number of visual tasks, for example, in office work, concerns stationary, flat, uncoloured objects, such as letters and figures. The speed, the accuracy, and the ease with which we can distinguish these objects depend—apart from the lighting—on many factors, such as: (1) the degree to which we are familiar with the objects (e.g. reading routine); (2) the configuration in which the object appears (e.g. word image); (3) our expectations regarding those configurations (e.g. familiarity with the terminology); and (4) the shape (e.g. the printing type).

When we leave these subtle factors out of consideration the visibility of an object under certain lighting conditions depends mainly on: (1) the size of the smallest detail to be perceived ('critical detail'); (2) the contrast with its background; and (3) the period of time that it is shown.

The following criteria for the power of vision ('visual functions') correspond with the above factors: (1) *visual acuity*; this is the reverse of the smallest perceptible detail; (2) *contrast sensitivity*; this is the reverse of the smallest perceptible contrast; and (3) *the speed of perception*; this is the reverse of the period of time necessary for a perception.

It appears that according to these three criteria, the eye—within practical limits of interior lighting—functions better as the luminance[1] of the background (for example, the sheet of paper; in experiments, often a screen of uniform luminance) is increased [FIG. 23]. In the case of a given reflectance of the background and adequate direction of the light this means

that vision is better as the lighting level is raised. A reference curve on contrast sensitivity and other tools for evaluating visual performance were agreed upon by CIE (1972).

In simple eye-tasks maximum *visual performance* (the speed and accuracy of perception) will occur at relatively low levels,

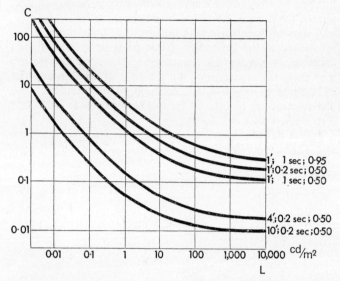

FIG. 23. Required contrast (*C*) as a function of background luminance (*L*) (Blackwell, 1967).
    Object: luminous disc; binocular vision; natural pupil; age group: graduate students.
    Parameters: size (minutes of arc); presentation time (seconds); chance of perception.

for example, 250–500 lux.[2] All kinds of usual work (reading, etc.), however, are taxing our visual power to such a degree that the optimal lighting levels are much higher than can be realized artificially with due observance of the requirements as regards quality, heat removal, and costs. So, from the point of view of visual performance, the highest level which can be realized without creating unfavourable secondary conditions is the best one. In other words, at least in the case of objects which are difficult to perceive (such as, for instance, small print, poor

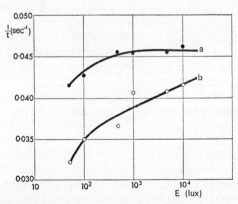

FIG. 24. Performance in a search task as a function of illuminance (*E*) (Muck and Bodmann, 1961).
    Task: finding two-digit numbers spread at random over a sheet of paper.
    Performance: reciprocal of average time needed (*t*).
    Size of numbers: 1·6 mm; 13 minutes of arc (critical detail: 2·6 minutes of arc).
    Curve *a*: contrast 0·93; $r_{paper} = 0.78$.
    Curve *b*: contrast 0·63; $r_{paper} = 0.11$.

[1] The luminance of an object is somewhat related to the 'brightness' we attribute to it. However, both concepts are not identical: objects with the same luminance may appear more or less bright according to other luminances in the surroundings, or to luminances which were in the field of view shortly before. For a diffusely reflecting surface (e.g. matt paper) the luminance is proportionate to its illuminance and its reflectance.
[2] 1 lux = 0·0929 fc

photocopies, pencil writing, etc.) we need more data than from this field of investigation for determining a scientifically justified level.

The above results of laboratory tests with regard to the effect of background luminance on the visual functions are supported by those of more realistic experiments, such as have been performed by Weston (1962) and by others [FIG. 24].

A start has been made with the investigation of some factors mentioned at the beginning of this paragraph, for example, concerning the extra time or extra illuminance required for the step from the sensation of the presence of an object to the recognition of its shape, as a function of the complexity and the number of objects to be distinguished (Meshkov and Faermark, 1967).

Effect of Age. Visual power largely depends on age [FIG. 25]. This is caused by the slackening of muscles and by changes

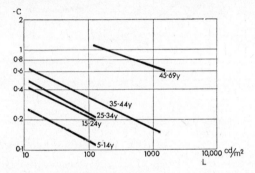

FIG. 25. Effect of age upon vision (Fortuin, 1951). Threshold contrast (C) as a function of background luminance (L). Landolt rings; opening 1 minute of arc; presentation time unlimited.

Parameter: age in years.

in the optical media, such as the lens and vitreous humour. The slackening of the muscles is a phenomenon of ageing in the conventional sense; the ageing of the optical media, however, starts before birth, namely at the moment that the blood supply to this organ stops.

Influence of Luminances in the Environment. 1. *Non-uniform Visual Field; Induction; Brightness Scales.* Investigation of the effect of light sources in the periphery of the field of vision on the foveal perception (called, *inter alia*, 'induction' or 'disability glare') has opened up the possibility to calculate contrast sensitivities etc. for any non-uniform field (Moon and Spencer, 1945; CIE, 1972; Bodmann, 1973).

Brightness scales show how the brightness impression caused by a certain luminance may be estimated quantitatively from the luminances in the visual field (Marsden, 1970; Kobayashi, 1970).

2. *Changing Visual Field; Adaptation.* The above phenomenon of induction relates to a stationary condition. Often the field of vision is not only structured but also varying, either owing to moving objects or because we look in various directions in succession, for example, when, during reading, we look up for a moment, possibly out of the window. When, in the latter case, we again look at our work our adaptation condition will have changed and a re-adaptation gradually occurs. The course of the contrast sensitivity in such adaptation and the phenomenon of after-images associated with it have been studied, *inter alia*, with a view to effective lighting

of entrances and exits of tunnels. They also play a part in the case of temporary darkening of lecture rooms for the projection of slides, etc. The effect can be described as a succession of adaptation conditions, characterized by different adaptation luminances (Schreuder, 1964; Boynton, 1969).

The Effect of the Incidence of Light; Contrast Rendering. The direction of incidence of light which so clearly plays a part in the perception of three-dimensional objects (shadow casting and modelling), also affects the visibility of flat objects. The effect, which is often underestimated, is illustrated in FIGURE 26. It should be borne in mind that this loss of contrast is a purely physical phenomenon (not entoptic as in the case of disability glare).

The effect of such a loss of contrast for the perception is equal to a loss of contrast sensitivity, either by direct glare or by a reduced background luminance. The practical consequence of the loss of contrast can therefore be expressed in terms of extra illuminance required.

It can be seen from FIGURE 23 that within the range of relevant luminances and sizes a loss of contrast of 1 per cent. may require about 15 per cent. extra illuminance for compensation (in order to have the same chance of seeing for a certain object within the same time of presentation). Contrast losses of 20 per cent. or more, with regard to the optimal situation, are no exception in offices, etc. A loss of 20 per cent. would require an extra illuminance which is three times the existing one; in other words, it means that only one-fourth of the illuminance is utilized. At best this effect would mean that the perception of

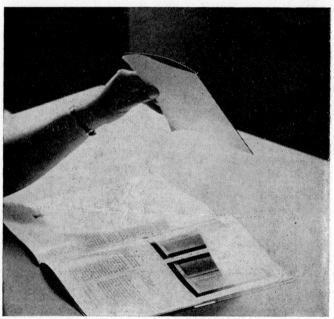

FIG. 26. Contrast loss due to specular reflections; 'less light, more sight'.

a certain object is more difficult; for an already critical object it may mean, however, that it can no longer be seen at all. Even when the object remains visible, an increased effort is required, delay and mistakes may occur.

COLOURED OBJECTS; COLOUR RENDERING

The appearance of coloured objects differs with the spectral composition of the light they receive. Though it is difficult to tell what is the *real* colour of an object, we can, and do, appreciate whether relevant colours have a *natural* appearance; in other words, whether the 'colour rendering' is adequate. Apparently, when making such a judgement we have some standard in our mind, though usually not explicitly. In many cases this standard is some form of natural light. However, daylight itself varies in spectral composition and therefore in colour rendering. Furthermore, in all kinds of ordinary situations we unconsciously use other standards: we have learned by experience to accept in certain circumstances appearances which differ very much from those in any kind of daylight.

The appearance is a result of our interpretation; it is apparently determined to a large extent by our expectations which, in their turn, depend upon the situation and upon the shapes we perceive.

According to a standardization by the *Commission Internationale de l'Éclairage* (CIE), the colour rendering qualities of light sources are characterized by the combination of: (1) the colour temperature of a relevant reference source; and (2) the index of colour rendering, *i*.

The colour temperature of a source is the temperature of the so called 'black-body',[1] at which the latter produces radiation of the same spectral composition as the source does. Colour temperatures are expressed in Kelvin (K), defined by T (K) = t (Centigrade) + 273.

The index of colour rendering, *i*, expresses the degree to which the colour-rendering qualities (according to measurement with a standard set of colour samples) approach those of the reference source. This degree is expressed in a scale where the reference source scores 100.

Sources with an index of ≥95 have a colour rendition which for all practical purposes may be considered equal to that of the reference source. The difference will be visible only by direct comparison. If $i = 90—94$ the difference will be noticed only by highly skilled specialists.

Specifying the colour index only makes sense when at the same time the reference source is characterized by its colour temperature.

Effort and Fatigue, Comfort and Discomfort in Vision

Criteria other than the possibility of visual perception have been used in the evaluation of visual situations.

1. One of them is the effort needed for a certain visual activity. Investigators in this field were faced with the problem of assessing effort. The usual solution was to assess symptoms of either 'visual' or 'central fatigue' at the end of the experiment. Variation in performance during the experiment has also been used as an indication (Khek and Krivohlavy, 1966). For a more direct assessment of effort, visual tasks were considered to require more effort the less they left the subject able to perform simultaneously, a second, non-visual task (Schouten *et al.*, 1962).

As far as optimum levels from the point of view of effort or fatigue have been shown significantly, they do not contradict the conclusion, drawn previously from visual performance tests, that, within practical limits of interior lighting, vision is better as the luminance of the background is increased.

2. Other investigations have concerned the subjective appreciation of levels (or background luminances) by occupants in field situations or by subjects in laboratory tests or simulated offices. According to the latter investigations, 1,000–2,000 lux must be considered optimal for usual work rooms. Optima are flat and depend upon experimental conditions (Fischer, 1970; Range, 1971).

3. The concept 'discomfort glare' is often met in appraisals of lighting situations. It has been defined as 'glare which causes discomfort, without necessarily impairing the vision of objects'. It covers a variety of sensations which may result from—absolutely or relatively—high luminances in the visual field. In order to 'prevent further complications' the effect of possible visual tasks upon the judgement has been left out of account. In spite of the loose definition, a fair amount of agreement exists about how to calculate the degree of discomfort glare from the luminance pattern. Some findings are shown in the following paragraphs on interior lighting.

INTERIOR LIGHTING
GENERAL REQUIREMENTS

An interior lighting system, either natural or artificial, generally has the dual purpose of providing: (1) adequate visibility of the specific eye tasks (such as small print, embroidery, facial expression); and (2) adequate visual impression of the environment (amenity).

In both respects a certain *quantity* of light will be needed, but the question whether the quantity is sufficient only makes sense provided that the light is of the right *quality*.

Requirements of quality can be classed as follows: (1) luminance patterns, including the limitation and possible avoidance of glare; (2) direction, including ratio of diffused to direct light and the angle of incidence of the direct light.

On the directional characteristics of the lighting depend: (2a) Contrast rendering, i.e. the limitation of specular reflections causing loss of contrast and visibility [see p. 90]. This is of special importance for the visibility of flat tasks (reading, etc.). (2b) Modelling, i.e. the appropriate rendering of three-dimensional shapes, be it as a part of the specific task or as a part of the environment.

(3) Colour and colour rendering. (4) Degree of constancy.

Apart from visual requirements, lighting provisions should be such that they meet *general requirements* as regards safety, avoidance of annoyance from noise or excessive heat, and as regards possibilities for maintenance.

The aspects mentioned above have to be considered equally in the case of artificial and of natural lighting, as well as in the case of combination of the two systems.

ARTIFICIAL LIGHTING OF WORK ENVIRONMENTS[2]

Limitation of Glare; Luminance Patterns

Discomfort Glare. A method has been developed by the American Illuminating Engineering Society for the computation of the *visual comfort probability* (VCP) for a certain installation, i.e. the percentage of people who will consider the glare not worse than on the *border between comfort and discomfort* (BCD).

---

[1] i.e. a body absorbing all incident radiation; a small opening in a closed vessel or furnace is a good approximation.

[2] The paragraphs marked * largely apply to daylighting as well. Much applies to other environments as, for example, schools. As regards specific environments, the reader is referred to the list of further reading.

Various simplified methods have been developed, of course with some sacrifice as regards accuracy or range of applicability: the British 'glare index' system, the American 'scissors curve', the method recommended by the International Labour Office (1965), and Söllner's method, shown in FIGURE 27. A

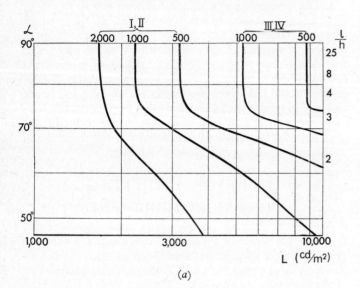

(a)

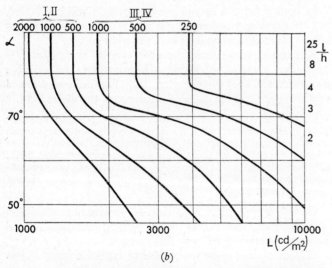

(b)

FIG. 27. Permissible luminance (*L*) of fittings for tubular fluorescent lamps as a function of the radiant angle (α) with the downward vertical, or as a function of the ratio of the length (*l*) of the room and its height (*h*), measured from eye level (Söllner c.s.).

Roman numerals correspond to classes of rooms as regards visual requirements [see TABLE 36].
Parameters: illuminance on the working plane (lux).

(a) Applies to fittings with no side radiation, e.g. recessed fittings, irrespective of the direction of mounting and to fittings with side radiation which are installed parallel to the direction of view.
(b) Applies to fittings with side radiation, installed at right angles to the direction of view.

compilation of the various methods has been given by Einhorn (1971).

As can be shown by glare evaluations, the use of unscreened fluorescent lamps should be restricted to rooms with low requirements as regards vision and amenity, or relatively high rooms (length and width less than twice the mounting height

of the fittings above eye level). Sometimes joists may offer sufficient screening.

For luminous ceilings the luminance at angles ⩾45 degrees with the normal should be limited to 500 cd/m². (According to American standards about 800 cd/m² would be permissible.)

Indirect discomfort glare caused by reflection of light sources should be controlled by avoidance of glossy surfaces. Especially in the case of large windows, the use of curtains or blinds at night is recommended in this respect. Apart from possible indirect glare from reflected light sources, they may prevent an unfavourable luminance pattern caused by the darkness outside. Moreover, if a light colour is chosen they contribute to the level and to directional qualities.

Disability Glare; Induction. It is improbable that installations will cause direct disability glare to a person looking on a horizontal task. Especially in low or deep rooms, however, inadequate luminances of light sources may impair vision in other directions. The effect can easily be assessed by screening the eyes by hand against direct light from the lamps: the improvement in vision may be tremendous.

Further Recommendations as Regards Luminance Patterns.* In order to avoid fatigue and discomfort by sudden or frequent re-adaptation, some limitations are to be set to luminance differences encountered when we look or move from one place to another. A rule-of-thumb method is generally applied—that the luminance of the visual task and its immediate surroundings should not differ by more than a factor 3, and those of the visual task and the periphery (e.g. floors and walls) should not differ by more than a factor 10.

This rule is founded on an assumption as regards just tolerable losses in contrast sensitivity or visual acuity as a result of incomplete adaptation when we are looking around. It is to be understood that large luminance ratios resulting from eye movements would cause repeated adaptation, and therefore eye fatigue.

The impression from everyday experience is that, for desks, etc., the factor 3 in the first part could be exceeded without objection: desk reflectances as low as 0·07 will not cause visual problems.

Contrast Rendering *

An important and often neglected aspect of a lighting situation is its contrast rendering. It is often underestimated to what extent, and with what consequences for task visibility and visual comfort, lighting situations may differ in this respect. The phenomenon of loss of contrast by specular reflections, interfering with adequate vision, is best known from the experience with glossy magazines. However, such reflections are not restricted to glossy surfaces. More subtle effects with dull paper, due to its texture, may also cause eye strain and fatigue.

The visual effect of loss of contrast of printed or pencil text as a result of specular reflections was shown quantitatively in a previous paragraph. It follows from that consideration that it makes little sense to specify lighting levels (required or attained) unless some account is given of the degree of contrast rendering, preferably in quantitative terms, e.g. 'contrast rendering factor' (CIE, 1972).

The effect can easily be checked in practical situations by shielding the light from sources in questionable positions [FIG. 26] or by turning a piece of printed matter in various directions.

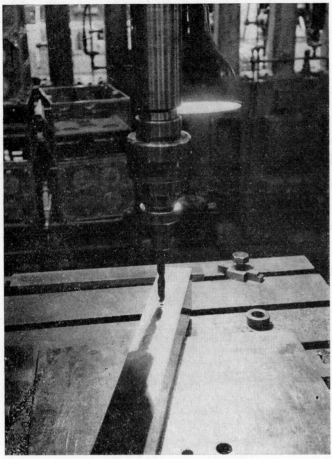

FIG. 28. Improved contrast by specular reflections.

In some situations, especially with three-dimensional objects, the effect may be used to enhance visibility [FIG. 28], but for flat tasks such as reading it should be avoided as far as possible.

Recommendations for the limitation of contrast losses are: (1) Adequate shielding of light sources, taking into account usual viewing angles towards desk tasks, etc. Matters are still complicated by the fact that many reading tasks and the like in

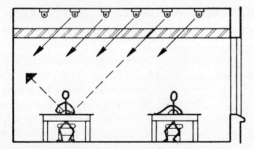

FIG. 29. Shielding of lamps, such that specular reflection towards the eyes is prevented (Lowson, 1965).

offices are not in a horizontal plane. An example of adequate shielding is given in FIGURE 29. (2) Adequate mutual arrangement of the light sources and desks [FIG. 30]. (3) Adequate amount of diffuse light, by using materials with high reflectance for the finish of ceiling and walls. (4) Use of large sources with

low luminance. (5) Use of polarizing materials in luminaires or in luminous ceilings. However, for the time being, its practical possibilities are limited.

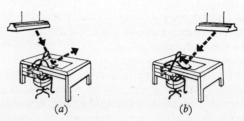

FIG. 30. Adequate (a) and inadequate (b) mutual arrangement of desks and luminaires (Lowson, 1965).

(a) Specular reflections away from the eyes; (b) specular reflections towards the eyes.

Modelling, Shape Rendering ★

Both for the sake of visibility of specific eye tasks, especially three-dimensional objects, and for that of an adequate general visual environment a certain degree of 'modelling' is required, to be caused by the interplay of light and shadow. Unless sufficient attention is paid to this aspect, shadows may be either too 'soft' or too 'harsh'.

Until recently no quantitative data about this aspect were available, so that it had to be dealt with only in a qualitative way. According to a rule of thumb the illuminance on a vertical plane should be at least $\frac{1}{4}$ of that on the horizontal plane. Lynes et al. (1967) examined which degrees of modelling are considered 'preferable' or within 'acceptable limits'. They showed that this qualitative aspect can be analysed in quantitative physical terms ('vector-scalar ratio'). Further research is needed, however.

Colour

Requirements as regards the colour of the light will as a rule originate from the two points of view mentioned earlier: (1) the specific eye tasks, related to the work to be performed; and (2) the amenity of the room.

From both points of view it is not merely the colour quality of the light that counts but also the colour pattern of walls, objects, etc. For an adequate visual environment both these factors have to be matched carefully. This requires mutual consultation and understanding between the designer of the colour pattern and the lighting designer.

The Colour Pattern.★ The appreciation of the colour pattern of a room will differ for various individuals. Cultural differences in this respect, affected by climate, tradition, or fashion, may easily be found. In spite of this, the following is considered to apply more or less generally.

According to their psychological effect, colours may be classified into a scale from 'warm' (e.g. red, yellow) to 'cool' (e.g. bluish-green, blue). Warm colours are recommended where a 'cool' impression is to be avoided (e.g. reception rooms or a room receiving little sunshine). Cool colours, on the other hand, are recommended where a suggestion of coolness may contribute to the amenity. Other psychological effects are the tendency of saturated and warm colours to appear closer, and of cool tints to appear more distant than they are. To a certain extent this offers possibilities for psychological 'correction' of unfavourable room proportions. Analogous effects are reached by colour contrasts: a pattern of very different colours makes a room look smaller; a more delicate pattern with soft contrasts contributes to the impression of space.

Apart from their influence upon the apparent size of a room and its warmer or cooler character, colours may contribute to a quiet impression in the case of minor contrasts of unsaturated and cool colours or, on the other hand, to vivacity in the opposite case. In this respect size and location of the coloured surfaces are important factors. It is often advised, especially in higher latitudes, that for the sake of a harmonious environment saturated colours be restricted to small surfaces.

A start has been made with experimental analysis of colour preferences for various environments (Judd, 1969; Inui, 1969).

The Colour of the Light. When speaking about the colour of the light we generally do not mean saturated colours, but various shades (e.g. yellowish, reddish, or bluish) of more or less 'white' light as produced by various light sources. Our appreciation of the colour of the light depends upon the lighting level. More yellowish or reddish light of incandescent lamps or 'warm white' fluorescent lamps is preferred at low and moderate levels respectively. At the levels used in modern offices incandescent light will, as a rule, be considered too yellowish. For exceptionally high levels, as for example, 3,000 lux, 'white' or even 'daylight' fluorescent lamps are preferred to the 'warm white' type.

Colour Rendering. Requirements of colour rendering may concern: (1) adequate appearance of the colour pattern of the environment; (2) adequate appearance of certain objects (e.g. textiles, paints or foods in stores); and (3) the possibility of distinguishing slight differences within a certain colour (e.g. judging human complexion in medicine).

In terms of the recent standardization by the International Commission on Illumination (CIE) practical requirements may be illustrated as follows:

TABLE 33

Requirements of Colour Rendering

Examples of rooms (or activities)	Colour temperature of the reference source required in K*	Required colour rendering index
Rating colours of textile, tobacco, paint, colour prints, etc.	6,500–7,400	90
Medical test or treatment†, art galleries, printing shops	ca. 4,000	90
Offices and workshops, stores, storehouses where goods have to be classed according to colour	ca. 4,000	80
Food stores, reception and conference rooms	ca. 3,000	80
Corridors, staircases, storehouses	ca. 3,000	50

* Colour temperatures [see p. 89] are expressed in Kelvin (K); $T(K) = t\ (^\circ C) + 273$.
† 3,200 K is preferred in case of relatively low lighting levels.

Bellchambers (1971) has shown that interiors with 'improved colour' fluorescent lamps, equal visual satisfaction is gained at lower levels than with 'high efficiency' lamps. The effect is such that to a fair extent it compensates for the lower efficiency

(provided, of course, that the illuminances are sufficient for the visual tasks). Preliminary findings by Rowlands *et al.* (1971) suggest that above a minimum level of say 300 lux, the use of lamps with good colour-rendering at the same power per unit area as high efficiency lamps, will despite the difference in illuminance, not result in reduced visual performance. According to this hypothesis, for which further evidence is needed, good colour rendering might be obtained without increased cost.

Constancy

Complaints about flicker of fluorescent light are still to be heard occasionally. Hopkinson and Collins (1963) found that the degree of discomfort from flicker increased with the size of surfaces (e.g. drawing desks) and with luminance. It increased rapidly when the frequency decreased below 70 c/sec. Gradina (1966) showed an effect of flicker upon general and visual fatigue from performance of a difficult visual task.

The basic fact underlying the cause of flicker in fluorescent light and its prevention, is that the gaseous discharges follow the alternations of the electric current. A current of 50 Hz causes 100 discharges per second. For most eyes this frequency is too high to be perceptible. If the coating of fluorescent tubes were indeed only fluorescent, their radiation would show the same alternations. However, they are 'phosphorescent' (i.e. emitting light after being irradiated) to such an extent that the gap between two subsequent discharges is overlapped. The ends of the tube are critical as regards causation of flicker, because of the fact that the electrodes change roles only once in a cycle, thus causing a change of the so-called 'dark space' from one end to the other with a frequency of only 50 c/sec.

People differ in sensitiveness to flicker. Generally speaking, however, complaints will usually be prevented by: (1) adequate combination of control gear for each pair of lamps, 'lead-lag circuits'; (2) installing tubes so that their adjacent electrodes are oppositely connected with the supply; (3) shielding the ends of the tube; and (4) replacement in due time, as flicker occurs more often with old tubes.

Absolute elimination of flicker is, of course, an additional advantage of the use of high frequencies (about 10,000 c/sec.), as is occasionally practised for the sake of improved output. In such installations special attention is required to the prevention of noise (high pitches).

Miscellaneous Health Aspects of Artificial Light

It still happens that certain visual and other discomfort is attributed to fluorescent light. There is no evidence, nor any reason to expect, that by its spectral composition it might be harmful to the sense of vision or in any other respect. Incidentally, increased eye fatigue and conjunctivitis have been found which disappeared when the people were working with incandescent light. However, it could be shown in such cases that the symptoms were not caused by the spectral composition of the fluorescent light, but by an inadequate application, for example, unfavourable incidence of the light resulting in excessive need for visual effort.

Levels of Illuminance

For many years the 'illuminance on the workplane' has been considered the most important characteristic—if not the only one—to specify a lighting installation.

Consequently, much attention was paid to the required illuminance, as may be shown from the great number of investigations in this field, and from the many highly specified recommendations for various activities. As far as attention was paid to other aspects of lighting, it was often the even distribution of illuminance over the workplane that was considered next.

At the same time, only rarely attention was paid to the real plane in which the work was situated, let alone to the question whether the work was two-dimensional at all. As a rule the—often imaginary—plane at 0·80 or 1·00 m. above floor level was considered to be the workplane.

Nowadays a shift in emphasis is to be noticed towards the other aspects, which have been discussed so far. Various reasons for this trend will be clear from the previous paragraphs. For example, in many instances the required quantity of light is not determined by the specific job requirements but by requirements of amenity; the illuminance on the workplane is not an adequate criterion for this aspect. Even with regard to task visibility, the effect of other aspects (e.g. the degree of contrast rendering and possibly modelling) is so dominant that it makes only sense to specify levels, provided that the quality is specified with corresponding accuracy.

As is illustrated in TABLE 34 below, recommended levels for the same job show remarkable differences for various countries.

The unavoidable arbitrariness in recommendations is often disguised by choosing the levels to be recommended according to a certain degree of visibility of the task, e.g. 'at least 90 per cent. relative visual performance' or '99 per cent. visual accuracy or chance of seeing'. The choice among such percentages might be determined by specific aspects of the task, e.g. the consequences of mistakes. As this is not practised, it merely reflects in a disguised way the current perceptions as mentioned above.

In TABLE 36 the Dutch recommendations on lighting levels are given as an illustration. As compared with other recommendations, the levels are neither extremely high nor extremely low. They are only defined for four classes of rooms and within a large margin. Further specification was considered neither necessary nor justified.

Apart from class IV ('rooms not continuously used for work') there are three classes. Because of the trend towards more administrative jobs and more automation, a large and growing number of workrooms fall within class II ('general offices and the like'). The recommended levels (of 500–1,000 lux) for this class were considered those levels which, according to the present-day lighting technique, can be reached within reasonable limits of quality (e.g. limitation of glare and heat), on the one hand, and cost (under conditions in the Netherlands), on the other.

Class I contains jobs with higher requirements as regards eye task. Here further specification of levels would be misleading as long as this cannot be done for other aspects which are at least as critical.

TABLE 34
Comparison of Recommended Levels (Lux)

	France 1961	Germany 1963	United Kingdom 1961	Sweden 1962	U.S.A. 1959	U.S.S.R. 1959 (fluoresc.)
1. Workshops:						
Rough	200	60–120	150	300	500	100–150
Extra fine	1,500	600–1,000	1,500	4,000	10,000	750–3,000
2. Offices	300	120–500	300	300–1,000	1,000–1,500	200–300

Moreover, as is illustrated in TABLE 35, a large increase is to be seen during the course of years.

TABLE 35
Recommended Levels (Lux) in the United States for Fine Assembly Work

1910	1916	1925	1945	1952	1959
50	100	250	500	1,000	5,000

The explanation for these large differences according to country and time is as follows:

Optimum levels, as regards amenity or visual performance [p. 87] are such that, more often than not, the cost of realization with due regard to visual and thermal comfort are prohibitive, so that a compromise is required. Actually the choice is not merely a matter of visual performance or comfort on the one hand and cost on the other; it also depends on expectations as regards the effects of lighting upon morale, productivity and—last but not least—prestige, and on the value attributed to the various factors mentioned. Recommendations are more or less self-fulfilling anticipations for a certain country and period as regard such compromises.

Class III contains rooms for work with less requirements as regards eye task. At the same time, a lower level of amenity is usually accepted here. This is a matter of convention and partly related to the fact that in these environments (usually very large, high rooms with low reflection factors) higher levels than 250–500 lux, if possible, would be too expensive.

TABLE 36
Classification of Rooms and Recommended Levels
(Netherlands Foundation for Illumination, 1967)

Class	Description	Examples	Recommended illumination
I	Details up to the limit of vision have to be observed for long periods at a stretch	Fine drawing work, precision tool making, ready-made clothing industry, miniaturization in electronic industry	1,000 lux or over*
II	Rooms or activities not covered by classes I, III, or IV	Normal reading and writing work, classroom, conference room, office, engineering fitting shop, car assembly, washrooms, toilets	500–1,000 lux
III	Observation of small details not usually necessary	Stores, forge, engineering workshop	250–500 lux
IV	Rooms not continuously used for work	Storage rooms, garage	125–250 lux

* If necessary by means of general lighting supplemented with local lighting.

The levels specified are those, averaged over that part of the room in which work is regularly performed and over the normal period of use of the lamps. A ratio of minimum to maximum illumination of at least 0·7 is recommended. Allowance was made for the presence of workers up to 65 years of age. This does not exclude, however, the possibility that some may need additional local lighting.

For windowless rooms, relatively high levels are recommended. In the Soviet Union, for example, an extra illuminance of 30–50 per cent. is recommended where people are working in time shifts, and 100–200 per cent. in case of the traditional working day. (It should be kept in mind that normal levels recommended in this country are moderate.) In the Dutch recommendations, shown above, a minimum of 500 lux is recommended for rooms without daylight.

The basic idea is that in daylit rooms illumination levels may considerably exceed the minimum design levels. Thus with the same design value the actual levels would be larger in the daylit rooms. It is necessary to compensate for this effect in rooms with artificial light only, if it were only for the impression when one enters the room.

Artificial Lighting During Daytime

In a large and increasing number of cases artificial light is used during daytime, be it exclusively or combined with daylight. Daytime use of artificial lighting offers broader possibilities than natural lighting only, in the following respects: (1) adequate lighting conditions (luminance pattern, levels, incidence, colour, evenness, and, if desired, constancy); (2) economy (building cost, running cost, utilization of building site and inner space, e.g. higher buildings, deeper rooms, lower ceilings) and (3) various other aspects of design (climate control, protection from traffic noise, construction).

Neglecting the fact that in all kinds of daylit work-rooms artificial lighting is used more during the day than it is at night, it is common practice that first the architect designs for daylight exclusively and later on the design for artificial lighting is made as if it were intended for use at night only. It is a requirement for good building design that the first sketch is based on an optimum decision as regards the relative contribution of natural and artificial lighting during daytime. This requires early co-operation of architect, lighting engineer, and other specialists.

In the history of building, the possibility of artificial lighting in daytime is only recent. In such a recent development, caution is required against prejudices, be they conservatism or modernism. For nearly all types of room it makes sense to consider the pros and cons of alternative daytime conditions for lighting and vision. The result may be anywhere between the extremes of 'natural light only' and 'windowless room'. The existing data (e.g. van Noort, 1965) do not show any general physiological reason for restriction. However, there are psychological reasons: visual contact with outside is appreciated to such an extent that, as regards rooms for regular and continued use, windows should not be given up lightly (see p. 96, Daylighting and Windows).

On the other hand the application of artificial light, even in rooms with ample daylight, shows that its contribution to vision and amenity is appreciated as well. Therefore a well balanced combination of windows and artificial lighting may deserve consideration (e.g. for workrooms, classrooms, and wards with more than 6 m. in depth).

Important aspects in such integrated design are the luminance pattern, the incidence of the light, and the colour matching. The adaptation luminance during daytime may be high, for example, because of the high luminances seen through the window. With the same illumination an object may look less bright in daylight than it does in artificial light, and visibility of objects and people may be insufficient by day [Fig. 31 (a)]. Therefore, as regards the *luminance pattern*, the paradox should be considered that the more daylight that is admitted, the more artificial light is needed [Fig. 31 (b)].

Harmonizing the *incidence* of artificial light with that of daylight does not necessarily mean that the two directions should coincide, because the artificial light may compensate short-comings of the daylight in modelling and reflections. Neither is it necessary, as has been thought, that the *colour* of artificial light is as close as possible to that of the daylight. Some types of fluorescent lamps (namely with a colour temperature ⩽4,000 K and a colour rendition index ⩾80) harmonize with daylight and are suited for use at night as well. However, reflectances of walls, etc., should also be considered. Incandescent lamps are less suited for combined use with daylight, not only because of their colour characteristics but also because of their relatively low luminous efficacy.

Lighting in Relation to other Environmental Factors

A trend exists towards *integrated design*, dealing with visual, thermal, and acoustical conditions as interrelated aspects of the environment. From the lighting angle attention is called to the following consequences: (1) output of lamps is improved by better control of their temperature; (2) heat from lamps in central parts of the building may be utilized in peripheral parts; and (3) integrated design contributes to a rational decision as regards window sizes and artificial lighting levels.

Full discussion of integrated physical environments is beyond the scope of this chapter. The reader is referred to 'Fundamentals of physical environment' in CIE Proceedings (1971).

Attention is called to another trend towards an integrated approach to the environment: a tendency to supplement the ('psychophysical') search for simple physical criterion, expected to account for people's responses to specific environmental factors, with a ('psychological') search for their feelings and behaviour with respect to the (visual and spatial) environment (e.g. a room or building) as a whole. The trend is characterized by an increased interest in field studies (including observation and 'open ended' questions). (Bitter, 1967; van Ierland, 1970; Markus et al., 1972.)

Finally there is a trend towards an integrated concern for the environment in a broader sense, including the control of available energy and other resources (Dorsey, 1973; Kovach, 1973). This may imply that some recommendations and practices reported in this chapter will have to be reconsidered.

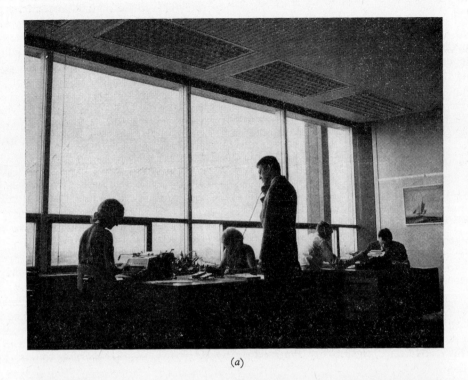

(a)

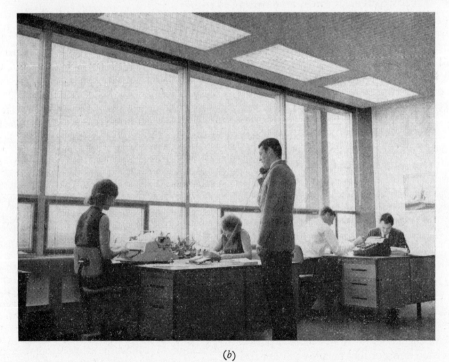

(b)

FIG. 31. 'The more daylight is admitted, the more artificial light is needed.' (Visual impressions simulated in photographs.)

DAYLIGHTING AND WINDOWS
Function and Needs

We do not depend any more on daylight for *lighting our work*. By the present standards the level that can be achieved with daylight is inadequate in a great and increasing number of situations. The belief that daylight would be 'better for the eyes' than artificial light is rather popular. Virtually no facts are known as yet to corroborate this view.

Neither is there much evidence that daylight in interiors is irreplaceable with regard to its *biological effects*. It may be questioned whether people in interiors would profit from it, because of the low daylight levels indoors and because of the nearly complete absorption of ultra-violet radiation by window glass. However, Bochenkova (1968) concluded from a comparative study of groups performing similar jobs that 'operators in premises without natural light developed some changes of arterial pressure and non-specific immunity'.

There is a fair agreement among experts that nowadays the main functions of the window are of a psychological nature. Consequently, the needs in this respect are not universal, but they depend upon climate, culture, designation of the rooms and habits of the occupants. The dominant need is for visual contact with the outside world. Beyond that, and again dependent on circumstances, daylight and possibly sunlight are appreciated for their abundance, their colour and directional qualities and their variety.

With regard to the above, experiences with windowless buildings are relevant. It can be argued (Manning, 1963) that people do work in windowless factories, artificially lit offices, department stores and underground railways without, it seems, suffering any ill effects or causing any difficulties for their employees which can be attributed to the artificial conditions, but this does not seem to be the whole story. Complaints have been reported by Mikhailova and Sviridov (1967) after a survey in seventy-two factories. Van Noort (1965), after a study in seven European countries, reported that 'sometimes workers had complained, but that in the majority of such cases the cause of the complaints was to be found in other circumstances'. He concluded that further and more profound investigation might perhaps reveal unfavourable physical or psychological effects of continued work in artificial environments, but that up till now there was no evidence of this kind.

Though favourable experiences have been reported about some experimental windowless school rooms, there is some factual support for the criticism they meet: it has been shown from drawings, that children in such schools were more concerned about windows than those in traditional school rooms (Karmel, 1965).

In small rooms used for regular stays for an extended period of time, a window is needed in order that people shall not feel locked-in or restricted in their contact with the outside world.

Questions remain with regard to the appreciation of 'vision strips'—relatively small windows, designed to provide an outside view only, which are not expected to contribute essentially to the lighting—in artificially lit work rooms. Experiences differ, presumably not only according to design but also according to circumstances such as culture, type of work and workers, atmosphere within the organization, etc.

It has been suggested that a series of vertical vision strips may be preferable to the normal horizontal type, as they offer the possibility of seeing all relevant parts of the outside scene, which is essentially structured horizontally.

Ne'eman and Hopkinson (1970) found for work rooms with permanent artificial lighting that the permissible minimum window size did not depend upon photometrical conditions (such as daylight factors) but upon the angle from which relevant outside objects are seen.

With regard to the required penetration of sunlight into various rooms within dwellings, data have been gathered in Sweden, the United Kingdom, the Netherlands (Bitter and van Ierland, 1967) and Switzerland (Barrier and Gilgen, 1970). Evidence was found for human adaptability in this respect: preferences appeared to be affected by the situation to which people were accustomed. For many people, it is essential for a night's rest that any natural or artificial light is kept out of sleeping rooms.

Spaces for *recreation* are, generally speaking, designed for temporary use. In many cases spaces without daylight or windows are accepted as a matter of course; however, in the case of gymnasiums or indoor sports windows are sometimes recommended. The windowless building is, however, usually to be preferred here, because of better control of luminances in the numerous directions of vision (not to mention its advantages with regard to the cost of air conditioning and the prevention of condensation) (Van Ierland, and van de Linden, 1970).

Codes and Recommendations

Recommendations for Minimum Daylighting. Many rules or recommendations with regard to natural lighting or windows for houses, schools, offices, or factories concern a certain *minimal access of natural light*. Often their original purpose is to ensure that during the normal daytime, or a certain percentage of it, the lighting level at work is at least equal to a certain value, for example, that which is (or once was) recommended for the type of work.

Apart from the fact that many lighting levels which are now recommended cannot, or only for a few hours, be guaranteed with daylight, the value of this effort is but relative for the following reasons:

1. The lighting level is not a warranted criterion for the visibility of the task, unless accompanied by a criterion for the quality of the light. Under certain circumstances the illuminance at which an object is clearly visible in the evening in artificial light can be insufficient during the day, because in the latter case one is adapted to higher luminances than in the evening. In other circumstances, particularly in daylight from one side, less light will be needed, because the contrast rendition is more favourable than in artificial light.

2. The lighting levels, and also the luminances of the light sources, may increase during daylight (still apart from direct sunlight) to a multiple of the design value. Depending on the spatial constellation, this may be an advantage or a disadvantage from the visual point of view.

3. In many situations natural light becomes less important as the provision with artificial light becomes better and cheaper.

Apart from town planning codes, in terms of minimum distances and maximum heights of building, etc., recommendations of this kind, specified according to purposes for which the rooms are to be used, may be framed in the following terms:

1. *Proportion of Glass Area to Floor or Façade Area.* In the past rules have been drawn up in terms of the proportion of glass area to floor or front area. These criteria have the advantage of a terminology which is conventional to architects, which makes it easier to check during the design of the building, or in existing buildings, whether the regulation has been complied with. Generally speaking, however, these proportions do not form a suitable criterion for the lighting level on the working plane, because these levels depend, in addition, on: (1) the shape of the room; (2) location and shape of the openings for daylight; (3) the kind of glazing; (4) the pollution of the window; (5) obstructions; and (6) reflections, either 'external' from obstructions or 'internal' from ceiling, walls or floor.

Application of the criterion is therefore justified only in more or less specified situations as regards the factors mentioned.

2. *Daylight Factor.* The daylighting levels of an interior depend upon the greatly varying lighting circumstances outside. Under certain conditions the interior lighting levels are proportional to the exterior illuminance under an unobstructed sky. On this basis the daylight factor (d) in a point of a plane has been defined as 'the ratio of the illuminance (E) on the given plane at that point, and the simultaneous exterior illuminance (E_0) in a horizontal plane from the whole of an unobstructed sky of assumed or known luminance distribution. Direct sunlight is excluded from both interior and exterior values of illuminance'.

The daylight factor is usually expressed in percentages:

$$d = \frac{E}{E_0} \, 100 \text{ per cent.}$$

It follows from this definition that the daylight factor at a point may be computed for: (1) various planes; actually it is only used for a horizontal plane at the height of 0·80 or 1·00 m. ('working plane'); (2) for various luminance distributions of the sky.

As a rule, the daylight factor has been used for conditions of the densely overcast sky. The luminance of a point of this sky is independent of its azimuth. Therefore, the daylight factor under this sky condition is independent of the orientation of the light opening. The 'densely overcast sky' may be considered to represent an unfavourable condition as regards sky light, which meanwhile, at least in the temperate region, occurs with such a frequency that it is relevant.

All factors mentioned in our criticism of the proportion of glass area to floor area as a criterion are taken into account in the determination of the daylight factor. In this respect the daylight factor is a considerably better criterion for the access of daylight than the relative amount of glass. Probably due to its abstract nature and the rather complicated calculation, it is not generally favoured by designers. Simplified presentation of results of calculation for certain classes of rooms partly meets this objection.

3. *Sky Factor.* The sky factor at a given point inside a building is the ratio of the illuminance on a horizontal plane at the point, due to the light received directly from the sky, to the illuminance due to an unobstructed hemisphere or sky of uniform luminance, equal to that of the visible part of the sky. The sky factor, therefore, does not depend on variable circumstances such as reflectances of interior and surroundings. It is merely a geometric quantity ('configuration factor') From the practical point of view it has the advantage over the daylight factor of a simpler calculation. However, it is not a substitute for the daylight factor for those interested in levels of daylighting: these may differ considerably in points with equal sky factor. For rooms within a specific category, e.g. classrooms which fit certain standards of shape and size, it is possible, however, to use as a criterion for the access of daylight the (average) sky factor in one or more well-defined points.

4. *Window Sizes for Specific Types of Rooms.* Krochmann (1964) translated recommended minimum daylight factors into window sizes, necessary to meet the recommendations in various designs (as regards proportions, sizes, reflectances). Thus their observation is enhanced by using a terminology which is familiar to those who should be primarily interested, such as designers and building inspectors.

Recommendations for Adequate Daylighting. Other recommendations are given with a broader object in view, namely to promote an adequate natural lighting, both qualitatively and quantitatively or possibly an adequate natural component for a combination of daylight and artificial light.

In this respect two kinds of criteria can be distinguished:

1. *The Daylight Factor.* When the exterior lighting levels change, with certain exceptions, both the interior levels and the luminance of the window will change equally; the change in luminance of the visible external objects (sky or obstructions) can have a large effect on the adaptation.

On account of this fatc it was initially expected that the daylight factor could not only give information about lighting levels but would also be a criterion for the adequacy of luminance ratios during daytime, however much the lighting conditions outside might change. However, this does not generally apply to such an extent that widely varying situations could be mutually compared by means of the daylight factor: the same value of the daylight factor can be effected in situations which from a visual point of view are completely different.

More relevant information is, of course, provided by the separate components of which the daylight factor consists, i.e. the contribution of the direct light from the sky and that of internal and external reflections. When using these quantities, which, however, is not done in codes, the step to the following class would be only a minor one.

2. *Multi-dimensional Criteria.* The requirements for adequate natural lighting of a room with a certain designation can, in general, not be formulated by a simple criterion, such as the daylight factor at a given point, or not even by a curve showing its relation to the distance to the window. Only a complex criterion will suffice, namely the luminance patterns in the room under various relevant sky conditions. In this respect the general recommendations for interior lighting apply, except for certain modifications, which will be briefly discussed below.

The window is often a source of glare, even disability glare, especially in high buildings, where there is an almost unobstructed view of the sky. As regards discomfort glare, at least at moderate levels, people are more tolerant with respect to windows than they are with respect to artificial lighting.

Some results of experiments by Hopkinson *et al.* (1967) were:
1. The luminance of the window has a greater effect on the senses than the size of the window. One can expect a bigger

improvement when curtains or light-absorbing glass are used than when the size of the window is reduced.

For an appreciable improvement, a decrease in the transmittance from 0·9 to about 0·3 is essential. However, the illuminance on the job would then be reduced to one-third of its value as well. Possibly the use of absorbing glass for a part of the window is the optimal solution.

2. The position of large sources is of little significance. A large window, for example, in the side wall of a schoolroom, causes almost as much discomfort glare as one in the wall facing the children.

3. Windows in two adjacent walls have advantages because they increase each other's surround luminance and thereby reduce the glare. Skylights may also be useful in this respect.

4. Gradual changes in luminances reduce the liability of discomfort glare; therefore, broad dark window-frames and rods should be avoided and light, preferably splayed recesses should be used (20–25 cm. deep and inclined at 30 degrees to the normal to the window).

5. Interruptions of large windows by bars, etc., cause extra discomfort.

Recommendations for Insolation and Shading. It will be understood from the paragraph on significance of insolation that for the time being standards and recommendations, be it for a minimum or an optimal insolation, cannot claim a broad scientific foundation. At best they are based on some follow-up of existing situations and, therefore, possibly biased with convention and current prejudices.

With this restriction the reader is referred to local recommendations. The experience usually underlying them should not be neglected without good reasons. On the other hand, they should not block the possibility of well-controlled experiments.

Without any restriction it is recommended—as may be found in many regulations for schools, workshops, etc.—that means, either permanent or controllable, be provided to prevent direct sunshine upon the eye task and to prevent glare from direct sunlight.

Sun control of interiors is applied mainly for the prevention of: (1) undesired heat; (2) undesired light (brightness or contrast); damage to goods.

As regards those means for protection from sunshine, which are effective from the first—and very important—point of view, we only mention them, the interested reader being referred to the literature on air conditioning. They are: (1) adequate arrangement of the building site; (2) adequate orientation; (3) limitation of glass surfaces; (4) external shading devices (fixed or movable); and (5) heat-reflecting glasses.

In those cases where primarily control of sunlight is needed and heat control is of little or no importance, *curtains* and *venetian blinds* (internal or between double glazing) apply. They offer the possibility that sunlight control is adapted to local and immediate needs.

Venetian blinds contribute to an adequate light distribution by their diffusing effect. However, just like curtains, they have the disadvantage that their use has to be adapted again and again to the changing position of the sun. Furthermore, in rooms used by a number of people simultaneously controversy may occur as to their optimal use.

So called 'grey' or 'tinted' glasses have a relatively large absorption of visible radiation as compared with heat-absorbing or heat-reflecting glass. They may contribute to a better brightness pattern as regards sky light. But, generally speaking, they will not provide sufficient protection from sun glare.

PUBLIC LIGHTING
INTRODUCTION

Until quite recently outdoor activities practically had to stop at sunset. It was only by the grace of the invention of electric lamps that, after dark, the streets and roads could be used to any extent by others than robbers and brigands. Consequently, from the outset the aim of public lighting was, and often still is, the promotion of public safety. About mid-century, however, the increasing pressure of motorized road traffic began to require a completely different type of road network, lighting included. Gradually, public lighting and traffic lighting grew to be synonymous, its main purpose now being to enable the traffic to proceed speedily and securely at night. In this section, we will deal in brief with the specific lighting requirements issuing from contemporary traffic conditions. Obviously, the requirements are directly related to the traffic itself, and can be derived from the fact that a car driver does need a great deal of visual information about his direct environment in order to be able to drive his car in an appropriate manner. The visual information concerns primarily the presence and position of other cars, and further the run of the road and the visibility of the road surface itself, including all obstacles that may endanger or hinder the flow of traffic. From this it follows that the driver himself (or rather his vehicle) must be visible to all other road users; and furthermore the driver should be able to trust his path to be free when he perceives no obstacle.

Translated into lighting terms, these requirements lead to the following four criteria of quality for road lighting installations:

1. The lighting level must be such that even small objects are visible. This requirements pertains to the visibility of the road itself, its borderlines, road markings, and details of objects that may offer danger, including other vehicles.

The lighting level can quantitatively be expressed in the average road-surface luminance. (The concept luminance has to do with the amount of light emitted or reflected by a surface; its definition is given at the end of this chapter).

2. The lighting must be uniform and not patchy. Particularly, isolated dark spots have to be avoided, as objects might disappear in them. This is quantified by the ratio between the minimum and the average road-surface luminance.

3. The lighting must cause no glare or dazzle. This can be expressed quantitatively in the 'Glare Mark', a numerical value associated with the degree of discomfort caused by glare, and in the 'equivalent veiling luminance' that quantifies the disability effects.

4. The course of the road must be discernible well in advance. This requires good visual guidance. At present, no quantitative measure exists.

It is generally accepted that the first criterion (the luminance level) is the most important of the four. The reason for this is threefold: primarily, the adaptation level, and thus the visual performance, is determined mainly by the road luminance; secondly the road surface forms the most important part of the background for obstacles on the road, and thirdly the road serves as a frame of reference for moving vehicles.

PUBLIC LIGHTING VERSUS VEHICLE LIGHTING

Under normal weather conditions the four criteria quoted above can be met in day-time [FIG. 32]. The need to fulfil these requirements at night also is apparent from the fact that in many cases night-time traffic is just as intense as day-time traffic. To meet them at night-time, two different methods are available—lighting by means of headlamps mounted on the vehicles, and stationary road lighting (public lighting).

Using the high (long, or country) beam of headlights on a

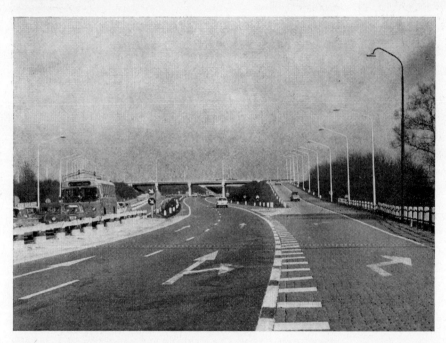

road without other traffic, the four criteria are met only to a meagre degree. True, glare is totally absent, but the road itself is only partially lighted. Obstacles will stand out as a light silhouette on a dark background only when they reflect light well. This implies, for example, that dark-clad pedestrians are poorly visible. Safe and reasonably fast traffic is possible under these conditions, but the safety margin, which is often ample during the day, is reduced considerably.

When one has to switch over to the low (dipped or passing) beam to avoid blinding others, like, for example, pedestrians, the situation changes distinctly for the worse, primarily because the field of view is restricted to a short range directly in front of the car. When oncoming motorized traffic is encountered the glare-free situation mentioned above no longer exists, because the other drivers must also be allowed to see the road. Due to the glaring headlights of the oncoming cars, visibility is again drastically reduced. Much work has been done to find the best compromise between visibility and glare; for intense traffic the safety margin offered by this compromise is, however, small indeed, as many accidents prove. In such situations the most promising solution is the installation of good public lighting, which permits the traffic to proceed with-

out hindering the other traffic with undue glare. Thus, the decision to install public lighting is closely related to the traffic volume; traffic intensity, however, is not the only factor which determines whether or not road lighting should be installed, since many local and regional factors are also involved. An alternative, particularly for roads that carry moderately heavy traffic, may be found in the application of polarized light for headlamps. These, and related problems are discussed in O.E.C.D. (1971).

THE LUMINANCE LEVEL

Contrary to the light from vehicle headlamps public lighting usually renders obstacles as dark silhouettes against as relatively

FIG. 32. Under normal weather conditions sufficient visual information is presented in the day-time.

bright background [FIGS. 33 and 34]. This observation has several far-reaching consequences for the design of lighting installations. First, it must be the main objective of the installation to render the road surface—which forms the most important portion of the background for obstacles—as bright as possible or, more precisely, the average road-surface luminance should be high.

As mentioned above, the luminance entails the light reflected from the surface and perceived by the eye of the observer-car driver. Thus, the way the light is reflected by the road surface is of prime importance. Now, drivers usually look well ahead—at least they should. When thus observed, however, normal road surfaces reflect the light more or less like a mirror. This implies, of course, that light that is emitted in a direction opposite to the direction in which the driver himself looks, contributes best to the road-surface luminance. This effect is known to all drivers, who will have noticed that the illuminated patch in front of oncoming cars seems much brighter than the patch in front of their own car. In fact, especially on a damp road surface, that other patch may seem one hundred times as bright! Under normal conditions of public lighting the difference is not that large; still, a considerable gain in

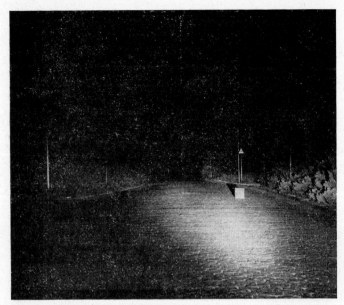

FIG. 33. Lighting from headlamps of vehicles reveals objects as light silhouettes against a dark background.

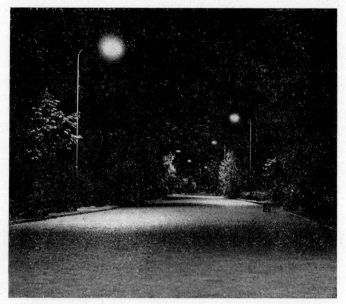

FIG. 34. Public lighting usually reveals objects as dark silhouettes against a relatively bright background.

'luminance-yield' may be obtained by directing most of the light *against* the direction of traffic. Thus, the road surface is an integral part of the lighting installation.

TABLE 37

Recommended minimum values of road luminance, uniformity and glare restrictions for roads when public lighting is needed.

Types of road	Luminance			Glare restriction
	$\bar{L}$	L min./$\bar{L}$ (overall)	L min./L max. (lengthwise)	G
Rural roads (motorways, trunk roads, etc.) . .	2	0·4	0·7	7
Urban roads				
motorways .	2	0·4	0·7	7
main arterial roads . .	2	0·4	0·7	7
main roads .	2	0·3	0·6	6
secondary roads	1	0·2	0·5	5
residential roads	Average horizontal illuminance E > 5 lux.			

(Adapted from draft Recommendations for the Netherlands.)

For different types of traffic routes specific values of the road-surface luminance are recommended. A summary of the draft-recommendation for the Netherlands is given in Table 37. The given values agree with the international recommendations of the C.I.E. (1974).

THE LUMINANCE PATTERN

The fact that, in public lighting, most obstacles are seen as dark objects against a bright background has another important consequence. Since not only large objects like other cars must be visible but also things like stones, etc. the presence of large,

dark areas on the road surface is not acceptable. That is, even in the darker areas the luminance must be sufficient to reveal these small objects. With this in mind minimum values of the road-surface luminance could be arrived at. Still, there is another consideration: a road that is uniform enough to render all dangerous obstacles perfectly visible, may yet be unacceptable, because it fails to allow the driver to orient himself. A solution is the introduction of two separate measures of non-uniformity: the overall measure expressed in the ratio between minimum and average luminance, and the length-wise measure, expressed in the ratio between the minimum and maximum point luminances on the line straight ahead of the driver [see TABLE 37].

Wet surfaces of a fine texture exhibit nearly complete specular reflection. The resulting luminance pattern is usually unacceptably non-uniform. The most promising solution available is the application of coarse, open-texture surfaces that permit moisture to drain easily. These surfaces are to be preferred anyway because they are less slippery than smooth surfaces.

When the light distribution of the lanterns and the reflective properties of the surface are known, both the luminance and the non-uniformity may be calculated (Schreuder, 1967).

GLARE

As said before, a high road-surface luminance may result from an installation that throws most of the light against the direction of traffic, particularly in combination with a smooth, shiny surface. Apart from the fact that such surfaces are mostly very slippery when wet, and that usually the resulting non-uniformity of the luminance pattern is quite unacceptable, the main objection to such installations is the resulting degree of glare. The adverse effects of glare from high-intensity street-lighting lanterns can be twofold: first, the glare proper, or disability glare, which reduces or even totally obstructs observation, and secondly, the feeling of disturbance (or discomfort glare) that may be quite pronounced even under those conditions where disability glare is not yet apparent. Numerous experiments have indicated that under most street-lighting conditions the restriction of discomfort glare is the more critical of the two. Both kinds of glare, however, should be reduced as far as possible. Consequently a glare rating system has been designed that allows the assessment both of the degree of discomfort glare restriction (Glare Mark) and of the equivalent veiling luminance (Adrian and Schreuder, 1971).

VISUAL GUIDANCE

In a way, the visual guidance represents a functional criterion of quality rather than a technical one like the three

study. Here we will restrict ourselves to some points of special interest.

Rural Roads. Rural roads that carry only little traffic normally remain unlighted. Special care must be given, however, to crossings in such roads, as they tend to constitute points of great danger. It is customary, therefore, to light such crossings. If this is done, the lighting should not be restricted to the crossing alone, but all roads leading towards the crossing must be lighted over a distance of at least several hundred feet. Rural roads with heavy traffic are lighted according to similar principles as urban roads, be it that the restriction of glare should be more stringent because a background of house-fronts, etc. is missing.

Urban Roads. Urban roads must always be provided with

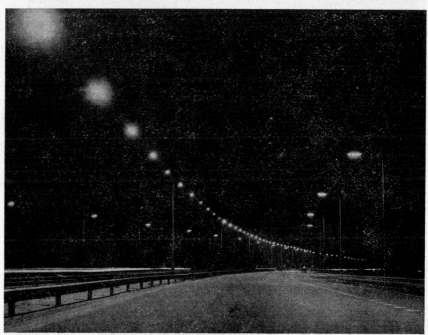

FIG. 35. An example of excellent visual guidance.

others. As such, it cannot be expressed simply in a quantitative way. On the other hand, it is one of the main objectives of the lighting installation to provide information on the run of the road well in advance. A good visual guidance is therefore indispensable. An example of excellent visual guidance is pictured in FIGURE 35; it may be observed that the visual guidance is provided not only by the row of lanterns but also by the road surface, the road markings, and the guard-rails. General rules for good visual guidance cannot be given; very much depends on the 'feel', the skill, and the imagination of the street-lighting designer.

APPLICATIONS

The way in which the rules of a practical art such as illuminating engineering can be put into practice is not easily described. Practice, and practice alone, can teach the exact manner in which to apply the general, theoretical rules.

The interested reader is referred to the many textbooks on public lighting (e.g. de Boer *et al.*, 1967; Waldram, 1952) in which the whole field of public lighting is discussed in great detail, and which list relevant references for further

public lighting; if they carry heavy traffic for obvious reasons and if they carry but little traffic (and during the small hours) for reasons of public safety. The recommendations given in TABLE 37 outline suitable installations. These recommended installations permit the motor traffic to proceed without their headlights, that means using their sidelights (parking lights) only, provided of course these lights meet reasonable specifications.

Motorways. Motorways are designed as dual-carriageway roads, with limited points of access and are restricted to fast traffic only. Usually, either a maximum or a minimum speed limit, or both, are imposed. Many motorways can be allowed to remain unlighted, provided effective glare fences are installed in the central reserve. On heavily used motorways, however, the situation is different, especially when the carriageways include more than two lanes each. In such cases the visual situation may be very complicated. Motorway lighting is an important means for increasing the quality of the road system in general. In particular it has important safety value during adverse weather conditions (fog, heavy rain, etc.).

Traffic Junctions in Motorways. Access and exit ramps on motorways constitute very critical situations from the point of view of visual information. As a rule, they must be very well lighted, even if the motorway itself does not carry such heavy traffic, and is consequently unlighted. Naturally, lighting conditions are even more critical when the access and exit ramps belong to a junction of two or more motorways. In fact,

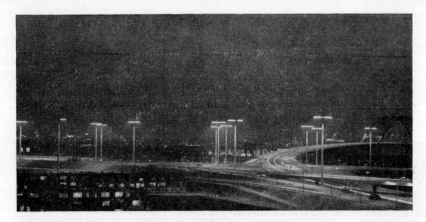

1. A 'black hole' effect should be avoided at the tunnel entrance, thus allowing the approaching car-driver to look well into the tunnel when he is still outside. This is possible when the luminance in the tunnel entrance is at least 0.1 that of the surroundings outside the tunnel.

Fig. 36. The lighting of a complex traffic junction by means of floodlights mounted on high towers.

most of those junctions present very complex traffic situations, often involving three or even four different pavement levels. This type of junction calls for a special type of lighting. Usually a whole area is covered with an intermingling cluster of roads at different levels, and the most convenient lighting system is then the adoption of floodlights mounted on a relatively small number of high towers, which may be well over 40 m. in height [Fig. 36].

Tunnels. Tunnel lighting is most critical during the day,

2. Ample time (about 15 sec.) should be provided for the adaptation of the sensitivity of the eye to the lower luminance level in the interior of the tunnel.

3. Disturbing flicker due to longitudinal spacing between the light sources should be avoided. The obvious solution is a continuous-line lighting system.

4. During the day the luminance level in the interior of tunnels with heavy traffic should be at least 15 cd/m.^{2}, and preferably 20 cd/m.^{2}.

An example of good, modern tunnel lighting is given in Figure 37.

APPENDIX

MEASUREMENT

From the large field of photometry we only mention possibilities for the assessment of those quantities which are the most relevant for the health officer.

He should be warned that not only the use and calibration but also the choice of the instrument requires some photometric knowledge and experience. In addition, he should be aware of the risk of misleading himself by measuring only those characteristics of a lighting situation which may be measured easily (e.g. illuminance levels), while neglecting other characteristics which may be less easily determined but which are more relevant.

The Measurement of Luminances

Two kinds of photometers are to be distinguished:

1. **Visual.** In visual photometers a visual field is divided into two parts. The luminance of one part is the one to be measured (or a known fraction of it). The other part is illuminated by a source within the instrument.

The measurement consists of matching the brightnesses by means of a control mechanism and subsequently reading the required adjustment of the latter on a scale, calibrated in luminances.

2. **Photo-electric.** Photo-electric instruments contain a

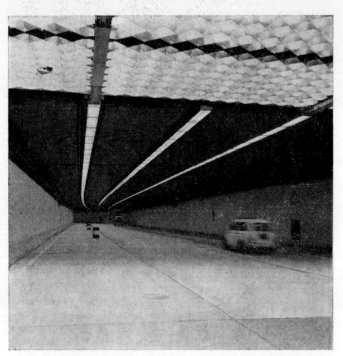

Fig. 37. An example of good, modern tunnel lighting.

because it is hardly possible to light a tunnel as brightly as a sunlit open road. Good visual conditions can be ensured, however, when the following rules are obeyed. More details are given by Schreuder (1964).

photosensitive receptor, which reacts to light either by releasing (in case of a selenium cell) or by modifying (in case of a photomultiplier) an electric current. In the latter case this current is amplified. Readings are made on a micro-ammeter calibrated in units of luminance.

Instruments with photomultipliers require frequent and careful calibration. Instruments with selenium cells will, under practical conditions, operate with restricted precision. However, provided that they are calibrated, for example, once a year, errors will not exceed tolerable limits for practical purposes within the field of interior lighting.

Measurement of Illuminance

Usual meters for illuminances ('levels') are photometers of the type with a selenium cell. Care should be taken that the radiation is evaluated according to its luminous efficacy and

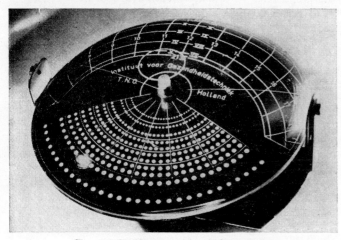

FIG. 38. Sky factor and insolation meter.

that measurements are corrected for all angles of incidence ('cos φ correction').

Some photometers with selenium cells are suitable for both luminance and illuminance measurements within practical ranges of interior lighting by the use of interchangeable parts. Instruments of this type will probably be the most convenient for the health officer interested in interior lighting.

Measurement of Reflectance

Measurement in the strict sense of reflectances requires instruments and skill such that we must refer to photometric literature. However, the reflectance of more or less diffusing materials as used in interiors can be estimated with amply sufficient accuracy by comparison with a series of samples, as for example, the 'Munsell Value Atlas'.[1]

Measurement of Natural Lighting

Assessment of the daylight factor implies that indoor and outdoor levels are measured simultaneously (or at least nearly so), and that subsequently one is expressed as a fraction of the other. To simplify this procedure the E.E.L.-B.R.S.[2] daylight photometer has been developed, by means of which the daylight factor may be read immediately.

[1] Munsell Color Co., Baltimore, MD, U.S.A.
[2] Developed by the British Building Research Station and manufactured by Evans Electro Selenium Ltd.

The problem of finding a place to measure the outdoor illuminance (E_0) under an unobstructed sky is avoided by making use of the fact that for the (standard) overcast sky E_0 is known when the luminance of a given point of the sky is known.

FIGURE 38 shows a simple instrument for the measurement of the sky-factor. By means of a transparent convex mirror, the unobstructed part of the sky is seen simultaneously with a diagram consisting of dots, each dot representing a contribution of 0·1 per cent. to the sky-factor.

Measurement of Insolation

The same apparatus [FIG. 38] allows, after proper orientation, readings at any moment of the times of insolation in the course of the year for a specific point of a room. For this purpose it is provided with a diagram showing the sun's path for the 21st day of each month.

There are several variants of this principle (Pleyel; Tonne); the instrument shown is that of TNO, the Netherlands. It can be supplied with diagrams for every latitude. The apparatus is used, for example, in the evaluation of existing dwellings (slum clearance) or to examine the need for shading.

PREDETERMINATION

It would require much technical background information to describe the various methods for calculation of lighting levels and luminances, either from natural or artificial lighting. However, the health officer should be aware of the fact that the essential characteristics of any situation (town plan, building, room) as regards daylight, insolation, and artificial lighting can be predicted very closely, so that disappointments need not occur. For most purposes, simple routine procedures, graphical methods and practical tools are available.

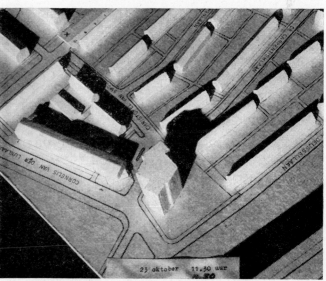

FIG. 39. Model study of insolation.

As regards daylighting, the climate is a factor to be considered in the choice of the method for predetermination (Hopkinson, 1963).

In *dry tropical regions*—or in tropical regions where the dry period is considered to be the critical one for the design of the building—the calculation is simplified by the fact that outdoor illuminances on horizontal and vertical surfaces, resulting from skylight and reflected sunlight, may be considered to be the same all over the day.

In humid tropical climates, or where this is considered to be the critical design condition, where daylighting depends mainly on direct and reflected skylight, accurate daylight calculations would make little sense because of the ever-changing sky conditions. Here the lumen method is appropriate.

Calculations of the daylight factor and its components were developed in and for regions with a *temperate climate*, where the densely overcast sky is considered to represent more or less a minimum condition of daylighting, which at the same time occurs so frequently that it makes sense to design for this condition.

Model studies may be useful for visualizing insolation [Fig. 39], especially in town planning, or for daylight prediction in complicated situations (Kittler, 1959).

SHORT EXPLANATION OF PHYSICAL TERMS

Spectral Luminous Efficacy; Luminous Flux; Lumen

An electric lamp transfers an input of electrical energy (e.g. 150 watts) into an output of electromagnetic radiant energy (radiant flux). The larger part of this energy is of such wavelengths as are not perceived by the eye, which is sensitive only to wavelengths of about 400–800 nm.[1] The sensitiveness of the normal eye, or in other words the 'spectral luminous efficacy' (expressed in lumen/watt), of the radiant energy has its maximum with 555 nm (green). If the radiant energy emitted is evaluated according to the luminous efficacy of the various wavelengths, it turns out that, for example, an ordinary 150-watt incandescent lamp renders a 'luminous flux' of about 2,500 lumen (1 lumen corresponds to $\frac{1}{680}$ watt, emitted at 555 nm).

Evaluation of radiant energy according to the visual efficiency-$(V_\lambda)^-$ curve for the CIE standard observer made it possible to describe lighting stimuli in one numeral instead of spectral distributions. However, it should be kept in mind, that these numerals and the corresponding units (lumen, lux, candela) apply only as far as the standard observer applies: they make no sense with respect to plants, animals, colour-blind persons, or other than 'light adapted' normal eyes (photopic, day or cone vision; luminance > 0.03 cd/m^2).

A provisional standard visual efficiency curve (V_λ–curve) has been defined for rod (scotopic) vision. The transitional region (mesopic vision) requires closer attention.

Luminous Intensity; Candela

As a rule, the flux of a light source will not be distributed evenly over the space. It is here that the notions '*solid angle*' and '*luminous intensity*' come in. Just as we may divide a plane around a point in angles, we may divide the three-dimensional space around a point in larger or smaller pieces, called '*solid angles*'. Just as we use the radian ($\approx 57°$) as a unit of angle in a plane surface, we use the 'steradian' (sr) as a unit of solid angle. By the definition of the steradian the total space around a point counts 4π, i.e. about 12.6 steradians.

The (luminous) *intensity* of a source in a certain direction

may now be defined as the 'flux per steradian' in that direction. The unit of intensity is therefore the 1m./sr called 'candela' (cd).

If the luminous flux of the above lamp was distributed evenly over the space its intensity in any direction would be $\frac{2500}{12\cdot6} = 200$ cd.

Illuminance; Lux; 'Square Law'; 'cos φ Law'

The 'illuminance' at a point of a surface is the luminous flux received there per unit of area. Accordingly, illuminance is expressed in lm./m.^{2}, called lux.

With increasing (e.g. doubled or trebled) distance from a point source the same flux will be distributed over a correspondingly (4 or 9 times respectively) larger area. This implies that the illuminance on a plane perpendicular to the direction of incidence of the light is inversely proportionate to the square of the distance ('square law').

In case of oblique incidence (angle φ with normal) the same flux is distributed over a larger area resulting in a correspondingly smaller illuminance; the effect is proportionate to the cosine of the angle of incidence ('cos φ law').

Reflectance, Transmittance

The *reflectance* or 'reflection factor' of a body is the ratio of the luminous flux reflected to the luminous flux received. Reflectances may be given either for specific wavelengths ('spectral reflectance') or for white light ('total reflectance'). They may relate to specular (direct) or to diffuse reflection. Analogous distinctions are made as regards transmittance. The (diffuse) reflectance of matt white paper is about 0.9.

Luminance; cd/m.^{2}

The 'luminance' of a light source (or lighted object) in a certain direction is defined as its intensity in that direction per unit of 'apparent area' (i.e. the projection of its area in the direction of view).

According to the above definition, luminances are measured in cd/m.^{2}. The luminance, for example, of a fluorescent tube may be, 5,000–8,000 cd/m^2., depending upon the direction in which it is seen.

Some surfaces, called Lambert surfaces, have the characteristic that their luminance is the same for all directions, which means that—practically speaking—they appear equally bright, if seen from various directions.

The luminance of a diffusely reflecting surface, e.g. a piece of matt paper, is proportionate to its illuminance (E) and its reflectance (r)

$$L = C \times E \times r$$

It can be shown that in metric units $C = \frac{1}{\pi}$, therefore

$$L = \frac{E \times r}{\pi}$$

For example, in case of $E = 700$ lux and $r = 0.9$

$$L = 200 \text{ cd/m.}^2$$

---

[1] 1 nm. (nanometer) $= 10^{-9}$ m. $= 10^{-9} \times 3.28$ ft

Contrast

The luminance difference (ΔL) between an object (e.g. a character) and its background (paper) is often expressed in proportion to the luminance of the background (L_b). The value $C = \dfrac{\Delta L}{L_b}$ is called the *contrast* of object and background. Often object and background will have the same illuminance. In that case, apart from specular reflection, $C = \dfrac{\Delta r}{r_b}$, where r is the reflection factor.

The term contrast is also used in another, subjective sense: the difference in appearance of two parts of a field of view, seen simultaneously or successively.

REFERENCES AND FURTHER READING

References have largely been restricted to recent titles, where, as a rule, further references will be found.

General

Commission Internationale de l'Eclairage (CIE) (1971) *Proceedings*, XVII.

Illuminating Engineering Society (I.E.S.) (1972) *Lighting Handbook*, 5th ed., New York.

Vision

Adrian, W. (1969) Die Unterschiedsempfindlichkeit des Auges und die Möglichkeit ihrer Berechnung, *Lichttechnik*, **21**, 2A.

Blackwell, H. R. (1967) The evaluation of interior lighting on the basis of visual criteria, *Appl. Opt.*, **6**, 1443.

Blackwell, H. R., and Smith, S. W. (1970) Additional visual performance data for use in illumination specification systems, *Ill. Engng*, **65**, 389.

Blackwell, O. M. and Blackwell, H. R. (1971) Visual performance data for 156 normal observers of various ages, *Journal of IES*, **1**, 3.

Bodmann, H.-W. (1973) Visibility assessment in lighting engineering, *Journal of IES*, **2**, 437.

Boyce, P. R. (1973) Age, illuminance, visual performance and preference, *Light. Res. Techn.*, **5**, 125.

Boynton, R. M., Rinalducci, E. J., and Sternheim, Ch. (1969) Visibility losses produced by transient adaptation changes, *Ill. Engng*, **64**, 217.

Commission Internationale de l'Éclairage (1972) *A Unified Framework of Methods for Evaluating Visual Performance Aspects of Lighting*, CIE publication No. 19, Paris.

Fortuin, G. J. (1951) Visual power and visibility. *Philips Res. Rep.*, **6**, 251.

Khek, J., and Krivohlavy, J. (1967) Evaluation of the criteria to measure the suitability of visual conditions, CIE—P 67-19.

Kobayashi, A. (1970) Apparent brightness scales, *Trans. A. I. Japan*, 91.

Marsden, A. M. (1970) Brightness–luminance relationships in an interior, *Light Res. Techn.*, **2**, 10.

Meshkov, V. V., and Faremark, M. A. (1967) Lighting and quantitative parameters of visual tasks, CIE—P 67-21.

Moon, P., and Spencer, D. E. (1945) The visual effect of non-uniform surrounds, *J.O.S.A.*, **35**, 233.

Muck, E., and Bodmann, H. W. (1961) Die Bedeutung des Beleuchtungsniveaus bei praktischer Sehtätigkeit, *Lichttechnik*, **13** (10), 502.

Schoutcn, J. F., Kalsbeek, J. W. H., and Leopold, F. F. (1962) On the evaluation of perceptual and mental load, *Ergonomics*, **5**, 251.

Weston, H. C. (1962) *Sight, Light and Work*, 2nd ed., London

Ultra-violet Radiation

Dantsig, N. M., Lazarev, D. N., and Sokolov, M. V. (1967) Ultra violet installations of beneficial action, CIE—P 67-20.

Thorington, L., and Parescandola, L. J. (1967) Ultra violet emission from light sources, *Ill. Engng*, **62**, 674; **63**, 41.

Various Effects of Visible Radiation

Assenmacher, I. (1966) Influence de la lumière sur certains rythmes physiologiques, *Lux*, 505.

Burner, M. (1966) Influence de l'éclairage sur le comportement de l'être humain dans son travail, *Z. Präv.-Med.*, **11**, 345.

Goromosov, M. S. (1968) The physiological basis of health standards for dwellings, *Wld Hlth Org. Publ. Hlth Pap.*, No. 33.

Grand, Y. le (1965) L'éclairage de demain, *Lux*, 267.

Logan, H. L. (1967) The relationship of light to health, *Ill. Engng*, **62**, 159.

Ott, J. (1965) Effects of unnatural light, *New Scientist*, **429**, 294.

Sausville, J. W. *et al.* (1971) Blue lamps in phototherapy of hyperbilirubinemia, *Journal of IES*, **1**, 112.

Wurtman, R. J. (1968) Biological implications of artificial lighting, *Ill. Engng*, **63**, 523.

Artificial Lighting of Interiors

General

British Lighting Council (1970) *Interior Lighting Design Handbook*, 3rd ed., London.

Discomfort Glare

Einhorn, H. D. (1971) Glare facts and formulations, *CIE, Compte Rendu*, XVII.

Contrast Rendering

Illuminating Engineering Society (N.Y.) (1973) The pre-determination of contrast rendition factors, R.Q.Q. Report No. 5, *Journal of IES*, **2**, 149.

Colour and Colour Rendering

Commission Internationale de l'Éclairage (1965) Method of measuring and specifying colour rendering properties of light sources, CIE publication No. 13.

Inui, M. (1969) Colour in the interior environment, *Lighting Research and Technology*, **1**, 86.

Judd, D. B. (1971) Choosing pleasant colour combinations, *Lighting Design and Application*, **1**, No. 2, 31.

Combined Use of Artificial and Natural Light

Commission Internationale de l'Éclairage (1971) Committee Report E. 3.2.

Fischer, D. (1973) A luminance concept for working interiors, *Journal of IES*, **2**, 92.

Fischer, D., and Kebschull, W. (1971) Tageslicht und Kunstlicht und ihre gemeinsame Konditionierung in der Beleuchtungstechnik, *CIE, Compte Rendu*, XVII, p.71.13.

Ne'eman, E., and Hopkinson, R. G. (1970) Critical minimum window size, *Lighting Research and Technology*, **2**, 17.

Integrated Design

Commission Internationale de l'Éclairage (1971) *Compte Rendu*, XVII, Committee Report E 1.6.

Dorsey, R. T., Clark, G. W., Kaufman, J. E. *et al.* (1973) Energy utilization in lighting, *Lighting Design and Application*, **3**, 5.

Fisher, W. S. (1971) Integrated environment, U.S.A. and European practice, *CIE, Compte Rendu*, XVII.

Miscellaneous Aspects

Barthès, E. (1966) Bases expérimentales pour un conditionnement lumineux, *Lux*, 477.

Bellchambers, H. E. (1971) Illuminations, colour rendering and visual clarity, *CIE, Compte Rendu*, XVII, p. 71.25.

Gradinà, C. (1966) Influence de la lumière scintillante fluorescente, *Arch. Mal. prof.*, **27**, 869.

Inui, M., and Miyata, T. (1973) Spaciousness in interiors, *Lighting Research and Technology*, **5**, 103.

Kovach, E. G., ed. (1973) *Technology of efficient energy utilization*, N.A.T.O., Brussels.

Lynes, J. A., Cuttle, C., and Burt, W. (1967) Beyond the working plane, C.I.E.—P 67-12.

Range, H. D. (1971) *Lichttechnik*, **23**, 356.

Rowlands, E. *et al.* (1971) Visual performance in illuminance of different spectral quality, *CIE, Compte Rendu*, XVII, p. 71.36.

Work Environments

American Standards Association (1965) *American Standard Practice for Industrial Lighting*, New York.

Illuminating Engineering Society, The I.E.S. Code (1973) Recommendations for lighting building interiors, London.

International Labor Office (1965) Artificial lighting in factory and office, C.I.S.—information sheet 11, Geneva.

Netherlands Foundation for Illumination (1967) Recommendations for interior lighting.

Other Environments

Antes, J. (1970) Bibliography of hospital illumination, *Guthrie Clin. Bull.*, **40**, 96.

Ierland, van, J. and Linden, van der, A. (1970) Light and night sporthalls, (Dutch, with English summary), *Electrotechniek*, **48**, 325; Publ. no. 338, TNO—Research Institute for Environmental Hygiene, Delft (The Netherlands).

World Health Organization (1966) Public Health aspects of housing in the U.S.S.R., *Wld Hlth Org. Chron.*, **20**, 10.

Daylighting and Windows

General

Commission Internationale de l'Éclairage (1971) *Compte Rendu*, XVII, Committee E. 3.2, Progress Report.

Daylighting Committee of the Illuminating Engineering Society, New York (1962) Recommended practice of daylighting.

Hopkinson, R. G. (1966) *Daylighting*, London.

Hopkinson, R. G., ed. (1967) Sunlight in buildings, Proceedings of C.I.E. Conference, Rotterdam (The Netherlands).

Needs and appreciation: Windowless Rooms

Bitter, C. and Ierland, van J. (1967) Appreciation of sunlight in the home, Publ. no. 242, TNO—Research Institute for Environmental Hygiene, Delft (The Netherlands).

Bochenkova, T. D. (1968) Working conditions in industrial buildings, devoid of natural lighting (Russ.), *Gig. Tr. prof. Zabol.*, (1), 10.

Hollister, F. D. (1968) The problem of windowless environments, *Res. Pap.*, No. 1, Greater London Council.

Markus, T. A., Brierly, E. and Gray, A. (1972) *Criteria of sunshine, daylight, visual privacy and view in housing*, Glasgow.

Mikhailova, V. N., and Sviridov, E. I. (1964) Survey of lighting in industrial windowless buildings (Russ.), *Svetotekhnika*, **10** (6), 13.

Noort, H. R. van (1965) Effect of daylight upon the health of the workers, Council of Europe.

Predetermination

Chauvel, P., Dourgnon, J., and Dogniaux, R. (1963) Abaques pour la détermination de la composante directe du facteur de lumière du jour, Centre Scientifique et Technique du Bâtiment, Paris.

Commission Internationale de l'Éclairage (1970) International recommendations for the calculations of natural daylight, Document No. 16 (E. 3.2) Daylight: (Simplified method, full reference of other methods).

Dogniaux, R. (1966) Comfort lumineux de l'habitat, *Lux*, 426.

Hopkinson, R. G., and Plant, C. G. (1966) L'éclairage naturel et la prédétermination de l'éclairement dans les locaux tropicaux, *Lux*, 436.

Kittler, R. (1959) Historical review of methods and instrumentation for experimental daylight research by means of models and artificial skies, *C.I.E., Compte-rendu*, XIV, 319.

Krochmann, J. (1964) Zur Frage der vereinfachten Tageslichtberechnung, *Gesundheitsingenieur*, **85**, 47.

McGervan, D. (1965) Miniaturization in daylight prediction, *Light and Lighting*, **58**, 256.

Narasimhan, V., and Saxena, B. K. (1971) Luminance and illumination from clear skies in the tropics, *CIE, Compte Rendue*, XVII, p. 71.01.

Ogiso, S. (1965) Study on daylight sources, *J. Fac. Engng Univ. Tokyo*, **28**, 103.

Rennhackkamp, W. M. H. (1967) Sky luminance distribution in warm arid climates, C.I.E.—P 67-01.

Discomfort Glare from Windows

Hopkinson, R. G. (1971) *Glare from Windows*, Dept. of the Environment, London.

Public Lighting

Adrian, W., and Schreuder, D. A. (1971) A modification of the method for the appraisal of glare in street lighting. Paper presented at the XVII Session of the Commission Internationale de l'Éclairage, Barcelona.

Commission Internationale de l'Éclairage (1974) International Recommendations for the Lighting of Public Thoroughfares, Paris, C.I.E. (Publication No. 12) (Second Edition, in press.)

de Boer, J. B. *et al.* (1967) *Public Lighting*, Eindhoven, The Netherlands, Centrex.

Organization for Economic Co-operation and Development (1971) *Lighting, Visibility and Accidents* (Paris, OECD).

Schreuder, D. A. (1967) The theoretical basis of road-lighting design, Chap. 3 in de Boer, *et al.*, 1967.

Schreuder, D. A. (1964) *The Lighting of Vehicular Traffic Tunnels*, Eindhoven, The Netherlands, Centrex.

Waldram, J. M. (1952) *Street Lighting*, London.

Photometry

Keitz, H. A. E. (1967) *Lichtberechnungen und Lichtmessungen*, Eindhoven, Holland.

Walsh, J. W. T. (1965) *Photometry*, 3rd ed., New York.

8

NOISE IN RELATION TO HEALTH

T. FERGUSON RODGER

Recently, especially since the advent of civil jet-engined aircraft, there has been much agitation about the noise nuisance. Our environment exposes us to sights which are unwelcome but we can readily avoid them; we can turn our head away or shut our eyes. With noise we are usually more captive, although some biological adjustment is provided in the damping by the stapedius muscle, which protects the ears to a slight extent from sudden sharp changes in intensity.

Our auditory equipment is so constructed that sounds which are unfamiliar and might threaten danger automatically arouse us to vigilance, and in a noisy environment when the process of discriminating between the familiar and the unfamiliar is continuous, relaxation and sleep are hard to attain. The intrusive sounds which arouse us need not, however, be loud—they can also include faintly heard sounds, such as the neighbours' radio or a dripping tap. Indeed, the only acceptable definition of noise is unwanted sound.

MEASUREMENT OF NOISE

Noise is measured by meters which register the *sound pressure level* of the noise (s.p.l.). This is a physical and objective measure on a scale which is expressed in decibels (dB). Decibels represent ratios between sound pressure levels and are dimensionless unless they are related to a datum. The datum or reference level, unless another is specifically stated, can be assumed to be a sound pressure of 0·0002 dyne/cm.^{2} which represents the weakest sound which can be heard. Decibels are calculated as follows:

$$n \text{ dB} = 20 \log \frac{P_1}{P_2}$$

where P_1 is the measured s.p.l. and P_2 the datum s.p.l. (usually 0·0002 dyne/cm.^{2}). The dB scale is logarithmic; an increase of 10 dB in a sound-level meter reading corresponds to a ten-fold increase in the energy, while an increase of 3 dB corresponds approximately to a doubling of the sound energy.

Loudness

Two sounds which have the same sound pressure level may not appear to have the same loudness. Loudness depends not only on sound pressure level but also on frequency, i.e. the pitch of the noise. As a rule, sounds are composed not of pure tones but of a number of frequencies combined. In order to measure loudness a judgement must be made by persons listening to the noise, and it has been found in this way that consistent judgements about the relative loudness of sounds can be made and a scale of loudness level produced. The equivalent loudness of a sound is measured by the sound pressure level of a standard pure tone of specified frequency which is assessed as the modal value of the judgement of normal observers as being equally loud.

'In practice, this means that a standardising laboratory, such as the National Physical Laboratory, measures the loudness of a sound by presenting it to a group of observers alternately with variable-intensity pure tones of 1,000 cycles/sec. (Hz), judgements of loudness being made (in specified listening conditions) until equality is reached. The sound pressure level (s.p.l.) of the pure tone at balance is the measure of the loudness—and the unit in which the result is expressed is called the phon. This is a slow and expensive way of measuring the loudness of sounds and is used only for fundamental research' (Robinson, 1961).

A sound-level meter can be used constructed to resemble the performance of the human ear and to allow for the fact that the human ear is much less sensitive to very low or very high pitched sounds; for certain kinds of noise its pointer readings will correspond roughly with subjective assessments of loudness. It is known as a sound-level meter with A weighting and decibels registered on it as dBA.

Noise levels of some typical sounds (quoted from Report of Committee on Noise, 1963):

Noise source or environment	Sound level (dBA)	Relative loudness (sones)
Room in a quiet London dwelling at midnight	32	—
Soft whisper at 5 ft.	34	1·6
Men's clothing department of large store	53	7
Self-service grocery store	60	10·6
Household department of large store	62	11·3
Busy restaurant or canteen	65	13
Typing pool (9 typewriters in use)	65	15
Vacuum cleaner in private residence (at 10 ft.)	69	17
Inside small saloon car at 30 m.p.h.	70	24
Inside small sports car at 30 m.p.h.	72	—
Inside small sports car at 50 m.p.h.	75	—
Inside compartment of suburban electric train	76	26
Ringing alarm clock at 2 ft.	80	34
Loudly reproduced orchestral music in large room	82	—
Printing-press plant (medium-size automatic)	86	56
Heavy diesel-propelled vehicle about 25 ft. away	92	111

Note: These figures are given merely as a rough guide; they are for the most part single measurements, and might be expected to differ by several decibels if repeated in similar situations.

As can be seen, the sound levels given, although they arrange the noises in rank order of loudness, give no real indication of their relative loudness. Relative loudness is much more clearly indicated by using *sones*, a measure derived from the *phon* by the formula sones $= 2^{(\text{phons} - 40)/10}$.

The sound energies to which the human ear responds are very small indeed compared with physical energies utilized in machines and most electrical circuits. At the level of the weakest perceptible sound the excursion of the ear drum is only about $\frac{1}{10}$ of the diameter of the hydrogen molecule. Even at high noise intensities, the energies involved are still comparatively small, and Glorig (1958) has expressed this graphically when he stated that it would require 100,000 men shouting at the top of their voices to equal the energy that we use to cook an egg.

HEARING LOSS DUE TO NOISE

It has been known for centuries that workers employed in processes which involve high levels of noise during their working day eventually become hard of hearing. This was described by Ramazzini in *De morbis artificum* in 1713 as occurring in those who hammered copper and who 'became hard of hearing and if they grow old at this work, completely deaf'. After the Industrial Revolution exposure to loud noise became much more frequent, deafness in boilermakers was described by Barr (1886). Since then deafness has been shown to occur in numerous other occupations, in weaving, forging, punch-press operating, foundry work, blasting, using circular saws, shipbuilding, bell ringing, using high-frequency drills in dentistry, operating earth-moving equipment, driving combine harvesters, using automated office equipment, and servicing aircraft jet engines.

Damage to hearing can also occur suddenly through gross mechanical effects in the ear produced by sound waves of very high intensity such as occur during an explosion. This phenomenon is known as acoustic damage or acoustic trauma. This is an exceptional event which need not be considered further here.

In assessing loss of hearing due to noise it is necessary to try to exclude the loss of hearing which occurs through age alone (presbycusis). In sample populations it has been found that at equal ages men tend to have poorer and more variable hearing than women, and their loss of hearing usually occurs earlier. The differences between the sexes could well be explained by men being more frequently exposed to noisy occupations and to military service. Since the noise in our environment, in our city streets, for instance, has now risen to a level at which damage to hearing can occur, the question arises how far the loss of hearing due to age is compounded with loss of hearing due to noise. Rosen (1964) attempted to answer this question by an expedition to the Mabaans people who live in a remote area in the Sudan near the Ethiopian border. They live at the Late Stone Age level, they have no guns, hunt and fish with spears, and in their dances they do not use drums but pluck five-string lyres and beat a log with a stick. 'The sound level in the villages is below 40 dB on the C-scale of the sound-level meter except perhaps at dawn when a domestic animal makes itself heard'. There are occasional thunderstorms during part of the year with one or two claps of thunder. There are some noisy productive activities, such as beating palm fronds with a wooden club, but the absence of hard reverberating surfaces, such as walls, ceilings, floors, and hard furniture, reduces the intensity of the noise, which, under these conditions, is about 73–74 dB at the worker's ear. The highest noise levels

(100–104 dB) the expedition encountered were when the villagers were dancing and singing, peaking when there were shouts to 106–110 dB. This kind of festival activity occurs mainly in the spring and very little during the rest of the year. When the population were examined audiometrically there was very little loss of hearing through age, and even in the seventh and eighth decades the level of hearing was equal to what is found in Western populations in the first two decades. In other respects also the Mabaans age more slowly, and they tend to live longer than people in the West. They have no vascular hypertension, blood-pressure levels remain almost the same throughout life, and they do not have coronary artery disease or duodenal ulcer. They have little atherosclerosis and few psychosomatic diseases, and this Rosen concludes is due to their having extremely little stress and strain in their lives. Rosen is careful to point out that the intactness of their hearing in later life may not be entirely due to the absence of noise, it may be related to a general absence of degenerative changes in the tissues.

Hinchcliffe (1959) compared the hearing of a rural and urban population in the age groups 55–64 and 65–75. He found that there was a mean hearing loss of 18 and 25 dB in the rural population in these two age groups; the corresponding loss in the urban population was 45 and 49 dB, which suggested that presbycusis is related to noise exposure.

Similarly, Glorig and Nixon (1962) examined a group of people in America of various ages who had always lived and worked in an unusually quiet environment and who had never suffered even moderate acoustic trauma. Their hearing was superior to that of the general population as sampled at the Wisconsin State Fair; the population who were examined at the Fair were predominantly those who lived and worked in industrial areas.

We are left with the presumption, to put it no higher, that quite apart from any effects which may be due to annoyance, modern urban noise may lead to a steady diminution of hearing throughout life. From this viewpoint alone public health authorities should concern themselves with all the sources of noise in the environment.

TEMPORARY AND PERMANENT THRESHOLD SHIFT

Temporary threshold shift (TTS) refers to any loss of hearing from which the ear recovers; TTS regularly follows exposure to loud noise, and recovery may take only a few seconds or several days. In estimating the effects of noise the TTS induced by the noise is significant because it indicates that a change in the hearing mechanism has followed the noise and because it is further assumed that any noise which produces TTS will with prolonged exposure also produce *permanent threshold shift* (PTS). Workers exposed to high levels of noise have TTS at the end of their day's work from which they usually recover by the following morning or after the weekend. TTS is probably due to metabolic changes in the cochlea, and failure to return to the normal biochemical state before further exposure takes place may be of importance in the development of permanent hearing loss.

Atherley (1964) found that in young textile workers the period of rest from 17.00 hours on Friday to 08.00 hours on

Monday was insufficient to allow complete recovery of hearing to take place. The present vogue among young people for loud music during their leisure hours could play a part in prolonging temporary hearing loss and add to the danger of permanent hearing loss.

The TTS which follows exposure to noise is most marked about half an octave above the noise causing the shift, and the PTS is also more marked at a higher frequency than the noise which induces it. In the usual run of noisy occupations the initial loss affects the perception of sound at about 4,000 Hz. The loss at first passes unnoticed because communication by speech is not much affected at this frequency. With further exposure the hearing loss increases and spreads to adjacent frequencies. When 3,000 Hz becomes affected the worker will begin to have difficulty in hearing what is said to him and will complain of deafness. The extent of the hearing loss also varies with the frequency of the noise, the higher the frequency, the greater the effect on hearing. Noises of an impulsive character, i.e. from banging or hammering, have been considered to be particularly detrimental to hearing.

Damage Risk Criteria

It is important to attempt to assess the risk of damage to hearing which will follow exposure to any given noise. This depends on so many factors that it is difficult to estimate. Among these are:

1. The intensity of the noise measured in decibels.
2. The distribution of the energy of the noise over the octaves of the noise spectrum.
3. Whether the noise is intermittent or continuous.
4. The average length of exposure per working day.
5. The expected duration of the occupation.

The damage a noise does to hearing, it has been suggested, is determined by the total energy incident on the ear over a given time and is proportional to the product of its intensity and the duration of exposure; in this respect it can be compared with radiation damage and, indeed, dosimeters have been contrived to measure the total noise above a given level experienced by a worker during the day. By and large, noise is not held to be injurious unless it exceeds 85 dB in intensity.

However, the level of noise as measured by a sound-level meter does not give sufficient information about the effect of the noise. Since noise is much more damaging at higher frequencies, it is necessary to discover how the noise is distributed through the various frequencies. To do this, apparatus is used to measure the noise energy at the mid-point of a series of octaves. The International Organization for Standardization (1963) has tentatively proposed the use of noise-rating curves which take into account the level of noise in several frequency bands, noise-rating numbers identify the curves. Applying experimental data to the noise-rating curves, intermittency of exposure and total duration of 'on' time during the working day can be taken into account in calculating the risk of damage. While the conclusions reached in this document are tentative and provisional and not as yet well supported by experimental data, they are a useful guide to modern thinking.

Burns and Littler (1960) have proposed that for exposure to broadband noise for eight hours per day, five days per week, for a working lifetime, hearing conservation measures should be instituted if the noise in any of the frequency bands reaches the level shown in the following table:

TABLE 38

Frequency band (Hz)	Sound pressure level value (decibels)
37·5–150	100
150–300	90
300–600	85
600–1,200	85
1,200–2,400	80
2,400–4,800	80

They do not consider that it is possible to stipulate sound pressure levels for frequencies outside the bands specified in the table, as there is insufficient knowledge of the effects of noise at these frequencies. Nor are the criteria applicable to impulsive noise or noise containing intense pure tones which may be damaging at somewhat lower levels. They also think that, using the above criteria, certain slight losses of hearing might be suffered after long periods of daily exposure, and that in view of the differences between individuals, a few susceptible people might suffer significant losses at noise levels below those quoted.

The British Medical Association have stated that they believe 'that there is general acceptance of the view that working conditions involving continuous exposure throughout working hours for a prolonged period to noise whose intensity exceeds 85 dB in any octave band in the speech frequency range (250–4,000 Hz) may cause permanent damage to hearing'.

Glorig (1962) has suggested that 'for habitual exposure to continuous (non-intermittent) steady noise that is "on" more than five hours a day, hearing conservation measures should be initiated where the sound pressure level in any octave band exceeds International Standards Organisation Noise Rating number 85'. Noise-rating number 85 allows the following octave band levels.

Octave mid-frequency	63	125	250	500	1,000	2,000	4,000	8,000
Sound pressure level (dB) approx.	103	96	91	87	85	83	81	79

Kryter (1950) suggests as a damage-risk criterion allowing any exposure which on average does not produce a TTS of more than 10 dB measured (by audiometry) 2 minutes after exposure at 1,000 Hz, more than 15 dB at 2,000 Hz, and more than 20 dB at 3,000 Hz and above.

According to work described by Ward (1960), the hearing level at 4,000 Hz after ten years of daily exposure to a specific noise is, in general, numerically equal to the temporary hearing level measured 2 minutes after the cessation of 8 hours continuous exposure to the same noise. More research will be required to test this generalization.

It may sometimes be necessary to make a very rough estimate of the effect of a noise before using instruments for more accurate measurement. If a noise is loud enough to make conversation difficult even when shouting at a distance of

30 cm. from the listener's ear detailed instrument studies are indicated.

The last factor which was mentioned as having to be taken into account is the expected duration of the occupation. Some occupations are followed for a life-time because they depend on skills which are acquired over a period of many years. In these cases a man entering an occupation in his teens can be expected to remain in it until retirement. Such a man is exposed to greater risk of hearing loss than one who is employed, for instance, in an engineering trade, where for relatively short periods of his working life he may be working in a noisy environment. It follows that special attention has to be paid to methods for conserving hearing in occupations such as weaving and boilermaking.

Individual Susceptibility

The findings in the preceding paragraphs on the effects of noise on hearing are based on averages over a large number of individuals, but it is important to realize that not everyone develops the same hearing loss with equal exposure. Some susceptible persons develop impairment quickly, although it is believed that with prolonged exposure differences between individuals tend to disappear, and even in susceptible individuals industrial noise rarely, if ever, causes total deafness. Those persons who are particularly susceptible to hearing loss are often aware that noise disturbs them more than it does others. They can suffer from nausea and vertigo after exposure to loud noise.

Attempts have been made to identify the susceptible individual by assuming that the likelihood of permanent damage is proportional to the amount of TTS produced by the noise to which the individual is occupationally exposed. On this assumption regular audiometric examinations during the initial period of employment are advised to allow susceptible individuals to be identified. The amount of variation in individual susceptibility was shown in one investigation in Royal Naval Flying Deck personnel in which the mean hearing loss after nineteen months was 3–4 dB, but in 10 per cent. of the men there was a 10–15 dB loss in the range of the lower speech frequencies.

Speech Interference Level

Effective communication by speech is necessary in most occupations for efficiency and to prevent accidents. Interference in communication by speech is a masking process; in other words, background noise raises our hearing threshold for speech. When communication by speech becomes difficult the extent to which the hearing threshold is raised is described as the speech-interference level and is expressed in dB. Discontinuous noise often produces less interference with communication than expected, because gesture and repetition can make good the gaps in what is actually heard. Using a sound-level meter with network A, which is designed to simulate the response of the human ear to sound, the speech-interference level can be taken in general as about 55 dBA. This is the lowest level at which background noise can occur in offices and committee rooms, lecture rooms and educational institutions without seriously interfering with speech. It is also the level at which telephone conversation can normally be conducted without undue difficulty.

Reduction of the Risk to Hearing

Logically the best way to reduce the risk to hearing is to reduce the noise at source or so to contrive the lay-out that the worker is insulated as far as possible from the noise. The other, and on the whole, easier method to apply, is to protect the ears. Two forms of protection are used; ear muffs, which are heavy, bulky, and conspicuous but, on the whole, comfortable, or ear plugs, which are easily available commercially and which, if carefully used, are effective, but which tend to be uncomfortable, and their use is therefore apt to be neglected.

If efficient types of either ear plugs or muffs are worn continuously Burns and Littler (quoted in Noise Report, 1963) suggest the following levels of noise exposure as being allowable:

TABLE 39

Frequency band (Hz) (i)	With ear plugs (dB) (ii)	With ear muffs (fluid seal type) (dB) (iii)
37·5–150	110	120
150–300	110	115
300–600	110	118
600–1,200	110	125
1,200–2,400	110	122
2,400–4,800	110	125

They point out, however, that the figures which they give are based on laboratory results, and in practice the degree of protection may be less than is indicated, which suggests that for safety the levels given in columns (ii) and (iii) should be fixed a little lower.

In very high levels of noise, such as when mechanics are working near jet engines, both plugs and ear muffs are sometimes used to gain fuller protection. But with this intensity of noise bone conduction becomes significant, and ear protection by itself is not sufficient. In these cases helmets can be used, and the face should also be covered.

It is difficult to persuade workers to use protective devices, and a programme of education for workers to emphasize the need for protection will usually be necessary. Where ear plugs are used, it is better to use individually moulded plugs, which, although more expensive, are generally more effective and more comfortable to wear.

From time to time a check should be made of the effectiveness of the devices, which tend, for instance, to become loose in use; this has to be done by audiometry, measuring the attenuation afforded by the device. If workers are exposed to exceedingly high noise levels, e.g. working on jet engines, they may have pain through vibration of the bones, and are more ready to use protection in order to avoid the pain. It is, perhaps, unnecessary to state that workers with infected discharging ears should not be asked to use ear plugs, and their removal from the noisy environment may become necessary.

PSYCHOLOGICAL AND EMOTIONAL EFFECTS OF NOISE

This section might have been headed the effects of noise on mental health, but since the evidence for effects on mental health are slender and, on the other hand, annoyance caused by noise is often great, it is better to speak simply of emotional and psychological effects.

One of the disturbing effects of noise already mentioned is the effect of noise on communication by speech. This necessarily has widespread effects on human relationships, particularly when communication is an essential part of the activity of those exposed to the noise. Noise in schools near London Airport causes frequent interruption of class teaching, and one inspector was of the opinion that this had resulted in the standards of work in one school near the Airport being well below average.

Effects on Performance of Tasks

On a common-sense basis one knows that loud noise has a detrimental effect on the performance of tasks and that for efficient study and concentration, the quieter the environment the better. The architecture of libraries and court rooms has always taken this into account. One would think it would be easy, therefore, to confirm by experiment the effects of noise on concentration and on the efficient performance of tasks, but this is difficult to demonstrate under laboratory conditions.

Broadbent (1951 and 1957) has, however, been able to show two ways in which work is affected by noise. First, if a man is concentrating on a task depending on a high degree of vigilance, when he has to respond, for instance, to the appearance of a faint light on a gun-sight, he will take longer to respond under noisy conditions. Secondly, when working on a task which allows no break for rest momentary errors and aberrations will occur more readily in noise. Broadbent explains such errors by suggesting that under noisy conditions there are brief interruptions or 'blinks' in the flow of information between the ear and the brain. He has been able to show that these effects occur outside of the laboratory in a normal working environment even in people who are accustomed to the noise. He was able to demonstrate these effects on efficiency only at a very high level of noise (90 dB). The effects of noise on performance he found depend on the state of the person and the nature of his task. If fatigue is setting in and the task is of an undemanding and routine kind loud noise may act as a stimulus and errors may diminish. If, on the other hand, the task is of a very exacting kind and workers are keyed-up the effect of a loud noise may be to make them jittery and produce more errors.

It will be noticed that the level at which the effect of noise on the performance of tasks can be clearly demonstrated (90 dB) and the level at which damage to hearing occurs (85–90 dB) are more or less the same. That this may be the natural or biological limit to noise which should not be exceeded is suggested by the fact that in experiments on mice it was found that when exposed to a level of 90 dB they preferred, and learned, to move from one side of a cage to the other when their movement activated a switch which reduced the noise. It is probable that in a natural environment a level of 90 dB would be only rarely encountered, in thunderstorms, for instance, and that we are not, therefore, naturally equipped to tolerate higher levels. It may be that now that we are encountering much higher levels in our daily lives the annoyance we express is self-preservative.

Noise as a Stimulus

But before discussing annoyance further it should be mentioned that noise can be enjoyed and sought after for itself, and not only noise which is appreciated because of its musical quality but for its non-specific stimulant effect, which, Broadbent (1960) has shown, can arouse tired workers to improved performance. It is now well known that animals have an appetite for stimulation; they will work hard and learn tasks if they are rewarded by receiving an electrical current through electrodes implanted in the brain or, as has been shown in chimpanzees, by having a television programme switched on. Eysenck (1966) has drawn attention to the fact that if, by using a questionnaire, people are separated into those who show the characteristics of extroversion and those showing the characteristics of introversion, then their reaction to noise differs significantly. The extroverts are those who have a low level of internal stimulation, and accordingly seek stimulation from their environment, whereas introverts, who are more contemplative, are highly aroused internally and avoid external stimulation. In an experiment by Weisen, quoted by Eysenck, when the extroverts were seated in a dark and silent room and could, by pulling a lever at a fast rate, produce bright light and loud music they chose to do so, whereas introverts placed in a brightly lit room with loud music chose to darken the room and shut off the noise. It is probable, therefore, that in the population there are extroverted people who do not object, and may actively seek a noisy environment, and, on the other, the introverted, who prefer quiet. Moreover, it has been found that the older people are, the more likely they are to be of the introverted type, and will consequently dislike noise. Of those people living near London Airport where a survey was made, 10 per cent. of those interviewed in the area of the lowest level of noise were very much annoyed by the noise of aircraft, whereas in the areas with the greatest intensity of noise, and where the noise of aircraft occurred most frequently, 20 per cent. showed no annoyance.

Loudness and Fear

But if loud noise can sometimes be sought after as a stimulant more usually it is unpleasant, and when it occurs unexpectedly it can arouse fear. Watson (1920) made children afraid of toy animals by presenting them to the child simultaneously with a loud noise. It was stated in evidence given to the Committee on Noise that young children living near London Airport often displayed extreme fear when they heard the noise of jet aircraft; this was presumably an innate and unlearned natural response. Adults, on the other hand, showed a fear reaction only infrequently, and usually when they were awakened from sleep, when it might be assumed that the unlearned instinctive response of childhood came to the surface. In the evidence given to the Committee it was also suggested that the peculiar character of jet aircraft noise, which has a screeching or screaming quality, caused it to be more objectionable.

Habituation

Over the past twenty years we have learned that there is an arousal mechanism in the nervous system which increases or reduces tension and alertness in proportion to the sensory stimulation to which the organism is exposed. A new or un-familiar sound will produce an arousal of the nervous system, even if it is of low intensity, but when this sound is repeated this effect will die down. Some sounds, however, which are significant to the subject, like the rattling of a saucer of milk to the cat or the baby's cry to the sleeping mother, will main-tain their capacity to exert a strong arousal effect. Through conditioning, there are many sounds in the environment which can act in this way, and these can be a cause of annoyance when they tend to arouse an individual from sleep or disturb him.

Intrusion on Privacy

Perhaps the most specific cause of annoyance is intrusion on the privacy which we enjoy as human beings, the quiet to indulge in our own pursuits, the enjoyment of home or garden in leisure moments. The resentment felt is comparable to the territorial reaction shown by animals. When territory is invaded it arouses aggressive activity, and this may be why annoyance is caused when a noise intrudes on our private enjoyment. We are annoyed when noise intrudes on our thoughts, when it distracts us from pursuing our own purposes, or sometimes even when it reminds us that there are other groups of people with aims different from our own who are enjoying a party in a neighbouring house when we are trying to go to sleep. Most complaints which are made about the nuisance of noise have this character.

A more or less continuous noise, through a masking effect, can paradoxically reduce the disturbance caused to the indi-vidual. For instance, in a quiet corridor of a hospital when patients are trying to sleep, even a whispered conversation by the nurses may cause annoyance, whereas in another part of the hospital, where a noise from a ventilation shaft, for in-stance, gives a raised level of noise the nurses' conversations would pass unnoticed. To eliminate the effects of unexpected intrusive sounds a source of noise which is continuous and evenly spread through all the frequencies, so-called 'white' noise, can help concentration, since adventitious sounds will be submerged in the masking noise. For this reason a noise of this kind is sometimes used in such places as reading rooms.

COMMUNITY ACTION

In many parts of the world community action is being taken against noise problems (Goodfriend, 1969; Kaye et al., 1971; Lancet, 1969, 1970; Port and City of London, 1969; Smith, 1970).

Recent studies have shown that permanent serious loss of hearing can take place in discotheques even after 2 hours' ex-posure, and 'rock and roll' musicians are at special risk; this is of real importance because it must be seriously affecting the health of many young people throughout the world (Dey, 1970; Speaks et al., 1970).

American industry is now seriously concerned about the problems of permissible noise exposure levels due to the legislation passed on 20 May 1969 by the United States Labour Department on specific safety and health regulations and standards (Fox, 1970; Schneider et al., 1970). Federal regulations under the Canadian Labour Safety Code will shortly be published (Smith, 1970).

The Noise Abatement Society (1969) recently summarized the law concerning noise as it concerns the United Kingdom, but clearly much more needs to be done. The effects of super-sonic aircraft on health have yet to be determined, but are being closely watched both in the United States and in Europe.

On 28 May 1970 the British Government published a White Paper (H.M.S.O., 1970) which placed restrictions on aircraft noise at airports and banned sonic booms over land; it also made checks necessary for noise from heavy road vehicles. The problems are discussed in two leading articles in Nature (1970a and b). Government concern over this question is shown by the fact that the Department of the Environment in the United Kingdom has established a Noise Advisory Council which in turn has set up a working group to study the effect of flight routeing near airports on aircraft noise (H.M.S.O., 1971). Sufficient data now exists to develop community noise control programmes.

REFERENCES

Abroi, B. M., Nath, L. M., and Sachai, A. N. (1970) Noise and acoustic trauma. Noise levels in discotheques in Delhi, *Indian J. med. Res.*, **58**, 1758.

Atherley, G. R. C. (1964) Monday morning auditory threshold in weavers, *Brit. J. industr. Med.*, **21**, 150.

Barr, T. (1886) Enquiry into the effects of loud sounds upon the hearing of boilermakers and others who work amid noisy surroundings, *Proc. roy. phil. Soc. Glasgow*, **17**, 223.

Beales, P. H. (1965) *Noise, Hearing and Deafness*, London.

Bell, Alan (1966) Noise. An occupational hazard and public nuisance, *Wld Hlth Org. Publ. Hlth Pap.*, No. 30.

Broadbent, D. E. (1951) The twenty dials and twenty lights test under noise conditions. A.P.U. 160/51, The Psychologica Laboratory, Cambridge, England.

Broadbent, D. E. (1957) Noise and behaviour, *Proc. roy Soc. Med.*, **50**, 225.

Broadbent, D. E., and Little, E. A. J. (1960) The effects of noise reduction in a work situation, *Occup. Psychol.*, **34**, 133.

Burns, W., and Littler, T. S. (1960) Noise, in *Modern Trends in Occupational Health*, Chap. 17, London.

Burns, William (1973) *Noise and Man*, 2nd ed., London.

Catlin, F. I. (1965) Noise and emotional stress, *J. chron. Dis.*, **18**, 509.

Dey, F. L. (1970) Auditory fatigue and predicted permanent hearing defects from 'rock and roll' music, *New Engl. J. Med.*, **282**, 467.

Dougherty, J. D., and Walsh, O. L. (1966) Community noise and hearing loss, *New Eng. J. Med.*, **275**, 759.

Eysenck, H. J. (1966) Personality and experimental psychology, *Bull. Brit. Psychol. Soc.*, **19**, 62:1.

Fisk, D. J. (1973) The problem of traffic noise, *R. Soc. Hlth J.*, **93**, 289.

Fog, H., and Jones, E. (1968) Traffic noise in residential areas. Report 36, National Swedish Institute for Building Research and National Swedish Institute of Public Health, Stockholm.

Fox, M. S. (1970) Medical aspects of the industrial noise problem, *Industr. Med. Surg.*, **39**, 241.

Glorig, A. (1958) *Noise and Your Ear*, Modern Monographs in Industrial Medicine, I, New York.

Glorig, A., Ward, W. D., and Nixon, J. (1962) Damage risk criteria and industrial deafness, in *The Control of Noise*, the National Physical Laboratory Symposium, No. 12, Londonl H.M.S.O.

Goldsmith, John R., and Jonsson, Erland (1973) Health effects of community noise, *Amer. J. publ. Hlth.*, **63**, 782.

Goodfriend, R. S. (1969) Community noise problems, origin and control, *Amer. industr. Hyg. Ass. J.*, **30**, 607.

Hinchcliffe, R. (1959) The threshold of hearing of a random sample rural population, *Acta oto-laryng. (Stockh.)*, **50**, 411.

H.M. Government (1970) *The Protection of the Environment*, White Paper, H.M.S.O., London.

International Organisation for Standardisation (1963) Draft Secretariat proposal for noise rating with respect to conservation of hearing, speech communication and annoyance. (ISO/TC43 (Secretariat 194) 314.)

Kaye, G. *et al.* (1971) Our Street. A study of noise, *Med. J. Aust.*, i, 643.

Kryter, K. D. (1950) The effects of noise on man, *J. Speech Dis., Suppl.* 1.

Kryter, K. D. (1971) *The Effects of Noise on Man*, New York.

Kryter, K. D. (1972) Non-auditory effects of environmental noise, *Amer. J. publ. Hlth.*, **62**, 389.

Lancet (1969) Leading article, ii, 1289.

Lancet (1970) Leading article, i, 928.

Lang, Judith and Jansen, Gerd (1970) The Environmental Aspects of Noise Research and Noise Control (Euro 2631), Copenhagen.

Lord, P., and Thomas, F. L., ed. (1963) *Noise Measurement and Control*, London.

Nature (1970a) Booms banned; exhaust exempted, **226**, 889.

Nature (1970b) Is supersonic transport worth the noise?, **227**, 873.

Noise (1963) Final Report of the Committee on the Problem of Noise, London, H.M.S.O.

Noise Abatement Society (1969) *The Law on Noise*, London.

Noise Advisory Council (1971) *Aircraft Flight Routeing near Airports*, H.M.S.O., London.

Port and City of London (1969) *The Quiet City Campaign*, Health Committee Report, London.

Robinson, B. W. (1961) Noise: its causes, effects and abatement, *Roy. Soc. Hlth J.*, **81**, 81.

Rosen, S. *et al.* (1962) Presbycusis. Study of a relatively noise-free population in the Sudan, *Ann. Otol. (St. Louis)*, **71**, 727.

Rosen, S. (1964) High frequency audiometry in presbycusis. A comparative study of the Mabaan tribe in the Sudan with urban populations, *Arch. Otolaryng.*, **79**, 18.

Rylander, R., ed. (1972) Some boom exposure effects. Report of a workshop held in Stockholm 1971, *J. Sound and Vibration*, **20**, 477.

Sataloff, J. *et al.* (1969) Hearing loss from exposure to interrupted noise, *Arch. environm. Hlth*, **18**, 368.

Schneider, E. J. *et al.* (1970) The progression of hearing loss from industrial noise exposures, *Amer. industr. Hyg. Ass. J.*, **31**, 368.

Smith, L. K. (1970) Noise as a pollutant, *Can. J. publ. Hlth*, **61**, 475.

Speaks, C., Nelson, D., and Ward, W. D. (1970) Hearing loss in 'rock and roll' musicians, *J. occup. Med.*, **12**, 216.

United States Environmental Protection Agency: Report to the President and Congress on Noise, Dec. 31, 1971, Document NRC 500.1.

Ward, D. W. (1960) The relation between temporary threshold shifts and permanent threshold shifts. 8th Annual Report of Annual Meeting of Armed Forces Committee on Hearing and Bio-acoustics, Washington, D.C.

Ward, W. D., and Fricke, J. E., eds. (1969) Proceedings of the American Speech and Hearing Association Conference on Noise as a Public Health Hazard, Washington D.C.

Watson, J. B., and Rayner, R. (1920) *J. exp. Psychol.*, 3, 1.

World Health Organization Regional Office for Europe (1971) Report of a Working Group on Noise Control (Euro 3901), Copenhagen.

9

WATER SUPPLY, SANITATION, AND DISPOSAL OF WASTE MATTER

F. E. BRUCE

Introduction

It has long been recognized by public health workers that no country can have a satisfactory state of public health if the fundamental requirements of an adequate, safe water supply and properly controlled disposal of human and other waste products have not been satisfied. These requirements became acute in the industrialized countries during the nineteenth century and were met by the construction of major engineering works for the collection and distribution of water, by the adoption of the water-carriage system of excreta disposal, and by the development of techniques of treatment of water and wastes which are now firmly established. These methods have been extended in varying degrees to most countries, but two-thirds of the world's population, urban as well as rural, still have to depend upon simple and often crude and insanitary means of satisfying their basic needs.

Whereas countries with well-developed water supplies and waste disposal systems have been able to reduce the incidence of intestinal and other waste-borne diseases almost to vanishing point, these diseases are still a major cause of sickness and death over much of Africa, Asia, and South America. A formidable amount of work requires to be done to remedy this situation, but present constructional progress is in many countries unable even to keep pace with the increase in population, let alone catch up on the backlog. The fact that urban populations are increasing much more rapidly than rural indicates that the greatest benefit will be obtained by pressing forward with water supplies and waste disposal schemes in the larger cities and towns, where well-engineered major works are necessary on health grounds and can be justified economically. At the same time, all countries have problems in rural areas where simple schemes can be quite satisfactory if they are carefully planned and subsequently maintained.

The elimination of water- and waste-borne diseases is not the end of the public health engineer's task, for the progress of science and technology has brought many new chemical hazards into the water-waste field, which can be countered only by devising fresh techniques and even re-thinking some well-established ideas.

HEALTH CONSIDERATIONS

Many specific water- or waste-borne diseases and toxic hazards are discussed in more detail in other chapters, but it may be useful to summarize the principal ones here, in order to indicate the variety of paths involved and hence the multiplicity of points towards which attention must be directed.

In most of the diseases of interest here, the infective agent, whether bacterium, virus, protozoal cyst, helminth egg or larva, is discharged, often in enormous numbers, in human faeces or, in some instances, in the urine. The subsequent route to a new human host may be direct, through the ingestion of faecally contaminated water (as in cholera, typhoid, paratyphoid, bacillary dysentery, infective hepatitis, amoebiasis, etc.) or soil or vegetation (as in ascariasis and trichuriasis), or it may involve an intermediate host such as fish (fish-tapeworm) or cattle or pigs (taeniasis or cysticercosis). In other diseases, entry to the new human host is by penetration of the skin, e.g. schistosomiasis (from contaminated water with a snail as intermediate host) or hookworm (from contaminated soil).

Contaminated water also features in the transmission of dracontiasis (guinea-worm disease) in which worm larvae are discharged through the skin of a sufferer and develop in an intermediate host, the crustacean Cyclops, which may be swallowed when the affected water is drunk.

Control of the transmission of water-borne diseases requires either: (1) the rigid prevention of contact between human wastes and water sources; or (2) where such prevention of contact is not possible, effective means of treatment of the wastes, the water, or both. Under any circumstances it is naturally desirable to work to alternative (1), and this should certainly be a guiding principle in rural areas where reliable treatment facilities cannot be easily ensured. In more urbanized and industrialized areas, where uncontaminated water sources are difficult to find, the emphasis shifts to alternative (2).

Many of the diseases mentioned above can, of course, be transmitted also by personal contact, by flies or by contaminated food. This fact, together with the existence of the soil-borne diseases and others which do not involve drinking water, emphasizes the need not only for the protection of water supplies, but also for properly controlled disposal of bodily wastes.

Harmful concentrations of chemical substances in water do not often arise from purely natural causes. In some areas the natural fluoride content is enough to produce dental fluorosis and possibly more serious effects, though these appear to require predisposing conditions such as malnutrition (World Health Organization, 1970a). The nitrate content of natural water is unlikely to reach a level at which it might cause methaemoglobinaemia in babies unless it is enriched by fertilizers, farmyard seepage or sewage effluents. Most reported cases of methaemoglobinaemia have been associated with water affected by farming operations.

Water passing over ore-bearing geological formations may

dissolve sufficient toxic substances such as lead or arsenic to constitute a hazard if used for water supply, but there is no evidence that such conditions occur at all frequently. In recent years, however, evidence has accumulated to show a tendency for the incidence of cardiovascular diseases to be higher in areas served by soft water than in hard water areas (Stitt, Clayton, Crawford, and Morris, 1973). A causal relationship has not yet been proved.

Most toxic substances in water are derived from industrial process effluents (whether direct or by way of sewage effluents) or from agricultural operations such as the use of pesticides, sheep-dips, etc. Not only may such materials make it impracticable to use the water for potable supplies, but they may kill bacteria, fish and intermediate organisms and so deprive a river of its power of natural self-purification.

The main threats to health arising from solid wastes lie in the attraction of waste food and other organic matter to flies, rodents and birds which may disseminate diseases (not normally originating from the waste itself) such as the intestinal infections, plague, typhus and salmonelloses. There is little evidence of any more direct transmission of human disease through solid wastes (Hanks, 1967).

However, the increasing quantities of toxic solid wastes and sludges from industrial processes which now have to be disposed of give rise to dangers of water and soil pollution and of accidental poisoning, especially of children and animals. Two recent Government reports (Ministry of Housing and Local Government, 1970b; Department of the Environment, 1971) have recommended that a more comprehensive control should be established over the disposal of all forms of solid waste.

THE WATER CYCLE

Water in nature passes through the hydrological cycle, in which it is evaporated by the energy of the sun from the surfaces of the ocean, lakes, rivers and moist ground, and is later precipitated as rain, snow, hail or dew. On reaching the ground part of the precipitation returns to the atmosphere by evaporation or by transpiration by plants, part percolates into the ground and the remainder flows over the surface to form streams which eventually carry it back to the sea.

At each stage of the cycle, changes occur in the quality of the water, that is, in the nature and amount of dissolved and suspended substances which it contains. Evaporation frees it of all these substances, but in its passage through the atmosphere and over the ground surface, the water dissolves gases, minerals, and organic materials and carries in suspension fine particles derived from soil and vegetation. It also develops a complex interdependent population of bacteria, algae, protozoa, and larger plants and animals. Water which has percolated into the ground beyond the soil layer is usually fairly free of living organisms, organic matter and suspended solids, but may be rich in dissolved minerals as well as containing gases of decomposition such as carbon dioxide and hydrogen sulphide.

An additional stage in the hydrological cycle is interposed by human use. Water is collected as rain, surface run-off, or groundwater, used for a variety of purposes and then returned to the cycle as sewage effluent, industrial waste waters or other discharges, usually into rivers or the sea, but sometimes into the ground and to some extent by evaporation.

For the proper protection and management of water resources the whole cycle of natural water circulation, with the added effects of human intervention, must be considered. Balances have to be struck between the use of the valuable carrying and cleansing properties of flowing water and the preservation of its quality by the adoption of more advanced and elaborate methods of treatment for effluents and water supplies.

SOURCES OF WATER SUPPLY

Rain Water

In some places, such as Bermuda and Gibraltar, where no satisfactory surface or ground water supplies exist, rain water is collected from the roofs of individual houses, or from large paved catchment areas. The collecting surfaces should be maintained in a clean condition and adequate enclosed storage provided.

Surface Water

The quality of water in a river deteriorates as it flows from source to mouth, though the quantity increases, and the flow becomes more uniform. Impounded reservoirs on the upper reaches may thus provide pure water which can be conveyed through gravity aqueducts to the area of consumption with a minimum of treatment. Water taken from the lower reaches of a river usually has to be pumped and requires complete treatment, though relatively little storage may be necessary and the expense of a large aqueduct is saved.

Ground Water

Water which soaks into pervious geological formations, such as gravel, sand, alluvium, and limestone, may be extracted through dug wells or boreholes.

Dug Wells. These are excavated as open vertical shafts, lined with brick, cast iron, or concrete. They may range in size from the simple village well 1 or 2 m. in diameter and 5 or 6 m. deep, to major shafts up to 6 m. in diameter and 100 m. or more in depth. The yield is sometimes improved by driving horizontal tunnels or adits at suitable depths.

Boreholes. Boreholes up to 0.6 m. in diameter are drilled by percussion or rotary tools, mechanically operated. They are lined with steel or other tubing, and since they generally penetrate to deep water-bearing strata which are overlain by impervious beds, the water is protected from surface or sub-soil pollution.

Pumps must be installed in deep dug wells or boreholes except where the pressure of the water is sufficient to force it to the surface, producing a flowing artesian well.

For small water supplies from sandy or alluvial ground *tube wells* 50–150 mm. in diameter may be constructed by direct driving of a tube fitted with a driving point and a screen at its lower end. These are practicable for depths up to about 25 m.

Springs. Springs are natural flows of water which occur where the ground water is brought to the surface at the junction of pervious and impervious strata, or through fissures or faults in the rock. They often yield water of excellent quality, but the flow may vary seasonally.

Infiltration Galleries. These are tunnels driven near river beds to collect ground water. Because they lie below river level they can give a steady yield of water which has undergone natural filtration in passing through the ground.

Sea Water

As it becomes increasingly difficult and expensive to meet the demand for fresh water, so the use of de-salted sea-water will become more competitive and more widely adopted. It is no longer confined to arid countries and sea-going ships. Methods of desalination are referred to later in this chapter.

Reclamation of Effluents

The re-use of sewage effluent after it has been discharged to, and diluted by, a river has been a commonplace occurrence for many years, as, for example, in the River Thames. The more direct use of effluents for industrial purposes, e.g. for power station cooling water, has also been practised on a considerable scale. More recently, methods have been developed for the purification of sewage effluents to a standard at which they can be used as drinking water. There have, as yet, been few examples of practical application, but the procedure may be expected to figure in the water economy in the future.

REQUIREMENTS OF WATER

The amount of water required daily for the maintenance of life is about 2 litres but much greater quantities are required for other domestic activities, such as washing, cooking, laundry, and the flushing of water-closets. The total quantity used for these purposes depends upon the ease of obtaining the supply, as the following table suggests:

NATURE OF SUPPLY	DAILY CONSUMPTION PER PERSON
Drawn by hand from outside well . .	20 litres
Piped to single tap in house . . .	45 litres
Piped to sink, wash-basin, bath, and water-closet, with domestic water-heating system	150 litres or more

The use of water for washing-machines, garden watering, and other purposes adds to these requirements. In many British cities daily consumption averages from 180 to 230 litres per person, while in some countries demands of over 450 litres per person per day are common.

Water must also be supplied for public purposes, including fire-fighting and street-cleansing.

Water requirements for industry vary widely. Small industrial users may be supplied by the local water authority, but larger consumers usually obtain their own supplies from rivers, wells, or other sources.

MEASUREMENT OF WATER QUALITY

The quality of water and its suitability for particular purposes are assessed by carrying out physical, chemical, biological, and bacteriological examinations.

Physical Quality

The colour, turbidity, taste, and odour of a water are measures of its acceptability or attractiveness to consumers. They do not necessarily indicate whether or not water is safe to drink.

Chemical Quality

A knowledge of the chemical quality of a raw water is necessary as a guide to its suitability for use, and to reveal and measure any undesirable contamination. It provides a basis for deciding the method of purification. Regular chemical analysis must also be carried out to check the effectiveness of treatment processes. Similarly, chemical analysis is used to follow the progress of purification of sewage and to measure the quality of the effluent. Some of the main chemical constituents and their significance are summarized below.

Chlorides. These are present in most natural waters. A sudden increase in concentration may indicate pollution by sewage, since human urine contains about 5,000 mg. of chlorides per litre.

Nitrogen. Nitrogen determined in various forms (*organic, albuminoid, ammonia, nitrite,* and *nitrate nitrogen*) measures the progress of bacterial decomposition of organic matter in sewage and natural waters.

pH. This is a measure of the hydrogen ion concentration and indicates whether a water is acidic (pH below 7), neutral (pH 7), or alkaline (pH above 7). In conjunction with *alkalinity* (caused by hydroxides, carbonates, and bicarbonates), *carbon dioxide* and other constituents the pH value serves to indicate whether a water is likely to be either corrosive or scale-forming.

Dissolved Oxygen. Oxygen dissolved in water is used by aerobic bacteria in the oxidation or organic matter, and is especially significant in rivers receiving discharges of sewage or other organic effluents. Heavily polluted waters may become devoid of oxygen and hence offensive through the release of hydrogen sulphide. Fish require a dissolved oxygen concentration of from 30 to 50 per cent. of the saturation value.

Biochemical Oxygen Demand. The biochemical oxygen demand (B.O.D.) of sewage or other polluted water measures its organic content in terms of the oxygen required for bacterial oxidation. The standard test measures the oxygen taken up in five days at 20° C.

Permanganate Value. The permanganate value, or oxygen absorbed, is a measure of the organic matter oxidized by potassium permanganate under standard conditions.

Suspended Solids. These are determined by filtering a sample of water or sewage, and give a guide to the efficiency of sedimentation and other treatment processes.

Hardness. This is caused mainly by salts of calcium and magnesium, which form scale in boilers and precipitate curd from soap, though not from synthetic detergents. It is determined colorimetrically.

Other chemical constituents, including toxic metals and salts, may have to be determined in assessing the suitability of a water for supply.

Recommendations on quality standards for drinking water have been published by the U.S. Public Health Service (1962) and by the World Health Organization (1970b and 1971).

Biological Quality

Growths of algae, protozoa, and other organisms are found in most bodies of surface water. The algae in particular are capable of rapid multiplication at certain seasons, and may cause difficulties in water supply by blocking filters and producing tastes. Regular microscopic examination, in conjunction with chemical analysis, enables the water biologist to foresee such developments so that preventive action can be taken.

Bacteriological Quality

Routine bacteriological examination of water is devoted mainly to detecting and enumerating coliform organisms. The presence of *Escherichia coli* is taken as indicating definite faecal pollution of either human or animal origin. Other coliform organisms may indicate more remote faecal pollution (Department of Health, 1969b). Tests for faecal streptococci and *Clostridium perfringens* may provide confirmatory evidence of faecal pollution, while colony counts at 37° C. and 22° C. are used to assess the general bacterial quality of a water. Tests for pathogenic bacteria such as *Salmonella typhi* are not done as a routine.

The *membrane filter* technique is now widely used in the bacteriological examination of water. It is labour-saving, gives rapid results, and permits early investigation of the source of any unfavourable bacterial counts.

WATER TREATMENT

Since natural waters are often polluted to a greater or lesser extent, they must be purified to make them fit for human consumption or for other desired purposes. Water for drinking must be made safe by the removal of pathogenic organisms and dangerous chemicals. It should also be made attractive to the consumer by the removal of visible suspended matter, colour, and any substances producing taste or odour.

The principal treatment processes are straining, sedimentation, filtration through sand (with or without the help of chemical coagulation), and disinfection. Other forms of treatment, e.g. softening or iron removal, may be necessary on economic grounds. Water for industrial purposes often requires further special stages of treatment.

Straining

Water collected from a river is drawn through an intake provided with a coarse bar screen to hold back sticks and other floating objects. Finer solids, including leaves and small fish, may then be removed by straining through mechanical screens in the form of rotating drums, discs, or continuous bands. These are cleaned by jets of water playing on the moving screen as it emerges from the water. In the *microstrainer* the straining medium is a woven stainless steel fabric with apertures down to 0.015 mm. which can remove a large proportion of algae.

Sedimentation

When water is stored in an impounding reservoir it is clarified to some extent by the settling out of silt and other solids. Non-impounded waters, e.g. from lowland rivers, may also be clarified by sedimentation in storage reservoirs or in smaller tanks having a detention period of a few hours.

The simplest type of sedimentation tank is a rectangular concrete tank through which the water flows continuously from one end to the other. When coagulants are used, as described below, or when water is softened with lime, a vertical-flow, hopper-shaped tank is often preferred [FIG. 40]. The chemically treated water flows upward at a carefully controlled rate, and the flocculent solids form a suspended *sludge blanket*

which traps the finer particles. The clarified water is collected over weirs at the top. A more elaborate development is the sludge contact type of tank, which incorporates chambers for the addition and mixing of the chemicals.

Coagulation

Many waters contain much fine suspended matter which cannot be removed by simple sedimentation. Others are naturally coloured by colloidal suspensions of organic acids derived from vegetation. They may be treated by addition of chemical coagulants which react with the alkalinity in the water to form flocculent precipitates. By the neutralization of surface electric charges and by physical trapping of the finer particles these flocs facilitate the clarification of the water by sedimentation and rapid sand filtration.

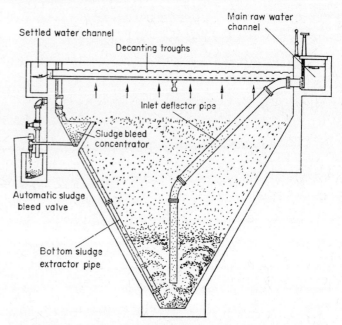

FIG. 40. Vertical-flow sludge blanket type of sedimentation tank. (By courtesy of Paterson Candy International Ltd.)

The most commonly used coagulant is aluminium sulphate, whose action is sometimes aided by small additions of other chemicals, including sodium aluminate, 'activated silica' and the synthetic polyelectrolytes. Iron salts are also useful coagulants.

Sand Filtration

With the possible exception of disinfection, filtration through a bed of sand is the most widely used method of purifying water. Two main types of sand filter are in use, the 'slow' and the 'rapid' filter.

Slow Sand Filters. Slow sand filters are beds of sand from 0·6 to 1 m. deep and covering an area of up to 0·4 ha per bed. The sand rests on layers of graded gravel, which lies over a system of brick, tile or concrete underdrains. The water to be filtered is fed on to the top of the sand, and passes slowly downward through the sand and gravel into the underdrains. These are connected to main collecting channels or pipes which lead to a filtered water tank. The normal rate of filtration is about 2·4 m.³ of water per m.² of filter surface per day.

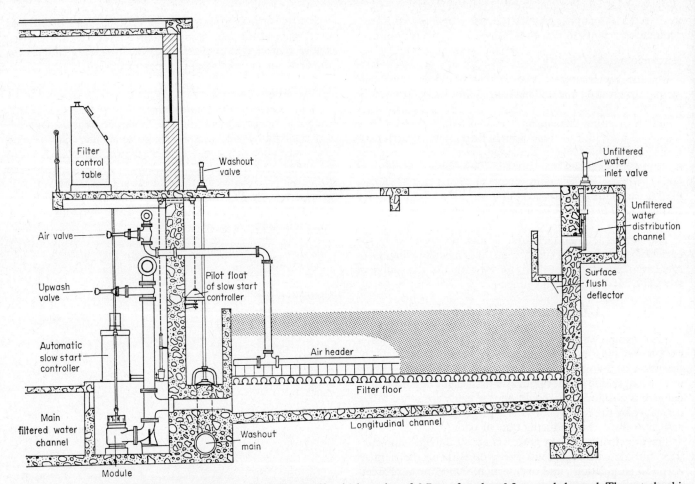

FIG. 41. Section of a rapid gravity sand filter. In this design the filter bed consists of 0·7 m. of sand on 0·3 m. graded gravel. The waterlevel is about 1·4 m. above the sand during filtration. To wash the filter, the water is lowered to the level of the weir to the left of the bed. Compressed air is admitted to the underdrains and produces intense agitation of the sand. This is followed by an upward flow of water to carry the dirt away through the washout main. (By courtesy of Paterson Candy International Ltd.)

The main work of a slow sand filter is done on the surface, where a slimy layer of bacteria, algae, protozoa, worms, and insect larvae develops. Besides trapping very fine suspended matter from the water, including bacteria, this living layer effects considerable chemical improvement by oxidizing organic matter. With the growth of the surface layer, however, resistance to the passage of water increases until it becomes necessary to clean the filter. This is done by draining the water down and scraping off the top 10–25 mm. of sand, either by hand or with mechnical equipment. The filter is then put back into service, but it is not fully efficient until the surface film has again developed. Cleaning may be necessary at intervals of two to twelve weeks, according to the amount of impurity in the water. When successive cleanings have reduced the depth of the sand to about 0·5 m. it is built up again with sand that has been thoroughly washed.

Rapid Sand Filters. These differ from slow sand filters in using rather coarser sand through which the water is filtered at a rate of from 100 to 150 m.³/m.² per day. The area of filter required to treat a given flow of water is therefore only about one-fiftieth of that needed for slow filtration. The beds are constructed either as gravity filters within open-topped concrete boxes [FIG. 41], or as pressure filters completely enclosed in steel cylindrical shells. Washing is carried out at

intervals ranging from a few hours to two or three days according to the rate of blockage of the filter. It is done by passing an upward flow of water through the sand bed to loosen and carry away dirt. This process may be assisted by compressed air, mechanical agitation, or surface jets of water.

Rapid sand filters do not have time between washings to build up a surface biological layer. They are usually preceded by chemical coagulation, and the coagulation floc to some extent takes the place of the biological layer as a trap for fine solids and bacteria. These filters are less effective in the removal of bacteria and in the chemical improvement of water quality than slow sand filters. They are, however, much more widely used for municipal water supplies because of the smaller land area required, and because final disinfection can be relied on to ensure the bacterioligical safety of the finished water.

Filtration Through Other Materials

Small water supplies may be clarified in enclosed filters in which a layer of fine *diatomaceous earth* is built up by the pressure of the water on the outside of a cylindrical metal former. The water passes inwards through the layer, and when the diatomaceous earth becomes blocked with dirt it is flushed out of the container by reversing the flow of water.

The *ceramic candle* filter uses a hollow cylinder of unglazed porcelain through which the water is passed from the outside. If the candle is cleaned frequently by scrubbing and boiling it can give filtered water of high bacterial purity. Some filters of this type are impregnated with a silver salt which, by releasing small concentrations of silver ions into the water, provides disinfection as well as filtration.

These filters are useful for domestic supplies and for emergency or field use.

Disinfection

It is common practice nowadays to disinfect water before distributing it to consumers, whether or not it has required filtration or other treatment. Filtration, operated with care, can reduce the bacterial content of water by from 95 to 99·9 per cent., but disinfection aims at a complete kill of pathogenic bacteria and of the coliform indicator organisms. It is not intended to effect complete sterilization. It should be noted that the concentrations of disinfectant normally applied in waterworks practice are not sufficient to kill amoebic cysts, nor are they effective against certain viruses.

Chlorine. Chlorine is by far the commonest disinfecting agent. On large works it is supplied compressed as a liquid in cylinders or drums. It is released from these as gaseous chlorine through measuring devices (*chlorinators*) and then dissolved in small quantities of water which are injected into the main body of water. The chlorinators are either adjusted manually or controlled automatically to supply chlorine at a rate proportional to the flow of water. On small works chlorine is applied as a solution of sodium or calcium hypochlorite or as bleaching powder.

Chlorine reacts with other substances in water, and its combination with ammonia (present in polluted waters from the breakdown of nitrogenous organic matter) to form chloramines is particularly important. The chloramines are very much weaker bactericides than uncombined chlorine, but their persistence and their smaller tendency to react with other substances gives them some advantage in extended distribution systems or long aqueducts. Addition of an excess of chlorine destroys the chloramines, and at the point where these disappear—the *break point* [FIG. 42]—practically no chlorine, either free or combined, is left in the water in a bactericidal form. Any chlorine added beyond the break point is available as *free residual chlorine* with full bactericidal power. In modern practice the dose of chlorine is controlled, often through automatic equipment, so as to maintain a small residual of free chlorine, e.g. 0·2 mg./litre, after a contact period of $\frac{1}{2}$–1 hour. Alternatively, a larger residual is achieved (*superchlorination*), followed, after a contact period, by *dechlorination* with sulphur dioxide or other chemical, so that no objectionable taste is left in the water.

Satisfactory chlorination requires complete mixing of the chlorine with the whole body of water and an adequate contact period, preferably not less than half an hour, before consumption. The bactericidal power of chlorine is improved at higher temperatures and at lower pH values. Since chlorine gas is highly toxic, precautions are necessary in the lay-out and operation of chlorination apparatus.

Ozone. This is the only other disinfectant which has achieved much use in public water supplies. It is generated by passing clean dry air between electrodes to which a high-frequency, high-voltage electric current is applied. The issuing air, containing 1 to 2 per cent. by weight of ozone, is injected or diffused into the water to be treated.

Ozone is a powerful bactericide, which kills rapidly and is more effective against spore-forming organisms than chlorine. It is less affected by variation of temperature or pH. Excess ozone soon comes out of solution, leaving no residual, but this fact commends it to those who do not like drinking 'medicated' water. It oxidizes colouring matter and gives the water a sparkling bluish appearance.

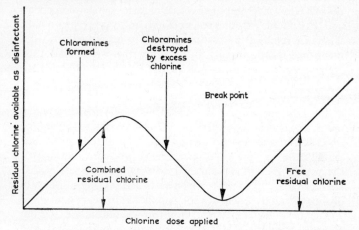

FIG. 42. Addition of chlorine to water containing ammonia. The curve shows the formation of chloramines, their destruction by further quantities of chlorine, and the establishment of free residual chlorine beyond the break point.

Ozone disinfection is considerably more expensive than chlorination, and until recently has been used in relatively few plants outside France, where it has always been widely favoured. The process has, however, gained some ground in the past few years.

Other disinfecting agents used for special purposes or for treating small quantities of water include certain compounds of chlorine, bromine, or iodine, ultra-violet light, and small concentrations of silver. Mention should also be made of boiling, which will kill all types of pathogens, and is indispensable in emergency.

Softening

In softening public water supplies, lime is added to precipitate the calcium and magnesium salts as calcium carbonate and magnesium hydroxide. Sodium carbonate is also added if non-carbonate hardness is present. The sludge is removed by settling and filtration.

Alternatively, the *ion-exchange* method of softening can be used. The water, which must be free of suspended matter, is passed through a bed of granular ion-exchange material, which has the property of exchanging sodium ions from its surface for the calcium or magnesium ions in the water. When the exchange capacity of the material is exhausted it must be regenerated by passing a brine solution through the bed to reverse the exchange process.

This principle is used in domestic water softeners.

By an extension of the ion-exchange process water for industrial use may be *demineralized* and converted to the equivalent of distilled water. This is done by passing it first through a cation-exchanger which replaces calcium, sodium, and other metallic ions with hydrogen ions. The acids thus produced are then completely removed in a bed of anion-exchange material.

Removal of Iron and Manganese

Iron and manganese may occur in ground water, where they go into solution under conditions of low dissolved oxygen, high carbon dioxide, and low pH. Similar conditions may be found in the bottom layers of a lake or reservoir. The metals are undesirable in water supplies because of taste and staining effects and the possible encouragement of iron bacteria in water mains. They are removed by oxidizing them to insoluble ferric and manganic forms, usually by aerating the water, and then filtering out the resulting precipitates.

Fluoridation

The addition of fluoride ions to water supplies to give an optimum concentration between 0·7 and 1·2 mg./l. (depending upon climate and on other dietary intake) as a protection against dental caries is now a well-established procedure throughout the world. It is of proven effectiveness, and no satisfactory alternative to this controversial measure has yet been shown to give comparable benefits to the population in general.

The most suitable and convenient chemicals are sodium fluoride, sodium silicofluoride, and hydrofluosilicic acid, and the equipment used to feed them into water is generally similar to that used for other water treatment chemicals. Usually, however, additional safeguards are introduced to control the dose within narrow limits. Precautions must be taken to protect workers handling fluoride chemicals, especially those in powdered form.

Experience of fluoridation in Britain has been described in official reports (Department of Health, 1969a) and in several technical journals.

Desalination of Sea-water

Methods of de-salting sea-water have been the subject of intensive research in recent years. The multi-stage flash distillation method has emerged as the most successful at present, but progress is being made with other methods such as freezing and reverse osmosis.

The heavy power requirement of desalination plants has encouraged their construction in conjunction with nuclear power stations where surplus energy is available or in oil-producing countries where power is relatively cheap.

Less saline water may be made potable by the process of electrodialysis through semi-permeable ion-exchange membranes.

DISTRIBUTION OF WATER

After treatment, water is distributed to consumers through a network of mains of cast iron, steel, asbestos, cement, rigid PVC, or (in smaller sizes) flexible polythene. Service reservoirs, either at ground level or in the form of elevated water towers, are sited at suitable points where they will maintain adequate pressure in the mains and will afford protection against interruption of supply, or a reserve for fire-fighting. They should be covered and water-tight to prevent contamination and algal growth.

Domestic supplies are taken from the mains by lead, iron, or copper service pipes, controlled by a stopcock at the boundary of each property. In most parts of Britain the service pipe feeds a storage cistern placed in the roof space, and all appliances within the house, except for one tap in the kitchen connected directly to the service pipe, are supplied from this cistern. By this means a reserve of water is held in the house, and the pressure on the plumbing fixtures is kept low and constant. In some areas, however, and in many other countries domestic storage cisterns are not used, and all supplies in the house are fed directly from the service pipe.

With few exceptions, domestic water supplies in Britain are not metered, and payment is usually based on the rateable value of the premises.

Back-siphonage in plumbing systems may occur when pressure is reduced through the closing of a valve, bursting of a pipe, or very heavy draw-off. If at the same time there is a submerged inlet at a higher level in the same plumbing system, e.g. an open or leaking tap dipping below water level in a basin, water from the latter will be drawn back into the piping and may reach other consumers. Backflow into the public mains cannot take place from an appliance which is supplied through a storage cistern at atmospheric pressure.

Some units of hospital equipment, e.g. instrument sterilizers and bed-pan washers, offer particular risks of spreading infection should back-siphonage occur, and special precautions must be taken in the design of the plumbing system.

SEWERAGE

A sewerage system is known as a *combined* system if it carries both foul sewage, i.e. wastes from houses and other buildings, and surface water from rainfall in the same set of pipes. A *separate* system has one set of sewers for foul sewage and another for surface water, which is thus kept free of human wastes and can be discharged direct to watercourses. The *partially separate* system also has two sets of sewers, but some rain water from roofs and surroundings of houses is allowed to flow into the foul sewers.

Because the volume of surface water to be carried in times of storm is very much greater than the volume of foul sewage, it is normal practice for combined systems to incorporate *storm sewage overflows*, from which a mixture of surface water and foul sewage may be passed direct to a river. In this way the sewage treatment works is kept to a reasonable size, but the overflow can cause serious pollution of streams. For this reason new sewerage systems are usually designed on the separate principle. Storm sewage overflows have been the subject of a recent report (Ministry of Housing and Local Government, 1970a) which considers pollutional effects as well as improved design.

Materials for pipe-sewers include glazed vitrified clay, concrete, asbestos-cement, rigid PVC, pitch-fibre and, for additional strength, cast iron or steel. Improved flexible joints permit rapid laying of sewers with less risk of subsequent damage through soil movement. Larger sewers are usually built of concrete cast in place, sometimes lined with hard engineering bricks.

Sewers are laid as far as possible on gradients which will ensure gravity flow with no accumulation of solid deposits, but pumping is sometimes necessary. Manholes are provided every 100 metres or so to permit inspection and cleaning of the sewers.

Quantity of Sewage

The quantity of domestic sewage is generally a little less than the quantity of water supplied, some having been lost by evaporation, garden watering and other uses. To the purely domestic flow must be added any wastes entering the sewers from industries. There may also be appreciable infiltration of ground water into the sewers through faulty joints or cracks, especially in an old system. The amount of surface water varies from nothing to perhaps 30 or more times the volume of foul sewage.

The average daily flow arising from domestic and industrial sources and from infiltration, without any surface water, is known as the *dry weather flow* or D.W.F. It has been normal practice in Britain to design sewage treatment works to handle volumes up to three times D.W.F.

In British towns the D.W.F. is generally between 140 and 220 litres per person per day. The actual rate of flow varies from hour to hour, from perhaps 30 per cent. of the average in the early hours of the morning to a daytime peak of 150 per cent., depending on the nature and size of the town and on the pattern of industrial discharges. The strength of sewage varies in a similar way, the low flow during the night being composed mostly of water from leaking taps or appliances and infiltration of ground water.

SEWAGE TREATMENT

Domestic sewage consists of water containing only about $\frac{1}{4}$ per cent. of its weight of dissolved and suspended solid matter. Much of this matter is organic and will rapidly be decomposed by bacteria with the consumption of oxygen and the creation of offensive conditions. Its content of intestinal organisms makes sewage a potentially dangerous mixture. For these reasons, treatment processes are applied to convert it to a liquid effluent and a sludge which can be disposed of safely and without nuisance, into rivers or the sea, or on the land.

Industrial waste waters vary in composition over a vast range, some containing mainly inert solids, others high concentrations of organic matter, and yet others a great variety of chemicals which may be inorganic or organic, natural or synthetic, toxic or non-toxic. Some of these wastes can with advantage be accepted into the public sewers for dilution and treatment with the domestic sewage. Others may be discharged direct to rivers. In either case some form of pre-treatment, e.g. sediment-ation or chemical neutralization, may be necessary.

The principal sewage treatment processes comprise *primary* or physical treatment to separate solids from the liquid, and *secondary* or biological treatment in which organic substances are broken down and stabilized by bacterial action. These two main stages, in a properly designed and operated plant, are able to yield an effluent which meets the standards recom-mended by the Royal Commission on Sewage Disposal (1912). These 'Royal Commission Standards' (biochemical oxygen demand not to exceed 20 mg./l. and suspended solids 30 mg/l.,

with modifications in certain circumstances) have served as a guide in Britain and elsewhere for 60 years. However, more stringent standards have increasingly to be applied nowadays, e.g. where a large sewage treatment works discharges its effluent into a small stream. In such cases a *tertiary* treatment process, such as sand filtration, microstraining or filtration through plots of land, becomes necessary.

The sludge removed from the sewage by sedimentation may also be given physical treatment (de-watering, filtration or incineration) with or without prior biological treatment in the form of anaerobic digestion.

Chemical coagulation may be used to assist sedimentation or sludge treatment.

Screening

The first step in the treatment of sewage is the removal of the larger solids by passing it through bar screens with openings from 20 to 100 mm. placed across an open channel. In small works the screenings are raked from the screen by hand and disposed of by burying. In larger works the screens are kept clean by mechanical rakes or brushes, and the screenings are often cut up by shredders or disintegrators and returned to the sewage flow, to be removed by sedimentation. An alternative to screens and shredders is the comminutor, a device with a slotted drum which rotates in the sewage flow and cuts and screens the solids in one operation.

Grit Removal

Some sewages contain substantial amounts of fine granular material, especially those derived from combined sewerage systems, which carry grit from roads. It is desirable to remove this material, which otherwise causes heavy wear in pumps and tends to settle out and cause difficulty in later treatment pro-cesses.

A common method is to allow the sewage to flow along a channel at a controlled velocity of about 0·3 m./s. This velocity is low enough to permit the heavy mineral solids to settle, but is high enough to carry the lighter organic solids forward. The grit which settles out in the channel is removed periodically and may be washed free of organic matter to allow it to be dumped on waste ground without causing nuisance.

Other grit removal devices use mechanical or hydraulic means to improve the separation of mineral and organic solids.

Sedimentation

The main process of primary treatment is sedimentation to remove as much as possible of the organic solids from the liquid. The tanks used employ the same principles as those de-scribed above for the treatment of water. They may be rect-angular, with horizontal flow, hopper-shaped, with vertical flow, or circular, with radial flow from the centre of the peri-phery. Some tanks incorporate slow-moving paddles to en-courage flocculation of the solids, which thus acquire increased settling velocities. Mechanical scrapers move the settled sludge to hoppers. from which it is drawn off either continuously or at frequent intervals to prevent its becoming septic.

The period of retention in sedimentation tanks may be from 2 to 8 hours and the process removes 50–60 per cent. of the suspended solids and about 40 per cent. of the B.O.D. of the incoming sewage.

Biological Treatment

The biological treatment of sewage involves essentially the oxidation of suspended and dissolved organic matter by aerobic bacteria which develop naturally in the human wastes. Carbonaceous matter is converted, through simpler molecules, to carbon dioxide and water, and nitrogenous material to ammonia, nitrites and nitrates. The work of the bacteria is supplemented by fungi, algae, ciliate protozoa, insects, and worms.

The earliest form of biological treatment was carried out by passing sewage over the surface of the land. Besides purifying the sewage *land treatment*, or '*sewage irrigation*', provides both water and nutrients for growing plants. Stringent public health precautions are necessary, and crops are usually restricted to those suitable for forage. Land treatment requires large areas, up to 4 ha. per 1,000 population, according to the type of soil and method of operation.

Attempts during the latter part of the nineteenth century to concentrate the effects of land treatment into smaller areas led, by way of various intermittent filtration or contact processes, to the method of continuous biological filtration through coarse media. This process now shares the field of aerobic sewage treatment with the activated sludge process, introduced in 1914.

Biological Filtration

Biological filters (also known in Britain as 'percolating filters' and in America as 'trickling filters') are beds of broken stone, slag, gravel, or other material, generally from 25 to 75 mm. in size, and from 1 to 3 m. deep, over which settled sewage is sprayed from rotating or travelling distributors [FIG. 43]. A

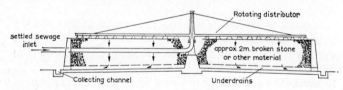

FIG. 43. Diagrammatic section of a biological filter for the treatment of sewage.

slimy film of aerobic bacterial and other organisms (the 'zoogleal' film) develops on the surface of the stones, and in trickling downward through the bed the sewage gives up much of its organic content to the film and receives back soluble salts produced in the oxidation process. Free access of air through the filter is essential. The filters are followed by final settling or *humus tanks* to remove the particles of the zoogleal film which slough off the stones periodically. The humus is generally returned to the primary sedimentation tanks, from which it is removed for treatment with the primary sludge.

When treating normal domestic sewage, filters are dosed at 0.4 to 2 m.³ of sewage per m.³ of bed per day, according to the strength of the sewage. These rates permit the treatment of sewage from up to 100,000 persons per hectare of bed 2 m. deep. A complete biological filter plant reduces the B.O.D. of the raw sewage by between 85 and 95 per cent.

By using the principle of *recirculation*, i.e. returning some of the filter effluent to mix with the sewage coming on to the filter,

it is possible to achieve considerably higher rates of treatment, though with a lower degree of purification. Another method of increasing the capacity of percolating filters is by *alternating double filtration*, in which the sewage passes through two filters in series, the order of the filters being reversed at intervals of one or more days. Thin sheets of plastic material with specially formed corrugations may be used in place of normal filter media to form deep filters which can treat sewage or industrial effluents at high rates within a very small base area.

The Activated Sludge Process

The activated sludge process differs from biological filtration in the fact that the bacterial population is kept suspended by continuous agitation within the liquid instead of being

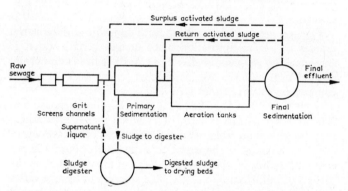

FIG. 44. Flow diagram of a typical activated sludge plant, incorporating digestion of combined primary sludge and surplus activated sludge.

established on the surface of solid media. The plant consists either of a long continuous channel, or of a series of chambers through which the sewage passes while it is being aerated. There are broadly two systems of aeration: the *diffused air* system, in which compressed air is introduced through porous plates of various designs or through perforated pipes, and the *surface aeration* system, which depends upon vigorous agitation by rotating paddles or brushes. The aeration tanks are followed by settling tanks in which the sludge is removed and the clear purified liquid overflows for discharge as the final effluent. Most of the sludge is returned to be mixed with the incoming settled sewage at the beginning of the aeration tanks. Thus there is a continuous circulation of activated sludge, i.e. solids consisting largely of bacteria and protozoa which are kept active by the constant replenishment of their supplies of food and oxygen [FIG. 44].

The activated sludge process can produce a higher-quality effluent than percolating filters. It requires less space, but more mechanization and skilful operation. Because the activity takes place beneath the surface, there is less trouble from smell and fly-breeding, and the method is less susceptible to low winter temperatures. It is, however, more likely to be upset by variations in sewage quality, especially by sudden inflows of toxic industrial wastes.

A simple, cheap form of the activated sludge process is the *oxidation ditch*, in which a surface paddle keeps the sewage circulating round a shallow ditch of oval shape in plan. This method has been found valuable in the treatment of organic industrial effluents.

Self-contained 'package' plants on the activated sludge

principle can be used for treating small sewage flows. They usually incorporate both aeration and settling compartments in a single structure.

Oxidation Ponds. These provide a simple, economical, and efficient means of treating sewage where space is available and there is ample sunlight. The sewage, after sedimentation, flows through one or more ponds, about 1 m. deep, in which algae produce by photosynthesis the oxygen required for bacterial oxidation of organic matter.

Sludge Treatment

The solids removed from primary or final sedimentation tanks are drawn off as liquid sludges containing from 90 to 99 per cent. water. Many methods are available for reducing this high water content and for converting the solids to a condition in which they may be used or disposed of harmlessly.

The most profitable form of sludge treatment is *anaerobic digestion*. The sludge is pumped daily into enclosed digester tanks in which anaerobic fermentation proceeds with the production of gas comprising about 70 per cent. methane and 30 per cent. carbon dioxide. In Europe and North America 0·03 m.^{3} of gas is produced per day for each person served by the treatment works. In countries where the diet is predominantly carbohydrate the quantities of sludge and gas produced may be twice as much. Sludge gas has a calorific value rather higher than that of coal gas, but lower than natural gas, and can generally provide all the power required for pumping, air compression, electricity generation, and heating on a modern activated sludge plant. The gas may also be compressed and used as vehicle fuel. For most effective digestion and gas production the digestors are heated to about 35° C.

Digestion converts much of the organic solids to gas and soluble matter, and so reduces the quantity of solids to be handled eventually. Digested sludge is a black liquid with a tarry odour and is more amenable to subsequent de-watering than undigested sludge. In recent years many works have encountered difficulty in the digestion of sludge as a result of increased quantities of detergents and other synthetic chemical residues. If this trend continues greater importance may be attached to other forms of treatment, such as filter pressing.

Apart from digestion, the main object of sludge treatment is to dewater it so that it can be handled as a relatively compact moist solid rather than a much greater volume of liquid with a low solids content The following processes are used and may be applied to either raw or digested sludge:

1. AIR DRYING by passing liquid sludge on to open-air, or sometimes covered, beds of sand, clinker, etc. Part of the water evaporates and part percolates through the bed to underdrains, leaving sludge with 50–60 per cent. moisture. This can be lifted by spades and handled as a solid.

2. LAGOONING, i.e. storing sludge in open basins some metres deep to allow settlement of the solids. Clarified liquid may be drawn off, and the solids are eventually dug out.

3. FILTER PRESSING, by which moisture is squeezed out through a filter cloth by mechanical pressure.

4. VACUUM FILTRATION, in which water is extracted by applying a vacuum to the inside of a filter drum rotating partially submerged in a trough of the sludge.

Chemical conditioning is necessary to prepare the sludge for the latter two processes.

After drying by any of the above methods, sludge may be further dried by heating.

Sewage sludge contains useful nitrogen and phosphorus, and although rather deficient in potassium, it forms a moderately good fertilizer. Undigested primary sludge contains grease and is odorous, but digested sludge and undigested activated sludge are easier to apply to land, and their humus content improves soil texture. In suitable circumstances sewage sludge may be composted with municipal refuse.

Where sludge cannot be used either as fertilizer or for composting, or, in a few cases, for recovery of by-products, it is usually tipped for land reclamation, dumped at sea, or incinerated.

TREATMENT OF INDUSTRIAL WASTE WATERS

Industrial waste waters are treated by methods basically similar to those used for domestic sewage. Additional processes, such as chemical neutralization or precipitation, ion exchange, centrifuging and evaporation may be used to prepare an effluent for discharge into a river or sewerage system, or for the recovery of useful materials (Klein, 1966).

Liquid radioactive wastes present special problems of disposal (Glueckauf, 1961). Low activity wastes, often in large volumes, are discharged to sea or into rivers where adequate dilution is available to bring the resultant activity below the permissible limits. High-activity wastes, which usually arise in smaller volumes, are concentrated by evaporation, chemical precipitation, filtration, or ion-exchange to give either concentrated solutions or solid sludges. These are then stored indefinitely to allow the activity to decrease naturally or dumped in sealed containers into deep parts of the ocean. Radioactive wastes from hospitals, laboratories, and commercial users of isotopes can generally be discharged safely to public sewers, but control must be exercised over rates of discharge, and storage may sometimes be necessary to permit some decay of activity.

Solid radioactive wastes may be incinerated, buried, stored, or dumped in the ocean. Radioactive gases, smoke, and dust are filtered and possibly subjected to other treatment before being discharged through high stacks giving adequate atmospheric dilution.

RURAL WATER SUPPLY AND EXCRETA DISPOSAL

The supply of water and the disposal of sewage or excreta often pose more difficult public health problems in rural than in urban areas. The reason for this is that shortage of money and the lack of trained operators necessitate the use of the simplest possible installations, and treatment processes are often out of the question.

An essential requirement for the success of rural sanitation programmes is the co-operation of the local population in ensuring that the facilities provided are properly used and maintained. This is made easier if the designs take into account not only the needs, but also the customs, of the people. Participation in the siting, design, and construction of wells, latrines, etc. can give a sense of proprietorship and pride rather than suspicion of works imposed by some outside body.

Responsible authorities should, where possible, organize regular visits of inspection to ensure that facilities such as well-pumps and septic tanks are maintained in good condition.

Pollution of Ground Water

Since surface water sources are easily contaminated and treatment is rarely practicable, small communities commonly depend upon ground water as their source of supply. The

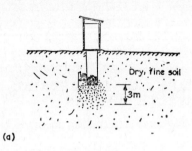

(a)

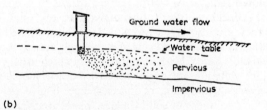

(b)

FIG. 45. Bacterial pollution of soil and ground water.
    (a) Limited travel of pollution in a fine-grained uniform dry soil above the water-table;
    (b) Pollution carried by the flow of ground water.
(By courtesy of the World Health Organization.)

ground is also the natural medium for the disposal of human excreta, so there are obvious risks of dangerous pollution of the ground water.

In assessing these risks, a few principles may be borne in mind. Seepage from excreta deposited in the ground *above* the water table will be mainly downwards, with little sideways spread. Under such conditions it has been observed that intestinal bacteria die off, or are filtered out, within two or three metres, and that this distance decreases in the course of time. If, however, the seepage is direct into the ground water, or reaches it within one or two metres, then bacterial contamination is likely to be carried laterally by the natural flow of ground water and may travel as far as 20 or 30 metres, depending on the rate of flow of the ground water and the permeability of the soil [FIG. 45]. Here again, the distance travelled is found to decrease as an equilibrium becomes established. Dissolved chemical substances can be carried for considerably greater distances.

It is important, therefore, in siting wells and latrines, to take account, as far as may be possible, of the depth of the water table below the surface and the direction in which the ground water flows. It should be remembered that the water table will

rise in wet weather and, where there is doubt, it is wise to assume that seepage from a latrine does reach the underground water. A well should be sited on the upstream side of a latrine, manure heap or other source of pollution, but even so the depression of water level in a heavily pumped well may draw water against the natural direction of flow.

The above comments apply to uniform subsoils such as sand and alluvium. In fissured limestone, chalk, or other formations, bacterial pollution may travel quickly for distances of several hundred metres. Guidance on the siting of wells and latrines is given by Wagner and Lanoix (1958, 1959).

Water Supplies

Dug wells should have an impervious lining to a depth of at least 3 m. and a concrete paving 2 m. wide round the head of the well to drain surface water away. They should preferably be covered by a slab through which a hand pump passes, but if this is not done a curb 0·5 m. high should be built round the top of the well to keep out surface water and dirt. In such a case it is better to have a single communal bucket on a windlass than to encourage the dipping of a variety of individual vessels.

Drilled wells and driven tube wells offer less chance of contamination than dug wells because of their lining, but it is desirable to surround the top 3 m. of the lining with concrete, and to provide a surface platform so that surface water cannot find a path down the outside of the lining [FIG. 46].

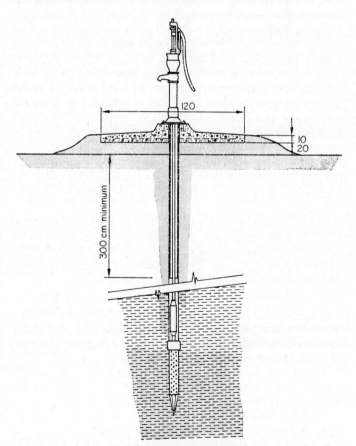

FIG. 46. Driven tube well, showing protection against entry of surface water, and use of submerged well pump. Dimensions are in cm. (By courtesy of the World Health Organization.)

Hand pumps for wells should, where possible, be of the type in which the working cylinder is submerged below water level. This type does not require priming, an operation which is necessary from time to time with the cheaper suction or pitcher type of pump, and which may introduce polluted water to the well.

Springs are often found at the junction of pervious and impervious strata or in fissured limestone. They should be protected from surface water (e.g. by an intercepting ditch) and enclosed in a concrete box-like structure forming a small collecting basin with a screened outlet pipe.

In default of more suitable sources, *rain water* may be collected from house roofs by means of gutters discharging into storage cisterns. The collecting surface should be of impervious material such as corrugated iron, asbestos-cement, or slates and the gutters should be of ample size to minimize

watertight and allow sewage to soak away into the subsoil. They therefore impose a heavy pollution load on the ground water and should be used with caution.

Septic tanks are frequently used to treat sewage from small groups of houses, hotels, institutions, and similar places. They are watertight tanks in which solids settle and are left for several months before removal. Some degree of anaerobic digestion occurs. The liquid effluent from a septic tank is of very poor quality and should be given secondary aerobic treatment on small biological filters or on suitable areas of land.

Where the water-borne system of sewage disposal is not possible, reliance must be placed on excreta disposal by means of latrines.

The *bucket latrine* or *conservancy* system requires a well-organized service for emptying buckets and disposing hygienically of the contents by burying, composting, or, as is sometimes

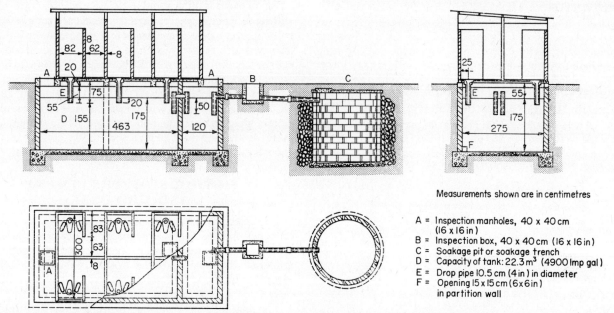

FIG. 47. Public aqua-privy built by UNRWA in refugee camps. (By courtesy of the World Health Organization.)

losses. Even so, losses due to splashing, evaporation, and overflowing are inevitable, and the amount collected may be only from 40 to 60 per cent. of the total rainfall.

Water Treatment

As previously noted, treatment of rural water supplies is rarely practicable and the emphasis should be on finding unpolluted sources and protecting them. However, occasions arise when some form of treatment is essential. Processes which can be adapted to simplified construction and operation are sedimentation, slow sand filtration, hypochlorination, and aeration (Wagner and Lanoix, 1959). However, money spent on treatment equipment will be wasted unless reliable, trained operators are available.

Excreta Disposal

In areas having piped water supplies but no sewerage system water-borne sewage may be discharged to cesspools or to septic tanks. *Cesspools*, in British practice, are watertight storage tanks which require to be emptied regularly.

Leaching cesspools, which are used in some countries, are not

possible, conveyance to a sewage treatment works. Modern equipment, including hard rubber buckets with tight-fitting lids, and specially designed vehicles, has made this service less obnoxious and hazardous than formerly, but the necessity for handling is a serious disadvantage, and the system is losing favour.

The *pit latrine* comprises a pit, at least 1·5 m. deep, preferably a good deal more, covered by a squatting plate or slab and seat. It provides storage for solid excreta, the liquids soaking into the soil. When the contents are within 0·5 m. of ground level the pit should be filled in with soil and a new pit dug.

The *borehole latrine* may be constructed in suitable ground by drilling a hole about 0·4 m. in diameter and 6 m. or more deep, penetrating the ground water. The solids undergo anaerobic digestion in the water and are thus reduced in volume. The ground water is, of course, grossly polluted, and siting in relation to water supply wells must be very carefully considered.

The *aqua-privy* is an impervious tank constructed immediately below the squatting plate or seat and kept filled with water so as to act as a septic tank. An overflow permits the effluent to soak away into the ground [FIG. 47].

The *pour-flush latrine* or *water seal latrine* may be basically either a pit or a borehole latrine or an aqua-privy. The special feature which gives it its name is a slab incorporating a water trap. After use a bucketful of water is poured in to flush the trap clean and to maintain the water seal. Odours and fly-breeding are thus prevented.

Chemical closets, in which caustic soda or a coal-tar preparation is poured into the container to disinfect the contents and to liquefy the solids, are useful for camp or domestic use in areas where the supply of chemicals presents no difficulty, but they are too expensive and troublesome for general village sanitation.

SOLID WASTE DISPOSAL

The disposal of solid refuse arising from normal domestic activities is, of course, a universal problem, but many countries are also meeting difficulties in dealing with wastes from industrial processes, especially those which are toxic or in other ways potentially harmful. For this reason some consideration is given here to both groups of wastes.

Quantities and Composition of Solid Wastes

Domestic Refuse. The production of domestic refuse in Britain averaged about 250 kg. per person per year in 1968 and is expected to increase to 285 kg. by 1980 (Department of the Environment, 1971). The corresponding compositions are as follows:

	(Percentages by weight)	
	1968	Estimated 1980
Dust and cinders . .	22	12
Vegetable and putrescible .	18	17
Paper	37	43
Metal	9	9
Rags	2	3
Glass	9	9
Plastics . . .	1	5
Unclassified . .	2	2
	100	100

The main trends, which have been going on for many years, are seen to be a reduction in dust and cinder, as solid fuel is replaced by other means of domestic heating, and increases in paper and plastics—mostly in the form of packaging. These changes are accompanied by a reduction in density and a considerable increase in the total volume of refuse.

These figures are averages for Britain and there are appreciable regional variations. Other countries show variations from the above quantities and composition, depending upon living standards, climate, and customs. In less developed rural areas, organic waste usually forms a larger proportion of the total.

Other Solid Wastes. The waste produced by trade and commercial organizations is generally similar in nature to domestic refuse, but is likely to contain larger proportions of paper and packaging materials. Wastes from industrial processes are mainly relatively inert, but also include materials which are toxic or inflammable. Much industrial waste is in the form of sludges. There appear to be no reliable figures for the total quantities of industrial solid wastes which have to be disposed of, but the Working Party on Refuse Disposal (Department of the Environment, 1971) estimated that the total may well be much greater than the quantity of domestic refuse.

Special arrangements may have to be made for the disposal of large items such as furniture, domestic appliances and vehicles. In Britain, the Civic Amenities Act (1967) requires local authorities to provide facilities for disposing of such items.

Recovery of Waste Materials

Several constituents of solid wastes have commercial value, though the market for some materials, e.g. glass, can fluctuate widely. Where the cost can be justified, separate collection of useful materials is preferable to separation from the mixed refuse.

Waste paper is pulped and used in the manufacture of board and some types of paper. Ferrous metals are compressed into bales and returned to steel mills and some non-ferrous metals may be worth recovery, even in small quantities. Food wastes can be concentrated by heating under pressure to provide animal food, while organic wastes in general may be composted. Textiles can be made into new cloth, felt or linoleum, glass can be melted and re-used, and bones can be processed to make grease, glue, fertilizer, and animal food. Dust and cinders are useful as covering material for tipped refuse, and the latter have enough calorific value to enable them to be used as fuel.

METHODS OF TREATMENT AND DISPOSAL

The choice of method of solid waste disposal is governed by economic and geographical considerations, such as the size and character of the area of collection, the cost of transport, the availability of suitable sites for tipping or incineration (having regard to visual and pollutional aspects) and the extent to which materials may be recovered.

The final method of disposal is nearly always by tipping on land, whether this is applied to the crude wastes, or to the smaller volumes resulting from incineration, pulverization, baling, or composting. In 1966–67, 90 per cent. of the refuse disposed of by local authorities in England was tipped directly on land with no pre-treatment and 8 per cent. was incinerated. Since that date the proportion incinerated has increased to about 15 per cent., and the trend towards incineration is likely to continue.

Controlled Tipping

When crude or pulverized refuse is tipped on land, strict precautions must be taken if unsightliness and nuisance are to be avoided. Controlled tipping (known in America as 'sanitary land-fill') has been practised in Britain for many years in accordance with recommendations set out by the Ministry of Health in 1931. Revised recommendations have been proposed (Department of the Environment, 1971).

The principle of controlled tipping is to place the refuse in well-compacted layers not more than 2·5 m. deep and to seal all exposed faces of each day's tipping with at least 0·25 m. of inert or non-putrescible material such as soil or ashes. The refuse is thus sealed into small cells in which organic material is broken down first by aerobic, and then by anaerobic bacteria. In the early stages heat is generated and temperatures of 60–65° C. may be maintained for two or three weeks. Proper sealing prevents the danger of spontaneous combustion, keeps down smells and reduces rat and fly breeding, though the use of insecticides and rat poison may sometimes be necessary. Industrial solid wastes may be tipped in the same way though care should be taken that dangerous or objectionable wastes (e.g. animal carcases) are well surrounded by other material. Possible risks of water pollution must be studied and special precautions are required if putrescible refuse is tipped into bodies of water such as old gravel pits.

Properly controlled tipping is not unsightly or offensive, and is of great value in the reclamation of low-lying or irregular areas for agriculture, playing fields, or parks at low cost (Bevan, 1967).

Separation

Mixed solid wastes can be sorted by a sequence of mechanical or hand operations. Dust and cinders are first removed through screens of selected aperture sizes, and ferrous metals, mainly food cans, are lifted out by electromagnets. Other recoverable materials must be picked off a moving belt by hand. Where crude, unsorted refuse is burnt in modern mechanical-grate incinerators, ferrous metals can be extracted magnetically from the incinerator residue, and there are prospects that mineral-processing techniques may be applied to these residues to separate non-ferrous metals.

Incineration

The fixed-grate forms of incinerator which have been used for nearly a century could not operate satisfactorily if fed with mixed wastes containing much dust and incombustible material. In recent years, several designs of continuous-feed, moving grate incinerators have been developed, and are increasingly used to burn crude unsorted refuse. Clinker, ashes and incombustible solids are collected in water below the grate and removed for tipping. In large installations the flue gases are washed and the fine grit removed by electrostatic or other precipitators to minimize atmospheric pollution. In some areas the heat from incinerators is used for district heating or electricity generation.

Pulverization

Pulverization of solid wastes is done either by a battery of heavy hammers rotating inside a robust casing, or by a less violent process of attrition inside a rotating drum fitted with blades. In the latter form the addition of water facilitates the shredding of paper and cardboard, but tougher materials are not broken down.

Pulverization produces a fairly uniform material of small particle size which can be tipped more compactly than crude refuse and is less attractive to flies and rodents. It provides better conditions for bacterial decomposition, especially when the wet method is used, and this is an advantage in both tipping and composting.

Composting

The organic portion of domestic refuse is suitable material for aerobic composting, especially if mixed with liquid sewage sludge to give the necessary moisture and nitrogen. The refuse is preferably pulverized and non-compostible material removed, though the latter process is sometimes left until after the composting stage.

Composting can be done in open heaps, windrows or shallow open pits, the material being turned over from time to time for mixing and aeration. Larger installations incorporate enclosed chambers in which more efficient composting is achieved by forced aeration, controlled moisture addition, and mechanical turning by means of rotating drums or tipping floors.

Under good conditions, temperatures of up to 70° C. are reached and pathogenic bacteria are destroyed, though the simpler composting methods are less reliable in this respect.

Compost made from municipal refuse is a useful soil conditioner and contains moderate amounts of nitrogen and phosphorus. The possible presence of toxic substances should not be overlooked. In Britain it has not been wholeheartedly accepted by farmers, who generally find chemical fertilizers more convenient. In countries where refuse has a large organic content, and chemical fertilizers are less easy to obtain, composted refuse can make a valuable contribution to soil structure and fertility.

Baling

Since refuse as collected is a loose mixture of low density, any form of compression can lead to a saving in the size and number of vehicles required for transport and in the land space needed for tipping. Several systems of compression are available, including static plants using hydraulic rams to produce dense bales, and screw mechanisms inside collecting vehicles.

Other Methods of Handling Refuse

The *Garchey* system of refuse disposal is applicable to blocks of flats and other large buildings, and obviates the need for the usual methods of storage and collection. The refuse falls through a water-flushed chute from each flat to a central collecting station, where surplus water overflows to the sewers. More water is extracted centrifugally, and the refuse is then incinerated or carried away for tipping.

Garbage grinders are electrically-driven devices fitted in kitchen sinks. Organic refuse passed through them is cut up and is carried along the sewers for treatment with sewage. Food containers and other refuse must still be disposed of by normal methods.

A more fundamental development, of which one or two examples already exist, is the conveyance of refuse from houses by pipeline, under a suction generated at a central collecting station. Here the refuse may be incinerated or tipped, or it may be pulverized and discharged into sewers for treatment with the municipal sewage. The implications and economics of such a system have not yet been fully explored.

The disposal of solid waste is covered by a model code of practice (WHO Regional Office for Europe, 1973).

REFERENCES

Bevan, R. E. (1967) *Notes on the Science and Practice of the Controlled Tipping of Refuse*, Institute of Public Cleansing, London.

Department of the Environment (1971) *Refuse Disposal*, Report of the Working Party on Refuse Disposal, London, H.M.S.O.

Department of Health and Social Security (1969a) *The Fluoridation Studies in the United Kingdom and the Results Achieved after Eleven Years*, Reports on Public Health and Medical Subjects No. 122, London, H.M.S.O.

Department of Health and Social Security (1969b) *The Bacteriological Examination of Water Supplies*, Reports on Public Health and Medical Subjects No. 71, 4th ed., London, H.M.S.O.

Glueckauf, E., ed. (1961) *Atomic Energy Waste: Its Nature, Use and Disposal*, London.

Hanks, T. G. (1967) *Solid Waste/Disease Relationships: A Literature Survey*, United States Public Health Service Publication No. 999–UIH–6, Washington.

Klein, L. (1966) *River Pollution*, Vol. 3, *Control*, London.

Ministry of Housing and Local Government (1970a) *Technical Committee on Storm Overflows and the Disposal of Storm Sewage: Final Report*, London, H.M.S.O.

Ministry of Housing and Local Government (1970b) *Disposal of Solid Toxic Wastes*, Report of the Technical Committee on the Disposal of Solid Toxic Wastes, London, H.M.S.O.

Ministry of Housing and Local Government (1970) *Taken for Granted*, Report of the Working Party on Sewage Disposal, London, H.M.S.O.

Stitt, F. W., Clayton, D. G., Crawford, Margaret D., and Morris, J. N. (1973) Clinical and biochemical indicators of cardiovascular disease among men living in hard and soft water areas, *Lancet*, i, 122.

Wagner, E. G., and Lanoix, J. N. (1958) Excreta Disposal for Rural Areas and Small Communities, *Wld Hlth Org. Monogr. Ser.*, No. 39.

Wagner, E. G., and Lanoix, J. N. (1959) Water Supply for Rural Areas and Small Communities, *Wld Hlth Org. Monogr. Ser.*, No. 42.

White, J. B. (1970) *The Design of Sewers and Sewage Treatment Works*, London.

World Health Organization (1970a) Fluorides and Human Health, *Wld Hlth Org. Monogr. Ser.*, No. 59.

World Health Organization (1970b) *European Standards for Drinking-Water*, 2nd ed., Geneva.

World Health Organization (1971) *International Standards for Drinking-Water*, 3rd ed., Geneva.

Rural Water Supply and Excreta Disposal

Assar, M. (1971) *Guide to Sanitation in Natural Disasters*, W.H.O., Geneva.

Ross Institute (1968) *Rural Sanitation in the Tropics*, Ross Institute Bulletin No. 8, London.

Ross Institute (1971) *Small Water Supplies*, Ross Institute Bulletin No. 10, London.

Solid Waste Disposal

Flintoff, F., and Millard, R. (1969) *Public Cleansing*, London.

Gotaas, Harold B. (1956) Composting: Sanitary Disposal and Reclamation of Organic Wastes, *Wld Hlth Org. Monogr. Ser.*, No. 31.

Stirrup, H. L. (1965) *Public Cleansing: Refuse Disposal*, Oxford.

World Health Organization (1972) Solid wastes disposal and control, *Wld Hlth Org. Chron.*, **26**, 147.

World Health Organization Regional Office for Europe (1973) Model code of practice for disposal of solid waste on land, *Wld Hlth Org. Chron.*, **27**, 439.

FURTHER READING

The following references are suggested (in addition to those given above) for further reading on the subjects discussed in this chapter. Most of the publications listed give further references to more detailed topics.

General

Southgate, B. A. (1969) *Water: Pollution and Conservation*, London.

World Health Organization (1966) Water Pollution Control: Report of a W.H.O. Expert Committee, *Wld Hlth Org. techn. Rep. Ser.*, No. 318.

World Health Organization (1967a) Treatment and Disposal of Wastes: Report of a W.H.O. Scientific Group, *Wld Hlth Org. techn. Rep. Ser.*, No. 367.

World Health Organization (1967b) *Control of Water Pollution: A Survey of Existing Legislation*. Reprinted from *International Digest of Health Legislation*, 1966, **17**, 629–834.

World Health Organization (1968) Water Pollution Control in Developing Countries: Report of a W.H.O. Expert Committee, *Wld Hlth Org. techn. Rep. Ser.*, No. 404.

World Health Organization (1969) Problems in Community Wastes Management, *Wld Hlth Org. Publ. Hlth Pap.*, No. 38.

World Health Organization (1973a) Reuse of waste water, *Wld Hlth Org. Chron.*, **27**, 492.

World Health Organization (1973b) Basic sanitary services: WHO programmes for the advancement and transfer of knowledge and methods in community water supply and waste disposal, *Wld Hlth Org. Chron.*, **27**, 430.

World Health Organization (1973c) Scientific aspects of marine pollution, *Wld Hlth Org. Chron.*, **27**, 433.

Quality of Water

American Public Health Association (1971) *Standard Methods for the Examination of Water and Wastewater*, 13th ed., New York.

World Health Organization (1974) Disposal of community waste water. Report of a WHO Expert Committee, *Wld Hlth Org. techn. Rep. Ser.*, No. 541.

World Health Organization Regional Office for Europe, Copenhagen.
(1971) *European Standards for Drinking Water* (Euro 0664).
(1972) *Automatic Water Quality Monitoring* (Euro 3119W).
(1972) *Accidental Pollution of Inland Waters* (Euro 3015W).
(1973) *Analytical Methods in Water Polution Control* (Euro 3110(1)).
(1973) *Hazards to Health and Ecological Effects of Pollution in the North Sea* (Euro 3128(1)).
(1973) *The Hazards to Health of Persistent Substances in Water* (Euro 3109W(1) and annexes).

Water Supply and Treatment

Cox, Charles R. (1964) Operation and Control of Water Treatment Processes, *Wld Hlth Org. Monogr. Ser.*, No. 49.

Holden, W. S., ed. (1970) *Water Treatment and Examination*, London.

Skeat, W. O., ed. (1969) *Manual of British Water Engineering Practice*, 4th ed., London, The Institution of Water Engineers.

World Health Organization (1973d) Water quality, trace elements and cardio-vascular disease, *Wld Hlth Org. Chron.*, **27**, 534.

Sewerage and Sewage Treatment

Bolton, R. L. and Klein, L. (1971) *Sewage Treatment; Basic Principles and Trends*, 2nd ed., London.

Central Office of Information (1970) *Water Pollution Control Engineering*, London, H.M.S.O.

Imhoff, K., Muller, W. J., and Thistlethwayte, D. K. B. (1971) *Disposal of Sewage and Other Water-borne Wastes*, 2nd ed., London.

IO
FOOD HYGIENE

MORLEY PARRY

THE THEORY AND SCOPE OF FOOD HYGIENE PROBLEMS

The terms food hygiene and food poisoning are not complete antonyms. Food hygiene can provide most of the answers to food poisoning problems, but study of the practicalities of food hygiene must inevitably be very much wider than an attempt to prevent a repetition of known food-poisoning incidents.

From the moment of harvest, extraction, capture, or killing, all food used by man is subject to processes of deterioration. Of itself, this natural tendency towards eventual putrefaction does not necessarily set free, in the food, poisonous substances that are a hazard to the health of the consumer.

The distinction between what will give rise to such a hazard and what will not is, however, so fine that control of this process of deterioration must be the basis of any programme for achieving positive food hygiene. To this must be added positive controls, based on information gained through earlier successful work, aimed at limiting the effects of outbreaks of food poisoning.

In a situation where each consumer produces all his individual food needs the hazards, which could arise from acceleration of the food-deterioration process, will have little or no public significance. Even the smallest possibility of handling errors, however, which increase the deterioration rate, becomes of vital importance when food is produced by one person for another to eat.

The true, present, fact in relation to food supplies in developed countries is that efficient and safe distribution of food from producer to consumer has become the only safeguard both against hazard arising from that food and the very real prospect of mankind starving amid abundance. Without the practice of food-protection techniques civilized man, in the modern world, would be denied food.

The consumer can no longer easily produce and always prepare his own food. It has to be brought to him and increasingly laid on his table absolutely ready for immediate consumption. This has the effect of making it imperative that man is no longer dependent on seasonal distribution of any foods. Seasonal production largely remains constant, but modern needs demand that there is always a fully balanced food supply available whenever and wherever it is needed. This means that there must be increased handling and processing of most foods. It also means that the possibility of handling error is increased and that the results of any such error, in terms of health hazard from the food, assumes not only an individual but also a national and international significance. In every language there is a word for 'food poisoning' or even 'upset stomach'. Man needs therefore to know exactly how to

use or delay or accelerate these natural processes of food deterioration to suit his own wishes. He must also be certain that every action taken with food will be such as will not introduce a hazard to the consumer. The need for positive food hygiene is thus self-evident and universal. The methods by which it is successfully achieved must everywhere follow a similar basic pattern, but the actual methods used in any local scale need to be worked out so as to fit with the proper pattern of life within that locality. Basically the methods used must be aimed at right techniques of food handling being observed by the right person at the right time in the right place. The methods must be widely accepted as reasonable, sensible, and economic, and as a result of these virtues, become *built in* to all food premises, all food processes, and, most important, into the minds of all people.

To achieve this end the food-trade worker and the food-hygiene officer need to have a basic understanding of all food-trade production, process, and distribution methods. The aim must be to control, effectively and quickly, any factor which either adversely affects food distribution or which exposes the consumer to an unnecessary, preventable, health hazard when the food is eaten. It is a confusion of thought therefore, against such a background, to regard food-hygiene precautions as a policy to be considered and implemented as an antidote to diagnosed and recorded cases of food poisoning. To develop this argument let it be assumed that precaution was, in any given year, always taken by all persons at all times. Theoretically it would follow that in that year there would be no recorded cases of food poisoning. An inference might then be drawn that there was no problem and that food-hygiene efforts could be slackened. In truth the very reverse would be the case. Food-hygiene effort would need to be increased in order to retain this freedom from disease.

Here is a completely factual, practical example. The ice-cream trade in the United Kingdom was originally quite haphazard and not fully organized along lines that encouraged food hygiene. Through the history of the trade there were quite frequent occasions when ice cream was the food which carried bacterial contamination as a result of mishandling or poor processing. Outbreaks of food poisoning occurred and were attributed to this food, after laboratory investigation of the product, and close public health inspection of the places where the trade was carried on. The Report of the United Kingdom Ministry of Health, for the year ending 31 March 1946, has an almost laconic paragraph reading, 'Of the staphylococcal outbreaks ... Ice cream was responsible for three large outbreaks affecting several hundred persons: the same phage type of staphylococcus was found in the ice cream and in the vomit of many of the patients. In all three ice cream outbreaks there was a delay of 18–24 hours between the preparation and freezing of the mixture.' Laconic this paragraph may be, but it underlines that there was investigation of both the product and the process. The following year the Ministry of Health report said, 'The epidemic of typhoid fever at Aberystwyth resulted in 104 cases in the town and 105 cases in patients who had left the town or were secondary patients elsewhere. The source of infection was an ice cream maker-vendor, who was a urinary carrier of Vi-phage type C. This epidemic showed the urgent need for regulations controlling the manufacture and pasteurisation of ice cream. Regulations accordingly, were published in draft in October, 1946, and came into force in April, 1947.'

These 'Ice Cream (Heat Treatment, etc.) Regulations, 1947' described an approved method of ice-cream manufacture and demanded that the product should be 'protected from contamination at all times'. The requirements as to the actions of food handlers engaged in the ice-cream trade (and, in fact, food handlers in general), and as to the hygienic construction of food premises, and their maintenance in that clean condition, were reinforced by the Food Hygiene Regulations, 1955. Since 1955 ice cream *has not once* been under the remotest suspicion, in England and Wales, of any connexion with one single case of food poisoning. The trade has been reorganized, food hygiene is now paramount in every action of every ice-cream trader. But, and this is the point, both the trade and the administration know that this absence of notified illness means extra effort to maintain this high position in the food-supply industry rather than an excuse to relax vigilance.

Positive food hygiene, therefore, relates to all foods and all food handling at all times. The problem is to control the development of deterioration and to prevent any unintended acceleration of that process by unwanted contamination of the food. In this context the word contamination must be taken to mean the unintentional introduction, by any causal agent, of anything into food that was not in that food at the moment of harvesting, extracting, catching, or killing, plus the positive removal of any part of the food which in the natural state would cause hazard to the consumer. There are easy examples of this removal of recognized hazard. Perhaps the most widely understood is the recognition of the fact that food animals are subject to disease and the rejection, for human consumption purposes, of any carcasses or parts found to be so affected on ante- or post-mortem inspection.

Completely natural commencement of food deterioration may be, for instance, as a result of the continuation of internal enzyme action within the food. Consider, in this respect, the germination of food seeds, the sprouting of potato tubers, and the improvement of the tenderness of meats by allowing carcasses to set properly after slaughter and to 'hang to bloom condition'. There are instances, as in the ripening of fruits, where man waits for a known and a given point in these catalytic processes before regarding certain foods as acceptable for use. Again, the completely natural starting of food deterioration may result from bacterial activity. This may follow from natural bacterial activity within the food itself, as in the separation of cream from stored milk by the action of lactic acid bacilli, or from introduced bacterial activity. By this is meant deliberately introduced bacterial activity, as in the production of yoghourts and margarines. These are foods changed to human acceptance form as a result of the introduc-

tion of controlled bacterial 'starters'. These starters are usually small quantities of the same or similar foods already in process towards controlled decomposition. Some food trades now use, however, artificial or synthetic 'starters'. These are easier to control with exactitude. It is also worth underlining that man occasionally accepts limited bacterial decomposition in some foods as a method of making the texture or the taste of the final food more acceptable to his special palate idiosyncrasies. Instances are in the production of cheeses like Limburger, or the flesh of 'game' birds. These are often eaten in a state of partial decomposition, without ill effect, by the *conditioned* consumer. People who eat these specialized foods literally *teach* their digestive tracts to accept and deal with the 'unsound' condition of these foods. On a wider scale every man learns to live with the bacterial flora of his own digestive tract, and in most cases the bacterial flora of the digestive tract of any people, such as his own immediate family, with whom there is regular and intimate contact. But at no time is uncontrolled or unintended introduced bacterial activity, or any other form of contamination, acceptable to any man. It does not always follow that the hazard is sufficient to cause death or even a serious degree of illness, but it is true to say that in every such case there is some degree of food intoxication. This may be so simple, in medical terms, as to need no treatment, but in most of these cases the sufferer is incapacitated or disinclined to follow his normal mode of life.

These are the considerations of food safety and food-trade economics that so greatly widen the scope of the term 'food hygiene'.

FOOD-HYGIENE POLICIES

The bald fact is that food poisoning occurs, that it is preventable, and that even one case, recorded or not recorded, is one case too many. There must, of course, be an increased and specialized drive towards applying corrective food-hygiene policies and techniques when cases of food poisoning occur. But the true scope of food hygiene is by no means limited by the considerations of food bacteriology. Theoretically, bacterial contamination can be prevented from becoming a food hazard by rendering sterile the food or the food-handling environment. This could, in some cases, be achieved by treatment of the food as, for instance, the modern production of sterile milk packed in aseptic conditions. This is a process that introduces no new or extra ingredient to cows' milk but which renders the milk sterile by controlled application of heat coupled with immediate cooling and packing. Thus treated, the milk will keep sweet, without refrigeration, provided the sealed pack is intact, for 6–12 months. Only a decade ago it was an achievement to keep raw milk for 48 hours and pasteurized milk for 5–6 days. Similar freedom from bacterial activity and hazard could be achieved by the boiling of foods or immersion of food-contact surfaces in boiling water. Yet again there are chemical sterilants that can be applied to sterilize the surfaces with which food comes into contact. But the bulk of the foods can never be chemically sterilized and remain acceptable for human consumption. Neither can all foods be boiled or pasteurized and remain palatable. More often than not the huge bulk quantities of food concerned (and the nature of the food) prevent the application of these safeguards. On other occasions the initial contamination occurs so soon and is so much an unavoidable part of obtaining the food that keeping food hazard in check is all that can be hoped. For those and other cogent reasons the bacteriologist alone cannot ever provide the total answer to food-poisoning problems, and it is certain that laboratory routines will never be capable of defining the effective limits of positive food-hygiene work. The effective food-hygiene team must include many experts, agronomists, biologists, chemists, entomologists and economists, histologists, right on through the gamut to zoologists. The thoughts and ideas of all these workers need to be collected, medically evaluated, and then turned into day-by-day food-trade fact and practice by intelligent management guided, and sometimes forced, by trained officers of central and local authorities.

Inferences from Recorded and Investigated Cases of Food Poisoning

It must be made clear that food poisoning or food intoxication can result from many causes. It may result from eating foods containing inorganic chemicals which are unacceptable to the human digestion. One such case arose in 1965/6 in Morocco when mineral engine oil was fraudulently introduced into cooking oils and about 10,000 people suffered from paralysis.[1] A similar outbreak was reported from Syria in 1973 due to the same cause, with 100 cases of paralysis (World Health Organization, 1974c). It may be as a result of eating poisonous plants or of consuming parts of animals that are in themselves poisonous. It is important that medical practitioners should be aware of these sources and the symptoms they produce, which may influence diagnosis. Such incidents, however, are not types of food poisoning with which the food hygienist is directly concerned. The guide to illnesses which are truly within the definition of food poisoning in the present context is the list of food-borne diseases that are now 'notifiable' by general medical practitioners in the United Kingdom. The Public Health (Infectious Diseases) Regulations, 1968 (which replaced the Infectious Diseases Regulations, 1953) call for the notification, *inter alia*, of typhoid fever, paratyphoid fever and other *Salmonella* infections, dysentery and staphylococcal infection likely to cause food poisoning. The regulations also demand that if a medical officer of health (of the local authority) has reason to believe that a person engaged in any connexion with the preparation and handling of food or drink for human consumption may be a carrier of typhoid fever, paratyphoid fever or other *Salmonella* infection, or of dysentery or of staphylococcal infection likely to cause food poisoning, he (the medical officer) *shall* (must) report the fact to the local health authority, and a notice may be given in writing to the responsible manager of the food business calling for all assistance to be given for the full medical examination of that suspect person.

Notifications are now made under the terms of Section 48 of the Health Services and Public Health Act, 1968, and the doctor making the notification is paid a small fee for complying with the legal demand.

The system is that on diagnosis the doctor in attendance officially informs the medical officer of health of the local authority district. That officer makes inquiries in an effort to locate the source of the illness and in turn notifies, once weekly, the incidence of food poisoning to the Registrar General. The Ministry of Health tabulates statistics and, when help is needed and asked for, assists in the epidemiological work necessary to define, limit, or prevent a recurrence of such an illness.

Food poisoning, in this context, is limited to explosive illness with any gastro-intestinal nausea or vomiting symptoms attributable to pathogenic bacteria in foods eaten by the patients. The task of the food-hygiene workers is to find the food or food-handling environment that was at fault.

While the medical work, including treatment of the patient, is assisted by the positive phage typing or identification of the particular pathogenic bacteria implicated, such information is not always vital to the food-hygiene worker, concerned with general clean food practice. Even with the possibility of the full examination of all likely causal agents, there are some food-poisoning incidents which cannot be definitely attributed to one given cause. There are also gastro-intestinal nausea and vomiting symptoms which result from a miscellaneous group of short sickness conditions and for which medical and bacteriological science has not yet produced definitions. Positive food hygiene, therefore, is based on general bacteriological facts which influence or dictate the handling or processing methods which can or cannot be countenanced in the distribution of food.

Micro-organisms

The policies to be aimed at by the food-hygiene worker are clear. The need is to contain the bacterial growth by application of processes which will remove or reduce the available warmth or the moisture and in all cases to produce food-handling conditions which prevent bacterial transference.

Other useful bacteriological facts are: (1) some bacteria (autotrophic) mainly live in soil and thrive on inorganic media; (2) bacteria which thrive on organic media, such as human food, are termed heterotrophic. Within each of these two categories there are four subdivisions:

1. Thermophilic bacteria. These are bacteria with the greatest resistance to ranges of heat below sterilization temperature (normally 100° C.). Sterilization temperature must therefore be applied for sufficient time if they are to be destroyed. Normally 'medical' sterility demands boiling for 30 minutes, but the nature of certain food makes it necessary to reduce this time. Thus what can only be described as 'commercial' sterility is applied, and in this the final palatability of the food is the first and unavoidable consideration. An illustration of this application of commercial limitation of sterility is the difference between sterilized milk—which gets a 'nutty' flavour not acceptable to all consumers—and pasteurization of milk. In earlier days milk pasteurization was by positive hold above 79·5° C. for 30 minutes followed by immediate cooling below 70° C. Modern practice is to raise the milk to 83° C. for up to 5 seconds and to cool the milk to 7° C.

Thermophilic bacteria are demonstrably able to grow at 55° C. and even up to 5° or 6° above this temperature in some food and processing circumstances. Some foods are not suitable for treatment at these high temperatures, and thus it is not always possible to destroy these organisms.

2. Mesophilic bacteria are those which multiply at tempera-

---

[1] Due to the detergent tricresyl phosphate contained in the oil.

ture ranges between 5° C. and 45° C. In this group are found the majority of bacteria which cause human disease. Coupled with the first group, and including temperatures above the 55° C. optimum of the thermophilics, the clear fact emerges that positive food-hygiene work must concentrate on holding foods, not capable of processing and sealed packaging, outside the temperature range 5° C. and 66° C. But obtaining a temperature below 4·5° C. in most temperate climates involves the application of some form of mechanical refrigeration. This is not always either economic or practicable with large consignments of bulk foods, and is very difficult in bulk food transport. The achievement of a temperature of 10° C. is more often more easily and economically possible. The effective temperature danger range is therefore generally agreed to be between 10° C. and 66° C. This does not preclude the use of methods with certain selected foods whereby those foods are held below 4·5° C.

3. Psychrophilic bacteria are those organisms which are able to thrive and multiply best at 20° C. or below. Their presence in foods makes the correct use of refrigerated storage a necessity. Some of these bacterial types are capable of ready multiplication at 0° C. Even lower temperatures, down to −5° C., are resisted by some psychrophilic bacteria, and they can continue to multiply in these conditions. Fortunately these types of bacteria are rarely pathogenic. They are, however, the organisms that generally cause commercial food spoilage. Their presence in foods, however, influences processes which aim at holding and marketing food supplies distributed in a frozen state.

4. Viruses. For a coverage of this subject see World Health Organisation (1973b).

Oxidation of Foods

Bacteria can also be classified by whether or not they need oxygen. Those that do use oxygen are termed aerobes, and are said to exist in aerobic conditions. Food-hygiene methods of dealing with bacteria of this type must obviously be such as will allow foods to be effectively stored in conditions which reduce oxidation of the foods. An instance of this is the modern process of storing dehydrated foods in sealed packs into which an artificially induced nitrogen atmosphere has been deliberately introduced. Bacteria which can thrive only in oxygen-free conditions are called anaerobic. These include the clostridia. Where a food process includes the canning, bottling, or sealed packaging of the treated foods the final conditions are anaerobic. Thus the foods need to be as free as possible of bacterial contamination before processing. The general food-handling environment in a food-canning factory therefore becomes as important, possibly even more important, than the actual heat-treatment process itself.

The pH of Foods

The acid/alkali balance of foods also has a bearing on the limitation of bacterial activity in or on the food. Bacteria multiply best towards neutrality (pH 7), with growth rates decreasing as the pH of the growth medium moves to either end of the scale. The decline is always more accentuated on the acid side of neutrality. Instances of foods that can be protected from bacterial multiplication by an increase of acidity are pickled onions and marinated herrings. At the other extreme full

strong sugar is highly alkaline and almost totally free of bacterial multiplication problems. The pH factor can, of itself, often be the decider in considering whether or not certain made-up foods need to be heat processed. For instance, the manufacture of iced lollipops from fruit syrups, water sweeteners, and flavours must include a pasteurization technique if the pH is above 4·5, and need not be so treated for a pH below that figure.

Spores

Bacteria are also classified as being resistant to adverse conditions if they can form spores. Prominent among these are clostridia, and there are also some aerobic bacteria which have this capability. In this form there is increased resistance to heat and drying.

Knowledge of this condition can be used to define acceptable food-processing techniques. Meats being canned thus need high temperature, above 120° C., retort conditions—in household terms, pressure cooking—if sterility of the products is to be made certain. This, once more, stresses the importance of the over-all food-handling environment up to the moment the food is processed. It also underlines the need for careful storage without damage to the food after such processing. This resistant capability of the bacteria is also a decisive factor in considering the time element in the application of heat techniques to food. This includes all forms of cooking. The killing off of any bacterial population within foods is not immediate on the application of heat, and experiment and trade experience must be relied upon to dictate the time that individual foods need for effective heat treatment. Imperfectly cooked meats or improperly heated 'warmed-up' foods are potentially more hazardous than well-cooked foods. One must stress the vital need for a clean food-handling environment so as to prevent initial contamination of food from any source.

Toxins

Some bacteria, in normal growth and decline activity, produce toxins. Toxins which form an integral part of the bacterial cell (endotoxins) are resistant to heat to a marked degree, and it is into this group that most pathogenic bacteria fall. The need for complete thorough cooking of food is thus again made plain.

Botulism, however, is a special form of food poisoning due to the toxin of Clostridium botulinus. The organism is anaerobic, and in spore form can withstand boiling for 200 minutes. Food processes need to hold a temperature of 120° C. to achieve destruction of these spores. The organisms cannot grow at a pH of 4·5 or below.

Botulism is rare these days, because processers and distributors know that the endotoxins and exotoxins concerned may be inactivated by salting (adding nitrates) plus effective cooking. Food processing on a commercial scale is now so well operated as to practically remove this hazard altogether. Sensible and proper cooking, even, for instance, home cooking, uses oven temperatures around the 205° C. mark as normal heat.

Moulds and Yeasts

In a similar manner the food-hygiene worker can afford to largely dismiss the poisoning hazards from moulds and wild yeasts. The presence of such organisms is a clear indication that all is not well with the food-handling environment, but they are not, of themselves, a prime food-poisoning consideration. In order to set the food-handling techniques right, therefore, it is as well to keep in mind some facts about these forms of contamination. Moulds and wild yeasts are both simple cell micro-organisms. The spore forms of moulds are resistant to adverse heat and moisture conditions and are freely airborne. Their presence, when detected, is thus an obvious indication of fault in the over-all food-handling environment. For their comparatively slow growth moulds and yeasts, being completely aerobic, do require some moisture and oxygen. They do not flourish at temperatures above 30° C. unless there is a compensating high degree of relative humidity, but they will thrive, occasionally, at temperatures equivalent to 10° C. of frost with a reduced relative humidity. The clear inference from this is that food storage must always be clean and dry, unless it is a process designed to induce palatability by deliberate, controlled, mould growth in the selected food. Bacteria, moulds, and yeasts, the micro-organism contaminants of foods, are a highly specialized study, but the same simple rule of great value to the food-hygiene worker continually emerges quite clearly. Food must be kept clean, covered, in controlled heat, and in controlled conditions of relative humidity.

Animals and Food Pests

Animals, rodents, and insects which can carry and excrete pathogens provide further reasons for the application of food-hygiene routines. There is no doubt but that the toleration of insect and rodent infestations and unnecessary animal contacts widens the risk of spread of pathogens. The task of the food-hygiene officer is to prevent or reduce these food hazards even where there is no obvious direct route between food-handling process and patient. Pests and animals must therefore be rigorously excluded from food rooms.

It must be seen that an understanding of these facts is necessary for the correct evaluation of food-handling methods and processing techniques, but of themselves, these facts about contaminants actively solve few problems. They have to be translated into food-trade terms, and in so doing emphasis increasingly falls on the need to have reliable food processes. Before processes are studied it is necessary to look at another aspect of the investigation of notified incidents of food poisoning.

THE MOST PREVALENT ILLNESS CONDITIONS

The name, type, and classification of bacteria involved in any given case of food poisoning will allow comparison between outbreaks to be made and thus reduce the guesswork in any deductions made from the given epidemiological facts. In the years since food poisoning first became legally notifiable in the United Kingdom in 1939 the main groups of bacteria implicated have been: (1) the salmonellae; (2) the staphylococci; (3) the clostridia; and (4) a miscellaneous group [see Chapter 16].

Outbreaks of Disease

In England and Wales the steps to be taken by medical officers of health in the investigation and control of food poisoning are set out in the Ministry of Health pamphlet Memo/188/Med, which, as all official publications, is obtainable from Her Majesty's Stationery Office. This publication says, *inter alia*, that:

'At the onset of the investigation it may be possible to prevent further cases by stopping the sale of suspected foods and by recovering unconsumed foods already sold. The foodstuff or one of its ingredients may be primarily infected and the infection may survive cooking. A primary infected article may contaminate equipment and lead to secondary infection of other articles or food products. The amount of noxious material which survives cooking may be so small that no harm would result from immediate consumption. Inappropriate or incorrect storage, however, including misuse of refrigeration and bad handling, can lead to such growth of organisms as will cause frank disease. An infection introduced by food handlers can survive and multiply in products such as cream, imitation cream, custards and table sweets, cold meats, meat products, soups and gravies which can easily become dangerous under adverse conditions of domestic storage although they would remain sound and comparatively free of risk, if properly stored in well equipped premises.'

With the appropriate details of the source and distribution channels of the suspected food coupled with efficient collection of samples, of food, faeces, vomit, etc., for laboratory examination it is then possible to correctly study the incident and draw correct conclusions as to the possible cause.

From investigations of this kind, coupled with the comparison work of the Food Hygiene Salmonellae Reference Laboratory of the United Kingdom Public Health Laboratory Service, it is possible to list the foods most usually involved and the contaminants most frequently incriminated. Some fifty bacteriological laboratories now operate in the United Kingdom, all freely available to carry out investigations for the assistance of the local public health authorities.

It was at one time considered, due to the difficulty in obtaining comparison foods where publicly sold meals were concerned, that it would be helpful to the bacteriologist if caterers were encouraged to retain one full meal from every service for sampling purposes. This meal would be kept in a refrigerator for two to three days ready to be taken to the examining laboratory for immediate analysis when incidents of food poisoning are notified. This is, at best a theory that may have some use in limited catering exercises, such as a once-a-day school-meal service, but it is completely impractical in busy, full-scale, catering operations.

Notification

While many cases of food-borne infection are notified, an even greater number of food-borne illnesses are acknowledged to be so minor in character that the patients recover before needing medical attention. There are also incidents that are secondary to other illnesses. It is doubtful therefore whether 100 per cent. notification can ever be achieved, anywhere at any time. The officially recorded cases in England and Wales rose to a peak of some 20,000 in 1,961 outbreaks in 1955/56. Since then there has been an irregular downward trend to an average of 12,000 people concerned in 3,000–4,000 outbreaks. This indicates that there are more 'sporadic' incidents than previously and the investigations showed that the foods most involved were (not in order of implication): (1) cooked meats; (2) gravy; (3) improperly reheated 'left-over' meals; (4) eggs; (5) table sweetmeats; (6) soups and stews; (7) prepacked foods, dried and otherwise packed; (8) imitation creams; (9) pies and 'made-up' meats; (10) processed, including home-cooked, foods improperly stored. This directs the attention of the food-hygiene worker to the facts of food distribution and processing Without that knowledge it is not possible to draw the correct preventive lessons from any investigated incident. The food alone is rarely suspect. The food plus the environment, including the handling and the processing, are always demonstrably the area of investigation. The most frequent causes of what can now be called environment failure are known to be: (1) incorrect processing of food; (2) incorrect storage of food; (3) incorrect maintenance and cleaning procedures; and (4) bad personal hygiene by food handlers.

But personal hygiene cannot be observed by food handlers unless the facilities exist to allow the workers to remain clean and the processes are such as themselves make the maintenance of clean conditions easy.

THE PROCESSING, DISTRIBUTION, AND SALE OF FOOD

It is universally understood that, while mankind may hope to produce more food, even using, as protein sources, materials which have not previously been considered for human consumption purposes, the real answer to the world food-supply situation must lie in man's ability to keep foods already in production in proper condition and away from attack by other forms of life. Materials now being considered as possible large-scale protein sources include, for instance, processed grass cuttings, the leaves of trees, and controlled 'mould' growths on crude oil. All of these will bring changed processing techniques that will need to satisfy food-hygiene controls before they can come into commercial use. Like all other foods, these new sources will be subject to what may be termed natural internal 'off' conditions and to 'introduced' hazard which will follow incorrect food-handling techniques.

One of the first of man's discoveries about food was that it was possible to increase the yield from his husbandry and to improve the quality and profitability of the end-product by protecting foods at source from attack by disease and pests. A modern example of this is that good veterinary medicine and sensible animal husbandry have, within the last fifty years, reduced the incidence of diseases transmissible to man both in relation to the meat and the milk yield of cows. From a position where the incidence of disease symptoms in both milk and meat was a commonplace, progress has been definitely established to a point where the detection of such conditions as bovine tuberculosis on post-mortem inspection is quite rare, and no incident directly linking processed milk supplies with food-borne disease has been recorded in the United Kingdom for more than twenty years. This progress has had to be helped all along the way by the imposition and acceptance of public health controls. The same type of progress has been seen in the changes in the fishing industry, although there the main impetus comes from the need of the fleets to go farther afield for their catches and still bring fish to port in a marketable condition. It was also found, and accepted, that growing crops could be increased in yield and made more resistant to attacks of pests and plant diseases by selection of seed strains. In this area, however, success did not fully come from normal husbandry methods. There was need to supplement the protection by an increasing use of chemical insecticides and fungicides. These may occasionally introduce their own related food-contamination problems. Often the very mention of the addition of chemicals to foodstuffs can arouse deep feeling and alarm in some people. The truth of the situation in regard to the world food supply is either that chemical additives in the form of pesticides, weed controllers, and preservatives are used or the mass of people of the world will starve.

The use of a food additive to the advantage of the consumer is justified when it serves the following purposes:

1. To maintain the nutritional quality of a food.
2. To enhance the keeping quality or stability with resulting reduction in food wastage.
3. To make foods attractive to the consumer in a manner, which does not lead to deception.
4. To provide essential aids in food processing.

The use of food additives is not in the best interests of the consumer if they are used:

1. To disguise the use of faulty processing and handling techniques.
2. To deceive the consumer.
3. When the result is a substantial reduction of the nutritional value of the food.
4. When the desired effect can be obtained by other good manufacturing processes which are economically feasible.

With regard to item (4) there is clearly a need for continued research to ensure that, as and when technologically possible, food should be processed without the use of additives.

While certain production techniques will influence food quality, there is no food-processing technique that will put what the consumer calls 'quality' into any food where such a degree of quality did not originally exist. The quality improvement (which is closely allied to the 'cleanness' of the product) has to be in the foods from the first moment of production. In the light of modern food marketing and distributing conditions this became a vital food-supply necessity. The food processer using closely controlled processing techniques needs constant good-quality supplies from the producer if he is to sell goods with safety and acceptability throughout the markets of the world.

Most of the food processes now in use are modernized versions of the long-known principle that the rate of food deterioration can be delayed by keeping the food 'clean'. This means protecting the food from those matters which can contaminate it. It means using the knowledge that effective control of the temperature of most foods allows those foods to be effectively stored until needed for eating. It means using the knowledge that controlling the relative humidity of food stores reduces wastage and consumer hazard. The modern, and unavoidable, much publicized emphasis on food processing has led in some quarters to the mistaken belief that all food research is aimed at inventing or designing new methods of food processing and preservation. This is not the fact. Food has to be distributed, and it cannot be distributed with safety or economy unless it arrives in proper condition at its destination. The underlying aim of all food processing is therefore either to remove existing hazards from the food or to limit the uncontrolled process of deterioration already outlined above. An example of the removal of hazard from a food has been given above in the heat treatment of milk by pasteurization or sterilization. Yet another has been stated as the removal of possible handling hazards from ice cream by the pasteurization of the mix before freezing.

Underlying every process through which food is taken on its way to the table, there is the need for methods of checking the efficiency of the handling methods or the process itself. This means legal controls on the processes which may be employed and sanctions against those who use the wrong process or incorrectly apply the right process. It also means a set of test and evaluation techniques which include the physical and organoleptic assessment of the food, the chemical analysis of the food, and the bacteriological 'grading' of the food.

The description 'bacteriological grading' is used deliberately in this context, for there were some early attempts to set down arbitrary rules, on which judgements on the safety of food were to be made, based on a count of the bacterial activity within the food. This was a 'colony' count made on a culture plate and known as a 'total plate count'. The figures were, in fact, produced empirically rather than by an absolutely dependable scientific process, and as a result proved to be as often misleading as they were useful. A later and far more reliable technique has been to estimate bacterial activity by the rate of reduction of substances such as methylene blue, when that substance is put in contact with the food. This 'time reduction' rate can then be expressed as a bacterial grade of the food under test. The 'grade' results are then used as guides to judgement both of the food under test and the efficacy of the processing methods.

The aim of modern food research, therefore, is to ensure that all the processes and handling techniques to which food is subjected are such as ought and need to be employed and are safe and certain in operation. Some processes call for very special handling precautions before the food is treated; all the processes call for a total public health control of the food environment. Such food processes as are now employed are all internationally practised, and there is little doubt that from the engineering and mechanical viewpoint every effort has been made, and continues to be made, to render the process foolproof. This throws into sharp perspective the need to ensure that the housing and the siting of the necessary mechanical aids to food handling are such as will add to the hygiene of the food. It must be certain that the maintenance of the equipment is correct and that the actions of machine minders are based on hygiene rules. A totally clean environment is vital for correct food processing.

Food processes now used include:

PROCESS	EXAMPLE	REMARKS
Applied Heat		
Boiling	Cooked meats	Product must go forward to purpose-designed sealed packaging or a clean, correct temperature-controlled environment.
Pasteurization	Milk, egg products from the shell	Must go forward to sealed packaging which in turn needs a controlled-storage environment.

PROCESS	EXAMPLE	REMARKS
Applied Heat (contd.)		
Sterilization	Canned soups	Must go forward to or be treated by retorting in sealed packaging.
Smoke curing	Fish	Actually the application of the hot products of the combustion of the heat-raising fuels. Must go forward to a clean storage environment.
Applied Heat Intended to Change the Nature of the Food		
Evaporation to concentrate	Sweetened tinned milk	Needs sealed or relative humidity controlled storage environment.
Evaporation to powder form	Cold-mix ice-cream	First pasteurized. Must go forward to humidity-controlled storage and needs bacteriological checks on subsequent handling.
Removal of Heat		
Refrigeration	Meat, jellies	Actually a method of storage rather than a true process.
Removal of Heat and Sublimation of Water Content		
Accelerated freeze drying	Complete make-up meals, such as meat and rice	Sealing in packs into which an artificial 'nitrogen atmosphere' has been pumped is part of the process. Utterly dependent on the control of the humidity of packing and subsequent storage.
Controlled Removal of Heat		
Freeze drying	Complete whole meals. Fruits, etc.	Needs temperature-controlled storage (below 0° C.).
Quick freezing	Fruit, vegetables	Needs temperature-controlled storage (below 0° C.).
Deep freezing	Cod-liver oil	Needs temperature-controlled storage (below minus 5° C.).
Extraction		
Pressure or centrifuging	Cod-liver oil	Needs sealed packaging.
Grinding		
Milling	Flour	Needs protection from contamination and pest infestations.

Many food processes are combinations or variations of those listed, but it cannot be over-stressed that every process depends for success on the original food being of acceptable quality and on the finished product going forward to a clean form of controlled distribution and sales environment that will prevent contamination of the foods after treatment.

The same conclusion is drawn from a study of chemical and biological food processing. The processes are mainly divisible into actions applied before the material is in normal food form and actions applied after the food is in normal distribution and sales form.

Chemical Action Processes (applied before the material is in food form) include:

PROCESS	EXAMPLE	REMARKS
Spraying of growing crop with insecticides, fungicides	Apple trees	Ripe fruit can carry some residue.
Colouring and flavouring	Fruit jellies	Need careful packing and checks on addition.
Fat extending and 'improving'	Baked bread	Need clean handling.

Biological Action Processes (applied before the material is in food form) include:

PROCESS	EXAMPLE	REMARKS
Antibiotic treatment of feeding stuff	Food from meat animals	Needs special assessment at post-mortem inspection.
Antibiotic injection hormones	Caponized fowls	Need special assessment at post-mortem inspection.

These food treatments are undoubtedly food processes, in that they call for the application of specialized inspectorial tests and techniques before the finished product can be eaten. They also depend on the final environment being clean if the foods are to be eaten with safety.

Biological Action Processes (applied to food as offered for eating) include:

PROCESS	EXAMPLE	REMARKS
Fermentation	Beers, wines	Needs special packing.
Souring	Cheese	Needs clean storage.
Flavouring	Game	Needs clean handling away from other foods.

Chemical Action Processes

These include the use of all accepted and legalized food additives, but there are also natural processes that change the chemistry of the food and produce similar, albeit slower, results. Examples are:

PROCESS	EXAMPLE	REMARKS
Pickling (addition of acid)	Onions	Needs special packaging.
Salting	Fish	Needs special display conditions in relation to other foods.
Anti-oxidizing	Cooking oils	Needs special packaging.
Bleaching	Confectionery	Needs controlled storage.
Preserving	Jams	Needs special packaging.

Irradiation is now a possible form of food processing. As yet this is practised commercially in only a few countries. For example, the North American countries allow the treatment of food seeds and potato tubers to prevent germination in storage. This type of food process would require a specialized testing system, as it does not fit into any of the above groupings. It is, in itself, a physical process but not one designed to produce any physical changes in the food which are recognizable on organoleptic examination. Its action would be to bring about chemical, biological, and bacteriological changes in the foodstuffs, for while irradiation does totally kill bacteria, it does not totally end enzyme activity in the food. There is no doubt that this process could be used with absolute success in removing the bacteriological hazards from most foods. For this reason it is being pressed as a treatment to be adopted to deal with foods shown to be what the bacteriologists call reservoirs of infection. Before this can happen, however, there remains a

great deal of investigation to be carried out to assess the side-effects of the treatment. It can be summed up as certainly the most positive of positive food-hygiene actions on the bacteriological side of food handling, but it has been shown that only first-quality goods react as the experts expect. The opposite, and well-founded, argument is that, starting with such quality of food, good, sensibly applied usual food-hygiene actions by all persons will produce equally good results without any possible side-effect at all and without the use of irradiation techniques.

All these food processes are designed to 'protect' the food for marketing and distribution purposes. It follows that in so doing they reduce or totally prevent health hazards, provided they are correctly carried out and the total food environment is hygienic.

CATERING

Consideration must now be given to food catering in the widest sense of that term. This must include the preparation and provision of foods and meals for sale, and the wholesale and retail distribution of foods. For the present purpose these count as processes, for they are all based on a combination of some of the above outlined methods or on the handling of the products of those processes. During these stages the food is frequently widely and necessarily in contact with human hands and with work surfaces. In this aspect of the distribution of food the emphasis on food cleanliness shifts from the food itself to the people who handle the food and the utensils and the equipment with which the food comes into contact before being eaten. It is here that the danger of contamination can be greatest. It is here that the greatest food protection effort needs to be made by everyone.

Specialized Production and Processing

Thus far it has been possible to consider situations where the production of a major food is followed by a processing of that major food supply to facilitate distribution to the consumer. It is now necessary to consider situations where the production and processing are so much the one a part of the other as to make them, in effect, one action. Milk supply is an example of this. It is also necessary to consider major food production, where none of the processes outlined above are used, but where the preparation of the food for distribution can, of itself, be designated a process. An example is the killing and dressing of food-animal carcasses. For present purposes mention will be made of milk, meat, eggs (out of the shell), ice cream, and shellfish.

All these widely distributed foods have two factors in common. Either the presence of initial contamination with spoilage and/or pathogenic bacteria is so inevitable or unavoidable that they must be subject to specialized, strictly enforced control laws or they are media in which contamination is especially hazardous if unchecked. The Food and Drugs Act, 1955, now operative in England and Wales (the latest of a long history of food-control laws which started to appear on the Statute Book as long ago as 1482) gives direct powers to the Central Government to make specialized control regulations for products in this category.

Milk. In its raw state, as taken from the cow, milk is

naturally infected with bacteria. It is, at the temperature when taken, an excellent culture medium for a considerable range of micro-organisms. Fortunately this situation is totally changed if the milk is cooled to 10° C. as soon as possible after milking time, and the product can easily be rendered safe and free from spoilage organisms by several heat-treatment methods which enhance rather than reduce its usefulness and consumer palatability. These treatments, now in use in the United Kingdom and the majority of countries in the civilized world, include pasteurization, sterilization, and ultra-heat treatment. The entire process of milk production, and of necessity the production of some milk products such as fresh dairy cream, is now controlled, from udder to delivery-for-use point, by the Milk and Dairies (General) Regulations, 1959. These Regulations are the latest in a long history of such controls, and are themselves under constant review as exact knowledge increases and new safeguarding processing methods are designed and used. They set down rules for every action in milk production from the construction of milking houses to the shape, size, and closure of the bottle or carton in which milk is now made available to consumers. Such detail cannot be paraphrased, and the whole of this legislation must be studied by any food-hygiene worker concerned with milk hygiene. Two points only need now be stressed. First, that no person can purchase raw milk in the United Kingdom unless it be at his own specific choice and free request. Broadly speaking, all milk is required to be heat processed in one of the legally acceptable forms, but if, for any personal reason, any person actively desires to have raw milk, then, on a deliberate request, he can be so supplied. Even then, that raw milk must be cooled (10° C.) immediately after being taken from the cow udder. The incidents of food-borne disease in the United Kingdom in recent history which have been attributable to milk have all been connected with such raw-milk purchase and the use of raw milk untreated apart from cooling. The control regulations apply to all milk handling up to the point of retail sale and use. There the food-hygiene controls do not cease, but fall once again under the general principles of food-hygiene law. Methods of testing the bacteriological conditions of milk and the efficiency of processing are: (1) the resazurin test; and (2) the methylene-blue test.

When methylene blue or resazurin is added to milk the bacteria present take up oxygen and change the colour of the introduced dye. Methylene blue becomes increasingly colourless as bacterial activity increases. Resazurin changes through a colour spectrum from blue to pink. The speed of the change shows the bacteriological content of the milk. Milk which has been pasteurized fails if the reduction period is 30 minutes or less, but there are special times and considerations for methylene-blue reduction, which range to 4 hours in summer weather and $4\frac{1}{2}$ hours in winter.

Meat. Similar specialized control regulations also apply to the killing and skinning of food animals in abattoirs and slaughterhouses. The last of a long series of such regulations are the Slaughterhouses (Hygiene) Amendment Regulations, 1959. As with milk, these laws are under constant review and cannot be paraphrased, because they cover in such detail all matter from the lairage of the cattle to the removal of trade wastes, the delivery into trade of the meat, and the actions of abattoir personnel with regard to their clothing and instru-ments. The design and construction of abattoirs is controlled, as are the killing and dressing procedures, and special regard is paid to the early and complete separation of all incdible by-products from edible products and the outlawing of the practice of using fouled wiping cloths for the removal of visible dirt or manure contamination from carcasses. These control regulations are available for study from H.M.S.O. The meat and meat products are subject to these controls until the moment they leave the abattoir, and they then become subject to the general food-hygiene laws in the distributive trade and general food-hygiene practices in the hands of the consumers.

Eggs. It is known that eggs have a natural bacterial content. This is a minor consideration in hen eggs but a major problem in duck eggs. By its feeding and living habits the duck (and similarly the goose) produces eggs that have a considerable likelihood of carrying pathogenic bacteria. The problem can be overcome in hen eggs by most normal and known methods of cooking, but in the duck egg the boiling time for real safety has been demonstrated to be 10 minutes or more. The real contamination problems with eggs, however, arise from cracked eggs, eggs removed from the shell for obvious commercial purposes, such as large-scale baking, and from the manufacture of egg yolks in bulk, egg white (albumen) in bulk, and egg yolk/white melange for bulk sales in packed forms. Sometimes the egg products are dried, occasionally they are formed into specialized trade-use powders, and on other trade occasions they are bulked and packed in cans and frozen for transport purposes from country to country. So much evidence built up of high bacterial contamination of eggs, removed from the shell, in all of these trade-use forms that there is now a total legal control in the United Kingdom under the Liquid Egg (Pasteurisation) Regulations, 1963 (H.M.S.O.), *q.v.* When these products get into normal food-trade distribution they, like eggs in the shell, fall within the terms of general food-hygiene law and production. The test for the efficiency of the pasteurization of these egg products is the alpha-amylase test. An amylase is an enzyme that hydrolyses starch and glycogen to maltose, but alpha-amylase breaks down starch without proceeding to the maltose condition.

Ice cream. This is a product that was originally considered a milk product. In its early history it was literally a frozen custard of eggs and milk, but modern ice cream is a product with its own standing in the food trade. Some 50 million gallons are eaten in the United Kingdom every year, and the basic ingredients are now skimmed-milk powder, animal and vegetable fats, emulsifiers, setting agents, and flavours. This industry is very rigorously controlled in the United Kingdom and, it must be said, with the wish and total co-operation of the ice-cream trade. The relevant laws are the Ice-Cream (Heat Treatment, etc.) Regulations, 1959 and 1963, *q.v.* (H.M.S.O.). Broadly speaking, these laws are a description of acceptable pasteurization and distribution processes, and all ice cream must now be pasteurized at one stage or another of its progress from raw ingredients to consumer. Additionally, the product on sale is subject to general food-hygiene law and practices, and the test now used, on an informal basis only, is the methylene-blue test described above. This must be an informal test in relation to ice cream, as it is basically a test for milk at normal temperature, while ice cream is not a full milk product except in specialized production to limited amounts, and in any case the product has to be thawed before the test can be applied, and the test thus does not really judge the condition of the product as actually consumed.

Shellfish. Shellfish are occasionally implicated as the cause of outbreaks of food poisoning, and it has been necessary to have special control regulations to cover their collection, cleansing, and treatment before sale to the public. The methods, generally speaking a period of self-cleansing 'laying' in pure potable water, apply to oysters and cockles in particular and are found in the Public Health (Shell-Fish) Regulations, 1934 and 1948 (H.M.S.O.), *q.v.* Once the shellfish are collected and treated and passed into trade or distribution, they fall under the general food-hygiene laws and practices.

Mussel poisoning is discussed in World Health Organisation (1973*a*).

Laws

Inasmuch as it has not been possible to set down the above paragraphs without reference to food-hygiene laws, it would be as well at this stage to list the existing control legislation with a direct food-hygiene connotation now extant in the United Kingdom.

1. The Food and Drugs Act, 1955
2. The Food Hygiene (General) Regulations, 1970
3. The Food Hygiene (Docks, Carriers, etc.) Regulations, 1960
4. The Food Hygiene (Markets, Stalls and Delivery Vehicles) Regulations, 1966, and the Amendment Regulations of the same year
5. The Milk and Dairies Regulations (General), 1959
6. The Slaughterhouses (Hygiene) Regulations, 1958/59
7. The Ice-Cream (Heat Treatment, etc.) Regulations, 1959/63
8. The Public Health (Shell-Fish) Regulations, 1934/48 (under amendment)
9. Byelaws for the handling, wrapping and delivery of food in the open air
10. Public Slaughterhouses Byelaws, 1956

FOOD TRANSPORT

The term food distribution repeatedly occurs as the theme of practical food hygiene is developed, and it is therefore necessary to have clearly in mind that there are food supplies that depend entirely upon specialized forms of transport. These are basically economic considerations, but they have effect on the spoilage and safety of the food conveyed. Instances of specialized transport are the design of refrigerated ships, as has been mentioned above, and the design of insulated and refrigerated road vehicles for the conveyance of frozen foods. In other cases the actual conveyance is part of a food-processing technique, as when green bananas are loaded and allowed to ripen on the journey overseas. The construction rules for such conveyance containers by road, rail, or sea are extremely detailed, and students wishing to look further would do well to study the publication, *Temperature Controlled Food Transport*, of the Royal Society of Health, London. The principles involved are that the design and materials will not be such as will contaminate the foods, and will, of themselves, permit and aid the easy cleaning of the container. Perhaps the more important consideration, however, is the efficiency of the insula-

tion against temperature change that needs to be built into all these conveyors. This is judged on obtaining a carriage temperature range such as:

> Chilled meats of all types −1° C. to +1° C.
> Fresh sausages, cooked meats.
> Cured meats, bacons, etc., +2° C. to +7° C.
> Cooked pies, pastry products cheese, +7° C. to +10° C., etc.
> Dairy produce, +4° C. to +6° C.
> Fruit and vegetables (excluding bananas), +7° C. to +10° C.
> Bananas, +10° C.
> Quick-frozen foods, −15° C.

The efficiency of the insulation and construction methods is capable of being assessed from a formula which need not bother the food hygienist except in so far as it is concerned with the 'K' factor. This is soon, internationally, likely to be the stated efficiency rating of such containers. The insulating efficiency will be internationally expressed as a 'K' factor degree. The definition of 'K' factor is the laboratory value of the thermal efficiency of the insulation material at average true operating temperatures.

The basic requirements for all food transport are:

1. Food cargoes should be packed only into vehicles designed for that purpose.
2. Unless packaged foods only are carried, the design should include some method for the observance of personal hygiene by the operators.
3. The container should be clean before loading starts.
4. The cleaning of the container or vehicle should follow a set routine that has been worked out having regard to the food and the nature of the delivery process.
5. The correct facilities, for instance, hot water, detergents, sterilants, and cleansing tools, must be readily available when cleaning is undertaken.
6. The personnel should always observe personal hygiene and be clean in their clothing and their methods of handling foods.

The materials most used for food-vehicle and food-container construction are: high-gloss glass fibre, reinforced plastic panels, non-marking aluminium alloys, plastic-covered steel sheet, heavy-duty steel plate, welded light-metal alloys, aluminium alloys, and galvanized steel sheet.

All of these are best cleaned by steam or hot water, but there are occasions, when these are not readily available, when correct strength sterilants (dependent on the processes and circumstances and the food) may be used. The growing practice of close packing the individual product to prevent any direct food contact with the bodywork is commended, and for this purpose it is noteworthy that large sisal-paper 'envelopes' are now available that cover most of the internal space of road and rail vehicles. These are known as 'liners', and are expendable after single use.

DISTRIBUTION METHODS AND SALES TECHNIQUES

Distribution methods and sales techniques also need to be understood if the achievement of the clean food environment is to be made possible. People still take small quantities of food to market, but basically the foods of the world are bulk distributed by using knowledge of correct packing methods that allow the food to travel, or by the use of cartage methods that assist in keeping the food in proper condition. Examples are the construction of refrigerated ships to convey meat from Australia and New Zealand to England, and the export of prepared foods, such as meat spreads and pastes, in sealed glass jars from England to America. The food-hygiene rules that have to cover all food operations must therefore cover the design and construction of vehicles, ships, and containers, and must dictate the handling circumstances that must obtain at any time of on-loading and off-loading. The materials used for packaging must be such as will safeguard the hygienic nature of the product, and not such as will allow the leaching (or chemical transference) of hazardous materials from the pack to the product. Sales techniques are changing so rapidly that any full description is made almost impossible, but two factors must be stressed. The first is the increase in the packing of individual food purchases in a pre-sealed and often pre-cooked form. This is the basis of many supermarket sales, and it is a technique that cannot succeed without the correct amount of food refrigeration, good lighting, and clean food storage. The second is the rather more subtle technique of 'artificial' underselling. This phrase will need explanation. Suppose that a given trader can sell 500 chickens with ease on any given sales day. In the old trade outlook such a trader would have 500 chickens on display, 200–300 in stock, and 500 in the delivery arrangement. In artificial undersell the trader would never have available more than 450 chickens. These would be delivered to his store as a fresh supply every day. But he would always be fifty short of his potential sales. This would mean that he would: (1) sell out every day and need no storage for stock; (2) need no refrigerated storage to keep the held stock fresh; (3) never have to make sure to sell old stock before starting on the new stock, which is always in demand; (4) create a justifiable reputation for clean food handling; (5) cut his general overheads by more than the lost profit on the 50 chickens which could have been sold but were not.

The Advance Preparation of Meals

A sales method, or merchandizing technique, that, in theory, could be avoided or made absolutely without hazard is the advance preparation of meals cooked ready to eat. This is a catering practice that is forced upon many, if not most, large-scale caterers in the United Kingdom. When it is understood that some 10,000,000 people, for instance, are all seeking a quick hot meal in the Greater London area between 11.30 a.m. and 3.30 p.m. it must be understood that advance preparation of meals is the only workable and economic method of meeting this demand. So the caterer gets the food ready and awaits the customers. Meat joints are cooked many hours in advance, sliced, and left until needed. The meal is then reheated for service. Theorists deplore this practice. Fact makes it unavoidable. The practical food hygienist accepts that the practice must go on and demands: (1) efficient cooling of the ready-cooked meat or meal; (2) temperature-controlled storage—below 10° C. while being kept; (3) a time limit on the store period (say 16 hours); and (4) efficient reheating above 100° C. before service. This is the technique that has, especially for

home catering use, developed into the frozen packed ready meal. These ready meals are bought and reheated in homes for consumption by families with income or work-time needs that make other cooking methods less attractive. Where meat or meals are plated ready for service only an hour or two before being eaten the hygienist looks for hot store cupboards which are above the 66° C. range and reheating above 100° C. for at least 20 minutes unless one of the newer infra-red or microwave cooking ovens is used.

If the time of holding for service is reduced to 30 minutes or less, then the hygiene safeguard lies solely in the temperature of the hot-plate store cupboard being above 66° C. Inasmuch as the limited-time hot-meal demand in the Greater London area has been instanced, it is worth noting that caterers there must follow such principles quite effectively, for the notified cases of food poisoning—against such a huge potential number of people at risk—is an almost negligible statistic, and even then the recorded events occur more frequently from *home*-prepared and reheated foods inefficiently stored in home kitchens.

Cleaning and Washing Up

Washing up of crockery and eating utensils is another special sales method that has to be accepted as inevitable. Theorists may speak of single-service disposable materials, and there are limited occasions when those may, with success, be used. Nevertheless, the main eating habits of most people will involve crockery, glassware, and utensils that will be used, cleaned, and used again by different people. This is true also of home eating. Efficient, clean washing up is therefore essential. In this context the term washing up covers all the actions of cleaning crockery, glassware, cutlery, utensils, and cooking pans. Washing up by hand, properly done, can be as efficient as by machine, for individual attention can be given to taking out of service cracked crockery and chipped utensils. Additionally the washer-up can make sure that lipstick stains, congealed food, etc., are fully removed.

The accumulation of dirty utensils should be avoided, for the longer they are left, the more difficult they become to clean.

Any process of good washing up will be made ineffective if the articles, when washed, are not stored in a clean place. There should be adequate reserves of crockery and utensils to avoid hurried work at rush-hour periods.

Preliminary Scraping. As soon as possible after use the dirty articles should be taken to the washing-up room, sorted into their various categories and sizes, and stacked. During this process food residues should be scraped or tipped off into the refuse containers. The object of this scraping is to keep the washing-up water as free as possible from food particles. This scraping should be done by a wooden spoon, a blunt knife, or other implement which will not scratch the crockery; or it can be done by running water, provided the solids are caught in a strainer and not washed down to clog the drain-pipes.

Liquid residues in cups, tumblers, and soup-plates should be emptied away at this stage.

The crockery and utensils are then washed in water at a temperature of at least 60° C. to which a detergent has been correctly added. This water should be changed as soon as it becomes dirty, and this is where machines have the advantage as the water is constantly changing. The 'wash-up' material is then placed into a sterilizing rinse in wire baskets in water at least 77° C. and immersed for at least 2 minutes. If water above 77° C. is used this time can be reduced. If water below that temperature is used, then a suitable chemical sterilant must be added. The materials being washed are then given a final rinse in clean cold water and stacked to drain. The slogan for all washing up is 'scrape, wash, rinse, stack, store'. If wiping cloths must be used they should be clean at the start and preferably used with chemical sterilant. The cloths themselves become impregnated with sterilant as wiping up proceeds. In some cases disposable paper wiping towels may be used, but these are not really practicable in large-scale operations.

Refuse Disposal. This paragraph really refers to all refuse in food premises, but it is opportune to introduce it here, inasmuch as the scraping of meal plates has been mentioned. There will be trade refuse in every food premises and kitchen refuse in every home. Keep it in covered bins away from all edible food, and get it out of the premises at the first opportunity.

The Sale of Food in the Open Air

It is simply wild fancy to hope that food sales in open markets will cease or consist of parcelled food and single-use equipment. The hygiene worker has therefore to devise methods of food handling in those circumstances which match the best 'indoor' techniques. Let the example be personal hygiene. Small portable hand-washing facilities are now available for these purposes. They consist basically of containers holding 2–4 gallons of hot water or tanks which can be connected to motor-vehicle engines from which the water is heated. Other designs utilize Calor or butane gas for water heating. Where food cooking is practised in the open air—as, for instance, in 'hot dog' trolleys—the special design, in good-quality stainless steel, is a trolley that has lids so arranged as to keep the cooking food completely covered until the moment of service to the customer.

Fish. Fish and shellfish pose two merchandising problems that must be accepted and faced. First, the peeling of prawns, shrimps, scampi, etc., must be by hand after cooking, and secondly, the sale of *fresh* fish in inland towns means boxed fish transport or special iced-compartment vehicles.

The first problem is how to ensure regular, good hand washing and how to make the provision of facilities to allow this to happen. The second is the efficient boxing and icing of fresh fish in transport. Plastic-lined wooden boxes are good, but aluminium boxes are preferable. These should be cleaned before packing, and sufficient ice or solid ice (solid CO_2) included to keep the fish fresh and cool.

Boned Meat. Many food-trade processes start with the boning out or carving of meat. This is essentially a hand operation. Even when machines are used the piece of meat needs to be put into place or held in position by the hand of the worker. These hands must be thoroughly clean at all times, and all work surfaces must be regularly sterilized. Soft woods must not be used. Permanent wooden work-surfaces should be avoided. In their place there should be stainless steel of good gauge and quality, or pressurized rubber nylon pads or disposable wooden boards.

Side Tables, Cream Cakes, etc. In catering there is real need for side-service tables, and they must be allowed, but they must be placed so as to avoid contamination of the food by any person or other agency. Cream-filled cakes should always be held below 10° C.

CLEANING ROUTINES

All merchandising techniques produce the need for specialized designed cleaning techniques to fit the trade or selling circumstances. Here is an example of such a routine. This is designed for the bakery trade, but all other trades can be studied and routines of similar calibre designed.

ROUTINE CLEANING CHART

Equipment or area	Routine to follow	Frequency of cleaning
GENERAL GOODS STORE		
Walls and shelves	Sweep and/or vacuum clean.	Frequently and regularly
	Wash down with hot water containing detergent.	At least once a week
Floors	Sweep and/or vacuum clean.	Frequently and regularly
	Wash down with hot water containing detergent.	Daily
ISSUING STORES		
General	Sweep and/or vacuum clean. Wash any surface that comes into contact with food with hot water containing detergent.	Daily
Walls and shelves	Wash down with hot water containing detergent. Walls can be hosed with 'live steam' if facilities exist.	Frequently and regularly
Floors	Wash down with hot water containing detergent or hose with 'live steam' if facilities available.	Daily
EQUIPMENT		
Utensils and supply vessels	Wash with hot water containing detergent, rinse and dry or wash out with 'live steam' if facilities available. If the utensils, etc., are used for meat, cream, imitation cream, or egg the hot water should contain detergent with sterilant.	At least once a day, more frequently if the process requires
Measures and pans	Clean thoroughly, wash with hot water containing detergent, rinse, and dry. If the measures and skips are used with meat, cream, imitation cream, or egg the hot water should contain detergent with sterilant.	Frequently and regularly
Ventilation ducts and fans	Brush and/or vacuum clean outside surfaces of ducts and metal fitments.	When cleaning the walls of the appropriate store
	Wash down with hot water containing detergent.	Regularly in other parts of the premises.
	Clean inlet screens and filters in the same way.	At least once a week

Equipment or area	Routine to follow	Frequency of cleaning	Equipment or Area	Routine to follow	Frequency of cleaning
EQUIPMENT (*contd.*)			**EQUIPMENT** (*contd.*)		
Storage tanks (not completely sealed)	Drain tank. Wash interior with hot water containing detergent. Rinse thoroughly and run off. When refilling first run off sufficient water to dispose of any residues.	At least once every 6 months	Scale pans and measures	Remove deposit or spillage. Wash with warm water containing detergent, rinse, and dry. If the pans and measures are used with meat, cream, or egg the water should contain detergent with sterilant.	Frequently and regularly during use At the close of every working period and at any change of trade operation
Brining tanks	Scrape, scrub, and wash with hot water containing detergent. Rinse thoroughly. Alternatively, wash out with 'live steam' if facilities available.	Before refilling	Knives, etc.	Wash in water at 43·5° C. or above or in warm water containing detergent with sterilant. Rinse and dry. Replace in purpose-built racks (preferably metal) attached to fixed equipment.	After use
Bulk egg-storage tanks	Wash out with cold water to remove residues. Wash with hot water containing detergent with sterilant. Rinse thoroughly with cold water.	Before refilling	Wooden trays	Scrub with the grain in warm water containing detergent. Rinse and dry. Wash with warm water containing detergent with sterilant. Rinse and dry. If the trays are used with meat, cream, imitation cream, or egg products the water should contain detergent with sterilant. Alternatively, wash by machine in hot water (above 43° C.).	Frequently and regularly Trays to be used must be clean or cleaned ready for the start of every working day
Blocking, forming, and stamping machines	Dismantle, degrease, and clean thoroughly. Immerse dismantled parts in boiling water or swab thoroughly with warm water containing detergent. Rinse, dry, and reassemble.	Frequently and regularly			
Homogenizers	Dismantle, wash working parts in warm water and detergent. Rinse with sterilant, rinse with clean water, reassemble.	At the close of every working period			
Whisks and cooling utensils	Clean thoroughly and scrub in water at 43·5° C. or above, immerse in warm water containing detergent with sterilant. Scour, rinse, and dry.	After every period of use	Wiping materials and cloths	(*a*) Use expendable material. OR (*b*) Keep in suitable chemical sterilant between uses and boil after changing.	(*a*) Discard into suitable containers conveniently placed (*b*) Change several times a day
Conveyor belts	Clean off dropped materials. Swab with warm water containing detergent. Clean surface of rollers.	Frequently and regularly during use At least once a day At least once a day	Savoy bags (icing bags)	Turn inside out, wash away surplus cream. Scrub inside and out with warm water containing detergent with sterilant, rinse in hot water. Boil for 5 minutes if material is suitable. Scour and sterilize nozzles. Rinse and dry.	After use
Proving and baking tins	Clean thoroughly.	When necessary			
Proving trolleys	Wash with hot water containing detergent, rinse, and dry.	Frequently and regularly during use			
Dough and pastry mixers	Remove spillage and extruded food. Clean thoroughly and wash with warm water containing detergent. Rinse with cold water and dry.	Frequently and regularly during use At the close of every working period	**EXTERIOR** Drains	Remove grease-trap inserts and clean. Wash out body of trap with hot water containing detergent with sterilant. Renew filter material.	Frequently and regularly
Flavours, essences, and colour containers	Clean the outside of containers.	Each time they are used	Open drainage channels	Remove any surface grit and scrub grids and channels with hot water containing detergent with sterilant.	At the close of every working day
Pastry boards and icing tables	Keep clean during use. Remove all traces of flour or sugar deposit. Immerse boards in boiling water and scrub, or scrub with warm water containing detergent with sterilant. Always scrub wooden surfaces with the grain.	At the close of every working period	Dustbins	Wash out with hot water and soda or a detergent solution and invert to dry. Alternatively, wash out with 'live steam' if facilities available.	After each emptying

Equipment or Area	Routine to follow	Frequency of cleaning
VEHICLES		
Surfaces, receptacles, and equipment, or parts of equipment that touch food	Clear crumbs and spillage during use.	Frequently
	Clean thoroughly.	Every day
	Surfaces soiled only with flour dust or non-fatty crumbs can be brushed out.	
Remaining parts of the interior of the vehicle and interior equipment	Wash with warm water containing detergent.	At least once a week

THE LOCATION AND DESIGN OF PREMISES, EQUIPMENT, AND UTENSILS

Premises

There are basic similarities in the construction of all premises where food is handled. These are found whether the premises be a small home kitchen, a small food shop, or a huge food factory. The use of good construction principles, and of materials that assist the maintenance of cleaning routines, thus become major factors in obtaining practical food hygiene. These principles are very clearly expressed in agreed Codes of Practice that have been worked out by health officers and food traders in the United Kingdom. An example of such a code, in general terms, is given below. Extra paragraphs need to be added for specific trade reasons, and copies of such codes, with specific paragraphs, can be obtained from Her Majesty's Stationery Office. The codes at present available are:

Code 3. Hygiene in the Fish Retail Trade.
Code 4. The Hygienic Transport and Handling of Fish.
Code 5. Poultry Dressing and Packing.
Code 6. Hygiene in the Bakery Trade and Industry.
Code 7. Hygiene in the operation of coin operated food vending machines.
Code 8. Hygiene in the Meat Trades.

Additionally there is the publication *Clean Catering* (H.M.S.O.), which is in fact a code for the caterer expanded into a complete booklet.

Before the 'Example' code is read it is necessary to indicate some general principles in regard to the siting and location of food premises and the correct allocation of working space for food handlers. Badly located sites hinder the proper observance of basic food-hygiene ideals, and as such they should, in theory, be avoided. Where it is not possible to obey this precept, all cleaning and food-handling routines should be carefully worked out to compensate for site and location difficulties. Adequate water supplies, lighting services, and ventilation must always be available. The immediate surroundings should be examined for the presence of noxious trades and practices. An unpleasant smell is not so important as whether the air is charged with smoke or other dirty particles, or whether the surroundings contain potential or actual breeding-grounds for rats or harmful insects.

If prospective premises form part of a large building the location of the water supply and other common services should be examined; and it should be ascertained whether the sanitary conveniences and wash basins to be used by the staff are conveniently sited and adequate in number. Attention should be given to the facilities for handling and storing foodstuffs and to the routes by which the foods reach the establishment and the refuse is removed. The inward route, at least, should be under the trader's own control; dark and potentially dirty passages and alleyways should never be used as food rooms.

Underground food rooms present special difficulties. It is important that their windows should not open on to areas or forecourts so narrow that dirt of noxious matter can be kicked, thrown, dropped, or blown into uncleanable recesses or even on to the food. Underground premises may be liable to flooding and drainage backflow, and they also need special ventilation and lighting. Premises where food is stored need to be cool and dry.

All food-handling or service premises should be extensive enough to allow all work chores to be carried out without congestion on the lines of work flow. Food handlers should never be crowded at work-tables or have to queue for the use of food-cleaning or washing facilities or facilities for personal hygiene. At the same time the premises should not be so large as to entail unnecessary walking about by workers. Food handlers have been observed to neglect hygienic practices if they involve additional walking, waiting, or working uncomfortably close to a colleague. There must be sufficient table and shelf space to allow used and unused utensils to be kept apart from each other and from food in course of preparation.

Food-preparation and washing-up rooms or zones should occupy a space equal to approximately half the sales area, but rather more than this is necessary in very small establishments. Every food establishment should contain a room used solely as a food work room not less than 8 ft. (2·43 m.) in height and with a minimum floor area of 100 ft.² (9·3 m.²) clear of furniture, fittings, and stored goods. If more than three people are employed in the room there should be an additional 33 ft.² (3 m.²) of floor area similarly clear for each person above three in number.

The greater the distance over which food has to be carried, and the more often it has to be handled, the greater the chance of its becoming contaminated. Therefore, the ideal to aim at is to have everything moving forward in orderly progression—from delivery area to sales area.

Temperature and Relative Humidity. As this section proceeds the terms 'cool' and 'dry' will increasingly occur, and it is therefore useful to explain those terms.

Cool is actually coupled with the idea of hot food being piping hot. At first glance that may seem a contradiction in terms, but it is understandable when it is made clear that the object is to keep foods outside the danger range of temperatures 10°–63° C. There is a range of food, such as bread, pastries, etc., that may be within this range with safety. There are other foods which need to be always in sub-zero conditions, such as frozen foods and ice-creams. One of the greatest problems facing the food-hygiene worker is the ready plated meal held until the consumer arrives and kept for this purpose in so-called 'hot' cupboards, which are usually found to operate around 37° C. Plated food so held for 30 minutes has almost become the equivalent of a laboratory culture plate if there is original bacterial contamination of the plated meal. The aim must therefore be to keep food cool or piping hot, in hot cupboards above 63° C.

Relative humidity is the degree of available moisture in the air at any given temperature, and it is evaluated by taking contrasting readings of two thermometers, one kept dry and the other with its bulb covered by a wick immersed in water.

Lay-out. The lay-out should be planned with a clear idea of the purpose of every part of the food premises. A goods entrance, separate from the customer's entrance, is essential for hygienic planning. The most convenient arrangement is for this goods entrance to open from a yard so situated that delivery vans can pull right up to the door of the building. The yard should have an impervious and even surface, a water standpipe, tap and washing-down hose, raised and covered accommodation for refuse bins and swill bins, and adequate drainage. If solid fuel is used the store should be in the yard, and bulk oil fuel should be kept completely separate from any food or utensil store.

Vegetable and Root-crop Storage. If root crops and uncleaned farm produce are being handled on any food premises they should be stored in a purpose-designed room which should be near the goods delivery point and is cool, dry, well ventilated, and large enough to allow for orderly storage. It is convenient in this room to arrange that water used for washing down drains to a gulley. Thus the room is best planned with an entrance direct from the yard—which will keep some dirt off the rest of the premises. Vegetables require ventilation. They should be stored on racks—preferably wire or metal—so arranged that air can circulate freely under and around them. The racks should be high enough off the ground so as not to be readily accessible to vermin. Potatoes and root vegetables should normally be stored in sacks as delivered; but if they have been bagged in wet weather they may be subject to disease, and they should be turned out, aired, and examined. The defective ones should be removed at once. Other fresh vegetables should be used the day they are received. If this is impossible they should be emptied out on to the racks, but new deliveries should not be emptied on top of older ones. Stored vegetables should be inspected frequently and thoroughly, as decay spreads rapidly. Near the entrance of the premises should come the dry food store, which should be flyproofed by fixing removable screens over windows and door openings; in addition, the walls should be treated with residual insecticides. The room should be dry, well lit and ventilated, and at least 7 ft. 6 in. (2·3 m.) high. This room should be used exclusively as a store, and therefore an internal water supply is not essential, but water for cleaning should be close at hand. Prepacked deep-frozen vegetables received into stock mean that sub-zero holding cabinets must be available. These cabinets should be such as allow for rotation of stock, and have a plainly marked effective loading line above which stock should not be placed. Rooms where food is 'worked' should never be used as thoroughfares to other parts of any building, and it is an advantage to study the processes and 'zone' the areas of floor space allocated to each. This, as a reduction of cleaning problems, is to be preferred against a multiplicity of small work-rooms. Full advantage should always be taken of natural lighting and existing mains services supplies, and the real aim should be to achieve cleanliness and supervision rather than pure design symmetry.

Siting of Equipment. All food equipment should be so placed as to allow room for cleaning around and behind, as well as in front. Where equipment and cupboards and store places are 'built in' the object must be to have them free of unnecessary ornamentation and finished to an even surface with surrounding wall surfaces or floor surfaces to obviate uncleanable ledges and areas.

Personal Hygiene Facilities. Sanitary accommodation must be provided for the staff, and should also be provided for customers. It is usually inconvenient for the same accommodation to be used both by staff and customers, except in quite small establishments. In larger establishments it is more satisfactory to combine the staff conveniences in a group with the staff washrooms and cloakrooms. It is important that the sanitary accommodation available to workers should be readily accessible. Although no general rule can be laid down, no worker should have to go more than thirty steps from the room where he is working to reach sanitary accommodation. The compartment containing the sanitary convenience should be separated from any working room and from the dining-room by an intervening ventilated space and should be well lit; this point is most important, as otherwise it may not be properly cleaned. There should be separate sanitary accommodation for each sex, with separate approaches.

There should be fully equipped wash-hand basins within any compartment containing sanitary conveniences or close to them, for example, in the intervening space referred to above.

The basic requirements of sanitary accommodation—ready accessibility, good light, and proximity to washing facilities—can be fulfilled in many different ways; only after consideration of all the circumstances can a decision be made on whether the provision in a particular instance is suitable and sufficient.

Where there is no water supply or when a water-carriage sewage-disposal system cannot be used for other reasons—for example at fair-grounds or at remote tourist centres—some form of chemical closet is needed. Whichever type is used should be fitted with a cover or otherwise constructed so that the contents are protected from flies. Care must be exercised to see that the equipment is kept as clean as possible. It should be situated as far from the food room as reasonable, and it should have hand-washing facilities adjacent.

It is never impossible to provide hot water, soap, nail brushes, and towels. Wall-cabinet roller towels which present each user with a fresh surface or, alternatively, paper towels for single use are preferable. Electric hot-air hand driers are also available.

Water Supply and Hot-water Apparatus. Ample and immediately available supplies of both hot and cold running water are essential. Where the food establishment occupies part of a building, it is desirable for it to have its own independent hot-water supply. All water used for food preparation and cooking, for drinking, for washing-up, and for cleaning utensils and surfaces with which food or utensils may come in contact should be public-supply-main water or of equivalent quality. Rain-water, river water, well water, and water from other non-purified sources should be used only for such outdoor purposes as washing down yards and swilling out dust-bins, except on the advice of the local health department.

It is not advisable to economize over water taps and piping. All sinks, wash-hand basins, and other fixed receptacles should receive their water supplies direct from taps appropriately placed. For internal piping copper is best; and where the course of the piping is not dictated either by the existing mains and tanks or by the siting of sinks and other appliances, it is worth while to give some thought to its arrangement. Pipes tend to collect dust, and horizontal or sloping overhead pipes are not only difficult to clean but may also accumulate moisture, which drips on to the food.

Whenever possible, pipes should either be run outside the kitchen (for example, under the floor or above the ceiling) or else they should be sunk into the wall. When they must come into the open they should for preference run vertically rather than horizontally, bringing the water straight down to the tap from the overhead pipes or straight up from the supply beneath the floor. In any case, they should be held at least 2 or 3 in. (5–8 cm.) away from the wall by pipe clips, so that they can be cleaned all round and do not create crevices in which insects or vermin may breed. If cold service pipes have to be run at high level they should be lagged to prevent condensation and the dripping which results.

Hot-water pipes should be lagged to conserve heat and so reduce the consumption of fuel. The methods of lagging pipes and storage tanks is important, as cases have occurred of mice burrowing into soft lagging and nesting in it. Pipes should be protected with a fine wire mesh to prevent this, and the lagging round tanks should be enclosed with materials which cannot be gnawed.

Hot Water. Many water-heating systems produce water which, although hotter than the 43·5°–48·5° C., which is about the most that normal human hands can stand, is never as hot as the 77° C. necessary for the proper sterilizing rinse of crockery, cutlery, and utensils. Such systems are satisfactory enough in smaller establishments which can carry out the sterilizing by steam or by water heated as required for sterilization purposes. Larger establishments which have a constant demand for washing-up water at 77° C. should be careful to ensure that their systems can provide water at 77° C.

Wash Basins. Workers should be encouraged to wash their hands both after visiting the sanitary convenience and whenever necessary during the course of work. They should not use the wash-up sinks for this purpose, as this may infect the sinks with germs which can later find their way on to food. Moreover, the sinks will usually not be free at the time when hands need to be washed. Accordingly, wash-hand basins with hot and cold water laid on, and with good lighting overhead, should be provided in or adjoining the food room and also in immediate proximity to the sanitary conveniences.

Sinks. Sinks and draining boards should have a smooth, hard, even surface, and are best constructed of porcelain-finished fireclay, non-corrosive metal (for example stainless steel), vitreous enamel or plastic, with one-piece tops welded to the sinks. Porcelain sinks are satisfactory if in good repair; but wooden sinks and draining boards harbour germs in the cracks and joints. Aluminium sinks scratch easily, are not robust, and are difficult to keep clean.

Sinks used for washing up should be small enough to ensure frequent replenishing with hot water but large enough to take the largest dishes comfortably. For washing pots and pans galvanized-iron sinks are suitable, as they are robust and withstand heavy cleaning.

It is desirable to have the sink fitted with a spray hose for washing down the sink and draining boards, and with a removable strainer in the waste pipe for trapping crumbs, tea-leaves, etc. A built-in, but removable refuse container is also an advantage.

The number of sinks required will necessarily depend largely on the trade. In general, it may be said that fish should never be washed in the same sink as vegetables, and a separate sink should therefore be reserved for fish. The meat-preparation room also needs a separate sink. All these sinks should have hot and cold water laid on.

Drains. Drains should be adequate to remove all waste water without risk of flooding. Normal-sized drains are 4 in. (10·2 cm.) in diameter. These are large enough to deal with a considerable flow of drainage, and may be suitable for some food establishments; but many establishments will need 6-in. (12·7-cm.) drain pipes. Grease traps are valuable because they prevent grease from congealing in the drain pipes. The grease tray should be removed regularly and washed out.

Many establishments have channelling covered with steel grids round the grease-producing areas. The tops of these grids and the channels themselves are likely to become dirt-traps unless they are very regularly cleaned. They are difficult to clean. Drainage should be adequate to remove all waste water without risk of 'pooling' at gully traps.

Materials. All materials used in the construction of food premises should be such as will, of themselves, assist in the task of maintaining the premises in a proper state of cleanliness. For example:

Outer yards should be paved with—
    (a) Hard-rolled tar macadam.
    (b) Hard-surfaced concrete.
    (c) Concrete-based cement-rendered surfaces.
    (d) Tiles (earthenware) set to tight joints.
    (e) Stone setts with flush joints, set in cement.
    (f) Flagstones with good hard cement.

Interior work floored should be—
    (a) Granolithic.
    (b) Terrazo.
    (c) Quarry tiles.
    (d) Quarry tiles incorporating non-slip elements.
    (e) Specialized plasticized floor tiles.
    (f) Hard cork lino over flush-fitted wood.
    (g) Surfaced-tight jointed hardwoods.
    (h) Oiled and sealed hardwoods.
    (i) Oil-dressed cement floors treated with silicate of alumina when laid.

Interior room floors where no heavy work is carried out and where the public are allowed for service or shopping should be—
    (a) Specialized plasticized floor tiles.
    (b) Hard cork lino over flush-fitted wood.
    (c) Surfaced-tight jointed hardwood.
    (d) Oiled and sealed hardwoods.
    (e) Where the sales action demands rugs or carpeting these should be of a quality that will withstand regular daily vacuum cleaning or surface cleaning.

Walls of food rooms should be—
    (a) Plastered and painted, two or three coats lead-free paint.
    (b) Tiled (ceramics or earthenware).
    (c) Sheeted with plastic laminate.
    (d) Sheeted with metal sheet (not galvanized).
    (e) Tiled with plasticized polyurethane tiles or the like.

Ceilings should be—
    (a) Plastered but not painted. They are designed when plastered to act as a heat-absorbing area, and painting of this plaster leads to increased problems of condensation in rooms where steam rises freely.

Woodwork, where wood has to be used, should be—

(a) Hardwood.
(b) Other woods given added protective surfacing such as two or three coats of lead-free paint.

Brickwork—

All brickwork of food premises (excluding outside walls) should be finished with fair face. That is, without uneven mortar joints.

CODE OF PRACTICE (EXAMPLE)

It is now practicable to set down an example of a code of practice which will equally apply to the construction and conduct of all food premises. In setting down the paragraphs it is inevitable that some of the items specified will also be the subject of food-control law. The agreed construction principles are, however, good sense in any food-handling circumstances.

1. The walls of food rooms made from permanent materials should be smooth and impervious.

2. Walls should be in good repair and be finished in a light colour.

4. Flaking paints and non-washable powder paint colours (distempers) should not be used.

5. Tiles are advantageous, and there should be rounded angles at floor level.

6. Ceilings should be in good repair, of even surface, and either porous or specifically insulated according to the process carried out.

7. Ventilation canopies should be fitted wherever excess steam is generated.

8. Such canopies should be of rust-proof materials.

9. Floors should be even, surfaced, and impervious to moisture.

10. Where frequent washing down is needed the floor should gently slope to a drain.

11. Pipes coming through walls, floors, or ceilings should be fitted in a manner that prevents ingress of insects through gaps.

12. All floors should be cleaned at least once a day.

13. Internal woodwork should be reduced to a minimum and should be of a design that makes cleaning easy. Wood should not (with the possible exception of butchers' blocks and special food-cutting surfaces) be used for food work surfaces.

14. Doors should be fitted so as to prevent insects and rodents gaining access.

15. Windows should be of plain glass, and the window-sills sloped so as to stop them being used as 'unofficial' shelves. Where cooked meat and processed made-up foods are displayed the windows should be refrigerated.

16. All lights should be placed to a planned illustrated pattern to fit the work process. The scale of lighting should never fall below 25 *lumens* per ft.² (formerly termed foot-candles or lamberts) at any work surface.

17. Ventilation must be worked out to suit the process, but some degree of mechanical ventilation is needed in most food rooms. Recall that the danger range starts at 10° C. This is approximately normal British Spring/Summer heat, and thus it is ALWAYS SUMMER IN MOST WORKING FOOD ROOMS ESPECIALLY IF COOKING IS CARRIED OUT THEREIN.

18. Ventilation should aim at minimum of 20 changes of air per hour.

19. The heating systems needs to be planned to fit the process and the ventilation system, and must have relationship to the needed relative humidity.

20. Any outdoor yards or paving used in connexion with the food business should be of an even impervious good-condition surface.

21. Separate tools should be used for cutting raw foods, especially meats and cooked foods.

22. Where wooden work surfaces have to be used they should be cleaned to a special routine, and will best be sterilized by washing with sodium hypochlorite in a correct solution that will be advised by the makers.

23. Degreasing is as important as sterilizing, and correct detergents should be selected and properly used.

24. Premises should be inspected regularly for the presence of rodents and insects, and domestic animals should be banished from food rooms.

25. Adequate storage for food and all utensils should be provided and kept in a good state of repair to prevent accidental contamination or contamination by insects, rodents, etc.

26. Refuse should be moved regularly and completely from food rooms and stored under cover and kept dry as possible until final removal from the premises.

27. Refrigerators should be purpose built and correctly used. Full regard must be to aid the food and the special needs of that food when correctly kept.

28. Meat should be hung or placed in containers or on special cleanable pallets.

29. Products should be kept at their correct temperatures and not indiscriminately taken into and out of that temperature ambient.

30. Refrigerators should be defrosted and cleaned regularly.

31. Food should not be placed on sale display in the direct rays of the sun or where any atmospheric contamination may occur or where persons may contaminate it.

32. Hands should be kept off food as far as possible, and where the trade-needs make handling necessary, then the hands should, indeed must, be clean.

33. Rabbit skinning, dressing poultry, and the like should never be carried out on the same surface as other food preparation, and the hands should be washed between every such operation.

34. Food for animals and pets should be handled absolutely separately from human food.

35. Delicatessen and meat products should be very carefully displayed and screened from contamination at all times.

36. All meat and meat products should be kept at below 10° C. until cooked.

37. Gelatines and gravies should not be kept in a ready-to-serve or use state from one day to the next.

38. All equipment should be purpose designed, and so should all utensils. Only correct utensils and equipment should be used, and they should be of correct materials and shape to make maintenance and cleaning easy.

39. All machine and container doors should be tightly fitting, and panels intended to be removed for cleaning or maintenance access should be gasketed to keep out insects and to prevent other forms of possible contamination of contents.

40. There should be a minimum of inaccessible internal surface that can be reached for cleaning. All the materials used should be non-toxic.

41. All machines or equipment delivery tubes, pipes, and chutes should be subject to a reasoned-out *in situ* chemical sterilization routine.

42. All liquid container machines and equipment should be fitted with anti-overflow devices.

43. Equipment designed to achieve set temperatures should have indicator thermometers to show their working efficiency.

44. Light should be arranged so that all working parts of any machine or equipment can be examined for cleanliness.

45. Precise cleaning instructions should be worked out and known to all operatives for all machines, equipments, and utensils.

THE ACTIONS OF PERSONNEL AND THE SPECIAL CARE OF CERTAIN FOODS
(INCLUDING INFESTATION PREVENTION)

A high standard of personal cleanliness is demanded from all food handling personnel at all times. They must refrain from finger licking, head scratching, nose picking, touching festering cuts, and blowing into paper bags or sucking from the ends of icing bags. They should never touch animals and then touch food without first washing their hands. They must wear designed, clean, washable overclothing and head coverings, and the wearing of good footwear is to be encouraged, as the tired worker is a careless worker.

All new entrants to any food trade should be given food-hygiene training so that they understand why there are rules and why they should want to obey them. Hand washing is of prime importance, and this means a good scrubbing of the finger-nails, which should be short. All personnel must learn to report to their supervisors at once if they are ill in any way. It will be for the supervisor, after medical advice, to decide on the next action. This applies to the housewife as a food handler, although she often cannot leave her home duties. At such times it is vital for her to take extra care.

The housewife should buy only from obviously clean shops and sales places. She should make sure she gets the food home clean and stores it properly when it is there. All food handlers, wherever they are, should cover all cuts and sores with clean waterproof dressings and be careful about coughing and sneezing. Any left-over foods that are to be reheated for consumption must be kept clean, cool, and covered. The washing up of articles of crockery is a vital link in the clean-food chain, and it should be carried out with hot water and detergent with frequent changes of that water. It is preferable if wiping cloths are not used, but where they are indispensable, then the cloths must be absolutely clean.

STORAGE OF FOOD AND CHECKS AS TO CONDITION

No food should ever be stored directly on to a floor. The proper storage of food means the use of properly designed containers at all times. The type of food usually dictates the kind of container, and the containers should always be placed so that they can be inspected and kept clean. The storage should be systematic and such as will allow proper use-rotation of stocks and purchases.

A considerable number of insect pests need to be guarded against in all food rooms, but the position is acute in food-storage rooms. The pests that have to be combated are:

In Dry Food Rooms: Insects and Mites

Warehouse moth, of which the grubs attack a wide variety of food, such as chocolate, raw cocoa beans, cereals, cereal products, dried fruit, spices, and nuts. Mill moth, which attacks flour.

Australian spider beetle, of which the grubs feed on almost any food. Biscuit beetle, of which the grubs attack cereal products, including flour, biscuits, and breakfast cereals.

Food mites may appear as a conspicuous growth or brownish dust around the bags or boxes of food. They require a fairly high humidity. Further information and methods of control may be found in the Ministry of Agriculture Fisheries and Food Advisory Leaflet No 483, *Insect Pests in Food Stores* (H.M.S.O.).

Bacon and ham is liable to be attacked by the larder beetle and the maggot known as 'cheese skipper'. Further information and methods of control may be found in Ministry of Agriculture, Fisheries and Food Advisory Leaflet No 373, *Insects Infesting Bacon and Hams* (H.M.S.O.).

Rats and mice are sources of infection, and their presence in food premises cannot be tolerated under any circumstances. There are many palliative measures which are extremely effective, but the true answer is to remove possible nesting and breeding areas from the premises and the surrounding areas. Cats and dogs should not be used in food premises to keep down rodent infestation; the one is as great a source of possible contamination hazard as the other. If poisons are used they should be kept separate from foodstuffs. Flies are also controllable using residual insecticides, of the DDT type, and by fly-proofing the entrances and windows. The usual flies are the house fly, the blue bottle (which feeds and lays eggs on meat), the vinegar fly, which lays eggs and thrives on unwashed milk bottles and lives on decaying fruit. Also included are cockroaches, which are the creatures of dirty uncleaned corners, and ants, which are not necessarily so. Both are difficult to dislodge, but the roach is killed by DDT and BHC insecticide, while the ants are kept down by scrupulous cleanliness and plenty of powdered residual insecticide. Wasps and other flying insects can only be effectively dealt with by having good screening to windows and ventilation inlets.

Good cleaning routines will always go a long way towards preventing or cleaning up any form of infestation on a food premises.

Storage of Special Food: Milk and Milk Products

Fresh milk, if received on the day it is to be used, should be stored in a cool room or at least in a cool place. Milk which is to be retained on the premises overnight should be put into cold storage, preferably immediately on delivery. Bottles should not be opened until the milk is about to be used. The tops and sides of milk bottles should be wiped with a clean cloth before the caps are removed.

Milk delivered in considerable bulk in bottles calls for adequate storage space, and a storage bay should be specifically set aside for this purpose. This bay should not be used for any other food or container storage. It should be the milk store. If bulk milk has to be used from a delivery churn, then have a plain round-rod, steel, double tripod constructed which will rock forward when empty and allow two internal inclined knobs to engage with churn handles. When rocked back into place the churn is then lifted free and swings forward to allow supplies to be run off into catering receptacles, thus doing away with the dipper.

Milk powder should not be reconstituted nor condensed milk diluted until required for use, and then only in the required quantities. If any has to be stored overnight it should be placed in the cold store in a covered container.

Butter (and other fats, including margarine) should normally be stored in the refrigerator, but small quantities held in the larder for use during the day should be stood (wrapped in greaseproof paper) on a marble or stone slab. Cheese keeps best in ventilated storage—for example, a cabinet with perforated metal sides—and should not be stored in the refrigerator. Whole or half cheese, particularly when new, and blueveined, curd, or cream cheese, should be turned over daily, and excessive moisture should be scraped or wiped off. Cheese should not be removed from its binding or wrapping, nor should it be cut until it is required for use. Cheeses which have been creamed for spreading must be used the same day.

Milk, butter, and cheese should be kept away from fruit, fish, oils, pickles, and other strong-smelling commodities which may taint them.

Frozen Foods and Similar Commodities

The actual needs of the business in relation to temperature-controlled storage require to be properly studied and provision made for deep-freeze storage, that is at ranges down to $-10°$ C., cold storage at $-5°$ to $0°$ C., chill storage at $2°$–$3°$ C., and cool storage below $10°$ C. It is not possible to have one piece of equipment to cover all these ranges.

The use of deep-freeze food will probably necessitate the use of thawing areas and/or thaw/cook ovens which cook by micro-wave electricity.

Meat and Meat Products

Meat should always be kept in stores capable of being temperature controlled. Sawdust on the floor of a meat store is unhygienic and outmoded; it becomes mixed with the dirt, and blown or kicked or moved to finally settle on the meat. Trays, washed regularly, and at least once daily, should be used to catch blood drips.

Manufactured meat products can be a source of danger, and should be stored with the utmost care. Raw meats, e.g. sausages, joints, and minced meat, should be kept in the refrigerator, the minced meat being spread out; cooked meats, e.g. brawn, pressed meats, tongue, meat sandwiches, and meat pies, should be stored at temperatures below $10°$ C. Only the quantities required for immediate use should be moved to the food-preparation room, and these should be served promptly.

Bacon in the piece is a comparatively poor breeding-ground for harmful germs, provided it is kept dry; it should therefore be hung in a cold, dry, unrefrigerated place, protected from dirt and insects by a fine-meshed net covering. Sliced bacon should be wrapped in transparent film and kept below $10°$ C. It is best stored, for short periods of up to 2 days, in the part of the refrigerator which gives a temperature of from $0°$ to $2°$ C. Ham should be treated in the same way as meat, but it is possible to store whole cured hams as described above for bacon in the piece.

Fish, Fruit and Canned Goods

Fresh fish and thawed frozen fish deteriorate rapidly, and should not be held for more than a day or two. They should always be stored in the refrigerator away from other foodstuffs which might be tainted by them—if not in a separate compartment, then in lidded trays used only for fish. Lightly smoked fish such as kippers, finnan haddocks, etc., can be left a little longer, but nevertheless should likewise be stored in a refrigerator separately or in lidded trays. Frozen fish should be stored at the lowest temperature below $0°$ C. available in the refrigerator, but only for a few days at such temperatures as are likely in many cases to be available. For longer periods (weeks) the storage temperature must be not higher than $-20°$ C. Heavily smoked and/or cured fish, such as 'red' herrings, salt cod, and salt pickled herrings, need only chill storage, say $-2°$ to $+2°$ C. for quite long periods.

Fresh fruit should be stored apart from other foodstuffs. Citrus fruit and apples are particularly liable to taint other food. Fruit requires dry, cool, and well-ventilated storage, with air circulating all round above and below. Fruit should be inspected frequently, as mould spreads rapidly on it; any mouldy fruit should be removed to the rubbish bins or swill tubs at once. High stacking of vegetable and fruit should be avoided, as this crushes the lower units and renders them liable to mould growth and rapid deterioration.

Canned goods should be stored in a cool, clean, dry place, preferably in their original cartons. The stock should be frequently inspected, and blown, rusty, and split cans should be referred to the local public health food inspection department, without whose sanction the contents should never in any circumstances be used for human food. Some vacuum-packed foodstuffs (for example, coffee) often present a blown appearance, although the contents are safe for consumption. The containers of all canned goods which include syrup, water, or oil should be periodically turned upside down on the shelves. Once the can is opened, the contents should be treated similarly to fresh food of the same kind.

Flour and Other Cereals

These should preferably be stored in metal containers protected from rats, mice, insects, damp, and casual damage. Such bins should have rounded corners, and should be small and light enough for frequent and thorough cleaning, including upending for drying. The lids should be tight fitting, preferably hinged, and self-closing. The best material for such bins is vitreous enamelware, but this is expensive; the best substitute is galvanized iron, which requires very careful cleaning. There should be sufficient surplus containers for each type of food so that they can be emptied in rotation, and thoroughly cleaned out and dried each time they are emptied. A scoop should be kept in each container, as these foodstuffs will readily deteriorate if dipped into with damp scoops, or worse still, with damp hands.

Jellies, trifles, custards, and similar sweets should be made up on the day they are to be served, and kept in a cool place until stored in the refrigerator.

Dried egg should be stored in its original container, and the contents of any damaged containers should be regarded with suspicion. Reconstitution should be confined to the quantity required for immediate use. If any has to be retained, even for an hour or so, it should be carefully covered and put in the refrigerator, for stored reconstituted dried egg used in lightly cooked egg dishes has been responsible for many outbreaks of food poisoning.

Egg Liquid in Bulk

All utensils used for mixing egg constituents should be thoroughly cleaned and sterilized before being used for any other cooking and catering purpose, and storage of these products should be at temperatures below 12° C. Dried foods (freeze dried included) must be stored in a dry atmosphere.

Refrigerators

The object of refrigeration is to keep foods in good condition, and this is achieved by allowing a good circulation of cold air currents around all the food in the refrigerator. It should, therefore, never be packed full, and needs to be regularly defrosted and cleaned. All perishable foods keep better at low temperature, but there are many foods and many food packagings that make refrigeration unnecessary. These include accelerated freeze-dried foods, vacuum-packed foods, and sealed canned and bottled goods. Foods which should go into the refrigerator include meat, poultry, game, fish, shellfish, prepared meat dishes, gravy, soups (not canned), custards, ice-creams, and synthetic food fillings. The door of the refrigerator should not be opened more often than is absolutely necessary.

All food on display where it may be contaminated by careless persons needs to be effectively screened.

All food wrappings need to be clean and themselves stored in clean places until needed for use.

LEGISLATION AND CONTROLS

All food-hygiene workers must be prepared to deal with the willing and the over co-operative as well as the reluctant and non-co-operative. There will always be a minority in opposition, and this minority itself is capable of division into those who do not believe in the ideas put forward and the rather more difficult group of those who do believe in the ideas but refuse to practise them because they have been put forward by people they do not accept. This underlines the need for fair and proper law designed to make everyone follow the trend to higher standards which have become accepted by the majority. The raising of food-handling standards is a continual process dependent for its its speed of success—or indeed for its lack of forward momentum—only on the readiness with which the food handlers can accept the sense and reasonableness of the demands that have been made of them.

The responsibility for a safe food supply has been devolved by Parliament upon elected local authority councils since the nineteenth century. These councils have had, for some long period, the statutory obligation to employ health officers. Today there is no person or place in the United Kingdom which is outside the immediate executive district of the councils, and their health officers are fully scientifically and technically trained, and in addition to their own training and experience have the widest possible facilities for consultation and exchange of information and advice. Basically it is the duty of the Ministry of Health to channel this information, advice, and consultation to the right quarter, but local officers enjoy complete freedom to consult and advise as they wish.

The law provided to back the rightful and proper public-health demands of the enforcing authority or its employed officers must have a format that allows for progress and invention. It must never be a form that makes for difficulty in the development and ready introduction of new handling and trading techniques.

Take the cleanliness of food utensils as an example. In this case the law needs only to ask for a final finished clean article ready for use; there is no need to outline the cleaning process. Indeed, to do so would limit the legal draftsmen to known processes and necessitate exemption provisions for areas and circumstances which already call for deviations in those known processes. Add to this the sure knowledge that every day brings new chemicals and new applications of techniques of chemistry or physics and it will be seen that 'directive' law would always be in a state of 'amendment' while 'permissive' law would encourage progress. In short, the law sets the target, the path can be chosen within proper limits by the person to whom the law applies.

The format considered necessary is:

1. A national empowering act which gives—

(a) power to enter and inspect;
(b) power to regulate sanitary conditions and to allocate responsibility between employer and employee;
(c) sanitary authorities power to prosecute offenders;
(d) power to take samples of foodstuffs (chemical, physical and bacteriological);
(e) power to properly constituted authority to be given knowledge of processes and ingredients;
(f) power to prepare food standards (and ready power to amend these);
(g) rights of appeal by traders to independent authorities (such as magistrates and other courts); and
(h) allows for universal application throughout the nation and sets a scale of penalties for contravention.

This is the general form and content of the United Kingdom Food and Drugs Act, 1955, which follows a long history of such legislation since the early nineteenth century. The basis of enforcement is that the prosecution 'proves' the offence and that it shall always be a defence to prove that 'all due diligence' was used provided that physical and constructional demands were observed. The 'reasonableness' of prosecution must be that the hard offender gets his punishment while the 'accidental' offender is not left with a sense of grievance against the principles of hygiene. It is bad for the offender to dislike the law, but it is very bad for the offender to be left with a strong dislike of the ideas behind the law. There are bound to be trades or food commodities which cannot be subjected to one set of hard-and-fast national rules. Indeed, present-day laboratory techniques could not produce such rules which would ensure complete freedom from food-borne diseases. This being the fact, then there is need for:

2. A set of Food Hygiene Regulations which:

(a) set a general pattern in somewhat greater detail than the National Act;

(b) set a like pattern for particularized trades or food-handling activities, i.e. transport, warehousing, display;

(c) clearly define the duty of employers to provide structural cleanliness facilities;

(d) clearly indicate the duty of employees to produce results which follow correct use of provisions made or their use;

(e) specify some standard of lay-out and fitment; and

(f) specify overall constructional minima.

In the enforcement of the demands of such regulations there must be a formula whereby the enforcing officer can make reasonable allowance for extenuating circumstances. The officer will be fully and properly trained, and his training will fit him to evaluate circumstances and their effects. If such officers are used only to enforce inflexible rules, then not only is their training invalidated but the success of any long-term education policy is jeopardized. There must, therefore, be tolerance by regular report to the sanitary authority and their approval of all enforcement action. Such regular local sanitary authority consideration of enforcement action will indicate the need for yet a third stage of law. That is:

3. The local by-law which will take account of:

(a) special local health conditions;

(b) special local trade needs; and

(c) special local enforcement possibilities or the lack of such possibilities.

Thus the law pattern can be summarized as that which sets the laboratory technique fairly face to face with proper trade techniques and allows a national pattern to be clothed in detail by regulations, and tailored to suit each particular locality by by-laws and with a sufficiency of officers appointed to properly enforce the provisions.

It is obvious that food traders must recognize that any piece of food-control legislation must confer rights, including rights of appeal, as well as laying obligations on them. Basically all food law is designed for the general protection of the customer from fraud or health hazard. It is not designed to make food fads, fallacies and fancies, or unnecessary fears into rules that must be inflexibly followed. Thus the law must properly influence the selling of food, and good merchandising methods must properly influence the law form.

This axiom is plainly stated in Section 2 of the Food and Drugs Act, 1955, by the words:

'If a person sells to the prejudice of the purchaser any food . . . which is not of the nature, or not of the substance, or not of the quality . . . demanded by the purchaser he shall, subject to the provisions of the next following section, be guilty of an offence.'

Section 3 makes it plain that the honest and straightforward trader is given as wide a protection as that given the customer. The trader is offered immediately available forms of defence against prosecution if he can prove that none of his actions were fraudulent by intent or that what has happened to the food is an unavoidable consequence of collection or preparation.

It is in respect of the avoidable consequences of collection or preparation that the pattern of merchandising is most influenced by the words of the law. In the United Kingdom a period has now been reached in which most foodstuffs are nationally distributed and most problems arise from queries by national marketing operators. The traders ask for guidance and advice which will help them completely to obey the law, and range from queries on the detail of food processes and food ingredients to questions on equipment, packaging and handling methods, lay-out of sales premises, and acceptable sales techniques.

The trader when inquiring is, of course, anxious to remove his and his company's actions from the jeopardy of the law. He seeks not to escape, but to obey, the law so that he can trade free of harassment and give his attention to holding and attracting customers. There is not much small business left in the food-distribution field in the United Kingdom today. This does not mean that there are no traders with small premises, small stocks, and small turnovers. Indeed, it is the fact that there are more shopkeepers and more workers in the food industries than has ever before been the case. Most of these small shops, however, are distribution centres for national and brand merchandise. They are therefore truly independent in choice of stocks, but almost wholly dependent on national distributors for quality of stocks.

The growth of companies engaged in national food distribution has meant that vast amounts of money are involved in the background of every retail sale. Here is an example. It is generally agreed in the broiler-chicken industry that the capital cost of premises from incubator to packing station stands at not less than £1·50p per head of stock handled. This means that producing 100,000 head of broiler chickens (this being about the average per plant) on the 3 months' handling cycle calls for a capital outlay of at least £150,000. Outlay of this magnitude can be made profitable only by a constant production flow involving four or five changes of poultry stocks, or at least half a million chickens, per year. This depends on someone selling half a million chickens a year, and such constant sales depend in large measure on each customer getting a product which is consistent. It is, in passing, debatable whether the customer is getting the chicken of her true choice and desire in this operation, but it is unquestionable that she is getting a consistently good product. Similar heavy capital involvement now occurs in every food industry. One national brand ice-cream company has more than £5 million invested in one factory and distribution centre.

In operations on this huge scale fraud or attempts at fraud become more of a hazard (economically) to the producer than they are likely to be to the consumer. Conversely, any food-hygiene failure at the production end increases the hazard of illness and the geographical distribution of the cases concerned. The concentration of effort, therefore, must be on avoiding careless food handling during collection, preparation, and distribution.

POINTS AND DISCUSSION

Many occasions arise, and will continue to arise, when it seems that the theory and practice of food hygiene are in direct contradiction. It is in such situations that the thoughtful food-hygiene worker is at his best. This comes from the fact that there is always a rational and sensible view-point that will emerge from an unbiased examination of the actual circumstances obtaining at the time under consideration. Here are some examples:

It is obviously right for foodstuffs to be covered against possible air-borne contamination. But foods often need to be displayed in a state where they are absolutely ready for immediate consumption but cannot, with sense, be so covered—on a side table in a cold-buffet restaurant, for example. Attempts at providing temporary removable covers of plastic foil and the like are rather pointless, for these covers, themselves, have to be handled excessively and put down while the food is served and then replaced. This is an example of the embroidery of food hygiene. All that is needed here is for the side-table food to come from a clean kitchen, be cleanly handled when set out, and then to be kept at as low a temperature as possible until service. Caterers have long known this, and they frequently decorate their cold-buffet tables with 'ice' statues. These not only enhance the display they also keep the temperature down, and are infinitely preferable to pieces of transparent pliofilm draped untidily over the foods.

A similar display in the open air, however, or on a mobile sales van or in a busy sales shop would need some form of durable transparent cover that would allow space only for the hands of the server and no other 'open' area. Having mentioned the hands of the server, it is relevant to go on to say that there are some foods that have to be manually handled. No machine will bone a chicken, for instance, and if there were such a machine it would probably be almost impossible to clean. Much better, therefore, to accept that there are times when the human hand has to touch the food and then to ensure that that hand is a clean hand. There is little virtue in the 'genteel' handling of foods when that situation arises. The crooked little finger and the forefinger and thumb-hold add nothing to food care. It is preferable to see the food handler acting as a food craftsman and really handling the food with confidence born of trade ability and utter personal cleanliness.

Smoking comes into the same category. It is illegal for food handlers to smoke in food rooms, and there are those who would extend this to the consumer. In the context of food hygiene it is understood that whenever the word 'smoking' is used this really refers to all use of tobacco, including so-called herbal smoking mixtures, snuff, and chewing tobacco. Various explanations are put forward for the ban. Experts have waxed lyrical over the dangers of falling tobacco ash, over the saliva, over the placing of half-used cigarettes where they may get into food, etc. The real fact is that smoking is a habit that can be quite untidy in respect of its used portions, and untidiness has no place in a properly run food room. At the same time the service areas of restaurants or cafeterias or a licensed public-house are technically food rooms, and to many people the 'smoke' after the meal or the drink is part of the pleasure of the visit. Their indulgence cannot therefore be lightly banned. It may be possible to do so on general health grounds (as in the campaign against lung cancer) or on fire-risk arguments, or it may only be possible to try to provide sufficiently large ashtrays to ensure that they do not dirty the sugar or complicate the washing-up problem by having too many cigarette ends in the saucers.

The presence of pet dogs in food rooms and food shops is another endless point of discussion. Truthfully the dog has no place in such areas. But if a straightforward legal ban were to be imposed, then there would be two immediate complications. First, there would be the creation of difficulty in relation to blind persons using guide dogs. Strictly speaking, trained dogs are not one whit less likely to be voiders of salmonella than any other canines. So the law would have to exclude such dogs. This exclusion could only be based on the fact that they are 'trained' animals. The way is thus open to exempt all trained animals, and this would result in a situation of farce when it came to local-officer enforcement. Far to be preferred is the requirement that the food trader shall not ever put food in any place where it is likely to be exposed to the *risk* of contamination. Mark that phrase. It is extremely wide in its application— the *risk* of contamination—and it is a cornerstone of the Food Hygiene General Regulations, 1955 *et seq*. The second complication comes to the trader who may have stray dogs entering his premises against his wishes and desires. If the law made an outright ban, then such a trader, who may well have placed all his food wares where they could not possibly be contaminated, would be in jeopardy. He would face a technical prosecution for matters that would in absolute fairness be quite outside his control. Such proceedings do not encourage good food traders, they only make disgruntled food handlers. Far better, therefore, to have the food properly placed for sale and a notice asking customers not to bring dogs into food rooms with them.

Food law thus becomes a network of advice notes for both trader and administrator. Perhaps the most viable example is the United Kingdom Milk Industry.

There are official Acts, Orders, and Regulations which describe or prescribe almost every action of the dairyman. They cover him from the time when the health of the cow is tested by veterinary officers of the Animal Health Service to the washing of the udders prior to milking; from the design and siting of equipment down to the method of placing the foil cap on the bottle, and the time and area of delivery of the milk to the householder. These laws are in considerable detail, and yet proof that the multi-million-pound milk industry has not found them irksome or a bar to trade is shown by the fact that nearly twenty-five years ago the Milk Marketing Board formed, jointly with representatives of producers and distributors, a Milk Quality Control Committee. This Committee administers a voluntary scheme to test all milk sold to the Board by wholesale contract. Assessment of the marketability of the milk is based on the 10-minute resazurin test (*q.v.*).

The abolition of the designation 'TT' and the high standard of product-dependability reached by the milk industry are factors that have led the Ministry of Agriculture, Fisheries and Food to propose amendments and withdrawals of some controls from the Milk (Special Designations) Regulations. The Milk Marketing Board and its producers and distributors now operate a scheme for the control of hygienic milk quality which, as a trade action, replace any controls withdrawn by the Ministry.

In the beginning the need was to remove pathogenic organisms from the milk. The right and easily applied answer to this, pending improvements in herds and herd conditions, was the pasteurization of the bulk milk. Pasteurization succeeded in reducing very greatly the health hazard, and also gave the dairyman much needed distribution time. Keeping quality was improved, and from this came the easy answer to the trade problem of moving milk from low-population production areas to densely populated consumption areas.

There is not any milk-processing dairy anywhere in the United Kingdom which does not record the processes to which milk is subjected, and test and assess the final quality of the product. It is plainly true that while the industry has helped to formulate the law, the law has very greatly moulded the industry.

The ice-cream industry also plainly demonstrates the effect of food law on the structure of a food trade. The Ice Cream (Heat Treatment, etc.) Regulations control all the processes and, with section 16 of the Food and Drugs Act, places control to a great degree on marketing methods. There is no doubt that, while prepacking of ice-cream was readily adopted by distributors as a useful handling method capable of close economic control, this method had its initial impetus from the demand of the regulations that ice-cream must be 'protected from contamination at all times'.

The present design of soft-serve ice-cream dispensers can also be directly attributed to the influence of food law. There has been a spectacular increase in this form of trading, but it is not a new idea. Soft-serve ice-cream machines were available to manufacturers in 1947. They had basic constructional faults which made cleaning difficult and effective sterilization of the freezer barrel almost impossible. The impact of the Heat Treatment Regulations and the introduction of the methylene-blue test, with the consequent grading of ice-cream, were such that machines of this type ceased to be made and did not reappear until 1960/61 in a completely new engineering form. The new form, while not solving all cleaning and sterilization problems, at least lends itself to the operator following cleaning and sterilization routines which will safeguard the product and the purchaser.

NEED FOR INTERNAL TRADE CONTROLS

Many other examples of the direct influence of law on the food distributive trades will come to mind whenever one considers the various regulations governing additives, colours, preservatives, and other aspects of food trading. There still remains the possibility of hazard introduced by personal behaviour of the food handler or the incorrect maintenance of premises and equipment. It is to cover these matters that the Food Hygiene (General) Regulations and other specialized food-hygiene regulations and by-laws were made (see list).

One of the urgent needs of the food manufacturers and distributors has, therefore, become some form of self-criticism and effective internal control. From the need to meet this problem has come the establishment and development of food-industry quality-control sections. Once the principle of self-imposed quality control had been established in the major food industries, its development has been spectacular.

It is worth noting that the food industry has of its own accord divided quality control work into the setting of standards and the attainment of those standards. The industry has recruited considerable personnel from local health departments to staff the sections of quality-control departments whose duty it is to see that the standards decided upon are attained and maintained.

From small beginnings intended to check the type and suitability of raw materials purchased for processing and distribution, the quality control sections have usefully spread their work. Many are today engaged on work as diverse as advice on crop husbandry and the amount of lean meat produced per pound of food consumed by selectively bred pigs and cattle.

There are undeniably purely industrial needs for quality control, but the need to remove trading from the jeopardy of the food law is a major factor both in the establishment of these sections and their undeniable success. If there is a fault inherent in quality control, then it is that such controls incline towards standardization of the controlled products. There is quite widespread and often necessary adverse customer reaction to this degree of standardization with some products. One would expect milk to be the same consistency every day of the year, but one would not really welcome such unvarying consistency in the 'taste' products, such as fish, meat, and vegetables.

STANDARDIZATION EFFECTS

The effects of making all foods bland or totally bacteriologically safe by sterility are seen in the obvious adverse consumer reactions in relation to that, for instance, called disparagingly 'modern bread'. Obviously this is a better and safer product. The standardization of additives and ingredients to assure value for money spent is a different issue to the question of ensuring safety from health hazard by standardization of the product.

The sale of sausages under national distribution brand-marks is a good example. In 1963/64 it was said that the sale of sausages of all types now approached 400,000 tons or *nine thousand million sausages per year*.

This huge sale entirely depends on the quality of the goods at the time of retail sale, and the distributors concerned have been forced to devise special wrapping and delivery methods that will ensure that the goods arrive in good condition. The size of this undertaking can be properly understood only when it is realized that one national distributor is recorded as having more than 55,000 sales outlets. All metropolitan and large town shops have a daily delivery, and even shops in the smallest village get a delivery every third trading day. This means special packs, special delivery vehicles, and special contracts with British Railways. From the point when this delivery is effected, the keeping quality depends on the speed of retail sale and the care given to the product by the retailer. This is simply another way of saying that the trade utterly depends on the exercise of good food-hygiene practice at all times. Similarly, there are very few food traders now doing small-scale production of articles such as butter, margarine, and other groceries and provisions. The present-day supermarkets and stores, some of which offer 400 types of goods, rarely produce more than one or two of the foodstuffs they put on sale. Apart from some who boil hams, there are few retail grocers and provision merchants who do otherwise than hand over to the customer goods packed by other persons at some centralized production plant.

Thus all food law needs to be drafted in common application form and to be individually re-assessed in the light of actual circumstances obtaining at the time of inspection. This makes it imperative that no textbook should attempt to be dogmatic on the *application* of the law, but that the reader should be guided as to the intention of the relevant sections of the general law, while specific sets of regulations be read in the full official text at all times. For that reason only the relevant sections of the Food and Drugs Act and the paragraph headings of three sets of food-hygiene by-laws are now discussed.

RELEVANT SECTIONS OF LAWS: FOOD AND DRUGS ACT, 1955

Section 1. Offences in the preparation and sale of injurious (to the consumer) foods.

Section 2. A general protection for the purchaser of foods.

Section 4. Power for the government to make regulations about the composition of foods.

Section 8. Punishments for the sale of unfit food.

Section 9. Power to examine and seize suspected food.

Section 11. Power of authorized officer to examine food in transit.

Section 13. Power of the Government to make regulations for securing the observance of sanitary and cleanly practices and conditions in food handling.

Section 14. Power of the magistrates' courts to disqualify caterers not obeying the law on food hygiene.

Section 15. Power of local authorities to make by-laws as to the handling and sale of food.

Section 16. The registration of certain food-manufacturing and sales premises (ice-cream, sausages, potted, pressed, pickled, and preserved foods).

Section 17. Power of Government to make Section 16 more widely applicable. (*Note:* This has never been used, to date, as since the Act was promulgated, the Food Hygiene Regulations have been made and are held to offer more effective control and sanction than registration procedures.)

Sections 18–19. The methods of application for and the refusal or revocation of registrations of food premises under Section 16.

Section 21. Power to make regulations to license vehicles similar in effect to extending Section 16 to the registration of food vehicles, etc. (Not used to date. See note on Section 17 above.)

Section 22. Special provisions governing the sale of ice-cream from stalls, etc.

Section 23. Prevention of spread of disease by the sale of suspect ice-cream.

Section 25. Provision of shellfish cleansing tanks.

Sections 28–48. Controls over milk, dairies, and cream substitutes.

Section 61. By-laws for the control of food markets.

Section 62–79. Powers to license and control slaughterhouses and abattoirs.

Section 82. Calls for the Government to set up a Food Hygiene Advisory Council. Such a Council has operated extremely successfully in England and Wales since 1956. In Scotland and Northern Ireland such Councils were formed some years later, but are similarly successful at this time.

Section 86. The definition of 'authorized' officers, including any medical officer and any public health inspectors in local-government employ.

Sections 89–99. Provisions for the sampling and analysis of foods (chemical and bacteriological analyses).

Sections 100–105. Powers of authorized officers to enter food premises, etc. and enforce the Act and Laws made under the Act.

Schedule 7. Describes sampling procedures.

The Food Hygiene (General) Regulations, 1970

Regulation 2 gives definitions. In consequence, for example,

(*a*) A catering business means a business wholly or *partly* engaged in the supply of food for human consumption.

(*b*) A food handler includes any person carrying out or assisting in the carrying out of any operation in the preparation, transport, storage, packaging, wrapping, exposure for sale, service, or delivery of food and includes the cleaning of articles or equipment with which food comes into contact.

Regulation 6. Prohibits food trading from insanitary premises.

Regulation 7. Demands the cleanliness of all equipment and utensils.

Regulation 8. Prohibits or restricts domestic food handling for later sale.

Regulation 9. Sets out the demands that ensure that food shall be protected from contamination at all times. Specifically banning smoking and the use of tobacco in food rooms.

Regulation 10. Demands personal cleanliness from food handlers, including their persons and their clothing.

Regulation 11. Demands that persons handling open food wear clean and washable overclothing while so engaged.

Regulation 12. Describes acceptable methods of food carriage and wrapping.

Regulation 13. Demands notification of illness by food handlers.

Regulation 14. Prescribes certain aspects of soil drainage systems.

Regulation 15. Describes acceptable water cisterns.

Regulation 16. Demands correct maintenance of sanitary accommodation.

Regulation 17. Demands effective potable water supplies.

Regulation 18. Demands the provision of wash handbasins.

Regulation 19. Demands provision of first aid materials.

Regulation 20. Demands accommodation for clothing not used in food handling.

Regulation 21. Demands facilities for washing food and equipment.

Regulation 22 and 23. Deal with effective lighting and ventilation.

Regulation 24. Food rooms not to be used as sleeping rooms.

Regulation 25. Cleanliness and repair of food rooms.

Regulation 26. Prohibits the accumulation of refuse.

Regulation 27. Outlines the storage and sales-display temperature of meat, fish, gravy, imitation cream, egg or milk foods in catering premises, but lists acceptable exemptions such as 'canned foods', 'pastry', etc. The limits are below 10° C. or above 66° C. Accepts time limits on display for sale.

The Food Hygiene (Docks, Carriers etc.) Regulations, 1960

Apply most of the above provisions in the specialized handling environments of docks and warehouses and carriers' premises.

The Food Hygiene (Markets, Stalls and Delivery Vehicles) Regulations, 1966, and The Food Hygiene (Markets, Stalls and Delivery Vehicles) (Amendment) Regulations, 1966

These are summarized as an example of special-circumstances regulations. All relevant regulations should be read in full, but as a guide, it is sufficient at this time to say that the Markets, etc., Regulations apply to delivery and open-air sale of food all the basic demands of the General Food Hygiene Regulations. The major interest must centre around the first schedule to those regulations, where certain methods of food packaging are stated as acceptable in deciding whether a food is 'open' or 'packed' in relation to the *provision of hand-cleaning* fitments on vehicles and stalls. These are given as:

FOOD	PACK
Butter, margarine and fat .	Any total enclosure of greaseproof paper or foil
Meat (not cooked) .	Any total wrap of cloth, hessian, and jute or of paper or film
Fish	Any total enclosure of greaseproof paper or film
Vegetables . . .	Any box, bag, sack, string container, or pliable film pack
Flour goods . .	Any total enclosure
Ice-cream . . .	Any total enclosure of paper foil cardboard, carton, or cup

While many of the regulations repeat those of the General Regulations sections to be especially noted are:

Regulation 4. Prohibits the use of insanitary stalls or vehicles.
Regulation 5. The construction of stalls and vehicles to be in good repair. Land on which markets are held to be clean and the store sheds and garages, whether or not holding food, to be clean.
Regulation 7. The removal of unfit food from fit food and all food to be protected from contamination.
Regulation 10. Describes acceptable transport methods.
Regulation 13. Demands identification of the trader and his vehicle or stall.
Regulation 14. Maintenance of sanitary accommodation at market-places.
Regulation 16. Wash-hand basins to be provided.
Regulation 17. First-aid material to be provided.
Regulation 18. Facilities for washing and sorting food and equipment to be provided.
Regulation 21. Describes acceptable methods of covering food stalls.
Regulation 23. Describes acceptable methods of transporting meat.

By-laws for the Handling and Sale of Food in the Open Air

These cover the same ground as the regulations already discussed, but being locally made by the responsible health authority, they usually add words to suit local necessities. In no case do they override the national regulations, but they are useful adjuncts thereto, as, for example, the description of contamination.

In regulations the word contamination is not closely defined, as it must meet all known, and some as yet unknown, eventualities.

In by-laws the words are:

Protect the food from dust, dirt, mud, filth, dirty water, animals, rodents, flies, insects, and other sources of contamination, including contamination by other persons.

The term 'other persons' in this context means someone not within the legal definition 'food handler', and can include customers in shops and eating places.

FOOD HYGIENE EDUCATION AND INSPECTION TECHNIQUES

The food hygienist cannot escape the task of critically assessing all practices and needs in his trade or work location and thus deciding the work priorities. For instance, propaganda efforts to persuade people to wash are valueless until the facilities to wash exist conveniently.

No organization for raising food-handling standards can be set up until such assessments are undertaken and local priorities known. A true knowledge of the people concerned is also a vital necessity.

AGENCIES CONCERNED

THE AGENCIES CONCERNED IN THE UNITED KINGDOM ARE:

The Department of Health and Social Security (DHSS), the Ministry of Agriculture, Fisheries and Food (on all general policy issues, specialized food technology information, and mass educational aids).

The Public Health Laboratory Service (on all bacteriological issues).

The Public Analyst and the Government Chemist (on all chemical issues).

The Health Education Council (on all adult education aids and mass teaching media).

The various Public Health Organizations (such as the Royal Society for the Promotion of Health).

The National organizations representing food traders.

THE OVERALL EXAMINATION OF PROBLEMS IS VESTED IN:

The Department of Health and Social Security (and allied Ministries) for—

Notifications.

Distribution of cases.

Methods of obtaining statistical information that can be of value.

Public relations possibilities including press, radio, and television.

The efficiency of existing law and the need for new powers.

The efficiency of the work of local councils and their officers.

National problems concerned with the supply of materials.

The design of easy-clean machinery.

Inspectorial techniques and technological advances.

The production of teaching aids and literature.

Two committees have been set up to deal with the medical aspects of food:

1. Committee on the medical aspects of chemicals in food and the environment.
2. Committee on the medical aspects of food policy.

The Public Health Laboratory Service examines—

Notifications of food infections.

Relevant bacteriological data.

Type of bacteria.

Distribution of bacteria in foods.

Possibilities of bacterial standards. (To date none are used as legal standards in the United Kingdom although there are agreed informal standards on which the laboratory service directors base advice.)

Investigation of cleaning power of bactericides and sterilants and their application to food-handling machinery and techniques.

The Public Analyst examines—

The chemical properties of foods *vis-à-vis* bacteriological dangers.

The possibilities of standards (a great number of exact chemical composition standards are now legally enforced in the United Kingdom).

The cross contamination of foods and packaging (leaching).

The optimum storage methods and conditions.

The temperature controls of foods and food-preserving methods in general.

The Health Education Council is concerned with—

The market for propaganda material.

The form of propaganda material.

The production of such material.

The distribution of such material, including all teaching aids, film strips, books, pamphlets, explanations of law, etc.

The organization of 'in-service' training for food workers.

The Professional Public Health Organizations examine—

The training of inspectorial personnel.

The collection and dissemination of information among workers.

The interchange of technological information.

The need and possibility of food-handler training and the provision of courses.

The production of teaching aids and propaganda material.

Representations to Ministries on the need for changes in laws.

The protection of the professional standing of the Health Officer and liaison with trade organizations.

The National Organizations of Food Traders examine—

The economic costs of any changes. Methods of holding costs within trade finance.

The standing of the food trader *vis-à-vis* the law and the protection of his right to appeal against harsh decision or incorrect application of legal powers.

The increasing of liaison between traders and enforcement authority.

The production of teaching aids and the use of craft lessons to assist food handling.

The production of principles of good business and statements of trade ethics.

The availability of materials and personnel to achieve food hygiene and the representation to Parliament of special trade needs or earned concessions.

It is worth noting at this point that in the United Kingdom the original teaching and propaganda film was Government produced in 1948/49. Since that date all the subsequent films have been produced without Government money by groups of traders and local government officers or food trade supply firms.

The Local Public Health Authority examines:

Number of food premises.

Type of food premises.

State of repair.

Presence or absence of facilities for cleanliness (including lighting, heating, water, drainage).

Inspectorial personnel requirements.

Storage of records and 'running' surveys, where information is regularly added.

Prospects of teaching aids being used.

Incidence of needs for prosecutions.

Provision of good standards in public buildings as an example, etc.

CONSULTATION

The matching of ideas and the interchange of knowledge must be free and frequent if food hygiene is to be a reality. It must be remembered that the health officer can study a trade only within the limits of the degree of co-operation extended to him by the trader. This may be supplemented by official sources of trade information. The consultations may range from single man-to-man talks to large-scale ministerially inspired conferences. At root these are all quite similar. They must all aim at showing the one man to the other as a sensible and reasonable being.

From such consultation in the United Kingdom come such ideas as:

The preparation of codes of practice agreed and supported by government, local government, and trade. (These deal with fine points of detail of structure and food-handling technique that cannot be covered in any general law.)

The distribution of teaching aids to points and areas where they will produce the best results.

The production of laws that are universally respected when promulgated, and thus likely to be obeyed.

The reduction of the element of unwillingness to accept ideals and standards.

Changing the feeding habits of people, from what is scientifically or aesthetically wrong, is a hard chore. An attitude of mind has to be changed. Everything must be 'explained'.

Explanation is by:

Individual talks.

Meetings with specific groups.

Community meetings.

Pamphlets, booklets, handouts.

Posters.

Pictures of people, akin to the viewer, in 'correct' situations.

Press articles (including magazines).

Prosecution of offenders.

Publicity of statistics about wasteful costs of food infections.

Radio and television programmes (both specialized and those in which the reference is deliberately 'accidental').

Exhibitions.

Merit awards.

Dissemination of information to engineers and supply houses.

Dissemination of information on new trading techniques (including storage, preparation, and sales).

Regular assessments of all actions and progress under the above and a publication of findings.

It should always be remembered that the average food handler will never become a lawyer or a bacteriologist or even a public health specialist. People accept best an understanding statement made in their own work or trade terms and most readily take to a good-humoured explanation, even one that makes them laugh. The correct timing of explanations is the real key to success. Never talk to people or at people—always talk with people. Make them equal in the task, and they will play their part.

There is no more glib phrase than the phrase 'we will educate them', no phrase is easier to say and harder to make into reality.

The tasks in food-hygiene education are:

Educating customers to expect and demand the right standards. This cannot be done without producing those standards in the home in everyday life.

The education of authority and employer into making correct structural provision to make food hygiene possible.

The education of customer and food handler to respect and use those facilities.

The education of children at school age into correct food-hygiene actions, although such actions are in some degree contrary to those of their parents.

The education of incidental workers (such as transport and warehouse workers).

The education of all ancillary trades into the mental attitude of giving some consideration to hygiene in all they do, viz. the engineer designing a machine capable of being cleaned.

The education of builders into the values and attributes of new materials.

The education of all into the values and economics of routine cleaning.

The dissemination of ideas (which includes the health officer being receptive to trade ideas).

The establishment of standards and the educational effect of well-chosen and well-presented prosecutions of offenders.

The problems of food poisoning and the achievement of positive food hygiene therefore may have bacteriological and medical overtones, but they are fundamentally problems of people, places, and practice. They thus depend on good management, sensible workers, and a readily available well-informed inspectorate.

The true technique of inspection is to create a position in which advice is sought by the inspected. Thus the inspector must be qualified and must have had training in public relations. There must be some immediate method by which the inspected can assure themselves that the inspector does not exceed his duties. This does not imply that every inspection leads to appeal to higher quarters. The best situation would be one in which those inspected were equally qualified or trained with the inspector. This is not likely to be the factual situation, and put bluntly the truth is that the degree of knowledge of the right to appeal must increase in direct ratio with the ignorance of those inspected. In practice, this leads to no appeals being made and to very ready acceptance of the inspector's work. Thus there is great need for that work to be sensible and practicable.

In the same way as central government consults and uses national organizations, the inspector uses local groups or sects. He uses them for the purpose that they themselves decided brought them together; he only grafts on his ideas. For instance, a local school would have some success if there were a series of talks on food hygiene. There is, however, more success, as a rule, if the teaching of reading happened to repetitively present food-hygiene facts, or the teaching of mathematics included problems concerned with lost work hours and wasted effort due to food poisoning. The inspector needs to know all about the local schools, religious centres, sports groups, acting or singing groups, in short, any possible natural combination of citizens. He then must get to know the leaders of those groups and activities and directly seek their help in putting over his message.

Inspectors must be available and constantly present in every community, and there must be an up-to-date and constant record of his work. In cases of punishment for contravention it is the general attitude in the United Kingdom to present the defendant as a basically good citizen who has slipped from grace. This is an attitude that creates the best reaction, and thus there are few deliberate second offenders in public health matters. Whatever the legal power, whatever the extent of the problem, the answer lies in the individual action—the inspector's task is to make food hygiene mean something individually to all.

ENTRY INTO E.E.C.

Great Britain entered the Common Market at the beginning of 1973 and this has had profound effects on Food Hygiene legislation regarding for example food additives and regulations, the import and export of meat, now being taken over by the WHO/FAO Codex. Details are discussed in a leading article in the Royal Society of Health Journal (1973), and also in a report from a symposium on meat hygiene and the E.E.C. (Royal Society of Health Journal, 1974).

INTERNATIONAL ACTION

The joint FAO/WHO Expert Committee on Food Additives is concerned with assessing the toxicity of additives, contaminants, pesticide residues etc. whilst the Food Standards Programme draws up International Food Standards. Since 1961 the Expert Committee has evaluated some 400 international food additives. Food can be grossly contaminated through the use of fungicides containing mercury, but more recently it has been shown that fish can be contaminated with methyl mercury leading to a form of poisoning that is irreversible. This is the so-called Minamata disease reported from Japan. The prescribed level of mercury in fish is laid down at 0·5 p.p.m. In 1972, an outbreak of mercury poisoning occurred in Iraq due to the treatment of seed with mercury (World Health Organization, 1974d). A conference on this subject was held in Baghdad in Novermbe 1974.

Other WHO programmes are concerned with the Codex Alimentarius and with a Food Virology Programme with reference centres in Brno (Czechoslovakia) and in Madison (U.S.A.). (World Health Organization, 1973 and 1974).

FURTHER READING

Christie, A. B., and Christie, M. C. (1971) *Food Hygiene and Food Hazards*, London.

Collins, C. P. (1963) *Food Hygiene—Ashore and Afloat*, London.

Dack, G. M. (1956) *Food Poisoning*, Rev. ed., Chicago.

Desrosier, N. W. (1963) *The Technology of Food Preservation*, 2nd ed., Westport, Conn.

Dewberry, E. B. (1959) *Food Poisoning*, 4th ed., London.

Graham-Rack, B., and Binsted, R. (1964) *Hygiene in Food Manufacturing and Handling*, London.

Harvey, W. C., and Hill, H. (1952) *Food Hygiene*, London.

Hobbs, B. C. (1953) *Food Poisoning and Food Hygiene*, London.

Joint FAO/WHO Expert Committee on Food Additives (1972) 15th and 16th Reports, Geneva, *Wld Hlth Org. techn. Rep. Ser.* No. 488 and 505.

Longree, K. (1967) *Quantity Food Sanitation*, New York.

Lu, F. C. (1973a) Toxicological evaluation of food additives and pesticide residues. The role of WHO and FAO, *Wld Hlth Org. Chron.*, **27**, 43.

Lu, F. C. (1973b) Wholesomeness of foodstuffs; the role of WHO, *Wld Hlth Org. Chron.*, **27**, 245.

Ministry of Health (1968) *Clean Catering*, London, HMSO.

Ministry of Health and Ministry of Agriculture, Fisheries and Food (1959–   ) *Food Hygiene Codes of Practice*, Nos. 3–8, London, H.M.S.O.

O'Keefe, J. A. (1958–66) *Bell's Sale of Food and Drugs*, 13th ed. and service pages, London.

Parry, M. (1963) Food laws and their influence on merchandising, *R. Soc. Hlth J.*, **83**, 179.

Parry, M. (1964) Food protection 1965, *Publ. Hlth Inspector*, **73**, 103.

Parry, M. (1971) Cleaner food and how to get it, Report 1, in *Second Symposium of Members of Parliament Specialists in Public Health*, Council of Europe, Stockholm.

Pearce, E. (1967) *Environmental Health and Hygiene*, 2nd ed., London.

Royal Society of Health Journal leading article (1973) Mercury and other metals in foodstuffs, *R. Soc. Hlth J.*, **93**, 58.

Royal Society of Health Journal (1974) Effect of EEC directives on meat (3 articles), *R. Soc. Hlth J.*, **94**, 3, 6, 12.

Tressler, D. K., and Evers, C. F. (1957) *The Freezing Preservation of Foods*, 3rd ed., Westport, Conn.

Ward, E. W. (1971) *Food Inspection*, London.

Williams Amphlett, H. (1973) Preservatives in food, *R. Soc. Hlth J.*, **93**, 92.

World Health Organization. Regional Office for the Western Pacific (1962) *Report on the Seminar on Food Sanitation*, Manila.

World Health Organization (1968) Report of a WHO Expert Committee with the Participation of FAO on Microbiological Aspects of Food Hygiene, *Wld Hlth Org. techn. Rep. Ser.*, No. 399.

World Health Organization (1969) Pesticide Residues in Food. Report of the 1968 Joint FAO/WHO Meeting, *Wld Hlth Org. techn. Rep. Ser.*, No. 417.

World Health Organization. Regional Office for Europe (1971) *Report of a Seminar on Food Hygiene*, Warsaw, 1970.

World Health Organization (1972) *1971 Evaluation of some Pesticide Residues in Food*, W.H.O. Pesticide Residues Series, No. 1, Geneva.

World Health Organization (1973a) Paralytic shellfish poisoning from mussels, *Wld Hlth Org. Chron.*, **27**, 33.

World Health Organization (1973b) WHO food virology programmes, *Wld Hlth Org. Chron.*, **21**, 210.

World Health Organization (1973c) Pesticide residues in food: Report of a joint FAO/WHO meeting, *Wld Hlth Org. techn. Rep. Ser.*, No. 525.

World Health Organization (1974a) Mercury as a food contaminant, *Wld Hlth Org. Chron.*, **28**, 8–11.

World Health Organization (1974b) Public health aspects of antibiotics in feedstuffs, *Wld Hlth Org. Chron.*, **28**, 38.

World Health Organization (1974c) The work of WHO in 1973, *Off. Rec. Wld Hlth Org.*, **213**, 57.

World Health Organization (1974d) Intoxication due to mercury-treated seed, *Wld Hlth Org. Chron.*, **28**, 248.

World Health Organization (1974e) Toxicological evaluation of certain food additives with a review of general principles and of specifications.

Seventeenth Report of the joint FAO/WHO Expert Committee on food additives, *Wld Hlth Org. techn. Rep. Ser.*, No. 539.

World Health Organization (1974f) Report of the 1973 joint FAO/WHO meeting, *Wld Hlth Org. techn Rep. Ser.*, No. 545.

World Health Organization (1974g) Fish and shellfish hygiene. Report of a WHO Expert Committee convened with FAO, *Wld Hlth Org. techn. Rep. Ser.*, in the press.

World Health Organization. Regional Office for Europe (1971) *Report of a Seminar on Food Hygiene*, Warsaw 1970 (Euro 0389), Copenhagen.

World Health Organization. Regional Office for Europe (1974) *Report of a Working Group on Harmful Residues in Food for Human and Animal Consumption*, Bremen 1973 (Euro 3604), Copenhagen.

II

NUTRITION AND PUBLIC HEALTH

G. R. WADSWORTH

SOME GENERAL CONSIDERATIONS

The study of nutrition is becoming an integral part of training for students of public health. However, there is some confusion about the nature and scope of the subject. In particular, there is division of opinion about the necessity for knowledge by students of nutrition of the chemistry and biochemistry of the substances supplied to the body from foods. Some believe that such knowledge is not essential, although the student who possesses it may derive added interest from his studies. In public health, however, a knowledge of practical, rather than theoretical, issues is of dominant importance.

In this chapter an attempt is made to indicate some of the principles which are involved, some of the complexities of the relationships between the diet and states of health and some of the responsibilities of health authorities in regulating what people eat. Dogmatism, which often conceals ignorance, has been avoided as far as possible in order that the student may appreciate the many important questions in human nutrition at present unresolved, and which suggest research projects that might be useful.

There are decisions which each person must make for himself and his immediate dependents to avoid disease and to preserve comfort. There are many conditions, however, which are imposed upon people because of chance or deliberate action by others. Very often, decisions made by the few have widespread effects on the many. Both circumstances apply to the food which people eat. In the first instance, the kinds and the amounts of food consumed are the choice of the individual. But this choice may be restricted because of the particular foods which can be bought or grown. Restricted supplies of some foods or abundance of others may be the results of governmental policies or of commercial interests. In addition, the composition of a food when it is consumed may be different from that in its original state.

Changes in composition of foods may be the result of procedures designed to preserve them from spoilage, or may be incidental to methods of farming and technical processing. Thus, nutrients may be removed or added and foreign chemicals may gain access. The individual has little or no choice about the availability or the particular composition of many of the foods that he has to consume. Health authorities therefore have the responsibility of ensuring that all members of the community can get the foods necessary for the maintenance of health, and as free as possible from harmful substances.

A particular example of the dependence of one person on others is the baby. The baby itself has no choice about its diet. The materials put into it are the choice of the mother; she, herself, may be influenced by others, by circumstances, by administrative policies or by commercial activities. Food in-

take at the earliest stage of life should be of the greatest concern to health workers. This is particularly so because there is reason to believe that variations in the diet and the ingestion of some materials, for example herbal medicines, at this time may be of serious consequence.

The scope of the subject of nutrition in public health embraces a knowledge of what people eat, the main reasons for the use of particular diets, the main components of foods, the poisonous substances which may be present in food, the amounts and kinds of food needed for optimal health, and the methods which can be used to control the diet of the whole community and of different classes of individual in it. Adequate discussion of all these topics would require at least one whole book; more space would be needed if the discussions were extended to include the organization of nutritional activities in the public health service. In this chapter only some indications relevant to these main topics can be given; some important subjects, for example fats and vitamins, have not been included. However, sources of extensive and detailed information will be found in the bibliography. Among the references are some which deal essentially with practical issues.

Food and Health

Disease is the result of interaction between the physiological mechanisms of the body and harmful agents. But reactions to the same agent can vary considerably between individuals. There are many striking examples of hazardous circumstances in which only a proportion of the population at risk showed signs of disease. The particular manifestations of the same disease may be different, for example in the foetus, the pregnant woman, and the man. Some variations in susceptibility and clinical effects of disease are due to variations in the state of nutrition and in nutritional requirements. Hence, a knowledge of nutrition is important for those who study the nature of disease and how to preserve health. Furthermore, some constituents of the diet may themselves be noxious and cause disease.

Information required by those responsible for nutrition may be available only in the form of average figures derived from limited inquiries. Interpretation of average figures must be cautious for a number of reasons. For example, not everyone in a locality is exposed equally to prevalent harmful agents so that, on average, direct causes and effects are obscured. Again, more than one hazard may be present at the same time. For example, information may be available that a certain proportion of a community is infested with hookworm. In the same community a proportion also have anaemia. One possible conclusion is that the anaemia was caused by ankylostomiasis. However, more detailed information might show that not all those with hookworms have anaemia, and that not all with anaemia have hookworms. Perhaps in that community inadequate diets alone, hookworm infestation alone, and both together were *each* a cause of anaemia. In order to overcome problems of disease, there is probably always a need to examine a sufficient number of individuals in different ways and to include assessments of their diet and nutritional status.

Average figures are often used, and may indeed be the only information available, to assess adequacy of food supplies. Here again, caution is needed in their interpretation. The average quantity of food available gives no indication of its relative distribution between different sections of the community nor between individuals. There are many instances in

mental conditions and various effects in the individual and in the community.

Conditions in which supplies of food are adequate and the community is prosperous and healthy are relatively infrequent. So also are those conditions in which states of ill-health can be defined as specific diseases. By far the most usual condition is one in which ill-health is common but cannot be assigned a specific diagnosis. In such circumstances measurement of the rate of growth of children and of mortality rates in early life become of great significance in nutritional practice. Proper growth is inhibited by diets which are inadequate in quantity or quality; inadequate nutrition, although not revealed by

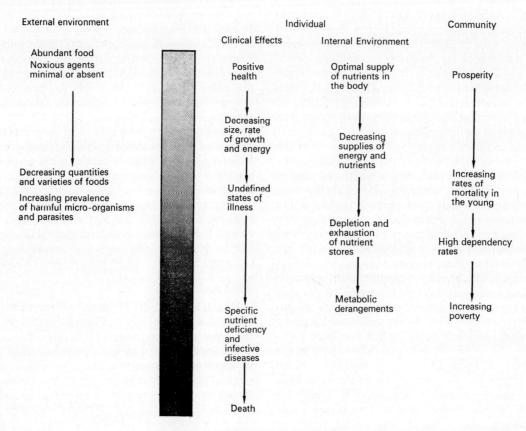

FIG. 48. Diagrammatic representation of associated features in the environment, the individual and the community.

which administrators have been complacent about the nutritional status of the population for which they are responsible, because average amounts of food seem to be satisfactory. But within these populations many people had too little food, and some had too much. Sometimes nutritional standards are regarded as satisfactory because of the results of very few, and sometimes isolated, surveys which may have been made many years previously. Important trends over a number of years, and seasonal variations, are thus ignored. No health administration should be without continuing sources of information about the amounts and kinds of food available for human consumption, and about the distribution of foods between different parts of the country and between different classes of the community.

As the diet decreases in amount and in the number of foods it contains, signs of ill-health begin to appear. FIGURE 48 is an attempt to show the relation between deterioration in environ-

clinical signs, seems to increase susceptibility to infectious diseases in children and to cause undue mortality from them. Systematic collection of records of growth is uncommon; even when information about growth of children is available it is rarely collected from schools and health centres and used by health authorities. Charts showing age–specific death rates and rates of growth of adequate samples of the child population should be on display constantly in the offices of those responsible for the nutrition of people. The information must, of course, be accurate and up to date.

Growth of Populations

People may be short of food because there are too many of them or because there is not enough production of food. The alarming rate at which the number of people in the world is increasing has led to vigorous attempts to limit the extent of human reproduction to avoid disastrous malnutrition. These attempts seem to be justified because agricultural production is being increased too slowly and, in fact, in some places has shown a decrease in recent years. Attempts to limit the rate of increase of the population are apparently counteracted by successful reduction in mortality rates, especially among children, as a result of the control of malaria and other diseases. However, in countries which are now prosperous improved standards of health and marked reduction in child mortality rates were followed by voluntary restriction of family size. Such a pattern can be discerned in other countries today. In any case, no problems are solved by allowing high mortality and morbidity rates to continue. Much sickness in a community and appreciable loss of child life aggravate poverty by causing high dependency rates and by other means.

As already stated, family size can be limited in some communities by spontaneous choice on the part of married people. However, there are fears that such a natural course of events takes too long to alleviate malnutrition which is already occurring and to prevent more severe shortages of food in the future. Therefore, limitation of birth rate is being attempted by the use of contraceptive devices. At present, much use is being made of preparations of hormones which can be ingested by women. There is evidence that when these preparations are taken continuously over a long time untoward effects may occur. Among these is an interference with the metabolism of the amino acid, tryptophan, which can be prevented by the vitamin, pyridoxine. Results of tests suggests that some women, when taking contraceptive hormones, must receive at the same time regular doses of pyridoxine. The side-effects of contraceptive pills, although seen so far in only a small proportion of women at risk, suggest the need for caution in using them, and suggest that other means of limiting the number of people to be fed and of increasing the production of food must not be neglected.

Animal life forms part of the human environment and animals compete with humans for food. Although the world is short of food, man fosters this competitive element. Each year hundreds of millions of dollars are spent in buying foods for pet cats, dogs, and birds. Wild birds and animals, particularly rodents, destroy large amounts of food intended for human consumption. At the same time very little has been done to exploit wild life for human food. Little attention seems to be given to the ecology of human life within the whole animal kingdom. Eventually, control of animal life may become imperative in the interests of human well-being or even survival.

Adaptation

Nothing in life is static; all natural processes are in a continuous state of change. In many parts of the world man lives for part of the year in a cold environment and for the remainder of the year in a warm, or a hot, environment. During the course of time man has changed his habits of work, and the growth of urbanization has altered his social and environmental conditions considerably. From time to time the human body is exposed to influences of potential harm, and, unless he is to succumb, man must make adjustments in his physiological mechanisms. The ability to survive under varying conditions depends on adaptation; beyond the range of adaptation, however, survival and avoidance of disease can be achieved only by control of environmental factors. Little has been done to explore the limits of adaptation to noxious conditions, including restriction of the diet, but information about them is important in predicting the effects on the human race of probable supplies of food in the future and in making plans accordingly.

FOOD AND HUMAN REQUIREMENTS FOR FOOD

Food is any material ingested by mouth and from which the body obtains the chemical substances, which are known as *nutrients*, required by the metabolic processes on which life depends. The composition of foods is often regarded as simple; people refer commonly to 'carbohydrates', 'protein foods' and so on. In fact, apart from some fats and sugars, the materials which make up the diet are complicated in their physical and chemical structures. No product of nature which is used as a food in its original form consists of only one substance. In spite of extensive analysis in laboratories since the last century, much still remains to be discovered about the disposition and the chemical and physical states of different nutrients in foods. Furthermore, some chemicals of known or possible biological importance are present in foods in such small amounts that their detection and measurement are only now becoming possible. The nutritional value of food can be modified by cooking and by the presence of other foods eaten with it. In addition, the exact composition of many dishes, for example 'curries' and 'stews', is not known, Therefore, there is a need for assessments of the nutritional value of whole meals in the state in which they are eaten. Such analyses have been rare.

Knowledge about the nature and amounts of all the substances which are ingested is becoming increasingly difficult to obtain. One reason for this difficulty is the access to foods of chemicals used in agriculture and food technology. Such chemicals may be present in the diet long before methods have been devised to detect their presence or measure their amounts. There is also the possibility that chemicals added to soils or foods may interact with substances naturally present so as to produce new chemicals of unknown composition or activity.

The concept of health cannot be defined easily, and from one point of view it is philosophical. Criteria for defining optimal health have not yet been agreed. In the meantime, the suggestion is made here that these criteria could be: a reasonable span of life, say 70 years, an ability to withstand the common stresses of life, for example infective disease, and the ability to adapt to a certain range of environmental conditions. Adequacy of the diet can be assessed by the extent to which it allows fulfilment of these criteria. The student will appreciate that much epidemiological and other forms of investigation are required in this context. Present standards for an adequate diet must be regarded as tentative.

Those who are responsible for agricultural and other policies which affect the nutrition of people must have guidance from nutritionists. This guidance takes the tangible form of tables of 'recommended dietary allowances'. They represent the opinion of committees who have considered the best information available at the time. Much of this information is that obtained from dietary surveys among groups of people, most of whom are assumed to be 'healthy'. The inference is that the diet which people actually consume is that which their bodies require. There are obvious objections to this inference. Furthermore, dietary requirements are given in average amounts and must be interpreted accordingly. Average requirements are sometimes regarded as minimal requirements for individuals. As a consequence those who consume less than the average have been considered to be malnourished. Actually, of course, in a large population about half the people will consume less than the average, and about half will consume more than the average. Average figures must be applied only to groups and not to individuals. This seems to be obvious, but, unfortunately, misinterpretation and misuse of average figures for dietary requirements and for the results of dietary surveys often confuse deliberations in which Medical Officers of Health are involved.

A diet which consists of a mixture of animal and vegetable products when consumed in sufficient quantity will supply all the nutrients required by the human body. As the variety of foods in the diet becomes less, there is an increasing liability for deficiencies to arise. Thus, a simple guide to assess quickly the possible existence of nutritional problems is the number of foods commonly being used. Adequate diets are composed from foods selected from each of the main groups. These groups are: meat, fish, eggs and milk; fruits and vegetables; mature seeds and nuts; starch-rich tubers and roots; and grain products. Unfortunately, the growing number of mixtures prepared on a commercial scale, especially for infants, leads to difficulties in assessing and advising about the intake of different nutrients. In this situation there is a danger that some nutrients, for example vitamin D and fats, may be consumed to excess.

Requirements of the Body for Energy

The proportions in different foods of water and solid material vary considerably. Hence, the weight of a portion of a food does not reveal its nutritional value. In practice, amounts of food are expressed according to the number of Calories that would be obtained from them. The Calorie is a unit of heat, so that to speak about the ingestion of a certain number of Calories is not really sensible. Nevertheless, the phrase is justified by convention and convenience. Unfortunately, many people refer to Calories as if they were discrete nutrients separate from other constituents of the diet, especially proteins. The student should remember that the word 'Calories' is merely a short and convenient way of saying 'the total amount of nutritional material'. He should also remember that proteins, fats, and carbohydrates all contribute to the Calories of the diet.

The unit used in nutrition is the large Calorie; this unit is one thousand times the small calorie, and to avoid confusion some authorities prefer the term 'Kilo-calorie'. Recently the International Organization for Standardization has recommended that the *joule* (J) be used as the unit of energy instead of the calorie. The joule is defined in terms of the basic units of mass, length, and time, and it is a direct measure of energy whereas the calorie is an indirect measure.

The value of a food as a source of energy, as determined in a calorimeter, may differ from the energy actually obtained from it by the body after ingestion. There are a number of reasons for discrepancy between the theoretical and the actual, or bio-

logical, energy values of foods. One reason is that not all materials which undergo combustion, and hence release heat energy, in the calorimeter can be digested and absorbed by the body. A common observation is that some people who ingest much food do not become obese, whereas others on the same intake gain body fat. This difference may be due to an increase in metabolic rate by some people, when the amount of food absorbed into the body is more than the amount needed. Such people 'burn up' extra food and excrete the products of metabolism. Other people may convert extra food to fat which is retained in the body. Information about energy metabolism in relation to food intake by different people must be obtained by the use of costly and complicated apparatus. Very few investigations of this kind have been made, so that details of the biological turn-over of energy by the body, and its variations with different physiological and pathological states are largely unknown. At present, ideas about the relationship of the amount of food intake and the state of the body are based on rather crude observations.

Too Little Food

When the amount of food in the diet falls below a certain level there is loss of body weight and less ability to do work. Mental effects are also found causing irritability and, later, apathy. When food intake by the adult falls below about 1,600 Calories a day, deficiency of protein will probably occur. At still lower levels of intake deficiencies of vitamins, especially riboflavine and niacin, will be probable. When the amount of food is less than 1,000 Calories a day death is soon inevitable, and will be hastened by physical exertion. The amounts of food quoted would apply to groups of people; some individuals may show ill-effects sooner or later than others when their intake of food is small.

Too Much Food

Increase in body size usually ceases on reaching adult life, although in some communities a progressive increase in weight with advancing age is common, especially in women. Gain in weight during childhood is due to proportionate acquisition of a number of materials, but in adults the major increase is in the amount of fat. How far change in weight in adult life is physiological is not known. Therefore, a 'normal' weight at any particular age cannot be postulated. When deposition of fat becomes excessive, 'overweight', that is to say appreciable departure from the mean weight of members of the whole population, becomes apparent. Actually, overweight people are not always excessively fat. Some who appear to be too fat are not overweight. Overweight is a general term; obesity, however, is a specific term which means a relative disproportion of fat to the total amount of material of which the body is composed. There is reason to suppose that if *overweight* and *obesity* were clearly differentiated some confusion about the relationship between body weight and disease would be resolved. However, excessive weight, of whatever type, is a result of eating more food than is required for physiological reasons.

In communities where conditions of life are stable, there is a sensitive relationship between the mean amount of food ingested and the mean body weight of large groups of adults. Thus, determination of the mean body weight from time to time provides a very useful index of the average food consumption, and hence of nutritional status. Measurement of food intake is difficult and subject to large errors. Records obtained at suitable intervals of the body weight of factory workers or inmates of prisons or other institutions can, therefore, be most useful to the public health nutritionist.

The effects of overweight can be judged both in the individual and in groups. The person who is grossly overweight may be disabled for mechanical reasons, for example in travelling in crowded public conveyances. A disproportionate size of the abdominal contents may embarrass breathing and in extreme cases can precipitate heart failure. Other conditions, such as inguinal hernia and arthritis may be more likely with excessive body weight.

Experiments have been made in which normal men have taken excessive amounts of food and diminished their physical activity. Much weight was gained and at the same time there were changes in the activities of endocrine glands. Induced changes in the hormonal balance, with consequent changes in metabolism, may help to explain the association of obesity, cardiovascular, and other diseases.

Examination of average records from large populations reveals an apparent association between excessive body weight and some pathological conditions [TABLE 40]. The interpretation of these statistics may not always be straightforward. For example, in cancer and tuberculosis, weight at the time of death will have been seriously depleted and will be quite different from the weight at the time that the pathological process began. Again, there are many exceptions to the average. For example, an appreciable number of men who die of cardiovascular disease are of average weight or less.

TABLE 40

Some Principal Causes of Death among Men and Women Rated for Overweight (Mayer, J. (1958) *Borden's Rev. Nutr. Res.*, 19, Pt 3, 35)

Cause of death	Men Percentage actual, of expected deaths	Women Percentage actual, of expected deaths
Organic heart disease, disease of coronary arteries, and angina	142	175
Cerebral haemorrhage . .	159	162
Chronic nephritis . . .	191	212
Diabetes	383	372
Cirrhosis of liver . . .	249	147
Appendicitis . . .	223	195
Biliary calculi . . .	206	284
Auto accidents . . .	131	120

The layman usually judges overweight on aesthetic grounds, and the fat person becomes an object of ridicule. The efforts of many women to keep their body size and shape within certain limits can be ascribed to a desire to be physically attractive. Such aims are guided, perhaps in subtle ways, by standards set by public figures and by artists. These are not scientific criteria, but science has not yet provided an alternative guide which can be accepted generally.

Reduction of body weight, or slimming, has become a subject of wide discussion. Sometimes marked limitation of intake of food has led to illness and death. Dissemination through radio, newspapers, and magazines of the idea that slimming is desirable may cause undue worry and expenditure on special preparations of foods and medicines by large numbers of people. Therefore, public health authorities should provide suitable guidance to the public on this matter.

Energy Requirements: Theoretical Considerations

The true needs of the body for a supply of energy can be determined by measuring the amount of oxygen used in a known time, or the amount of heat being lost. There is a quantitative relationship between oxygen consumption, heat production, the work done internally and externally by the body, and the potential energy in the diet. Simultaneous measurements of oxygen consumption and physical activity show that energy expenditure is a function of the type of person, the type of activity, the conditions under which the activity is performed and the duration of each kind of activity. There is thus a very wide range of energy requirements by different individuals and from time to time. The appetite varies so as to control the intake of food according to energy needs. However, this physiological control is not precise.

The pattern of food intake and energy expenditure is changing with time. In primitive society much physical effort is needed to procure food, for example in hunting. In modern, sophisticated society not only can food be obtained with little effort, but also it is available in attractive forms. Conditioned reflexes associated with the ingestion of food may thus be stimulated too frequently and in the absence of a real need for food. The precise physiological mechanisms associated with appetite, and in particular the factors which influence them, have not yet been elucidated fully. The hypothalamus is an important centre which is involved. This part of the brain forms a link between the nervous and endocrine systems, and its activities can be modified by numerous circumstances in the body. There is reason to believe that the function of the hypothalamus in promoting hunger or satiety can be modified by habit. When food intake is restricted the desire to ingest food can decrease, and 'an appetite that grows with what it feeds on', although alluding to a different circumstance, seems to be true also in a gastronomic sense. Results of exploration of the effect of different levels of feeding early in life, when functional characteristics of the central nervous system are being established, in determining the pattern of hypothalamic reactions to the intake of food might prove to be important.

Body size is also an important factor governing food requirements. The larger a person's body, the more metabolic tissue is present. Excessive fat in the body may lead to an increased metabolic rate, because although fat itself is metabolically inert, the cells which contain it are not; their metabolic activity seems to be influenced by the amount of fat they contain. Increase in weight, although usually due to deposition of fat, is accompanied by an increase in cell mass. In the course of wasting both fat and metabolic tissue are lost. Metabolic rate is often expressed in terms of surface area of the body. Oxygen consumption per unit surface area tends to remain constant, so that the absolute amount of metabolic activity, reflected in oxygen consumption, increases with body size because surface area increases correspondingly. The increase in metabolic activity is the result of an increase in the amount of metabolic tissue and also to an increase in metabolic rate of unit amount of tissue. In semistarvation there is an absolute fall in metabolic rate of non-fat tissue, and in obesity an absolute increase. In addition to metabolic effects associated with endocrine change, to which reference was made above, overweight, by increasing the amount of metabolism and energy turn-over, may impose extra work on the cardiovascular and other systems of the body. Evidence for the involvement of the cardiovascular function in the response of the body to overweight is a fall in blood pressure when obese people lose weight.

During physical activity body weight influences energy requirements. This can be understood by considering the amount of energy needed to lift a heavy body up a flight of stairs compared with that needed to lift a light body. However, actual studies have not always verified clear relationships between body weight and energy expenditure. In some forms of external work body weight shows no correlation with energy expenditure; in other activities, although there is a correlation, very wide individual variations in the association are found. One reason for such discrepancy is a difference between individuals in the efficiency of conversion of energy to work. Obese people may perform the same movements as thin people with less consumption of oxygen. This seems to be due to larger muscles in the obese and the fact that their muscles have more practice in moving weight. Another factor of importance in relation to food requirements is the amount of movement performed during everyday life. People who are overweight, including the obese and women late in pregnancy, may be less active than those who are smaller in size.

The potential value of foods as sources of energy can be obtained from tables of food composition in which values derived from calorimetry have been corrected arbitrarily to allow for losses incurred during digestion, absorption, and metabolism. In group studies there is close agreement between average intake of energy in the form of food and average energy expenditure. But, as already stated, there is much individual variation. If the amount of food requirement is important in relation to health, there is a need for much more information about actual food intake and actual energy turn-over in individuals. There is also a need for information about the biological energy value of different diets in relation to the individual, feeding habits, the presence of disease, and other circumstances.

The orthodox view is that there is a simple and direct relationship between energy expenditure and intake of food, and that the type of food is not important. However, this simple relationship may be complicated by the metabolic characteristics of the consumer and by the nature of the diet. For example, some obese people are inefficient in their metabolic use of carbohydrate but can metabolize fat freely. These people can lose weight on a diet rich in fat, although excessive in its energy value. There is also a difference in the metabolic history of different kinds of carbohydrate. Fructose, glucose, and starch, from which glucose is released on digestion, have different effects on fat metabolism. Effects of the constitution of the diet on metabolic processes can also be modified according to the respective amounts of energy being supplied from fat in the body and from the diet. An illustration of this is a variation in the fatty acid composition of human milk according to the amount of food being ingested, the proportion of the total energy derived from fat in the diet and body fat,

and the fatty acid composition of these fats. Thus, when examining the diet in relation to body weight, characteristics of the individual, and the diet, apart from its energy value, must be considered.

The amount of food needed by an individual will depend upon the factors discussed above; a distinction must be made between these needs and the size of the body which is desirable. When a person who is too large lives at first on a restricted diet he will be in a state of undernutrition relative to his present needs. As a consequence he will experience hunger, lassitude, and other effects. If these symptoms are ignored and the diet continued, there will ensue loss of weight due to a decrease in the amount of water, fat, and to a lesser extent other materials from the body. As a consequence, the need for energy will diminish because the amount of metabolic tissue will be less and there will also be a reduction in the absolute metabolic rate. At this stage the amount of food required to maintain energy balance will be less than it was before reduction in body size. Subjective symptoms of hunger should then disappear. When loss of weight is excessive, as in starvation, appetite may be lost to such an extent that the food needed to sustain life is not consumed.

Requirements of the Body for Protein

Too Much Protein. During the early part of the present century there was much speculation about the optimum amount of protein needed for health. Much controversy was resolved, however, when the amino acid composition of proteins was discovered. At the same time, interest in the quantitative aspects of dietary protein diminished and a number of questions relevant to this remain unanswered.

The adult deals with excessive intake of protein in various ways. Efficiency of utilization decreases as intake of nitrogenous materials increases so that a higher proportion is excreted. Nearly all of the ingested protein which is not utilized in the body is excreted as urea in the urine. However, the body seems to hold a reserve of protein; whether this represents a distinct compartment or a relatively labile part of the ordinary tissue–protein is not known. There is evidence that the extracellular, extravascular fluids and blood can supply protein to the rest of the body if required. Whether by excretion, deposition in reserve depots or in other ways, the adult can apparently cope with all probable levels of dietary protein. During early life the situation is different. The child seems unable to control utilization of nitrogen efficiently, so that the more nitrogenous material that is given by mouth the more is retained in the body. There is also evidence that the size of the foetus, and hence its protein content, is influenced directly by the amount of protein available to it. Much nitrogenous material is taken up into the products of growth; growth can thus be regarded as a form of excretion from the internal environment. The rate of growth is influenced directly by the quantity of protein ingested, and there is cessation of growth when the intake of protein falls below a critical level. When growth ceases in this way there will be an accumulation of materials present in the body fluids which usually pass into newly formed structures. The alternative route of excretion for these materials is through the kidney, but renal function early in life is not fully developed and consequently cannot effectively get rid of excessive amounts of some substances, for example calcium and phosphate. When the concentration of protein in the diet is raised the rate of growth increases. This effect is apparent when babies are fed on cow's milk in place of human milk. As the rate of growth increases more materials are abstracted from the internal environment. Thus, rate of growth modifies the immediate environment of the tissues, and the rate of growth is influenced by the level of protein in the diet. There is thus a theoretical basis for the supposition that too much, as well as too little, protein might have deleterious effects in the very young.

Too Little Protein. By feeding animals on diets in which the concentration of protein varies, pathological states can be produced. When the quantity of the diet, whatever its composition, is severely restricted a condition comparable to *marasmus* in children results. Ingestion of enough of a diet in which the amount of protein relative to the amount of the other constituents, that is to say the concentration of protein, is low results in a state comparable to *kwashiorkor* in humans. The concentration of protein is expressed conveniently in terms of the proportion of the total potential energy of the diet which is represented by protein. The total energy is expressed as Calories and the energy from protein as the protein-Calories. The index of protein concentration in the diet is thus the protein-Calories as a percentage of the total Calories. The nutritional value of the diet in relation to protein can be indicated by the protein-Calories *per cent.* together with the biological value of the protein, which is a function mainly of its amino acid composition. Combining these two factors, the term *net dietary protein-Calories per cent.* (NDpCal%) is derived.

By analogy with the results of experiments on animals some conditions of protein depletion in children can be termed *protein-Calorie deficiency diseases.* These conditions would correspond to those described by the clinical term *kwashiorkor.* When protein depletion is part of the result of starvation, the term *marasmus* is applicable. The syndromes described by the term kwashiorkor can thus be regarded as the result of too low a *concentration* of protein in the diet, or to an excessive concentration of non-protein materials, usually carbohydrates.

There is confusion about the use of different terms which are used to describe similar clinical states of malnutrition. There is also inconsistency in describing such conditions according to definite criteria. For example, 'protein-Calorie deficiency' is often used to indicate simultaneous inadequacy of protein and quanity of food, that is to say Calories. Use of the term in this way is at variance with the original concept on which it was based. The terms 'protein malnutrition' and 'protein-Calorie malnutrition' are undesirable. They suggest that protein and Calories have a positive action in causing malnutrition. Agreement was reached some years ago (*Sixth Report of the Joint FAO/WHO Expert Committee on Nutrition,* 1967) that the alternative term for kwashiorkor and marasmus should be 'protein-Calorie deficiencies'.

Protein Requirements: Theoretical Considerations

In the normal adult, whose diet and physical activity are stable and who is free from disease or other forms of stress, a condition of nitrogenous balance is present. This means that the total amount of nitrogenous material ingested by mouth is balanced by the total losses of nitrogen. This condition of equilibrium is sometimes assumed to indicate nutritional adequacy of protein. However, in a body depleted of protein, nitrogenous equilibrium may persist. Only during periods of progressive depletion or progressive acquisition will an imbalance between gains and losses of nitrogen be found.

The provision of adequate amounts of protein is a function of total quantity and of the type and relative amounts of amino acids absorbed from the diet. There are eight amino acids which must be obtained from food: relative, or complete, absence of any one of them is incompatible with health or perhaps life. Knowledge about the 'essential amino acids' has been obtained by the use of synthetic diets using pure amino acids in place of protein, which are therefore different from ordinary diets. The results of these experiments, which were costly and difficult to undertake, have been accepted as the best estimates of amino acid requirements. Moreover, they provided an explanation for differences between the nutritional values of different kinds of protein.

Much current theory about protein requirements of the human body is based on experiments using synthetic and semi-synthetic diets. Usual diets differ from those used in such tests. The availability of amino acids from dietary protein depends upon their release by digestion from foods. The presence of particular amino acids established by chemical analysis of a food does not reveal the extent of the release nor of the proportions of different amino acids present at the mucosal surface of the intestine through which absorption takes place. Absorption of amino acids is influenced by concentration and sometimes by competition between different amino acids and other substances. The biological value of proteins in the diet will depend upon the extent to which they provide essential amino acids which are absorbed and utilized in the body. Requirements for amino acids vary with age, physiological states and pathological conditions. Thus, the biological value of a particular protein can vary with the individual who consumes it.

Ideally, the nutritional value of a diet in terms of protein would be determined by the extent to which ingestion of the diet itself provided nitrogenous material for metabolic processes. Humans cannot be used routinely for such tests; instead laboratory animals, especially rats, are employed. Tests on living animals show the amount of nitrogen actually utilized and retained in the body. This actual nutritional value thus takes account of such factors as digestibility of the foods which provide nitrogenous material, the presence in the lumen of the intestine of materials which either enhance or inhibit absorption of amino acids and the metabolic state of the consumer. Tests are preferably performed using whole diets, because the nutritional value of dietary protein can be affected by the quantity of the diet and the nature of other substances in it.

NUTRITION AND THE ENVIRONMENT

The environment of the body consists of all external and internal materials and circumstances. These include the soil, the atmosphere, food, endocrine levels within the body, and, in the first stages of life, the uterus and its blood supply. Modification of any internal or external factor to which the body is exposed can raise nutritional problems. For example, impaired intestinal synthesis of vitamin B_{12} occurs in ruminants which feed off land deficient in cobalt. This results in deficiency of vitamin B_{12} in the tissues and excreta of the animals, and a diminished supply of it for man. Harmful materials in soil, selenium, for example, or radioactive strontium, can gain access to cereal grains used as food. A great many other examples could be given, but special mention will be made here only of the environment of the foetus and the presence of noxious chemicals in foods.

Nutrition of the Foetus

The adult can select the amount and type of food which enters the body; the foetus cannot do so. The foetus must accept the particular mixture of nutrients and other substances, for example hormones, present in the blood of the mother. The placenta normally allows substances needed by the foetus to pass through, and inhibits those that might be harmful. The foetus is thus dependent upon the nutrient constitution of the maternal blood, the uterine blood flow and the function of the placenta. Changes can occur in each of these and, by interfering with the normal flow of nutrients, may prove disastrous. Temporary and perhaps minor defects in the supply may be of particular consequence in embryonic life when mitotic activity is high, and a single cell may represent potentially a large portion of the fully developed body.

Much interest has been taken in the experimental production of congenital abnormalities in animals. Lesions can be produced by a number of noxious influences, and the particular effects depend on the stage of embryonic or foetal life when the influence is present. Deficiencies of different vitamins in the mother's diet can lead to congenital abnormalities in the offspring. However, the concentration of a vitamin in the mother's blood can be influenced by factors other than the diet. For example, pyrexia causes depression of the level of vitamin A in plasma. Such a depression could presumably diminish the amount of the vitamin passing to the foetus. Furthermore, diminished flow of blood through the placenta limits the supply of materials to the foetus. This may explain why congenital abnormalities occur more frequently when the mother has toxaemia, because toxaemia is associated with considerable reduction in uterine blood flow.

Considerable attention is being given to the function of the placenta in relation to the condition of the foetus. The concept of 'placental insufficiency' has been invoked to explain the birth of babies whose weights are considerably less than that expected for the gestational age. These 'small-for-dates' or 'dysmature' babies show signs suggestive of malnutrition. Perhaps the most important consequence of placental insufficiency on the foetus is permanent retardation of mental development subsequent to birth. There is uncertainty about the aetiology of placental insufficiency. One possibility is a deficiency of folate at an early stage of pregnancy, although this is controversial.

The relationship between the diet of the mother and foetal development may, therefore, be complicated by the presence of other factors. Furthermore, the nature of the diet of the mother may not affect the foetus primarily, but secondarily to an initial effect on the placenta. In addition, any influence acting directly on the foetus or placenta need only be temporary to produce permanent effects. Thus, a vitamin deficiency present for perhaps a few days early in pregnancy, although impossible to detect, may have serious consequences.

Observations on whole communities indicate that the nutrition of the mother influences the outcome of pregnancy. In places where diets are poor the average birth weight is comparatively small, premature births are common and the neonatal mortality rate is high. Again, however, the interpretation of these observations may not be straightforward. For example, neonatal death rate is influenced to a considerable extent by obstetric services. In poor communities these services are usually limited or may not exist.

Critical stages in the development of both temporary and permanent teeth take place during intra-uterine life. There is evidence that the diet of the mother during pregnancy can influence the state of the teeth of her child during its first years of life [FIG. 49].

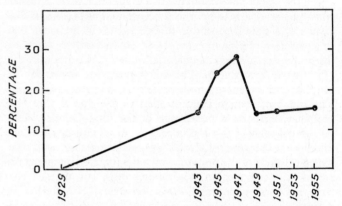

FIG. 49. Incidence of freedom from caries in five-year-old London children in different years. (From May Mellanby, Helen Coumoulos, Marion Kelley, and Gwenneth Neal (1957), *Brit. med. J.*, **2**, 318.) Freedom from caries was higher in children born in 1942, and this may have been a reflection of the consumption of a more satisfactory diet by their mothers during pregnancy.

Chemicals in Foods

In the past, malnutrition has often been accepted as the outcome of dietary deficiencies. The idea of positive harmful effects of materials present in foods, although accepted in Ancient Greece, has been given serious consideration only in recent times. Harmful substances may have been added by man, but sometimes they are intrinsic components of the natural food. Whether these substances are harmful or not, may depend on characteristics of the consumer. For example, *favism*, due to exposure to, or ingestion of, the bean *Vicia faba*, occurs only in those who are sensitive to it. Many foods contain poisons, for example acetylandromedol in some samples of honey, cyanide in cassava, alkaloids in yams, and many others. However, preparation and cooking usually destroy such poisons and relatively few people are known to have been affected by them. Perhaps of greater significance, because of its widespread occurrence, is a reaction by some people to wheat protein leading to intestinal malabsorption.

An important problem, which is likely to increase as time goes on, is contamination of food with extraneous chemicals. These may be accidental or deliberate additives. Insecticides are now used widely in agriculture and often get into foods. Some are fat-soluble and are retained in the body after ingestion and gradually accumulate. Demonstrable amounts of DDT have been found in human tissues, including the placenta, but no ill-effects due to its presence have been identified.

In the course of time an increasing number of chemicals are liable to gain access to the human body. The question arises whether the presence of foreign substances in the tissues is already causing suboptimal health, and whether their continued presence over many years may eventually produce overt pathological changes. Much attention is being given to the situation by research teams, health authorities, and the World Health Organization. Assessments are, however, very difficult to make and firm guidance is not usually possible at the present time. The Medical Officer for Environmental Health should keep himself informed of latest developments and must take action to prevent obvious contamination of foods with poisonous substances.

Recent developments in agricultural practice are causing increased access to foods of harmful micro-organisms. Poultry, pigs, and cattle which are reared intensively in enclosed spaces ('factory farming') are liable to harbour salmonella, brucella, and other organisms which can cause disease in humans. Spread of such organisms may be through eggs, milk, or meat. Freezing and modern forms of packaging and marketing can still allow viability of organisms in foods. Harmful bacteria in the deeper muscles of large birds have been found to survive cooking under some conditions. Dust from factory farms is disseminated over long distances because of the action of extractor-fans used in ventilating the buildings. The dust may contain viruses and bacteria.

Antibiotics are used commonly in foods for livestock, and may also be given to animals for therapeutic purposes. Their use in agriculture can lead to ingestion of small amounts of antibiotics by humans over long periods of time, a possible consequence of which is the development of sensitivity. Subsequent exposure to antibiotics of sensitized people can lead to serious reactions including death due to anaphylactic shock. Furthermore, continued use of antibiotics in the rearing of livestock can lead to the multiplication and dissemination of organisms which are antibiotic-resistant.

Thus, although modern practices may lead to greater efficiency in food production, they may at the same time produce new threats to health [see also CHAPTER 10].

NUTRITION AND HUMAN ADAPTATION
Climate

Man is a homeothermic animal; his body may increase its production of heat in conditions of cold, and may decrease it in warmth. There are mechanisms which control loss of heat from the body so as to keep the central temperature constant. This control may involve change in metabolic rate and consequently a change in food consumption. When there is an increase in the quantity of heat produced in the body, there is an increase in the amount of material being oxidized and a need to replace it from the diet. Although this concept is reasonable, in fact, little is known about the actual effect of climate on food intake under optimal conditions. In many tropical countries food is scarce, and the amount consumed is small for this reason. The small amount of information available suggests that people in very cold climates eat no more on the average than those in hot countries. But, again, the amount consumed may be limited by availability. Dietary surveys have usually been made in Arctic regions only during open seasons when physical activity is high

and foods are more plentiful. The results, therefore, do not reflect the average conditions throughout a whole year. Furthermore, the high level of energy expenditure caused by wearing extra clothing and carrying personal loads for long distances on foot explain the relatively high intakes of food which have sometimes been observed. There is evidence that in hot climates extra food is needed to supply the energy used by physiological mechanisms which prevent a rise in body temperature. Quite apart from physiological mechanisms of control, the actual climate in which the human body lives (the 'microclimate') is controlled by clothing, housing, and artificial cooling or warming; in addition the rate and duration of physical activity can be adjusted appropriately at will.

So far, considerations of the effect of climate on food requirements have been based mostly on theoretical evidence. The enormous problem of deciding the amount of food needed now and in the future for the whole human race demands realistic information obtained from studies made directly on people living under ordinary conditions of life.

When there is a sudden fall in climatic temperature appetite is increased and may lead to ingestion of more food than is needed for nutritional reasons. This stimulation of appetite seems to be temporary. The increasing use of air-conditioned houses and restaurants in the tropics raises the question of whether, because many people are now eating in a cold climate and living mostly in a hot climate, they are eating too much food. The use of air-conditioning or transfer to a cool climate in the treatment of debilitating disease in the tropics may be justified in so far as the appetite is stimulated and intake of food increased.

Altitude and Space

When man ascends to a high altitude by climbing or flying, special nutritional problems arise. In mountaineering, as in polar exploration, there is a high output of energy. The necessity of carrying food leads to the use of concentrated materials of light weight. These may be unappetizing and lead to an inadequate intake of food and possibly failure of a project. Altitude can cause cravings for specific foods and, until acclimatization occurs, to diminished appetite. At this stage energy requirements are met by body tissues which become depleted as shown by considerable and rapid loss of weight.

An adequate supply of carbohydrate seems to be necessary for mental and neuromuscular efficiency during aerial flight. However, there is no evidence that special diets for pilots are necessary. But while errors of judgement, syncope, and decompression symptoms continue to occur without apparent reason further investigation of optimal diets for pilots is justifiable.

Intensive studies are being made of the effects on metabolism of travel in space. The results of these studies are not readily available but they are being used to devise suitable diets for astronauts.

Nutrition and Adaptation to Injury and Disease

Infective disease always accompanies poverty and malnutrition. The situation is complex. For example, poverty and lack of food can result in migration and congregation of people so that dissemination of infection is aggravated. There are examples to show that those who are severely malnourished succumb more readily to infections which have little serious effect on those who are well nourished. However, variation between strains of micro-organisms responsible for disease, degrees of immunity, and the genetic characteristics of people, may obscure the effects of nutrition on the clinical manifestations and the outcome of infection. But there is sufficient evidence from animal experiments and from observations on human patients to show that nutritional status is important in this context. Application of modern techniques is providing more specific information in this field. For example, the size and activity of the thymolymphatic system, which is important in defending the body against infective disease, are diminished in children who are malnourished.

Studies on patients have established that during stress due to trauma, surgical operation, or disease there is a change in metabolism. This change results at first in a 'catabolic phase' in which there is excessive loss of nutrients from the body. In particular, there is an appreciable negative nitrogen balance which cannot be reversed by increasing the intake of protein. The excessive loss of nitrogen is inevitable and an essential part of the reaction of the body to the onset of stress. In the absence of a catabolic phase because of previous depletion of body tissues, healing is delayed and incomplete. Using this knowledge, the diets needed by sick people can be composed on a rational basis. Repletion of deficiencies of nutrients in the body by special feeding before surgical operations leads to better results. An adequate intake of protein is important in the healing of pressure-sores. There is evidence that repletion of protein deficiency is necessary for the healing of fractures and the resolution of tuberculous lesions. Diets in convalescence, and those for the chronic sick, must provide adequate amounts of protein to make up for losses incurred by diminished appetite and excessive catabolism during the initial stages of illness. Sick people are usually at complete or partial rest so that their requirements for energy may be relatively low. Their appetite must not be satisfied by fluids or carbohydrates at the expense of meeting their requirements for protein.

GROWTH

If nutrition is to be a science, precise measurements must be applied to various aspects of the relationships between diet and the form and function of the human body. So far exact measurements, comparable to those made in other fields of science, have not usually been possible in relation to the nutrition of people under their ordinary conditions of life. One exception to this is the measurement of the rate of growth of children.

Growth is important in nutrition because the rate of change in the size of a child provides objective evidence of nutritional status. Except in rare instances where there are hormonal or genetic abnormalities, the rate of growth is influenced sensitively by the amount and the quality of the diet. However, to be of use the measurements involved must be made very accurately. Accuracy is not difficult to attain in measuring the size of a child of, say, 25 kg. in weight or 125 cm. in height. But the dimensions in question are not these absolute ones, but *differences* between individual children or from time to time in the

same children. On the average, children of about 10 years of age gain 5 cm. a year in height. Significant differences in nutritional status would cause a change in this rate so that quantities to be detected would be less than 5 cm. a year, or less than about 0·4 cm. a month. Differences of this order may have to be detected when comparing the heights of different children at a particular time. A comparable range of differences in weights would be about 0·25 to 3·0 kg. These quantities could easily be distorted or annulled by changes in posture, the weight of clothes and changes in the weight of clothes due to their moisture content, careless observation, and other factors.

Children may increase their height and weight disproportionately and relative differences between gains in height and weight will result in the development of various shapes of the body. Variations in shape and composition of the body seem to be significant in relation to predisposition to particular diseases. Such variations are susceptible to modification by the diet. Therefore, the study of types of physique and the history of their development are of considerable interest to the nutritionist. However, in nutrition, the important issue is not the study of the phenomena of growth and development, which belong to the science of anthropology, but the study of how growth and development are modified by the diet.

There are technical difficulties in making visual records of relative changes in height and weight in relation to each other and a number of complicated systems have been devised for the purpose. A comparatively simple method was used successfully for many years in the Applied Nutrition Unit of the Colonial Office in Britain. This method is described here.

Children of school age increase their height on the average by approximately the same amount each year. Change in height can therefore be depicted by a graph using an arithmetical scale. Increase in weight is a result of gain in size in three dimensions and may be compared to the pattern of increase in size of a sphere. Thus, linear plots of change in weight cannot be made on an arithmetical scale. In fact, a close approximation to a linear progression is found by plotting changes in weight with age on a semilogarithmic graph. When, therefore, heights and weights are to be charted on the same graph a different scale has to be used for each dimension. In order to construct these scales and at the same time to provide a standard pattern of growth against which to assess the rate of growth of a child or of a group of children, the procedure is as follows:

1. Using arithmetical graph paper plot the mean heights against the corresponding mean weights of children chosen as a standard.

2. From this graph draw up a table in which mean weights in whole numbers, selected at appropriate intervals, are set against the corresponding mean heights. The purpose of (1) and (2) is to obtain whole numbers for the weight scale, because fractional numbers would be difficult to place on a scale. Fractional numbers on the height scale can be placed without difficulty, however.

3. Mark off on the ordinate of an arithmetical graph, or on a strip of card or plastic material, the series of weights and corresponding heights in the table.

4. Using the abscissa of the arithmetical graph for change in

Mean age (years)	No.	Weight (kg)	Height (cm)
6½	348	8.5	113.2
7½	579	20.9	120.2
8½	466	22.8	123.9
9½	383	24.9	128.5
i0½	339	28.1	134.3
11½	292	31.5	139.8
12½	188	35.3	144.8
13½	116	41.1	153.5

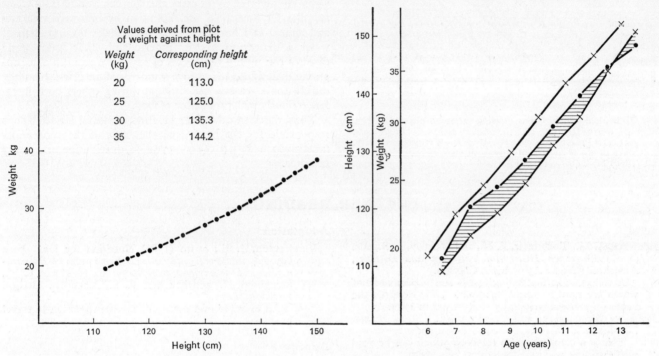

Values derived from plot of weight against height

Weight (kg)	Corresponding height (cm)
20	113.0
25	125.0
30	135.3
35	144.2

FIG. 50. Plotting changes in height and weight on the same graph. Construction of standard scales and growth of standard children. Comparison of standard pattern of growth with that of boys in Sarawak.
Left
Construction of standard scales for height and weight taken from Iowa Standards. [Baldwin, B. T. (1925) *Amer. J. phys. Anthropol.*, **8**, 1.]
Right
Pattern of growth of Chinese boys in Sarawak compared with Iowa standard. [Wadsworth, G. R. (1963) *Sarawak Museum Gaz.* **xi**, 307.]

age, plot the heights and weights against age for the standard group. A single line will result because the scales have been made so that values for height and weight at a particular age correspond.

5. On the same graph, and using the same scales, plot the heights and weights of the children under examination. Unless the size and change in shape are identical in the unknown and the standard group, different lines for changes in height and weight will be found. When children are lighter for a particular height than are those in the standard group, the line for weight will be placed lower on the graph than that for height. Reversal of the position of the respective lines would indicate children who were relatively heavy for their height. According to whether lines for change in height or weight are above or below the line for the standard, an assessment can be made of whether the children of the study are relatively large or small. The slope of the lines representing changes in height or weight indicate whether the rate of growth of the children is slower, similar or faster than that of the standard group.

An illustration of the method is given in FIGURE 50.

Standardization of symbols used in the graphs allows immediate interpretation. For example, height can always be represented by a dot (●) and weight by a cross (×); vertical hatching between lines for height and weight can indicate relative lightness for height, and horizontal hatching relative heaviness for height. In FIGURE 50 Chinese boys up to the age of 12½ years were relatively light, but at 13½ years they were relatively heavy. At all ages the Chinese boys were smaller in height and weight than the standard group, although the rate of change in size was approximately the same as that in the standard group.

An illustration of how the method of providing a visual record of the pattern of growth can be applied to identify the early onset of different shapes of the body is given in FIGURE 51.

There is a temptation to interpret relative heaviness as 'fatness'. However, records of height and weight by themselves do not give any information about body composition. The results of simultaneous measurements of skinfold thickness will assist in differentiating between obesity and overweight due to other causes [see also CHAPTER 35].

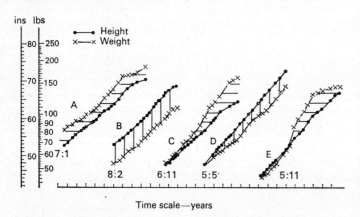

FIG. 51. Individual growth charts showing variety of physique types. A. Chronic overweight; B. Chronic underweight; C. Progressive overweight; D. Progressive underweight; E. Transient obesity. Figures refer to age in years and months at start of record. [Grant, M. W. (1966) *Med. Offr*, **115**, 331.]

WATER

In this chapter attention has been given to various aspects of food and human nutrition. Foods, however, cannot be produced in the absence of water, and foods which are most valuable in providing protein, namely those from animals, require much more water for their production than do vegetable foods. Continuous ingestion of water by humans is essential for life.

There is much concern about present and future shortages of food; actual and potential shortages of water are more serious. With the rapid growth of urbanization enormous quantities of water are diverted to industry and this can lead to insufficient supplies for household use. Pollution by industrial effluents and animal and human excreta often make the ingestion of water a danger to health. Enteric and other water-borne diseases can nullify the effects of expensive and difficult programmes designed to improve standards of nutrition. Flooding during some seasons and drought during others both interfere seriously with production of food.

Thus, the Medical Officer for Environmental Health who is responsible for the nutritional standards of the community must give attention to the conservation, distribution, and purity of water.

FURTHER READING

General

Beeuwkes, A. M., Todhunter, E. N., and Weigley, E. S., eds. (1967) *Essays on History of Nutrition and Dietetics*, American Dietetic Association, Chicago.

   A collection of fascinating essays and papers some of which are now historical 'landmarks', for example the paper on pellagra written by Goldberger in 1929.

Davidson, Sir Stanley, and Passmore, R. (1972) *Human Nutrition and Dietetics*, 5th ed., Edinburgh.

   This is a comprehensive textbook which can be read easily without previous specialized knowledge.

King, M. (1966) *Medical Care in Developing Countries*, Nairobi.

   This is a most useful practical manual which includes sections on nutritional problems in the context of clinical practice.

McHenry, E. W., and Beaton, G. H. (1963) *Basic Nutrition*, 2nd ed., London.

   The senior author, who for thirty years had experience of research and teaching of nutrition, states that this book was written for students in colleges, universities, and schools of nursing. It is a clear and comprehensive textbook.

Macy, I. C., Ershoff, B. H., McCay, C. M., Simonson, E., Schneider, H. A., and Samuels, L. T. (1951) *Nutrition Fronts in Public Health*, Proceedings of the Nutrition Symposium held at Yale University, 1950, National Vitamin Foundation, New York.

   Deals with a number of nutritional topics including nutrition and the process of ageing.

Thomson, W. A. R., and Garland, J., eds (1968) *Diet and Nutrition*, Symposium issue of the *Practitioner*, **201**, 283.

   A collection of essays on trace elements in health and disease and other nutritional topics written for the general practitioner.

World Health Organization (1973) *The Health Aspects of Food and Nutrition*, 2nd ed., Western Pacific Regional Office, Manila.

   Contains much detail of practical issues, including administration of nutritional activities, surveys, indicators of nutritional status, and sample recipes.

Adaptation

Vanderveen, J. E., *et al.* (1968) Nutrition for long space voyages, in *Fourth International Symposium of Bioastronautics and the Exploration of Space*, eds. Roadman, C. N., Strughold, H., and Mitchell, R. B., Aerospace Medical Division, Texas.

   An example of a metabolic study in relation to travel in space.

Appetite

Code, C. F., ed. (1967) Control of food and water intake, in *Handbook of Physiology*, Vol. 1, Section 6. Alimentary Canal, American Physiological Society, Washington, D.C.

   A complete review of all aspects of the subject including discussions on palatability, feeding habits and their origins, the regulation of the intake of water, and local and central mechanisms associated with ingestion of food.

Dietary Requirements

Department of Health and Social Security (1969) *Recommended Intakes of Nutrients for the United Kingdom*, London, H.M.S.O.

   The most recent document of this kind to be published. It contains references to other similar publications from other countries.

Durnin, J. V. G. A., and Passmore, R. (1967) *Energy, Work and Leisure*, London.

   A comprehensive, precise, and readable account of the amounts of energy used in all kinds of everyday activities.

Joint FAO/WHO *Ad Hoc* Expert Committee (1973) Energy and Protein Requirements, *Wld Hlth Org. techn. Rep. Ser.*, No. 522.

   This account is generally accepted as the basis for calculation of the food requirements of communities.

Dental Disease

Wadsworth, G. R. (1963) A survey of the relationship between diet and dental disease, *Dent. Hlth*, **3**, 8.

   A general review.

Fat

Brown, H. B. (1971) Food patterns that lower blood lipids in man, *J. Amer. diet. Ass.*, **58**, 303.
  This paper contains a useful review of the many different kinds of fat in the diet.

Sinclair, H. M., ed. (1958) *Essential Fatty Acids, Proceedings of the Fourth International Conference on Biochemical Problems of Lipids*, London.
  A symposium of a relatively new aspect of nutrition.

Foods

Anderson, T. A., and Fomon, S. J. (1971) Commercially prepared strained and junior foods for infants, *J. Amer. diet. Ass.*, **58**, 520.
  An examination of the variation in the constitution of commercial preparations for infant feeding. The results show that in conditions of modern life the mother may need special knowledge about nutrition in the interests of her infant.

Brink, M. F., Balsley, M., and Speckman, E. W. (1969) Nutritional value of milk compared with filled and imitation milk, *Amer. J. clin. Nutr.*, **22**, 168.
  Much detail is given of the compositions of whole cow's milk and different preparations of milk.

Cameron, A. G. (1971) *Food—Facts and Fallacies*, London.
  Straightforward discussions about the colour of bread, fluoridation of water supplies, food additives, and other topics related to nutritional problems in a sophisticated society.

Fox, A., ed. (1971) *Hygiene and Food Production*, Edinburgh.
  A collection of papers which discuss problems of food hygiene under modern conditions of farming. Of particular value to the public health officer responsible for control of nutrition and food supplies.

Grist, D. H. (1953) *Rice*, London.
  Detailed descriptions, including one on the disposition of nutrients in the grain of this important food, are given in Chapters 4, 14 and 15.

Lang, K. (1970) Influence of cooking on foodstuffs, *Wld Rev. Nutr. Diet.*, **12**, 266.
  A comprehensive review of the results of cooking of foods on their chemical constitution, vitamin losses, damage to protein, and enhancement of nutritional value.

Pyke, M. (1964) *Food Science and Technology*, London.
  An informative book, clearly written and well illustrated. A useful review for the medical officer not familiar with food science.

Standal, Bluebell R., Bassett, D. R., Policar, Purification B., and Thom, M. (1970) Fatty acids, cholesterol, and proximate analyses of some ready-to-eat foods, *J. Amer. diet. Ass.*, **56**, 392.
  A study of some processed foods, the results of which showed that different commercial products of the same material do not always have identical nutrient contents.

Wadsworth, G. R., and McKenzie, J. C. (1963) The potato with special reference to its use in the United Kingdom, *Nutr. Abstr. Rev.*, **33**, 327.
  A review which emphasizes the complex structure and the nutritional and economic implications of a 'simple' food.

Food and Nutrition Policies and Administration

Berg, A. D., and Levinson, F. J. (1969) A new need: the nutrition programmer, *Amer. J. clin. Nutr.*, **22**, 893.
  A discussion about the aims of nutritional policies and of the various ways in which malnutrition might be prevented on a community scale.

Lamont-Havers, R. W. (1968) Trends in human nutrition research, *J. Amer. diet. Ass.*, **52**, 300.
  A summary of the numerous projects involving nutrition and officially sponsored in the United States. The paper is a useful guide to health officers in deciding about nutritional activities, and the need for specialized research centres is illustrated. Activities are classified into three groups: normal nutrition; nutritional disorders; nutrition in specific diseases and states of stress.

Scott, M. L. (1953) *School Feeding: Its Contribution to Child Nutrition*, FAO Nutritional Studies No. 10, Rome.
  A practical consideration with a brief synopsis of school feeding programmes in different parts of the world.

Wadsworth, G. R. (1971) International work in nutrition: applied nutrition programmes, *J. trop. Med. Hyg.*, **74**, 211.
  A discussion about the objectives, organization, and content of the ANP, which is the usual form of nutritional project sponsored by international agencies.

Growth

Beal, V. A. (1969) Breast- and formula-feeding of infants, *J. Amer. diet. Ass.*, **55**, 31.
  One of the few objective studies of the diet in relation to growth during the first two years of life.

Grant, M.W. (1964) Individual variations in the rate of growth of children between the ages of five and fifteen years, *Med. Offr*, **112**, 37.

Grant, M. W. (1966) Juvenile obesity—chronic, progressive and transient, *Med. Offr*, **115**, 331.
  These two papers illustrate the practical use of the method described in the present chapter of charting growth. They provide valuable information about the different patterns of growth of children who were observed over a number of years.

Tanner, J. M. (1962) *Growth at Adolescence*, 2nd ed. London (reprinted 1969).
  A detailed review of growth of children, especially at adolescence.

Infant Nutrition

Gairdner, D., ed. (1965) *Recent Advances in Paediatrics*, London.
  Contains sections relevant to the nutritional state of the newborn and a detailed review of the pathological and biochemical changes found in kwashiorkor.

Toverud, K. V., Stearns, G., and Macy, I. G. (1950) *Maternal Nutrition and Child Health*, Bulletin No. 23, National Research Council, Washington, D.C.
  A world-wide survey of the knowledge at the time of writing of the nutritional status of the mother and its effect on the child. There are over 1,000 references.

Jelliffe, D. B. (1968) Infant nutrition in the tropics and subtropics, 2nd ed., *Wld Hlth Org. Monogr. Ser.*, No. 29.

Minerals

Underwood, E. J. (1962) *Trace Elements in Human and Animal Nutrition*, 2nd ed., New York.
  This is the standard work on the subject.

Nutrition and Disease

Johnston, J. A. (1953) *Nutritional Studies in Adolescent Girls and their Relationship to Tuberculosis*, Chicago, Ill.
  An important longitudinal study of protein and calcium metabolism in tuberculosis.

Puffer, R. R., and Serrano, C. V. (1973) *Patterns of Mortality in Childhood*, Washington.

Scrimshaw, N. S., Taylor, C. E., and Gordon, J. E. (1968) Interactions of nutrition and infection, *Wld Hlth Org. Monogr. Ser.*, No. 57.
  A comprehensive and authoritative review.

Wadsworth, G. R. (1971) Nutritional disorders: ischaemic heart disease, in *Medical Progress 1970/72, The British Encyclopaedia of Medical Practice*, ed. Richardson, Sir John, London, p. 204.
  An examination of present information about nutritional factors which may be involved in the aetiology of ischaemic heart disease.

Walker, W. F., and Johnston, I. D. A. (1971) *The Metabolic Basis of Surgical Care*, London.

Discussions on various physiological and biochemical mechanisms which are involved in the reaction of the body to disease and surgical operation. There is a special section on intravenous feeding and other aspects of nutrition in clinical practice.

Mönckeberg, F. (1973) Malnutrition and mental capacity, *Bol. ofic. sanit. panamer.* (English ed.), **7**, 93.

Nutrition Education

Beeuwkes, A. M. (1965) Nutrition education, *Wld Rev. Nutr. Diet.*, **5**, 1.

A comprehensive review of the subject.

Clements, F. W. (1956) *Report of an International Seminar on Education in Health and Nutrition, Baguio, 1955*, FAO Nutrition Meetings Report Series No. 13, Rome.

A valuable account which is still relevant to present-day problems.

Ritchie, J. A. S. (1967) *Learning Better Nutrition*, FAO Nutritional Studies No. 20, Rome (reprinted 1969).

A practical handbook for the public health worker.

Williams, P. C. (1965) *Suggestions for Speakers and Standards for Slides*, Institute of Biology, London.

A useful guide for those who, like public health nutritionists, have to speak to groups of people. The paper appeared originally in *Inst. Biol. J.* and copies are obtainable from the Institute of Biology, 41 Queen's Gate, London S.W.7.

Poisons in Foods

Belsey, M.A. (1973) Favism, *Bull. Wld Hlth Org.*, **48**, 1.

Jo Kian Tjaij, Djohan Aziz, Tjut Irawati, and Sahat Halim (1971) Accidental oral poisoning in two hospitals in Medan, *Paediat. Indones.*, **11**, 47.

A rare account of an outbreak of poisoning due to cassava.

Liener, I. E. (1969) *Toxic Constituents of Plant Foodstuffs*, New York.

An account of the many natural constituents of plants used as foods which are known to have adverse effects on health. Particular attention is given to products used to prevent deficiency of protein, for example, soya bean. Ways of eliminating poisons from foods are described.

Roe, F. J. C., ed. (1970) *Metabolic Aspects of Food Safety*, Oxford.

This book consists of papers on physiological and biochemical mechanisms involved in the metabolism of food and extraneous chemicals. Useful for reference purposes. See also references to CHAPTER 10.

Population, Sociology, and Economics

Banks, A. L., ed. (1954) *The Development of Tropical and Subtropical Countries, with Particular Reference to Africa*, London.

This report of an informal seminar contains much useful discussion on practical problems related to the improvement of standards of nutrition. The contribution of B. S. Platt on 'Food and its Production' will be found of particular interest.

Cipolla, C. M. (1962) *The Economic History of World Population*, Harmondsworth.

A small book which contains important analyses of total supplies of energy and energy requirements of the whole world, in the context of which requirements for food must be assessed.

Greaves, J. P., and Hollingsworth, D. F. (1966) Trends in food consumption in the United Kingdom, *Wld Rev. Nutr. Diet.*, **6**, 34.

An analysis of official records which illustrates how the kinds and amounts of foods consumed change with time.

Potts, M. (1971) Against nature: the use and misuse of birth control, *Med. Gynaec. Sociol.*, **5**, 6.

The author gives the history of the use of hormones in birth control and discusses the balance between population size, consumption of resources, productivity, and pollution.

Russell, Sir John (1954) *World Population and World Food Supplies*, London.

This book considers the special problems faced by different countries and gives many examples of how difficulties have been overcome and productivity increased.

Spengler, J. J. (1968) World hunger: past, present and prospective, *Wld Rev. Nutr. Diet.*, **9**, 1.

A review of the past history and future possibilities about the population of the world and its supply of food. Useful commentary notes and references are appended.

Pregnancy

Beal, V. A. (1971) Nutritional studies during pregnancy, *J. Amer. diet. Ass.*, **58**, 321.

A statistical analysis of the results of a study, which lasted 20 years, of associations between gain in weight of the mother during pregnancy and other maternal characteristics with the size at birth of the child.

Council on Foods and Nutrition: American Medical Association (1958) *Nutrition in Pregnancy*, Symposium IV, Chicago.

Contains detailed records of food intake, blood changes, weight gains, and other characteristics obtained from groups of women in the United States.

Protein

Allison, J. B., and Fitzpatrick, W. H. (1960) *Dietary Protein in Health and Disease*, Springfield, Ill.

This book explains clearly the basis for the assessment of the nutritional value of protein in food.

Platt, B. S. (1962) Proteins in nutrition, *Proc. roy. Soc. B*, **156**, 337.

A description of the many pathological changes produced by depletion of protein in the experimental animal.

Platt, B. S., Miller, D. S., and Payne, P. R. (1961) Protein values of human food, in *Recent Advances in Human Nutrition*, ed. Brock, J. F., p. 351, London.

An explanation of the concept of *net dietary protein–Calories per cent*.

Porter, J. W. G., and Rolls, B. A., eds, (1973) *Proteins in Human Nutrition*, London and New York.

Vitamins

Harris, L. J. (1955) *Vitamins in Theory and Practice*, 4th ed., London.

A readable and comprehensive account of the vitamins.

Water

Ferrando, R. (1969) The water problem, *Wld Rev. Nutr. Diet.*, **11**, 4.

A review of the water resources of the world, water requirements, water pollution, the use of water in agriculture, and modern techniques for obtaining increased supplies of water.

Publications of the World Health Organization

Committees are convened, sometimes at regular intervals, by the WHO to discuss nutritional problems. Summaries of the discussions are published. The publications are small, clearly written and they represent the opinions of world authorities. A list of some of these reports of particular value to the student of nutrition in public health is given here.

Prevention and treatment of severe malnutrition in times of disaster (1951) *Wld Hlth Org. techn. Rep. Ser.*, No. 45.

Calcium requirements (1962) *Wld Hlth Org. tech. Rep. Ser.*, No. 230.

The public health aspects of the use of antibiotics (1963) *Wld Hlth Org. techn. Rep. Ser.*, No. 260.

Expert committee on the medical assessment of nutritional status (1963) *Wld Hlth Org. techn. Rep. Ser.*, No. 258.

Medicine and public health in the Arctic and Antarctic: selected papers from a conference (1963) *Wld Hlth Org. Publ. Hlth Pap.*, No. 18.

Physiology of lactation (1965) *Wld Hlth Org. techn. Rep. Ser.*, No. 305.

Protein requirements (1965) *Wld Hlth Org. techn. Rep. Ser.*, No. 301.

Nutrition in pregnancy and lactation (1965) *Wld Hlth Org. techn. Rep. Ser.*, No. 302.

Methods of planning and evaluation in applied nutrition programmes (1966) *Wld Hlth Org. techn. Rep. Ser.*, No. 340.

Requirements of vitamin A, thiamine, riboflavine and niacin (1967) *Wld Hlth Org. techn. Rep. Ser.*, No. 362.

Nutritional anaemias (1968) *Wld Hlth Org. techn. Rep. Ser.*, No. 405.

Requirements of ascorbic acid, vitamin D, vitamin B_{12}, folate and iron (1970) *Wld Hlth Org. techn. Rep. Ser.*, No. 452.

Joint FAO/WHO Expert Committee on Nutrition (1971) *Wld Hlth Org. techn. Rep. Ser.*, No. 477.

Evaluation of food additives; specifications for the identity and purity of flood additives and their technological evaluation; some extraction solvents and certain other substances; and a review of the technological efficacy of some antimicrobial agents (1971) *Wld Hlth Org. techn. Rep. Ser.*, No. 462.

Food fortification; protein–calorie malnutrition (1971) *Wld Hlth Org. techn. Rep. Ser.*, No. 477.

Nutrition: a review of the WHO programme in nutrition (1972) *WHO Chronicle*, **26**, 160, 195.

Nutritional deficiencies (1973) *WHO Chronicle*, **27**, 355.

Energy and Protein requirements (1973) *WHO Chronicle*, **27**, 481.

Is there a protein problem? (1973) *WHO Chronicle*, **27**, 487.

The problem of malnutrition (1974) Bengoa, J. M., *WHO Chronicle*, **28**, 3.

Stanbury J. B., *et al.* (1974) Endemic goitre and cretinism: public health significance and prevention, *Wld Hlth Org. Chron.*, **28**, 220.

12

HEALTH HAZARDS OF IONIZING RADIATIONS AND RADIOACTIVE SUBSTANCES

JOHN C. COLLINS

Introduction

The siting of nuclear power stations and the testing of nuclear weapons in the atmosphere excite intense inquiry about the ensuing status of the public health. Interest in this branch of public health is sharpened not only by remembrance of the devastating effects of the small atomic bombs dropped over Hiroshima and Nagasaki but also by a realization that the problems are unique, in that they endanger future generations as well as the present. For these reasons, such exceptional attention is often given to radiation problems that there is danger of losing a proper perspective by which the risks may be judged and compared with more established and conventional risks.

The public health profession is pressed frequently to provide a simple explanation of the hazards, in a branch which spans medicine, physics, chemistry, engineering, and the law. However, it is only within the recent past that the development of controlled fission for electricity generation, of uncontrolled fusion in nuclear weapons, and of the use of radioisotopes in medicine, industry, and research have expanded so rapidly that public health authorities must take serious cognizance of the issues involved. Experience is limited, therefore, and much has yet to be learned, particularly in the areas of special public health concern, where interest centres on the existence of thresholds and the effects on human tissues of chronic radiation exposure at low dose-rates.

RADIOISOTOPES AND THEIR RADIATIONS

A radioisotope is denoted by its chemical name followed by its mass number, which is the total number of protons and neutrons in the nuclei of the isotope. Strontium-90 is one of a number of isotopes of the chemical element strontium, and it has a mass number of 90. There are seventeen other isotopes of strontium; five of them are stable, that is non-radioactive, and occur in the natural environment, and the rest are radioactive and may be produced artificially. Strontium-89 is radioactive, and with strontium-90 is produced by the fission of uranium-235 or plutonium-239. It appears in fall-out, therefore, and the ratio of strontium-89 to strontium-90 indicates the age of the fall-out since the fission occurred, because strontium-89 has a short half-life and strontium-90 has a long one.

The hazard likely to arise from an isotope will depend upon the types of radiations which it emits, the energies at which they are emitted, and the quantity of the isotope. Radioisotopes emit one or more of the three types of radiation known as alpha, beta, and gamma radiation. Some isotopes emit all three, others only one or two. In general, alpha radiation does not present any external radiation hazard, since the alpha particles are not able to penetrate human skin. However, the particles lose their energy very rapidly in a short track length, and alpha emitters are particularly hazardous if taken into the body and assimilated in body organs. Beta radiation can present an external radiation hazard, because most beta particles are able to penetrate human skin, but they are shielded with relative ease, and may be completely stopped by only a quarter inch of perspex. Beta emitters also are particularly hazardous if metabolized in the body organs following ingestion or inhalation. Gamma radiation creates the most serious external radiation problem, and several inches of lead are required to stop gamma radiation altogether. Gamma radiation from sources within the body is relatively less hazardous.

The energy at which the radiations are emitted is also a guide to the potential hazard of a radioisotope. Alpha radiation is always emitted at specific energies and, though this is usually of the order of 5 megaelectronvolts (MeV) per alpha particle, there are a few isotopes which emit alphas at higher energies. Beta radiation, on the other hand, is emitted in a spectrum of energies as shown in FIGURE 52, and the energy quoted for beta

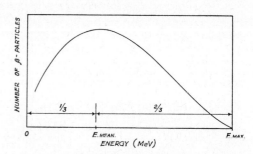

FIG. 52. Typical spectrum of β-particle energies.

radiation is the maximum of that spectrum. The mean energy of emission, which is used in calculating radiation dose-rates, may be taken as one-third of the maximum energy. Strontium-90 is a 'pure' beta emitter and does not emit alpha or gamma radiations. It has a quoted beta energy of 0·54 MeV. This is the maximum energy of the beta-particle spectrum emitted, and the mean energy is 0·18 MeV. Gamma radiation is emitted like alpha radiation at specific energy levels. The energy range is from a few keV (1 keV = 10^{-3} MeV) to 3 or 4 MeV and occasionally higher.

The quantity of radioactivity associated with an isotope is given by the rate at which its nuclei disintegrate and release the radiations. The standard quantity is known as the curie, which is commonly abbreviated to Ci. This is defined as a disintegration rate equivalent to 37×10^9 disintegrations per second (or 2.2×10^{12} disintegrations per minute). A curie of radioactivity is a large quantity and is likely to present considerable risks. It is necessary, therefore, to use units denoting small fractions of the curie, such as the millicurie (1 mCi = 10^{-3} Ci), the microcurie (1 μCi = 10^{-6} Ci), and the picocurie (1 pCi = 10^{-12} Ci). In public health work the picocurie is used frequently, but analysis of samples with these very low levels of contamination is difficult. A picocurie is equal only to 2.2 nuclear disintegrations per minute, and these may have to be detected against an instrument background of 10 counts per minute.

As the disintegration of a quantity of radioactive material continues, its radioactivity becomes less. The length of time after which only one-half of the original activity remains is known as the half-life. Each isotope has its own characteristic half-life, which is constant and cannot be altered. Thus, if it is possible to measure the half-life of an unknown contaminant with sufficient accuracy the isotope can probably be defined with confidence. For example, strontium-89 has a half-life of 51 days and strontium-90 one of 28 years. Half-lives vary from fractions of a microsecond up to millions of millions of years.

The decay of a radioisotope causes its conversion into another isotope of a different chemical element. It is usual to refer to the 'parent' isotope and its 'daughter' products in a decay chain. When the first daughter is also radioactive it, too, will decay, though with its own characteristic radiations and half-life. The final product of the decay chain will be stable, that is non-radioactive.

$$\text{Radium-226} \xrightarrow[1620 \text{ y}]{\alpha\beta\gamma} \text{Radon-222 (gas)} \xrightarrow[3.8 \text{ d}]{\alpha\gamma}$$

$$\text{Polonium-218} \xrightarrow[3.1 \text{ m}]{\alpha\beta} \text{Lead-214} \xrightarrow[26.8 \text{ m}]{\beta\gamma} \cdots \longrightarrow$$

$$\text{Lead-206 (stable)}$$

FIG. 53. Decay chain with half-lives of radium-226.

FIGURE 53 shows part of the long decay chain of the naturally occurring isotope radium-226. Occasionally, as in the production of radon-222, a daughter may be in gaseous form, even though both its parent and its own daughter are solid. Particular care must then be taken to provide good ventilation of any storage place.

$$\text{Strontium-90} \xrightarrow[28 \text{ y}]{\beta} \text{Yttrium-90} \xrightarrow[64.2 \text{ h}]{\beta} \text{Zirconium-90}$$

$$\text{(stable)}$$

FIG. 54. Decay chain with half-lives of strontium-90.

Equilibrium between parent and daughter is established when the daughter decays as fast as it is formed. FIGURE 54 shows the decay chain of strontium-90, an isotope formed artificially in nuclear fission. The yttrium-90 daughter in this chain builds up to 99 per cent. of its equilibrium concentration after $2\frac{1}{2}$ weeks, and there is then as much yttrium-90 activity as there is strontium-90 activity.

The radiotoxicity of an isotope is dependent not only on its physical half-life but also upon its biological half-life. The biological half-life is defined as the period of time in which one-half of the radioactivity absorbed in the human body would be excreted. The combination of the physical and biological half-lives is known as the effective half-life of an isotope, and this is calculated from the equation:

$$\frac{1}{T} = \frac{1}{T_r} \times \frac{1}{T_b}$$

where
T = effective half-life;
T_r = physical half-life;
T_b = biological half-life.

When either T_r or T_b is short compared to the other, then it will predominate in the above equation and the effective half-life will be close to the shorter value.

THE PRODUCTS OF NUCLEAR FISSION

When uranium is fissioned by slow neutrons, as in the core of a nuclear reactor or in the detonator to the hydrogen bomb, about 200 fission products are produced, all of which are radioactive. FIGURE 55 gives the distribution of fission products

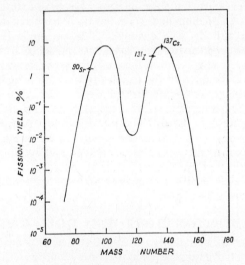

FIG. 55. Fission yield spectrum.

by mass number and shows that strontium-90, iodine-131, and caesium-137 are all produced in relatively large proportions. These three isotopes are of particular importance.

Strontium-90 is important because it tends to follow calcium through the food chains and accumulates in bone, whence both its own beta radiation and that of its daughter yttrium-90 can irradiate the bone marrow. It may therefore be a contributory factor in the induction of leukaemia. Because bone cells have a relatively slow rate of turnover, strontium-90 lodged in human bone may be regarded as being permanently sited, and it will irradiate the bone marrow for the remainder of the individual's life. The biological half-life of this isotope in the bone is thus long as well as its physical half-life, and there will be virtually no elimination from the site of deposition.

Iodine-131 is important in fresh fission products because it is deposited on grassland, whence it is easily ingested by grazing cattle and transferred to the milk supply. When taken into the body by infants drinking cows' milk about one-half accumulates in the thyroid. At the age of 6 months not only is a human drinking more milk (about one litre) than at any other subsequent time in life but also the ratio of thyroid mass to total body mass is a minimum. Any iodine deposited in the thyroid will effect the maximum amount of damage by irradiation from the beta particles. However, iodine has a short radioactive half-life of 8 days and, though the biological half-life in the thyroid is 138 days, the resultant effective half-life of 7·6 days means that elimination is fairly rapid.

Caesium-137 presents yet another problem, in that it is distributed uniformly throughout body tissues and will therefore contribute to the irradiation of the gonads as well as of the bone marrow. This isotope is thus of genetic significance, and is a principal contributor to the genetic damage in a population irradiated by fall-out. It has a long radioactive half-life of 30 years and a biological half-life in the total body of 70 days.

Neutrons released in fission produce radioisotopes by being absorbed into the nuclei of stable atoms. Activation products are thus produced, and these can form a substantial part of the total contamination in a fall-out cloud. It is apparent that some nuclear weapons tests produce considerably less fall-out contamination than do others. A 'clean' bomb is said to be one in which the proportion of fission detonator power to total fusion power is a minimum and which has been detonated at a considerable altitude. The quantities of fission products and of activation products from irradiated dust and debris are thereby kept low. At a high altitude the activation products are reduced considerably and with the fission products are forced by the heat of the explosion into the stratosphere. Here they are held in the circulating wind streams, and they filter through to the troposphere only slowly. The transfer from stratosphere to troposphere occurs with greater rapidity in the spring than at other times of the year. For this reason, and because at this time cattle are turned on to rapidly growing pastures, fall-out levels in milk tend to rise in the months of May and June in the Northern hemisphere.

RADIATION DOSE AND DOSE-RATE

A quantity of radiation energy absorbed in a quantity of tissue is a radiation dose. Units of dose are expressed, therefore, as an energy density, that is as energy per unit mass. The unit used is the rad (r), which is defined as the dose delivered by the absorption of 100 ergs per gram of absorbing medium. A smaller unit of dose representing one-thousandth of the above unit is the millirad (mr), and dose-rates are commonly expressed as millirads per hour (mr/h). The absorbing medium should be specified.

The early unit for measurement of dose was the Roentgen (R), which is defined in terms of the ability of gamma or X-radiation to ionize air. It is therefore an exposure dose which would be received by a person standing in the position in air where a measurement or a calculation has been made. It can be shown that 1 milliRoentgen (mR) = 0·87 mr in air = 0·95 mr in tissue.

The absorbed dose in millirads is only an expression of the physical dose, and does not describe the amount of biological damage which is likely to ensue. This will be dependent on the 'linear energy transfer' of the radiation which gives the density of deposition of energy per unit length of track. It is necessary, therefore, to specify a dose equivalent with the unit 'rem', which is an abbreviation for 'rad equivalent in man'. This dose equivalent is obtained by multiplying the absorbed dose (mr) by a quality factor corresponding to the linear energy transfer of the radiation. Thus Dose Equivalent (mrems) = Absorbed Dose (mr) × Quality Factor (QF). In practice, QF = 1 for all gamma and beta radiations except the low-energy beta radiations from tritium, for which QF = 1·7. For alpha radiation QF = 10. Thus an absorbed dose from alpha contamination within the body may be considered to be ten times as hazardous as an equivalent absorbed dose from beta–gamma contamination.

In order to calculate the radiation dose-rate from a radioactive source it is necessary to know the isotope, the energies of the radiations which it emits, and their frequencies. Frequencies are quoted in physical tables as a percentage against each of the known energy values. The procedure is to obtain a mean effective energy of emission by weighting each separate radiation energy by the frequency with which it is emitted and by summing the total of these weighted frequencies. For example, the effective beta and gamma energies of iodine-131 are calculated as follows:

β Energies			γ Energies		
MeV	Per cent.	Effective MeV	MeV	Per cent.	Effective MeV
0·25	2·5	0·007	0·08	2·2	0·002
0·33	9·3	0·031	0·28	6·3	0·018
0·61	87·2	0·532	0·36	79·0	0·284
0·81	0·7	0·006	0·64	9·3	0·060
			0·72	2·8	0·020
		0·576			0·384

$$\text{Mean effective } \beta \text{ energy} = \frac{0\cdot576}{3}$$
$$= 0\cdot19 \text{ MeV}$$
$$\text{Effective } \gamma \text{ energy} = 0\cdot38 \text{ MeV}$$

The simplest case for calculating the radiation dose from a radioactive source is that which obtains when the source is at a point. The following formulae give the approximate dose-rates 1 metre from a point source of beta and gamma activity respectively:

$$D_\beta = 30 \text{ C}$$

where D_β = beta dose-rate at 1 metre (mr/h);

   C = beta activity (mCi).

It will be seen that no energy term is included in the above formula. This is because beta radiations do not penetrate far in tissue and all their energy is deposited. The greater their range, however, the greater is the mass of tissue irradiated and the energy deposition per unit mass remains reasonably constant.

$$D_\gamma = 0\cdot6 \text{ C E}$$

where D_γ = gamma dose-rate at 1 metre (mr/h);

   C = gamma activity (mCi);

   E = effective gamma energy (MeV).

If the above two-point source equations are used in practice, even when the activity is distributed somewhat, then the result obtained will give an overestimate of the radiation dose-rate and will thus err on the side of safety. The dose-rate at any distance other than 1 metre may be estimated by using the inverse square law. Thus $D\gamma$ at x metres $= (D\gamma$ at 1 metre$)/x^2$.

An alternative method of estimating directly the gamma dose-rate from a point source is to use the specific gamma ray constant for the isotope. Values for the constant may be found in the standard texts, and are quoted usually in Roentgens per millicurie per hour at 1 centimetre. The inverse square law may be used as above to obtain the dose-rate at other distances.

NATURAL BACKGROUND RADIATION

The addition of small quantities of radioactive isotopes as contaminants in the environment does not bring radioactivity into the environment for the first time. There has always been a natural level of background activity due to radioactive elements present in the rocks and soil of the earth, some of which are taken up into food crops and are dissolved into drinking-water supplies. We are concerned to ensure that the addition to this natural background by artificial isotopes discharged in waste, or arriving by fall-out from nuclear weapons tests, should not increase the natural levels beyond such as are tolerable to our populations. However, it must be remembered that some degree of contamination has always existed, as has some small degree of external irradiation of man.

The background radioactivity to which we are subject arises from two principal sources. First, there is the gamma radiation emanating principally from the potassium, uranium, thorium, and radium compounds and their daughter products in the earth's crust and in the soil. The radium decaying to radon and the thorium decaying to thoron release their radioactive daughters into the atmosphere, so that there is a general level of natural radioactive 'pollution' which we breathe from day to day. The gamma radiation from the soil varies in intensity from place to place, depending on the actual composition of the soil and rocks. As shown in TABLE 38, the older igneous rocks of the earth tend to have greater concentrations of radioactive material than the more recent metamorphic and sedimentary deposits.

The rocks are broken down by weathering to form the soil, and our crops growing in the soil become naturally contaminated. The contamination is principally in the form of potassium, since in all natural potassium 0·01 per cent. is of the radioisotope potassium-40. This is a beta–gamma emitter with a half-life of 10^9 years. Some radioactive carbon-14 is also present, formed by the action of cosmic radiation on atmospheric nitrogen. Carbon-14 is a pure beta emitter with a half-life of 5570 years. Our food supplies are thus contaminated naturally, and we ourselves become radioactive by metabolizing this potassium and carbon, and to a lesser extent some radium and uranium. We carry with us, therefore, an internal burden of radioactive contamination which contributes to our total radiation dose.

The second source of natural radiation exposure is the cosmic rays incident upon earth from outer space. They are attenuated by the earth's atmosphere, and at high altitudes, where the atmosphere is thin, cosmic radiation dose-rates are much higher than they are at sea-level. TABLE 41 gives the variation in gonadal dose-rates with altitude. There is also a small variation in cosmic radiation exposure between the equator and the poles of the earth, to which the cosmic radiation particles are attracted. The sea-level dose-rate is about 4 per cent. higher at the poles than at the equator.

TABLE 41
Background Radiation

Source	Radiation	Radioisotope	Dose-rate to gonads (mrems/y)	
			Typical values	Possible average
Igneous rock	γ	Potassium-40 Thorium Uranium Radium $\}$	40 40 20	45
			Total: 100	
Sedimentary rock	γ	As above	Total: 20	
Internally deposited isotopes	$\beta\gamma$	Potassium-40 Carbon-14 $\}$ Radium $\}$	19 1	20
			Total: 20	
Cosmic radiations	Neutrons and charged particles	*Altitude (ft.)* Sea-level 5000 10,000 20,000 50,000	35 50 100 400 4000	35
			Grand total:	100 mrems/y

Assimilation of carbon-14 from the atmosphere into growing trees has made it possible in recent years to establish a method of dating articles made from old timbers. The specific activity of the carbon in the timber (pCi carbon-14/g. total carbon) at the time the tree was felled is known, since growing timber contains a fixed proportion of carbon-14. After felling, the ratio of carbon-14 to total carbon in the wood decreases in accordance with the half-life decay of the carbon-14. By measuring the new specific activity of the timber which is to be dated, the decay time can be calculated, and this is the age of the wood.

LIMITATION OF BIOLOGICAL RISKS OF IRRADIATION

The exposure of an individual to radiation produces risks which are different in character to those arising from exposure of the population. A clear distinction must be drawn between the somatic and the genetic risks. FIGURE 56 shows how the risks may be subdivided and how this leads to the derivation of the various upper limits of radiation dose used in radiological control. Subdivision of the somatic risks characterizes the biological effects produced by acute and by chronic exposures and reflects the ability of tissue to repair a moderate degree of radiation damage. Genetic damage, whether by mutation or by chromosome breakage, is considered irreparable, and the probability of a specified effect appearing in a subsequent generation is dependent on the total radiation dose received, whether by acute or by chronic exposures.

The assessment of likely damage to a population, or of the probability of harm to an individual, would be obtained ideally from a graph relating the risk-rate of a specified biological effect to the radiation dose absorbed in man. There is considerable experience of the somatic risks of acute exposure; this has

irradiation of human tissue results in some energy deposition in the cells, and this must produce at the least a local effect. There is also some probability that a further effect may be induced either in an organ or in the body itself.

The International Commission on Radiological Protection (I.C.R.P.) specify radiation doses to the whole body and to different organs, which should not be exceeded. Their recommendations are exclusive of doses received from natural background and from exposure to medical diagnosis or therapy.

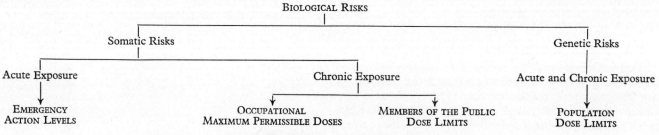

FIG. 56. The limitation of biological risks.

been obtained from the follow-up studies of the survivors of the two Japanese atomic bombs and from studies of those who have been involved in serious reactor accidents. As a result, emergency action levels may be specified, such as those used in civil defence or in pre-planning for reactor emergencies. These are maximum levels for use only under accident conditions by rescue workers who may be able to save life without themselves becoming casualties from exposure to very high doses. By contrast, evidence of the somatic risks of chronic exposure is very limited and is confined to a few specific occupational circumstances in which there appears to have been a definite relationship between exposure under working conditions and a subsequent clinical effect attributable to the radiation. The occupational maximum permissible doses are set at such levels that there is a negligible probability of employees being affected by exposure during their work. The dose limits for individual members of the public are set at one-tenth of the occupational doses, because the latter are not under the special medical supervision required for workers in the atomic energy industries.

There is no human experience of the genetic effects of radiation because the use of radioisotopes and the development of nuclear fission have not been continuing for long enough on a scale which could reveal adverse effects in the population. The gaps in our knowledge are partly filled by inference from the results of animal experiments, which provide tentative values for doubling doses (doses which double the probability of a specified effect) and some evidence that there is no threshold dose below which harmful mutations will not be produced. Thus the smallest dose may cause a genetic mutation, and this will carry a very high probability of being harmful. For this reason and because the mutation will increase the genetic load in future generations for whom we have a special responsibility, population genetics are of overriding importance. They provide the most limiting conditions on the uses of ionizing radiations and govern the establishment of population dose limits used in the control of exposure of the general public.

Dose limits and maximum permissible doses cannot be regarded as absolutely safe working limits. Even low-level

The former are unavoidable, and the benefits of the latter are so great as to outweigh by far the risks incurred. The Commission recognizes that 'any departure from the environmental conditions in which man has evolved may entail a risk of deleterious effects. It is therefore assumed that long continued exposure to ionising radiation additional to that due to natural background involves some risk.' Since man cannot dispense with the use of the radiations, risks must be balanced against benefits. The maximum permissible dose is therefore one which carries a negligible probability of serious somatic or genetic damage, either to an individual or to a whole population.

The Commission's recommendations fall into two parts. First, there are the limiting organ burdens and the associated body burdens of the isotopes, which are calculated from the permissible organ doses using available radiobiological data. This part of the recommendations is fundamental. Secondly, there are the limits for concentrations of radioisotopes in drinking water and in air, which are derived from the model of a standard man. These values are to be used with judgement according to circumstances, and form the basis of calculating the 'derived working levels' of radioisotopic contaminants in the environment.

GENETICALLY SIGNIFICANT DOSES

A genetically significant dose is the average dose per head of a population up to the mean age of child bearing, usually taken as 30 years. It may be calculated for certain known exposures in the United Kingdom as follows:

Background radiation:

Average gonadal dose 100 mrems/y × 30 y = 3 rems

Medical exposures:

Average gonadal dose 19 mrems/y × 30 y = 0·6 rems

The I.C.R.P. has recommended that the genetically significant dose from all other sources of exposure shall not exceed 5 rems. It is emphasized that this is to be an average through the whole population and must include the received bydoses workers occupationally exposed in the atomic energy industry, who may be receiving substantially more than 5 rems by the age of 30. In order that the average per head of population shall not exceed this figure, it is necessary to limit the exposure of the general public to a more restrictive value. For purposes of setting maximum permissible doses and dose limits, the population is divided into three categories. The contributions of each to the genetically significant dose of the whole population may be calculated by assuming that their maximum permissible gonadal doses are attained as follows:

1. Occupational Workers

Employment in this category not normally commenced before age 18. Maximum permissible cumulative dose governed by the expression $5(N - 18)$ rems, where N is the age in years.

Expression implies a maximum permissible dose =
$$(5 \text{ rems/y} \times 12 \text{ y}) = 60 \text{ rems by age 30.}$$

If this category is restricted in number to 2 per cent. of the population, its contribution to the population genetically significant dose = $0.02 \times 60 = 1$ rem.

2. Adult Workers not Directly Engaged in Radiation Work

Employment in this category not normally commenced before age 18.

Maximum permissible dose = 1.5 rems/y giving a limit of
$$(1.5 \text{ rems/y} \times 12 \text{ y}) = 18 \text{ rems by age 30.}$$

If this category is restricted in number to 3 per cent. of the population, its contribution to the population genetically significant dose = $0.03 \times 18 = 0.5$ rem.

3. General Public

Dose from internal contamination limited to 0·01 of dose to occupational workers.

Contributions to the population genetically significant dose =
$$0.01 \times 5 \text{ rems/y} \times 30 \text{ y} = 1.5 \text{ rems.}$$

Dose from external irradiation to be kept to a minimum Allowance for contribution to genetically significant dose = 0·5 rem.

The total of these separate contributions to the genetically significant dose of the population represents the average dose per head from all sources of radiation and = $1 + 0.5 + 1.5 + 0.5 = 3.5$ rems. This is below the I.C.R.P. recommended maximum dose of 5 rems, and thus leaves a factor of safety.

MAXIMUM PERMISSIBLE DOSES AND DOSE LIMITS

Control of occupational radiation levels is easier when dose-rates are expressed in millirems per hour. For occupational workers an average annual maximum permissible dose of 5 rems may be represented as 100 millirems per week on the basis of a 50-week working year. Assuming exposure throughout a 40-hour week, this becomes 2·5 millirems per hour. Similarly, for the adults not directly engaged in radiation work, 1·5 rems per year becomes 30 millirems per week or 0·75 millirems per hour.

Maximum permissible doses for occupational workers and dose limits for individual members of the public are given in TABLES 42 and 43. These values may be adjusted to suit short

TABLE 42
Maximum Permissible Doses
(Excluding natural background and medical exposures)
Occupational Workers

Part of body	Rems per 13 weeks	Rems per year	Remarks
Whole body, gonads, blood-forming organs	3*	5†	With a max. permissible cumulative dose of 5 rems (age in years—18)
Other internal organs, eye lenses	8	15	
Skin, bone, and thyroid	15	30	
Hands, forearms, feet, and ankles	38	75	

* Limited to 1·3 rems/13 weeks for women of reproductive capacity.
† For design purposes, whole body exposure rates in the working environment shall not normally exceed:

5 rems per year, or
100 millirems per week, or
2·5 millirems per hour

TABLE 43
Dose Limits
(Excluding natural background and medical exposures)
Members of the Public

Part of body	Rems per year	Remarks
Whole body, gonads, blood-forming organs	0·5	1·5 rems/y* for adult workers not directly engaged in radiation work
Other internal organs, eye lenses	1·5	
Skin and bone (except of hands, forearms, feet, and ankles) and thyroid	3·0	1·5 rems/y to thyroid of children up to age 16
Hands, forearms, feet and ankles	7·5	

* For design purposes, whole body exposure rates shall not normally exceed:

1·5 rems per year, or
30 millirems per week, or
0·75 milirems per hour

periods of exposure. Thus, if the whole body exposure of an occupational worker was known to be limited to 2 hours per week theoretically it could be received at the rate of 50 millirems per hour. However, the I.C.R.P. emphasize that maximum permissible doses are maximum values and recommends that 'all doses be kept as low as practicable, and that any unnecessary exposures be avoided'.

RADIATION EXPOSURES OF THE GENERAL PUBLIC

In Western Europe and the United States the medical use of X-rays and radioisotopes is by far the most important man-made addition to the genetically significant dose of a population. The use of diagnostic X-rays for routine chest examination is now very commonplace, and the benefits which accrue to the public health far outweigh the risks incurred from irradiation. The doses received from therapeutic uses of X-rays and gamma rays are very much higher, but a relatively small number of patients are treated in this way. The over-all contribution to the genetically significant dose arising from medical exposures is shown in TABLE 44. It amounts to about 20

TABLE 44

Genetically Significant Dose-rates from Medical Exposures

Procedure	U.K. (1958) (mrems per year)	U.S.A. (1964) (mrems per year)
Diagnostic . . .	14	55
Therapeutic . .	5	7
Total . . .	19	62

per cent. of the natural background radiation in the United Kingdom and about 60 per cent. in the United States.

The entire surface of the world is now covered with fall-out from the nuclear weapons tests that have taken place in the last 20 years, and it is impossible for the public to avoid ingestion and inhalation of some degree of artificial radioactive contamination from this source. In addition, gamma-emitting isotopes deposited on the ground will produce external irradiation and must also be taken into account in assessing the genetically significant dose. A reservoir of the long half-life (long-lived) fission products remains in the stratosphere, and these isotopes will percolate through to the troposphere in the course of the next few decades. These will continue to be a source of contamination in the next generation. Fortunately, the number of nuclear weapons detonated up to early 1972 has not yet produced levels of environmental contamination causing a serious public health risk. TABLE 45 gives the dose com-

TABLE 45

Estimated Dose Commitment to United Kingdom population 1966–2000 from Weapons Tests Fall-out

Source	Bone marrow (mr)	Gonads (mr)
Strontium-90	40	—
Caesium-137	50	50
Carbon-14	13	13
Short half-life isotopes . .	17	17
Total	120	80

mitment from 1966 to the year 2000 from all nuclear weapons tests. The table shows that the genetic dose commitment during this period is of the same order as the natural background radiation in any single year. The genetically significant dose-rate from this source in 1963 was about 12 mrems per year, but with the abandonment of atmospheric testing by the major nations, this figure had dropped to 3 mrems per year in 1966, and was still at this level in 1972.

The general public should not be allowed unrestricted access to atomic energy establishments, and proper security pro-

cedures should ensure that they do not receive external radiation exposure from this source. However, all industries produce waste materials, and low-level radioactive waste is discharged both into the atmosphere and into rivers and the sea by chemical plants and laboratories engaged in radioisotope work. These discharges are made under the strictest control, but there is, nevertheless, at least a degree of risk that very small quantities of radioactive contamination may enter the diet through the contamination, for example, of fish or food crops. These risks are kept to the lowest possible order by the enforcement of the most rigorous administrative and technical controls. High-level radioactive wastes, such as are produced at nuclear fuel processing plants are treated and stored permanently on site, in order to ensure absolutely that there can be no risk to the public health.

The radiation doses received by occupational workers contribute to the population's genetically significant dose, because the mutated genes in this small group will be passed ultimately to the whole population by intermarriage. On the assumption that the average gonadal dose-rate to occupational workers is 0·5 rem per year and that in neither the United Kingdom nor the United States is this group yet more than 0·1 per cent. of the total population, the maximum genetically significant dose-rate from this source is 0·5 millirem per year.

A very large number of radioactive consignments is now transported daily by road, rail, sea, and air and through the postal services. They are packaged and labelled in accordance with the recommendations of the International Atomic Energy Agency, which are incorporated in agency regulations specific to the mode of transport. The various regulations are designed to ensure that, in the event of a serious accident, there is only a remote risk of contamination or serious radiation exposure to any member of the public or of the transport agency's staff. Relatively few of the consignments are of large quantities of radioactivity, such as irradiated nuclear fuel elements or multi-curie irradiation sources, and in these cases extra precautions are taken, both with regard to the packaging and also in the pre-planning of the route that the transport vehicle will follow. In many countries emergency plans have been drawn up for action following an accident to a vehicle carrying radioactivity. The risk of an accident to a road vehicle is now high, and the emergency plans for isolating the area of the accident and dealing with localized contamination have already been put into practice in many places. It is essential that such plans be made.

There are a number of additional sources of possible exposure of the public to ionizing radiations, all of lesser significance than those so far described. Television sets operating at high voltages emit X-rays, though the highest dose-rates are to be found at the back of the set, rather than at the front. Manufacturers of the sets are recommended to ensure that the dose-rates shall not exceed 0·5 mrem per hour on the outside surface of equipment to which maintenance engineers shall have access. Colour television, operating at even higher voltages, creates more of a problem than does black-and-white television. A further source of intense X-irradiation of the public is the use of shoe-fitting fluoroscopes, sometimes called pedoscopes. These are generally the subject of strict design control and should incorporate a time-limiting device to switch off the X-ray beam after about 5 seconds. This should ensure that the doses received by the customer and the fitter are within the limits recommended by I.C.R.P. for members of the public. The use of radioactive material and X-rays in schools and colleges is now very widespread in many countries, and the potential hazards are considerable. The experimental work undertaken by the children should be supervised very closely by persons experienced in radiological protection, and the safe storage of radioisotopes should be the special responsibility of a member of the school staff. Additional irradiation may arise from luminous watches and clocks and from the use of instruments and devices incorporating small quantities of radioactivity. TABLE 46 summarizes the total genetically significant dose to a population.

TABLE 46

Summary of Approximate Genetically Significant Dose-rates (United Kingdom 1972)

Source	Dose-rate (mrems per year)
Natural background	100
Medical uses of radiations . . .	19
Weapons fall-out	3
Occupational exposure	0·5
Miscellaneous (television, shoe-fitting, schools, etc.)	0·1

NUMERICAL EVALUATION OF RADIATION RISKS

Maximum permissible doses and dose limits are prescribed by sound judgement rather than by scientific precision. They must be interpreted and used, therefore, with equal professional judgement according to the circumstances. However,

tries to a figure of some 200 deaths per million per year in shipbuilding.

Workers occupationally exposed to radiation must accept the conventional risk-rate appropriate to their form of employment. Our present problem is to consider by how much the risk may be increased due to the radiation. Most radiation work is carried on under conditions where the conventional risk-rate is low, probably at around 30 deaths per million per year. A trebling of the rate to 100, on account of the radiation hazard, would probably be unacceptable. Equally, any requirement that the additional rate should be zero cannot be met if radiation work is to be continued. It seems likely that an additional rate of one-third, or about 10 deaths per million per year, would be a reasonable and acceptable figure. This would ensure that the total risk was still low by comparison to many other industries not engaged in radiation work.

Experience at Hiroshima has shown that the induction of leukaemia is a major somatic component of all radiation fatalities. The limited amount of statistics available on leukaemia suggests that a dose of 1 rad, received by a statistically large population in the course of 1 year, may cause 1 or 2 extra cases of leukaemia per million for some 10 or 20 years following the exposure. This gives a total of about 20 additional cases per rad received in any 1 year per million people exposed. The average occupational exposure in the United Kingdom and in the United States is about 0·5 rad per year. Assuming this to be an upper estimate of whole body dose, the expected number of additional cases of leukaemia among radiation workers would be $20 \times 0.5 = 10$ cases per million exposed. These cases would be spread over a 20-year period following 1 year's exposure. This figure is the same as that suggested as being an acceptable risk-rate. The natural incidence of leukaemia in the population is about 50 cases per million per year, so that

TABLE 47

Radiation Risk-rates

Risk	Natural incidence	Upper estimate of additional incidence per rad whole body dose	Percentage increase in risk-rate		
			Per rad per year	To occupational workers at 0·5 rad per year av.	To general public at 0·1 rad per year av.
Leukaemia	50/million per year	20/million per year	40	20	4
All fatal malignancies (including leukaemia) . . .	2200/million per year	40/million per year	1·8	0·9	0·2
First-generation visible genetic defects . . .	15,000/million live births	20/million live births	0·1	0·05	0·01

even the lowest dose received at the lowest dose-rate entails some risk and, therefore, it is necessary to consider what is a permissible somatic risk in normal occupational employment and a permissible genetic risk to the general public.

It would be ideal to be able to refer quantitatively to precise estimates of the risks incurred in using ionizing radiations. Available information on dose–effect relationships is very limited, however, and only the most tentative risk estimates can be made. Our primary concern is with the possibility of occasional fatalities, and here the annual accident statistics in industrial employment provide a perspective. Published figures for the light industries show a fatality rate of about 30 deaths per million per year, with the rate rising through other indus-

the radiation-induced cases would represent an increased risk to occupational workers of 20 per cent.

The increased risk-rate to occupational workers due to all fatal malignancies, including leukaemia, may be estimated assuming an average whole-body exposure of 0·5 rads per year. Available information suggests that a dose of 1 rad to a large population might lead to a further 40 total cases above a natural incidence of 2,200 per million per year. As shown in TABLE 47, this would produce an increased risk-rate of 0·9 per cent.

Considering the genetic risk to the whole population, whole-body irradiation of parents amounting to 1 rad may increase the incidence of first-generation visible genetic defects by 20 per million live births. The natural incidence of first-generation visible genetic defects is 15,000 per million live births, and the additional load in the population due to radiation exposure at the rate of 0·1 rad per year would therefore be 0·01 per cent. Further genetic defects would be expected to appear in subsequent generations, though many would not be visible, and their rate of production as a result of a single exposure to radiation would become progressively lower.

It is against risk estimates such as these that the benefits of a nuclear power programme and of the uses of radioisotopes in medicine, industry, and research must be weighed. The risks are small in comparison to the natural incidence of similar effects in the population, and they should be compared further with other risks inherent in modern life, such as the risk of leukaemia from the inhalation of diesel fumes or the fatality risk of driving on modern highways. The possible hazards in operations involving ionizing radiations, such as the disposal of radioactive wastes and the transport of radioactive materials, must be judged against a perspective of other known risks.

LEGISLATION

The principal public health problem associated with the development of nuclear energy and the use of radioisotopes is undoubtedly in the disposal of the inevitable radioactive wastes which arise. In the United Kingdom a special Act of Parliament, The Radioactive Substances Act, 1960, controls the accumulation and disposal of radioactive wastes. The Act requires that users of radioactive substances shall register with the Department of the Environment before radioisotopes are brought on to their premises. The Act requires also that users shall have specific authorizations for the disposal of any radioactive wastes, whether solid, liquid, or gaseous.

For small-scale disposals, such as those from colleges and research laboratories, the authorization is likely to permit disposal of liquid waste into the municipal sewerage system. Conditions under which the authorization is granted will specify the total quantity of activity which may be discharged in a given period of time. Taking into account the available dilution, a maximum concentration of 10^{-4} microcuries per millilitre may be allowed in the sewer. Solid radioactive waste will be required to be buried in the local refuse tip in quantities which are limited by the volume of waste in which the radioactivity is dispersed. The conditions placed on disposal of solid radioactive waste in this way are that quantities in approximately 0·1 cubic metres of refuse shall not exceed 100 microcuries of isotopes with half-lives greater than one year, or 1 millicurie with half-lives less than one year but including tritium and carbon-14, which are considered to be of relatively low radiotoxicity. Further conditions may limit the dose-rate on the outside surface of the container to a maximum of 20 millirads per hour and stipulate that the radioactive waste shall be buried immediately under not less than 2 metres of other refuse. Small quantities of gaseous waste are generally allowed to be discharged to the atmosphere without restriction on quantity. The outlet point must be sited so that there can be no serious inhalation risk by persons on the ground or inside buildings to which the effluent plume might have access through open windows.

When the quantities permitted be to disposed of to local authority services are too limiting, users in the United Kingdom have the opportunity of disposing through the National Disposal Service. This is operated for the Department of the Environment by the United Kingdom Atomic Energy Authority. Upon receipt of an authorization the user delivers his waste to one of the Authority's establishments. A charge is made for the final disposal.

Legislation covering the transport of radioactive materials has now been fully developed in the United Kingdom. Practice follows the recommendations of the International Atomic Energy Authority (I.A.E.A.). Statutory legislation covering transport by road came into force in 1970 following publication of two Statutory Instruments made under the Radioactive Substances Act, 1948. The Carriage by Road Regulations, 1970, impose on consignors, carriers, and drivers certain prohibitions and requirements, particularly in relation to the packaging and labelling of radioactive material. The Road Transport Workers Regulations, 1970, require that carriers apply special precautions for the protection of their employees and establish a scheme of work to the satisfaction of the Licencing Authority for specially regulated transport operations. The British Railways Board have published regulations on radioactive consignments within their Dangerous Goods Regulations. Regulations for the carriage of radioactivity by sea are specified in the *Blue Book*, a publication issued by the Board of Trade and covering the whole range of dangerous goods. Carriage by air is subject to the over-all regulations of the International Air Transport Association. The carriage of radioactivity by the postal services is under the jurisdiction of the General Post Office, who may lay down more stringent conditions than those of the I.A.E.A., because of the possibility of consignments of radioactivity coming into close proximity with undeveloped photographic film. The Post Office Regulations are published annually in the *Post Office Guide*.

All packages for transport of radioactivity are designed to restrict the radiation dose to the general public and to porters who may be handling them and to provide strength to withstand a severe accident. Special labels which are recognized internationally are used, in order that staff of the transport agencies can recognize the degree of risk involved in handling the various consignments and may be able to follow their instructions.

Radiological protection of persons exposed in the course of their employment is controlled by statutory legislation under the Factories Acts. Maximum permissible radiation doses are based on the recommendations of the International Commission on Radiological Protection. The Ionizing Radiations (Sealed Sources) Regulations, 1969, specify general conditions of work with sealed sources, including the methods by which radiation doses shall be recorded, the frequency with which radiation monitors shall be calibrated, and the manner in which leakage tests on the sealed sources shall be carried out. The Ionizing Radiations (Unsealed Sources) Regulations, 1968, specify the particular conditions under which work with unsealed sources may be undertaken and the special precautions required. These regulations under the Factories Acts are administered by H.M. Factory Inspectorate of the Department of Employment.

The work of the United Kingdom Atomic Energy Authority is authorized by the Atomic Energy Authority Act, 1954, by which the Authority was established. This Act, which is administered now by the Department of Trade and Industry, imposes upon the Authority the absolute obligation to ensure that no ionizing radiations from its premises cause 'any hurt to any persons or any damage to any property'. A similar obligation is required also of the operator of any nuclear plant licensed under the Nuclear Installations Act, 1965. This Act requires that any critical assembly shall be licensed prior to construction and operation.

Other legislation and codes of practice in the United Kingdom which may be the concern of the Public Health Authorities include the requirements by the Home Office for the use and operation of pedoscopes in shoe shops, the recommendations by the Department of Education and Science on the control of exposure of schoolchildren undergoing advanced science courses, guide lines from the Ministry of Health on the exposure of members of the public attending scientific exhibitions where radioisotopes are displayed or used, and separate codes of practice for use in the medical and dental professions, in teaching and research, and by the veterinary profession.

A HISTORICAL SUMMARY

Several detailed reports on the damaging effects of X-rays had been published by 1898. It was not until about 1925, however, that the first maximum permissible dose was established. It was measured in days and was fixed as the exposure time which would result in one-thousandth of the erythema dose.

The concept of a physical dose was evolved by 1932, and in this year external doses from X- and gamma radiation were limited to 100 milliRoentgens per day. This figure was based on the experience of three technicians in a New York hospital who had been working for fifteen years with radium gamma rays without incurring observable damage. By 1936 there was ample evidence that bone sarcomas in a group of luminous dial painters were being induced by radium ingested as much as 20 years previously. It was noticed that none of the dial painters who had ingested less than 1·2 microcuries of radium was affected, and the maximum permissible body burden of radium was fixed therefore at 0·1 microcurie.

By 1949 radiations were being used both in medicine and by industry which were far more penetrating than the medium-voltage X-rays for which the 1932 limit had been designed. Accordingly, it was decided that the maximum permissible dose to the bone marrow and other critical organs should be reduced to 300 milliRoentgens per week, though the maximum dose to the skin was allowed to remain at 600 milliRoentgens per week.

In 1956 the I.C.R.P. recommended a further reduction in the permissible dose to the gonads and blood-forming organs to the values given in TABLE 39. The new recommendation that the cumulative dose should be limited by $5(N-18)$ implied an average dose over a working lifetime of 5 rems per year, which was equivalent to 100 millirems per week. The permissible genetic dose was thus fixed at 60 rems and the lifetime dose at 200 rems.

In 1973 WHO set up an International Reference Centre for Environmental Radioactivity, working in close liaison with the International Atomic Energy Agency (see Shalmon, 1973).

The increasing number of people who may be exposed to radiations has been responsible in recent years for more cautious attitudes in radiological protection, and particular attention has been given to the establishment of maximum permissible population doses. In industrially developed countries there is now no one likely to escape irradiation extra to the natural background. The whole subject is under continuous and careful scrutiny with research programmes on the effects of chronic exposure at low dose-rates being of special interest. Until more is known about the biological effects produced at these low levels and, in particular, whether thresholds exist, we have a duty to keep our exposures at the lowest possible levels.

FURTHER READING

Abbatt, J. D., et al. (1961) Protection Against Radiation, London.

Collins, J. C. (1960) Radioactive Wastes—Their Treatment and Disposal, London.

Eisenbud, M. (1963) Environmental Radioactivity, New York.

Food and Agricultural Organization (1964) Agricultural and Public Health Aspects of Radioactive Contamination in Normal and Emergency Situations, Rome.

Fowler, E. B., ed. (1965) Radioactive Fallout, Soils, Plants, Food, Man, New York.

Gibson, R. (1966) The Safe Transport of Radioactive Materials, London.

Hine, G. J., and Brownell, G. L. (1956) Radiation Dosimetry, New York.

International Atomic Energy Agency (1961) Radioactive Waste Disposal into the Sea, Safety Series No. 5, Vienna.

International Atomic Energy Agency (1963) Disposal of Radioactive Wastes into Fresh Water, Safety Series No. 10. Vienna.

International Atomic Energy Agency (1965) Regulations for the Safe Transport of Radioactive Materials, Safety Series No. 6, Vienna.

International Atomic Energy Agency (IAEA) (1973) Dosimetry in Agriculture, Industry and Medicine, Vienna.

International Commision on Radiological Protection (1959) Permissible Dose for Internal Radiation, Publication 2, London.

International Commission on Radiological Protection (1964) Report of Main Commission, Publication 6, London.

International Commission on Radiological Protection (1965) Handling and Disposal of Radioactive Materials in Hospitals and Medical Research Establishments, Publication 5, London.

International Commission on Radiological Protection (1966) Principles of Environmental Monitoring Related to the Handling of Radioactive Materials, Publication 7, London.

International Commission on Radiological Protection (1966) The Evaluation of Risks from Radiation, Publication 8, London.

International Commission on Radiological Protection (1966) Report of Main Commission, Publication 9, London.

Komarov, E. (1973) Chromosomal aberrations as a biological indicator of the effects of radiation and other environmental hazards, Wld Hlth Org. Chron., 27, 466.

Lapp, R. E., and Andrews, P. L. (1954) Nuclear Radiation Physics, London.

Loutit, J. F. (1962) Irradiation of Mice and Men, Chicago.

Medical Research Council (1960) The Hazards to Man of Nuclear and Allied Radiations, Cmnd. 1225, London, H.M.S.O.

Medical Research Council (1966) The Assessment of the Possible Radiation Risks to the Population from Environmental Contamination, London, H.M.S.O.

Ministry of Health (1964) Code of Practice for the Protection of Persons against Ionising Radiations arising from Medical and Dental Use, London, H.M.S.O.

Ministry of Housing and Local Government (1959) *The Control of Radioactive Wastes*, Cmnd 884, London, H.M.S.O.

Ministry of Labour (1964) *Code of Practice for the Protection of Persons Exposed to Ionising Radiations in Research and Teaching*, London, H.M.S.O.

Morgan, K. Z., and Turner, J. E. (1967) *Principles of Radiation Protection*, New York.

Price, B. T., *et al.* (1960) *Radiation Shielding*, London.

Royal Society of Health (1973) *Radiation Levels in Air, Water, Food*, London.

Russell, R. S. (1966) *Radioactivity and Human Diet*, London.

Shalmon, E. (1973) The WHO International Reference Centre for Environmental Radioactivity, *Wld Hlth Org. Chron.*, **27**, 463.

United Kingdom Atomic Energy Authority (1966) *The Radiochemical Manual*, Amersham.

United Nations. Reports of the United Nations Scientific Committee on the Effects of Atomic Radiation, 1962, 1964, 1966, New York.

United States Department of Health, Education and Welfare (1960) *Radiological Health Handbook*, Washington, D.C.

World Health Organization (1958) Mental Health Aspects of the Peaceful Uses of Atomic Energy, *Wld Hlth Org. techn. Rep. Ser.*, No. 151.

World Health Organization (1960) Medical Supervision in Radiation Work, *Wld Hlth Org. techn. Rep. Ser.*, No. 196.

World Health Organization (1961) *Diagnosis and Treatment of Acute Radiation Injury*, Geneva.

World Health Organization (1962) Radiation Hazards in Perspective, *Wld Hlth Org. techn. Rep. Ser.*, No. 248.

World Health Organization (1963) Public Health Responsibilities in Radiation Protection, *Wld Hlth Org. techn. Rep. Ser.*, No. 254.

World Health Organization (1965) Public Health and the Medical Use of Ionising Radiation, *Wld Hlth Org. techn. Rep. Ser.*, No. 306.

World Health Organization (1965) *Protection of the Public in the Event of Radiation Accidents*, Geneva.

World Health Organization (1972*a*) Report of a Joint IAEA/WHO Expert Committee, Medical uses in ionizing radiation and radioisotopes, *Wld Hlth Org. techn. Rep. Ser.*, No. 492.

World Health Organization (1972*b*) Health legislation: protection against ionizing radiation. A summary, *Wld Hlth Org. Chron.*, **26**, 516.

World Health Organization (1973*a*) Report of a Joint IAEA/WHO Expert Committee, Medical radiation physics, *Wld Hlth Org. techn. Rep. Ser.* No. 390.

World Health Organization (1973*b*) Specifications for the quality control of radioactive pharmaceuticals, *Wld Hlth Org. Chron.*, **27**, 364.

World Health Organization Regional Office for Europe (1972) Report of a Working Group on the Health Effects on Personnel of Ionizing Radiations and other Physical Factors, The Hague 1971 (Euro 4701), Copenhagen.

13

HUMAN PROBLEMS IN AIR AND SPACE TRANSPORTATION

P. HOWARD

AVIATION

Commercial airlines compete fiercely for the privilege of transporting increasing numbers of people over long distances at great speeds and at high altitudes. They select those aircraft that seem best suited to their needs in terms of range, pay-load, cost, and ease of operation. Passengers choose particular flights for a variety of reasons, of which convenient times of departure and arrival, patriotism, previous personal experience, and the reputation of the airline itself are but a few. For both the operators and the travellers, however, the prime consideration is usually economy; lower running costs should mean a reduction in fares which leads to heavier bookings and hence to yet more economic operation. It is as axiomatic that safety and (relative) comfort shall be assured as that the cabin shall have windows; these facilities are 'designed-in' to all aircraft and can be taken for granted by all concerned. Indeed, the existence of human problems associated with flight tends to be forgotten, and may never be consciously realized by the passengers. This fact is a considerable tribute to the aircraft designers, whose efforts have largely conquered the deficiencies of the environment in which aircraft travel. But although the precise form in which the remedies are dispensed is decided by engineers, the prescription of them must be a medical responsibility, based upon an understanding of the nature and effects of the stresses of flight.

The branch of environmental medicine which deals with such matters may properly be called aviation physiology, because the greater part of its practice is concerned with ensuring that normal people are maintained in a physiologically normal state. If this aim is successfully achieved, the clinical problems of aviation medicine are greatly eased, for air travel then imposes no greater strain upon the invalid than does any other form of transportation, and it may often impose much less. This chapter describes some of the stresses of which more than 200 million passengers, in varying states of health, each year remain in blissful ignorance. It also touches lightly upon special problems of military aviation and of space flight.

Pressure and Altitude

The barometric pressure falls with increasing altitude, at first rapidly and then at a progressively slower rate [TABLE 48]. At 18,000 feet it is one-half of the standard pressure of 760 mm. Hg; at 27,000 feet it has fallen to one-third, and at 33,000 feet (a representative operating altitude for jet airliners) it reaches one-quarter of the sea-level value. At 65,000 feet, which is the cruising height of supersonic transport aircraft, the total

atmospheric pressure is only 42 mm. Hg, or approximately 5½ per cent. of that at the ground.

These changes of pressure are not accompanied by a significant alteration in the composition of the air, at least up to the altitudes of interest to general aviation. The partial pressure of oxygen in the inspired gas remains at about one-fifth of the

TABLE 48

Pressure/Altitude Characteristics of the Standard Atmosphere

Altitude above sea-level (ft.)	Barometric pressure (mm. Hg)	Inspired oxygen tension (mm. Hg)
0	760	160
2,000	707	148
4,000	656	138
6,000	609	128
8,000	565	119
10,000	523	110
12,000	483	102
14,000	447	94
16,000	412	87
18,000	380	80
20,000	349	73
22,000	321	67
24,000	295	62
26,000	270	57
28,000	247	52
30,000	226	47
32,000	206	43
34,000	188	39
36,000	171	36
38,000	155	33
40,000	141	30
50,000	87	18
60,000	54	11
65,000	42	9

total, but the oxygen tension in the alveoli falls disproportionately with ascent. This is because the partial pressures of water vapour and of carbon dioxide in the alveolar gas are essentially unaffected by outside events—they exert partial pressures of 47 mm. Hg and about 40 mm. Hg, respectively. Before calculations of alveolar oxygen tension are made, the total pressure must be adjusted to take account of these other gases. For example, at 10,000 feet the barometer reads 523 mm. Hg, of which 110 mm. Hg is attributable to oxygen. Saturation of the inspired gas with water vapour reduces the total effective pressure to 476 mm. Hg, and the oxygen component to 100 mm. Hg. The latter represents the 'space' available to be shared between oxygen and carbon dioxide in the lung; if the CO_2 tension remains at its normal value, the oxygen tension will be 60 mm. Hg, compared with the 103 mm. Hg normally present at sea-level. At greater heights the effect is even more striking. At about 50,000 feet, where the barometric pressure is 87 mm. Hg, the alveoli can contain only water vapour and carbon dioxide, while at 63,000 feet the total air pressure is the same as the water vapour tension; at this altitude the lungs are filled with 'steam' and tissue fluids begin to boil at body temperature.

Oxygen Lack

Although the alveolar oxygen tension falls in parallel with the decline in barometric pressure (it is lower on a wet day than on a fine one, even at sea-level), altitudes of a few thousand feet give rise to no significant symptoms of oxygen lack in sedentary passengers. Some impairment of night vision can be demonstrated at a height of only 4,000 feet, but it is of minor importance, even for pilots. By the time 10,000 feet is reached, the oxygenation of the arterial blood is appreciably reduced, and this height forms a convenient physiological limit, beyond which the effects of hypoxia become increasingly severe. Individuals vary widely both in their susceptibility and their responses, but the early symptoms are commonly light-headedness, euphoria, and a feeling of drunkenness, progressing to stupor. Prolonged exposure to altitudes above about 22,000 feet results in unconsciousness, and the tolerance time becomes shorter at greater heights, falling eventually to a constant value of approximately 15 seconds. Severe hypoxia leads to circulatory collapse which, if the cause remains untreated, ends in death.

Acute exposure to moderate altitudes calls forth compensatory changes. Respiration increases in rate, or in depth, or in both, and the resulting fall in the partial pressure of carbon dioxide in the alveoli allows the oxygen tension to rise, though only slightly. The reduced pressure of CO_2 in the blood shifts the oxygen dissociation curve to the left (the Bohr effect), permitting a greater degree of saturation to be attained at a given oxygen tension. However, the increased affinity of the haemoglobin for oxygen also hinders delivery to the tissues, which may therefore suffer from hypoxia despite an adequate perfusion with well-oxygenated blood.

All the ill-effects of hypoxia can be prevented, or reversed, by the administration of oxygen at an appropriate concentration. The aim should be to maintain the partial pressure in the alveoli at a level close to 100 mm. Hg, and this can be achieved by a progressive enrichment of the inspired air during ascent. To sustain sea-level conditions within the lungs, the oxygen concentration must be increased to about 30 per cent. at 10,000 feet, to 50 per cent. at 20,000 feet, and to 80 per cent. at 30,000 feet. A limit is reached at about 33,000 feet, for at that altitude even pure oxygen barely suffices to preserve a normal tension in the alveoli. In practice, no added oxygen is considered necessary for flights up to 10,000 feet, except at night. If a similar degree of hypoxia is accepted throughout the altitude range, the upper limit to which 100 per cent. oxygen may safely be used increases to 40,000 feet. This provides the easily-remembered and useful rule that, other factors being equal, breathing pure oxygen at 40,000 feet is physiologically equivalent to breathing air at 10,000 feet.

Effects of Pressure Change

If hypoxia were the only problem associated with altitude, the task of the aircraft engineer would be greatly simplified, for he would need only to add the correct proportion of oxygen to the cabin atmosphere. Unfortunately, the fact that gases obey Boyle's law introduces other difficulties. The volume of a perfectly elastic closed container increases as the surrounding pressure is reduced; thus, an ideal balloon holding a litre of air at sea-level will expand to a capacity of 2 litres at 18,000 feet and to 10 litres at 53,000 feet. If the container is not completely distensible, the increase of volume will be limited, and the resulting difference of pressure between the outside and the inside will be manifested as a rise of tension in the wall. During descent these changes will, of course, be reversed. The gas-containing cavities of the body are all imperfectly elastic, and some of them are able to communicate with the environment only through valves or sphincters. Troubles may arise in these structures during either the ascent to, or the descent from, altitude.

A tiny bubble of gas trapped beneath a dental filling can, for example, produce excruciating pain when the ambient pressure is reduced. Similarly, the expansion of gas in the gut can cause bloating and abdominal pain if social inhibitions do not allow the excess volume to be voided. In both these cases relief is rapidly obtained when the barometric pressure is restored to normal.

As the gas in the cavity of the middle ear expands during ascent, it forces open the flap valve at the lower end of the Eustachian tube and flows freely into the nasopharynx. In the subsequent descent, however, the valve closes and gas is trapped in the middle ear. As it contracts, a pressure differential is built up between the mouth and the ear, causing deafness and pain. If steps are taken to ventilate the cavity (by yawning or swallowing) at a stage when the pressure difference is low, the condition can easily be remedied, but equilibration becomes increasingly more difficult as ground-level is approached and the rate of increase of pressure rises. Rapid recompression from very high altitudes can even lead to rupture of the drum. The process of 'clearing the ears' is made more difficult if the mucous membranes are swollen by a cold or by Eustachian catarrh. Congestion may also affect the ostia of the paranasal sinuses, producing either complete closure or valvular obstruction, which may give rise to pain during ascent or descent respectively.

The tissues of the body contain in solution all the gases of the atmosphere. Oxygen and carbon dioxide are active and freely diffusible, and rapidly reach a new equilibrium when the environmental pressure changes. The physiologically inert gases, especially nitrogen, are less mobile and tend to have a higher solubility in structures such as fat and tendon which are poorly supplied with blood. If decompression exceeds a certain critical value, and particularly if it occurs rapidly, nitrogen is released from these tissues more quickly than it can be removed by the circulation, and appears as bubbles of gas. Depending upon the site, size, and fate of the bubbles, a number of different syndromes may result, which are grouped together under the generic name of decompression sickness. They range in severity from mild and localized pain in the region of one or more joints (similar to the 'bends' experienced by divers returning too rapidly to the surface) to gross neurological impairment and circulatory collapse which may prove fatal. As a rule, all signs and symptoms of decompression sickness disappear rapidly upon descent to a lower altitude, but will recur earlier and with increased severity if a second exposure to low barometric pressures is then permitted. Occasionally, a return to sea-level is followed a few hours later by delayed secondary collapse, which may progress rapidly to death if it is not treated energetically.

The obvious way of preventing the ill-effects of pressure change and of oxygen lack is to restrict the altitude to which air travellers are exposed. This may best be done by means of a pressurized cabin in which compressed air, usually derived from the engines, is employed to maintain a constant pressure in the passenger and crew compartments, irrespective of the altitude of flight. In most civil airliners the cabin pressure is at first allowed to fall as the aircraft climbs, but with increasing height enough pressure is added to hold the effective cabin altitude at about 6,000 feet. For a cruising height of 40,000 feet, this requires a differential pressure of about 9 lb. per sq. in. to be maintained between the outside and the inside of the aircraft. For a short-range airliner operating at 25,000 feet, a pressure differential of 6 lb. per sq. in. suffices to keep the cabin altitude at a comfortably safe level. The temperature and humidity of the air used for pressurization must be adjusted (as received from the source it is both hot and dry) and frequent changes are necessary to preserve the illusion of freshness.

Failures of the pressurization system or of the structural integrity of the fuselage are rare events, but if one or the other should occur the occupants of the cabin will be subjected to an altitude close to that at which the aircraft is flying. A large cabin will take many seconds to decompress completely unless the defect is catastrophically great, and the physical effects of a very rapid change of pressure are therefore unlikely to be prominent. The situation represents a real emergency for passengers and crew alike, however, for unless oxygen is immediately made available, severe hypoxia will develop. The pilot will, of course, initiate a descent at the maximum safe rate, but it may take several minutes to reach a height at which oxygen is no longer needed. For this reason, high-flying transport aircraft are fitted with a barometrically controlled system which automatically drops an oxygen mask in front of the face of each passenger should the cabin altitude rise unduly. In addition, masks connected to an independent oxygen supply are always to hand on the flight-deck for use by the crew.

For military aircraft, in which the wearing of oxygen masks is acceptable as a routine, the requirements for cabin pressurization can be less stringent. The limit is set more by the need to prevent decompression sickness than by considerations of hypoxia, and effective cabin altitudes of up to 25,000 feet may therefore be permitted. This means that the differential pressure in an aircraft flying at 40,000 feet need be only about $2\frac{1}{2}$ lb. per sq. in., although in many cases provision is also made for a higher pressure, 'cruise' setting. To avoid unnecessary wastage of oxygen, the cabin is pressurized with air, and the gas delivered to the mask is enriched only to the extent dictated by the actual cabin altitude. If a decompression occurs

above 40,000 feet, where even pure oxygen is insufficient for the maintenance of normal physiological function, the gas is automatically supplied at an appropriate positive pressure, thus 'supercharging' the lungs with oxygen. Protection against extremely high altitudes, in excess of about 55,000 feet, requires the use of some form of pressure suit, because conditions at such heights are physiologically equivalent to those of space itself.

Speed and Acceleration

The human body has no mechanisms for the direct appreciation of its own rate of travel. Assessments of speed are made from visual clues (such as the relative motion of external objects) and from the noise and vibration that are inseparable from any method of transportation. Information from these senses can be grossly misleading. Changes of speed or of direction, however, involve accelerations, for which the threshold of perception is very low. It is convenient to classify accelerations according to their duration; tolerance for those lasting for less than one second depends largely upon the structural strength of the body, while those which last for a longer time primarily affect cardiovascular function. Two special cases must also be considered, namely, vibrations, and angular or rotational accelerations.

SHORT-DURATION ACCELERATIONS

An acceleration of short duration is experienced at the moment of touch-down of an aircraft, when its rate of descent reaches zero. (Strictly, a reduction of speed should be called deceleration, but the physical and physiological effects are the same.) In normal circumstances the occupants of the aircraft will feel no more than a slight bump as the undercarriage contacts the runway, but in violent landings or in crashes a series of very large forces may be encountered. The energy absorbed in crushing or buckling of the aircraft structure will attenuate the loads applied to the passengers and thus increase their chances of survival, but the risk of injury can be further reduced if certain precautions are taken. These include the securing of potential missiles such as loose pieces of luggage and, more important, the proper restraint of the passengers themselves. It is vital, but not sufficient, to ensure that seat-belts are securely fastened. Injuries caused by striking the head on the seat in front must be avoided by the adoption of a correct posture, as described in the airline safety leaflet. However, protection against deceleration really begins with the design of the aircraft and its equipment, for neither harnesses nor postural precautions can be of much avail unless the seat itself is of adequate strength and firmly attached to the cabin floor. It has been demonstrated beyond doubt that injuries and fatalities in aircraft crashes can be drastically reduced by the use of properly stressed rearward-facing passenger seats. This is because forward decelerations are most commonly encountered in crashes, and aft-facing seats permit the weight of the body to be distributed over the large area of the seat back. Flexion of the trunk over a narrow belt is also avoided. Nevertheless, there has been considerable reluctance on the part of the airlines to incorporate aft-facing seats, although they are fitted as standard equipment on all passenger transport aircraft in the Royal Air Force. In passing, it should be pointed out that neither better seats nor any other improved form of crash provision will be fully effective in saving lives unless due provision is made for rapidly evacuating the cabin. This involves a sufficiency of clearly-marked emergency exits and, particularly in the case of large aircraft, ancillary devices such as escape chutes. It also requires that the crew and cabin staff should be calm, efficient, and well-versed in the emergency procedures.

Very brief accelerative forces are of importance to military aviation in a different context, for they are applied by the ejection seats which offer the only chance of escape from a crippled high-performance aircraft. An explosive charge, often supplemented by a rocket motor, projects the seat almost vertically upwards from the cockpit to a height that varies with the speed and altitude of the aircraft, but which may amount to several hundreds of feet. Automatic devices later release the man from the seat and open his parachute, imposing other but smaller forces. The initial acceleration of ejection is applied in the vertical axis of the spine to a healthy body which is firmly strapped to a strong and rigid seat; conditions very different from those obtaining in a crashing airliner. Even so, the forces involved sometimes exceed the limit of tolerance, and minor degrees of vertebral injury are not uncommonly seen after ejection.

LONG-ACTING ACCELERATIONS

Accelerations of long duration occur during normal take-off and landing runs, but they most frequently accompany changes in the direction of the flight path. During turns, they constitute centrifugal forces of the same type as those produced by the more exhilarating fairground machines, but they are usually of smaller degree. In civil aviation the centrifugal forces imposed are so little different from the normal gravitational pull of the earth that they rarely attract notice on their own account; passengers may become aware of the rotation or banking attitude of the aircraft, but not of the small increase in weight induced by the change of direction.

High-performance military aircraft are required to perform flight manoeuvres at high speeds and with small radii of turn. In these circumstances the forces generated may exceed that of gravity by a factor of five or more, and have profound effects upon the cardiovascular system. A progressive failure of the blood supply to the retina leads to impairment of vision, starting in the peripheral fields and spreading to the centre until the classical syndrome of 'black-out' occurs. With longer exposures or at higher accelerations the cerebral blood flow becomes inadequate, and unconsciousness follows. Some protection can be achieved by voluntary measures, such as straining and tensing the muscles of the limbs, but external pressure applied to the legs and abdomen provides a more effective remedy, by raising the blood pressure and by preventing the pooling of blood. The anti-G suit, which consists essentially of a pair of trousers inflated automatically to a pressure proportional to the centrifugal force, is based on this principle.

ANGULAR ACCELERATIONS

Angular accelerations occur when speed and direction change at the same time as, for instance, during a steepening turn. They are of importance in the production of illusions of motion (a feature that they share with some forms of linear accelera-

tions) and in the genesis of motion sickness. Particularly violent sensations are also evoked by complex accelerations, such as those arising when the head is rotated while the aircraft is performing a turn, a loop, or a roll.

Many types of illusion have been described and named, but only two of the more important disturbances will be mentioned here. They are:

1. The oculogyral illusion, which follows exposure to angular forces and consists of the apparent rotation of stationary objects. After recovery from a spin, for example, the pilot of an aircraft in level flight may experience the illusory sensation of rotation in the opposite direction, leading him to take potentially disastrous 'corrective' action. The illusion is especially likely to occur at night, when the misleading information from the semicircular canals is not moderated by an external frame of visual reference.

2. The oculogravic illusion also results from stimulation of the vestibular system, but its origin lies mainly in the otolith organs. In its most typical form it consists of a false perception of attitude in the vertical plane, or pitch axis. The acceleration that results from applying more power to an aircraft in level flight gives rise to a sensation of climbing; in an otherwise dark visual field a reference light will appear to move downwards. Similarly, a reduction of speed gives an erroneous sensation of diving. The oculogravic effect is not, however, confined to straight and level flight, but may arise whenever a prolonged acceleration is applied. In some manoeuvres it may co-exist with the oculogyral illusion, thus increasing the probability that inappropriate remedial action will be taken.

Habituation to these illusions is slight, and the only safeguard against them is an absolute reliance on instruments, acquired and maintained by constant practice.

Motion sickness is inevitably associated with all forms of transport, but it is now a relatively minor problem in aviation. Apart from psychological factors, which may be very strong, the predisposing causes of motion sickness include the labyrinthine and visual stimulation produced by repeated angular accelerations. Such forces can result from random rotational movements of the head during flight through a turbulent atmosphere. Present-day jet aircraft cruise at altitudes well above the weather, but they may be required to climb or descend through rough air, and occasional areas of 'clear air turbulence' are encountered even at great heights. In these circumstances, a small proportion of passengers will develop symptoms. The incidence may be increased by environmental factors, such as heat, noise, 'stuffiness', or unpleasant odours, and, of course, by the presence of other sufferers.

Prevention is the key to the treatment of motion sickness. Experienced travellers who are susceptible to the condition often have a sovereign remedy of their own, but hyoscine hydrobromide is undoubtedly the most effective drug. It may be administered alone, or as a proprietary preparation in combination with amphetamine or other medicaments. For less sensitive patients, and for those who find the side-effects of hyoscine objectionable, antihistaminics can provide an acceptable alternative, and cyclizine is among the best of these. The important point is that measures should be taken at least 30 minutes before flight, for once motion sickness has developed drugs can be of little help. The best that can be done for an established case is to provide warmth for the body and ventilation for the head. The head should be supported, and unnecessary movements avoided. Prostration severe enough to require more active treatment is, fortunately, very rare.

A small but significant number of aircrew suffer from airsickness at some point in their career; usually at an early stage of their flying. Natural selection eliminates the more susceptible before they complete their training, and the remainder habituate rapidly to vestibular stimulation. They may, however, occasionally feel unwell when travelling as passengers through bad weather.

Fitness for Air Travel

At one time travel by air was something of an adventure for invalids, but it is now fully recognized that it can be a life-saving measure, offering greater speed and comfort than can be offered by any other form of transport. In general, there are very few cases of illness for whom air travel is unsafe, but certain patients cannot be accepted by commercial airlines for aesthetic or social reasons; even these can, if sufficient justification exists, be carried in specially chartered aircraft. A publication entitled *Medical Criteria for Passenger Flying* (*Scheduled Commercial Flights*), prepared by a joint committee of the American Medical Association and the Aerospace Medical Association, gives a comprehensive guide to the subject, and further advice on individual cases can be obtained from the Senior Medical Officer (Passenger Section) of the British Airways Joint Medical Staff, London Airport.

Conditions debarred because of the distress that they might cause to other passengers include open wounds, incontinence, severe burns, and all infectious diseases, as well as such potentially antisocial states as major epilepsy, alcoholism (either chronic or acute) and noisy or violent forms of mental illness.

Cases of gastro-intestinal disease or recent abdominal surgery must be considered carefully; the main dangers are the distension caused by the expansion of gas, and the possibility of vomiting. Anti-emetics should be given prophylactically to patients suffering from such conditions, and also to diabetics and women in advanced states of pregnancy. The latter are usually accepted by airlines up to and including the thirty-fifth week; some companies will also carry pregnant women in the last month provided that labour does not appear to be imminent. Deliveries in flight are by no means common, but they do occur, and present no serious problems to a well-trained cabin staff.

Some conditions, although acceptable in themselves, merit special review before permission to fly is granted. For example, cardiac diseases in which the integrity of the cardiac muscle or blood supply is in doubt should be considered with caution. They include coronary occlusions less than three months old, severe angina pectoris, and congestive cardiac failure. Even the moderate reduction in oxygen tension associated with low cabin altitudes imposes on the heart a load which must be avoided whenever possible, and the flight regime must be taken into account when an assessment of fitness to travel by air is made. If the cardiac muscle has recovered functionally, there should be no contra-indication to flying.

In pulmonary diseases the problem to be considered is the reduced ventilatory capacity of the lung, which might lead to an undue susceptibility to hypoxic conditions. Following an attack of lobar pneumonia, a minimum of four weeks should elapse before flying is permitted. If a large volume of tissue has been inactivated or removed, for example by lobectomy or pneumonectomy, three months should be allowed for recovery. In the case of a pneumothorax, flight may be permitted one week after refill, provided that the lung is at least three-quarters expanded. However, the possible consequences of a mediastinal or diaphragmatic shift produced by gas expansion should not be forgotten. The best guide to fitness for air transportation is the exercise tolerance, and it is generally true that a patient who can walk to an aircraft and climb the steps without dyspnoea will not be distressed by flight.

Flying is contra-indicated when the red cell count is below $2\frac{1}{2}$ million per cubic millimetre or the haemoglobin is less than 50 per cent. of normal. If air travel is essential, anaemic patients should be transfused to increase the haemoglobin to at least 65 per cent. Blood dyscrasias and cases of malignancy recently treated with cytotoxic drugs also constitute contra-indications, because of the possibility of haemorrhage under conditions of lowered oxygen tension. For a similar reason, conditions in which the function of the liver is grossly impaired should not travel by air.

Diabetes is no bar to flying, provided that the patient is well stabilized and there is no associated severe cardiovascular disease. The patient should be reminded of the importance of eating at normal 'physiological' intervals rather than being guided by local clock time, which may change by several hours in a long flight between continents.

Patients in the terminal stages of illness may usually fly without detriment, but because of the legal administrative difficulties that arise should they die *en route*, cases of doubt should not be accepted for air travel.

Commercial airlines expect that a certain number of their clients will be ill or invalid when they embark, and that a very small number will develop or reveal some totally unrelated condition during flight. The provisions made include emergency oxygen supplies, a range of common drugs, and a staff trained in advanced first aid. Most carriers will also provide special facilities to meet the requirements of individual cases, if due notice is given. The increasing use of air ambulances and of casualty evacuation services is adequate testimony to the safety and convenience of air transportation for the seriously ill and the wounded.

Immunization

The speed of modern air travel is so great, and the frequency of flights so high, that large numbers of passengers are each day widely dispersed throughout the world from areas where communicable diseases are endemic. In comparison with the incubation of, say, smallpox, international flight times are very short, and a single planeload of people recently exposed to that disease could wreak havoc in a number of countries before they themselves developed overt signs. It is now generally accepted that this risk applies only to smallpox and yellow fever, and it is against these diseases that international regulations are primarily directed. Most countries will not allow passengers from certain areas to enter unless they are in possession of valid certificates of vaccination against smallpox; the number of countries insisting upon immunization against yellow fever is smaller. Primary vaccination is reckoned to provide acceptable immunity only after eight days in the case of smallpox, and after ten days for yellow fever, but re-vaccination is considered to be immediately effective against both diseases. Many airports provide facilities for the re-vaccination of travellers who have forgotten either to carry their international certificates or to keep them up to date.

Certain countries regularly require evidence of vaccination against cholera from passengers travelling via India and the Far East, and temporary regulations may also be introduced to safeguard against the spread of other epidemic diseases. Special provisions may have to be made to deal with the mass move-ments of pilgrims, refugees, and displaced persons, but the normal traveller on a recognized air route is unlikely to come into contact with plague, typhus, or relapsing fever, all of which could pose a potential threat.

Even when immunization is not mandatory, travellers are well advised, for their own protection, to seek inoculation against local hazards. For example, typhoid is a universal disease, and as such its spread cannot be curtailed by vaccina-tion or increased by the movements of unprotected people. Nevertheless, the uncertainty of sanitary precautions abroad makes it desirable for passengers to be immunized in advance.

Malaria is widely spread throughout the world, and any traveller who goes to, or passes through, an area where it is prevalent should take appropriate precautions, in the form of mosquito netting, insect repellent, and prophylactic anti-malarial drugs such as chloroquine and primaquine.

Hygiene in Aircraft

The Committee on International Surveillance of Com-municable Diseases stressed the importance of maintaining high standards of drinking water and food in aircraft. Ref. Article 14 of the International Health Regulations. It also approved the use of resmethrin and bio resmethrin aerosols for aircraft disinfection (World Health Organization, 1974, pp. 3–5).

Supersonic Passenger Flight

In most respects, the human problems associated with super-sonic airliners are no different from those of flight at lower speeds. Moreover, what new factors there are do not arise from travelling at two or three times the speed of sound, but from the fact that supersonic aircraft can only be operated eco-nomically at very high altitudes—typically between 60,000 and 80,000 feet. The amount of ozone in the atmosphere increases with increasing height to reach a maximum at about 95,000 feet, and at the cruising altitude of Concorde the concentration may reach 10 parts per million. The requirement for the cabin atmosphere specifies an upper limit of 0·1 parts per million of ozone, so that it would not be permissible to pressurize the passenger and crew compartments with untreated ambient air. Fortunately, the heating of the gas produced by the pressuriza-tion equipment causes most of the ozone to dissociate into oxygen, but as a second line of defence catalytic filters are also installed in the system.

A perfectly fitting mask delivering pure oxygen provides protection against hypoxia only to an altitude of 40,000 feet, and would be quite inadequate in the event of a cabin pressure failure at the cruising height of a supersonic airliner. Pre-cautions must therefore be taken to ensure that, even in an emergency, passengers are never exposed to extreme altitudes.

Because this problem was appreciated at the design stage, it has been possible to incorporate pressure control systems powerful enough to limit the cabin to a maximum of 25,000 feet under almost all foreseeable conditions, whatever the out-side altitude. At this height, of course, conventional passenger oxygen equipment is quite satisfactory provided that it is properly used.

At great heights, atmospheric shielding against cosmic radiation is lost, but the hazard to supersonic passengers is negligibly small. A transatlantic crossing at 65,000 feet will give a total exposure that is only a small fraction of the radia-tion dose involved in a chest X-ray, and even the aircrew who make many such journeys each year are not seriously at risk. The radiation flux may, however, be considerably increased at times of solar flare activity; should such an event occur, descent to a lower altitude might be required.

Pollution of the stratosphere by supersonic aircraft could also affect health indirectly. The emission of nitrogen oxide could lead to a depletion of ozone and set up a skin cancer hazard whilst the emission of sulphur dioxide could affect the earth's climate.

SPACE

In terms of the physiological and medical problems involved, manned space flight is simply an extension of conventional air transportation. The facts that it is available only to a privileged and carefully selected few; that they can be trained for months or even years to fly a single machine under exacting conditions in a vehicle designed to be of maximum efficiency and minimum weight, without much regard for comfort; and that no great importance needs to be attached either to timetables or to expense, all permit the solutions adopted to diverge from those currently used in aircraft. However, the basic principle remains that the traveller must be protected against stresses imposed by his environment. In space, these stresses are different in degree from, but with one exception of the same kind as, those encountered in flight through the atmosphere. This section briefly indicates some of the differences.

Acceleration

To achieve the speed required for orbital flight, or the still greater velocity necessary for journeys to the moon or planets, relatively high accelerations must be applied for a period of several minutes. Similarly, large forces are generated by the loss of speed associated with re-entry through the earth's atmosphere at the end of the flight. The effects of acceleration on the cardiovascular system can be largely avoided by ensuring that the forces are applied in the chest-to-back direction. The body must be supported in a form-fitting couch, and attention must be paid to the position of the arms, legs, and head if a semblance of comfort is to be maintained. Movements of the limbs become impossible during launch and re-entry, and difficulty in breathing results from the effort of expanding a 'heavy' chest, but the accelerations experienced lie well inside the limits of physiological tolerance for a properly aligned and supported man.

Cabin Conditioning

The requirement for an adequate partial pressure of oxygen is the same for an astronaut as for an airline passenger. A space capsule is, however, a totally sealed cabin, the atmosphere of which must be maintained from within. The simplest solution, adopted by the American authorities, is to pressurize the cabin with pure oxygen to an equivalent altitude of about 27,000 feet, where the inspired oxygen tension is about 250 mm. Hg. This is considerably above the normal level, without being high enough to entail the risk of oxygen toxicity. In Soviet flights, on the other hand, space cabins have been filled with air at sea-level pressure; an arrangement that is more complex and expensive of weight, but which provides more physiologically normal conditions.

The carbon dioxide produced by metabolism must be removed from the atmosphere, and lithium hydroxide or a similar alkaline absorbent is currently used for this purpose. An activated charcoal filter is also desirable, to capture other gases and offensive odours.

Heat is an important waste product of human and of electrical activity, and the thermal load is increased by solar irradiation of the cabin. In the vacuum of space, heat cannot be lost by convection or conduction, although some of the incident energy can be re-radiated at longer wavelengths. Thermal balance thus relies upon the provision of sizable heat exchangers, involving the evaporation of waste water into the surrounding void.

In a totally reliable sealed cabin, astronauts could travel comfortably and safely without the need for special clothing. For certain hazardous phases of flight, such as re-entry, it is advisable that they should be protected against the consequences of a failure of the system, by wearing space-suits. The same is obviously true for all operations outside the spacecraft or on the surface of the moon. The suit must incorporate most of the protective features of the cabin itself, supplying pressure and oxygen, and permitting the removal of carbon dioxide and heat. At the same time it must be sufficiently flexible to allow free movement of the body and limbs, and comfortable enough to be worn for long periods of time.

Weightlessness

The state of weightlessness exists whenever a spacecraft is in orbital flight or coasting towards its objective, when the sum of all the external forces acting upon it is zero. The immediate physiological effects are slight, because all the vital functions of the body are independent of gravity. Special measures are needed to overcome some of the physical consequences of weightlessness, such as the refusal of liquids to pour, but these pose relatively minor engineering problems.

There appears to be an undue susceptibility to motion sickness in weightless astronauts, despite careful selection and training. It is probable that in the absence of information from the otoliths, which normally respond to gravity and other linear forces, stimulation of the semicircular canals by angular accelerations leads to an exaggerated response, manifested as disorientation, nausea, and even frank vomiting. More usually, the symptoms are mild, and as with other types of motion sickness, habituation is rapid.

Weightlessness produces changes in cardiovascular function which do not become apparent until after the return to earth. They then result in orthostatic intolerance, shown by abnormal responses of the arterial blood pressure and heart rate when an upright posture is assumed. In a severe case, the astronaut may faint when he is tilted passively towards the vertical. Tolerance is regained in a few days, the time required being related to the duration of the exposure to weightlessness. The mechanism of the 'deconditioning' is obscure, but several factors seem to be involved. They include a loss of muscle tone from inactivity in the spacecraft, and a reduction in the normal reflex constrictor response to the pooling of blood in the legs. The former can be prevented by a regimen of graded exercises in flight, and the extent of the latter can be somewhat ameliorated by various techniques designed to induce the periodic distension of the peripheral vascular bed.

A further consequence of space flight is the mobilization of minerals from the bones. The condition is akin to the osteoporosis seen in patients who are confined to bed for long periods of time, and in astronauts it probably results from a combination of weightlessness and inactivity. A slightly surprising feature is that the loss of calcium is not confined to the bones that are normally weight-bearing; the entire skeleton appears to be affected to a greater or lesser degree. The dynamics of the process are not well understood, but it is known that the demineralization can be curbed by increasing the calcium content of the diet.

At the present time, manned space flight is an expensive and restricted form of transportation, but one with an enviable record of success and of safety. As in the case of general aviation, these features depend upon the ability of engineers to provide a tolerable environment as specified by physiologists. Further alleviation of the human factors inherent in both types of travel will result from a narrowing of the compromises that both disciplines are currently forced to accept.

FURTHER READING

Barbour, A. B., and Whittingham, H. E., eds (1962) *Human Problems of Supersonic Flight*, Oxford.

Bergin, K. G. (1956) Contra-indications to air travel, in *British Encyclopaedia of Medical Practice Interim Supplement*, **167**, 6.

Committee on Medical Criteria of the Aerospace Medical Association (1961) Medical criteria for passenger flying, *Arch. environm. Hlth*, **2**, 124.

Gillies, J. A., ed. (1965) *A Textbook of Aviation Physiology*, Oxford.

Henry, J. P. (1966) *Biomedical Aspects of Space Flight*, New York.

McFarland, R. A. (1953) *Human Factors in Air Transportation*, New York.

Randel, H. W., ed. (1971) *Aerospace Medicine*, Baltimore.

Robinson, Douglas H. (1973) *A History of Aviation Medicine*, London.

World Health Organization (1974) *Annual Report of the work of WHO for 1973*, Geneva.

14

AIR POLLUTION AND HEALTH

P. J. LAWTHER

Introduction

The history of man's concern about the effects of polluted air on his health and comfort is long. There are descriptions of suffocation by smoke and fumes in the classical literature, and legislation against the use of coal because it was 'prejudicial to health' is found in England as early as 1273. John Evelyn's famous pamphlet *Fumifugium, or the Smoake of London Dissipated*, addressed to Charles II, merits study by anyone interested in pollution, since it contains observations on the nature, effects, and abatement of pollution which, today, are strangely accurate. Populations grew with the Industrial Revolution, and pollution became more intense as emissions from homes and factories increased. During the nineteenth century the problem was examined, recommendations made, and laws passed, but the modern intense concern with pollution is due largely to a series of episodes of fumigation in towns with associated increases in mortality; the greatest of these, and the most effective as a stimulus to research and legislation, was the London 'smog' of December 1952.

New sources of pollution, especially the motor vehicle and modern chemical industry, have been responsible for new problems and heightened anxiety, until today there can be few aspects of 'public health' which are the subject of so much intensive research and debate. Much of the work is bad; much of the debate is emotional; much of the anxiety is ill-founded. A proper review of the study of the effects of air pollution on health can be made only in a large book, and the essay which forms this chapter will of necessity be sketchy. An attempt is made, however, to demonstrate the complexity of the nature and effects of pollution so that the problem may be seen in perspective among the many lesser and greater hazards to the health of the public. The literature on the subject is by now enormous; if this essay were to be annotated properly in the conventional manner the references would occupy almost as much space as the text of the chapter. Excellent technical textbooks, bibliographies, and periodical reviews exist, and reference should be made to the list appended. Some important air pollutants cannot be dealt with here; air-borne radioactivity is a topic which demands separate and very detailed treatment, as does pollution by spores, moulds, and bacteria.

Sources

There is no reasonable definition of pure air; in addition to oxygen, nitrogen, the rare gases, and water vapour, the 'natural' atmosphere contains carbon dioxide, oxides of nitrogen, ammonia, ozone, salt particles, and many other compounds derived from volcanoes, forest fires, vegetation, and rotting organic matter.

But the commonest pollutants of town air arise from the combustion, complete and incomplete, of fuels, especially coal and oil. When any hydrocarbon fuel is burned in an inadequate supply of air, smoke, consisting mainly of carbon, will result. Coal smoke, probably the oldest, and in Britain the commonest, pollutant of the air in towns, is more complex: if soft coal is burned in the old-fashioned British open grate the pollutant emitted at first is an aerosol of tar droplets as the 'volatile matter' is distilled off; some of it, together with coal-gas, then burns with a smoky flame, which consists of greasy carbon. Only later when all gas and volatile matter have been burnt or given off does the coal burn cleanly with the emission of carbon dioxide and water. Sulphur dioxide with small amounts of sulphur trioxide are given off if the coal contains sulphur compounds (usually pyrites and complex organic compounds).

When coal is burnt in industrial furnaces the emission of tarry aerosols is avoided by proper stoking. Carboniferous smoke is then the common sign of inadequate combustion, and can be avoided by proper design and operation. With the higher temperatures occurring in industrial furnaces the proportion of sulphur trioxide in the total sulphur oxide emissions is increased somewhat. Some of this may condense as sulphuric acid on smuts on the internal surface of the stack, to be emitted during soot blowing or whenever the flue velocity is great enough to detach them.

Particles of ash and grit may be emitted from industrial furnaces because they are carried up the stack by the relatively high efflux velocity of the flue gases. These mineral particles are usually large and fall out near the source unless, of course, they are previously trapped by mechanical or electrostatic arresters.

The pollutants emitted from oil-fired plants again depend on the efficiency of combustion and on the amount of sulphur compounds in the fuel. Kerosene contains very little sulphur, petrol virtually none, diesel fuel for road vehicles (DERV) may contain about 0·4 per cent., and heavy fuel oil up to about 5 per cent. or even more (in general, the sulphur content rises with viscosity). The emission of ash is minimal, although the heavy fuel oils contain appreciable amounts of mineral matter, among which may be compounds of vanadium. Some coal is especially rich in compounds of chlorine and fluorine, the burning of which will lead to the emission of hydrochloric acid and hydrogen fluoride. Many trace elements may also be emitted.

The use of gas (coal-gas, gas from oil, or natural gas) leads to very little pollution. It is important, however, to remember that inadequate combustion of any carbon-containing fuel is accompanied by the emission of carbon monoxide, and most combustion processes if they occur at high enough temperatures result in the emission of small quantities of oxides of nitrogen derived either from nitrogen compounds in the fuel or from fixation of atmospheric nitrogen.

These latter compounds are of particular importance as pollutants from motor vehicles. The petrol (spark-ignition) engine usually burns a 'rich' mixture, i.e. fuel is burnt in a less than chemically adequate supply of oxygen, with the resultant emission of carbon monoxide (up to 11 per cent. of the exhaust gases in some phases of operation) and hydrocarbons, either as unburnt petrol or as petroleum compounds the molecules of which have suffered rearrangement or 'cracking'. The diesel engine (compression ignition) burns its fuel in a large excess of air, and if this is dispersed adequately in the cylinder no smoke or carbon monoxide ought to be formed. In normal operation a puff of faint smoke on starting or in response to sudden load is common, but the emission of black smoke (accompanied by carbon monoxide) is symptomatic of maladjustment, faulty operation, or wear.

In both types of engine fuel is burnt under high pressure and appreciable fixation of atmospheric nitrogen occurs, oxides of nitrogen, predominantly nitric oxide, being emitted in the exhaust gases.

Petrol contains additives to prevent premature detonation in the cylinder; tetraethyl or tetramethyl lead is commonly used, and some of this lead is emitted as oxide or halide in combination with salts added as 'scavengers'. Recently, additives to diesel fuel have been developed to lessen the tendency to smoke emission. These are usually barium compounds, the barium being emitted after combustion, usually in the form of barium sulphate.

Lubricating oil frequently contains additives which may be emitted from worn engines in which lubricating oil escapes through the piston rings to be burnt with the fuel.

Dispersion and Distribution

Much confusion arises when, in studying the clinical aspects of air pollution, undue weight is given to consideration of amounts of pollutants emitted from various sources rather than of the ground-level (or lung-level) concentrations in the air. Analyses and estimates of emissions are relevant only inasmuch as they may enable one to forecast the pollution at lung level or to plan to avoid it altogether.

The dispersion of pollutants from their source depends on several factors. Normally, in the atmosphere air temperature varies inversely with height, with the result that the air near the ground being warm rises and aids the dispersion of pollutants. Efficient dispersion, giving low ground-level concentrations, is helped by discharging pollutants from high stacks with high efflux velocity and plume buoyancy (obtained by good stack design and adequate temperature) and good air movement. The site of the source is of obvious importance.

Certain meteorological conditions give rise to temperature inversions in which, because of radiation cooling, cold air comes to lie beneath a layer of warmer air aloft. During such conditions, which may be diurnal and short lived or prolonged for several days, a lid is in effect put over a town and dispersion of pollutants grossly hampered unless they are emitted at such a height or with such velocity as to penetrate the ceiling.

Obviously the conditions favouring high ground-level concentrations are emission at low velocity from low sources, and when this occurs in sheltered places or in temperature inversions very high concentrations may be found. The coal fire, discharging its sluggish plume at low level, is the main cause of pollution at ground level in Britain, and coal smoke may often be seen rolling down roofs during temperature inversions. Fog frequently accompanies temperature inversions, and secondary atmospheric reactions can occur between pollutants in the stagnant air or in the fog droplets themselves; the oxidation of sulphur dioxide to sulphuric acid at such times is a reaction which might be of clinical significance.

The difference in dispersion patterns between high industrial sources and domestic emissions is of great importance when considering town planning and the siting of industry and power plants. All too frequently it is assumed that the effect on ground-level concentrations of pollutants from these two classes of source will be additive. In fact, during low-temperature inversions domestic sources will contribute overwhelmingly to the concentration at lung level, while industrial plumes, if the stacks are well designed, will pierce the inversion ceiling and make scant contribution to the amounts found below. These high sources come to earth during windy weather when background pollution from low sources is minimal, and contribute over short periods, and usually in varying places, to the ground-level concentrations. Obviously topographic factors are of great importance, and care must be taken in making general statements. Not infrequently the dispersion of a plume might be thought to be adequate from theoretical considerations, only to find later that a tall building is erected in its path. The subject is one to be considered not only by meteorologists but also by those versed in aerodynamics.

Usually, motor-vehicle exhaust gases disperse rapidly and are found only in very low concentrations when samples are taken even 50 m. from a busy street. Turbulence caused by vehicle movement aids dispersion. A notorious example of the consequences of inadequate dispersion on a grand scale is Los Angeles. In the Los Angeles basin there is a state of almost chronic temperature inversion, and the exhaust products from roughly 3 million motor-cars accumulate in the air above the city, where the hydrocarbons and oxides of nitrogen take part in photochemical reactions with ozone to produce a haze of powerful lacrimatory properties. Bright sunlight is an essential factor.

Sampling and Methods of Measurement

Concentrations of pollutants vary with time as well as in space, and methods of sampling must be selected according to the purpose of the measurements. Gross samples may be required for detailed chemical analysis; small samples collected at low velocity may be needed for microscopic examination of structure of particles; short-term or long-term samples of one or more 'indicator' compounds may be needed for epidemiological research; results from large networks of sampling stations may be needed for studies in dispersion or for purposes of town planning. Samples may be needed to assess long-term trends. For purposes of research finer and more specific methods than those used in general public health are needed.

Deposited matter, collected in settling jars, used to be the common index of air pollution, but since particles which fall out readily under gravity are usually too big to penetrate the respiratory tract, these measurements, though useful as indices of spoiling of amenity, are of no clinical value. Smoke and sulphur dioxide are usually measured and quoted as indices of pollution in towns where fossil fuels are burnt. Smoke measurements are indices of pollution by incomplete combustion, and sulphur dioxide is usually determined because of its corrosive properties and because it is suspected of causing respiratory disease. It cannot be stressed too strongly that reported concentrations of these two pollutants should, from a clinical point of view, be regarded only as indicators of much more complex constituents. It is impossible to give any rule about the number of sites needed to determine pollution in a town. Pollution will vary with patterns of fuel usage, topographical features, and with weather and climate. Obviously the greater the number of sites and the more frequent the measurements made, the more complex will the picture be. For many purposes one central site must suffice; in many large towns samples from five sites have given sufficient information for assessment of trends and for epidemiological research. In the British National Survey (Department of Trade and Industry) instruments are sited in selected towns to give readings characteristic of five types of district:

  Residential with high population density
  Residential with low population density
  Industrial
  Commercial centre of town
  Smoke control area (which may belong to any of the above
    four categories)

In the National Survey towns are placed in eighteen out of twenty-seven possible categories based on high, medium, or low domestic and industrial coal consumption and good, medium, and poor natural ventilation.

Smoke and sulphur dioxide may be measured with a simple daily sampler, in which air is aspirated by means of a small electric pump, through a filter-paper and then through a Drechsel bottle containing dilute hydrogen peroxide adjusted to pH 4·5. The air volume is measured by a gas meter. The air is sucked in through an inverted funnel as an elutriator, so that particles of effective diameter of less than about 20 μm. are sampled. Smoke ('permanently suspended matter') is determined by assessing the darkness of the stain and subsequent reference to a calibration curve of reflectivity against mass/unit volume (the validity is highly dependent upon the optical properties of the smoke sampled, and checks on calibration are needed frequently). Sulphur dioxide is usually determined by titration to pH 4·5 with dilute borax. Obviously the result obtained is in fact an estimate of net gaseous acids; the presence of other acid gases and ammonia will interfere with the result. The samples are taken over 24-hour periods: man-power can be saved by the use of eight-port samplers which automatically switch to a different filter and bottle each 24 hours. For purposes of research shorter periods may be used in times of high pollution. Instruments recording continuously or at determined variable intervals are available.

'High-volume' samplers, like commercial vacuum cleaners, are used for collecting comparatively large samples for chemical analysis or for gravimetric determination of particulate concentrations. The particulate matter is usually collected on glass-fibre paper, which is a highly efficient filter.

The use of the cascade impactor enables one to collect particles or droplets in four size ranges. In this instrument the air is aspirated through a series of jets of diminishing aperture so that the velocity of impingement of the particles increases in four stages. The particles are collected on microscope coverslips, which may or may not be treated with gelatine films containing reagents which enable something to be learned of the chemical nature of the particles. The examination and sizing of fog droplets is made easy by dyeing the coverslips with naphthol green, which is leached out when the aqueous droplets hit the slide. Sulphuric acid particles, as in droplets, appear as bright red zones if thymol blue is used as an indicator. Usually a membrane filter is added as a fifth stage of the impactor to catch very small particles. The electron microscope is used to study the minute structure of air-borne particles, and they may be collected for this purpose by means of a thermal precipitator. Air is drawn slowly over a hot wire flanked by coverslips mounted on brass blocks. The particles are deposited on the slips by thermophoresis, and can be transferred by various techniques for examination, shadowed or unshadowed, in the electron microscope. Among the gases determined frequently are carbon monoxide, oxides of nitrogen, and ozone. Physical methods, such as infra-red absorption, are convenient for the determination of carbon monoxide, and standard methods are published for the measurement of oxides of nitrogen. Ozone, a gas of importance in Los Angeles, is difficult to measure with any specificity (especially in the presence of other gases), and total oxidants are usually determined and quoted as an index of the ozone concentration. Aliphatic hydrocarbons are determined in some cities when 'photochemical smog' is important and methods for their measurements are either relatively simple and non-specific or complex and relatively specific. Polycyclic aromatic hydrocarbons, of interest because some of them are carcinogenic, may be measured after chromatographic separation, by fluorescence spectroscopy or ultra-violet absorption spectrophotometry. Vapour-phase chromatography, mass spectrometry, electron diffraction, and measurement of electron spin-resonance all have their place in research on air pollution.

Nature of Pollution

Pollution may vary in quantity and quality, and failure to pay enough attention to these distinctions and to the complexity of its physical and chemical nature has been responsible for much of the failure to understand its effects. That which accumulates during prolonged temperature inversions differs from the more usual day-by-day variety mainly by virtue of the fact that large increases in concentrations of many reactive pollutants, especially in the presence of water droplets, may interact with the formation of new compounds; already the oxidation of sulphur dioxide to sulphuric acid has been mentioned; ammonia and sulphur dioxide may interact; olefines, oxides of nitrogen, and ozone react with sunlight to form the lacrimatory peroxyacetyl nitrates of Los Angeles. Short-term variations in concentrations of pollutants depend largely on their rates of emission, and in Britain one sees a marked diurnal variation as domestic fires are lit. Concentrations in the so-called 'smogs' may be twenty times those found on average days, smoke being as high as 10 mg./m.^{3} and sulphur dioxide reaching 2 p.p.m.

Examination of particulate pollution with the light microscope or the electron microscope shows a great variety of types of particle. There are tar droplets from the distillation phase of coal fires, smoke particles, which are usually aggregates of varying degrees of complexity of minute (<0.1 μm.) spheres of carbon or polymers of high carbon/hydrogen ratio, particles of partly burnt fuel, which may be in the form of cenospheres; sodium chloride, ammonium sulphate, and a large variety of electrolytes are seen, and one frequently sees the characteristic sulphuric acid droplets. Occasionally fibres of asbestos may be identified.

Fog droplets vary greatly in size as the relative humidity approaches 100 per cent., diameters ranging from 1 μm. to over 50 μm. Most of the solid particles in town air are less than 1 μm. in diameter, and can be studied in detail only by use of the electron microscope.

A feature of the smoke aggregates which may be of clinical importance is their enormous surface-to-mass ratio; such great surface areas may be important for the adsorption, and subsequent oxidation, of sulphur dioxide during the inadequate combustion in the fire. Chemical analyses reveal the presence of a vast number of compounds. Inorganic compounds include metal sulphates, chlorides, and nitrates, as well as ammonium salts, fluorides, lead, and indeed almost every element, at least in trace amounts. The variety of organic compounds is even greater, and include amines, phenols, acids, heterocyclic compounds, and polycyclic aromatic hydrocarbons. These latter compounds are of especial interest, because some of them are carcinogenic. Tarry coal smoke is the richest source and, contrary to popular supposition, smoke from diesel vehicles is remarkably poor in polycyclic hydrocarbons; the exhaust products from petrol engines are richer than those from diesel vehicles, but traffic contributes remarkably little in comparison with the polycyclic hydrocarbons present in the air in coal smoke.

Gaseous pollutants include carbon dioxide and sulphur dioxide, carbon monoxide, ammonia, and oxides of nitrogen. The presence of relatively substantial amounts of nitric oxide (in comparison to nitrogen dioxide) may appear surprising in view of the ease and rapidity with which nitric oxide in large concentrations is oxidized to the brown nitrogen dioxide. The presence in the atmosphere of this free nitric oxide serves to underline the often forgotten fact that in considering the chemistry of air pollution we are dealing with compounds in extreme dilution; their reaction times are sometimes very slow, and such apparent 'incompatibles' as gaseous acids and bases can coexist, as do nitric oxide and oxygen.

Mention has been made of but a few of the particles and compounds found in polluted air. Two important facts must be borne in mind: the shape and size of many of the particulate pollutants will vary with changes in humidity because of the electrolytes they contain; it is not unreasonable to suppose that, among the crude classes of organic chemicals briefly mentioned above, there may be some complex substances, present in trace amounts, which have powerful pharmacological or biochemical properties which may be of great importance in the production of some of the clinical effects of pollution observed in man.

No specific mention has been made of pollution arising from chemical and metallurgical industry, nor from the dissemination of pesticides in agriculture.

Effects on Man

The effects of pollution are most clearly manifest during the intense fumigations which occur during prolonged temperature inversions over large towns in winter when much fuel is being burnt. The London 'smog' of 1952 is said to have caused at least 4,000 deaths, and less spectacular increases in mortality have been seen to accompany other 'acute' episodes. Not unexpectedly, the vast majority of the excess deaths occur among patients suffering from diseases of the cardiac or respiratory systems, among the very old and feeble and the very young. The ease with which variations in mortality with episodes of high pollution may be demonstrated depends on the size of the population under study, the number of susceptible people it contains, and, of course, the magnitude of the stimulus. In general, it may be said that the larger the population and the greater the percentage of sick and feeble people it contains, the greater will be the response to and association with a given amount of pollution. By the same token, perceptible increases in mortality will be seen to accompany smaller increases in pollution. This dependence of death rate on the number of susceptible people, though of obvious importance, is frequently overlooked, and in assessing trends (such as improvements in pollution following legislation) false conclusions may easily be reached; an antecedent influenza epidemic may remove a high proportion of susceptible patients, and the response of the population to subsequent high pollution might be expected to be less dramatic as a result. On the other hand, such an epidemic inevitably produces a secondary susceptible population of convalescents who, having survived the influenza, may in their weakened state succumb to high concentrations of irritant pollutants. Likewise weather has an important influence on mortality by virtue of the stress it may produce but also because it influences the rate of emission of pollutants. Winters differ greatly in respect of weather, and epidemics of infectious diseases and beneficial trends in death rates following reduction in pollution as a result of legislation can only be claimed by careful examination of long series of results.

The mechanisms by which episodes of high pollution produce increases in mortality are as yet unclear, inasmuch as the specific pollutant or combination of pollutants which cause the symptoms commonly seen among patients in times of high pollution have not yet been identified. There would seem to be no specific 'smog' syndrome and no specific pathological picture. Clinical signs of increase in airway obstruction are commonly seen; in some patients heart failure is precipitated or aggravated; in others sputum increases in quantity or alters in nature; yet again, some patients cough excessively. Air pollution in the concentrations found in 'smogs' is irritant, and the likely crude explanation is that deaths occur in patients who cannot tolerate any further stress of any kind, of which irritation of the bronchial tract is one variety. The results of some recent research suggest that in addition to its irritancy, particulate pollution contains substances which alter the growth of certain bacteria commonly found in the sputum of bronchitic patients, and this factor may be important.

In seeking the cause of death as a result of exposure to high pollution, morbid responses must also be considered. There are those ill people who escape immediate death from pollution to die later without being counted as victims; there are those who suffer exacerbations of their respiratory or cardiac disease and yet recover; and there are those who, having been free from symptoms until a 'smog', come thereafter to display symptoms and signs as though the stress had made manifest latent or early disease. Daily variations in the health of groups of bronchitic patients have been studied by use of various techniques in order to assess the effects of pollution in concentrations less intense than those found in 'smogs'. A very simple method has produced striking evidence that relatively small increases in pollution can produce deterioration in bronchitic patients: patients from chest clinics were asked to record in diaries by means of a simple code their own assessment of their health as departures from 'usual' or from how they felt the day before the diary entry. Deteriorations were seen to follow increase in smoke to 250 μg./m.^{3} together with sulphur dioxide over 500 μg./m.^{3} (0·175 p.p.m.). The mechanism by which these changes are produced is, again, obscure, and much experimental work on animals and man has been done in an effort to identify the noxious agent or combination of pollutants. The most likely explanation is that something increases airway resistance either by producing bronchospasm or by promoting hypersecretion of mucus. Because of its well-known action in high concentrations, sulphur dioxide has been suspect for many years, and more experimental work has been done on this gas than on any other.

Published work on this topic must be read with utmost caution. It will be remembered that the highest concentration of sulphur dioxide measured over an hour in London has been 2 p.p.m. Much of the work reported in the literature has been with exposures greatly (sometimes grossly) in excess of this, and among the papers published so far there is no good evidence of increases in airway resistance having been produced consistently by 2 p.p.m. The question of synergism is frequently mentioned, and much work has been done on the enhancement of the action of sulphur dioxide by the addition to the inhaled gas of 'inert' particles. The results obtained from some work on animals suggested that synergism did take place, but repetition of the experiments on man have negative results. The partial pressure on the atmosphere exerted by 2 p.p.m. sulphur dioxide is very small, and it may be thought that it is unreasonable to expect enough gas to go into solution in the respiratory tract to produce any effect. Attempts have therefore been made to make it more effective by bringing the gas to the mucosa in a more concentrated form by absorbing it on smoke aggregates or carbon particles. Again, results have so far been disappointing. The oxidation of sulphur dioxide to particulate sulphuric acid would seem to be an effective way of increasing the irritant effect of the gas, and again experimental inhalations of sulphuric acid mists in many laboratories have failed to produce relevant results so far. But it must be remembered that a given mass concentration of sulphuric acid in air can be presented in very many forms with respect to number and strength of particles and, moreover, the latter quantity will vary abruptly as the particle is inhaled to be diluted in the warm, moist air of the bronchial tree. Recently efforts to protect acid against rapid dilution on inhalation have been made, but so far without producing positive results. But this work is in its preliminary stages.

Smoke has been said to contain large numbers of complex organic compounds, and it may be more reasonable to seek among them substances of much greater pharmacological activity than the common 'chemical' irritants. Substances with histamine-like properties or compounds capable of potentiating the action of endogenously produced histamine, and other bronchoconstrictors and stimulators of glandular secretion are being sought.

Responses other than those which directly affect airway resistance need to be considered, and some apparently remote phenomenon such as disturbance of secretion or normal functions of pulmonary surfactant by inhaled pollutants may be the cause of death or exacerbation of disease. Throughout all our deliberations and experiments it is important to remember that many of those who respond unfavourably to high pollution have heterogeneous lungs in that ventilation/perfusion ratios may be abnormally distributed; in such patients functional change, such as bronchospasm or mucus hypersecretion, which would pass undetected and without doing harm in the normal subject might cause serious shunting of air to under-perfused parts of the lung with disastrous results. The vasoconstrictor response of the pulmonary arterioles to alveolar hypoxia may put a serious if not intolerable strain on the right heart. In other cases, where cardiovascular impairment is the main trouble, any stress to the respiratory tract might prove fatal or tip a patient into failure.

The importance of the search to identify the compounds responsible for death or exacerbation of existing disease is obvious; once identified, the steps to prohibit their emission or to neutralize them or their effects must be made. But an even more important and complex task is the assessment of the part played by air pollution in the production of disease.

Chronic bronchitis, with its all too common sequelae of emphysema and cor pulmonale, is commoner in towns than in country districts, and is especially prevalent in Britain. There are good reasons for the supposition that air pollution plays an important part in the genesis of the disease, but proof is difficult to obtain, since the problem is one of extreme complexity; chronic bronchitis, while relatively easy to define in its fully blown state, is a disease, or group of diseases, which has a long history, varied sequelae, and many causal factors. It is closely linked to social class, occupation, nutrition, housing, climate, allergy, infection, and many other factors, many of which are also related to pollution. Again, the scene has changed, and the fully-blown disease seen now differs from that seen before the widespread use of antibiotics; and there are all the complications attendant upon the problem of elucidating the cause of diseases which develop over many years. There are good reasons to believe that initiating factors which were important sixty years ago might have been replaced by new stimuli; in more recent disease, for example, neglect of childhood infections in the past may have been a potent initiating factor which may now have been displaced by cigarette smoking.

But it is first necessary to define the disease studied and to consider the hypotheses concerning its evolution. One of the major advances in this field has been the adoption of the Medical Research Council Questionnaire on Respiratory Symptoms by the use of which symptom complexes may be studied rather than diagnoses, thereby avoiding to some extent the confusion caused by the use of different diagnostic criteria. The use of such methods in epidemiological research enables prevalences to be studied in general and working populations and comparisons to be made on an international basis.

A common way in which chronic bronchitis develops has been described by Lynne Reid. In response to an irritant or some stimulus unidentified, the mucus-secreting glands and goblet cells in the bronchial tree are made to secrete more mucus than is normal and, if the stimulus persists, hypertrophy of mucus-secreting elements occurs, and inevitably some encroachment on the lumen of the conducting airways occurs, with resulting impedance of air flow, which may, however, be slight. This stage is manifest clinically as simple chronic bronchitis, by chronic cough with the expectoration of clear mucoid sputum. There is strong clinical, experimental, and epidemiological evidence that this change is commonly brought about by cigarette smoking, which is, after all, the most intense form of air pollution to which the smoker is subjected. Not all smokers get simple chronic bronchitis, and there is therefore some idiosyncratic factor. There is good reason to believe that if smoking is stopped the mucus hypersecretion also ceases and some regression of the hypertrophic changes occurs. Certainly symptoms abate.

All too often infection occurs and purulent sputum is coughed up. There are initially bouts of acute infection, but later the infection becomes chronic. With increasing airway obstruction disturbance of the lung architecture and function occurs, and frequently emphysema supervenes. Respiratory failure often occurs, and right heart failure is a common end point.

There are good reasons to believe that air pollution is one of the most important urban factors involved in the causation of this complicated infected chronic bronchitis, though few would claim that the transition from simple bronchitis is brought about solely by pollution. Studies of large numbers of children have shown that infection in the lower respiratory tract in infancy is more frequent in areas of high pollution, and this gradient is seen in both main social classes. Studies of sickness in postmen have supported the view that pollution plays an important part in causing the disease.

Some workers have claimed that the causal factor is sulphur dioxide or some like irritant in the air, but it seems improbable, in the light of industrial experience and experimental evidence, that this is so. Rather it would seem reasonable to seek some factor which would favour the initiation and persistence of infection. Interference with ciliary clearance mechanisms by the presence of excess mucus may be important, and recent experimental work has shown that particulate pollution, predominantly coal smoke, can both enhance and inhibit the growth of *Haemophilus influenzae in vitro*. The mechanism by which these changes are produced and the compounds responsible are complex and not yet elucidated, but may well be of great importance in the cause of this disease.

There would seem to be no doubt, therefore, that air pollution plays an important part both in producing exacerbations of existing disease and in the genesis of chronic bronchitis. The factors responsible are almost certainly many, varied, and complex.

Lung cancer is seen more commonly in towns than in country districts, and air pollution has often been blamed for this disease. The reasons frequently given are twofold: some research has shown there to be a close association between the incidence of lung cancer and pollution by coal smoke, and, as has been said earlier, coal smoke contains substances which are carcinogenic. Polycyclic aromatic hydrocarbons, especially 3:4-benzpyrene, are the carcinogens which have received most attention and blame. They are undoubtedly carcinogenic to skin of experimental animals, and the skin cancer seen in some occupations is undoubtedly due to members of this class of compound. Lung cancer has been produced in experimental animals by implantation of benzpyrene in the lung and by the administration of heavy doses intratracheally, generally in association with particulate matter. An excess of lung cancer is seen among some workers in the gas industry, though the increased prevalence is in no way proportional to the massive exposures received.

The relevance of 3:4-benzpyrene to the development of the modern epidemic of lung cancer is very dubious. Lung cancer has increased since the beginning of the century, at first in men, later among women; pollution of the air by coal smoke and its associated hydrocarbons was massive in the last century, and has been declining rapidly as lung cancer has been increasing. Furthermore, though parts of Britain show a close relationship between smoke pollution and lung cancer, this association is not constant, and indeed urban/rural gradients in lung-cancer mortality are seen in Scandinavian countries and other places where pollution by coal smoke is virtually nil.

It is necessary to postulate that a new carcinogenic factor began to operate at or about the turn of the century and involved men before women and probably town dwellers before those who lived in the country. Its influence has spread and continues to do so, so that lung-cancer mortality continues to increase.

The subject is complex, but there can no longer be any doubt at all that the factor of overwhelming importance is the smoking of cigarettes. Few texts, if any, are of greater importance in modern public health than the reports on smoking and health issued by the Royal College of Physicians and by the United States Surgeon General. As the results from more surveys and epidemiological studies, prospective and retrospective, become available the part played by urban air pollution is seen to dwindle, many modern workers think almost to insignificance. There remains the question of whether smoking potentiates or enhances the possible carcinogenic action of coal smoke, but there is no doubt at all that the cessation of smoking, the most intense and easily abolished personal form of air pollution, would produce a massive fall in the prevalence of lung cancer. This has ceased to be a matter of controversy.

There are, of course, other causes of lung cancer, knowledge of which is derived from study of occupational medicine. They include radioactivity, arsenic, chromates, nickel, and asbestos. Some of these are present in the ambient air and must not be ignored, but their presence cannot be said at most to contribute significantly to the modern rise in lung cancer nor, of course, could they explain the close association which exists between the number of cigarettes smoked and the incidence of the disease.

Asbestos is a mineral (or more accurately a group of minerals) which merits close study. In industry heavy exposure leads to diffuse pulmonary fibrosis, and among asbestos workers the lung-cancer rate was over ten times that seen in the general population. But more recently attention has been focused on the production, especially by crocidolite (blue asbestos), of mesothelioma of the pleura and peritoneum. The reason for mentioning this here is that it has been shown that exposure to very small quantities, even non-occupational, can produce the tumours after very long induction periods, and cases have been found in the vicinity of asbestos works. Asbestos fibres have been found in town air and, indeed, with the ubiquitousness of asbestos in modern products, it would be surprising if it were not found.

The modern rise in lung cancer is sometimes attributed to motor vehicles, especially to the inhalation of diesel exhaust, the reasons given being that they are new sources of pollution of town air and that exhaust products sometimes contain polycyclic hydrocarbons. There are insuperable objections to the suggestion that motor vehicles are the cause of the rise in lung cancer: the disease was already increasing rapidly long before the diesel vehicle was widely introduced around the late 1930s, and there is no evidence that lung cancer is more frequently seen among people who by virtue of their occupation are exposed to unusually high amounts of exhaust products of either diesel or petrol vehicles.

The motor-car is at present the object of intense interest and study in relation to its contribution to air pollution. Its importance has been greatest in places like Los Angeles, since the petrol engine is the prime source of the compounds which are transformed by light to form the intensely lacrimatory compounds in 'photochemical smog'. The olefinic hydrocarbons and oxides of nitrogen are of particular importance in this respect.

In other parts of the world it is the carbon monoxide emitted by petrol engines which has been the subject of much research. Because of its strong affinity for haemoglobin, comparatively small concentrations of carbon monoxide in air can lead to high concentrations in the blood; when equilibrium is achieved between 100 p.p.m. of carbon monoxide and the blood, 16 per cent. of the haemoglobin is bound as carboxyhaemoglobin, which is not only useless as a carrier of oxygen but also shifts the dissociation curve of oxyhaemoglobin to the left, and thus further impairs oxygenation of tissues. The rate at which equilibrium is achieved will, of course, depend on the minute volume respired, which will depend on the degree of exercise of the subject.

Degrees of saturation in excess of 20 per cent. are well known to produce symptoms ranging from headache, through inco-ordination and stupor, to death. Only in exceptional circumstances (working in badly ventilated garages or tunnels, or running a car with a leaking exhaust) would one expect to find such concentrations, but work has been directed to the study of the occurrence of carbon monoxide in streets and cars and in the blood of policemen and drivers, and to the examination of possible sub-sensory effects of concentrations which might be expected to result from exposure to traffic. Several surveys of carbon monoxide concentrations in street air in different countries reveal a remarkable consistency in results; mean concentrations of around 20 p.p.m. in busy streets are usual, with peaks of 100 p.p.m. not infrequent, and a peak as high as 360 p.p.m. has been measured. From these concentrations it is difficult to forecast blood concentrations likely to be found in exposed people, since they are so closely dependent on length of exposure and on activity. Sampling of blood is

therefore greatly to be preferred. Recent survey work has shown that even in policemen and others exposed to traffic fumes the commonest cause of high blood carbon monoxide is smoking. Saturations in excess of 4 per cent. are rarely found in non-smokers, whereas smokers commonly have 8 per cent. carboxyhaemoglobin saturations, and in some cases much higher values are found. It is important to remember that carbon monoxide from traffic and from smoking does not always produce additive effects; if the subject's initial blood carboxyhaemoglobin is below the value which it would be if he were in equilibrium with his surroundings, then any extra intake of carbon monoxide will hasten the time at which he achieves equilibrium. If, on the other hand, his pre-exposure carboxyhaemoglobin saturation percentage is higher than the equilibrium value, then he will lose carbon monoxide from his blood. Smoking may therefore hasten the achievement of equilibrium with high environmental concentrations.

The relevance of saturations of the order of 10 per cent. is that they might, by virtue of interference with cerebral oxygenation, impair perception or the performance of fine tasks and lead to errors of judgement or execution in such situations as driving in heavy traffic. Much work has been done on this question, but great caution is needed when interpreting the results. Many claims have been made that neurophysiological changes or impairment of perception have resulted from low saturation, but on close scrutiny of the published work it is often seen that technical inadequacies have invalidated the results. The most important and commonest failure is to ignore the strict need to use double-blind techniques in which neither the subject nor the experimenter are aware of whether the gas inhaled is air or air plus carbon monoxide. The results of experiments in which subject and experimenter know what gas is being administered are without value, and have already led to considerable confusion in the literature. At the present moment it is possible to say with certainty that comparatively low concentrations of carboxyhaemoglobin are associated with impairment of visual discrimination similar to that produced by the anoxia equivalent to breathing at altitude. Much work on this subject using strict double-blind techniques and carefully selected tests is in progress, and assessment of the relevance of carbon monoxide from traffic (and from smoking) must await the results. It is important to remember that diesel vehicles emit virtually no carbon monoxide.

Lead has been mentioned earlier. The maximum allowable concentration for 8-hour exposures of healthy people in industry is 200 μg./m.^{3}, and concentrations greater than 5 μg./m^3. in the air of busy streets have rarely been reported. The subject must, however, be kept under review.

Oxides of nitrogen from motor vehicles in heavy traffic do not approach the 5 p.p.m. industrial maximum allowable concentration, but, as already mentioned, are important in photochemical reactions, and may be catalysts for other secondary atmospheric chemical changes.

Abatement

Smoke may be abolished by increasing efficiency of combustion, and there is every reason, medical, economic, and aesthetic, to abolish it. There is no need to await the results of any research. Proper design of furnaces and grates and the use of correct stoking and firing techniques are effective in reducing the emission of smoke from coal in industry. Raw coal cannot, however, be burnt smokelessly on open domestic fires. Reactive cokes burn without smoke in the home, and the use of closed free-standing stoves for combustion of solid fuel has produced great improvement, as has the use of such alternative fuels as oil, gas, and electricity.

The problem of grit and dust emissions from industrial furnaces can be solved by the use of mechanical or electrostatic arresters.

The reduction of emission of sulphur dioxide is very difficult to achieve by means which are not economically impracticable. It may be achieved in domestic heating equipment by use of electricity or sulphur-free oil or gas, but in industrial usage the desulphurization of coal and oil is not yet economically feasible. Gas washing by various processes is practised in some power plants, but has the great disadvantages of being expensive and of cooling the flue gases, with consequent reduction of plume buoyancy. The use of dry scrubbing processes avoids much cooling, and such methods, with the erection of properly designed high stacks for efficient dispersion and dilution, are the ones of choice today. There is abundant published work on such techniques.

For domestic heating in new housing estates 'district' heating, in which hot water is piped from a central boiler house with an adequate stack, has much to commend it, and is not used enough in modern planning.

Means of abatement of pollution from motor vehicles is the subject of much discussion and research at present. Needs vary in different places. In Los Angeles and similar cities the important need is to reduce emission of hydrocarbons so that the formation of 'photochemical smog' may be avoided. Hydrocarbon loss from crankcase blow-by is easily prevented, but such devices as after-burners, catalytic converters in exhaust systems, or modified carburettor design and practice may also be necessary. In Great Britain and in most European cities hydrocarbons are usually of minimal concern, for the stability of air, high ozone content, and intense sunlight are not there to form peroxyacetyl nitrates in more than trace amounts on rare occasions. Any reduction in carbon monoxide concentration in petrol exhaust would, of course, be welcome if it could be achieved by economic means, and abolition of odour would be desirable on aesthetic grounds. The emission of black smoke from diesel exhausts is preventable by good maintenance and avoidance of over-fuelling. Regular inspection and servicing are invaluable, and the practice of derating engines has much to commend it. There may be a place for the use of anti-smoke additives. In both spark and compression-ignition engines there is much room for improvement in design.

There is no space for more than a brief mention of legislation. At the risk of appearing parochial, it is suggested that the British Clean Air Act 1956 and Alkali Act 1966 should be studied, since they are good examples of sensible, workable laws which aim to deal with problems which are capable of solution and are based on good evidence and sound economics.

The question of legislation against air pollution must be approached with great caution and regulations made only on the basis of sound reasoning and regard for the cost to the community of preventive measures. The paucity of medical evidence incriminating specific pollutants must be recognized and hazards clearly distinguished from nuisances. In develop-ing countries it is particularly important to retain a sense of perspective and priority, since frequently air pollution, while being 'fashionable', is often of low priority beside other serious problems of public health; to divert scarce technical man-power and resources would be dangerous.

In many parts of the world 'air quality criteria' are being laid down or their establishment contemplated. In some cases these can at best be of academic interest, since vagaries of climate and other conditions commonly produce variations in concentrations of pollutants of twenty-fold. All too often there is in the development of these 'maximum allowable concentrations for ambient air' no definition of the proportion of the population who must be completely protected against any stress at all times. Susceptibility varies even more than weather; and one cannot ignore economic facts. Uncomfortable questions must be faced; how much is a community prepared or able to pay for air, of what degree of purity, for what percentage of the year? In the face of the scarcity of good evidence and the high cost, some ambient air-quality criteria appear at best to be inspired guess-work and at worst pious nonsense.

Trends

With increased efficiency of combustion, the use of new fuels, and the operation of Clean Air Acts pollution by smoke is declining rapidly in Great Britain and elsewhere. With increasing fuel usage emissions of sulphur dioxide have increased, but much of the excess has been from power stations with tall stacks, and ground-level concentrations in Britain have actually declined despite increase in emissions. Further reductions which would result from widespread use of nuclear energy, natural gas, or desulphurized fuels would be most welcome.

Emphasis has throughout been given to the importance of studying pollution at lung level. There is, however, gloomy evidence of global trends; for some time there has been concern about the rise of concentrations of atmospheric carbon dioxide due to the rapid increase in combustion of carbon-containing fuels. There is now sound evidence that this increase in pollution is taking place, and the results enable atmospheric physicists to predict with fair accuracy the future rate of increase. Carbon dioxide is transparent to light from the sun but relatively opaque to infra-red radiation; it therefore produces a greenhouse effect—short-wave sunlight comes through the atmosphere, heats the earth, which emits some of the energy as long-wave radiation which is not allowed to escape, and as a result the atmosphere is getting hotter. The consequences are obvious. But there is more recent evidence that the contamination of the upper atmosphere by sulphur compounds, such as ammonium sulphate crystals and perhaps sulphuric acid, is filtering off some ultra-violet radiation and producing a change opposite in sign to the carbon dioxide. These are interesting long-term problems.

Air pollution, discussed but briefly here, is complex in nature and effect, never beneficial, often unpleasant, costly in terms of material damage, and is sometimes fatal in high concentrations. It causes disease and can make life less joyful. It is worthy of careful study.

Efforts are being made in many countries to obtain data that will enable the health risks associated with atmospheric pollution to be assessed and the situation improved (World Health Organization, 1974).

REFERENCES AND FURTHER READING

Alkali, etc. Works Order (1966) S.I. No. 1143, London, H.M.S.O.

Central Office of Information (1973) *Towards Cleaner Air*, London, H.M.S.O.

Clean Air Act (1956) London, H.M.S.O.

Clean Air Act (1967) Chimney heights, 2nd ed. of the 1956 Clean Air Act Memorandum, London, H.M.S.O.

Clean Air Act (1968) London, H.M.S.O.

Commins, B. T., and Waller, R. E. (1967) Observations from a ten-year study of pollution at a site in the City of London, *Atmospheric Environment*, **1**, 49.

Committee on Air Pollution (1954) The final report of the Beaver Committee, London, H.M.S.O.

Davies, C. N., ed. (1961) Inhaled Particles and Vapours, I. Proceedings of an International Symposium organized by the British Occupational Hygiene Society, Oxford, 29 March–1 April 1961, Oxford.

Davies, C. N., ed. (1967) Inhaled Particles and Vapours, II. Proceedings of an International Symposium organized by the British Occupational Hygiene Society, Oxford, 28 September–1 October 1965, Oxford.

Douglas, J. W. B., and Waller, R. E. (1966) Air pollution and respiratory infection in children, *Brit. J. prev. soc. Med.*, **20**, 1.

Evelyn, J. (1661) *Fumifugium or the Smoake of London Dissipated*, National Society for Clean Air, reprinted 1961.

Green, H. L., and Lane, W. R. (1964) *Particulate Clouds, Dusts, Mists and Smokes*, 2nd ed., London.

Hepple, P., ed. (1972) Lead in the environment, *Proceedings of a Joint Institute of Petroleum and British Occupational Hygiene Society Conference*, London.

Izmerov, N. F. (1973) Control of air pollution in the USSR, *Wld Hlth Org. Publ. Hlth Pap.*, No. 54.

Izmerov, N. F. (1974) Principles underlying the establishment of air quality standards in the U.S.S.R., *Wld Hlth Org. Chron.*, **28**, 256.

Lawther, P. J., Waller, R. E., and Henderson, M. (1970) Air pollution and exacerbations of bronchitis, *Thorax*, **25**, 172.

Lawther, P. J., Martin, A. E., and Wilkins, E. T. (1962) *Epidemiology of Air Pollution*, Report on a Symposium, *Wld Hlth Org. Publ. Hlth Pap.*, No. 15.

Meetham, A. R. (1964) *Atmospheric Pollution: Its Origins and Prevention*, 3rd ed., Oxford.

Ministry of Health (1954) Reports on Public Health and Medical Subjects, No. 95. Mortality and morbidity during the London fog of December 1952, London, H.M.S.O.

National Society for Clean Air (1966) *Sulphur Dioxide: An Examination of Sulphur Dioxide as an Air Pollutant*, London.

Newhouse, M. L., and Thompson, H. (1965) Mesothelioma of pleura and peritoneum following exposure to asbestos in the London area, *Brit. J. industr. Med.*, **22**, 261.

Pitts, J. N., and Metcalf, R. L. (1971) *Advances in Environmental Science and Technology*, 2 vols., New York.

Reid, Lynne McA. (1967) Bronchial mucus production in health and disease, in *The Lung*, ed. Liebow, A., Baltimore.

Royal College of Physicians (1971) *Smoking and Health Now.* Summary of a report of the Royal College of Physicians on smoking in relation to cancer of the lung and other diseases, London.

Royal College of Physicians (1970) *Air Pollution and Health*, London.

Stern, Arthur G., ed. (1968) *Air Pollution*, 3 vols, 2nd ed., New York.

Stewart, A. B. (1972) Co-operation in prevention of air and water pollution, *R. Soc. Hlth J.*, **92**, 3.

United States Department of Health (1966) *Carbon Monoxide.* A bibliography with abstracts, Public Health Service Publication, No. 1503, Washington.

United States Department of Health (1969) *Air Quality Criteria for Particular Matter*, Ap 49, Washington.

United States Department of Health (1969) *Air Quality Criteria for Sulphur Oxides*, Ap 50, Washington

United States Department of Health (1972) *The Health Consequences of Smoking*. A report of the Surgeon General, Washington.

United States Environmental Protection Agency (1971) *Photochemical Oxidants and Air Pollution: An Annotated Bibliography*, Ap 88, 2 parts, Washington.

United States Environmental Protection Agency (1972) *Biological Aspects of Lead: An Annotated Bibliography*, Ap 104, 2 parts, Washington.

Walton, W. H., ed. (1971) Inhaled particles and vapours III, *Proceedings of an International Symposium organized by the British Occupational Hygiene Society*, London, 16–23 September 1970, 2 vols, Woking.

Warren Spring Laboratory (1966) National survey of smoke and sulphur dioxide, Instruction Manual, Stevenage.

Warren Spring Laboratory (1967) The investigation of atmospheric pollution, 1958–1963, 32nd Report, London, H.M.S.O.

Warren Spring Laboratory (1972) *National Survey of Air Pollution, 1961–71*, Vol. 1, London, H.M.S.O.

World Health Organization (1963) *Air Pollution: A survey of Existing Legislation*, Geneva.

World Health Organization (1968) Report of Five WHO Scientific Groups. Research into Environmental Pollution, *Wld Hlth Org. techn. Rep. Ser.*, No. 406.

World Health Organization Expert Committee on Atmospheric Pollutants (1964) Atmospheric Pollutants, *Wld Hlth Org. techn. Rep. Ser.*, No. 271.

World Health Organisation (1969) Urban Air Pollution with Particular Reference to Motor Vehicles. Report of a WHO Expert Committee, *Wld Hlth Org. techn. Ref. Ser.*, No. 410.

World Health Organization (1972) Report of a Scientific Group: air quality criteria and guides for urban pollution, *Wld Hlth Org. techn. Rep. Ser.*, No. 506.

World Health Organization (1974a) The long-term effects of air pollution on health, *Wld Hlth Org. Chron.*, **28**, 12.

World Health Organization (1974b) Health aspects of environmental pollution control: planning and management of national programmes. Report of a WHO Expert Committee, *Wld Hlth Org. techn. Rep. Ser.*, in the press.

World Health Organization Regional Office for Europe (1973) *Report of a Working Group on the Long-term Effects of Air Pollution* (Euro 3114A), Copenhagen.

World Health Organization Regional Office for Europe (1974a) *Report of a Working Group on the Study of Chronic Respiratory Diseases in Children in Relation to Air Pollution, Rotterdam 1973* (Euro 3114(2)), Copenhagen.

World Health Organization Regional Office for Europe (1974b) *Manual on Air Quality Management in Europe*, in the press.

15

THE SPREAD AND CONTROL OF AIR-BORNE INFECTIONS

A. B. CHRISTIE

The air man breathes, though composed of gases, is peopled with masses of living organisms, and these move freely into and out of his respiratory tract. Mostly they are harmless, but many are pathogenic and, entering the airstream, either damage the respiratory epithelium or pass through it and cause disease in other parts of the body. In the first group are the acute or chronic respiratory infections; in the second many of the common and some of the uncommon specific fevers. The gross mechanism of transfer of infection must be the same in all—entry of the infectious agent into the respiratory tract; but the physiological and pathological results of such entry vary so widely that it is impossible to regard as a single group all the various respiratory infections. It is convenient to consider them under two heads, though within each group there is still much diversity:

1. Infections whose main effect is to damage respiratory epithelium and cause inflammatory reactions in some part of the respiratory tract, e.g. influenza and the common cold.

2. Infections in which, though the infective agent enters by the respiratory tract, it is conveyed through the bloodstream to other parts of the body and causes diseases not necessarily characterized by respiratory symptoms, e.g. rubella, meningitis, and smallpox.

THE RESPIRATORY TRACT

The respiratory tract is not a homogeneous confine. At different levels it provides conditions which vary as much as in any location in nature. Temperature, humidity, pH, viscosity, and cell type change markedly from the anterior nasal mucosa to the walls of the alveoli, and this affects the ability of the various inhaled organisms to survive in the respiratory tract (Christie, 1969). Thus, rhinoviruses flourish in the epithelium of the nasal mucosa, finding there ideal conditions with respect to temperature, pH, and oxygen supply, and causing the commonest of all human ailments, the cold. Lower down the tract, especially in the bronchioles and alveoli where the most obvious differences are a higher temperature and a lower oxygen tension, rhinoviruses are seldom found and rarely do any damage to the cells of the lower respiratory tract. By contrast, respiratory syncytial virus flourishes and causes severe and sometimes fatal infections in the lower part of the tract: higher up, it is much less often found and, when it is, causes only minor or trivial illnesses. *Haemophilus influenzae* is another organism which can cause severe inflammatory reactions in the lower respiratory tract: higher up, it is sometimes the cause of life-threatening acute epiglottitis, but above the pharynx it does not thrive and is rarely present in nasal secretions. Streptococci are often present in the throat, where they find conditions very conducive to a commensal existence, but are still able to cause an acute inflammatory reaction there, presumably when some subtle change in the conditions, immunological or environmental, takes place; they can, of course, spread to the lower respiratory tract, sometimes in the wake of a virus invasion but at other times on their own, and they can then cause, primarily or secondarily, severe streptococcal pneumonia. *Corynebacterium diphtheriae* finds in the tonsils and pharynx ideal conditions for multiplication and for the production of toxin; instead it sometimes settles on the larynx and upper trachea, but only rarely does it descend lower; when it does, it can grow rapidly and cause a suffocating bronchitis or bronchiolitis. Meningococci are fairly common inhabitants of the pharyngeal mucosa and may be present in over 50 per cent. of a population, causing no symptoms at all in the great majority, but in the unfortunate few spreading rapidly, not indeed to other parts of the respiratory tract, but out into the bloodstream and into the central nervous system. The oddest adaptations of all are perhaps those of the influenza viruses, for although they characteristically cause a mainly upper or middle respiratory syndrome, they may also cause on the one hand a mild coryza or common cold, or on the other an overwhelming and rapidly fatal pneumonia.

It is not suggested that the sites chosen or attacked by these many organisms are determined solely by the changing environmental conditions in the respiratory tract. Other factors play a part, of which age is one. Respiratory syncytial virus, for example, can cause fatal bronchiolitis in an infant, mild catarrh in an adult, or an acute exacerbation of symptoms in an elderly bronchitic. The effect of age may, of course, be no more than a reflection of immunological experience. Another factor is the external environment, for example the effect of cold on colds. This will be discussed more fully later, but here it may be said that the effect is by no means so obvious as is commonly believed. The season of the year is important, but again the effect is far from clear so that one may well recall the words of Hippocrates: 'Whoever wishes to investigate medicine properly should proceed thus; in the first place to consider the seasons of the year and what effect each of them produces, for they are not all alike, but differ much from themselves in regard to their changes'. These changes still puzzle us in spite of microbiological and immunological advances.

CLIMATE

There is a tendency among those who live in non-tropical climates to associate respiratory infections with cold and damp and other uncomfortable features of their temperature environment. The association undoubtedly exists, but it is perhaps not so close as at first appears, for the concept is based almost exclusively on man and his adaptation to environment, overlooking the fact that man may not be the most adaptable or even the dominant inhabitant of the environment. As far as respiratory viruses are concerned, there is ample evidence that they can flourish and spread in almost any external conditions of temperature and humidity. This is not surprising, for if they can multiply in the widely differing environmental conditions of the human respiratory tract, should one wonder that they can adapt to similar differences in the climate of the outside world? In other words, may not the whole world, from the point of view of a virus, be regarded as one vast global epithelium around which respiratory pathogens find conditions to which they adapt as readily as in man's respiratory tract? (Christie, 1971a).

Evidence that this is so is not lacking. In Trinidad, for example, since 1964 the main pathogens isolated from children with respiratory disease have been respiratory syncytial virus and para-influenza viruses, with a heavy incidence of both, but especially of respiratory syncytial virus, in infants under 6 months old. In one outbreak, 35 of 40 para-influenza isolates were from children under 2 years old, and a para-influenza virus was isolated from 53 per cent. of children with croup (Spence and Barratt, 1968; Bisno et al., 1970). Jennings and Grant (1967a and b; Jennings, 1968) studied the age distribution of haemagglutinin-inhibiting antibodies to influenza viruses in Jamaica, and found it very similar to that reported in other parts of the world with very different climates. In young Jamaican children they also found that adenoviruses, para-influenza viruses and respiratory syncytial virus had much the same incidence and effect as had been reported among nursery children in Chicago and Edinburgh (Beem, 1966; Aitken, Moffat, and Sutherland, 1967). Sutton (1965) carried out a longitudinal survey of minor illnesses in Trinidad children and compared his findings with those in English children. There was a higher incidence of minor respiratory infections among pre-school children in England, but otherwise the findings in the two different climates were strikingly similar. Differences in climate seemed in all these studies to have little effect on the ability of respiratory viruses to colonize the respiratory tract of man.

In Kenya, Strudwick (1962) carried out a morbidity survey in the Nyeri district of the Central Province and found that in infants under 1 year old the percentage of illnesses due to respiratory disorders was as high as 75 per cent. These illnesses occurred both in drought and in the rainy season, and the disease pattern was 'of a temperate rather than a tropical climate', a remark well illustrating the tendency to regard respiratory diseases as exceptional in the tropics. A longitudinal study of children in Gambia from birth to 18 months old showed that respiratory infections were very common incidents, infections of the upper respiratory tract being commonest in the first year of life and in the cool season, while the lower respiratory tract was affected more often in infants in the second year of life and in the rainy season (Marsden, 1964). Climate may have had some effect on this odd behaviour of respiratory viruses in both Kenya and Gambia, but its effect was certainly not to limit spread. In Lagos, Nigeria, serological surveys showed evidence of infection with influenza A virus in

70 per cent. of children aged 1 to 5 years, and in over 60 per cent. to 80 per cent. of adults, but infants under 1 year old seemed largely to have escaped. This was the case, too, with adenoviruses and respiratory syncytial virus, antibodies to the latter being found in 32 per cent. of children aged 1 to 5 years, but in only 6 per cent. of infants under 1 year old (Njoku-Obi and Ogunbi, 1966a and b). Apart from this last odd finding, the range of respiratory infections in Lagos was very similar to what has been found in serological surveys in many different regions of the world (Taylor-Robinson, 1965; Brown and Taylor-Robinson, 1966; World Health Organization, 1967).

Studies carried out among university students in the Philippines showed that 75 per cent. of first-year students had serological evidence of past infection with para-influenza virus type 3, and 25 per cent. of them with type 1 (Chan et al., 1963): most of the students had never left the islands so that these viruses must have been circulating freely in the Philippines. A study of respiratory infections in students at the University of the Philippines and the University of Wisconsin showed that these infections were the commonest causes of student admissions to hospital in both universities but whereas at Wisconsin they accounted for 30 per cent. of admissions, in the Philippines the figure was over 64 per cent. The hospital admission rate for respiratory infections among Philippine students was 49·4 per 1,000, but only 24·3 per 1,000 at Wisconsin (Evans et al., 1967). A later study in the Philippines showed very similar results (Evans and Espiritou-Campos, 1971). Clearly, the semi-tropical climate of the Philippines had no favourable effect on the incidence of respiratory infection as compared with the more temperate climate of Wisconsin. The same conclusion was reached in a Medical Research Council investigation into the incidence of respiratory infections among overseas students working in the United Kingdom. Most of the students came from tropical countries, but they did not suffer from more respiratory infections than their British colleagues, and appeared, in fact, to have had the same respiratory viral experience in their tropical homeland as if they had spent their early lives in the British Isles (Medical Research Council, 1964).

Where the climate is neither tropical nor temperate there is still evidence that respiratory infections can spread readily. In Eskimo children in Alaska, for example, acute respiratory disease has been shown to be the major cause of illness in the first year of life (Maynard et al., 1967), 35 per cent. of infants suffering one attack of pneumonia or bronchitis before the age of 1 year. Outbreaks of respiratory illnesses caused by respiratory syncytial virus and by influenza A2 occurred, and there was also serological evidence of infection with para-influenza viruses types 1 and 3, adenoviruses types 2 and 5, and several rhinoviruses, findings very similar to those reported frequently from regions with very different climates (Taylor-Robinson, 1965; World Health Organization, 1967). The study of the spread of respiratory infections in Arctic or Antarctic conditions has usually shown that when an infectious agent is introduced it can persist if the community is big enough to sustain its spread, but that in a small isolated community, cut off during the winter, it may die out (Holmes et al., 1971). The determining factor seems to be isolation, rather than climate, and when the isolation is broken by the arrival of a relief ship or plane new infectious agents are introduced, and these spread in the previously isolated community, irrespective of climate and weather (Paul and Freese, 1933; Cameron and Moore, 1968). There is no evidence, although observations are few, that the extreme cold leads to more severe illnesses from respiratory infections. In animal experiments it would appear that, whereas sudden exposure to cold may lower resistance to infection, mice adapted to cold over a period of weeks have less severe reactions to infection than control animals (Marcus et al., 1963; Marcus and Miya, 1964). In man, those coming in the relief ship to Antarctic stations have sometimes gone down with more severe respiratory illnesses than the men they were relieving (Taylor, 1960; Hedblom, 1961), and this suggests that in the exchange of viruses between the two parties, some factor or factors, perhaps not entirely immunological, must play a part. The prolonged exposure to cold may not be relevant at all, but at least it had no adverse effect on the resistance of the over-wintering party to viruses introduced by the relieving party. Yet the members of the over-wintered party, on returning to warmer climates, have sometimes gone down rapidly with respiratory illnesses, infected presumably by viruses or other agents they had not been in contact with during the Antarctic winter (Cameron and Moore, 1968). Environment is always complex, and the obvious elements may be the least important. As Cameron and Moore (1968) point out, for example, relative humidity inside the huts may have had more to do with the survival or transfer of viruses than the Antarctic cold outside. It is at least clear that, as far as climate is concerned, the agents of respiratory infection can survive in widely differing climatic conditions.

Isolation seems to be the main limiting factor to the spread of respiratory infections. In an isolated community, sufficiently small, respiratory infections are uncommon or not persistent, but they flare up when viruses are introduced from outside, as by the arrival of a ship or plane from an area more heavily populated with both human beings and viruses. This is true whether the climate be that of the Arctic or Antarctic, Tristan da Cunha (Shibli et al., 1971) or the tropical Western Caroline Islands in the Pacific. In this group of islands Yap and Guam are frequently visited by planes and ships, and when influenza A2 virus was introduced a mild epidemic followed. In other islands in the group, rarely visited by plane or ship, the introduction of the same virus caused a severe repiratory illness with an attack rate of 100 per cent. Some of the more remote islands escaped infection altogether, but it was their isolation not their climate that protected them (Brown, Gajdusek, and Morris, 1966).

COMMUNITY INFECTIONS

Studies of the spread of respiratory infections in urban families or institutions provide a contrast to the experience in remote tropical islands, for we are now dealing not with the rare or chance introduction of an infective agent but with frequent and repeated invasions of intimate communities by a variety of micro-organisms. The difficulty lies not in the search for pathogens, for they are all too easily found, but in the assessment of how they enter the community, how they spread, how long they persist, whether they cause illness and, if so, what is the influence of antibody and age. These questions are easy to state, less easy to answer, and it is, in fact, very difficult

to define the extent of the problem of respiratory infections in different communities and at different ages. Family studies have shown that respiratory viruses may be introduced by any member of the family, most often by the pre-school child, though the mother or father may also bring the virus into the home, depending on the nature of their occupational or social exposures to infection outside (Sturdy, Frood, and Gardner, 1971). The virus then spreads first to the youngest members of the family and later to older members, and the period of virus shedding and spreading in the family is short, often less than a week. The introduction of a virus usually causes illness in the youngest children, respiratory syncytial virus causing lower respiratory infection and para-influenza viruses mainly upper respiratory infections, but in the adults infection is often subclinical. In nurseries and infant schools a similar pattern is found, although because of the larger susceptible populations the period of spread is longer, though the outbreak peaks are still fairly sharp (Aitken, Moffat, and Sutherland, 1967; Pereira, Andrews, and Gardner, 1967). Hospital studies deal with selected populations, but they illustrate a similar role played by respiratory viruses in acute respiratory illnesses (Fransen, 1970; Mufson et al., 1970; Jacobs et al., 1971).

Bordetella pertussis is an organism which spreads readily only when contact is close. In the home children under 3 years old do not often escape infection if another child in the household is in the infectious stage of whooping cough. In nursery classes and nursery schools the disease spreads much less readily. This is in contrast to the rapid spread of, for example, measles in such institutions, and suggests that *B. pertussis* spreads mainly by direct droplet infection and close intimate contact, while measles can spread through the air of wards and classrooms and infect children at some distance from the primary source. In both these infections, measles and whooping cough, the immunity which follows an attack is long-lasting or permanent, but this is not true of infections with many of the respiratory virus infections mentioned above, for in these immunity seems often to be short-lived, and second or repeated attacks are common. With influenza such repeated attacks may sometimes, but by no means always, be ascribed to a change in the type of the infecting virus, but this is not true of respiratory syncytial virus infections. Second attacks with this virus are not uncommon, even within the first year of life, and the second is not always milder than the first attack: indeed, it is sometimes more severe, as if the first encounter with the virus leads to sensitization of the infant lung cells by reagin, and so to a severe reaction in those cells when next the child is infected with the virus; or it is as if antigen–antibody complexes form and cause cellular damage in the second attack. Whatever the pathogenesis of these severe reactions, they are factors which must be considered in any programme of vaccination against respiratory syncytial virus (Chanock et al., 1967, 1971; Parrott et al., 1967; Chin et al., 1969; British Medical Journal, 1970a; Gardner, McQuillin, and Court, 1970).

COMPOSITION OF POPULATIONS

According to its epidemiological experience, which will vary according to geography, age, social and economic structure, climate, but most of all to its degree of isolation, a community is composed at any one time of a mixture of three immunological types of persons with regard to any infection:

1. Immune persons: those who have acquired immunity from a previous infection or from active immunization by vaccine.

2. Susceptible persons, with no history of previous infection or immunization. This group will diminish as infection spreads from the third group.

3. Infected persons, who may be ill or symptomless but who will eventually be added to the numbers in the first group.

The proportions in the three groups may differ greatly according to the population and the infection being studied. Thus, in the most remote West Caroline Islands (Brown, Gajdusek, and Morris, 1966) the population with regard to influenza A2 virus is probably in Group 2, all susceptible and with no previous history of infection: introduction of the virus would rapidly transfer nearly all the members into group 3. It would be impossible to forecast how many infections would be overt and how many inapparent, although outbreaks in virgin populations tend to be sharp and severe, and some attacks might be fatal. Eventually most of the population would move with their acquired antibody into immune group 1, but in the absence of further introductions of virus and with rapidly waning antibody they would with time again pass into susceptible group 2. By contrast, the population in an infant nursery in a large Western city would, with regard to influenza, para-influenza and respiratory syncytial viruses, be divided mainly between groups 2 and 3, susceptible or already infected with one or other of the viruses, depending to some extent on the season of the year: a small number might be immune or partially immune to some of the viruses, and the introduction of one of the viruses would lead to a wave of respiratory illnesses in the nursery, most of them minor but a few severe, but many of the children would have inapparent infections: most of the children would move, at least temporarily, into group 1 with respect to the current virus, but the same movement in and out of the three groups would be repeated frequently, as one virus after another entered the environment. In a community of older persons, for example a military training establishment, illnesses due to respiratory infections would be expected mainly in incoming recruits (McNamara *et al.*, 1962; Buescher, 1967; Van der Veen, Oei, and Aberbanel, 1969). These young men have probably been exposed to, and become immune to, many of the infective agents that cause respiratory illnesses in childhood, but on entering the training camp two things happen; they meet infective agents they have not perhaps dealt with previously, but they are also exposed to stresses which in some odd manner affect their reaction to infection. The timing of inoculations against other diseases, for example, has seemed to influence the reaction of recruits to adenovirus infections (Pierce *et al.*, 1962). They become sharply ill; yet the same viruses passing through factory workers of similar age groups may cause little or no apparent illness (Christie, 1969).

There must be a reason for such odd epidemiological incidents, but it is not obvious and probably not immunological. The relationship between men and the other organisms which share his environment is never simple, and although one must attempt to classify and reduce to some intelligible order known elements of that environment, the attempt at classification may be too clumsy to include some subtle but all-important factor; and where man's respiratory environment is involved there are probably many such factors. One obvious difficulty is that whereas the number of infective agents is very large, the number of ways in which the respiratory passages can react to infection is limited. Irritation of the nasal mucosa by an infective agent provokes copious secretion, the discharge of which is the main characteristic of the common cold. In infected bronchi the secretion is more viscid and has to be removed by coughing, the main symptom of bronchitis. In the alveoli, the secretions coagulate and cause consolidation, with all the respiratory distress of acute pneumonia. These very different pathological pictures may be caused by any of a large number of micro-organisms, and the difficulty is not lessened by the fact that one micro-organism may cause different reactions at different sites at different ages (Christie, 1969); nor is it lessened by the fact that some patients are more effective shedders of virus than other, for no apparent reason. The one thing that is clear is that for any population the entry of a respiratory pathogen into the community and its passage through it is an epidemiological phenomenon the development of which cannot be predicted with mathematical precision.

MODES OF SPREAD

Where so much is unknown it may seem optimistic to define modes of spread, and indeed there are many uncertainties regarding the mechanism of transfer of the agents of respiratory infection. The possible aerial convection of smallpox virus, for example, is one of the great historical controversies of medicine, and is still unresolved. There appear, however, to be three possible modes of transfer, although in any one infection more than one may operate, and even a different one at different times. Cruickshank (1969) in the third edition of this book described the three classically accepted modes—direct droplet, direct air-borne, and indirect air-borne.

Direct Droplet

Moist droplets are expelled from the mouth and nose of an infectious patient and some of these droplets reach the respiratory mucosa of someone very near the patient. As Cruickshank (1969) pointed out, these droplets may be inhaled directly or may be conveyed on the hands or fomites. Some micro-organisms, such as meningococci, do not survive long outside the body, and such micro-organisms depend for their continued existence on this direct droplet transfer to another patient. Such transfer will obviously be easiest in confined spaces and be helped by overcrowding.

Direct Air-borne

Some of the droplets expelled from an infectious person are very small, dry rapidly, and remain suspended in the air, liable to be carried considerable distances by air currents. Such droplet nuclei probably explain the spread of measles and chickenpox across hospital wards, or even from one isolation cubicle to another in the same block. As Cruickshank (1969) emphasized, the micro-organism must be highly infective for man as it is likely to reach susceptible persons in very small doses in droplet nuclei.

Indirect Air-borne

When moist droplets are expelled from an infectious patient most of them fall on the floor or other surfaces, or on to blankets and clothing. Dusting, cleaning, and shaking may later raise a cloud of these dried particles into the air, and, provided the micro-organisms can survive drying, they can be inhaled and cause infection at some distance from the original source of infection. How great a hazard this method of spread is in hospital wards or other institutions is not clear, but it certainly cannot be discounted. In some diseases, for example psittacosis and Q fever, dust-borne infection is sometimes the only obvious method of spread, and this will be discussed later in this chapter. In other infections, for example streptococcal or staphylococcal infections, direct droplet, indirect, and direct air-borne methods of transfer may all play a part.

ACUTE RESPIRATORY SYNDROMES

The Common Cold

Everyone knows the symptoms of the common cold, but no one can define its aetiology. When controlled studies have been carried out, either cross-sectional or longitudinal, rhinoviruses are the infective agents most commonly isolated (Hamre and Procnow, 1963; Gwaltney and Jordon, 1964: Tyrrell, 1965a; World Health Organization, 1969). But almost any other respiratory pathogen can cause the same symptoms. In volunteer experiments rhinoviruses have again been shown to produce colds, although not with complete regularity. Mere exposure to infectious patients in the same room for hours on end has often failed to infect volunteers with colds (Andrewes, 1962; Tyrrell, 1965a and b), although when infectious material has been instilled directly into the nose a much higher rate of infection has been achieved. Such instillation may appear a crude attempt to simulate what happens in natural infection, but it may in fact be closer to what occurs than one would think (Christie, 1969). Rhinoviruses withstand drying very badly, so that wafted in droplet nuclei through a room they might soon lose their infectivity; in coarser, moist droplets they survive, and if such droplets land on someone's nasal mucosa, as they may well do when some infected person near by coughs or sneezes, they readily set up infection; this is not very different from the nasal instillation of infectious material. Volunteer experiments are made difficult for other reasons too; there are over 100 rhinoviruses, all of which may not be equally infectious for man, cultivation in artificial medium may reduce infectivity, and the presence of antibody in volunteers, although not perhaps preventing infection, may prevent the onset of symptoms (Taylor-Robinson and Bynoe, 1964). In spite of these difficulties it seems certain that most colds in man are caused by rhinoviruses, although the exact mechanism and the factors which determine infection may not always be clear.

One of these factors is the influence of weather, especially the effect of cold. The man in the street has no doubt that cold causes colds, but the scientific investigator has more difficulty in establishing any connexion. Volunteers have been exposed to cold and draughts by various methods: they have been left standing in draughts after hot baths, or in wet clothes after long walks, or even immersed in cold baths while being inoculated with infectious material, but in spite of such treatment they have not developed more colds than control volunteers (Dowling et al., 1958; Andrewes, 1962; Jackson et al., 1963; Douglas, Lindgren, and Couch, 1968). These experiments are crude when compared with the subtle alterations in pH, temperature, and other factors which affect the growth of viruses on laboratory media, and presumably in the cells of the human nasal mucosa, but at least they do not support the view that colds and draughts by themselves cause or induce colds. Yet colds are commoner in winter than in summer in temperate climates. It may be that the winter factor affects the virus rather than the host, and that the experiments with volunteers mentioned above are therefore irrelevant. Or it may be simply that cold weather drives man indoors and causes him to warm his house and so, by altering the environment, make it easier for the virus to pass in sufficient quantity from one host to another. In a semi-tropical country, Panama, Monto and Johnson (1967; Monto, 1968a and b) showed that colds were more frequent at the start of the rainy season; the mean temperature was 80° F. (26.6° C.) and did not fluctuate by more than 5° F., but the inhabitants stayed indoors because of the rains. The fairly stable outside temperature could scarcely have affected the host or the virus, but the environment indoors may have affected both.

Influenza

Influenza viruses are divided into three subgroups A, B, and C. Influenza A virus causes sharp epidemics or pandemics, influenza B virus tends to cause less severe, localized epidemics, and influenza C virus seems to cause mainly subclinical infection. One of the main characteristics of influenza A virus is change in antigenic composition. During an epidemic the strain breeds true, but between epidemics antigenic variation is constantly occurring. These variations may be too slight to affect the epidemic behaviour of the virus or the immune status of the population, but major antigenic shifts eventually occur which effect both. Thus, minor variants of influenza A virus caused repeated outbreaks of disease between 1933 and 1946, but then a major shift took place and the new virus was known as A1. This virus, with minor variation, continued to cause outbreaks until 1957, when a major shift to A2 caused the pandemic of that year. With minor variations in its antigenic composition this A2 virus continued to cause outbreaks until 1968, when a big antigenic variation occurred in the strain which first appeared in Hong Kong. Cross-neutralization with earlier A2 strains was still demonstrable in this new variant, so that it was not completely distinct from the original A2 virus and was therefore known as the A2/Hong Kong/68 virus, not A3; but the antigenic alteration was enough to make it unlikely that population immunity and previous A2 strains would afford protection against this new one (Miller, Pereira, and Clarke, 1971).

So it proved; yet the epidemic behaviour of the Hong Kong/68 virus and the response of different populations to it could not have been forecast. The virus was first detected in Hong Kong in July 1968 and reached a peak there later that month. By August it was already in Singapore, the Philippines, and other areas of South-East Asia. In September there was an explosive outbreak in Madras and the virus was already present in Australia and Iran. It reached the United States in early

September, produced a major outbreak in California early in November and rapidly spread widely through the United States. In Britain the virus behaved very differently. It was first isolated in England in August 1968, there was one school outbreak in September, but it was late in December before there was any sharp rise of cases in the general population. Even then, its spread was slow, and sharp outbreaks were still occurring as late as mid-March. Although the virus spread widely, its progress was slow and, because the load was spread over many months, there was no great pressure on hospital beds. The highest incidence was in children under 5 years of age. Outbreaks ceased after the end of March 1969, but the virus reappeared in the autumn. Contrary to what anyone could have forecast, it spread rapidly in the population, reaching dramatic peaks of incidence within a few weeks, and these ended abruptly. The highest incidence was in the elderly. The virus in both years was virtually the same, not more than 4 per cent. of the 1969–70 isolates showing any antigenic variation from the 1968–9 strain (Pereira and Schild, 1971). The experience of the population in 1968–9 might have been expected to protect it to some extent against the same virus in 1969–70, but this was certainly not the case. If other variables influenced the epidemic interaction between host and virus, what were those variables? Subtle differences in the weather may have been responsible, the degree of air pollution, or some unknown factor that increased the virulence of the virus or made infected patients more efficient shedders of virus. There may have been several such interacting variables (Miller, Pereira, and Clarke, 1971), but they were not detectable by ordinary epidemiological methods.

The pattern traced by the Hong Kong/68 variant of the A2 virus in its spread across the world is not typical of the behaviour of every influenza epidemic, but it does emphasize that, as in the case with the common cold, there are perhaps as many unknown as known factors which affect the spread of influenza virus in any population. As regards the mechanism of transfer from person to person it appears that this is by direct droplet spread from an infectious patient, although there is no obvious outpouring of infectious material as there is from the patient with the common cold. Where the virus lodges between epidemics is a matter for conjecture: it may persist in symptomless human carriers or in an animal reservoir. Influenza virus can certainly infect many animals, but transfer from animals to man has never been proved (World Health Organization, 1969).

Other Acute Respiratory Viral Infections

Influenza and the common cold, with all their epidemiological uncertainties, are yet in the main attributable to one of two main families of viruses: influenza viruses and rhinoviruses. With many other acute respiratory disorders this is not so, for there is a large number of viruses all able to cause infections, and most of them cause different illnesses at different ages. Respiratory syncytial virus, for example, appears to be a common infection at all ages, for the incidence of antibody in adults is high, yet it is mainly in the first 3 months of life that it causes severe illness (*British Medical Journal*, 1970a; Jacobs *et al.*, 1971): it is the commonest cause of bronchiolitis or pneumonia at that age. Possible explanations for the severe

reactions to respiratory syncytial virus in young infants have already been discussed [p. 202], but it remains an epidemiological or immunological puzzle. In the elderly the virus can be one of the rarer causes of acute exacerbations of chronic bronchitis (Somerville, 1963) but for the most part at other ages and in many different parts of the world, it causes mainly mild or unapparent infections (Kravetz *et al.*, 1961; Doggett, 1965; Taylor-Robinson, 1965).

Para-influenza viruses are also ubiquitous and cause a variety of respiratory illnesses from coryza to pneumonia, although most often, even in young infants, the illnesses are mild or inapparent; most city children develop antibody, often silently, to para-influenza type 3 virus before they reach 4 years of age (Chanock, Mufson, and Johnson, 1965). Para-influenza type 2 virus, on the other hand, may cause acute laryngotracheobronchitis, or croup, in young children. In adult volunteers the instillation of para-influenza viruses usually causes only rhinitis or pharyngitis (Tyrrell *et al.*, 1959). Adenoviruses, too, cause a wide range of illnesses, from a rare necrotizing pneumonia in infants (Hsiung, 1963; Becroft, 1967) to mild upper respiratory catarrh, but most infections are silent. Adenoviruses may run through a nursery causing a succession of minor respiratory illnesses, but in military camps they are often the cause of sharp, febrile, respiratory illnesses among recruits (McNamara *et al.*, 1962; Pierce *et al.*, 1962; Buescher, 1967; Van der Veen, Oei, and Aberbanel, 1969). Pharyngoconjunctival fever is a fairly distinct clinical condition occurring in institutions, which is usually associated with adenovirus infection (Parrott *et al.*, 1954; Kendal *et al.*, 1957), but in the main adenoviruses produce, like the other respiratory viruses, no characteristic illness.

The clinical pattern of illnesses caused by respiratory viruses is, in fact, mainly non-specific. The clinician may diagnose bronchiolitis in an infant, but he cannot be sure it is caused by respiratory syncytial virus infection; adenoviruses are sometimes the cause. He can diagnose croup, but he cannot say whether or not it is caused by a para-influenza virus, for other organisms are sometimes responsible. Pneumonia may be caused by an influenza virus, but also by an adenovirus, a para-influenza or even a Coxsackie or echovirus: very often, of course, the cause is not viral but bacterial. The common cold is usually caused by a rhinovirus, but almost any of the respiratory viruses can provoke identical symptoms, and pharyngitis, caused in about one-third of cases by streptococci, may be the main symptom of almost any respiratory virus infection. The problem of respiratory virus infections is one of definition: which virus causes which syndrome, at what age, and under what conditions of environment or climate. Such precise definition is obviously not attainable, yet, lacking such definition, the problems of specific prevention, especially by vaccines, are difficult to solve.

Pneumonia and Pneumonitis

In pneumonia, of whatever aetiology, there is consolidation of lung tissue and loss of diffusion surface. In infants and the elderly the consolidation has the patchy scattered distribution of bronchopneumonia; in older children and adults it is more localized as lobar pneumonia. The cause of lobar pneumonia is often the pneumococcus, but bronchopneumonia may be caused by a wide range of bacterial pathogens. To what extent viruses play a part in each type is uncertain. Viruses can certainly, especially in young infants, cause consolidation on their own, often in epidemic form (Hsiung, 1963; Becroft, 1967; Lang *et al.*, 1969), and they may well act in many cases of lobar and bronchopneumonia by first attacking the respiratory epithelium and altering it in some way so that pyogenic organisms can more easily invade it. This certainly seems the case in influenza when pneumococcal, staphylococcal or streptococcal pneumonia sets in after the first day or two of viral illness. Whether the pyogenic organisms are normal commensals of the patient with pneumonia or more invasive types spread by carriers is not known. If a rise in the carrier rate of invasive bacterial types were concerned in the spread of pneumonia, epidemics of bacterial pneumonia would be expected from time to time, but apart from the post-influenzal types these do not occur. The outbreaks of acute respiratory illnesses, including pneumonia, which occur among young recruits in military units are caused mainly by viruses (McNamara *et al.*, 1962; Buescher, 1967; Van der Veen, Oei, and Aberbanel, 1969), although when so many young susceptible adults are crowded together pneumococci and streptococci may also spread from one to another.

Among young children socio-economic factors seem to affect the incidence of pneumonia. Children in good homes probably suffer an equal number of respiratory infections, but they develop pneumonia less often than children in poorer homes (Cruickshank, 1969). It is not clear which factors cause this higher incidence among poorer children, whether housing, clothing, damp, malnutrition, or neglect. It is easy to say that any or all of these factors could lower a child's resistance, but what such lowering of resistance means in immunological terms is far from clear. It may well be that among poorer children there is more intimate contact with other children both inside and outside the home, and so more sharing of respiratory pathogens. In the elderly bronchitic, the respiratory epithelium has already been damaged through the years, and exacerbations, with consolidation of lung tissue, are readily induced by pathogens, both bacterial and viral (Lambert, 1968; Stenhouse, 1968). In these exacerbations there often appears to be a weather factor—damp, cold, or fog—but, as with the common cold [p. 203], it is difficult to determine the exact part which this factor plays.

Primary Atypical Pneumonia. *Mycoplasma pneumoniae* is a common respiratory pathogen and the commonest cause of primary atypical pneumonia. It spreads readily in families (Biberfeld and Sterner, 1969) and in military units (Forsyth, 1965): Mogabgab (1971) reported that during twelve years at an Air Force base in Mississippi at least half of all cases of pneumonia were associated with *M. pneumoniae* infection, and outbreaks of primary atypical pneumonia have been reported in civilian populations (Evans *et al.*, 1967). There seems no doubt that *M. pneumoniae* spreads freely during normal human contact but often causes only mild respiratory illness or inapparent infection (Lambert, 1968; Biberfeld and Sterner, 1969; Fransen and Wolontis, 1969). In the elderly bronchitic it can be one of the causes of acute exacerbations (Lambert, 1968).

Psittacosis. Although psittacosis in man is a generalized infection, the main assault is usually on the lungs and spread occurs by the respiratory route. The mechanism of infection is different from that of the respiratory infections so far discussed in that the organisms, of the genus *Chlamydia*, are spread mainly in dust from infected birds. The infection is not confined to the psittacine family: pigeons and many varieties of common birds, as well as poultry, are often infected. The organism is passed in the bird's faeces, urine, or nasal discharge; the debris in their cages becomes heavily contaminated and dust from this is inhaled by those who look after the birds (Barrett and Greenberg, 1966). Sometimes even momentary exposure is enough to transmit infection (Shaughnessy, 1955; Dew *et al.*, 1960; *British Medical Journal*, 1972). Although farmers do not appear to catch infection from their flocks, workers in poultry plants have often been infected, and here infection may come not only from feather dust but also from the handling of infected viscera (Bowmer, 1958; Rindge, Jungherr, and Scraggs, 1959). Petrels are eaten for food in the Faroe Islands and here again psittacosis has occurred among those plucking and preparing the carcasses (Bedson, 1940). Infection from man to man is uncommon but there have been several hospital outbreaks in which doctors, nurses, and other patients have been infected by sputum from a patient suffering from psittacosis (Haagen and Krackeberg, 1937; Olson and Treuting, 1944; Berman *et al.*, 1955; Barrett and Greenberg, 1966). Since restrictions on the importation of birds were removed in 1966, the number of cases has increased (156 cases known in 1972). *The Lancet* (1973) recommends that restrictions on the importation of birds should be reintroduced and that psittacosis should be made notifiable.

Q Fever. *Coxiella burneti*, the organism which causes Q fever, infects and spreads rapidly among domestic animals, especially cattle, sheep, and goats. Coxiellae are passed in milk, faeces, and urine, and also in uterine discharges: placentae are often heavily infected. The infection spreads widely among flocks and herds, and apparently across country from one herd or flock to another (Luoto and Pickens, 1961). Coxiellae can survive for months in the dried state, and in sheds and byres the concentration of dried coxiellae in the air may approach aerosol proportions (Christie, 1969) and few animals then escape infection. Man is probably fairly resistant to overt infection, although a good deal of inapparent infection occurs (Babudieri, 1959). Although there may be widespread infection among the farm animals in an area, outbursts of disease in man occur very sporadically both in time and place, and infectivity may be limited to one farmstead or one house and operate for only two or three days (*American Journal of Hygiene*, 1946; Robbins and Ragan, 1955; Stoker and Thompson, 1953). Perhaps some elusive environmental factor effects either the organism or the host at these times. Dust from straw used for packing has caused outbreaks of Q fever among those who unpacked (Harvey, Forbes, and Marmion, 1951); dust from a glue factory has appeared to infect passers-by (Marmion *et al.*, 1953); laboratory clothing has infected laundry workers (Stoker and Marmion, 1955); and dust from the wool of passing sheep has infected inhabitants of houses along the route in Italy (Babudieri, 1953). In all these instances infection was presumably conveyed by the inhalation of *Coxiella burneti* in the dust, but Q fever can also be contracted by drinking milk contaminated with the organism (Brown, Colwell, and Hooper, 1968).

GENERALIZED INFECTIONS

Smallpox and Chickenpox

The virus of smallpox enters the body through the respiratory mucous membranes and passes via the bloodstream to the cells of the reticulo-endothelial system, where it multiplies during the incubation period. Thereafter it spreads again through the bloodstream and reaches the cells of the respiratory mucous membranes and the skin, as well as most other organs of the body. On the mucous membranes and the skin it produces the typical lesions of the disease, and as these break down the virus escapes from the body. The lesions of the respiratory mucous membranes break down a little earlier than those on the skin, for they are more superficial, but the difference in time is a matter of hours not days and the patient with smallpox is not infectious before the rash appears on the skin, or for not more than 12 hours or so at the most. Virus has not been cultured from mouth washings in the first two days of the illness, and it is most profuse from the sixth to the ninth day; it has not been cultured after the twelfth day (Downie et al., 1961). All this accords with epidemiological findings that the smallpox patient is most infectious in the early stage of the disease and that the virus spreads readily by droplets to susceptible close contacts. The degree of infectivity of any one patient varies largely with the intensity of the rash. If a patient has a heavy skin rash he probably has many lesions on his mucous membranes and excretes a great deal of virus. If his rash is sparse, his mucous membranes are probably only slightly affected and little virus is excreted. Thus, one patient had a rash so discrete that it escaped detection; although she had many contacts during the infective period, she infected no one except her husband, who died of haemorrhagic smallpox (Christie, 1969).

Virus also escapes from broken-down skin lesions and crusts, and blankets, floor dust, and fomites are contaminated with virus from this source and also from fallen droplets. Virus-laden dust can then be inhaled, and there is no doubt that many patients, especially laundry-workers, have been infected in this way, without being in contact with a smallpox patient. Virus can be conveyed in air currents, at least through a building. In one outbreak in a hospital in Germany twenty patients caught smallpox: the original patient had been well isolated, but the virus was conveyed to patients in distant parts of the hospital along convection routes that were later demonstrated by smoke tests: exposure to the infected air for only 15 minutes was enough to cause infection in one patient (Wehrle et al., 1970). All this was within one building. This does not prove that in the outside air smallpox virus can be conveyed in sufficient concentration to infect people at a distance, but most doctors who have had to deal with smallpox outbreaks know of cases that are hard to explain in any other way (Christie, 1969).

Chicken-pox virus leaves the body in the same way as smallpox virus, but it is much less resistant to conditions outside. The virus of smallpox may survive in crusts in favourable conditions for as long as a year, but chicken-pox virus dies rapidly, and in experimental conditions it has not been possible to infect susceptible children with extract of crusts (Downie, 1965). The patient therefore becomes non-infectious soon after the lesions become dry, but in the early phase of the illness the virus is often wafted in air currents across a ward and can infect another patient at a distance.

Measles

The evolution of measles in a patient is similar to that of smallpox—entry by the respiratory route, multiplication in the body, and excretion by the respiratory mucous membranes. The patient is highly infectious for a few days before the rash appears, but antibody then builds up rapidly and within a day or two excretion of virus ceases. During the infectious period, virus is excreted in vast quantities from the respiratory tract and few susceptible contacts escape infection. Direct droplet spread takes place rapidly around the patient, but the virus is also conveyed rapidly across wards in droplet nuclei and cross-infection with measles is a common hospital experience. The virus can pass through the conjunctiva and this is probably a common route of infection (Papp, 1956; Christie, 1969). Some infants may acquire subclinical infection while still under the protection of maternal antibody (Wilson, 1962), and in school outbreaks there has sometimes been evidence that inapparent infection in one outbreak protects against infection in a later one (Cheeseman, 1950). But such inapparent infections, if they occur, are rare. The virus does not survive for long outside the body so that there is no danger of late or remote spread of infection.

While the infectivity of measles is very high in all types of population and environment, the results of infection vary greatly. In Britain and many other developed countries today measles has lost much of its severity, but the disease can still sweep through virgin populations with great ferocity (Bloomfield, 1958; Bech, 1962; Adels and Gajdusek, 1963). On the other hand, immunity is probably lifelong, and when measles has invaded an isolated community older members have been protected by immunity acquired in an outbreak over sixty years earlier. In developing or undeveloped countries measles may still cause serious complications and carry a fatality rate of up to 25 per cent. (Taneja, Ghai, and Bhakoo, 1962; Morley, Woodland, and Martin, 1963). These are factors which must influence any programme of prevention.

Rubella

The spread of rubella is similar to that of measles. It is usually regarded as being much less infectious, but this may well be due to the fact that very many infections are inapparent. In one outbreak, for example, 40 per cent. of over 100 patients with rubella had no rash, although virus isolation and antibody studies proved that infection had occurred (Brody et al., 1965; Sever et al., 1965), and there is no reason to doubt that this is the normal pattern of an epidemic of rubella. When serological studies have been made of women of child-bearing age in different areas, it has been found that as many as 85 per cent. of the women have at some time been infected, though many, perhaps most of them, have no recollection of having suffered from the disease; in other areas, the percentage has been lower. The importance of rubella lies, of course, in the ability of the virus to disrupt the process of organogenesis in foetal cells and so produce deformities in the full-term infant. The aim of prevention is to protect the women of child-bearing age who have not acquired antibody by previous exposure. The percentage of women may be quite low, but the total number is very high. As a result of the 1966 epidemic of rubella in the United States 20,000 defective infants were born. (Reimann, 1971; Dudgeon, 1973).

Whooping Cough

Whooping cough is a serious disease of infants and young children in whom, even if it causes no complications, it still interferes greatly with growth and development at a critical age. The agent of infection is *Bordetella pertussis*. One or two claims have been made for a viral aetiology (Connor, 1970; Pereira and Candelas, 1971); there is no doubt that respiratory viruses can cause spasmodic coughs, though whether they can cause the long drawn-out illness of whooping cough or outbreaks of the disease is much more doubtful.

Infection is by direct droplet spread and intimate contact [p. 202]. Stocks (1933) calculated that the risk of catching whooping cough from someone in the same house was seven times higher than from someone living next door, and the risk from someone next door was twice as high as from someone in another house in the same street. Maternal antibody crosses the placenta but does not protect infants against the disease, and the youngest infants often have the most severe attacks. Prevention must obviously be concentrated on the home.

Mumps

The virus of mumps is excreted in the urine and saliva of patients, but only the latter is concerned in the spread of the disease. The patient's saliva may contain virus from 6 days before the parotitis to 4 days after, and during that time the patient is highly infectious. The disease spreads readily in the home, but also in classrooms and in confined military quarters (Dermon and Le Hew, 1944). It has been shown by serological and virological studies during the outbreaks that a great deal of mumps infection, perhaps as much as 30 or 40 per cent., is inapparent (Maris *et al.*, 1946; Henle *et al.*, 1948). When this is taken into consideration, mumps must be regarded as a highly infectious disease. Because of its complications, especially orchitis and meningo-encephalitis, it cannot be regarded as a trivial one.

Diphtheria

Corynebacterium diphtheriae spreads from person to person mainly by droplet infection in close personal contact. In compact communities such as wards, nurseries, or classrooms, the environment can be come heavily contaminated and virulent *C. diphtheriae* have often been isolated on laboratory media from floor dust, but whether these dust organisms can infect healthy mucous membranes is not known. The number of infected persons often rises rapidly in institutional outbreaks and by the end of a week or ten days many of the inmates harbour the organism. Not all of them suffer from the disease: many become symptomless carriers, but when investigating such an outbreak it may be difficult to decide who are carriers and who are in the incubation stage of the disease. The policy must be one of strict isolation and observation and the intelligent application of all we know about susceptibility and immunity to the disease. There is no doubt that the disease is spread more by carriers than by case-to-case infection, and that nasal carriers are much more dangerous than throat carriers. The idea that nasal carriers always have nasal discharges or crusts in the nose is misleading. Such children are suffering from anterior nasal diphtheria and are easily detected clinically. The true carrier, by definition, has no symptoms or signs of the disease at all and can be detected only by bacteriological tests.

Streptococcal Infections

Streptococcal infections are spread in much the same way as diphtheria. The carrier again is the main vehicle, and the nasal carrier again more dangerous than the throat carrier. The dust around a case or a carrier is often heavily contaminated with streptococci, and such dust may spread infection in a ward, especially if it alights on an already damaged skin surface, such as a burn or a surgical wound, or on the mucous membrane of a patient's respiratory tract already altered by virus infection (Cruickshank, 1969). Cross-infection in wards can almost certainly occur in this way, although droplet infection from a case or carrier is much commoner. Streptococci can, of course, be carried on hands, instruments, or dressings from one patient to another unless strict asepsis is practised, and patients with streptococcal skin sepsis can be profuse shedders of the organism into the environment.

Scarlet fever, puerperal sepsis, erysipelas, and other streptococcal infections have in Britain all become less common and less severe over the last half-century. This decline in severity and incidence has to some extent coincided with the advent of the antibiotics and other antimicrobial drugs, but though these drugs may have affected incidence a little by helping to eradicate sources of infection, there is no evidence at all that they have had anything to do with the decline in severity of streptococcal infections. This must be due to some secular trend in the diseases, caused either by a change in virulence in the organism, an increase in the resistance of the host, or a more successful adaptation of the host-parasite relationship. The same has not occurred with diphtheria in Britain: the organism has been dislodged, probably in the main by immunization of the population, but when it gains an entry to a susceptible section of the population the diphtheria it causes is as severe as in the pre-immunization era.

The main importance of streptococcal infection is in the incidence of rheumatic heart disease and acute nephritis. Rheumatic heart disease is usually preceded by streptococcal infection of the throat but acute nephritis often follows infection of the skin with nephritogenic streptococcal strains. Both conditions are equally common in temperate and tropical climates (Paul, 1963; Back and De Pass, 1964; Iyer and Padmavati, 1965; Potter *et al.*, 1968; World Health Organization, 1971; Strasser and Rotta, 1973).

Meningococcal Meningitis

Almost traditionally, the spread of meningococcal meningitis has been linked with the number of meningococcal carriers and with the degree of overcrowding in a community (Glover, 1920). While it is true that these factors do appear to operate in some outbreaks, it has been shown that very high carrier rates may exist without any outbreak of disease, and that outbreaks can occur when the carrier rate is quite low (Dudley and Brennan, 1934; Vedros and Hottle, 1970). There must be other factors in the environment, the parasite or the host, which determine spread.

In the past, most outbreaks of meningococcal meningitis seem to have been caused by group A meningococci, while between outbreaks group B and others have colonized carriers. Around 1960 however, clinical disease caused by group B meningococci began to appear and has become more common. Many of these group B organisms are resistant to sulphonamides, whereas in the past most group A strains had been sensitive. The pattern has now changed even with group A strains, so that sulphonamides can no longer be depended on to eradicate the carrier state or to cure clinical disease. Penicillin resistance can be induced in the laboratory (Miller and Bohnhoff, 1947) and penicillin-resistant strains will probably appear in nature and greatly complicate the treatment of patients and carriers (Vedros and Hottle, 1970; Christie, 1972). These changes in meningococcal behaviour and incidence are but one example of the instability of the environment which man shares with micro-organisms and of which the most constant characteristic is change (Christie, 1972). This disease is a great scourge in Central Africa—the meningitis belt (World Health Organisation, 1973).

PREVENTION AND CONTROL

GENERAL

The air we breathe is a commodity over which we can have little immediate control. Food can be processed and water sterilized before we eat or drink, but we have no option but to breathe the air we find around us, and with it any respiratory pathogens it may contain. The concentration of such pathogens can to some extent be reduced by simple and obvious measures such as improving ventilation. Ghipponi et al. (1971) have shown, for example, that there is some correlation between the type of hut lived in by African tribes, the general bacterial content of the air inside and the incidence of cerebrospinal meningitis, and this finding is really very similar in nature to the relationship between overcrowding and meningitis which Glover (1920) reported in barracks in England, a relationship which we have seen was not absolute [p. 207]. The concentration of pathogens in the air can also be lessened by removing obviously infected persons from the environment, and this can be done in such diseases as smallpox, diphtheria, and measles. One difficulty is that the infected person has already spread the pathogens and infected others before he is detected. Another is that the obviously infected person is often not the only or main source of infection; this is true of the undetected diphtheria or streptococcal carrier or the missed case of modified smallpox. It is far more true of the multitudes of persons infected with respiratory viruses, many of whom are not ill at all or so slightly affected that interference with their normal activities is simply not practicable. It is, of course, common sense to advise that people with severe head colds or sore throats or the aches and pains of mild influenza should stay at home and not spread their viruses in buses, trains, and offices. It is common sense to advise that the elderly, the bronchitics, and the cardiac patients should avoid crowded places during epidemics. But it is not common sense, and it is in fact against all experience, to expect that these measures will have any measurable effect on the spread of respiratory infections through the community at large. When an influenza virus gathers epidemic momentum its progress is not halted by such feeble countermeasures by the population it invades.

None of this means that efforts should not be made to improve environment. While climate does not affect the incidence of respiratory infection [p. 204], we have seen that socio-economic factors do, and these act alike in city life and in African villages (Cruickshank, 1969; Ghipponi et al., 1971). Anything which raises the socio-economic level of a community is, then, likely to have some effect, if not on the intensity of spread of infection, then perhaps on the severity of the resulting illness: such factors might be improvement in housing and general amenities or in the standard of clothing and nutrition. Something might be done in military establishments to reduce the stresses on new recruits or to dilute their numbers with more salted men, but this is probably more easily said than done. The control of dust in dormitories and wards may check some of the spread of streptococcal and diphtheritic infection. In aviaries and cowsheds the suppression of dust may do a little to stop the spread of psittacosis and Q fever, although infection in these diseases is so capricious that any measures applied might easily miss the real avenue of spread. Under special conditions, such as an air-conditioned hospital unit, air filters may be installed to prevent micro-organisms entering, or ultra-violet light used to destroy any that get in, but such methods can have only limited application. In general, it can be said that every attempt must be made to reduce the load of micro-organisms in the inspired air in any environment, but it must be accepted that respiratory pathogens are hazards of the air we breathe and not easily dislodged from it by mechanical means. Lacking effective means of removing or destroying the parasites, we must rely for the time being on methods of immunizing the host against the parasite. These must now be briefly considered.

IMMUNIZATION PROGRAMMES

Respiratory Virus Vaccines

It is not possible here to deal in detail with all the aspects, theoretical and practical, of a respiratory virus vaccine programme: only an outline of the problems can be attempted. A full discussion is available in the Proceedings of the International Conference on Vaccines held in Washington in 1970 (Pan American Health Organization, 1971).

The main difficulty in seeking to immunize a population against respiratory virus disease is the great number of viruses concerned. Around 120 respiratory viruses can cause disease in man: the list includes influenza, para-influenza and respiratory syncytial viruses, coronaviruses, the rhinoviruses, and adenoviruses; Mycoplasma pneumoniae though not a virus can be added to the list. Even if one excludes rhinoviruses and selects of the remainder only those most commonly causing disease, there still remains a considerable load of antigenic material. A second difficulty is that immunity to infection with most of the agents appears to be short-lived, and may be counted in months rather than years. The difference between infection and disease must be borne in mind, although when one is considering control of spread of an infective agent in a community, infection may be just as important as disease: most adults, for example, do not become ill when infected with respiratory syncytial virus but they can shed virus and be a danger to infants. Age is of great importance with regard to respiratory virus vaccines, for, as we have seen [p. 204], the effects of infection vary greatly with age, and a vaccine suitable for infants would not be suitable for adults, and vice versa. Associated with age is the problem of harmful immune reactions produced by infection or immunization, the main example of which in this field occurs with respiratory syncytial virus vaccines [p. 204]. Perhaps the most fundamental difficulty concerns the nature of the protecting mechanism against respiratory virus infection, and there seems little doubt that in many instances respiratory secretory antibody is much more important than serum antibody (Kim et al., 1969). This raises the questions of whether parenteral injection of antigen can be expected to stimulate the production of secretory antibody or only of serum antibody, and, if the latter, whether such antibody can be expected to protect. It seems clear that parenteral injection of influenza vaccine does give protection against the disease, but whether antigen must be conveyed from the site of injection to the respiratory tract to stimulate secretory antibody is not so clear. In adenovirus infections, vaccine given orally in enteric-coated form does protect (Edmonson et al., 1966), although it does not induce secretory antibody, and it may be that some adenoviruses cause infection more deeply than on the respiratory mucosa and so encounter serum antibody (Chanock et al., 1971). Inhaled virus vaccines, on the other hand, seem to induce both secretory and serum antibody, and for that reason may be more promising immunizing agents. One helpful element in this otherwise difficult field is that, apart from the influenza viruses, most of the respiratory viruses are antigenically stable. Another is that, as has been fully discussed earlier [p. 204], the types of respiratory infections seem to be very much the same all over the world irrespective of climate. The composition of any vaccines, therefore, other than influenza vaccines, is likely to remain epidemiologically satisfactory for many years.

Composition of Vaccines

A composite vaccine for infants would need to include respiratory syncytial virus and the para-influenza viruses types 1, 2, and 3; such a vaccine, if successful, would prevent most of the severe respiratory virus infections of early infancy. The addition of adenoviruses types 1, 2, 3, 5, and 7 would further reduce the risks though adding to the load of antigen. For older children and adults influenza viruses A and B and *Mycoplasma pneumoniae* become more important causes of diseases and would have to be included in a composite vaccine, while respiratory syncytial virus could be omitted. Whether, for adults, the other components of the infant vaccine could also be dropped would depend on whether it is accepted that vaccine prevention is feasible only for serious respiratory disease or whether a maximum reduction of all respiratory infections is the aim. If the latter, adenoviruses types 14 and 21 would have to be added and, of course, antigenic material from all the rhinoviruses. Such a vaccine, as far as can be seen, is certainly not practicable, but some of the narrower polyvalent vaccines may well be. Trials with live enteric-coated mixed types 4 and 7 adenovirus vaccines have been successful in military recruits (Buescher, 1971; Chanock et al., 1971). Trial with inactivated mycoplasma vaccines have had some success (Mogabgab, 1971); but work with live

mycoplasma vaccines is still at the experimental stage. These experiments include the induction by chemical means of temperature-sensitive (ts) mutants of viruses and mycoplasmas, in the hope that such ts mutants will prove to be attenuated in virulence, still able to provoke immunity to wild strains, but unable because of their temperature-sensitivity to colonize and cause disease in the lower respiratory tract where the temperature is higher [p. 199]. Experiments in hamsters have been encouraging, and it may be along this or some related line that vaccines capable of inducing secretory antibody against respiratory viruses in man will be developed (Chanock et al., 1971).

Influenza Vaccine

Inactivated influenza vaccines have been in use now for many years, with varying success. There are several difficulties. The main one is to ensure that the composition of the vaccine with regard to antigenic components will match the epidemic strain of virus to which the vaccines are next exposed. Major antigenic shifts come at relatively infrequent intervals (e.g. 1946, 1957, 1968) and the minor shifts in between are not large enough to affect vaccine efficiency. Monitoring of new strains by WHO information centres gives warning of major and minor shifts although there may not always be time to prepare new vaccines in advance. But antigenic variation of influenza viruses is probably not unlimited and it may well prove possible, by careful selection of past and present strains and perhaps induced mutant strains, to produce a vaccine sufficiently multivalent to protect against future epidemic strains. A second difficulty is waning immunity, and it seems that herd immunity can be attained only by repeated annual vaccination. Such herd immunity will affect the spread of an epidemic strain only if a very high proportion of the population is vaccinated annually, and Davenport (1971) has shown that in military populations such herd immunity can be attained. The problem with civilian populations is the sheer weight of numbers, a staggering difficulty in highly developed countries, an almost insurmountable one in the underdeveloped. Even with the best available inactivated vaccines, protection rates above 70 per cent. have not always been reached, and such a rate is probably not high enough to prevent epidemic spread.

Live vaccines are still largely at the experimental stage; given intranasally as drops, sprays, or as snuff (Tyrrell and Beare, 1971) they may yet prove to be more reliable immunizing agents than inactivated vaccines. In the U.S.S.R. they have been used on a very wide scale (Smorodintsev et al., 1971). In the United Kingdom only inactivated vaccines have been released for general use. The official recommendations are that these should be used mainly to protect special groups such as patients with chronic chest, heart, or renal complaints, diabetes and other endocrine disorders, children or elderly people living in institutions in which rapid spread is likely, and doctors, nurses, and other health service personnel likely to be in contact with infected patients. This is a limited programme, unlikely to reduce epidemic spread, although capable perhaps of reducing the number of deaths. Vaccine is given on a fairly large scale to employees in factories and large stores as well, but the greatest impact on epidemic spread may come from the mass immunization of schoolchildren: this may become part of future policy. Influenza can be a fairly mild febrile illness, but in pandemic form it can slay more victims than have been killed so far in any world war.

Vaccines Other than Respiratory Virus Vaccines

Under this cumbersome title must be considered the vaccines available against the other air-borne infections discussed in this chapter—smallpox, measles, rubella, etc. The two main differences which simplify the production and use of these vaccines are that there is not the wild profusion of infective agents to deal with, and that immunity, once established, is long-lasting. They can accordingly be much more briefly considered.

Smallpox Vaccine. There is no doubt that vaccination against smallpox gives very great protection to the individual and that this lasts at least for several years. The only problem is to vaccinate a sufficient proportion of the world population, a problem at present being tackled with such success by the WHO smallpox eradication scheme that the disappearance of smallpox as a world epidemic disease is likely within a very few years. In 1973, smallpox was endemic in only four countries; India, Pakistan, Bangladesh and Ethiopia. In the western hemisphere, no cases had occurred since 1971, although in 1973 an outbreak occurred at St Mary's Hospital, London (Report of the Committee of Inquiry, 1974).

WHO Reference Centres continued their work in Utrecht and Toronto. During 1973, 400 batches of vaccine were tested. This represents the monitoring of more than 200 million doses of vaccine, which met the WHO standards for potency, stability and purity. In all, some 33 million doses of vaccine were distributed. More than 250,000 copies of WHO's diagnostic wall charts, smallpox recognition cards and teaching slides were distributed, in English and French (World Health Organization, 1974, p. 58).

Already, as a result, routine infant vaccination has been given up in the United Kingdom, United States, and elsewhere, for it is felt that the risk of serious complications of smallpox vaccination far outweighs the risk of contracting smallpox in these countries (*British Medical Journal*, 1970b). Trials of attenuated and inactivated vaccines are being carried out to try to reduce these complications, but it may well be that by the time these new vaccines are generally available the disease will have been eradicated by the old vaccines (Henderson, 1971; Kaplan, 1971).

Measles Vaccine. Live measles vaccine given by subcutaneous injection induces a high level of protection in the vaccinee. How long the protection lasts is not yet known but it is probably at least for several years. Inactivated vaccine also protects, but distressing reactions have occurred when vaccinees have later encountered live measles virus, either naturally or as a live vaccine: inactivated vaccine is no longer used. When vaccination has been used on a wide scale there has been a drop in the incidence of measles in the population, but it is now clear that a very high vaccination rate, over 80 per cent., is required if measles is to be eradicated from a population (Warin, and Mayon-White, 1971; Witte, 1971). While in some countries measles is as a rule a fairly mild disease, it cannot in any country be regarded as trivial. In some developing countries, Nigeria for example, it is still a leading cause of death, and a mass immunization campaign against the disease is one of the most urgent public health measures (Morley, Woodland,

and Martin, 1963; Foege, 1971.) Infants under 6 months are usually protected by maternal antibody; after that age most children are attacked by the disease, but the age at which they are attacked varies from country to country. In Nigeria, the median age of the disease is much lower than in Europe, and lowest in areas of high population density (Foege, 1971). Clearly, an immunization programme adapted to the epidemiological pattern in Europe would fail in Nigeria. The difficulty with measles vaccine is not in its protective efficacy, but in the organization of an immunization programme to reach the maximum number of susceptible children before they are exposed to the wild virus. Reactions from the live vaccine are usually mild, although convulsions and rare cases of encephalopathy have occurred in connexion with vaccination campaigns, but with improvements in vaccine production reactions are becoming less common. The risk is certainly acceptable in countries where measles is still a killing disease.

Rubella Vaccine. The aim with rubella vaccine is to protect the unborn child. If a susceptible pregnant woman is exposed to rubella in the early months of pregnancy there is no way of protecting the foetus against infection. Immune globulin is highly unreliable, and therapeutic abortion is the only certain method of preventing the birth of an infant with congenital rubella. This is not to say that abortion must always be carried out; that is a matter for the parties concerned to decide. It must be emphasized that most women of child-bearing age are already immune to rubella, as can be shown by serological tests, and abortion should not be considered until it has been shown that the pregnant woman lacks antibody from previous infection.

The aim of rubella prophylaxis is to render women immune before they become pregnant. There are several possible approaches. The first is to try to vaccinate all young children in an attempt to stop the circulation of wild virus in the environment of pregnant women. This has been the method initially followed in America, but it has not prevented the circulation of virus in adult communities, and it has been shown that vaccinees reinfected with wild virus do shed the virus although they may not develop symptoms of the disease (Horstmann *et al.*, 1970; Lehane, Newberg, and Beam, 1970). The second method is to vaccinate all girls between the ages of 11 and 13 years in the hope that their immunity will last long enough to protect them during their child-bearing years. This has been the method advised in Britain. The third method is to immunize susceptible pregnant women in the immediate post-partum period. This must obviously be only a subsidiary method. Rubella vaccine virus does cross the placenta and can infect the foetus; whether it can disrupt organogenesis is still uncertain. It is, however, obvious that the post-partum woman given live rubella vaccine must avoid conception for at least 3 months after vaccination. The problem of congenital rubella can certainly be solved. The best means of solving it has yet to be established.

Whooping Cough Vaccine. Whooping cough vaccines have had a varied career. In some countries, for example Czechoslovakia, vaccination campaigns have reduced the incidence to a very low figure. In Britain, after initial success, the vaccines failed to control the incidence. Two explanations for the failure in Britain are possible. The first is that the vaccines used did not contain a wide enough selection of

Bordetella pertussis agglutinogens, and that when a change in epidemic serotype took place in Britian the British vaccines gave little protection against the new serotype. The other explanation is that the British vaccines were simply not potent enough: they contained only 2 international potency units per dose while the recommended dose is 4 units. Both these explanations may be true, for a change in epidemic serotype in Britain certainly did coincide with increasing failure of the vaccines. Vaccines with 4 international units have been in use in Britain for some years now, but it is not yet clear whether the epidemic situation has changed. The subject of whooping cough vaccines has been covered in a recent review (Christie, 1971*b*).

Mumps Vaccine. Mumps is predominantly a disease of children and it is mainly when it attacks adults that it causes serious complications, of which the two most important are meningitis and orchitis. The essence of any mumps vaccination programme must therefore be to establish permanent immunity in vaccinees and to eradicate the virus from the community. Merely to shift the age incidence of the disease from children to adults could be disastrous. A live and a killed mumps vaccine have both been available for some years, but with neither has it been demonstrated that immunity established in the child lasts long enough to protect the adult. Killed vaccine has been used extensively in Finland to protect military recruits against mumps, and this is perhaps a more rational use of mumps vaccine (Penttinen, Cantell, and Poikolainea, 1969). Whether there is any danger of producing a hypersensitive state in the vaccinees, such as has occurred with respiratory syncytial virus and measles vaccine [pp. 204 and 210], is not known. For the time being, mumps vaccine can hardly rank for high priority in vaccination programmes (for review see Robbins, 1971).

Diphtheria Vaccine. The use of diphtheria toxoid over the last thirty to forty years has shown that the disease can be eradicated from a vaccinated population. In most developed countries the vaccine is given in a course of three injections during the first year of life, reinforced perhaps by a booster dose at school entry. The immunity is long-lasting but does decline with age, and a population may be built up in the course of years in which about 75 per cent. of the child population is immune and about 30 per cent. of the adult. Against such protection rates the reproduction rate of infection per case or carrier falls below one, and the disease dies out in the community (Smith, 1971). Continuation of this disease-free state depends on the maintenance of a high immunization rate among infants, probably at least 85 per cent. Unfortunately, when a disease disappears, enthusiasm for vaccination disappears with it, and there are probably few areas in Britain where the level of infant immunization approaches 85 per cent. and many are far below it. The result is bound to be a fall in the protection rates of children first and adults later, and the organism, if it gains entry, will spread in the community. Vigorous measures must then be taken to contain it; these include the detection and separation of the immune from the susceptibles, isolation of the infected, and active and perhaps passive immunization of susceptibles. In underdeveloped countries where the disease may still be endemic, these principles must be applied constantly, but eventually eradication of the disease lies with routine active immunization.

Meningococcal Vaccine. Very little attention has hitherto been given to the prevention of meningococcal infections by immunization, for prophylaxis by sulphonamides or penicillin has been much easier to apply. With the emergence of drug-resistant strains of meningococci, however, the possible use of vaccines has become important. Polysaccharide capsular antigens certainly provoke serum antibody, and when such vaccines have been used in military establishments they seem to have afforded considerable protection (Artenstein, 1971). The antibody which results is group-specific, although antibody formed by natural infection shows cross-reactions with heterologous groups of meningococci. A vaccine against group C meningococci, for example, gives no protection against group B; indeed, group C vaccinees may become carriers of group B meningococci or even develop group B meningitis. Obviously *polyvalent* group vaccines will be required to protect a community against meningococcal infection, but so far such vaccines are not available. Meningococcal vaccines may become more and more important prophylactic weapons, if drug-resistant meningococci become increasingly common.

ERADICATION

The aim of any programme of prevention must be eventual eradication of disease. With respiratory infections there are many epidemiological factors which must limit such expectation. Most obvious is the bewildering number of infective agents. With the means at our disposal—environmental improvement, vaccines, and drug prophylaxis—it is impossible to eradicate all respiratory infections, although each of these means can do something to reduce each of the infections. With regard to the acute respiratory virus syndromes the most promising candidate for eradication is influenza. The number of influenza virus strains is not infinite, and modern virological technique will probably be able to produce vaccines capable of dealing with any antigenic shift and of inducing the appropriate mucosal antibody in vaccinees. The problem then will be to immunize populations on a world-wide scale and to maintain the resulting immunity. This is perhaps an astronomical task but, in a moon-landing era, surely not an impossible one. On a smaller scale is the problem of respiratory syncytial and parainfluenza virus infections in infants, and of adenovirus infections in certain groups of adults, mainly military recruits. There is reasonable hope that these could be eradicated by improved and safer vaccines. Mycoplasma infections can probably be prevented by vaccines: the main difficulty is how and where to use the vaccines. Eradication of the common cold by any means yet at our disposal seems unlikely; the solution may lie with interferon-induction or some other means of adapting the host's defences to meet the array of rhinoviruses.

With the more specific generalized infections the outlook is far more promising. Smallpox may very soon be eradicated from the world, although constant vigilance may for ever be required to prevent its re-entry. Measles probably can be eradicated by mass immunization campaigns, but the measles virus will not readily give up the struggle for existence and continued immunization of infants will probably be necessary to keep it under control. It is difficult to forecast the future of rubella. It may continue to be a minor disease of young children and male adults, but the problem of congenital rubella should be overcome. Diphtheria has been virtually eliminated in many countries, and only administrative difficulties hinder its elimination in others; but complacency in face of a falling vaccination rate will almost certainly allow the disease to re-appear. Whooping cough vaccines are being improved and, given along with diphtheria vaccine, as they usually are, should lead to the disappearance of the disease, although constant watch must be kept on any changes in epidemic serotypes. When these more serious air-borne infections are under control attention might be given to the eradication of mumps [p. 207].

With regard to respiratory infections such as Q fever and psittacosis, an added difficulty is that these infections have alternative hosts in animals and birds. Experimental work has been carried out with Q fever vaccines (Wisseman, 1971) but, if a safe vaccine became available, the difficulty would be to know who required vaccination, for though infection is wide-spread in animals, disease in man is uncommon. The infection in animals is not of very great economic importance, so its elimination probably comes low in any veterinary disease eradication programme. With psittacosis the simple preventive measures taken by those who look after birds can do something to control the spread to man (*British Medical Journal*, 1972).

Streptococcal infections have to some extent solved their own problems, for at least in some parts of the world streptococci seem to have become less virulent for man. The main dangers remain acute rheumatism and acute glomerulonephritis, and to some extent these problems remain unsolved (Kuttner and Lancefield, 1970). Streptococcal infections of the pharynx should be treated with penicillin for ten days to eradicate streptococci, and children who have suffered one attack of rheumatic fever must be given penicillin daily for the rest of childhood to prevent further streptococcal infections—a rather clumsy prophylactic regime. Glomerulonephritis follows skin as often as throat infections and there is no way of detecting clinically when the infecting strain is a nephritogenic one; fortunately, nephritis does not recur with anything like the regularity of rheumatic relapses. Drug prophylactic measures have been mentioned in relation to meningococcal infections, and we have seen there that they have a declining role. Whether drugs or other antiviral agents will emerge as effective weapons against viruses and other agents of respiratory infection is im-possible to forecast. Amantidine, interferon and *N*-methylisatin β-thiosemicarbazone have as yet produced no dramatic break-through. There may be other antiviral agents on the way, a note of conjecture on which this chapter might very well end.

REFERENCES

Adels, B. R., and Gajdusek, D. C. (1963) Survey of measles patterns in New Guinea, Micronesia and Australia, with a report of new virgin soil epidemics and the demonstrations of susceptible primitive populations by serology, *Amer. J. Hyg.*, **77**, 317.

Aitken, C. J. D., Moffat, M. A., and Sutherland, J. A. W. (1967) Respiratory illness and viral infection in an Edinburgh nursery, *J. Hyg. (Lond.)*, **65**, 25.

American Journal of Hygiene (1946) Epidemic of Q fever among troops returning from Italy in the spring of 1945, II. Epi-demiological studies, *Amer. J. Hyg.*, **44**, 88.

Andrewes, Sir Christopher (1962) Harben Lecture. The common cold, *J. roy. Inst. publ. Hlth Hyg.*, **25**, 31, 55, 79.

Andrewes, C. H. (1967) The common cold: prospects for its control, *Med. Clin. N. Amer.*, **51**, 765.

Artenstein, M. S. (1971) Polysaccharide vaccines against meningococcal infections, in *Proc. Pan Amer. Hlth Org.*, p. 350.

Babudieri, B. (1953) Epidemiology, diagnosis and prophylaxis of Q fever, in Advances in the Control of Zoonoses, *Wld Hlth Org. Monogr. Ser.*, No. 25.

Babudieri, B. (1959) Q fever: a zoonosis, *Adv. vet. Sci.*, **5**, 81.

Back, E. H., and De Pass, E. E. (1964) Acute rheumatism in Jamaican children, *W. Indian med. J.*, **13**, 173.

Barrett, P. K. M., and Greenberg, J. M. (1966) Outbreak of ornithosis, *Brit. med. J.*, **2**, 206.

Bech, V. (1962) Measles epidemics in Greenland, *Amer. J. Dis. Childh.*, **103**, 252.

Becroft, D. M. O. (1967) Histopathology of fatal adenovirus infection of the respiratory tract in young children, *J. clin. Path.*, **20**, 561.

Bedson, S. P. (1940) Virus diseases acquired from animals, *Lancet*, **ii**, 577.

Beem, M. O. (1966) Acute respiratory illness in nursery school children. A longitudinal study of the occurrence of illness and respiratory viruses, *Amer. J. Epidem.*, **90**, 30.

Berman, S., Freudlich, E., Glazer, K., Abrahamov, A., Ephrati-Elizur, E., and Bernkoff, H. (1955) Ornithosis in infancy, *Pediatrics*, **15**, 752.

Biberfeld, G., and Sterner, G. (1969) A study of *Mycoplasma pneumoniae* infections in families, *Scand. J. infec. Dis.*, **1**, 39.

Bisno, A. L., Barratt, N. P., Swanston, W. H., and Spence, L. P. (1970) An outbreak of acute respiratory disease in Trinidad associated with parainfluenza viruses, *Amer. J. Epidem.*, **91**, 68.

Bloomfield, A. (1958) *A Bibliography of Internal Medicine. Communicible Diseases*, Chicago.

Bowmer, E. J. (1958) A human outbreak of psittacosis due to infected turkeys in poultry-processing plant, *Canad. J. publ. Hlth*, **49**, 27.

British Medical Journal (1970*a*) A puzzling respiratory virus, *Brit. med. J.*, **1**, 317.

British Medical Journal (1970*b*) Smallpox vaccination, *Brit. med. J.*, **2**, 311.

British Medical Journal (1972) Psittacosis, *Brit. med. J.*, **1**, 1.

Brody, J. A., Sever, J. L., McAlister, R., Schiff, G. M., and Cutting, R. (1965) Rubella epidemic on St. Paul island in the Pribilofs, 1963, 1. Epidemiologic, clinical, and serological findings, *J. Amer. med. Ass.*, **191**, 619.

Brown, G. H., Colwell, D. C., and Hooper, W. (1968) An out-break of Q fever in Staffordshire, *J. Hyg. (Lond.)*, **66**, 649.

Brown, P. K., and Taylor-Robinson, D. (1966) Respiratory viruses in sera of persons living in isolated communities, *Bull. Wld Hlth Org.*, **34**, 895.

Brown, P., Gajdusek, D. C., and Morris, J. A. (1966) Epidemic A2 influenza in isolated Pacific island populations without pre-epidemic antibody to influenza virus types A and B and the discovery of other still unexposed populations, *Amer. J. Epidem.*, **83**, 176.

Buescher, E. L. (1967) Respiratory disease and the adenoviruses, *Med. Clin. N. Amer.*, **51**, 769.

Buescher, E. L. (1971) Respiratory virus diseases: discussion, in *Proc. Pan Amer. Hlth Org.*, p. 132.

Cameron, A. S., and Moore, B. W. (1968) The epidemiology of respiratory infection in an isolated Antarctic community, *J. Hyg. (Camb.)*, **66**, 427.

Chan, V. F., Campos, L. E., Cenabre, L., and Guinta-Fanratiga, E. (1963) Viruses of the respiratory tract in Filippinos, I. Para-influenza types 1 and 3, *J. Philipp. med. Ass.*, **39**, 303.

Chanock, R. M., Kim, H. W., Vargosko, A. J., Deleva, A., Johnson, K. M., Cumming, C., and Parrott, R. H. (1961) Respiratory syncytial virus, 1. Virus recovery and other observations during 1960 outbreak of bronchiolitis, pneumonia and minor respiratory diseases of childhood, *J. Amer. med. Ass.*, **176**, 647.

Chanock, R. M., Mufson, M. A., and Johnson, K. M. (1965) Comparative biology and ecology of human viruses and mycoplasma respiratory pathogens, *Progr. med. Virol.*, **7**, 208.

Chanock, R. M., Smith, C. B., Friedewald, W. T., Parrott, A. H., Forsyth, B. R., Coates, H. V., Kapikian, A. Z., and Charpure, M. A. (1967) Resistance to para-influenza and respiratory syncytial virus infection—implications for effective immunization and preliminary study of an attenuated strain of respiratory syncytial virus, in *Vaccines against Viral and Rickettsial Diseases of Man*, Pan American Health Organization Scientific Publication No. 147, Washington, D. C., pp. 53–61.

Chanock, R. M., Kapikian, A. Z., Perkins, J. C., and Parrott, R. H. (1971) Vaccines for nonbacterial respiratory diseases other than influenza, in *Proceedings* (1971), p. 101.

Cheeseman, E. A. (1950) Epidemics in schools, *Spec. Rep. Ser. Med. Res. Coun.*, No. 271, London, H.M.S.O.

Chin, J., Magoffin, R. L., Shearer, L. A., Schlieble, J. H., and Lennette, E. H. (1969) Field evaluation of a respiratory syncytial virus vaccine in a pediatric population, *Amer. J. Epidem.*, **89**, 449.

Christie, A. B. (1974) *Infectious Diseases: Epidemiology and Clinical Practice*, Edinburgh.

Christie, A. B. (1971a) The public health importance of respiratory virus diseases in the developed and developing countries, in *Proc. Pan Amer. Hlth Org.*, p. 81.

Christie, A. B. (1971b) Immunization against whooping-cough, *Community Health*, **2**, 241.

Christie, A. B. (1972) Acute infectious disease, in *Medical Progress 1971–72*, ed. Richardson, Sir John, London.

Connor, J. D. (1970) Evidence for an etiologic role of adenoviral infection in pertussis syndrome, *New Engl. J. Med.*, **283**, 390.

Cockburn, W. C. (1973) Influenza in man and animals, *Wld Hlth Org. Chron.*, **27**, 185.

Davenport, F. M. (1971) Killed influenza virus vaccines: present status, suggested use, desirable developments, in *Proceedings* (1971), p. 189.

Dermon, H., and Le Hew, E. W. (1944) A mumps epidemic in a task force, *Amer. J. med. Sci.*, **208**, 240.

Dew, J., Mawson, K., Ellman, P., and Brough, D. (1960) Ornithosis in two railway guards: an occupational hazard, *Lancet*, **ii**, 18.

Doggett, J. E. (1965) Antibodies to respiratory syncytial virus in human sera from different regions of the world, *Bull. Wld Hlth Org.*, **32**, 841.

Douglas, R. G., Lindgren, K. M., and Couch, R. B. (1968) Exposure to cold environment and rhinovirus common cold. Failure to demonstrate effect, *New Engl. J. Med.*, **279**, 742.

Dowling, H. F., Jackson, G. G., Spiesman, I. G., and Inowye, T. (1958) Transmission of the common cold to volunteers under controlled conditions, III. The effect of chilling of the subjects upon susceptibility, *Amer. J. Hyg.*, **66**, 59.

Downie, A. W., St. Vincent, L., Micklejohn, G., Ratnakanna, N. R., Rae, A. R., Krishnan, G. N. V., and Kempe, C. H. (1961) Studies on the virus content of mouth washings in the acute phase of smallpox, *Bull. Wld Hlth Org.*, **25**, 29.

Downie, A. W. (1965) Chicken-pox and zoster, in *Virus and Rickettsial Diseases of Man*, Bedson, S. P., Downie, A. W., MacCallum, F. O., and Stuart-Harris, C. H., London.

Dudley, S. F., and Brennan, J. R. (1934) High and persistent carrier rates of *Neisseria meningitidis* unaccompanied by cases of meningitis, *J. Hyg. (Lond.)*, **34**, 525.

Dudgeon, J. A. (1973) The prevention of rubella, *Wld Hlth Org. Chron.*, **27**, 70.

Edmonson, W. P., Purcell, R. H., Gundelfinger, B. F., Love, J. W. P., Ludwig, W., and Chanock, R. M. (1966) Immunization by selective infection with type 4 adenovirus grown in human diploid tissue culture, II. Specific protective effect against epidemic disease, *J. Amer. med. Ass.*, **195**, 453.

Evans, A. S., D'ALessio, D. A., Espiritou-Campos, L., and Dick, E. C. (1967) Acute respiratory disease in the University of the Philippines and University of Wisconsin students: a comparative study, *Bull. Wld Hlth Org.*, **36**, 397.

Evans, A. S., and Espiritou-Campos, L. (1971) Acute respiratory disease in students at the University of the Philippines, 1946–49, *Bull. Wld Hlth Org.*, **45**, 103.

Foege, W. H. (1971) Measles vaccination in Africa, in *Proc. Pan Amer. Hlth Org.*, p. 207.

Forsyth, B. R. (1965) Etiology of primary atypical pneumonia in a military population, *J. Amer. med. Ass.*, **191**, 364.

Fransen, H., and Wolontis, S. (1969) Infections with viruses, *M. pneumoniae* and bacteria in acute respiratory illness, *Scand. J. infect. Dis.*, **1**. 31.

Gardner, P. S., McQuillin, J., and Court, S. D. M. (1970) Speculation on pathogenesis in death from respiratory syncytial virus infection, *Brit. med. J.*, **1**, 327.

Ghipponi, P., Darrigol, J., Skalova, R., and Cvjetanović, B. (1971) Study of bacterial air pollution in an arid region of Africa affected by cerebrospinal meningitis, *Bull. Wld Hlth Org.*, **45**, 95.

Glover, J. A. (1920) *Special Report Series Medical Research Council* No. 50, London, H.M.S.O.

Gordon, J. E., Wyon, J. B., and Ascoll, M. D. (1967) The second year death rate in less developed countries, *Amer. J. med. Sci.*, **254**, 357.

Gwaltney, J. M., and Jordan, W. S. (1964) Rhinoviruses and respiratory disease, *Bact. Rev.*, **28**, 409.

Haagen, E., and Krackeberg, E. (1937) Veroff a.d. Gebiete d. Volksgesundheits dienstes 48, Heft 423, 384; quoted by Shaughnessy, H. J. (1955).

Hamre, D., and Procnow, J. J. (1963) Virologic studies on common colds among adult medical students, *Amer. Rev. resp. Dis.*, **88**, No. 3, Pt. 2, 227.

Harvey, M. S., Forbes, G. B., and Marmion, B. P. (1951) An outbreak of Q fever in East Kent, *Lancet*, **ii**, 1152.

Hedblom, E. E. (1961) The medical problems encountered in Antarctica, *Military Medicine*, **126**, 818.

Henderson, D. A. (1971) Smallpox. The problem, in *Proceedings* (1971), p. 139.

Henle, G., Henle, W., Wendell, K., and Rosenberg, P. (1948) Isolation of mumps virus from human beings with induced apparent and inapparent mumps, *J. exp. Med. Biol (N.Y.)*, **88**, 223.

Holmes, M. J., Allen, T. R., Bradburne, A. F., and Stott, E. J. (1971) Studies of respiratory viruses in personnel at an Antarctic base, *J. Hyg. (Camb.)*, **69**, 187.

Horstmann, D. M., Liebhaber, H., Le Bouvier, G. L., Rosenberg, D. A., and Halstead, S. B. (1970) Rubella—reinfection of vaccinated and naturally immune persons in an epidemic, *New Engl. J. Med.*, **283**, 771.

Hsiung, C. C. (1963) Adenovirus pneumonia in infants and children: pathologic studies of 40 cases, *Chin. med. J.*, **82**, 390.

Iver, J., and Padmavati, S. (1965) Difficulties of rheumatic fever prophylaxis in Delhi. Results of a preliminary study, *J. Ass. Phycns India*, **13**, 89.

Jackson, G. G., Muldoon, R. L., Johnson, G. C., and Dowling, H. F. (1963) Contribution of volunteers to studies on the common cold, *Amer. Rev. resp. Dis.*, **88**, No. 3, Pt 2, 120.

Jacobs, J. N., Peacock, D. B., Corner, B. D., Caul, E. O., and Clarke, S. K. R. (1971) Respiratory syncytial and other viruses associated with respiratory disease in infants, *Lancet*, **i**, 871.

Jennings, R., and Grant, L. S. (1967a) Respiratory viruses in Jamaica: virologic and serologic study, I. Virus isolation and serologic studies on clinical specimens, *Amer. J. Epidem.*, **86**, 690.

Jennings, R., and Grant, L. S. (1967b) Respiratory viruses in Jamaica: virologic and serologic study, II. Haemagglutination-inhibiting antibodies to influenza A viruses in the sera of Jamaicans, *Amer. J. Epidem.*, **86**, 700.

Jennings, R. (1968) Respiratory viruses in Jamaica, III. Haemagglutination-inhibiting antibodies to type B and C viruses in the sera of Jamaicans, *Amer. J. Epidem.*, **87**, 440.

Kaplan, C. (1971). Smallpox. Vaccines; present status, suggested use, desirable developments, in *Proc. Pan Amer. Hlth Org.*, p. 144.

Kendal, E. J. C., Rodan, K. S., Riddle, R. W., Andrews, B. E., Tuck, H. A., and McDonald, J. C. (1957) Pharyngoconjunctival fever: school outbreaks in England during summer of 1955, *Brit. med. J.*, **2**, 121.

Kim, H. W., *et al.* (1969) Respiratory syncytial virus neutralizing activity in nasal secretion following natural infection, *Proc. Soc. exp. Biol. Med.*, **131**, 658.

Kravetz, H. M., Knight, V., Chanock, R. M., Morris, J. A., Johnston, K. M., Rifkind, D., and Utz, J. P. (1961) Respiratory syncytial virus, III. Production of illness and clinical observations in adult volunteers, *J. Amer. med. Ass.*, **176**, 657.

Kuttner, A. C., and Lancefield, R. C. (1970) Unsolved problems of the non-suppurative complications of group A streptococcal infections, in *Infectious Agents and Host Reactions*, ed. Mudd, S., Philadelphia.

Lambert, H. P. (1968) Antibody to *Mycoplasma pneumoniae* in normal subjects and in patients with chronic bronchitis, *J. Hyg. (Lond.)*, **66**, 185.

Lancet (1973) Leading article, ii, 1246.

Lang, W. R., Howden, C. W., Laws, J., and Barton, J. F. (1969) Bronchopneumonia with serious sequelae in children with evidence of adenovirus 21 infection, *Brit. med. J.*, **1**, 73.

Lawther, P. J., Waller, R. E., and Hudson, M. (1970) Air pollution and exacerbations of bronchitis, *Thorax*, **25**, 525.

Lehane, D. E., Newberg, N. R., and Beam, W. E. (1970) Evaluation of herd immunity during an epidemic, *J. Amer. med. Ass.*, **213**, 2336.

Luoto, L., and Pickens, E. G. (1961) A résumé of recent research seeking to define the Q fever problem, *Amer. H. Hyg.*, **74**, 43.

Marcus, S., Miya, F., Phelps, L. J., and Spencer, L. (1963) Influence of low ambient temperature on resistance of mice to experimental Coxsackie infection, *Arctic Aeromedical Laboratory Technical Documentary Report 62–65*; quoted by Holmes, M. J., *et al.* (1971).

Marcus, S., and Miya, F. (1964) Effect of different routes of challenge Coxsackie B virus on cold-stressed mice, *Arctic Aeromedical Laboratory Technical Documentary Report 64–2*, quoted by Holmes, M. J., *et al.* (1971).

Maris, E. P., Enders, J. F., Stokes, J., and Kane, L. W. (1946) Immunity in mumps, IV. Correlation of the presence of complement-fixing antibody and resistance to mumps in human beings, *J. exp. Med. Biol (N.Y.)*, **88**, 323.

Marmion, B. P., Stoker, M. G. P., McCoy, J., Malloch, R. A., and Moore, B. (1953) Q fever in Britain, *Lancet*, **i**, 503.

Marsden, P. D. (1964) The Sukuta project. A longitudinal study of health in Gambian children from birth to 18 months of age, *Trans. roy. Soc. trop. Med. Hyg.*, **58**, 455.

Maynard, J. E., Felty, E. T., Wulff, H., Fortuine, R., Poland, J. D., and Chin, T. D. Y. (1967) Surveillance of respiratory virus infections among Alaskan Eskimo children, *J. Amer. med. Ass.*, **200**, 927.

McNamara, M. J., Pierce, W. E., Crawford, Y. E., and Miller, L. F. (1962) Patterns of adenovirus infection in the respiratory diseases of naval recruits. A longitudinal study of 2 companies of naval recruits, *Amer. Rev. resp. Dis.*, **86**, 485.

Medical Research Council (1964) An investigation into respiratory illnesses in overseas and United Kingdom students. A report to the Medical Research Council's Committee on the aetiology of chronic bronchitis, *Brit. J. prev. soc. Med.*, **18**, 174.

Medical Research Council (1965) Medical Research Council Working Party on Acute Respiratory Viral Infections. A collaborative study of the aetiology of acute respiratory infections in Britain 1961–64, *Brit. med. J.*, **2**, 319.

Miller, C. P., and Bohnhoff, M. (1947) Studies on the action of penicillin, VI. Further observation on the development of penicillin resistance by meningococci *in vitro*, *J. infect. Dis.*, **81**, 147.

Miller, D. L., Pereira, M. S., and Clarke, M. (1971) Epidemiology of the Hong Kong/68 variant of influenza A2 in Britain, *Brit. med. J.*, **1**, 475.

Mogabgab, W. J. (1971) *Mycoplasma pneumoniae* vaccines, in *Proc. Pan Amer. Hlth Org.*, p. 117.

Monto, A. S., and Johnson, K. M. (1967) A community study of respiratory infections in the tropics, I. Description of community and observations on certain respiratory agents, *Amer. J. Epidem.*, **86**, 78.

Monto, A. S. (1968a) A community study of respiratory infections in the tropics, II. The spread of six rhinovirus isolates within the community, *Amer. J. Epidem.*, **88**, 55.

Monto, A. S. (1968b) A community study of respiratory infections in the tropics, III. Introduction and transmission of infection within families, *Amer. J. Epidem.*, **88**, 69.

Morley, D. C., Woodland, M., and Martin, W. J. (1963) Measles in Nigerian children. A study of the disease in West Africa, and its manifestations in England and other countries during different epochs, *J. Hyg. (Lond.)*, **61**, 115.

Mufson, M. A., Krause, H. E., Mocega, H. E., and Dawson, F. W. (1970) Viruses, *Mycoplasma pneumoniae* and bacteria associated with lower respiratory tract disease in infants, *Amer. J. Epidem.*, **91**, 192.

Njoku-obi, A. N., and Ogunbi, O. (1966a) Viral respiratory diseases in Nigeria. A serological survey, I. Complement-fixing antibody levels of influenza A, B and C and para-influenza 1, *J. trop. Med. Hyg.*, **69**, 81.

Njoku-Obi, A. N., and Ogunbi, O. (1966b) Viral respiratory diseases in Nigeria. A serological survey, II. Complement-fixing antibody levels of adenoviruses, respiratory syncytial virus, and psittacosis virus, *J. trop. Med. Hyg.* **69**, 147.

Olson, B. J., and Treuting, W. L. (1944) An epidemic of a severe pneumonitis in the Bayou region of Louisiana, I. Epidemiological study, *Publ. Hlth Rep. (Wash.)*, **59**, 1299.

Pan American Health Organization (1971) *International Conference on the Application of Vaccines against Viral, Rickettsial and Bacterial Diseases of Man*, Pan American Health Organization Scientific Publication No. 226, Washington, D.C.

Papp, C. (1956) Expériences prouvant que la voie d'infection de la rougeole est la contamination de la muquevose conjunctivale, *Rev. Immunol. Ther. antimicrob.*, **20**, 27.

Parrott, R. H., Kim, H. W., Arrobio, J. O., Canchola, J. G., Brandt, C. D., De Meio, J. L., Jensen, K. E., and Chanock, R. M. (1967) Experience with inactivated respiratory syncytial and para-influenzal virus vaccines in infants, in *Vaccines against Viral and Rickettsial Diseases of Man*, Pan American Health Organization Scientific Publication No. 147, Washington, D.C., pp. 35–41.

Parrott, R. H., Rowe, W. P., Huebner, R. J., Bernton, H. W., and McCullough, N. M. (1954) Outbreak of acute febrile pharyngitis and conjunctivitis associated with type 3 adenovirus infection, *New Engl. J. Med.*, **251**, 1087.

Paul, F. M. (1963) Study of acute nephritis in Singapore children, *J. Singapore pediat. Soc.*, **5**, 54.

Paul, J. H., and Freese, H. L. (1933) An epidemiological and bacteriological study of the 'common cold' in an isolated Arctic community (Spitzbergen), *Amer. J. Hyg.*, **17**, 517.

Penttinen, K. K., Cantell, P. S., and Poikolainea, A. (1969) Mumps vaccination in Finnish defence forces, *Nordsk. Med.* **81**, 685; quoted by Robbins, F. C. (1971).

Pereira, M. S., Andrews, B. E., and Gardner, S. D. (1967) A study on the virus aetiology of mild respiratory infections in the primary school child, *J. Hyg. (Lond.)*, **65**, 475.

Pereira, M. S., and Candelas, J. A. N. (1971) The Association of viruses with clinical pertussis, *J. Hyg. (Camb.)*, **69**, 399.

Pereira, M. S., and Schild, G. (1971) Antigenic variant of the Hong Kong/68 influenza A2 virus, *J. Hyg. (Camb.)*, **69**, 99.

Pierce, W. E., Still, W. T., Rytel, M., and Miller, L. F. (1962)

The relationship between routine inoculations and the incidence of respiratory disease in the naval recruits at Great Lakes, Illinois, *Annual Report to the Committee on Influenza of the American Forces Epidemiological Board*; quoted by Rytel, M. W. (1964) *Amer. J. med. Sci.*, **247**, 84.

Potter, E. V., Moran, H. S., Poon-King, T., and Earle, D. P. (1968) Characteristics of beta haemolytic streptococci associated with acute glomerulonephritis in Trinidad. *J. Lab. clin. Med.*, **71**, 126.

Riemann, H. A. (1971) Infectious diseases. Annual review of significant publications, *Postgrad. J. Med.*, **47**, 332.

Rindge, M. E., Jungherr, E. L., and Scraggs, J. H. (1959) Serological evidence of occupational psittacosis in poultry plant workers, *New Engl. J. Med.*, **260**, 1214.

Robbins, F. C., and Ragan, P. (1955) Q fever in the Mediterranean area: report of its occurrence in allied troops, 1. Clinical features of the disease, *Amer. J. Hyg.*, **44**, 6.

Robbins, F. C. (1971) Mumps: the problem, in *Proc. Pan Amer. Hlth Org.*, p. 216.

Sever, J. L., Brody, J. A., Schiff, G. M., McAllister, R., and Cutting, R. (1965) Rubella epidemic in St. Paul island in the Pribilofs, 1963, 2. Clinical and laboratory findings for the intensive study population, *J. Amer. med. Ass.*, **191**, 624.

Shaughnessy, H. J. (1955) Psitticosis (Ornithosis), in *Diseases Transmitted from Animals to Man*, ed. Hull, T. G., Springfield, Ill.

Shibli, M., Gooch, S., Lewis, H. E., and Tyrrell, D. A. J. (1971) Common colds on Tristan da Cunha, *J. Hyg. (Camb.)*, **69**, 255.

Smith, J. W. G. (1971) Bacterial diseases. Prevention and control by vaccines. Diphtheria, in *Proc. Pan Amer. Hlth Org.*, p. 316.

Smorodintsev, A. A., Alexandrova, G. I., Schwartzman, J. S., and Zhelova, G. P. (1971) Respiratory virus disease: discussion, in *Proc. Pan Amer. Hlth Org.*, p. 127.

Somerville, R. G. (1963) Respiratory syncytial virus in acute exacerbations of chronic bronchitis, *Lancet*, **ii**, 1247.

Spence, L., and Barratt, N. (1968) Respiratory syncytial virus associated with acute respiratory infections in Trinidadian patients, *Amer. J. Epidem.*, **88**, 257.

Stenhouse, A. C. (1968) Viral antibody levels and clinical states in acute exacerbations of chronic bronchitis: a controlled prospective study, *Brit. med. J.*, **3**, 287.

Stocks, P. (1933) Some epidemiologal features of whooping-cough, *Lancet*, **i**, 265.

Stoker, M. G. P., and Thompson, J. (1953) An explosive outbreak of Q fever, *Lancet*, **i**, 137.

Stoker, M. G. P., and Marmion, B. P. (1955) The spread of Q fever from animals to man. The natural history of a rickettsial disease, *Bull. Wld Hlth Org.*, **13**, 781.

Strasser, T., and Rotta, J. (1973) The control of rheumatic fever and rheumatic heart disease: an outline of WHO activities, *Wld Hlth Org. Chron.*, **27**, 49.

Strudwick, R. H. (1962) A morbidity survey conducted in North Tetu division of Nyeri district, Central Province, Kenya, *E. Afr. med. J.*, **39**, 536.

Sturdy, P. M., Frood, G. D. L., and Gardner, P. S. (1971) Viruses in families, *Lancet*, **i**, 769.

Sutton, R. N. P. (1965) Minor illness in Trinidad: a longitudinal study, *Trans. roy. Soc. trop. Med. Hyg.*, **59**, 212.

Sutton, R. N. P. (1965) Minor illness in Trinidad: a longitudinal study, *Trans. roy Soc. trop. Med. Hyg.*, **59**, 212.

Taneja, P. N., Ghai, O. P., and Bhakoo, O. N. (1962) Importance of measles to India, *Amer. J. Dis. Childh.*, **103**, 226.

Taylor, I. M. (1960) Medical experiences at McMurdo Sound, in *Cold Injury*, Transactions of the Sixth Conference, 1958, Fort Knox, ed. Horvath, S. M., Josiah Macy, Jr. Foundation, New York, p. 157.

Taylor-Robinson, D., and Bynoe, M. (1964) Inoculation of volunteers with H rhinoviruses, *Brit. med. J.*, **1**, 540.

Taylor-Robinson, D. (1965) Respiratory virus antibodies in human sera from different regions of the world, *Bull. Wld Hlth Org.*, **32**, 833.

Tyrrell, D. A. J., Bynoe, M. L., Petersen, B. K., Sutton, R. N. P., and Pereira, M. S. (1959) Inoculation of human volunteers with parainfluenza viruses types 1 and 3 (HA2 and HA1), *Brit. med. J.*, **1**, 302.

Tyrrell, D. A. J. (1965a) Symposium on the common cold, *Proc. roy. Soc. Med.*, **59**, 637.

Tyrrell, D. A. J. (1965b) *Common Colds and Related Diseases*, London.

Tyrrell, D. A. J., Peto, M., and King, N. (1967) Serological studies on infection by respiratory viruses of the inhabitants of Tristan da Cunha, *J. Hyg. (Camb.)*, **65**, 327.

Tyrrell, D. A. J. (1969) Some recent trends in vaccination against respiratory viruses, *Brit. med. Bull.*, **25**, 165.

Tyrrell, D. A. J., and Beare, A. S. (1971) Live influenza vaccine: an interim report, in *Proc. Pan Amer. Hlth Org.*, p. 96.

Vedros, N. A., and Hottle, J. A. (1970) Neisseria and neisserial infection, in *Infectious Agents and Host Reactions*, ed. Mudd, S., Philadelphia.

Van der Veen, J., Aberbanel, M. F. W., and Oei, K. G. (1968) Vaccination with type 4 adenovirus: evaluation of antibody response and protective efficacy, *J. Hyg. (Camb.)*, **66**, 499.

Van der Veen, J., Oei, K. S., and Aberbanel, M. F. W. (1969) Patterns of infections with adenovirus types 4, 7 and 21 in military recruits during a 9-year survey, *J. Hyg. (Camb.)*, **67**, 255.

Warin, J. F., and Mayon-White, R. T. (1971) Measles in a vaccinated community, *Lancet*, **ii**, 1034.

Wehrle, P. F., Posch, J., Richter, K. H., and Henderson, D. A. (1970) An airborne outbreak of smallpox in a German hospital and its significance in respect of other recent outbreaks in Europe, *Bull. Wld Hlth Org.*, **43**, 669.

Wilson, G. S. (1962) Measles; a universal disease, *Amer. J. Dis. Childh.*, **103**, 219.

Wisseman, C. L. (1971) Problems of rickettsial diseases and vaccines: desirable developments, in *Proc. Pan Amer. Hlth Org.*, p. 289.

Witte, J. J. (1971) Measles vaccination in the United States, in *Proc. Pan Amer. Hlth Org.*, p. 213.

World Health Organization (1967) Respiratory disease survey in children. A serological study, *Bull. Wld Hlth Org.*, **37**, 363.

World Health Organization (1969) Respiratory viruses. Report of a World Health Organization Scientific Group, *Wld Hlth Org. techn. Rep. Ser.*, No. 408.

World Health Organization (1971) Rheumatic heart disease in India, *Wld Hlth Org. Chron.*, **25**, 524.

World Health Organization (1973a) Report of a WHO Expert Committee on Smallpox: Smallpox Eradication in 1972, *Wld Hlth Org. techn Rep. Ser.*, No. 347.

World Health Organization (1973b) Cerebro-spinal meningitis, Wld Hlth Org. Chron., **25**, 524.

World Health Organization (1974) The work of WHO in 1973, *Wld Hlth Org. Off. Rec.*, No. 213.

World Health Organization Regional Office for Europe (1973) Report of a Working Group on Measles Vaccination, Algiers 1972 (Euro 1902), Copenhagen.

World Health Organization Regional Office for Europe (1973) Report of a Working Group on the Prevention of Rubella, Budapest 1972 (Euro 1901), Copenhagen.

16

EPIDEMIOLOGY AND CONTROL
OF WATER- AND FOOD-BORNE INFECTIONS

BRANKO CVJETANOVIĆ

INTRODUCTION

Water and food are ingested daily by everyone, and they may carry pathogenic micro-organisms which cause intestinal infections and intoxications. Failure to protect water and food from contamination by faecal matter, which can carry intestinal pathogens excreted by sick persons and carriers, is the cause of intestinal infections. While some infections are exclusively water- or food-borne, there are others, such as poliomyelitis and hepatitis, that can be spread at the same time by close contacts or droplets. There is practically no infection that cannot be transmitted by ingestion of contaminated water and food, and such incidental infections also occur in diseases which do not belong to the group of intestinal infections. In this chapter we shall consider in detail only those infections that are most commonly transmitted by water and food, and which represent an important public health problem.

A common pattern of water- and food-borne infections is that their maintenance in the community depends on an anal–oral circulation of micro-organisms due to the ecological conditions, and failures of sanitation and personal hygiene. Environmental conditions, social, cultural, and economic factors play an important role. Certain food habits, and the way water and food are kept, prepared, and consumed, in addition to personal cleanliness and the availability of facilities for the practice of hygiene in daily life, are the factors which determine the incidence of intestinal infections. They are therefore common in the underprivileged groups of the population. Poverty and lack of education foster the spread of intestinal infections, hence the reason why they represent an especially grave problem for the developing countries.

In fact, taken from a broad aspect, in the evolution of human society water- and food-borne infections are best brought under control by means of good planning, public education, and prosperity. However, in emergencies specific measures are used to bring water- and food-borne outbreaks under control rapidly, although the ultimate solution cannot be achieved until society reaches a high standard of community and individual hygiene which is associated with economic development. At present, enteric fevers and other intestinal infections are mainly diseases of poor and underprivileged people.

With the progress of sanitation and hygiene, water- and food-borne diseases are controlled, and people living in healthy environments, who respect the principles of personal hygiene, are not victims of intestinal infection—with the possible exception of a few who are neither poor nor deprived of facilities but who do not respect the principles of personal

hygiene. There are, of course, accidental infections in persons who are the victims of the unhygienic practices of others.

In *developing countries* all over the world, intestinal infections, namely enteritis, colitis, gastritis, duodenitis (reported as B36 under the *International Classification of Diseases*), are a leading cause of deaths in children under 4 years of age [FIG. 57]. It is

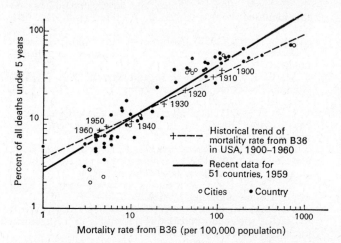

FIG. 57. Levels of health and mortality from B36. (B36 comprises gastritis, duodenitis, enteritis, and colitis except diarrhoea of the newborn.) [Cvjetanović, B. *et al.* (1965) *Milbank mem. Fd Quart.*, **43**, No. 2, 240.]

considered that high infant and young child mortality is an indicator of the low level of development of health services and of the low stage of general evolution of a community. High infant and child (under the age of five) mortality is correlated with the death rates due to intestinal infections associated with diarrhoea (B36), as shown on data collected from 51 countries during the last six decades [FIG. 57]. This correlation seems to be general. Many developing countries are now where the United States was at the beginning of the century in respect to infant and child mortality and diarrhoeal diseases. On the path to progress and development diarrhoeal diseases are gradually controlled. However, since many developing countries have still a long way to go, diarrhoeal diseases, which are the main cause of high infant and child mortality, will continue to be a problem of paramount importance for such countries.

In such areas intestinal infections in general are highly endemic; their incidence is more or less stable and maintained at a high level, with seasonal variations and fluctuations which are caused by migrations, pilgrimages, and other mass movements and happenings that disturb the usual pattern of daily life. In more prosperous areas, intestinal infections occur in small or larger outbreaks. Central water supplies and central food distribution—typical for modern society—when they accidentally fail in achieving hygienic precautions and standards, may be the cause of large explosive outbreaks. However, small outbreaks occur more often.

Food-borne outbreaks are not always caused by microorganisms of intestinal infections. For reporting purposes such outbreaks are considered as any illness caused by ingestion of pathogenic organisms or other noxious agents contained in polluted water or food, and affecting two or more persons at a time. However, there is one exception: a single case of botulism is considered as an outbreak. Typical food-borne outbreaks are usually caused by the following micro-organisms: *Salmonella, Shigella, Staphylococcus aureus, Clostridium botulinum, Clostridium welchii (perfringens), Bacillus cereus, Vibrio parahaemolyticus*, and enterococci (Lancefield group D streptococci). Infections with other enteropathogenic organisms such as *V. cholerae*, while often traced to the eating of contaminated food in certain restaurants, still do not cause typical food-borne outbreaks such as are known after 'church dinners' and marriage festivals, for example outbreaks of typhoid and other salmonelloses. A typical feature of food-borne outbreaks is that they strike many people at one time, but as mentioned above two associated cases are also considered to be an outbreak.

Diarrhoeal diseases, characterized by the diarrhoeal symptom or syndrome, which progresses from a few loose stools to severe dehydration and death, are of various aetiological origins. However, from a practical public health standpoint they can be considered as one broad epidemiological entity. Although their causation is different and often linked with malnutrition (Cruickshank, 1967; Gordon *et al.*, 1968) and a heavy load of helminths, they have some important common features. They attack mostly infants and young children, and thus the expression 'weanling diarrhoea' is often used (Gordon *et al.*, 1968). In fact, the infant is protected from this in the early months of life by being fed with mother's milk. As soon as he starts to take a variety of different food carrying various bacteria, his digestion is often upset by these bacteria and their toxins, resulting in diarrhoea. As a normal inhabitant of intestines, *Escherichia coli* often produces toxic substances that do not disturb adults, but cause diarrhoea in infants when present in great numbers (Gorbach, 1967). The young are particularly vulnerable before they adapt to their surroundings. However, only in a small fraction of children with diarrhoea can recognized pathogenic organisms be isolated. Diarrhoeal diseases should therefore be at least partly considered as a syndrome—perhaps part of a general adaptation syndrome— apart from such cases that are definitely proved to be caused by Enterobacteriaceae and other infectious agents. The poorest of the developing countries are those that suffer most (World Health Organization, 1964*b*).

Infantile gastro-enteritis which, like 'diarrhoeal diseases' has never been clearly defined, overlaps with other terms such as 'infantile diarrhoea' when diarrhoeal symptoms prevail, or 'summer diarrhoea' when it appears in epidemics in the summer. The variety of entities is due to:

1. Primary infectious origin.
2. Secondary sequelae or other non-intestinal infections, such as otitis media and respiratory infections.

3. Nutritional deficiencies and faulty feeding of infants.

While infantile gastro-enteritis is a 'summer' disease, there are also known episodes of rather violent 'winter vomiting disease' which, while attacking people of all ages is still predominant in infants. Its aetiology is unknown but viral infection cannot be excluded.

The mode of spread of intestinal infections through water and food varies to a certain extent from one infectious agent and disease to another. The survival of micro-organisms in water and food and their ability to multiply there and to produce toxin are important factors. This will not only depend on the quality of the micro-organisms but also on the water and food, the quality, the temperature, pH, and other factors. Finally, it will depend on food habits, whether food is eaten raw or cooked, whether the micro-organisms are killed or reach the body of the victim alive. There are also host factors such as immunity, gastric acidity, etc., which will determine whether man will be infected or not.

Infection takes place after ingestion of contaminated food or water. Whether an individual will be infected or not depends on many factors, such as the immune state, and the state of the gastro-intestinal tract. Hypochlorhydria will facilitate penetration of most micro-organisms and in particular *Vibrio cholerae*. A very important factor is the quantity of microorganisms (and/or toxin) which reaches the intestines. There is a certain minimum infective dose that is needed to trigger off infection. In some diseases, e.g. dysentery and typhoid, this dose is small, while in others, e.g. bacterial food poisoning and cholera, a great number of organisms are needed. The evolution of the clinical picture depends to a certain extent on the infective dose.

Epidemiological inquiries start with the establishment of a proper diagnosis supported whenever possible by microbiological and serological tests. The investigation of sources and ways of infection are essential in order to establish a clear picture of the evolution of the outbreak and to forestall its possible development. On the grounds of such inquiries, a clear picture of the cause of infection can be established, and it may be accordingly determined which control measures should be taken.

Control of intestinal infections with diarrhoeal symptoms has two aspects: one aspect is the immediate life-saving measures which are achieved through rapid treatment aimed at replacement of lost body fluids and establishment of electrolyte balance.

Treatment at present available for diarrhoeal symptoms is simple and effective. Modern therapeutic techniques for rehydration are able to save the lives of nearly all patients who report in time before irreparable damage is caused by fluid losses and acidosis. However, elimination of toxins which a number of water- and food-borne infectious agents produce is sometimes difficult. When treatment facilities are available, patients usually recover very quickly from the acute symptoms, but this does not mean that infectious organisms have been eliminated. To this purpose, antimicrobial drugs are administered. Antimicrobial drugs should, however, be considered only as the additional, secondary step in treatment. Their role in most of the typical diarrhoeal diseases which are of short duration is rapidly to eliminate, after clinical recovery, infectious germs and thus render the patient non-infectious to their surroundings, so that they can return to their homes and to normal life. However, in intestinal diseases in which lasting systemic infections occur, such as typhoid, prolonged treatment with antibiotics is needed. On the other hand they are of no value in salmonella food poisoning.

Most intestinal infections, in particular the so-called 'diarrhoeal diseases' are not systemic infections but are due to the pathogenic effect of the causative organisms on intestinal organs. There are specific features in each intestinal infection and in the degree to which they attack intestinal mucosa or other intestinal organs, as well as in the degree of their own penetration, or penetration of the toxins they produce, into the blood and other organs.

Thus treatment aimed at saving lives is an essential part of control measures.

Secondly, *preventative measures* against intestinal infections consist of important long-term measures such as sanitation, food control, and personal hygiene, which are the only means to eliminate intestinal diseases. Epidemiological investigations into the cause of an outbreak may indicate the need of applying some specific sanitary measure, such as chlorination of certain water supplies that become contaminated or elimination of contaminated shellfish. Specific measures comprise immunization against infections for which an effective antigen is available, such as anti-typhoid vaccine, or possibly chemoprophylaxis under some specific circumstances. However, the use of antibiotics for both treatment and prophylaxis may cause a rapid increase in the resistance of Enterobacteriaceae to the drugs used. The resistance transfer factor, that is transmitted so easily from one intestinal micro-organism of the same or a different species, has rendered many micro-organisms resistant to most of the commonly used antibiotics (Anderson, 1968). Feeding and treatment with antibiotics of animals, which carry salmonella, for example, have aggravated the situation. Numerous examples of indiscriminate use or rather abuse of antibiotics are known. In view of this, the use of antibiotics in public health practice must be well scrutinized, as the damage may be greater than the benefits. This is particularly true for certain intestinal infections for which prompt rehydration treatment is of paramount importance and antibiotic therapy of secondary significance.

Preventive measures such as immunization and sanitation should be used after careful consideration of numerous factors. One of the important factors that must be studied and determined concerns the high-risk groups. In general, these groups are composed of infants and children, but food handlers and certain other professions have also to be taken into account. The application of proposed preventive measures must be feasible and realistic, and the control programme should be medically and economically sound. It is nowadays an accepted principle to plan control programmes[1] after thorough cost–effectiveness and cost–benefit analysis of various possible control strategies. This is particularly necessary in the field of intestinal infections, which are so widespread and may be considered diseases of the masses and therefore require special attention in order to achieve the best results for the least expenditure.

The *economic aspects* of certain intestinal infections, e.g.

[1] See CHAPTERS 41, 42, and 46 on the planning of health services.

typhoid and cholera, warrant careful consideration in view of extensive international and internal food trade and tourist traffic. Failure to prevent contamination of food which is aimed at exportation (or meant to be consumed internally) and failure to protect the health and well-being of tourists may bring considerable economic loss. For countries which are developing tourism the measures to prevent contamination of food, of potable water and of the fresh-water and sea-water used for bathing are of great economic importance, as any outbreak of intestinal infections will limit tourist trade. On the other hand, rational use of funds for prevention of the disease will enable considerable saving, while the spread of infection would instead require heavy expenditure for treatment of the sick.

MAIN INTESTINAL INFECTIONS

We cannot examine in detail all intestinal infections, but only those which are the most important and most typical. Details of the natural history of each disease, its epidemiology, spread, and control, will therefore be given only in a few cases, but they will illustrate the most important aspects that are valid in general for most of these infections.

For reasons of simplicity and brevity, the most important of these diseases individually or as groups are listed in TABLE 49 with their main features given in a gross schematic way.

The data in TABLE 49 indicate that this group of water- and food-borne diseases are not in any respect compact and similar. In general they have one and the same common characteristic in that they are water- and food-borne, but they differ in many details concerning their aetiology, epidemiology, and control.

ENTERIC FEVERS

These infections comprise typhoid and paratyphoid and are caused by *Salmonella typhi* and *Salm. paratyphi* A, B, and C respectively. They are systemic infections of long duration and are distinct from local infections such as salmonella food poisoning which is characterized by short incubation and duration.

Typhoid Fever

This infection gives rise to a disease which is very serious, and in spite of presently available antibiotic treatment has high fatality rates in comparison with other water- and food-borne infections. The severity of this disease and its spectacular water- and food-borne spread require special attention, and typhoid fever will therefore be dealt with in some detail.

Causative Organism. *Salmonella typhi* is exclusively pathogenic for man. Primates such as chimpanzees can be infected but develop a form of the disease which is not comparable to that in man, either in its duration or its severity (Cvjetanović, Mel, and Felsenfeld, 1970). *Salmonella typhi* can survive well in water and in food. It can even multiply in food under favourable conditions. It can survive in the human body, and thus can spread from infected men and carriers to healthy susceptibles.

The Natural History of Typhoid. Invasion of the human body by *Salm. typhi*, its action in it, and its excretion and

TABLE 49

Main Water and Food-borne Infections

Infection	Causative organism	Source of infection	Mode of transmission	Incubation	Period of infectivity	Susceptibility, communicability, infectiousness	Distribution	Control
Typhoid	*Salmonella typhi*	Sick persons and carriers	Faecal matter in water, food, flies; 10^8–10^{10} *Salm. typhi* in 1 g. of faeces	7–21 days	From beginning of illness until recovery, during carrier state	General susceptibility, infectiousness depends on infective dose and immunity	Practically everywhere in the world	Sanitation, food and water control, health education, vaccination
Paratyphoid	*Salm. paratyphi* ABC	Sick persons and carriers, domestic animals for paratyphoid B	Faecal matter in water, food, flies infected eggs, meat	1–10 days				
Dysentery, bacillary	*Shigella dysenteriae, Sh. flexneri, Sh. sonnei*	Sick persons and short-term carriers	Faecal matter, food and water; 10^8–10^{10} *Shigella* in 1 g. faeces	1–7 days	During illness and carrier state	General susceptibility	All areas, warm climates more than others	Sanitation, food and water control, vaccination, chemoprophylaxis
Infectious gastro-enteritis	*Escherichia coli, Proteus* other organisms of unknown origin	Sick persons and carriers (animals)	Faecal matter, food and water	1–5 days	During illness and carrier state	General susceptibility, more in children	Ubiquitous, in all areas	Sanitation, food and water control, health education
Food poisoning	Salmonella, staphylococcus enterotoxin, *Clostridium botulinum, Cl. welchii*	Contaminated food containing toxins and/or pathogenic organisms	Food	2–36 hours	Non-existent	General susceptibility	Ubiquitous, in all areas	Food hygiene, personal hygiene, health education
Cholera	*Vibrio cholerae* classical and El tor vibrio	Sick persons and carriers short and long term	Faecal matter, food and water 10^7–10^9 *V. cholerae* in 1 g. faeces	1–5 days	5–14 days after beginning of the disease	Susceptibility general, low immunity	Endemic zones and larger areas during pandemics	Sanitation, food and water control, health education, vaccination
Enterovirus	Enteroviruses Echo, Coxsakie, polio	Sick persons and carriers	Faecal matter, food and water, but also contact	3–14 days	During illness and carrier state	General susceptibility, more in children	Ubiquitous, in all areas	Sanitation, food and water control, health education
Hepatitis	Hepatitis	Sick persons and carriers	Food, water, contact (blood, syringes for serum hepatitis)	1–3 months	During illness and carrier state	General susceptibility	Ubiquitous, in all areas	Sanitation, food and water control. For serum hepatitis boiling of syringes, control of transfusions
Amoebiasis	*Entamoeba histolytica*	Sick persons	Faecal matter, food and water	3 days— several months	During illness and carrier state	General but low susceptibility	Endemic areas of tropical and warm climates	Sanitation, food and water control, health education
Helminths	*Ascaris lumbricoides, Trichuris trichiura, Enterobius vermicularis, Echinococcus, Taenia*	Sick persons, infected people and animals	Infected persons and animals, then excreta, soil and contacts	2 days—1 month	During illness	General susceptibility	Ubiquitous, in all areas	Sanitation, food control

transmission to other persons, are the basis of the understanding of the natural chain of events in the epidemiology of the disease which in turn makes a basis for a sound control programme. After ingestion of an infective dose (I.D.) of *Salm. typhi*, which according to studies on volunteers (Hornick and Woodward, 1966) is between 10^4–10^5 organisms (for I.D. 25) [FIG. 58] but in nature is perhaps lower (Cvjetanović, 1957).

There are a number of factors which determine whether *Salm. typhi* will or will not infect an individual, e.g. the state of the intestinal tract, stomach acidity, presence of other flora, etc. (Hornick and Gregg, 1968). The infectious process begins in susceptible individuals by the penetration of micro-organisms through the intestinal mucosa into the lymph nodes. After an incubation period of one to three weeks, which it is believed depends partly on the amount of ingested micro-organisms, *Salmonella typhi*, which have multiplied in the lymph nodes, penetrate into the bloodstream and into the different organs including the spleen. Bacteriaemia and toxaemia due to the liberation of the endotoxin are produced and temperature, headache, and other symptoms result. The invasion of salmonella into small blood vessels in the skin causes the well-known 'rose spots'. While some micro-organisms at this early stage can pass into the stool, it is only after the wide-spread of organisms within the body and their invasion of intestinal lymph tissue and liver and kidney in the second and third week that they are readily excreted in the faeces and possibly urine, and the patient becomes a dangerous excretor of *Salm. typhi*. Accordingly, early laboratory diagnosis of typhoid should be attempted by blood culture, since coproculture and serological

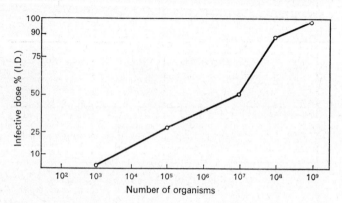

FIG. 58. Infective dose for man in typhoid fever (semi-log). [Data from Hornick and Woodward (1966) *Trans. Amer. cli. climat. Ass.*, **78**, 70.]

tests become positive only after another week or two. As soon as the diagnosis is made, antibiotics such as chloramphenicol or ampicillin should be given in small doses to prevent rapid liberation of endotoxin from killed bacteria, which would aggravate the clinical status. Recently many strains of *S-typhi* have become drug resistant and therefore their sensitivity should be tested to determine the drug of choice. After a few days the temperature should become normal and convalescence will begin after a few weeks, if complications, etc. do not appear in the meantime. During the illness in cases which are not treated or are inadequately treated, necrosis of Peyer's patches may occur and intestinal perforation result. Various organs can be involved during the course of the illness and possibly also after recovery.

When the clinical illness is over, the individual problem of the patient is solved, but not that of the community as the patient may continue to excrete the micro-organisms for shorter or longer periods of time irrespective of whether he was treated with antibiotics or not. He may become a temporary carrier for a few days, weeks, or months, or a chronic carrier who will carry and disseminate germs for years, even for the rest of his life. About 3–5 per cent. of infected people become long-term carriers and constitute the reservoir and source of infection for new outbreaks and sporadic cases. Often, *Salm. typhi* has been found accidentally in apparently healthy people (Watson, 1967) never suspected of being carriers. There must therefore be more carriers than is suspected, especially in endemic areas. The number of organisms that carriers excrete is large, ranging from 10^6 to 10^{10} per gramme of faeces, and they are excreted regularly rather than intermittently as believed earlier (Merselis *et al.*, 1964). Some people who have other infections and lesions, such as urinary schistosomiasis, tend to have very

high carrier rates of typhoid and excrete *Salm. typhi* in the urine (Saad El-Din Hathout *et al.*, 1966). There is no effective way of eliminating the carrier state in all cases by antibiotic treatment (Bullock, 1963) or even by removal of the gall bladder where *Salm. typhi* is often found. It is apparent that the treatment of typhoid with chloramphenicol often produces carriers as indicated in a study on a large group of female patients in Chile, where 7·4 per cent. of the patients were found positive (Armijo, Pizzi, and Lubos, 1967). In view of this, prevention of spread of infection from carriers to healthy men should be centred upon food and water control, cleanliness, and personal hygiene. Typhoid is often, and rightly, called the disease of dirty hands. In the history of typhoid in the United States, it is very well known that one particular carrier, a cook called 'Typhoid Mary', spread typhoid wherever she prepared food, due to her unhygienic habits. The lack of proper sanitary excreta disposal, of safe water supply and of protection of food from flies, and contamination from dirty hands are the causes of the spread of infection. As people become infected so the circle of infection is perpetuated.

The Epidemiology of Typhoid. Many of the notions and principles governing present-day epidemiology of the infectious diseases have been developed from the observation of typhoid outbreaks and the role of carriers. At present the epidemiology of this disease is so well known that it even allows formulation of mathematical models for the dynamics of typhoid fever (Cvjetanović, Grab, and Uemura, 1967). We have described above the natural history of typhoid primarily as far as individual patients is concerned. The natural process and the dynamics of typhoid in the community are, in fact, the same but involve masses of people, and therefore a quantitative description of the process has to be given. Endemic situations are determined by annual incidence rates that indicate frequence of transmission of infection. In endemic areas in developing countries an annual incidence of ten or even more per thousand is not infrequent, but in developed countries the rates of one case per 100,000 or even per 1,000,000 population are now common and indicate the great differences that exist in various parts of the world.

Epidemics in limited groups of populations are described in terms of the number of cases that occur in a certain span of time during which infection began and the outbreak developed and ceased. Simple graphical presentations of two typical explosive water-borne outbreaks of typhoid fever are given in FIGURE 59. In Split, Yugoslavia, in 1949 after heavy rainfall the ground in which defective water mains and sewers were laid was flooded, and a contact between faecal matter and drinking water was established. Over 600 cases of typhoid occurred in two months. Diarrhoeal disease of undefined aetiology appeared first, followed a few days later by typhoid. The rather slow evolution and decline of the outbreak was due to the fact that defective pipe lines continued to serve the population for a considerable period of time before the defects were discovered and proper measures taken to rectify the situation. The end of the outbreak was extended with a typical 'tail', which was not caused by water-borne infection since the water mains were repaired but by contact infection with cases and carriers. It is common for an explosive water-borne outbreak to be followed by a 'tail' of contact infections. The higher the standards of personal hygiene the longer will such a 'tail' be. The number of carriers created by such an outbreak is not negligible and they can give rise to further infections, thus increasing the level of endemicity.

Similarly, in Zermatt in 1963, after the water from a particular source which supplied Zermatt was contaminated, cases appeared among inhabitants and tourists. Four hundred and

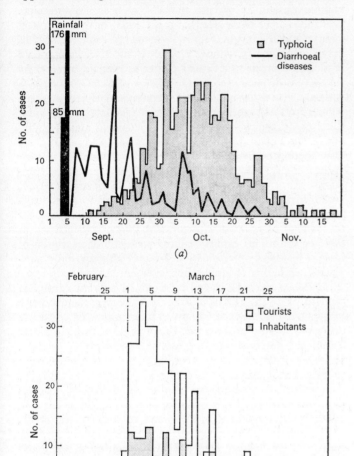

FIG. 59. Typical water-borne outbreaks of typhoid fever.
  (a) Split, Jugoslavia, 1948. [Cvjetanović, B. (1956) *Textbook on Principles of Epidemiology*, Zagreb.]
  (b) Zermatt, Switzerland, 1963. [Bernard, R. P. (1965) *J. Hyg.* (*Camb.*), **63**, 537.

thirty-seven cases occurred of which 260 were among tourists from the United States and European countries. Water-borne outbreaks among tourists are no exception, as during the tourist season many water supplies are overstrained and failures occur.

Epidemiological inquiries about each outbreak and case of typhoid are often revealing. They indicate the source of infection and reasons why the outbreak occurred giving an indication of the control measures which should be undertaken. Phage-typing of *Salm. typhi* in view of the differences that exist in the world (Nicolle, 1970), is a useful tool in the search for the source of infection. It was in fact the Central Public Health Laboratory in London which first gave the

alarm about the outbreak, after diagnosing typhoid in tourists who returned from Zermatt and undertaking phage-typing. It is often the case that tourists bring typhoid to England after visiting countries where this disease is endemic. Typhoid is therefore becoming more and more a tourist disease which calls for international co-operation in tracing the source of infection. Techniques are now available (Moore, Perry, and Chard, 1952) for the isolation and tracing of carriers, e.g. of paratyphoid, in cities through investigation of contamination of sewage at different points in the house or apartment where the person is shedding the pathogen.

The epidemic process can be described as quantitative changes in the classes of population that exist in each community. The population is divided into the susceptibles and the infected, and there are daily transitions from one group to another according to the dynamics of infection. Such transitions can be given mathematical expression and formulated into a mathematical model. Available electronic computer services facilitate working of the calculations to be made. Such a model can first be tested to see whether it fits the realities of life by verifying whether it can reproduce known epidemic and endemic situations. The dynamics of typhoid are presented on the flow chart in FIGURE 60 that shows the classes (X_1–X_{10}) of population as these refer to typhoid and the direction (→) and rate (R) of the transition from one class to another. The rate of new infection (RI) depends on the total number of infections to which the susceptible population (X_1) is exposed.

The flow chart [FIG. 60] is self-explanatory. At its right edge the stages of the above-mentioned natural history are indicated and the natural flow of events in typhoid in the community presented in the same order as it affects an individual case.

The stages an individual goes through from susceptibility to infection, incubation, illness (possibly resulting in death) carrier state, resistance, and back to susceptibility are the same as those the community goes through. However, on the flow chart the size of different groups is indicated (X_1–X_{10}) and the transition from one class and state to another indicated in a quantitative manner (R, RI). The rest of the application of the model is a matter of computation which, with the electronic computers and skill that are available, is not difficult nowadays.

Such models of typhoid epidemics and endemicity can be used to simulate and reproduce the natural course of typhoid but they can also show the results of interference with such a natural course. For example, the effect of an immunization or sanitation programme can be studied on such a model. In fact such a model gives excellent opportunities for evaluation of the relative effectiveness of various preventive measures and of various control strategies in the combat of typhoid. They greatly help in establishing rational, medically and economically sound, control programmes. We shall, therefore, consider the problem of typhoid control with the mathematical model in view to assist us.

Control of Typhoid Fever. This can be achieved by a general rise in sanitary standards, education, and socio-economic development. However, when facing the practical problem of developing control programmes in a community the health administrator is facing numerous constraints such as the available funds, priorities in the field of health, and in other fields of social and economic development. He is obliged to use

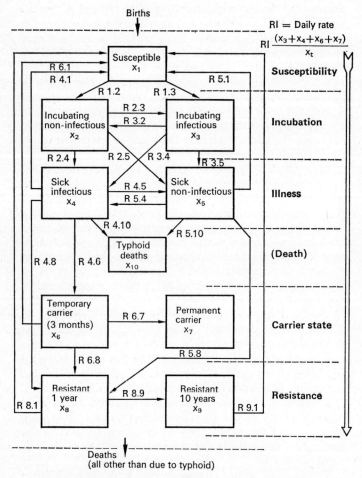

FIG. 60. Flow chart for epidemiological model of natural course of typhoid fever. [Cvjetanović, Grab, and Uemura, (1971) *Bull. Wld Hlth Org.*, **54**, 53.

the resources available in the most economical and profitable way. Accordingly, he should select from among available control measures one or more combined and apply these in the most efficient way possible. To this effect there is a need to develop an effective strategy for control of typhoid, using mathematical models.

For the control of typhoid, health education, sanitation, and immunization appear to be the most effective measures. Health education is always useful and it should go hand in hand with general education; every health authority is expected to give adequate support to it [see CHAPTER 49]. As far as sanitation and immunization are concerned they require closer examination in order to determine when and how they should be applied.

Immunization against typhoid is effective, as shown in controlled field trials with several types of vaccines (Cvjetanović and Uemura, 1965), of which acetone-inactivated and dried vaccine appear to be the most effective, with heat-killed phenol vaccine coming next. The protection given by heat-killed phenol vaccine is of somewhat lower degree and shorter duration than that of acetone vaccine. Two doses of either of these vaccines would protect 70–90 per cent. of the inoculated persons for the period of 5–7 years respectively. One dose is less effective and gives protection of a shorter duration, but if

for any reason a second dose is not given, one inoculation should nevertheless not be considered as wasted and useless. The immunization of children is apparently both more effective and more necessary than that of adults since the incidence in children is higher and they therefore represent a high-risk group. Typhoid vaccine can be combined with paratyphoid (A and B) vaccine and is known as TAB vaccine. Controlled field trials (Hejfec *et al.*, 1968) have shown that paratyphoid B antigen, if given in about the same quantity of micro-organisms as typhoid vaccine, is effective. Paratyphoid B vaccine protects to a similar degree as typhoid vaccine. As yet there is no such proof of the efficacy of *Salm. paratyphi* A antigen. The usual quantity of paratyphoid B and A component in TAB vaccine was earlier inadequate to immunize successfully against paratyphoid (Cvjetanović and Uemura, 1965). Since paratyphoid A is relatively mild and rare in most areas there is no reason for including it in a combined vaccine against enteric infection. Typhoid antigen can also be combined with other antigens such as DPT (Cvjetanović *et al.*, 1971). Since typhoid vaccine is highly effective, gives long-lasting immunity and costs little, it is a practical proposal for the control of typhoid in areas with high incidence where sanitary conditions cannot be improved in a short period of time. The effect of vaccination is rapid although only temporary, while that of sanitation is slow but lasting.

Sanitation has been shown to be effective in the control of typhoid. With the advent of water chlorination, the incidence of typhoid has dropped rapidly. Furthermore, its incidence decreased rapidly in those developed countries which widely introduced proper sewage disposal and water supply systems. However, strictly speaking, there have not been control trials to measure the effectiveness of various sanitary measures, but circumstantial evidence and studies on diarrhoeal diseases (Rubenstein *et al.*, 1969; Schliessmann *et al.*, 1958; van Zijl, 1966; Wolff and van Zijl, 1969) and cholera (Azurin *et al.*, 1971) indicate approximately the effectiveness of sanitary measures. Availability of a sufficient quantity of water and proper excreta disposal in houses considerably lowers the incidence of enteric infections. The effect of availability of water and excreta disposal in cholera is much more dramatic than in typhoid, but still one can postulate that proper excreta disposal would eliminate about 50 per cent. of infection. Proper excreta disposal is not possible on a large scale without water and therefore in practice these two measures must go together [see CHAPTER 9].

Planning of control measures can be improved by using mathematical models. Providing the effectiveness of vaccine and the coverage of the population is known, the model will be able to indicate the expected effect of mass immunization campaigns or an intensive and continuous immunization programme. The efficacy of a vaccination campaign reflects both the effectiveness of the vaccine and the coverage. As a departure point we may take the model that simulates the state of stable endemicity and study the effect of vaccination on an endemic situation. In FIGURE 61 the effect of a single mass vaccination and the effect of repeated immunization are presented in a graphic form. From the figure it can be seen that following single vaccination there is a rapid drop in incidence followed by a gradual increase of incidence and restoration to a new level of endemicity, which is nevertheless lower than the one

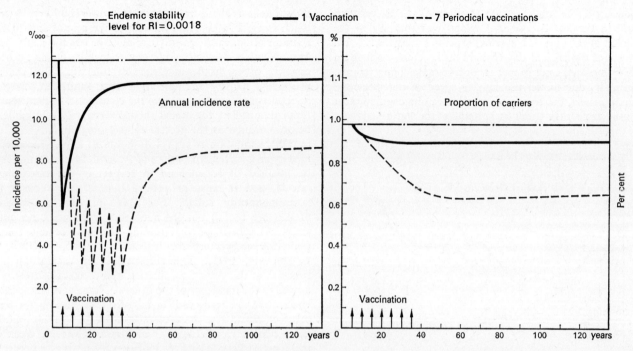

FIG. 61. Effect of a single and repeated mass vaccination on the dynamics of typhoid fever. Efficacy of vaccination = 60 per cent. [Cvjetanović, Grab, and Uemura (1971) *Bull. Wld Hlth Org.*, **45**, 53].

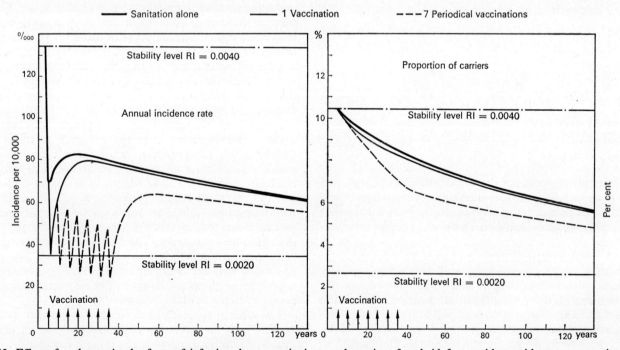

FIG. 62. Effect of a change in the force of infection due to sanitation on dynamics of typhoid fever, with or without mass vaccination. [Cvjetanović, Grab, and Uemura (1971) *Bull. Wld Hlth Org.*, **45**, 53.]

before immunization. This effect is due to a reduction in the number of carriers [see the right-hand part of FIGURE 61].

Similarly, the effect of repeated immunization is shown, which indicates that again, due to a diminution in the number of carriers, a long-term downward trend is obtained. These downward trends are observed in reality in developed countries. The effect of sanitation alone, and combined with

immunization, which is simulated by lowering the force of infection, is presented in FIGURE 62.

The rapid downward trend in the United States is shown in FIGURE 63. While typhoid is declining due to improvement of sanitation, namely water supplies and sewage disposal, foodborne salmonelloses are on the increase. The United States data showing continuous decline of typhoid are following predictions of the model, while levelling of the decrease in typhoid in the last decade in England was contrary to the prediction of the model. Nevertheless, closer study has shown that most of the present-day typhoid in the United Kingdom is due to imported cases in tourists or cases among immigrants. Accordingly, due to the present-day speed of transport and communications, the trends of infection in one country must be viewed against the wider background of the world situation.

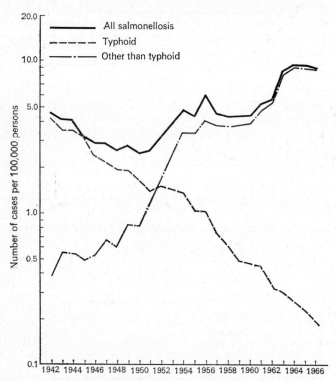

FIG. 63. Reported incidence of human salmonellosis, United States, 1942–66. [United States Department of Health, Education, Welfare, and Public Health Service (1967) *Salmonella Surveillance Annual Summary 1966*, p. 9.]

A mathematical model has shown that the effect of sanitation is constant and cumulative, thus resulting in continuous downward trends in morbidity. Consequently, from a long-term policy point of view, sanitation should be preferred to immunization.

Cost–benefit and cost–effect analysis are now absolute musts in planning of control measures. A cost–benefit analysis of three different programmes which have been worked out for Western Samoa, using a mathematical model, is presented in FIGURE 64. The effect and costs as well as benefits of (*a*) immunization alone, (*b*) sanitation (privy construction) alone, and (*c*) both combined are given in the graphs. However, these graphs, as well as any results of simulations with mathematical models, have to be critically examined and creatively applied. Computers do not relieve us of the obligation of using common sense. In the model [FIG. 64], vaccination is placed close to sanitation as far as cost–benefit is concerned and a decision is difficult. The effect of immunization is specific and vaccination only acts on typhoid, while sanitation has an effect on other intestinal infections and therefore gives additional benefits; accordingly, it should be preferred. However, instead of

monovalent typhoid vaccine, we can use combined vaccine (such as DPT + Ty) and thus lower the cost of anti-typhoid immunization. Consequently, for more or less the same cost of immunization we have additional benefits. Finally, various districts differ in the incidence of infections and the two measures, namely immunization and sanitation, may be selectively applied according to the conditions. In fact, simulations obtained by the model should serve only as a guideline before formulating the precise control programme.

While sanitation is always desirable in any civilized community and useful irrespective of typhoid, immunization must be justified by actual need in respect of the disease concerned, and it must be proved that it gives benefit and is economically sound. For this purpose mathematical models are useful, but are not necessary, since other much simpler methods of determining the cost–benefit balance point are satisfactory for orientation purposes (Grab and Cvjetanović, 1971). The cost–benefit of vaccination is a function of the cost of vaccination and the cost of treatment, as well as the incidence of the disease. Namely, funds spent on vaccination are recovered (or not) from savings on the treatment of cases. The more cases that are prevented, then the more benefit *re* treatment is obtained. However, when the incidence is very low, there will be very few cases prevented and therefore immunization will appear less beneficial from an economic point of view. From mathematical computations a simple nomogram has been developed which can help in indicating whether immunization is profitable or not. For this purpose incidence, costs of treatment per case, costs of protection, e.g. vaccination per person and per year, should be known for the infection concerned. A corresponding 45 degree slope indifference line is drawn (Grab and Cvjetanović, 1971), and any value that falls in the area to the left and lower part of this line indicates loss, and that in the right upper area indicates benefit. The same technique can be used for calculating and presenting on the nomogram cost–benefit of vaccination against other infections than typhoid such as cholera and tetanus which are presented in FIGURE 65. Similarly, the cost–benefit of other preventive measures such as sanitation can be presented. In FIGURE 65, ranges of different values are given for the three diseases presented. If an average value for the whole country falls in the loss area, this does not mean that particular data for a specific age group or group at high risk will not fall in the benefit area. The nomogram facilitates the distinction of such priority groups and communities. This simple method is only for rough orientation and for evaluation of short-term programmes, however. For long-term analysis it is necessary to use mathematical models.

The rational approach to the control of typhoid should be applied with the necessary adaptation for control of other intestinal infections prevalent in the same community.

Paratyphoid Fever

Paratyphoid fever caused by *Salm. paratyphi* A, B, and C is usually less severe than typhoid. Paratyphoid B is the most common variety and thus most important. Paratyphoid also affects animals, unlike typhoid which is strictly a human disease and is spread more often by foods such as milk and milk products contaminated by carriers, than by water [see CHAPTER 10]. Dried egg albumin and similar products can be

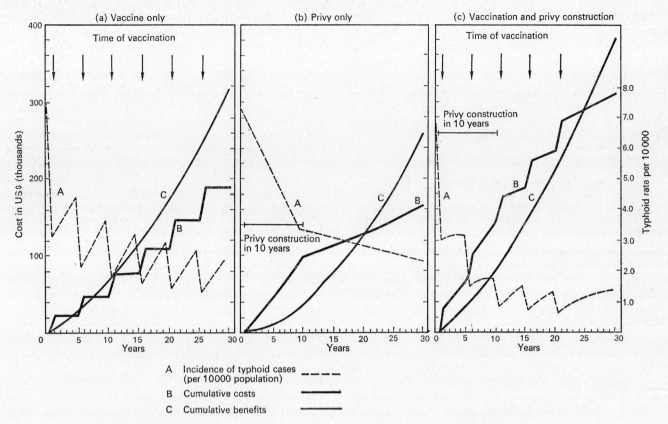

A Incidence of typhoid cases
   (per 10000 population) − − − −
B Cumulative costs
C Cumulative benefits

FIG. 64. Various typhoid control programmes; their impact on incidence of the disease and cumulative costs and benefits. [Cvjetanović, Grab, and Uemura (1971) *Bull. Wld Hlth Org.*, **45**, 53.]

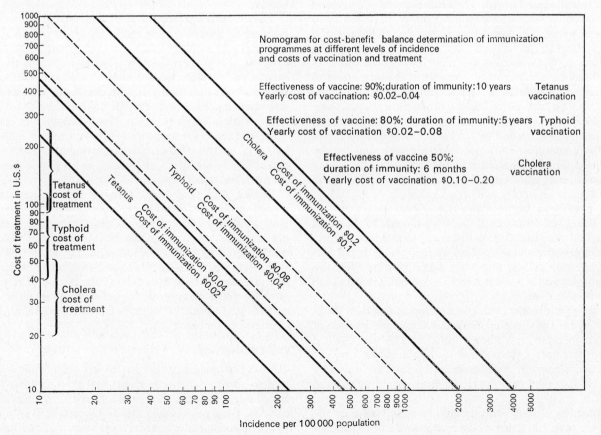

FIG. 65. Cost-benefit of immunization against typhoid, tetanus, and cholera. [Cvjetanović, B.]

contaminated and carry *Salm. paratyphi* B and other salmonellae.

The prevention and control of paratyphoid fever follows more or less the lines described for typhoid control. As indicated above there is an effective vaccine against paratyphoid B if given in a high enough dose, while there is no evidence that the paratyphoid A component of TAB vaccine is effective. Food control and sanitation are the most important measures in combating paratyphoid.

BACILLARY DYSENTERY

Bacillary dysentery is spread from man to man. Animals do not play a role in the spread of this infection. It is caused by *Shigella dysenteriae* (*shigae*), *Sh. flexneri* and *Sh. sonnei*. While *Shigella shigae* which caused a very severe illness was once common, it gradually gave way to *Sh. flexneri* and even later to *Sh. sonnei*. It seems that, as environmental sanitation is improving, shigellae that are able to adapt to the improved level of sanitation and spread under such conditions are emerging, and those that cannot are declining.

The *epidemiology* of bacillary dysentery and its spread are typical of water- and food-borne infections. Dysentery spreads rapidly and attacks groups of people, army units, and schools where food and water, the common sources of infection, are shared by many. Its appearance is violent and the duration of outbreaks usually short. However, epidemiological patterns may also depend upon the endemic situations. The spread of dysentery differs from place to place, and while it is usually due to poor sanitation and hygienic habits the spread of *Sh. sonnei* dysentery, however, among schoolchildren in the United Kingdom, where it is now common, was due to the use of a common towel in the lavatories and to contact with common lavatory seats. While bacillary dysentery in developed countries is due to defective hygiene and is mostly food-borne, infection in developing countries is due to direct contact. *Shigella flexneri*, and *Sh. shigae* too, are still prevalent and cause large outbreaks not infrequently due to the contamination of water. Poor personal hygiene and lack of environmental sanitation in developing countries contribute, together with flies, to the spread of dysentery in epidemic proportions, especially among infants and young children, and this represents one of the main killing diseases of infancy and early childhood.

The parallelism between the rise of the fly population, temperature, and dysentery in moderate climatic zones is well known. The same bacillary dysentery has its different features in various climatic and socio–economic set-ups. It is the prevailing infection and an important public health problem in developing countries while it is rare in communities with high standards of hygiene.

The use of antibiotics such as streptomycin and sulfa drugs in the treatment of dysentery has resulted in rapid increase of resistance to these and other antibiotics. The use of these drugs in chemoprophylaxis is not successful. As said earlier, rehydration therapy in severe cases is important and this may be all that is needed to bring relatively rapid recovery to the patient.

Symptomless carriers and very mild infections make up the majority of cases and therefore dysentery should be considered as one of those diseases with the 'iceberg phenomenon'. For this reason preventive measures are very important.

Control of bacillary dysentery as said above should be based on improved sanitation and personal hygiene (World Health Organization, 1964b). It has been shown that the incidence of shigelloses is lower in families which have better sanitary conditions, namely flush toilets inside houses and water on the premises (Stewart *et al.*, 1955). The quantity of readily available water seems to be the most important factor. Health education of the public is of great importance as well as strict control of food establishments and the personnel that serves in them. It should be ascertained daily, in each establishment, that food handlers who suffer from diarrhoea are excluded from working with food. Chemoprophylaxis is neither effective nor recommended in view of the presence of drug resistance among shigellas. Oral administration of live streptomycin-dependent strains (Mel, Cvjetanović, and Felsenfeld, 1970; Mel *et al.*, 1965, 1968) is effective, but immunity is strictly type-specific and the vaccine needs to contain several types of the microorganism, and in addition several doses are needed to obtain a high degree of protection. Vaccination will be more effective if at the same time gastric acid is neutralized. All such considerations makes vaccination an impractical procedure to follow for the protection of large population groups.

Infections Due to Pathogenic *Escherichia coli*

It has been shown that the majority of inadequately defined infantile gastro-enteritis is due to the species *Escherichia coli* which contains pathogenic types characterized by their particular O and B antigens: O25, O55, O86, O111, O119, B4, and B5.

These organisms spread among infants in nurseries and hospitals in particular. The spread by means of milk and food and also very often by dust and even possibly by air-borne droplets. They are extremely contagious but usually only infants and young children show symptoms. Outbreaks of *Esch. coli* are common both in developed and developing countries and are very difficult to control. There are no vaccines available nor can chemoprophylaxis be used effectively because it would be necessary to repeat it too often. The best means of control is strict aseptic nursing techniques and improvement of standards of hygiene in hospitals, particularly hospitals for young children.

Besides *Esch. coli* and *Proteus* organisms, certain other bacteria which are found in the intestinal tract are associated with diarrhoeal symptoms. Sometimes, especially in developing countries, such infections afflict children debilitated by malnutrition, such as kwashiorkor, and it is difficult to distinguish to what extent each of these two factors, malnutrition and infection, have contributed to the disease. There is still need for further study of the aetiology of infantile gastroenteritis and diarrhoeal diseases and the ways in which they can best be combated.

Food Poisoning

Food poisoning may be due to various chemical and infectious factors (micro-organisms and their toxins). We will consider here only the most common food poisoning caused by bacteria. Food poisoning is usually characterized by a sudden attack of abdominal pains, cramps, vomiting, and diarrhoea.

This usually happens a few hours or a day after contaminated food has been consumed. The bacteria multiply in food, especially when this is left at room temperature and not refrigerated, and they produce an enterotoxin. Food poisoning occurs in every country in the world and is mainly caused by staphylococci, salmonellae, and *Clostridium welchii* and *botulinum*. Salmonella, in fact, causes an intoxication and infection while others produce a toxin which causes the intoxication. The main features of food poisoning are given in TABLE 50.

TABLE 50

Main Features of Common Food Poisoning Due to Micro-organisms

Micro-organism	Feature	Incubation (hours)	Symptoms
Staphylococci (entero-toxin)	Intoxication with enterotoxin	2–6	Nausea, vomiting, prostration, severe abdominal pains, subnormal temperature
Salmonella	Infection and intoxication	12–36	Abdominal pain, diarrhoea, vomiting and fever
Cl. welchii	Intoxication	8–22	Abdominal pain and diarrhoea
Cl. botulinum	Intoxication	12–36	Diplopia, ptosis, husky voice, constipation

Chemical poisoning usually has a shorter incubation period apart from the staphylococci which produce a powerful enterotoxin.

Salmonellae

Salmonellae cause the majority of food poisoning outbreaks. *Salm. typhimurium* is a very common causative organism, but many other salmonellae also play a part. Their distribution and frequency in various parts of the world differ. An international system of salmonella surveillance based on national surveillance programmes is of assistance in establishing the link between the appearance of an unusual type of salmonella in the country and the importation of foodstuffs from certain parts of the world, where specific salmonellae are common among certain animal species. Pigs, cattle, and poultry are readily infected with salmonellae and so are meat, milk, and eggs. Meat (particularly processed minced meat such as sausages, pork pies, etc.) as well as powdered eggs (and cakes made from them), and fish meals, etc., are common sources of infection. Pasteurization and cooking are often not properly carried out to kill salmonellae. If the food is kept at room temperature non-refrigerated salmonellae multiply in it and man is exposed to tremendous infective doses when he consumes it. Many unhealthy practices that exist in restaurants, in the preparation and storage of food, add to the hazards of food poisoning with salmonella.

Staphylococcal Enterotoxin

Staphylococcal enterotoxin causes a very severe and immediate (3–6 hours) intoxication with a typical picture of vomiting, diarrhoea, prostration, and subnormal temperature.

Coagulase-positive *Staphylococcus aureus*, which is found in the nasal cavity of carriers, is present in nearly half the adult population and is also capable of producing enterotoxin. Staphylococcal skin lesions, especially those on the fingers of food handlers, represent a particular danger as staphylococci from such lesions reach food easily and multiply in it. The various meat products, and milk products (cream, ice-cream, custard) as well, are most often involved in large explosive outbreaks.

Clostridium welchii

Cl. welchii causes an intoxication that is slower in developing than that due to staphyloccoci, and is in fact sometimes combined with an infection. The outbreaks are associated with common meals provided by central kitchens which prepare meat usually arriving already contaminated from the slaughter-house. Further multiplication occurs when the meat is processed, left over for the next day to be eaten cold, or is inadequately heated.

Botulism

Cl. botulinum produces an extremely powerful toxin that can easily kill by its neurotropic action, paralysing certain cranial nerves, and by its action on other organs causing such symptoms as diplopia, husky voice, ptosis, and constipation. Being an anaerobe, *Cl. botulinum* multiplies readily in canned and inadequately boiled food. Spores of *Cl. botulinum* are found in the soil and can easily contaminate vegetables and fruit. However, tinned meat and fish have often been incriminated. Spores of *Cl. botulinum* are very resistant to heat, and this is why canned food can still contain live micro-organisms.

Control of Food Poisoning

Control of food poisoning caused by bacteria is possible only through the regular daily practice of strict control of the quality of the original food, proper food storage, thorough cooking and safe preparation of food products and their proper preservation. Education of the food handlers and caterers is essential as well as control of restaurants, slaughterhouses, packing plants and central kitchens in hospitals, schools, and other establishments. An important task is the control of food preparation and distribution during field trips, in tourist establishments and on other occasions where *ad hoc* arrangements are made which often prove deficient in many ways. As far as salmonelloses are concerned, close co-operation is necessary with veterinarians as these infections are in fact transmitted from animals to man [see CHAPTERS 10 and 22].

CHOLERA

At present we are in the midst of the seventh pandemic of cholera which started a decade ago in 1961, apparently originating in Sulawesi island in the Indonesian archipelago. To judge by past pandemics we are facing another decade at least in which we shall see the spread of cholera in countries with low standards of hygiene, with incursions of the disease into developed countries in the present-day climate of rapid travel, and in particular into less privileged communities in such countries. It is nowadays, therefore, necessary to consider cholera in more detail (Araoz *et al.*, 1970).

The epidemiological features of cholera are fascinating. While in the first part of this century classical *V. cholerae* was gradually retreating to its endemic foci in the delta of the Ganges and Brahmaputra, a new pandemic, the seventh in modern times, began in 1961. The present pandemic is due to the spread of *Vibrio cholerae* biotype El tor (so-called after the El Tor quarantine station in the Sinai peninsula, where the organism was first isolated). This organism is more resistant to environmental factors than the classical vibrio and it has a particular ability to spread rapidly, giving rise only occasionally to acute cases of cholera. Usually, El tor vibrio has already firmly established its foothold by the time the first severe cases appear. It is these biological characteristics of the causative organism on the one hand, and rapid travel with slow progress of

common method of spread in endemic areas is by contaminated food, explosive water-borne outbreaks are also known. Cholera travels with man, who is the only known host of this infection and its spread entirely depends on the movement of human beings.

While cholera is making progress and covering more and more territories nowadays, its effect is not so devastating as that of the past pandemic, for the simple reason that at present effective treatment is available which can save practically all sick persons who report for treatment within the first six hours of the onset of symptoms. However, the problem in many rural areas is how to reach treatment centres quickly when the nearest one may be as much as hundreds of miles away and there may be no transportation available. There is, as always, a

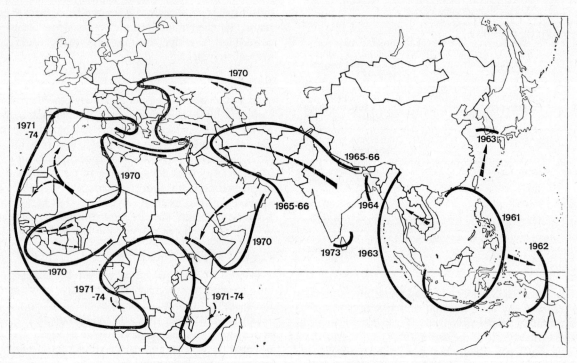

FIG. 66. Global spread of cholera 1961–74. [Cvjetanović, B.]

sanitation on the other that have produced the seventh pandemic and have given it its particular force. The discrepancy between the fast development of transport, and the advent of jet travel on the one hand, and the poor or even deteriorating standards of sanitation in any parts of the world has favoured the spread of cholera. Cholera has spread from South-East Asia to other parts of Asia; eastward and to the north first then turning towards the west to reach the Middle East by 1967 and the West Coast of Africa in 1970 briefly invading Europe in that and the following year. [FIG. 66]. Further spread to areas with low standards of sanitation in the Western Hemisphere is possible and quite probable.

The epidemiological patterns of cholera differ according to climate, population density, personal habits, etc. In endemic areas a seasonal increase is common. Yet, while monsoons in Bengal bring an end to the epidemic, the same monsoon rains mark the beginning of outbreaks in the Philippines. In endemic areas inter-epidemic periods are bridged by hidden ('iceberg phenomena') spread of infection among carriers. While the

gap between knowledge and the facilities to apply it. As a result of these difficulties in developing countries, fatality rates of 30–40 per cent. are not uncommon, while in well-established treatment centres the fatality rate is about 1 per cent. or lower. Treatment consists in the rapid replacement of rehydration fluid and establishment of electrolyte balance, which must be done quickly since patients lose body fluids rapidly due to the profuse diarrhoea, and severe dehydration quickly follows accompanied by acidosis and low blood pressure, finally ending in coma and death. Such severe cases, however, are not typical, they are in fact rare, mild cases being much more common. For one severe case there are about ten mild cases and up to a hundred symptomless carriers. Carriers are positive for a few days up to two weeks or so, while chronic carriers are rare. In fact, there has been only one well-recognized case studied, namely 'Cholera Dolores' from the island of Negros in the Philippines who is still a carrier after eight years of observation. The infection in the community is widespread through carriers, and cannot be controlled easily, especially in developing countries which are lacking in sanitary facilities. Cholera, like other intestinal infections, appears to be a disease of poverty and ignorance, which thrives where there is poor sanitation and low personal hygiene. Those belonging to the under-privileged classes are particularly exposed to the infection. The infection is spread through water and food as well as through close contacts with sick and carriers: outbreaks have been traced to contaminated water and food in restaurants. Bathing in polluted water and sea-water has also been incriminated. Certain customs such as the washing of dead bodies of persons who died of cholera and kissing them have been associated with the spread of the disease. Ritual ablutions and the defaecation habits of, for example, Muslim populations and Hindus, etc., are particularly dangerous; this is proven by the fact that practically all population groups in the world with such practices have now been infected with cholera.

John Snow first described the cause of the spread of cholera in London. The removal of the handle of the Broad Street pump is an example of specific action to control the disease. After more than a century it still holds that the provision of safe water and food is the cornerstone in the control of cholera.

Control of cholera lies in the domain of general socio-economic development accompanied by sanitation and education. However, where rapid action is required several specific measures are in use. Chemoprophylaxis with tetracycline and other antibiotics to which (except for streptomycin) *V. cholerae* is fortunately sensitive, has been used. The effect was claimed to be good but no one has yet succeeded in controlling large outbreaks with this measure alone.

Immunization with the killed vaccines that are available today is not very effective, since inoculation of routinely used vaccines protects about 50 per cent. of inoculated persons for a few months only. This immunity, which is partial but relatively high after inoculation, rapidly decreases and after six months has practically entirely vanished. Neither do two doses nor an increased amount of antigen give any greater protection. The immunization must be repeated every six months or at least once a year at the beginning of the epidemic season. Newer types of vaccine such as those containing adjuvant are more promising. Yet in spite of all limitations of immunization this is widely used, because people request to be vaccinated and the governments of affected countries are in favour of undertaking such spectacular action. Mass vaccination with jet guns is a spectacular way of demonstrating that some action is being taken. Much energy and resources are therefore invested and wasted on vaccination, while environmental sanitation is frequently left in a deplorable state. The value of sanitation is shown by the example of Japan, a country to which cholera has been brought repeatedly yet has never caused a single secondary case because of the high level of sanitation in the country. A controlled field trial in the Philippines proved the high effectiveness of water sanitation and excreta disposal as control measures (Azurin *et al.*, 1971). Sanitation is the only measure that can make a country non-receptive to cholera and the only measure that pays in the long run, as shown by cost–effect and cost–benefit analysis based on mathematical models similar to the one described earlier for typhoid. The rational use of funds for the control of cholera is of paramount importance, because developing countries have restricted resources and must make the best use of them. However, emotional factors play an important role in the formulation of strategies of cholera control on a national level. It is commonly accepted that the international health regulations (World Health Organisation, 1971) cannot alone prevent the spread of cholera, as their main purpose is to facilitate international travel and trade without exposing countries to undue risks of the introduction of cholera. However, the application and, even more so, violation of international health regulations often create hardships and economic losses due to imposed limitations of travel and trade, that in turn present another difficulty in the control of cholera at an international level. Cost benefit and cost effect analysis are essential in control (Abel-Smith, 1973).

The very existence of cholera and its spread in many areas is an indicator of the inadequacy of sanitation and personal hygiene, and should serve as a reminder that much more must be done to improve sanitary conditions in the world if we really want to bring cholera under control [see CHAPTERS 9 and 10].

AMOEBIASIS

Entamoeba histolytica, among other protozoa, can cause chronic disturbances of the intestinal tract. However, in areas with high standards of hygiene and adequate nutrition this protozoon does not cause clinical illness in spite of the fact that there might be up to 10 per cent. of persons who are carriers of the cysts of *E. histolytica*. In developing countries in tropical zones where nutrition is inadequate and sanitation poor, clinical symptoms are common. The roles of two distinct forms or races of *Entamoeba* as well as the role of intestinal flora in the pathogenesis of amoebiasis are not fully understood.

The spread of infection is maintained through shedding of the cyst in the environment where they can readily survive for weeks and months. The cysts can contaminate vegetables and fruits and be ingested with them. The use of night soil as fertilizer, which is common in some areas, particularly favours the spread of amoebiasis.

Control of amoebiasis lies in environmental sanitation, proper excreta disposal and personal hygiene. The thorough cooking of food and boiling of suspect water are necessary in areas with high incidence of amoebiasis.

OTHER PROTOZOAN AND HELMINTHIC INFECTIONS

Protozoa such as *Giardia lamblia* and *Balantidium coli* have been associated with the intestinal disorders and symptoms of diarrhoea. The number of these protozoa, the nutritional status of the infected people, and the influence of other factors such as intestinal flora play a role in the aetiology of diarrhoea ascribed to these two protozoa.

Helminths such as *Ascaris lumbricoides*, *Trichuris trichiura*, *Enterobius vermicularis*, *Taenia solium*, and *Trichinella spiralis* invade the human body via the oral route but do not necessarily all cause intestinal illness; neither are they strictly speaking water- or food-borne. Some of these diseases namely ascariasis, trichiuriasis, and enterobiasis are spread from man to man without intermediary hosts. Taeniasis and trichinellosis belong to the group of anthropozoonotic diseases. They are caused by ingestion of contaminated raw or inadequately cooked meat [see also CHAPTERS 10, 22, and 24].

The control of the above infections is again ensured by environmental sanitation, cleanliness, food control, proper cooking of meat, and personal hygiene.

The polio virus belongs to the group of enteroviruses. This virus, or rather its types 1, 2, and 3 of which type 1 is predominantly epidemic, has its normal habitat in the intestinal lymph nodes and is excreted abundantly in the faeces. However, in the early stages of the illness the virus multiplies very actively in the body and can be found in the oropharynx; from here it can spread by droplet nuclei by respiratory routes. Poliomyelitis is therefore only partly a water- and food-borne disease. Probably, the respiratory mode of spread is of more importance for communities with a high level of sanitation and the oral–intestinal route of spread more common in communities with low standards of hygiene. However, since the infection is very extensively spread it shows that its infectivity is very high. Yet only a few rare persons who are infected develop paralysis. It is possible that the presence of other intestinal flora, especially enteroviruses, plays a role. Muscular activity and trauma such as injections have been associated beyond any doubt with paralysis of the muscles concerned, while surgical operations (removal of tonsils) open the way to bulbar paralysis.

Control of poliomyelitis comprises sanitation and immunization. Immunization is performed with all three types of virus, contained either in killed or live vaccine. The immunization has greatly decreased paralytic polio in the world, and this infection which was at one time the public health problem number one in many countries has virtually come under complete control. This, of course, is true for countries where economic and health conditions enable regular mass immunization of the susceptible population. Due to the use of vaccine, the age of the susceptible population has considerably increased because of the lack of exposure to the natural infection in the younger age groups. Therefore, adults from areas where polio is under control, who travel to endemic areas, should be immunized. Children and pregnant mothers have to be specially protected by immunization. Immune gamma globulins are given to exposed persons who need to be protected quickly.

Sanitation in the prevention of polio requires stricter measures of safety than in the case of bacterial infection, since the polio virus is more resistant than bacteria. It can pass through filters and is resistant to chlorination. Otherwise, general measures which apply for other water- and food-borne diseases also apply to polio.

OTHER ENTEROVIRUS INFECTIONS

The most important viruses of this group besides polio are the Echo (Enteric Cytopathogenic Human Orphan virus) and Coxsackie viruses. There are many types of these viruses which have been associated with gastro-intestinal illnesses. There are more children with diarrhoea among those from whom the virus was isolated than among those who proved negative. While for Echo, especially certain of its types, there is a strong association with diarrhoeal disease, for other enteroviruses this is not the case.

Control of infections caused by enteroviruses is not a practical proposition. Incidence may be high but severity is not important enough to require immunization. Sanitation, which is not considered as a special measure to control these infections but rather to control intestinal infections of bacterial origin, does, however, have an effect on infections with enteroviruses.

Infectious Hepatitis

Catarrhal jaundice has been known for long, but isolation of the virus of infectious hepatitis and definite proof that it is the aetiological agent of catarrhal jaundice are still awaited. There are two viruses; one causes infectious hepatitis proper, which enters the body by mouth; the other causes serum hepatitis, which is introduced to the human body by injections, transfusions, or other direct contact of the infected blood of one person with the bloodstream of another person (see Pickles, 1939).

The spread of infectious hepatitis is commonly caused by contaminated food and water, but an acute illness spread by droplets is possible, and contact droplet infections are also described. Like other intestinal infections, its seasonal prevalence occurs in the autumn and winter, probably due to the consumption of contaminated fruit and vegetables and to outdoor living. In children, infectious hepatitis is associated with diarrhoea and in this way it may spread like other intestinal infections. Explosive outbreaks due to contaminated water, milk, shellfish, and various foods are known. Carriers also exist in hepatitis.

The control of infectious hepatitis depends upon the provision of safe water and food. The possibility of contracting infection by eating shellfish and by bathing in polluted seawater should not be neglected. In cases where such measures cannot be taken, for instance when travelling to low sanitation areas, immune gamma globulin may be given. The control of serum hepatitis requires strict aseptic precautions during surgery and injections, as well as the control of blood donors.

Water- and food-borne infections do not comprise only those which have been described in some detail here. Tuberculosis and tularaemia, for example, can be transmitted by food and water like many other infections which are commonly transmitted by other mechanisms [see also CHAPTER 25].

The most important common factor among all water- and food-borne infections is their control through sanitation and personal hygiene. With economic development and prosperity, sanitation will improve and thus the prospects for the effective control of water- and food-borne infections will be opened. However, nowadays many sanitary defects in developing countries, and even in some areas of developed countries, foster the spread of intestinal infections and require control measures in order to protect the population. Proper planning, execution and evaluation of control programmes in thus one of the important tasks of public health services.

REFERENCES AND FURTHER READING

Abel-Smith, B. (1973) Cost effectiveness and cost benefit in cholera control, *Wld Hlth Org. Chron.*, **27**, 407.

Anderson, E. S. (1968) *Ann. Rev. Microbiol.*, **22**, 131.

Araoz, J. de, *et al.* (1970) Principles and practice of cholera control, *Wld Hlth Org. Publ. Hlth Pap.*, No. 40.

Armijo, R., Pizzi, A., and Lobos, H. (1967) *Bol. Ofic. sanit. panamer.*, **62**, 295 (and in: *Bol. Ofic. sanit. panamer.*, English edition, Selections from 1967).

Azurin, J. C., *et al.* (1971) Effect of environmental sanitation in the control of cholera, *Bull. Wld Hlth Org.*, (in press).

Azurin, J. C. *et al.* (1974) Strategy of cholera control, *Wld Hlth Org. publ. Hlth Pap.* (in the press).

Bullock, W. E. (1963) *Amer. J. med. Sci.*, **246**, 42.

Cruickshank, R. (1967) *Med. Clin. N. Amer.*, **51**, 643.

Cvjetanović, B. (1957) *Vrijednost Cjepiva Protiv Trbušnog Tifusa*, Zagreb.

Cvjetanović, B., Grab, B., and Uemura, K. (1971) Epidemiological model of typhoid fever and its use in the planning and evaluation of antityphoid immunization and sanitation programmes, *Bull. Wld Hlth Org.*, **45**, 53.

Cvjetanović, B., Mel, D. M., and Felsenfeld, O. (1970) *Bull. Wld Hlth Org.*, **42**, 499.

Cvjetanović, B., and Uemura, K. (1965) *Bull. Wld Hlth Org.*, **32**, 29.

Cvjetanović, B., *et al.* (1972) Studies of combined quadruple vaccines against diphtheria, pertussis, tetanus, and typhoid. Reactogenicity and antigenicity, *Bull. Wld Hlth Org.*, **46**, 47.

Debré, R., *et al.* (1955) Poliomyelitis, *Wld Hlth Org. Monogr. Ser.*, No. 26.

Gorbach, S. L. (1967) *Gut*, **8**, 530.

Gordon, J. E., *et al.* (1968) *Arch. environm. Hlth*, **16**, 424.

Grab, B., and Cvjetanović, B. (1971) Simple method for rough determination of the cost-benefit balance point of immunization programmes, *Bull. Wld Hlth Org.*, **45**, 536.

Greenwood, M. (1935) *Epidemics and Crowd Diseases. An Introduction to the Study of Epidemiology*, London.

Hathout, Saad El-Din, *et al.* (1966) *Amer. J. trop. Med. Hyg.*, **15**, 156.

Hejfec, L. B., *et al.* (1968) *Bull. Wld Hlth Org.*, **38**, 907.

Hobbs, B. C. (1968) *Food Poisoning and Food Hygiene*, 2nd ed., London.

Hornick, R. B., and Gregg, M. B. (1968) in *Tice's Practice of Medicine*, Vol. 3, Hagerstown, Maryland, p. 1.

Hornick, R. B., and Woodward, T. E. (1966) *Trans. Amer. clin. climat. Ass.*, **78**, 70.

Mel, D. M., Cvjetanović, B., and Felsenfeld, O. (1970) *Bull. Wld Hlth Org.*, **43**, 431.

Mel, D. M., *et al.* (1965) *Bull. Wld Hlth Org.*, **32**, 633, 637, 647.

Mel, D. M., *et al.* (1968) *Bull. Wld Hlth Org.*, **39**, 375.

Merselis, J. G., Jr., *et al.* (1964) *Amer. J. trop. Med. Hyg.*, **13**, 425.

Metselaar, D., Dola, S. K., and Gemeri, W. (1973) Poliomyelitis: epidemiology and prophylaxis 2. Distribution of oral trivalent vaccines by lay volunteers, *Bull. Wld Hlth Org.*, **48**, 45.

Moore, B., Perry, E. L., and Chard, S. T. (1952) *J. Hyg.*, **50**, 137.

Nicolle, P., *et al.* (1970) *Bull. Acad. nat. Méd. (Paris)*, **154**, 481.

Nottay, B. K., and Metselaar, D. (1973) Poliomyelitis: epidemiology and prophylaxis 1. A longitudinal epidemiological survey in Kenya, *Bull. Wld Hlth Org.*, **48**, 44.

Pickles, W. N. (1939) *Epidemiology in Country Practice*, Bristol.

Pollitzer, R. (1959) Cholera, *Wld Hlth Org. Monogr. Ser.*, No. 43.

Rubenstein, A., *et al.* (1969) *Publ. Hlth Rep. (Wash.)*, **84**, 1093.

Rublin, F. L. (1973) Simultaneous multiple immunization, *Bull. Wld Hlth Org.*, **48**, 175.

Schliessmann, D. J., *et al.* (1958) *Publ. Hlth Monogr.*, No. 54.

Snow, J. (1855) *On the Mode of Communication of Cholera*, 2nd ed., London.

Stewart, W. H., *et al.* (1955) *Amer. J. trop. Med. Hyg.*, **4**, 718.

Watson, K. C. (1967) *Lancet*, **ii**, 332.

Wolff, H. L., and Zijl, W. J. van (1969) *Bull. Wld Hlth Org.*, **41**, 952.

World Health Organization (1960) Report of the Expert Committee on Poliomyelitis, *Wld Hlth Org. techn. Rep. Ser.*, No. 203.

World Health Organization (1964a) Report of the Expert Committee on Hepatitis, *Wld Hlth Org. techn. Rep. Ser.*, No. 285.

World Health Organization (1964b) Report of the Expert Committee on Enteric Infections, *Wld Hlth Org. techn. Rep. Ser.*, No. 288.

World Health Organization (1967) Report of the Expert Committee on Cholera, *Wld Hlth Org. techn. Rep. Ser.*, No. 352.

World Health Organization (1971) *International Health Regulations, 1969*, Geneva, pp. 31/34.

World Health Organization (1974a) Food-borne disease: methods of sampling and examination in surveillance programmes. Report of a WHO Study Group, *Wld Hlth Org. techn. Rep. Ser.*, No. 543.

World Health Organization (1974b) *Guidelines in the Laboratory Diagnosis of Cholera*, Geneva.

World Health Organization Regional Office for Europe (1973) *Report of a Conference on Cholera Control in Europe, Copenhagen 1971* (Euro 1401), Copenhagen.

Zijl, W. J. van (1966) *Bull. Wld Hlth Org.*, **35**, 249.

17

THE SPREAD AND CONTROL OF ARTHROPOD-BORNE DISEASE

H. M. GILLES

Many important diseases of man are transmitted by arthropods. An arthropod which acts as the agent of transmission or inoculation, or both, of the causative parasite of a disease is commonly referred to as a vector. The arthropod, however, also plays an important part in the life history of the parasite and is as important a host of the parasite as man and often more so.

Transmission of true arthropod-borne disease is biological, for an essential part of the life cycle of the parasite takes place within the body of the vector, during which cyclical change or multiplication or both may occur. The host in which sexually mature forms are found is known as the definitive host and that in which only immature forms are found as the intermediate host. This differentiation cannot, of course, be made in some cases, such as, for example, viruses, where sexually mature forms are not known. The period of time occupied by the developmental cycle in the vector is known as the extrinsic incubation period and is important epidemiologically, for only after its completion is the infection transmissible. The transference of the parasite to the new host may result either from inoculation by the vector, from contamination of the skin or mucous membrane by infective faeces excreted by the vector, or by its infective body fluids when crushed.

Biological transmission of a particular infection is normally specific and confined to one vector genus, sometimes to a single species. In the case of ticks and mites which do not undergo a complete metamorphosis during development the infecting parasite may be transmitted hereditarily (transovarially) from one generation to another.

Transmission of a disease may take place purely mechanically without the vector acting as a host to the parasite. Mechanical transmission can occur as a result of contamination of the legs, body, or mouth-parts of any insect with the infecting organism which may thus be carried to the person or food of another host. Mechanical transmission as opposed to biological transmission can be effected by widely separated genera.

ARTHROPOD-BORNE VIRUS INFECTIONS

Modern techniques of isolation and identification have revealed nearly two hundred viruses which are carried by arthropods, of which only a small proportion (about 70) produce clinically recognizable human disease. Most of these viruses have been classified, mainly by antigenic analysis, and the majority of the medically important ones have been placed in three groups.

Group A includes among others o'nyong-nyong, an African disease, chikungunya, and both eastern and western equine encephalitis. The latter two are primarily diseases of horses and birds, although other animals also may acquire the infection. The vectors are primarily culicine mosquitoes, but ticks and mites have also been incriminated. Infection of man is normally sporadic in incidence, but may become epidemic when the level of transmission is high. Chikungunya virus has been isolated from man and mosquitoes from widely scattered parts of tropical Africa extending south to Natal, and from India, Burma, Cambodia, and Thailand. In Uganda, the sum of evidence indicates an intensive epizootic in forest monkeys transmitted by *A. africanus* with incidental leakage to man by inefficient vector systems which alone could not maintain an outbreak.

Group B contains the most important arboviruses of man and includes yellow fever, St. Louis encephalitis, Japanese B encephalitis, Russian spring-summer encephalitis (and related infections). With the exception of the last these are mainly transmitted by mosquitoes.

Domestic fowl and wild birds are the main reservoir of St. Louis encephalitis infection; the vectors are culicine mosquitoes and mites, the former being responsible for transmission to horses and man. Human cases occur in the United States during the late summer and autumn, and the disease has also been recorded in Africa.

Russian spring–summer encephalitis and related infections are found under a variety of names in the U.S.S.R., China, Korea, central Europe and India, where it is called Kyasanur Forest disease. The natural hosts are goats, sheep, monkeys, and rodents, and transmission is effected by ticks of several genera. The type virus, however, is also excreted in milk, and man can acquire infection by the alimentary route.

Group C contains certain mosquito-borne infections so far recognized only in South America.

Prevention of the infections mentioned above can be effected in some cases by the use of formalin-inactivated vaccines. Control of the vector population where practicable will reduce the risk of infection. Steps can also be taken to avoid being bitten by vectors.

A number of arthropod-borne viruses infecting man, including sandfly fever and Colorado tick fever, do not fit into any of the groups so far described, which is indicative that other groups exist. Colorado tick fever is found in the United States, where small rodents are believed to be the normal hosts. Man, in whom it causes acute illness, becomes infected as the result of being bitten by the vector tick, *Dermacentor andersoni*.

The majority of arboviruses are zoonoses. Because infection usually produces prolonged immunity, attack rates in all age groups indicate the introduction of a new arbovirus; while disease confined to children implies reintroduction of a virus or overflow from a continuous animal cycle to susceptible humans. A computer-simulated model has been designed to express in quantitative terms the factors which play a role in the transmission cycle of an arbovirus.

Yellow Fever

Yellow fever is a disease which is enzootic in certain species of forest monkeys in parts of both Africa and South America. The vectors are *Haemagogus* spp. and *Aëdes leucocelanus* in

were reported from Nigeria, Ghana, Haute-Volta, Mali, and Togo.

Yellow fever does not occur in Asia or the Pacific region, though the urban vector is widespread.

Epidemic spread of the disease occurs only between 40° N. and 35° S. latitude, since a mean temperature of not less than 24° C. is necessary for the developmental cycle in the vector. The extrinsic incubation period lasts from 4 to 12 days. The incubation period in man is 3–6 days.

There are two main epidemiological forms of yellow fever. In the *urban type*, the mosquito vector is *Aëdes aegypti*, which

AFRICAN YELLOW FEVER

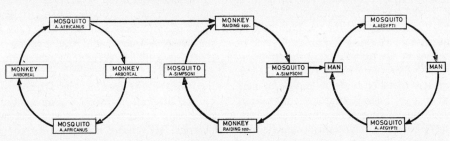

FIG. 67.

South America and *A. africanus* and *A. simpsoni* in Africa, which can convey the infection to man. The disease usually appears sporadically in man in rural areas, but can assume severe epidemic form in urban areas, where it is spread by *A. aegypti*. *A. africanus* has also been observed to bite at ground level by day, and *A. simpsoni* is sometimes present at canopy level by night. These reversals of behaviour by the two mosquitoes offer further opportunities for the transmission of infection from monkey to man.

The endemic zone in Africa approximately covers that part of the continent which lies between 15° N. and 10° S. latitude. In South America the endemic zone stretches from south of

SOUTH AMERICAN YELLOW FEVER

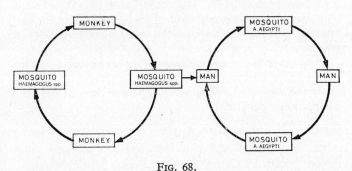

FIG. 68.

Honduras to the southern border of Bolivia and includes the western two-thirds of Brazil, Venezuela, Colombia, and those parts of Peru and Ecuador which lies east of the Andes. Certain towns are considered as not forming part of these zones provided they maintain continuously an *Aëdes* index not exceeding 1 per cent. This index represents the proportions of houses in a limited, well-defined area in which breeding places of *A. aegypti* are found. In 1969, epidemics of yellow fever

is primarily a domestic mosquito which breeds in or near houses, with the female preferring to lay her eggs in water collecting in artificial containers, such as old tins, etc.

The virus cycle is man–mosquito–man; this method of spread requires large numbers of susceptible hosts, and hence tends to occur in large towns. Villages, with frequent passage of people from one village to another, will also be suitable for this type of spread. Urban type yellow fever can be effectively controlled by anti-mosquito measures. *Jungle type* yellow fever may occur either in endemic or epizootic forms. In the endemic form, the disease, which is primarily one of monkeys, is almost constantly present, and sporadic cases of human infection occur from time to time. The primary spread of the virus is from monkey to monkey, via *A. africanus* in Africa and *Haemogogus sp.* in South America; both these mosquitoes live in the tops of trees. *Haemogogus species* will occasionally bite man, for example when a tree is felled, and South American jungle yellow fever is thus maintained. In Africa, however, there is another way in which jungle yellow fever virus can be transmitted from monkey to man. Certain monkeys have the habit of raiding crops, particularly bananas; another mosquito, *A. simpsoni*, occurs on the edges of forests, and becomes infected by biting infected raiding monkeys, and then later bites the farmer when he collects his crop. *A. simpsoni* thus acts as a so-called 'link-host' [FIGS. 67 and 68].

A life-long immunity follows recovery from the disease as well as from sub-clinical or unrecognized infections which comprise a large proportion of the total. There is evidence to suggest that the presence of extensive immunity to other group B viruses modifies the severity and spread of yellow fever. Clinical diagnosis should wherever possible be confirmed by laboratory tests. The virus can be isolated from the blood during the first three days of the disease. After the third day the mouse protection test can be used. This test involves demonstrating whether or not mice are protected from a challenge dose of the virus by antibodies in the patient's serum. A second protection test should be made some five days later. A significant rise of titre in the second sample would confirm the diagnosis, while an unaltered titre would only indicate an immunity due to a past infection or vaccination. Neutralization, complement fixation, or haemagglutination inhibition tests can also be employed, depending on the particular circumstances and the likelihood of previous exposure to other group B viruses. The interpretation of serological results is complicated by the cross-reactions that may occur with other members of group B. To confirm that the infection is due to yellow fever, the rise in HI, CF, and N antibodies should be greater for yellow fever virus than for other group B arboviruses. In the event of death an autopsy should be performed and the liver examined for the characteristic lesions. Where an autopsy is not possible a viscerotome may be used to obtain a piece of liver for examination.

Since the virus circulates in the blood during the first few days of the disease, a suspected case must be isolated for the first six days in a screened room or under a mosquito net. Steps should be taken at once to obtain laboratory confirmation of the diagnosis, but institution of control measures should not await results from the laboratory. Domestic contacts also should be isolated under screened conditions for six days, and the patient's house and all premises within a radius of 60 yards ($\simeq 55$ m.) should be sprayed with a residual insecticide.

In densely populated areas elimination of vector breeding must be undertaken at once. *A. aegypti* is a peri-domestic mosquito and will breed in practically anything that will hold water. This includes water containers such as jars and cisterns, as well as innumerable objects which may hold rain-water: defective gutters, old tins, jars and coconuts shells (often hidden in the grass), and the bottoms of small boats and canoes. These breeding foci should be reduced as far as possible by suitable measures; water containers covered or screened, tins and other rubbish buried, and so forth. This is unlikely to prevent all breeding, but it will simplify treatment of the remainder by regular oiling or by addition of insecticidal briquettes.

Residual spraying of the interiors of all houses and outbuildings or of all surfaces close to breeding places (peri-focal spraying) will reduce the *Aëdes* population rapidly. Epidemic transmission will cease when the *Aëdes* index is reduced to below 5 per cent.

Protection of scattered populations by vector control is, however, impracticable, and recourse must be had to vaccination of the whole community. This will afford protection for at least *ten* years. Two vaccines are available: the 17D strain maintained by passage in chick embryo and the Dakar strain maintained in mouse brain. This latter is prepared in a form which permits administration by scarification and is very suitable for use in scattered populations in rural areas. *Infants under one year of age should preferably not be vaccinated*, since encephalitis follows vaccination in this age group more frequently than in adults. Some countries do not require vaccination certificates in the case of infants.

The spread of the disease is controlled by requiring all persons entering or leaving an endemic area to be in possession of a valid certificate of vaccination. Those not in possession of such a certificate may, on arrival in a non-endemic area, be subjected to quarantine for a period of six days from the date of last exposure to infection or until the certificate becomes valid. A vaccination certificate becomes valid ten days after vaccination and remains so for ten years. A certificate of re-vaccination done not more than ten years after a previous vaccination becomes valid on the day of vaccination.

To prevent introduction of an infected mosquito into countries where the disease is absent but conditions exist for transmission, aircraft coming from the endemic zone must be disinsecticized (by insecticidal aerosol) as specified by the World Health Organization.

Dengue Fever

Dengue fever is widespread in urban areas in the tropics and sub-tropics and often appears in epidemic form. The virus, of which four main serotypes exist, circulates in the blood at the onset of symptoms and for a few days after. The incubation period is 4–7 days, and transmission is through species of *Aëdes*, usually *A. aegypti*, in which the extrinsic incubation period is 8–14 days. Infection confers immunity to the homologous strain for about a year. Diagnosis must be based on the clinical findings, intracerebral inoculation of blood in suckling mice, and other virological and serological tests. The only practical preventive measures are control of the vector by elimination of breeding places or insecticidal attack on the adults, or the prevention of mosquito bites by screening or repellents.

South and South-East Asia Haemorrhagic Fever

In recent years epidemics of dengue with haemorrhagic manifestations have occurred in the Philippines, Thailand, Malaya, Singapore, and India, and dengue viruses have been isolated from *Aëdes aegypti* during these epidemics. The outbreaks have had an urban distribution, with clinical cases clustered in the crowded poorer central districts of cities. The disease is usually, but not exclusively, seen in races of oriental origin, and the haemorrhagic fatal manifestations are usually confined to persons under 15 years of age, with a peak incidence in the 3–6 years group. The dengue shock syndrome (DSS) is the most severe manifestation of dengue haemorrhagic fever and it has been postulated that DSS occurs as a result of a second infection with a heterologous dengue virus and that an immunological mechanism is involved in the pathogenesis of the syndrome.

Some outbreaks of haemorrhagic fever have been caused by the arbovirus Chikungunya (Group A). In general, the clinical syndrome associated with chikungunya infection is milder than haemorrhagic dengue.

Japanese B Encephalitis

The majority of infections are inapparent or mild. The disease occurs in China, Taiwan, Korea, Japan, Malaysia, Singapore, India, and Sarawak. The most efficient vectors are *Culex tritaeniorrhynchus*, and *C. gelidus* and the preferred vertebrate hosts are birds and domestic animals, e.g. pigs; man being only an incidental host. The highest infection rates in man appear in populations which have close contact with both pigs and ricefields. The domestic pig is an amplifier host and is probably the main source of infection for man. The virus is spread from rural to urban areas by viraemic birds. There are two peaks of incidence—under 9 years and over 60 years.

Control of the vector mosquitoes is not practicable on a large scale. Isolation of pig sties from human habitats reduces the mosquito/man contact. Vaccination of domestic pigs has been tried in Japan but the success of such a measure is highly debatable.

Sandfly Fever

Sandfly fever appears epidemically over much of the tropics and sub-tropics, where it is transmitted by *Phlebotomus papatasii*. Recovery from the disease is followed by a long-lasting immunity to the homologous strain of virus. Sandfly breeding can be controlled to some extent by clearing piles of rubbish and mending cracked and dilapidated walls. The insects are particularly susceptible to DDT, and have been drastically reduced in many places by residual house spraying employed for the control of mosquitoes.

DISEASES DUE TO RICKETTSIAS

The typhus fevers are a group of infections caused by species of *Rickettsia* and transmitted by various arthropod vectors.

Epidemic Typhus

Epidemic typhus, caused by *Rickettsia prowazekii*, infects man only and is transmitted by the louse, *Pediculus humanus*. The disease occurs mainly in cold climates, but it may appear in the tropics at high altitudes and in deserts, and has been reported from every continent except Australia.

The incubation period is about nine days, and the louse becomes infected by feeding on a person with the disease from two days before symptoms appear until the end of fever. The rickettsias multiply in the cells of the louse midgut, and when these rupture the organisms are discharged in the faeces. Human infection follows contamination of breaches of the skin surface by infected louse faeces. The rickettsias can remain viable for months on dried louse faeces, and may possibly cause infection through the conjunctiva or by inhalation, as well as percutaneously. Recovery is followed by immunity, which persists for several years. In some patients the infection appears to remain latent after symptoms have subsided and to relapse some years later (Brill's disease). A clinical diagnosis is confirmed by the Weil–Felix reaction, in which *B. proteus* OX_{19} is agglutinated and also OX_2 to a lower titre, or more specifically by the complement fixation test using suspensions or extracts of the specific organism.

Isolation of infected persons is usually not practicable in epidemics. Delousing of the whole population with residual insecticidal powders is the principal control measure. This is carried out by blowing insecticide (commonly 10 per cent. insecticidal powder) with a dusting gun under the clothes next the skin over the whole body, the operation occupying only a few minutes. In some areas lice have become resistant to DDT, and other insecticides must be used, such as BHC or pyrethrum powder.

Vaccines containing attenuated strains of epidemic or murine rickettsias will give some degree of protection for about six months and may be used in endemic areas before seasonal transmission starts.

Murine Typhus

Murine typhus is essentially a rodent infection which appears sporadically in man. It exists throughout the world, and the organism, *Rickettsia mooseri*, is conveyed to man by the faeces of infected rat-fleas of the genus *Xenopsylla* or the rat-mite, *Bdellonyssus bacoti*. The Weil–Felix test gives the same reaction as in epidemic typhus. Control of murine typhus is rarely required, but if needed the anti-rat and anti-flea measures employed in plague will be effective.

Tick-borne Typhus

The rickettsias causing the various forms of tick-borne typhus infect animals primarily but may appear sporadically in man. These infections occur in all five continents, and there are antigenic differences between the strains of *Rickettsia* causing them. A number of genera of ticks convey infection to man from the animal host (rodents and dogs in the case of fièvre boutonneuse and probably South African tick-bite fever, and rodents in the case of Rocky Mountain spotted fever). Trans-ovarian passage of infection in the tick sometimes occurs. The Weil–Felix reaction shows a titre of agglutination of Proteus OX_{19} and OX_2 which is lower than it is in the louse- or flea-borne forms. Complement fixation is specific.

Control consists in avoidance of ticks by the use of protective clothing, the elimination of ticks, and, in the case of Rocky Mountain spotted fever only, immunization with a vaccine which protects for about a year. Isolation of patients is unnecessary. Ticks on dogs can be controlled by insecticidal powders such as dieldrin or benzene hexachloride.

Mite-borne Typhus

Mite-borne typhus (often known as 'scrub typhus') is present in eastern and southern Asia, some Pacific islands and Queensland in Australia. It is enzootic in wild rodents and the two most important vectors, the larvae of *Trombicula akamushi* and *T. deliensis*, convey the rickettsia, *R. tsutsugamushi* (*R. orientalis*), among rodents and also to man. In Indonesia the rat flea is the vector. The disease is very focal in distribution and transmission occurs in abandoned agricultural land and in forest fringes. Scrub typhus is endemic in the entire range of the Himalayas and can occur even at high altitudes (up to 3,840 m.). The seasonal occurrence of scrub typhus in Japan corresponds exactly with the time of appearance of each species of vector. Only the larval mites feed on the vertebrate hosts' blood, and the rickettsia persists through the nymph, adult, and egg stages into the larva stage of the next generation, which is thus infective. Man contracts the disease by exposure, i.e. walking or resting in infected foci, particularly after slight rain or heavy dew. The incubation period is 1–3 weeks, usually about twelve days. Recovery is associated with immunity to the homologous strain, the indigenous people as a rule being immune to the local strains. The Weil–Felix reaction gives agglutination mainly of Proteus OX*K* about the tenth day of the disease. *R. tsutsugamushi* (*R. orientalis*) can be recovered from the blood of patients during the febrile period and cultured in living tissue culture or in the yolk-sac membrane of developing chick embryos. A complement fixation test has been used for diagnostic as well as sero-epidemiological surveys. Indirect immunofluorescence employing smears of rickettsiae as antigens is a most useful addition to the other means of diagnosing rickettsial infections.

The main control measure is personal prophylaxis against the bites of the mites by rubbing or impregnating clothing with dimethyl or dibutyl phthalate, benzyl benzoate or benzene hexachloride. These kill the mites on contact. Particular care should be taken to treat those parts of the clothing giving access to the interior of the garment. The adult mites live in the surface soil, and they can be killed by spraying with heavy doses of dieldrin or benzene hexachloride ($\frac{1}{4}$–1 kg. per acre).

THE RELAPSING FEVERS

These treponemal diseases are transmitted either by the louse, *Pediculus humanus*, or ticks of the genus *Ornithodorus*.

Louse-borne Relapsing Fever

Louse-borne relapsing fever is usually epidemic and has the same geographical distribution as epidemic typhus. The louse becomes infected with *Borrelia recurrentis* while feeding on persons suffering from the disease during pyrexial periods. Ten to fifteen days later treponemata are present throughout its body fluids. Man contracts the disease when an infected louse is crushed and abrasions of the skin, or possibly mucous membrane, are contaminated with the body fluid. Immunity follows recovery and persists for one or two years. The clinical diagnosis may be confirmed by demonstrating the treponemata in blood taken during the pyrexial periods, either by dark-ground illumination or in stained thin films. Control consists in mass delousing, usually by residual insecticidal powders, as in epidemic typhus.

Tick-borne Relapsing Fever

Tick-borne relapsing fever occurs in all continents except Australia. The causal organism is morphologically identical with *Borrelia recurrentis*, but is called *B. duttoni* in tropical Africa and by a variety of specific names in other areas. The vector in tropical Africa is *Ornithodorus moubata*, which, together with *O. rudis* in South America, feeds primarily on man and lives in cracks and crevices in mud-built houses. The other vector species are not domestic in habit, and they feed primarily on rodents and other small mammals. The disease, therefore, is highly endemic where the vector is domestic in habit and very sporadic in areas where human contact with the tick is in open country or caves. Transovarial passage of the treponema occurs in the tick, which is long-lived. Infection is transmitted by contamination of breaches in skin surfaces with infected tick faeces or coxal fluid or by the bite. Humans entering caves, working in bush country, living in infected huts, or sleeping in rest houses in the vicinity of infected villages are liable to acquire the infection. The incubation period is 3–10 days, and recovery is followed by immunity lasting about a year. The diagnosis is established by demonstrating the treponemata in the blood during the pyrexial periods.

In areas where transmission is by non-domestic vectors control consists in wearing protective clothing, such as high-legged boots, or in using repellents. Domestic vectors can be controlled by treating the interiors of houses with benzene hexachloride or dieldrin. Spray treatments (usually suspensions) have been used in dosages ranging from 0·2 up to 6 g.

gamma BHC per square metre; the higher dosage will give protection up to a year or more. The most satisfactory control results from rehousing the people in buildings which provide no harbourage for ticks.

BARTONELLOSIS (OROYA FEVER)

This is a specific fever caused by the organism *Bartonella bacilliformis* and characterized by anaemia and a papular eruption (verruga peruana) on the skin and mucous membranes. The disease occurs only in South America in valleys on the slopes of the Andes. The organism is present in the erythrocytes and reticulo-endothelial cells of those infected, and it is taken up by species of *Phlebotomus* while feeding. In these it can be found in the midgut and proboscis, and when a susceptible person is bitten infection follows, usually in 3–4 weeks. The principal cause of mortality is a particular susceptibility of patients with Oroya fever to septicaemic infections with *Salmonella* organisms, commonly *Sal. typhimurium*. Recovery confers some resistance to re-infection, so that in endemic areas the disease is most prevalent in children. *B. bacilliformis*, a very small, pleomorphic Gram-positive coccobacillus occurring singly or in chains or clusters, can be demonstrated in thin blood films from infected persons and in biopsy of the skin lesions. The disease has been successfully controlled by applying residual insecticides to the interior of houses and outbuildings.

DISEASES CAUSED BY PROTOZOA

A number of clinically distinct diseases are caused by protozoa of the genus *Leishmania* which are transmitted by species of *Phlebotomus*.

Visceral Leishmaniasis

Visceral leishmaniasis or kala-azar, caused by *L. donovani*, is most prevalent along the Ganges and Brahmaputra rivers in India, but it is also present along the Chinese coast north of the Yangtse River and focally in the Mediterranean basin, the Sudan, Ethiopia, and Kenya. In South America the disease appears sporadically over a wide area with a high endemicity along the northern coast of Brazil.

The parasites occur in man in the reticulo-endothelial cells and in the blood. They are ingested by the sandfly, in which cyclical development occurs, terminating in 7–9 days with the production of leptomonad flagellates which invade the pharynx. When the insect feeds subsequently these infective forms are introduced, enter macrophages, and revert to the leishmania form. They are carried to the viscera, particularly the spleen and liver, where they settle, multiply, and cause enlargement of the organs. In a small proportion of cases of kala-azar, following the disappearance of the visceral lesions, the parasites re-invade the skin a year or two later, causing unsightly nodules or macules. These cases of post-kala-azar dermal leishmaniasis are resistant to treatment and provide an important reservoir of infection.

The incubation period ranges from two weeks to more than a year. The disease is most common in rural areas and the outskirts of towns. An animal reservoir exists in China and the Mediterranean basin (dog), in Kenya (rodents), in the Sudan (dogs and rodents), and in South America, (dog, fox, and cat), but man is the only reservoir in India. Epidemics of kala-azar often occur after outbreaks of debilitating disease or periods of privation. There is some evidence of resistance to subsequent infection, both visceral and cutaneous following recovery from kala-azar.

A number of species of sandflies have been proved as vectors in nature—*P. argentipes* in India, *P. chinensis* in China, *P. intermedius* and *P. longipalpis* in South America, and *P. perniciosus* in the Mediterranean. They live and breed in cracks and crevices in the soil and in stone walls. They have a short hopping flight, resting frequently, and rarely fly more than a hundred yards or so from their breeding places.

The diagnosis is established by demonstrating *L. donovani* in the blood or, more commonly in marrow from the iliac crest, sternum, or tibia, or in spleen puncture, or by culturing the organism. The aldehyde (formol gel) and antimony (Chopra's) tests are not specific, but a positive reaction supports a clinical diagnosis. The indirect fluorescent antibody technique has been successfully used in the sero-diagnosis of visceral leishmaniasis.

Control consists in identifying and treating infected persons, including cases of dermal leishmaniasis, and in attacking the sandfly. The breeding places of these insects in walls can be plastered over and the rubble of broken-down houses cleared away. *Phlebotomus* is susceptible to residual insecticides, which should be sprayed over the inner walls of houses.

Cutaneous Leishmaniasis

Cutaneous leishmaniasis is caused by local multiplication of *Leishmania* in reticulo-endothelial cells of the skin, resulting in single or multiple granulomata which break down to form indolent ulcers. The infection occurs focally and sporadically in dry zones of the tropics and sub-tropics throughout the world. Animal hosts, mainly dogs, are found naturally infected, and may form a reservoir of infection. Several varieties of cutaneous leishmaniasis have been described [see TABLE 51].

TABLE 51

Some Varieties of Cutaneous Leishmaniasis

Name	Parasite	Geographical distribution
Tropical sore	*L. tropica*	India, Mediterranean basin, Senegal, U.S.S.R.
Chiclero's ulcer; Forest 'yaws'	*L. mexicana*	Mexico, Honduras
	L. guyanensis	Guyana
UTA	*L. peruviana*	Peru
Pseudo-lepromatous	*L. pifanoi*	Venezuela
Diffuse cutaneous (DCL)	Unidentified	Ethiopia

The causative parasites are morphologically indistinguishable from *L. donovani* and are transmitted by vector species of *Phlebotomus* which feed on the skin lesions. Cyclical development of the parasite occurs in the vector, and a granuloma develops some 2–6 months after the infective bite. Autoinfection may cause further lesions.

Recent studies by Ashford *et al.* (1973) have shown that in Ethiopia cutaneous leishmaniasis is transmitted between rock hydrax by the sandflies *P. longipes* and *P. pedifer*. It is also postulated that man intrudes on this system but in no way

sustains it, and that the hydraxes are the only significant reservoir hosts.

Recovery confers substantial resistance to subsequent infection, and hence the greatest prevalence is in children. The diagnosis may be confirmed by demonstrating the leishmania in juice aspirated from the margin of the ulcer through intact skin. The leishmanin Skin test (Montenegro's) is positive in all cases except in those of the pseudo-lepromatous type, where it is variable. Control can be achieved by eliminating sandflies, as described above, and by dressing the ulcers to prevent infection of the vector.

Mucocutaneous Leishmaniasis

Mucocutaneous leishmaniasis or espundia is characterized by ulcerating granulomata of the skin and mucous membrane of the mouth and nose. The parasite, *L. braziliensis*, is indistinguishable from *L. donovani*. The disease is focally endemic in forest regions of Central and South America. It occurs mainly among men working in virgin forest, and an animal reservoir of infection (dog, rodents, fox) has been found. The disease is transmitted by sandflies. The diagnosis is established by recovery of leishmania in smears or cultures from tissue fluid or in biopsy of skin lesions or infected lymph nodes. An intradermal test (Montenegro's) is positive in most cases. Control measures are not practicable in such a sporadic disease, but concentration of isolated families into small villages in the forest will reduce contact with the sandfly.

Recent observations made by Lainson and Shaw (1970) in Brazil, have led to the belief that the name *Leishmania braziliensis* can only be used in *sensu lato* for what is probably a complex species, subspecies or races of *Leishmania* which may occur not only in different geographical regions but also in the same forest areas. Two distinct types of parasites were noted from both man and wild forest animals—a slow-growing organism which is probably responsible for mucocutaneous leishmaniasis in Brazil and a fast-growing strain which gives rise to skin lesions only.

TRYPANOSOMIASIS

African Trypanosomiasis

African trypanosomiasis is caused by either *Trypanosoma gambiense* or *T. rhodesiense*, and the infection is conveyed to man by the bites of flies of the genus *Glossina*, in which cyclical development of the parasite occurs. The disease is confined to that part of Africa lying between latitudes 10° N. and 25° S. *T. rhodesiense* infection is limited to Kenya, Tanzania, Uganda, Malawi, Zambia, Rhodesia, and Mozambique, while *T. gambiense* is more widespread, extending from West Africa through Central Africa to Uganda, Tanzania, and Malawi. There has been a marked resurgence of trypanosomiasis in Congo Kinshasa, while a recent epidemic of *T. rhodesiense* has been reported from Ethiopia.

The relationship between *T. gambiense* and *T. rhodesiense* is not clear; though morphologically similar, their clinical effects are not the same, and the infections are transmitted by different species of tsetse flies. They may be either different species or variants of a single species modified by passage through different vectors and hosts. The tsetse is infected by imbibing the parasites in the blood of the host, and the trypanosome then passes through a developmental cycle which terminates eighteen or more days later with the appearance of infective trypanosomes in the fly's salivary glands. These are inoculated when the tsetse feeds. Man is the principal host of both trypanosomes, but *T. rhodesiense* can also parasitize certain species of wild game, particularly the larger antelopes, in which symptomless infection results. Since the parasite has been known to persist over periods of years in depopulated areas, it is believed that on occasions an animal reservoir is epidemiologically important. No animal reservoir of *T. gambiense* is known.

Each species of tsetse has particular requirements in regard to climate and vegetation, which determine its distribution. All of them tend to concentrate seasonally in habitats offering permanent shade and humidity. The distribution of the fly thus varies with the season, and in addition it advances and

density that their normal agricultural and other activities eradicate the tsetse habitats. It is also possible to remove or alter the foci sheltering the fly during arid periods, and thus cause them to disappear; this must be done under the guidance of an entomologist who has studied the local vector species. A clearance of all trees and shrubs to a depth of a mile or more may be used to prevent extension of the range of the fly or to isolate a focus. Game extermination has proved successful in eliminating certain species of fly which depend on them. Residual insecticides have in some circumstances proved effective against certain vectors when sprayed from the air or at ground level on the trees and shrubs, and riverine species can be controlled or eliminated by a combination of insecticidal treatment of blocks of vegetation, applied at ground level, which are separated by cleared areas.

AFRICAN TRYPANOSOMIASIS

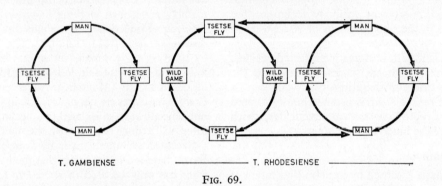

T. GAMBIENSE ———————————— T. RHODESIENSE ————————

Fig. 69.

retreats spatially at intervals of years. Population density affects the incidence of the disease, which is sporadic at densities below 20 per square mile, and is liable to become epidemic at densities up to 200 or so per square mile, above which it disappears because tsetse habitats are eliminated.

The incubation period is between two and three weeks. The disease can be spread by fly following man, traffic, or animals, or by the movement of infected persons. Endemicity results from intimate contact between the human and infected fly populations, and where this is high, epidemic spread may follow. The sex incidence varies according to occupation; where the fly is concentrated near watering points or on farms women tend to show a higher prevalence, but men are more commonly infected in occupations in the woodland-savannah.

The diagnosis is established by recovering trypanosomes in fresh or stained films of blood, in juice aspirated from the enlarged glands, or in cerebrospinal fluid. The serum levels of IgM, IgA, and IgG immunoglobulins are raised in both *T. gambiense* and *T. rhodesiense* infections. The fluorescent antibody test has been used in the serodiagnosis of African trypanosomiasis and antibodies have also been detected in the cerebrospinal fluid of patients with sleeping sickness.

Control is directed against the parasite in man or against the fly, and is commonly a combination of both. The survey of infected communities and treatment of all those found infected rapidly lowers the incidence and reduces the reservoir of infection. Chemoprophylaxis will give protection for some six months in individuals or communities. Control of the fly is effected most cheaply by concentrating the people to such a

American Trypanosomiasis

American trypanosomiasis, also known as *Chagas' disease*, is found in Central and South America. The parasite, *Trypanosoma cruzi*, is found in the peripheral blood as a trypanosome, and intracellularly in the tissues as a leishmanioid body. Triatomine bugs are the vectors. Two almost independent cycles of infection occur, one being in warm-blooded, wild animals—armadillos, opossums, monkeys, etc.—and the other in domestic infection of man, dogs, and cats. The vectors of the wild cycle have little contact with man, whereas those of the domestic cycle infest cracks and crevices in the houses in rural areas. Many species of triatomine bugs transmit infection, the most important domestic vectors being *Panstrongylus megistus*, *Rhodnius prolixus* and *Triatoma infestans*. The bugs, while feeding, imbibe the parasite, which, during a developmental cycle of 3–8 weeks in the bug's hind-gut, multiplies and develops into infective trypanosomes. During subsequent blood-meals the bug defaecates and the parasites are deposited on the skin, where they may enter through abrasions or mucous membranes, symptoms developing in 1–2 weeks' time. The trypanosomes may be found in stained thick blood films during the first week of infection, and trypanosomes or leishmanioid forms may be detected in fluid aspirated from the skin swellings (chagomas) at the site of entry of the parasite. Blood may be inoculated into white rats, which are later examined for the presence of parasites in their blood or tissues. A complement fixation test (Machado's) is specific in chronic cases, and on occasions xenodiagnosis is employed, i.e. feeding laboratory-bred vector bugs on the suspected case and then examining their faeces for infective trypanosomes 1–2 months later. Immunofluorescence has been used in the diagnosis of Chagas' disease.

Chagas' disease flourishes only where social and economic levels are low, and long-term control measures involve economic rehabilitation, in particular, better housing. Mud hovels with thatched roofs need to be replaced with houses of materials giving no harbourage to bugs. Residual insecticides, especially dieldrin (at 1·6 g./sq. m.) or benzene hexachloride (at 0·5 g./sq. m.), applied to floors, walls, and thatch will eliminate most of the vectors, but re-infestation occurs in a few months. Personal prophylaxis consists in avoiding sleeping in houses liable to harbour the vectors and in using bed nets. Transmission of *T. cruzi* by blood transfusion has been reported from Brazil, Venezuela, and Argentina. All potential donors should be tested by a complement-fixation reaction and rejected if positive.

FILARIASIS

Man is the definitive host of several filarial nematodes. Their embryos (microfilariae) are taken up by insect vectors when feeding on man. They pass through a developmental cycle lasting about a fortnight, at the end of which infective larvae are present in the proboscis. When the insect next feeds the larvae escape and pass through breaches of the skin surface into the tissues.

Bancroft's Filariasis and Malayan Filariasis

Wuchereria bancrofti is endemic throughout much of the world lying between the Tropics of Cancer and Capricorn,

Aëdes. The subperiodic form is associated with swamp forest, and it infects monkeys and other animals, and man as well; it also is carried by species of *Mansonia*. The infection is often confined to foci within the flight range of the vector. Elephantiasis develops in individuals in whom reaction to the worms causes the local lymphatics to become sealed, and in these cases the microfilariae cannot reach the blood stream.

A diagnosis is made by finding microfilariae in thick blood films, taken towards midnight in the case of worms with nocturnal periodicity. In stained films the arrangement of their nuclei permits a specific diagnosis to be made. Serological tests, such as a complement fixation test, a fluorescent antibody test, and a haemagglutination test, as well as an intradermal test, have all been used for diagnostic purposes and in epidemiological surveys. They are group-specific.

The infection may be controlled by attacking the vector mosquitoes or by reducing the human reservoir. Control measures may be taken against the aquatic stages of the mosquito by eliminating breeding places, using insecticides to kill aquatic forms or, in the case of *Mansonioides* mosquitoes, destroying by herbicides or hand collection the water vegetation on which the insect is dependent. Adult vectors may be controlled by residual insecticides applied to the inner walls of houses. *Culex fatigans*, a common vector, is naturally tolerant of DDT and strains resistant to benzene hexachloride and dieldrin have been reported. Organophosphorus insecticides can be used against the larval stages, which often breed in septic pits and drains near houses. The human reservoir of infection may be reduced by treatment of the infected population with diethylcarbamazine (*Hetrazan*), which abolishes or greatly reduces circulating microfilariae and kills some of the adult worms. Sharp reactions may follow the use of this drug when

BRUGIA MALAYI

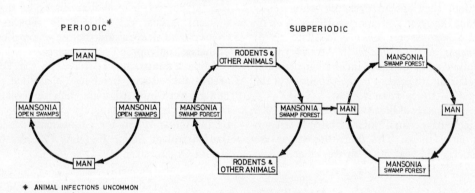

FIG. 70.

while *Brugia malayi* occurs only in parts of Asia. The worms live in the human lymphatics and lymph nodes, and the microfilariae pass into the peripheral blood, commonly appearing there nocturnally. In some of the Pacific islands the embryos of *W. bancrofti* show a diurnal periodicity, while some strains of *B. malayi* are subperiodic.

Many species of mosquitoes of several genera are natural vectors of *W. bancrofti* which infects man only. Periodic *B. malayi* infects man almost exclusively, and is associated with open swamps, lakes, and reservoirs; it is carried by certain species of *Mansonia*, and less commonly by *Anopheles* and

microfilariae are numerous. Spaced doses over a long period, e.g. 4–6 mg./kg. diethylcarbamazine citrate once weekly or once monthly for eight to twelve doses, have proved effective in South-East Asia against both forms of filariasis.

Loiasis

Loiasis has a focal distribution in the equatorial rain belt of Africa. The adult worms, *Loa loa*, live in man's connective tissues causing transient subcutaneous swellings (Calabar swellings). It produces microfilariae which commonly have a diurnal periodicity, and these pass into the peripheral circulation, where they are taken up by certain species of *Chrysops* flies. Development occurs in these resulting in the presence of infective forms in the proboscis some ten or more days later. When the fly feeds they break out, pass into the tissues through the puncture made by the bite, and become mature some six months later. The vector species, *C. silacea* and *C. dimidiata* mainly, breed in shaded marshy streams, and the female alone feeds on blood. The flies attack man in open spaces in the forest during the day-time. A tentative diagnosis can be based on the occurrence of Calabar swellings and eosinophilia, and on occasions the worm may be seen migrating below the conjunctiva or thin-skinned areas. Microfilariae can be demonstrated in stained thick films of the peripheral blood taken towards midday.

As in the case of Bancroft's filariasis, control measures are directed against the parasite in man and against the vector fly. Diethylcarbamazine clears microfilariae from the blood and kills the adult worm in recent infections, but it sometimes causes unpleasant reactions. The drug can be used as a chemoprophylactic at an adult dosage of 200 mg. twice daily for three successive days once a month. The fly may be controlled by clearing shade vegetation at breeding sites or by applying residual insecticides to the mud in the breeding places. Personal protection against bites of *Chrysops* can be effected by screening of houses and wearing long trousers.

Onchocerciasis

Onchocerciasis is caused by a filarial nematode, *Onchocerca volvulus*, which inhabits the subcutaneous tissues, giving rise to small tender nodules, which persist for years. It has a focal distribution in tropical Africa and in Mexico, Guatemala, Colombia, and Venezuela. The microfilariae migrate into and live in the skin, at first in the vicinity of the nodule but later, owing to accumulation, they spread over the whole body surface and even invade the eyes. The embryos are taken up by *Simulium* species (*S. damnosum* and *S. neavei* in Africa and *S. ochraceum*, *S. metallicum*, and *S. callidum* in America) while the fly is feeding. Following an extrinsic incubation period of 10–14 days, infective larvae are present in the proboscis of the fly and escape into man's tissues when it bites.

The vector species of *Simulium* breeds at altitudes of 2,000 ft. or more in the highly oxygenated water of hillside streams or at the edges of large rivers. The immature stages are attached to stones, sticks, and vegetation on the water, but in

the case of *S. neavei* they are found on the carapace of certain aquatic crabs in shady parts of the stream. Though some species of *Simulium* have a long flight range, the infection is mainly concentrated near the breeding sites, and thus tends to be focal. Man is the only known reservoir of infection.

The diagnosis can be confirmed by finding the microfilariae in superficial shavings of the skin removed by means of a scalpel or razor blade without causing bleeding. The skin snip is teased into fragments in a drop of saline, and active larvae can be seen under a low magnification of the microscope. In early cases snips should be taken from the vicinity of the nodule, but in old-established cases they may be taken from the outer surfaces of the ankle, calf, or buttock. The embryos may be distinguished from those of *Acanthocheilonema streptocerca* by examining films stained by Mayer's haemalum; *A. streptocerca* are smaller (20 μ, as compared with 35 μ for *O. volvulus*) and have a column of nuclei extending to the very tip of the tail.

Control is most commonly effected by attacking the vector. When the volume of the stream is not too large residual insecticides, as emulsions or miscible oils, may be added to the water above the highest breeding point in sufficient quantity to give a concentration below the lowest breeding sites of $\frac{1}{2}$–1 part of DDT per million. This is lethal to the developing forms. Treatment should be repeated for half an hour every ten days for three months in order to cover the life-span of the adult fly. Insecticides may be sprayed from aircraft on the vegetation around breeding places on alternate days for a period of three weeks in order to kill the adult *Simulium*. Removal of the subcutaneous nodules reduces the incidence of eye lesions, and mass treatment with diethylcarbamazine of all infected persons in the community kills the microfilariae and reduces transmission. This, however, is liable to cause sharp allergic reactions. Suramin kills the majority of adult worms, but the microfilariae disappear slowly. Personal prophylaxis against this vicious fly consists of wearing long trousers and sleeves, and the use of repellents (e.g. dimethylphthalate) on exposed skin surfaces.

A mass campaign was started in the Volta valley in 1974 against the disease, involving 10 million people of which 1 million were infected with onchocerciasis. Research goes on in the search for a suitable drug for chemotherapy; conducted by the Organization for Co-ordination and Co-operation in the Control of Major Endemic Diseases (OCCGE), (World Health Organization, 1974, p. 43).

FURTHER READING

General

Askew, R. R. (1971) *Parasitic Diseases*, London.
Brown, A. W. A., and Pal, R. (1971) Insecticide Resistance in Arthropods, *Wld Hlth Org. Monogr. Ser.*, No. 38.
Davey, T. H., and Lightbody, W. P. H. (1971) *The Control of Disease in the Tropics*, 4th ed., rev. Davey, T. H., and Wilson, T., London.
Edington, G. M., and Gilles, H. M. (1969) *Pathology in the Tropics*, London
Surtees, G. (1971) Urbanization and the epidemiology of mosquito-borne disease, *Abstr. Hyg.*, **46**, 121.
World Health Organization (1971) Alternative Insecticide for Vector Control, *Bull. Wld Hlth Org.*, **44**, 1–470.

World Health Organization Expert Committee on Insecticides (1971) Nineteenth Report, *Wld Hlth Org. techn. Rep. Ser.*, No. 475.
World Health Organization (1974) The work of WHO in 1973, *Wld Hlth Org. Off. Rec.*, No. 213.

Arboviruses

Brown, A. W. A. (1974) The safety of biological agents for arthropod control, *Wld Hlth Org. Chron.*, **28**, 261.
Catalogue of Arthropod-borne Viruses of the World. The subcommittee on information exchange of the American Committee on Arthropod-borne Viruses, *Amer. J. trop. Med. Hyg.*, (1970) **19**, Part 2, 1082.

De Moor, P. P., and Steffens, F. E. (1970) A computer-simulated model of an arthropod-borne virus transmission cycle, with special reference to chikungunya virus, *Trans. roy. Soc. trop. Med. Hyg.*, **6**, 927.

World Health Organization (1967) Arbovirus and Human Disease, *Wld Hlth Org. techn. Rep. Ser.*, No. 369.

Filariasis

Buck, A. A., ed. (1974) *Onchocerciasis: Symptomology, Pathology, Diagnosis*, Geneva.

Sasa, M. (1970) *Recent Advances in Researches on Filariasis and Schistosomiasis in Japan*, Tokyo.

World Health Organization Expert Committee on Onchocerciasis (1966) Second Report, *Wld Hlth Org. techn. Rep. Ser.*, No. 335.

World Health Organization Expert Committee on Filariasis (1967) Second Report, *Wld Hlth Org. techn. Rep. Ser.*, No. 359.

World Health Organization (1973a) Onchocerciasis programmes in Africa, *Wld Hlth Org. Chron.*, **27**, 540.

World Health Organization (1974) Third report of the expert committee on filariasis, *Wld Hlth Org. techn. Rep. Ser.*, No. 542.

Leishmaniasis

Ashford, R. W., Bray, M. A., Hutchinson, M. P., and Bray, R. S. (1973) The epidemiology of cutaneous leishmaniasis in Ethiopia, *Trans. roy. Soc. trop. Med. Hyg.*, **67**, 568.

Lainson, R., and Shaw, J. J. (1970) Leishmaniasis in Brazil, *Trans. roy. Soc. trop. Med. Hyg.*, **5**, 654.

World Health Organization (1971) Leishmaniasis, *Bull. Wld Hlth Org.*, **44**, No. 4.

Schistosomiasis

Wright, W. H. (1972) Economic impact of schistosomiasis, *Bull. Wld. Hlth Org.*, **47**, 559.

Trypanosomiasis

Miles, M. A., and Rouse, J. A. (1970) Chagas's disease—a bibliography, *Trop. Dis. Bull.*, Suppl. v, 67.

Mulligan, H. W. (1970) The African trypanosomiases, London.

World Health Organization Expert Committee on Trypanosomiasis (1969) *Wld Hlth Org. techn. Rep. Ser.*, No. 434.

World Health Organization (1973b) Trypanosomiasis in Kenya, *Wld Hlth Org. Chron.*, **27**, 368.

Yellow Fever

World Health Organization Expert Committee on Yellow Fever (1971) Third Report, *Wld Hlth Org. techn. Rep. Ser.*, No. 479.

World Health Organization (1973c) Report of the Expert Committee on yellow fever, *Wld Hlth Org. Chron.*, **27**, 499.

18

THE CONTROL OF MALARIA

G. SAMBASIVAN

Malaria is a protozoal disease caused by infection with parasites of the genus *Plasmodium*, transmitted in nature through the bite of infected mosquitoes of certain anopheline species. Exceptionally, direct transmission from man to man can occur following transfusion of infected blood, or through the common use of contaminated sryinges and needles as in the case of drug addicts. Instances of transplacental transmission of malaria parasites to the child have also been recorded when the mother has had clinical attacks of malaria during the later months of pregnancy.

Several species of malaria parasites have been identified in mammals, birds, and reptiles. There are four species of human malaria parasites: *Plasmodium falciparum*, *P. vivax*, *P. malariae* and *P. ovale*. Within each species are strains which differ in their virulence, their response to drugs, their infectiousness to certain species of anopheline vectors, and the immunity which they produce in man. Of the four species of human malaria parasites, *P. falciparum* and *P. vivax* account for the vast bulk of malaria in the world.

Although human malaria has been experimentally transmitted to some species of monkeys, extensive studies have failed to prove the existence of any animal reservoir of human malaria in nature. In this respect, malaria differs from yellow fever and plague in which animal reservoirs play an important role.

GEOGRAPHICAL DISTRIBUTION AND PRESENT STATUS

As an indigenous disease malaria is now mainly confined to the tropical and subtropical regions of the world [FIG. 71]. In the past it existed in the majority of the countries and since 1920 has been reported from as far north as Archangel (64° N.) in the U.S.S.R. and as far south as Cordoba (32°5′ S.) in Argentina. Even within the tropical and subtropical belts there are large areas which are naturally malaria-free because of ecological factors unfavourable to vector breeding, e.g. arid regions. In the Central and South Pacific regions certain islands such as Galapagos, Marquesas, Fiji, and New Caledonia have no anophelines and so are non-malarious.

Temperature is an important limiting factor in malaria transmission. *P. falciparum* requires a constant temperature of at least 20° C. for its development in the mosquito vector. 'The theoretical frontier of distribution of this species is 20° C. summer isotherm.' (World Health Organization, 1969.) The transmission of *P. vivax* and *P. malariae* can occur at somewhat lower temperatures. With the disappearance of malaria in recent years from Europe, the United States, and a number of areas in Asia, the geographical boundaries of *P. falciparum* and *P. vivax* now appear to be almost the same. *P. malariae*

has a wide but uneven distribution with very low prevalence, except in a few scattered areas in equatorial Africa. *P. ovale* is a rarity outside tropical Africa, where its prevalance seldom exceeds 5 per cent. of the malaria infections.

The boundaries of the spread of the disease have changed considerably during the past forty years. At present, large areas of the originally malarious regions have been cleared of the disease. In the less developed countries this has been mainly due to the malaria eradication campaigns undertaken by their governments. In the more developed countries the disappearance of the disease has been the result of a combination of favourable factors. The ecological changes consequent on the rapid socio-economic development of the past few decades in these countries had already reduced the sources of vector breeding and reduced the malaria potential. Furthermore, the efforts of the various governments in combating malaria were helped by the extensive network of health services that were already available, and by the active participation of a population motivated by a better awareness of their health needs. Yet, only twenty years ago it was estimated that each year some 300 million people suffered from clinical attacks of malaria and that it caused directly three million deaths annually. The major effect of endemic malaria is the chronic invalidity it produces, and the disease is recognized as a serious hindrance to economic development in the tropical and subtropical regions of the world. In many instances the malaria season corresponds with the periods of agricultural activity.

From recent reports received from governments, the World Health Organization reckons that, out of a total population of 1844 million[1] in originally malarious areas, malaria has been eradicated from areas with a population of 739 million of which nearly 52 per cent. are chiefly in Europe and North America and 48 per cent. in the tropical and subtropical regions, where a further 309 million population is now living in areas where transmission has been arrested. Published reports from the Republic of China and North Korea indicate that the prevalence of the disease has been considerably reduced in these countries. Nevertheless, over 400 million people still live in areas exposed to malaria risk. The disease continues to be highly endemic in tropical Africa and still constitutes a serious health hazard in several parts of Asia, Central and South America, and North Africa. While many areas of the world have been freed from indigenous malaria, the risk from imported cases is rising as a result of the increased volume and speed of international traffic. This presents a serious public health problem in areas where the vectors are present and conditions are favourable for the re-establishment of transmission. It is also a clinical problem in countries where, as a

[1] This figure does not include the populations of mainland China, North Vietnam, and North Korea.

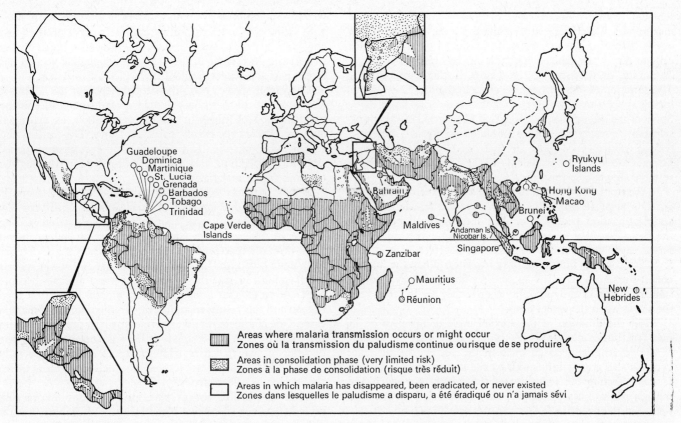

Fig. 71. Epidemiological assessment of status of malaria, 30 June 1971. [World Health Organization (1972) *Weekly Epidemiological Record*, No. 9.]

result of the disappearance of malaria for some years, the medical profession and the laboratory services are prone to miss the diagnosis. In the United Kingdom, between 1954 and 1969, there were 58 deaths from imported malaria (Shute, 1969).

LIFE-CYCLE OF THE MALARIA PARASITE

The principles and practice of malaria control are based on an understanding of the life-cycle of the malaria parasite and the factors influencing malaria transmission. The parasite has an asexual cycle (schizogony) of development in man, and a sexual cycle (sporogony) in the vector mosquito. In man the parasite undergoes two phases of development—the tissue phase called the exo-erythrocytic phase in the parenchymatous cells of the liver, and the erythrocytic phase in the red blood cells [FIG. 72].

The parasites that are injected into the blood through the bite of an infected mosquito are tiny spindle-shaped bodies 10/15 μ in length called sporozoites. In less than 30 minutes after the mosquito bite the sporozoites disappear from the blood and enter the parenchymatous cells of the liver, in which they grow into primary exo-erythrocytic (E.E.) schizonts, their cytoplasm and nuclei dividing repeatedly to form hundreds of daughter forms known as merozoites. After a few days when the E.E. schizont matures, the merozoites are discharged into the blood circulation, and each of them is capable of infecting a red blood cell. The average time required for the completion of the primary E.E. phase varies from about $5\frac{1}{2}$

days for *P. falciparum* to about 16 days for *P. malariae*. In the case of *P. vivax*, and probably in *P. malariae* and *P. ovale*, some of the merozoites from the primary E.E. schizont enter fresh liver cells and start a secondary E.E. phase. In *P. falciparum* there is only the primary E.E. phase and this may account for the absence of relapses in this infection.

The merozoite that enters a red blood cell grows into a

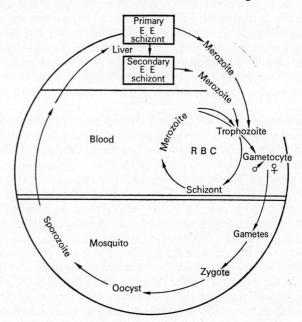

Fig. 72. Life cycle of the malarial parasite *P. vivax*.

schizont, with its nucleus and cytoplasm dividing to form merozoites. When the schizont matures, the red blood cell bursts liberating the merozoites which infect other red blood cells to repeat the schizogonic cycle in the blood until drugs, immunity, or death of the host stops further development. The duration of one schizogonic cycle in the R.B.C. is 2 days for all species except *P. malariae* in which it is three days. Some of the merozoites, entering R.B.C.s instead of becoming schizonts, develop into unsegmented sexual forms—male and female gametocytes. The further development of these gametocytes can take place only if they are sucked up by a suitable anopheline mosquito.

In the stomach of the mosquito the male gametocytes throw out fine flagellae (gametes) which enter the female gametes, and fertilization takes place. The fertilized cell penetrates the stomach wall of the mosquito and comes to rest under the serous layer where it develops into an oocyst, which after a few days contains thousands of sporozoites. When the mature oocyst bursts, some of the sporozoites find their way into the salivary glands of the mosquito whence they are injected with the saliva when the insect bites.

While the duration of the asexual cycle of the parasite in man (the intrinsic cycle) is determined mainly by the species of the parasite, the sexual cycle in the vector (the extrinsic cycle) is also greatly influenced by the temperature and other factors affecting the longevity of the vector. No species of malaria parasite can develop in the vector below 15° C. The optimum temperature for growth is about 28° C. and at this temperature *P. vivax* takes only 8 days to complete its development in the mosquito while at 16° C. it takes 55 days. *P. malariae* needs a relatively longer period for its development than the other species. At 24° C. the extrinsic cycle of this species lasts 24 days while it is 14 days for *P. falciparum* and 11 days for *P. vivax*.

MALARIA VECTORS

Out of over 300 known species of anophelines about sixty have been incriminated as vectors of human malaria in nature. The life-cycle of a mosquito covers four stages: egg, larva, pupa, and adult. Under favourable conditions the eggs deposited on water hatch in about 2 days, the larval stage lasts about 5–7 days, and the pupa about 2 days. Temperature is the main factor determining the length of these acquatic stages of the mosquito. The adult may live from a few days to a few months, the temperature and relative humidity influencing longevity. Adult mosquitoes are very vulnerable to dryness. Yet the adult can survive through hot and dry weather and through the cold season and maintain the species by adjusting the pattern of its behaviour and by adopting a depressed state of physiological activities. The longevity of the adult vector female is a factor of great significance in malaria transmission as even under favourable conditions no mosquito can transmit malaria until it has lived at least 10 days, for the completion of the extrinsic cycle of development of the parasite. The longer it lives after this period the greater are its chances of transmitting malaria.

Vector species also differ in their choice of water collections for oviposition. Some prefer sun-lit waters, others need more shaded locations. Some species require moving waters and others stagnant pools. Although most species prefer clean water, some can breed in polluted water and others need water with saline content. In planning malaria control projects and engineering works in the tropics, the lack of appreciation of these basic differences in the habits of anopheline vectors has in the past sometimes resulted in very costly mistakes.

The vector species also differ in the habits of the adults. A knowledge of this has now assumed special significance as the main method of attack in malaria eradication, as explained later, is directed against the adult mosquito. The feeding and resting habits and the flight range of adult vectors need special attention in planning anti-adult measures for interrupting the transmission of malaria.

It is only the female mosquitoes that bite, as the blood is needed for the development of their ovaries. With very few exceptions in nature most anophelines are night-biters. The degree of preference for human blood or for animal blood varies with the species of the vector. The greater the preference for human blood, the higher is the potential of a vector species for transmitting malaria. Sometimes, when animals become scarce, a vector that normally prefers animal blood may turn to man and this results in an increase in the number of malaria cases. One complete round of development of the ovaries from the blood meal to egg-laying is called a gonotrophic cycle, the duration of which varies with the species and is generally about 48 hours in the tropics and as much as twice or thrice that period in cold climates.

Most anopheline vectors rest inside houses for varying periods between successive blood meals. This habit is greatly influenced by ecological factors such as the type of house, the activity of the inhabitants, the availability of suitable outdoor resting places, etc. Flimsy houses exposed to draught and houses in which smoke is present do not afford suitable resting places for vectors. Vectors may feed on man indoors or outdoors depending on where people are during the vector feeding time, which varies from species to species and sometimes from season to season. The behaviour of a vector species is influenced by a combination of local ecological factors. The same species may behave differently in different ecological situations.

The effective flight range of a vector species is calculated as the distance from a breeding place that the females of the species travel in numbers sufficient to maintain transmission. This distance is much less than the maximum distance the vector can travel from its breeding place. In the tropics the effective flight range of vectors very rarely exceeds two miles and is often less than one mile. Generally, for the protection of an area in the tropics it is sufficient to extend vector control measures over a surrounding zone of a half to one mile. In temperate regions the vectors have a much longer effective flight range and this makes it necessary to extend the control operations over a wider area.

EPIDEMIOLOGY

Malaria is *endemic* in an area when over a succession of years there is a constant measurable incidence of cases due to natural local transmission. The term *epidemic* malaria is applied when the incidence of cases in an area rises rapidly and markedly above its usual seasonal level or when a number of infections occur in an area where there was no transmission previously. The most direct and reliable proof of malaria infection is the demonstration of malaria parasites in the blood. Indirect evidence is provided by the enlargement of the spleen, which is a cellular response of the body to malaria infection, and by the presence of malarial antibodies in the blood. In long-standing infections the splenic enlargement and the antibodies may persist for some time even after the infections have been cured. As a routine epidemiological method for assessing endemicity the measurement of malarial antibodies is at present impracticable as it involves sophisticated laboratory techniques. The detection of malarial antibodies by fluorescent antibody technique (F.A.T.) has recently been used as an effective method of screening blood donors in some countries. Spleen surveys and parasite surveys form the main basis for demarcating malarious areas except in areas of very low endemicity where a case-finding method may be required. In countries where there are other endemic diseases such as kala-azar or bilharziasis causing splenomegaly, it is obvious that spleen surveys cannot be used for demarcating malarious areas.

Spleen rate (S.R.), which represents the percentage of individuals of any particular age group with enlarged spleen, is used for classifying the different degrees of malaria endemicity:

Hypo-endemic—Spleen rate in children 2–9 years up to 10 per cent.

Meso-endemic—Spleen rate in children 2–9 years from 11 to 50 per cent.

Hyper-endemic—Spleen rate in children 2–9 years constantly over 50 per cent. Adult S.R. also high.

Holo-endemic—Spleen rate in children 2–9 years constantly over 75 per cent. Adult S.R. usually low.

The size of the enlarged spleens also gives an indication of the duration and intensity of transmission in the community. Spleen sizes are classified as follows:

Size I. Palpable only on deep inspiration.
    II. Spleen does not project below a horizontal line half-way between the left costal margin (in the mid-clavicular line) and the umbilicus.
    III. The lowest palpable part of the spleen between the lower limit of II and a horizontal line through the umbilicus.
    IV. The lowest palpable part of the spleen between the umbilicus but not extending below a horizontal line drawn half-way between the umbilicus and the symphysis pubis.
    V. The lowest palpable part of the spleen below IV.

The degree of splenic enlargement in a population can be calculated from the weighted averages as in the following example:

Number of persons examined: 100
Number with enlarged spleen: 50—composed of 10 spleen I, 20 spleen II, and 20 spleen III

Average enlarged spleen (AES) =
$$\frac{10 \times 1 + 20 \times 2 + 20 \times 3}{50} = \frac{110}{50} = 2 \cdot 2$$

Average spleen (AS) =
$$\frac{10 \times 1 + 20 \times 2 + 20 \times 3}{100} = \frac{110}{100} = 1 \cdot 1$$

In general, spleen surveys mainly concentrate on the age group 2–9 years which has the highest prevalence of spleno-megaly.

PARASITE SURVEYS

The main purpose of these surveys is the determination of parasite rates, i.e. the percentage of persons of any particular age group showing parasites in the blood at the time of the survey. In addition, parasite surveys are also used for finding out the prevalence of the different species of plasmodia and the density of parasitaemia. The percentage of individuals showing gametocytes in the blood—gametocyte rate—is also used in some countries as an epidemiological index.

Except in mass blood surveys, when blood samples from every person are examined, parasite surveys cover only a representative sample of the population. The sampling should therefore be planned with due regard to statistical requirements in order to ensure that the results actually represent the prevalence of infection in the population surveyed. Comparison of parasite rates taken at half-yearly or yearly intervals is the main basis for assessing the results of antimalaria measures. However, when the parasite prevalance reaches low levels, this method loses its sensitivity and will need to be replaced by case detection aimed at determining the incidence of infection.

Infant Parasite Surveys

In endemic areas infants form the non-immune section of the indigenous population and serve as a sensitive group for confirming the presence of transmission. Infant parasite rates, representing the percentage of infants showing parasites in their blood, also indicate the degree of transmission present in the locality. When repeated at monthly intervals infant parasite surveys provide valuable epidemiological information on the duration of the transmission season. A zero infant parasite rate, however, does not necessarily mean that there is no transmission in the rest of the community.

Examination of Blood Films

When a large number of blood films have to be examined in connexion with malaria control or eradication programmes, the routine practice is to use thick blood films and screen 100 microscopic fields which correspond to approximately $0 \cdot 2$ mm^3 of blood. To examine the same volume of blood by thin smear takes a much longer time which no large programme can afford. As a rule in malaria eradication programmes, a thick and a thin film are taken from each individual on the same slide, and the thin film is examined only when the diagnosis of the species of the parasite seen in the thick film is in doubt. The limitation of a single blood film examination should be borne in mind in interpreting the results. When the parasite density is below 15 per mm^3, the chances of missing parasites in a single examination are considerable. Recognition of malaria parasites in stained thick films requires specialized training, and this is an aspect of great practical importance in malaria eradication programmes.

Different methods of improving the detection of parasites are under investigation at present. These include fluorochrome staining of slides, the use of wide-angle objective which gives a better depth of focus and a wider field of vision, and the use of a simple hand-operated disc centrifuge for concentrating the parasites in the blood sample. For details of laboratory techniques, differentiation of parasite species, measurement of parasite density, etc., the reader should refer to the standard textbooks on malariology, e.g. *Practical Malariology* by Russell *et al.* (1963).

MALARIA RECONNAISSANCE

In countries where even the basic information on the distribution of the disease is lacking, one of the first activities to be undertaken is a malaria reconnaissance which is an extensive rather than an intensive survey carried out as rapidly as possible. As splenomegaly in children is readily recognizable and reliable evidence of endemic malaria, the survey is generally limited to the examination of children. In the interests of speed, wherever possible this is done in schools or other places where children can be assembled. Blood films are collected at the same time from those children showing splenomegaly, in order to ascertain the species prevalence and to confirm that the splenomegaly is of malarial origin. In areas where diseases such as kala-azar or bilharziasis are present, causing splenomegaly, the reconnaissance has to be based on parasite surveys. Confining the taking of blood films to those with splenomegaly also serves to prevent overtaxing of the laboratory facilities which are often very limited. As for the size of the sample to be examined, 5 per cent. of children under 15 is reckoned as a practicable objective (Christophers, 1949). The spleen rate and average enlarged spleen size obtained for each school or locality are entered in a map, and this could form the basis for a rough demarcation of malarious areas. Additional information on malaria distribution may be obtained from hospital and dispensary records. An understanding of the landscape features and ecological conditions associated with the breeding of the local anopheline vectors would also be valuable in identifying areas which are possibly malarious. The latest available census data and a map of the country showing the main geographical features, communications, and the location of schools should be obtained to facilitate the reconnaissance.

The limitations of the data collected through reconnaissance should be clearly understood. They are not sufficiently accurate to serve as baseline data for evaluating the results of subsequent control operations; but they could form the basis for stratifying the areas for more detailed malaria surveys. Besides showing the broad distribution of endemicity, the information gathered may also reveal communities in more urgent need of control measures.

MALARIA SURVEYS

Malaria surveys are investigations carried out for the collection of data and information necessary for planning, implementing, and evaluating antimalaria programmes. The scope of a survey depends on the objectives for which it is undertaken. When malaria eradication or large-scale malaria control is the objective, the survey should include the quantitative measurement of the disease prevalence and its seasonal fluctuations, as well as a review of the various factors related to man, vector, and the parasite that affect the epidemiology of the disease in the different geographical regions of the country. The survey report should also cover the history of malaria in the country and the results of any previous attempts at controlling the disease. A malaria survey cannot always be expected to indicate the most suitable method of interrupting transmission. From the facts gathered during the survey it is up to the malariologist responsible for planning antimalaria measures to decide on the most appropriate course of action. When the survey reveals lack of information on the response of malaria to the standard methods of control, it may be necessary to carry out pilot or research projects to obtain the required information. Unless some follow-up action is contemplated, malaria surveys are not indicated as the expense and the time involved in such surveys could be better utilized for other more useful health activities.

FACTORS AFFECTING THE ENDEMICITY OF MALARIA

The natural history of malaria in an area is the result of the interplay of various factors affecting the bionomics of man, the mosquito, and the parasite in the local environment. Man, as the source and the victim of malaria, influences in many ways the transmission as well as the persistence of malaria in an area. Racial and genetic factors, immunity, occupation, migration, etc., have a direct influence on malaria prevalence. The long period of carrier state when the parasite carrier is symptomless also plays an important part.

It is known that Negroes are naturally refractory to *P. vivax* infection. This genetic character is most marked in West Africa, where in many regions *P. vivax* cannot be found in the local Negro population. Another genetic factor that influences the severity of infection is the presence of haemoglobin S (sickle-cell trait). This abnormal haemoglobin which is common in some West African communities appears to slow down the multiplication of the parasite in the blood, thus lowering the severity of the disease.

In highly endemic areas, where the population is exposed to repeated infections, newborns during the first few weeks of birth show a much lower malaria rate than one would expect. This relative insusceptibility to infection is attributed to the passive transference of certain immunoglobulins (IgG) responsible for immunity from the mother across the placenta to the child. After this period, from six months to two years the infant is very vulnerable to acute malarial attacks. Thereafter, those who survive gradually build up acquired immunity which at first serves to modify the severity of clinical symptoms and later also to reduce the parasitaemia. In these communities the adults are able to tolerate varying degrees of parasitaemia without overt clinical symptoms. The immunity thus acquired is strain-specific. Thus, a person immune to a local strain of *P. falciparum* may be susceptible to a different strain of *P. falciparum* from another region. The strain-specificity of immune response appears to be less marked in *P. vivax* than in *P. falciparum*. It is recognized that immunity, once established, may last for about two years or more after the infection has been cured and transmission eliminated.

The fact that high endemicity is accompanied by a high level of immunity to the local strains of plasmodia accounts for the absence of great fluctuations in malaria incidence from year to year in such areas. Under these conditions malaria is said to be 'stable'. On the other hand, in areas of low endemicity with correspondingly low levels of immunity abnormal increases in vector breeding may result in epidemics of malaria. Malaria in such areas is often referred to as 'unstable malaria'. Immunity also affects the mortality rates. Deaths from malaria are more common in non-immunes during primary attacks, and may be as high as 25 per cent. in untreated *P. falciparum* infections.

In endemic areas occupations requiring persons to be out of doors at night carry a greater risk of contracting malaria, as the protective measures applied in houses are often impracticable in the open. Persons engaged in land reclamation, railway traffic staff, transport drivers, wood cutters, charcoal collectors in forests, fishermen, hunters, etc., in tropical areas fall under this category. Some of the activities of man also increase the malaria risk of an area by creating new breeding places for vectors. Construction of dams, embankments, irrigation systems, and other engineering works meant for economic development could seriously affect the health of the people if adequate measures are not taken to prevent the creation of new breeding places.

Seasonal migration of labour during the planting and harvesting seasons is a common practice in the tropics. This often coincides with the mosquito season, and the immigrants get infected with the local strain of malaria and on their return carry these strains back to their own province. The local population in turn also becomes infected with the strains imported by the immigrants. Nomads form a permanent migratory group with no fixed abode and serve as a source for the exchange of parasite strains. Migration by small or large groups is a cause of the spread of malaria. Moreover, war with its large-scale movement of troops and civil populations and the attendant disruption of normal civil services is a notorious cause of increase in malaria. There were sharp rises in malaria incidence during and immediately after the two world wars. In Italy, for example, the malaria hazard was greatly increased during the Second World War by the destruction of irrigation and drainage systems, the disruption of malaria control services, and the importation of large numbers of parasite carriers.

Among the environmental factors affecting the malariogenic potential in some situations, the level of the subsoil water table is important. In areas like Sind in Pakistan where the vector breeds in pools, a rise in subsoil water table through irrigation or flooding increases the malaria risk. On the other hand, in the Philippines the subsoil water level has no effect on vectors that breed in foothill streams.

The influence of altitude on malaria transmission depends on climatic factors as well as on the availability of suitable vector breeding places. The highest level of endemic malaria recorded is in the Andean region of South America. In Bolivia, endemic areas have been found at 2,500 metres (8,200 ft). Outbreaks of malaria can occur even at higher altitudes during periods of abnormally favourable climatic conditions. Garnham (1945) reported transmission of malaria at 2,600 metres (8,500 ft) in Kenya as a result of mosquitoes introduced into the area through road and rail transport. For practical purposes, however, malaria transmission is seldom a serious problem above 2,000 metres (6,500 ft).

The species prevalence and the strain of the parasites also influence the epidemiology of malaria in an area. Mention has already been made of the effect of temperature on the duration of development of the different species of parasites in the mosquito. In the development of the parasite in man, the incubation period, which is the interval between the infective bite and the onset of fever, varies according to the species of the parasite. It is approximately 11 days for *P. falciparum*, 14 for *P. vivax*, 15 for *P. ovale*, and about 3–4 weeks for *P. malariae*. These are subject to great variations; for instance, the incubation period of *P. falciparum* may vary from a minimum of 6 days to a maximum of 25 days. In temperate climates some strains of *P. vivax* show very prolonged incubation periods or latency extending to several months. Before malaria was eradicated from the Netherlands, infections acquired during the transmission season in the autumn used to cause an increase in malaria cases during the following spring.

In epidemics where both *P. vivax* and *P. falciparum* are present, the rise in case incidence starts with *P. vivax* to be followed later by *P. falciparum*. The epidemic wave due to *P. falciparum*, while rising to higher levels than that of *P. vivax*, tends to subside earlier. This sequence of events could be attributed to the larger carry-over of *P. vivax* infections through relapses from the previous year, to the shorter incubation interval of this species, mainly due to the early appearance of gametocytes in peripheral blood, and to the ability of *P. vivax* to complete its sporogonic cycle in the mosquito at a lower temperature than *P. falciparum*.

In the absence of fresh transmission, malaria is a self-limiting infection. Even without specific treatment, in the surviving patient the infection spontaneously dies out after a time. This life-span of infection varies with the species and the strain of the parasite. Most of the *P. falciparum* infections terminate in less than 1 year and *P. vivax* in about $2\frac{1}{2}$ years. For *P. malariae* no definite period can be fixed as relapses have been recorded as long as 20 or 30 years after infection. But *P. malariae* generally has only a very low rate of propagation. Even in *P. falciparum* and *P. vivax* some infections last longer than the periods mentioned above. However, experience from different parts of the world shows that in the absence of transmission most infections terminate within 3 years irrespective of the species of the parasite. This fact constitutes the basis of the modern practice of malaria eradication [see p. 252].

During the course of a malaria infection there are periods when the infected person exhibits no clinical symptoms while parasites are present in the peripheral blood. This carrier state, called asymptomatic parasitaemia, occurs between bouts of fever during an attack or between relapses sometimes separated by long periods. It may also occur prior to the onset of fever in a primary attack or as a terminal event before the extinction of an infection. In the later stages of an eradication programme, the detection of parasite carriers is important in areas receptive to malaria where vectors are present and climatic conditions are suitable for transmission. The infectiousness of a case to mosquitoes also depends on the age of the infection. Gametocytes of a long-standing infection are less infective to the vector than gametocytes of younger infections. In endemic areas the children show the greatest gametocyte density and form the major reservoir of infection.

Various factors related to the bionomics of the vectors have a profound influence on the epidemiology of malaria. The feeding, breeding, and resting habits, the longevity, the duration of the gonotrophic cycle, and the influence of temperature and humidity have already been mentioned. Rainfall, when associated with suitable temperature, plays a very important role. It is often the number of rainy days and the interval between them that are more important than the total annual rainfall. The effect of rainfall on vector breeding potential also varies according to the terrain. For example, heavy rains and flooding in the Punjab greatly increase the production of the pool-breeding vector *A. culicifacies*, while in Ceylon the same vector species increases when the rains fail and pools form in river beds. Thus, epidemics of malaria were associated with heavy rains in the Punjab and with drought in Ceylon although the vector species was the same in both areas.

A vector species, to be efficient, should have a definite preference for human blood, access to man in sufficient density and a long enough infective life after completion of the sporogonic cycle of development of the parasite. As a measure of the potential risk of transmission, it is the man-biting density of the vector that is more important than its over-all density.

Seasonal fluctuations in incidence are a characteristic feature of malaria and these are related to climatic factors. Even in areas of perennial transmission there are certain periods of the year when transmission is higher than at other times. In areas of low endemicity where malaria is unstable, epidemics may occur at intervals of about 5–7 years and spread to contiguous non-malarious areas. These cyclical epidemics have in the past been attended by high mortality. The causes of these epidemics could be traced to the concurrent occurrence of various factors favourable to increased transmission, such as increased density and longevity of vectors and low levels of communal immunity. Epidemics with no previous history of such episodes occur when the malaria potential of an area is raised as a result of invasion by new vectors or by the introduction of gametocyte carriers or infected mosquitoes. Severe epidemics of malaria followed the introduction of *A. gambiae* in Brazil in 1930 and in Egypt in 1942. Epidemics can also result from man's activities which increase vector breeding, as in the case of malaria epidemics associated with some irrigation projects.

METHODS OF MALARIA PREVENTION

Preventive measures against malaria aim at breaking the man–mosquito cycle of transmission. Their scope and objectives cover a wide range, from the protection of individuals to the eradication of the disease from the entire population of countries or large geographical regions.

Individual Protection

In malarious areas where no organized antimalaria operations for the protection of the community are in force, individuals have to rely on personal protective measures for the prevention of bites by infected mosquitoes and for stopping the development of the parasite in man by means of drugs.

The siting of houses away from the breeding places of vectors and from infected villages can greatly reduce the risk of infection. In tropical countries the Armed Forces, while selecting camp sites for tactical exercises, pay particular attention to ensure that the distance from the nearest village is beyond the effective flight range of the local malaria vectors.

Travellers in malarious countries should, as far as possible, avoid spending nights in local villages where the chances of contracting malaria are generally greater than in cities. Screening of houses and the use of bed-nets, protective clothing and mosquito repellents at night are additional measures to prevent mosquito bites. Fumigation has been a customary practice in malarious areas to keep off the mosquitoes. But now, with the advent of insecticides, more effective methods of reducing the chances of being bitten by infected mosquitoes are available. Various formulations of insecticides in aerosol dispensers or in liquid form can be used by individuals for spraying their sleeping quarters. Among the insecticides used for this purpose, one of the most useful formulations is the extract of pyrethrum. Mosquito repellents generally contain dimethyl phthalate, Indalone Rutgers 612, etc., as active ingredients and differ in the duration of their effectiveness against different species of mosquitoes. Most of the repellents last only for a few hours. A new compound, diethyltalnamide, is claimed to be effective for about 18 hours.

Drugs play an important prophylactic role against malaria. In fact, in many instances individual drug prophylaxis is the only effective and practicable method of preventing clinical attacks. The drugs generally used for this purpose are pyrimethamine (*Daraprim*), proguanil (*Paludrine*) and 4-aminoquinolines (chloroquine) and they act by interfering with the metabolism of the parasite at different stages of development. Pyrimethamine and proguanil, by their action on the primary exo-erythrocytic stage, also serve as causal prophylactics in *P. falciparum* infections, while chloroquine is the most effective drug for suppressing the development of the asexual erythrocytic forms of all species of the parasite. In some areas, the parasites show varying degrees of drug resistance, and this fact should be considered while selecting the suppressive drug for any locality.[1] The following is the usual suppressive regimen recommended for a non-immune adult weighing 150 lb.:

Chloroquine: 300 mg. base once or twice weekly, or 100 mg. base 6 days a week in areas of very intense transmission in Africa. The drug is always taken after a meal.
Daraprim: 25 mg. once weekly.
Paludrine: 100–200 mg. daily.

In order to ensure an adequate level of chloroquine in the blood, suppressive treatment should be commenced a week prior to arrival in a malarious area and continued throughout the stay. At the end of this period the drug regimen should be continued for a month more to effect the cure of any remaining *P. falciparum* infection. Any person who gets fever after returning from a malarious area should have his blood examined for malaria and if necessary get radical treatment for curing the infection [see p. 250].

Protection of Communities

Methods employed for the control of malaria in a community are directed either at the vectors through vector control or at the parasite in man through chemotherapy. The former aims at the prevention of the breeding of vectors or at their destruction in larval or adult forms.

---

[1] The World Health Organization periodically publishes in its *Weekly Epidemiological Record* the list of areas from which drug resistance in malaria parasites has been reported.

Prevention of Vector Breeding

Permanent elimination of the sources of vector breeding is the ideal method of malaria prevention. However, this is generally practicable only in cities and other areas of concentration of population, where breeding places are relatively few and the cost involved can be economically justified. In spite of its obvious limitations, source reduction could serve as a supplementary measure to other methods of malaria control in special situations.

Drainage and filling of breeding places and water management by means of fluctuating water levels by controlling the flow have been used in certain areas for reducing vector breeding. Extensive subsoil drainage has been employed in Malaya for controlling malaria and, at the same time, for reclaiming marshy lands for economic development. In Italy, even before the advent of modern insecticides, through a coordinated plan of land reclamation and colonization malaria was effectively controlled. For flushing out larvae of vectors such as *A. minimus* and *A. fluviatilis* breeding in moving water, automatic and hand-operated syphons have been used in the Philippines, Western Malaysia, and India. Naturalistic method which exploit the natural limiting factors of breeding have been successfully employed in controlling vector breeding. Against *A. umbrosus* in Western Malaysia and *A. leucosphyrus* in Sabah, which prefer shaded breeding places, clearance of overhanging vegetation has been used. In the tea estates of India *A. minimus* and *A. fluviatilis*, which prefer the grassy edges of sun-lit breeding places, the provision of shade by planting Mexican sun flower, lantana and other suitable plants has effectively controlled breeding. Tide gates and dykes have been used for changing the salinity of water and thus controlling vector breeding in seaside swamps. It is obvious that a knowledge of the breeding preferences of the local vector is essential for selecting the suitable method of control. Among the natural enemies of mosquito larvae used in mosquito control, the most important is the larvivorous fish. There are several kinds of small, hardy, surface-feeding fish that feed on anopheline larvae. *Gambusia affinis* and *Lebistes resticulatus*, known as guppies, have been extensively used in malaria control. *Gambusia* continues to be used as a valuable agent for controlling vector breeding, especially in areas where the adult vectors are not susceptible to DDT. In using *Gambusia* for anopheline control, it is important to ensure that the breeding places are periodically restocked with the fish until they are able to establish themselves.

Larvicides. The effectiveness of larviciding depends on the thoroughness with which it is applied to all breeding places at regular intervals, depending on the time taken for the completion of the aquatic stage of development of the mosquito. The laborious and repetitive nature of these operations is a serious limitation to its extensive use. The larvicides generally employed in anopheline control are mineral oils, Paris green, DDT and some organophosphorus compounds of relatively recent origin.

The oiling of breeding places has long been the mainstay of mosquito control. Oil forms a film on the water surface and kills larvae and pupae by suffocating and poisoning them. In addition, oil also destroys the marginal vegetation that provides shelter to larae. An effective larvicide should have a high toxicity to larvae and pupae, good spreading capacity with stable film formation, and a minimum of toxicity to fish and livestock. Local availability and cost are also important practical considerations. Diesel oil and crude oil alone, or in various combinations with kerosene and other materials, are generally used for larviciding. The spreading capacity and the effectiveness of oils can be increased by the addition of small quantities of emulsifiers or spreading agents such as triton X 100. As the spreading capacity also depends on the character of the water to be treated, it is important to carry out preliminary field trials prior to embarking on large-scale larviciding operations. For controlling vector breeding in wells, lead-free petrol has been extensively used in India.

The equipment available for the application of oil larvicides covers a wide range from a simple bucket and mop, and knapsack sprayers, to highly sophisticated and mechanized devices. In many countries in the tropics various improvised methods of applying oil larvicides using drip-cans, sawdust soaked in oil, etc., have been found effective for dealing with certain types of breeding places.

Paris green is a powder containing copper acetoarsenite. It is diluted with inert dust and applied with blowers. The particles of Paris green float on water and act as a stomach poison when ingested by larvae. Unlike oils, it does not kill pupae or very young larvae. At the dose at which it is applied the treated water is not dangerous to fish, cattle, or man. In the past, Paris green has been extensively used in the Americas and elsewhere for anopheline control.

DDT, which is practically insoluble in water, is used in an oily solution or emulsion for killing larvae. The great advantage in its use is that only very small quantities of the insecticide are required for effectively controlling breeding. When used with oil larvicides it is possible to effect substantial savings in oil. However, large-scale use of DDT as a larvicide is not recommended because of its long-term adverse effects on acquatic life.

Among the new organophosphorus compounds used as larvicides, abate is the most important. It is an effective larvicide and its toxicity to fish, animals, and man is very low. Hence it can be used for controlling breeding even in water used for drinking.

For details of the dosages, methods of application, etc. of larvicides the reader should refer to *A Text Book of Malaria Eradication* by Pampana (1969) and the *Field Manual for Antilarval Operations in Malaria Eradication Programmes* published by the WHO (1969*b*).

Imagocides. Even before the advent of DDT and other residual insecticides it was demonstrated that it was possible to control malaria by killing mosquitoes in houses with pyrethrum spray. The disadvantage of this method is that it has to be repeated at least once every week throughout the transmission season. On the other hand, residual insecticides, when sprayed on walls in houses, leave a deposit on the surface that remains lethal to mosquitoes for many weeks.

The ability of residual insecticides to interrupt transmission is due to the fact that most vector species rest on sprayed walls in houses before or after every blood meal, and thus pick up a lethal dose of the insecticide. As vectors in most malarious countries feed on alternate nights there are five chances of the mosquito getting poisoned with the insecticide before the lapse of 10–12 days required for the malaria parasite to complete its development in the mosquito.

The duration of effectiveness of the deposit varies with the insecticide used, the type of surface on which it is sprayed, and to some extent on environmental factors such as humidity. Insecticides are used as solutions, emulsions, or water-dispersible powders (w.d.p.). For porous surfaces such as mud or brick walls DDT w.d.p. is the formulation of choice. It is convenient to transport and easy to use, as the powder has only to be mixed with water to the required concentration before spraying. In the case of some mud walls DDT deposited on the surface gets drawn into the wall leaving the surface innocuous to mosquitoes. This phenomenon, known as 'sorption', is attributed to the physical character of the mud and is influenced by relative humidity. It is therefore desirable to carry out preliminary trials with the insecticide on local mud surfaces before embarking on large-scale spraying operations. The standard specifications for the various insecticide formulations used in vector control have been defined by the Expert Committee on Insecticides of the World Health Organization.

The insecticides used as imagocides in anopheline control belong to one of three main groups:

1. Organochlorines:
    e.g. (a) DDT (dichlorodiphenyl tetrachlorethane).
         (b) HCH (hexachlorocyclohexane) generally known as BHC.
         (c) Dieldrin.
2. Organophosphorus compounds:
    Malathion.
    Dichlorvos (DDVP).
3. Carbamates:
    Propoxur (OMS 33).

DDT is the most widely used residual insecticide for anopheline control. Its availability in the post-war period has been the most important single factor that has made it possible to eradicate malaria from large parts of the world. In fact, in tropical regions where DDT has failed to produce substantial reduction in transmission, eradication of malaria has become considerably more expensive and laborious. DDT has prolonged residual action under most conditions—three months to one year or more. Its toxicity to man and animals is low, it is easy to handle, and above all it is the least expensive of the residual insecticides. In view of these advantages, alternative residual insecticides are considered only when DDT is not available or is not effective due to technical reasons. On some vector anophelines DDT has an irritant effect which is a disadvantage if the vector, after biting, escapes before picking up a lethal dose of the insecticide.

In the control of malaria the persistence of DDT residue in sprayed houses is a great advantage. In its agricultural use, however, the persistence of DDT as an environmental contaminant has become a serious problem, as DDT accumulates in the food chain and adversely affects fish and some species of birds of prey.

HCH and dieldrin are also used in anopheline control. HCH generally has a shorter life than DDT—about three months. It has a fumigant effect and is lethal to mosquitoes even when they are not in contact with the insecticide residue. Dieldrin

is an effective insecticide, but has a higher degree of toxicity to man and hence is used only in special situations.

Organophosphorus insecticides are liquids unlike organochlorines which are solids. Malathion is the most commonly used insecticide of this group. It has a low toxicity to man. DDVP is a highly volatile insecticide which kills mosquitoes that come in contact with its vapour. It is particularly useful for controlling mosquitoes in closed spaces such as aircraft and barns, where there is little movement of air.

Among the carbamate insecticides propoxur (OMS 33) has been tried out in many parts of the world in malaria eradication. It is a very efficient residual insecticide, and it is reported to have an air-borne action that kills mosquitoes 10–30 metres outside sprayed houses for a few weeks after house spraying. The very high cost of using this insecticide is its main drawback. The WHO estimates that compared to DDT at the present market price the cost of using malathion or propoxur is 3·1 times and 8·5 times higher respectively.[1]

Vector Resistance to Insecticides

Experience in many parts of the world has shown that residual insecticides cannot be used indefinitely for vector control because of the emergence of resistance to the insecticide used. It was this fact that contributed to the urgency for achieving malaria eradication. Physiological resistance to insecticides is genetically inherited, and is not the result of exposure of individuals to repeated sublethal doses of the insecticide. The vector population contains individuals naturally resistant, and when the insecticide kills off the susceptibles the former progressively multiply to produce a pure resistant population. Thus, the selection of resistance is the result of insecticide pressure on the vector population. Two distinct types of resistance to organochlorines have been recognized. One relates to DDT and its analogues, and the other to HCH and dieldrin. DDT resistance does not cause resistance to HCH and dieldrin, and vice versa.

Antimalarials

Drugs play an important role in the control of malaria. Every malaria case cured is one less in the reservoir of infection in the community. According to the site of action in the developmental cycle of the parasite, antimalarials may be grouped as follows:

1. Causal prophylactics which act on the primary tissue forms, e.g. pyrimethamine (*Daraprim*) and proguanil (*Paludrine*).
2. Schizonticides acting on the asexual erythrocytic forms, e.g. 4-aminoquinolines (chloroquine and amodiaquine), mepacrine and quinine.
3. Gametocytocides which eliminate gametocytes from the blood, e.g. 8-aminoquinolines (primaquine).
4. Anti-relapse drugs which acts on the secondary tissue forms of *P. vivax*, *P. malariae* and *P. ovale*, e.g. primaquine.
5. Sporonticides which inhibit the development of the gametocytes in the vector, e.g. pyrimethamine and proguanil.

Pyrimethamine and proguanil are also schizonticides, but this action is less than that of chloroquine which is the drug of

---

[1] *Official Records of the World Health Organization*, No. 190, 1971, Appendix 14.

choice for the treatment of clinical cases. Chloroquine also destroys the gametocytes of all species of human plasmodia except *P. falciparum*.

In malaria control drugs are employed for suppressive treatment, presumptive treatment and for radical treatment. Suppressive treatment has already been mentioned under individual protection [p. 248]. Populations could be kept free from overt clinical attacks by the administration of schizonticides (chloroquine) and causal prophylactic drugs (pyrimethamine) at regular intervals. In actual practice this is possible only in populations under supervision as in the case of the Armed Forces, schoolchildren, labour groups engaged in construction works, etc., except when the drugs are mixed with the domestic supply of salt. Medicated salt has been used in Brazil, Guiana, Tanzania, and in Iran among nomads for controlling malaria. Before such a programme is undertaken in any area, however, it is necessary to study the food habits of the population and to ensure that there are no alternative sources of salt supply.

For the protection of communities, pyrimethamine has an advantage because it is excreted through the mother's milk thus providing some measure of protection to the infant. On the other hand, when used alone it has the disadvantage of producing parasite resistance.

Presumptive treatment consists of a single adult dose of 600 mg. chloroquine base and 50 mg. pyrimethamine administered to suspected malaria cases pending confirmation by blood examination. Its aim is to relieve symptoms and to prevent the case from serving as a possible source of mosquito infection. If malaria is later confirmed the infection is treated radically. Radical treatment of confirmed malaria infection is an essential activity in malaria eradication. The object is to eliminate the erythrocytic forms as well as the secondary tissue forms responsible for relapses. The standard course of radical treatment for *P. vivax*, *P. malariae*, and *P. ovale* consists of 1,500 mg. of chloroquine base given over a three-day period, followed by primaquine 15 mg. base daily for 14 days.

For *P. falciparum* infections too, the same course of radical treatment is followed, the primaquine acting as a gametocytocide. In India, for practical reasons the primaquine administration is limited to a 5-day period.

In recent years certain repository antimalarials have been tried out in the field. They are injected intramuscularly and by the slow release of the active base are expected to have prolonged action over several weeks. The original repository compound, CI–501 Camolar, which is derived from a metabolite of proguanil, had only very limited scope because of proguanil resistance. The later compound, CI–564, aimed at overcoming the resistance problem, is a combination of CI–501 and a sulphone (DADDS).

Drug Resistance

Even before the synthetic antimalarials were discovered it was known that some malaria infections did not respond to quinine treatment and some strains of parasites required much higher doses of the drug for treatment than others. Drug resistance as defined by the WHO is 'the ability of a parasite strain to multiply or to survive in the presence of concentrations of a drug that normally destroy parasites of the same species or prevent their multiplication'.

Drug resistance is primarily a problem related to *P. falciparum* infections. Since 1948, proguanil and pyrimethamine resistance has been reported from Malaysia, Indonesia, many parts of Africa, Venezuela, etc. At present, the importance of drug resistance is due to the finding of chloroquine-resistant cases of *P. falciparum* in countries undertaking malaria eradication. Although chloroquine resistance has been reported from Colombia, Brazil, Venezuela, Thailand, Malaysia, and Vietnam, this drug continues to be the mainstay in the field treatment of malaria in these countries as elsewhere. However, it is a serious problem to the clinician and it poses a potential threat to eradication in the affected areas. The importance of chloroquine resistance in eradication programmes depends on the extent of dependence on this drug for achieving eradication. If chloroquine has to be used in the attack phase for interrupting transmission, as insecticides alone cannot achieve it, the problem is of grave import to eradication.

Resistance is considered relative when the infection responds to increased doses of the drug and absolute when it is refractory even to higher doses. Chloroquine resistance is graded as RI when the initial asexual parasite clearance in the blood is followed by recrudescence, RII when there is reduction in parasitaemia but no clearance, and RIII when there is no marked reduction in asexual parasitaemia. For the treatment of chloroquine-resistant infection, quinine and pyrimethamine or pyrimethamine and sulphadiazine combinations have been found effective.

MALARIA—CONTROL AND ERADICATION

The scope and extent of antimalaria operations in a country depend on the resources available, the effectiveness of the antimalaria methods under local conditions, and the priority the government gives to the control of the disease. Where eradication is at present impracticable, the object should be to obtain the maximum reduction of malaria within the limits of available resources.

MALARIA CONTROL

The aim of malaria control is to reduce malaria. The extent of reduction to be expected varies according to the local circumstances. Under favourable conditions, a well-conducted malaria control programme should result in malaria eradication, as was the case with some developed countries in the temperate zone. Even large-scale malaria control may be beyond the present means of some countries. But there is no place where some measure of relief from malaria cannot be provided. In countries where the health infrastructure is non-existent or very rudimentary the least that can be done is to make antimalaria drugs—generally chloroquine—available to those who suffer from clinical attacks. This could be done through any government or private agency operating in the area. In India and in Italy one of the earliest organized antimalaria measures undertaken was the provision of quinine—the only effective antimalarial then available—to the population at a very nominal cost. As the health services develop, basic training in the control of malaria should be given to appropriate public health personnel. They could then organize limited vector control operations in towns and other areas of population concentration and economic importance. At the same time, certain vulnerable age groups, such as children and expectant mothers, could be protected by regular chemoprophylaxis through schools and maternal and child health centres. In intensely malarious areas, the very development of basic health services may be seriously hampered by malaria. In such areas it is obvious that the control of malaria should form one of the first public health activities. A very striking effect of malaria control is the dramatic reduction in infant mortality rates. In a town of 12,000 people in Northern Nigeria, three years of malaria control reduced the infant mortality rate from 137 to 66·7.[1] The methods of malaria control best suited to the area will have to be selected. Residual insecticide spraying of houses is generally the least expensive and most effective method of control. The fear of possible development of insecticide resistance of vectors should not stand in the way of extending the benefit of this method to the malaria-ridden communities of the tropics. As the aim is limited to the reduction of transmission, and not the total interruption of transmission, it may be possible to reduce the frequency of house spraying and thus minimize the selection pressure of the insecticide. After the health infrastructure has been established and the public health personnel have acquired some local experience in malaria control methods, the feasibility of a time-limited malaria eradication programme could be considered. In planning the development of malaria control operations leading to an eradication programme, it is important to specify targets for population to be protected, personnel to be trained, etc. Otherwise malaria control may drag on indefinitely.

In many of the still malarious countries projects for harnessing the resources of lakes and rivers for economic development are in progress. In order to prevent these projects from increasing the malaria hazard provision should be included in the construction plans for the elimination vector breeding places resulting from the project activities. There should also be provision for the protection of local populations and imported project personnel.

Control of Malaria Epidemics

A malaria epidemic is a public health emergency which calls for speedy and concerted action. The immediate objective is to stop transmission and provide treatment to those who suffer from clinical attacks. After testing the susceptibility of the local vectors to the residual insecticides that can be procured quickly, a suitable insecticide should be selected and house spraying organized to cover the entire area affected by the epidemic in as short a time as possible. When residual insecticides are not available as an alternative, pyrethrum spraying of houses repeated twice every week could be undertaken. Mass drug administration of the entire population with chloroquine and pyrimethamine, repeated at fortnightly intervals, is indicated if the proportion of clinical cases in the population is high. Recently, ultra-low volume aerial spraying of insecticides was employed successfully for the control of mosquito-borne encephalitis in the United States. This method, which depends on the dispersal of very small quantities of insecticides, may be of use in controlling epidemics of malaria in some situations where the houses are not very widely scattered.

[1] Malaria Service N. Nigeria (1955) *Information Bulletin* No. 3, Lagos.

ERADICATION

Feasibility Studies

The national decision to launch a malaria eradication programme should be based on a full understanding of its technical and operational feasibility. In most of the malarious countries, the total resources available for social and economic development are far less than the actual requirements. It is therefore important to relate the consequences of investment in malaria eradication to the other aspects of social and economic development. Concrete examples of the economic benefits of malaria eradication would strengthen the plea for such eradication. A feasibility study should cover the following aspects:

1. Adequacy of the existing knowledge of the malaria situation in the country.
2. Effectiveness of the methods of malaria eradication under local conditions.
3. Adequacy of available resources.
4. Prospects of sustaining achieved eradication.

An examination of the available information of the malaria situation should include the geographical spread, the intensity and the seasonal fluctuations in the incidence of malaria as well as the various factors related to man, the vector, the parasite and the environment that influence the local epidemiology of the disease. The effectiveness of the methods of malaria eradication depends upon technical and operational factors, and these should be examined separately for the various epidemiological regions of the country. Where interruption of transmission is not feasible, because of the behaviour of the vector or man, eradication is impracticable. The same is the case when essential activities such as house spraying, case detection and treatment cannot be carried out effectively because of civil unrest, insecurity, military operations, etc. A study of the resources should cover the man-power, the materials, and the money required for the project and relate these to the available resources, taking into account the needs of the current as well as the expected national priority programmes. External assistance has played a very valuable role in the global malaria eradication effort and this may continue in the future. However, in the eagerness to benefit from such assistance, if national priorities are ignored and obvious operational and technical problems glossed over, the programme can only result in disappointment to the government, to the assisting agencies, and to the personnel engaged in eradication. In examining the prospects of sustaining eradication, the plans for the development of health services, especially in the rural areas of the malarious parts of the country, and of epidemiological services for the control of communicable diseases should be considered. In malarious areas, where there is considerable movement of population across national boundaries, the prospects of achieving eradication and maintaining it are in danger unless there is a concurrent co-ordinated eradication programme on both sides of the border. The WHO has played a useful role in facilitating such inter-country co-operation.

'Malaria eradication implies the elimination of malaria parasites from the human population so that there is no resumption of transmission even in the presence of vectors.' Eradication of the vector is not necessary for the eradication of malaria. According to the WHO an originally malarious country may be considered as having eradicated malaria when adequate surveillance has not revealed any evidence of local transmission or residual endemicity for a consecutive period of three years, during the last two of which no large-scale anti-mosquito or antiplasmodial measures that could mask the detection of foci of infection have been undertaken.

The total elimination of the infective agent of a human disease is an objective that is obviously difficult to attain. The WHO Expert Committee on Malaria, in formulating the principles and the guidelines for malaria eradication, has stated that the existence of a few isolated infections (cryptic cases) is not inconsistent with the claim of eradication provided there is an adequate organization for eliminating them when detected. *P. malariae* infections, which sometimes persist for many years, have only very low infectivity and are therefore generally inconsequential from the point of view of eradication. To the purist, the term eradication used in this context may not be acceptable. However, to the sanitarian concerned with the health and welfare of the population the methods based on this concept of eradication have proved effective as evidenced by the large areas of the world already freed from endemic malaria. The important feature of an eradication programme is that when eradication is reached, routine repetitive anti-malaria measures can be discontinued without the risk of re-establishment of endemicity. However, this does not mean that one can forget about malaria at that stage. As long as malaria exists in some parts of the world and there are possibilities of importing infection, vigilance has to be maintained for recognizing cases and eliminating infection.

A malaria eradication programme is 'a special public health programme whose objectives are the ending of transmission of malaria, the elimination of infective cases and the prevention of re-establishment of endemicity' (World Health Organization, 1971a). This may be planned as a time-limited programme covering the entire malarious area of a country from the beginning or developed in stages starting with a part of the country. As already mentioned, in malarious areas where eradication is not practicable at present, control of the disease should be undertaken as an interim step towards the long-range goal of eradication.

The modern concept of a time-limited malaria eradication programme is based on the experience that during a period of three consecutive years, if transmission is interrupted the vast majority of malaria infections will undergo cure, natural or therapeutic, and the remaining infective reservoir could then be eliminated by case detection and treatment.

After preliminary studies have shown that eradication is technically, administratively, and operationally feasible, a plan of operation is prepared covering the four phases of an eradication programme—preparatory, attack, consolidation, and maintenance. The various activities to be undertaken in each phase are stated in the plan which serves as the basis for the long-term commitments of the government and any external agency assisting in the programme. The plan covers both the technical as well as the financial, administrative and personnel aspects of the programme.

It is important to recognize that 'malaria eradication is not an end in itself but a step towards general public health and welfare' (World Health Organization, 1957). The malaria eradication plan should therefore be an integral part of the national health plan within the over-all socio-economic development plan of the country. For the preparation of a malaria eradication plan of operations it is necessary to secure the collaboration of a public health administrator with experience in national health planning and an economist familiar with the fiscal policies of the government and the over-all socio-economic development plan of the country.

In a malaria eradication programme (MEP) which involves three biological entities, man, parasite, and the vector, it is impossible to lay down a rigid time-table for reaching the goal of eradication. The duration of the attack and consolidation phases in the plan should only be considered as an intelligent forecast based on available information and previous experience. The actual duration will depend mainly on the response of malaria to the measures adopted. In addition to the routine evaluation undertaken by the project staff, the plan should provide for a yearly independent assessment. Based on the results of these assessments the necessary modifications are made in the plan of operations. In some instances, this may call for changes in the organizational pattern or the inclusion of supplementary measures involving additional expenditure. The plan should therefore be sufficiently flexible to permit the adoption of essential modifications. In this connexion it should be borne in mind that if the changes proposed involve any substantial increase in expenditure they should be foreseen well in advance, as government funds are generally fully committed and new requests take at least a year before funds become actually available. The same applies to requests for additional supplies from external agencies assisting the government.

In the recruitment of personnel for malaria eradication, care should be taken to ensure that as far as possible they have the minimum educational qualifications that would facilitate their ultimate integration after appropriate training into the general health services. As eradication work is strenuous many programmes have suffered from a high turn-over of trained personnel. Long-term career prospects are essential for ensuring the stability of the service, on which depends the efficiency of staff performance and the attainment of the goal of eradication.

In countries in the tropical regions where transmission is intense over the greater part of the year, malaria eradication needs the undivided attention of a specialized service within the national health administration, with vertical lines of authority to ensure the efficient management of the programme. The technical direction of the entire programme should be vested in a central directorate even when the operations remain the direct responsibility of the different political and administrative divisions of the country. These special provisions for facilitating the efficient conduct of the programme should not be permitted to lead to the separation of the malaria eradication service from the general health services, whose active participation is vital to the achievement of the objective of eradication. It is also necessary to secure the co-operation of other departments such as education, agriculture, finance, defence services, etc. To this end inter-departmental committees should be set up at national and provincial levels.

In some countries in the subtropical and temperate regions, where transmission is limited to a few months of the year and the distribution of malaria endemic areas is spotty with large intervening non-malarious areas, it may be possible to under-take malaria eradication as a routine function of an integrated general health service, right from the beginning. Even in such cases, however, it would be necessary to have a small nucleus of staff experienced in malaria eradication at the centre to plan, guide and evaluate the programme.

The activities undertaken during each phase of a malaria eradication programme are briefly described below. FIGURE 73 shows the phases of the programme in relation to the epidemiological status.

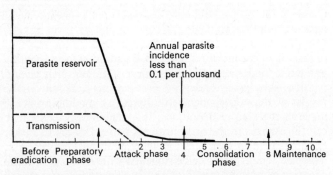

FIG. 73. Phases of malaria eradication and epidemiological status of malaria. [Adapted from World Health Organization (1963) Terminology of malaria and of malaria eradication, Report of a Drafting Committee.]

Preparatory Phase

This phase may take one or two years and include the following activities:

1. Geographical reconnaissance (G.R.) and detailed logistic planning. G.R. includes the numbering of houses, the taking of a house-to-house census of the population, preparation of maps showing communications, location of villages and houses, and the compilation of other facts that could facilitate field operations. The information gathered through G.R. is useful not only for malaria eradication but also for the planning of other rural health activities, and needs to be kept under constant review in order to include new houses, new settlement areas, etc.

2. Recruitment and training of personnel:

The training should be oriented to the actual duties to be performed. Professional staff can be trained at international training centres if suitable institutions are not available in the country.

3. Setting up of physical facilities such as headquarters, zone and sector offices, laboratories, warehouses, transport and equipment maintenance, workshops, etc., and the procurement of supplies and equipment.

4. Collection of parasitological and entomological data for the future epidemiological evaluation of the programme. The previous entomological findings relating to the seasonal prevalence of the vectors, their resting and feeding habits and their susceptibility to insecticides are verified. Even when the vector is susceptible to DDT it would be prudent to test and select an alternative insecticide that may be readily obtained should the vector later develop resistance to DDT. Information on social customs which may have a bearing on the application of malaria eradication procedures is also collected during the preparatory phase.

5. Health education and public relations:

This is an activity which should be continued throughout the programme. Every member of the eradication service has a health education role in the population to which he is exposed. The training of personnel should include the practical aspects of health education and public relations as an integral part of every major field activity, and should not be confined to a few lectures by specialists in health education.

Attack Phase

1. Application of attack measures:

The methods of interrupting transmission best suited to local conditions are selected on the basis of previous field trials. In general, DDT indoor residual spraying is the main method of attack. This is supplemented by chemotherapy to the extent practicable to hasten the depletion of the parasite reservoir. When transmission persists in spite of residual spraying, chemotherapy becomes even more important as an essential additional measure in all stages of the attack phase. The dosage and frequency of application of insecticide are based on local epidemiological requirements and not on any arbitrary formula. Within the same country the timing and frequency of spraying cycles may vary, according to the transmission season and certain social customs such as replastering of houses prior to certain festivals. In specific situations, such as urban areas where the vector breeding places are few and houses numerous, it would be more effective and economical to undertake larval control instead of house spraying which is often unpopular with urban populations.

2. Evaluation of the effect of attack measures:

In the earlier stages of the attack phase, when parasite rates are still high, the response of malaria to the measures applied is assessed primarily through comparing data of successive parasite surveys, the baseline data having been compiled during the last year of the preparatory phase. In programmes showing satisfactory response, the parasite rate at the end of the first year should fall to about one-sixth or at least to one-fifth of the original rates and continue to decrease at the same rate at the end of the second year of attack. These standards are based chiefly on experience in different parts of the world where *P. falciparum* was the dominant infection. They have also been found valid in a few countries where *P. vivax* was the main infection. When the parasite rate is more than one-fifth of the original rates after one year of attack, this is an indication of the persistence of transmission to a degree incompatible with the objective of eradication, and the underlying causes should promptly be investigated and appropriate corrective action taken. Simple causes for the failure should first be excluded before seeking more complicated explanations. In most instances the persistence of transmission is due to operational defects resulting in incomplete spray cover, or to the wrong timing of spraying cycles in relation to the transmission seasons. Non-immunes, such as expatriates and infants born after spraying, should show zero parasite rates if transmission has been interrupted. But the absence of infection among them does not necessarily mean the same in the rest of the population.

When the parasite rate falls below 5 per cent., this method of evaluation by comparing parasite rates from successive sample surveys loses its sensitivity and is therefore replaced by measurement of the incidence of infection by means of case-finding covering the total population. The case detection is carried out through regular house visits and through static centres such as hospitals, clinics, etc. This is further reinforced by enlisting the participation of voluntary collaborators. As it is impossible to blood film the entire population, and as malaria infection is invariably accompanied by pyrexia, fever, or a recent history of fever is used as a means of screening the population. For every fever case a blood slide is taken and single-dose presumptive treatment is administered. The laboratory services are expanded to cope with the increase in the number of blood slides.

Entomological observation to assess the response of the vectors to insecticide application is an important activity during the attack phase. Although it is not possible to obtain absolute proof of interruption of transmission through entomological methods, they may provide the earliest warning of lack of effectiveness in the attack measures. Regular observations are carried out in selected areas on the density of vector mosquitoes in sprayed rooms. Some vectors get irritated by DDT and escape before picking up a lethal dose from sprayed walls. Exit window traps are used for capturing escaping mosquitoes. If a significant number of the specimens captured from sprayed houses survive 24 hours it is an ominous sign. The age composition of the captured vectors also serves as a pointer to the degree of effectiveness of the insecticide. A marked increase in the proportion of parous (having laid eggs) to nulliparous specimens in the collections is further evidence that the insecticide may not be producing the desired effect. Throughout the attack phase standard tests are carried out periodically to determine the susceptibility of the vectors to the insecticide used. In case the vectors have developed resistance to DDT, consideration should be given to replacing it with an alternative insecticide.

As the parasite reservoir continues to decrease full surveillance is instituted. Besides case-finding and administration of presumptive treatment, this covers epidemiological investigation to determine the origin and spread of infections and the applications of remedial measures when necessary. The remedial measures for the elimination of foci of infection include radical treatment of positive cases plus insecticide spraying of houses in the affected locality for killing any infected mosquitoes that may be present. In some instances, mass drug administration of the local population may be necessary. Surveillance should be in operation at least one year before the end of the attack phase.

It should be noted that in malaria eradication the term surveillance covers not only epidemiological intelligence on the status of malaria but also action designed to eliminate foci of infection.

For effective surveillance the number of blood slides examined from fever cases in any given area should be at least 1 per cent. of the population during each month of transmission, and this activity should show adequate distribution in space and time, age, and sex. The validity of the surveillance data should be critically assessed. The data for each operational unit should be separately scrutinized in order to ensure that averages calculated for whole districts or provinces do not hide high parasite incidence in some localities. The field reports should be designed to show clearly the operational perform-

ance with regard to spraying, case-finding, etc., as well as the current epidemiological situation in each operational unit area.

When adequate surveillance shows that the annual parasite incidence is less than 0·1 per thousand of the population, routine insecticide spraying can be discontinued and the area can enter the consolidation phase. This decision is based on an independent assessment. Even with an annual parasite incidence of 0·1 per thousand, if the load of imported cases in any area is likely to be greater than could be dealt with by surveillance that area should continue to remain in the attack phase. Similarly, when abundance of efficient vectors and suitable climatic conditions for transmission enhance the malaria potential of an area the surveillance organization should be of a very high order of efficiency before withdrawal of spraying is recommended.

Consolidation Phase

1. The main activity during this phase is the continuation of surveillance activities throughout the project area. As there is no insecticide cover to prevent transmission, the chief concern is to reduce the chances of mosquitoes getting infected from the remaining few parasite carriers and from imported cases. The speed with which cases are detected and action taken to eliminate foci of infection therefore assumes even greater importance in the consolidation phase. At this stage the single-dose presumptive treatment administered to malaria suspects should contain a sporonticide (pyrimethamine) to render the case non-infective to mosquitoes. Every effort is made to reduce to the minimum the interval between blood-taking, laboratory diagnosis, and action to eliminate foci of infection. Stocks of insecticides, drugs, spraying equipment and transport are maintained at suitable places to facilitate prompt action for eliminating foci.

2. The full participation of the general health services in the surveillance activities, including the epidemiological investigation of positive cases and remedial action, is encouraged. Concurrently, a planned programme is instituted for the training of malaria eradication personnel for their future duties in an integrated health service and for the re-orientation of the general health service personnel in the vigilance activities for the prevention of re-establishment of transmission. In the later stages of the consolidation phase, the malaria eradication staff may be integrated into the general health services. This process could start with areas of low malaria risk and gradually extend to higher risk areas. Premature assignment of other duties to ME personnel and the withdrawal of key ME personnel could lead to serious setbacks to malaria eradication. It would be advisable to have a transition period between consolidation and maintenance, to try out in the field and evolve the type of integrated health service best adapted to the resources and to the local health needs.

When adequate surveillance has shown that there have been no indigenous cases of malaria for a consecutive period of three years the area could be considered for entry into the maintenance phase. The presence of a small number of isolated cases, or cases arising out of the first relay of transmission from a few imported cases, need not necessarily delay the entry into the maintenance phase provided there is effective machinery for the detection and prompt elimination of such foci. The final decision for entry into the maintenance phase is made on the recommendation of an independent assessment based on the status of malaria in the area, the degree of risk from imported infection, and the ability of the available health services to prevent the re-establishment of malaria transmission.

Maintenance Phase

The maintenance of achieved eradication is a responsibility of the general health services as a normal part of their communicable diseases control function. However, in tropical regions where the risk of re-establishment of endemicity is high, the central epidemiological organization as well as the peripheral echelons responsible for the control of communicable diseases will need to be suitably strengthened with personnel experienced in malaria eradication, in order to ensure the efficiency of the vigilance activities. The pattern of vigilance in an area will depend on the potential risk of malaria transmission. In tropical areas where vectors are present and chances of importation of infection great one should always be prepared to deal with sporadic episodes of localized transmission. For the successful maintenance of achieved eradication it is essential to provide the personnel, materials and the resources which can be mobilized at short notice to eliminate any resurgence of malaria.

At the invitation of governments claiming to have achieved eradication, the WHO makes provision to examine the situation, confirm malaria eradication, and enter the name of the country and the area from which malaria has been eradicated in the malaria eradication register maintained by the WHO. Thereafter, the governments concerned are expected to send periodic reports of the malaria status of these areas to the WHO for publication in the *Weekly Epidemiological Record*.

REFERENCES AND FURTHER READING

Black, R. H. (1968) *Manual of Epidemiology and Epidemiological Services in Malaria Programmes*, WHO, Geneva.

Boyd, M. F., ed. (1949) *Malariology*, Philadelphia.

Christophers, R. (1949) in Boyd, M. F., ed., *Malariology*, p. 836.

Garnham, P. C. C. (1945) *Malaria Parasites and Other Haemosporidia*, Oxford.

Gonzales, C. L. (1965) Mass campaigns and general health services, *Wld Hlth Org. Publ. Hlth Pap.*, No. 29.

Macdonald, G. (1957) *The Epidemiology and Control of Malaria*, London.

Pampana, A. (1969) *A Text Book of Malaria Eradication*, 2nd ed., London.

Peters, W. (1970) *Chemotherapy and Drug Resistance in Malaria*, London.

Russell, P. F., West, L. S., Manwell, R. D., and Macdonald, G. (1963) *Practical Malariology*, 2nd ed., London.

Shute, P. G. (1969) *Brit. med. J.*, **ii**, 781.

Shute, P. G. and Maryon, M. (1974) Malaria in England past, present and future, *R. Soc. Hlth J.*, **94**, 23.

World Health Organization (1957) Sixth Report of the Expert Committee on Malaria, *Wld Hlth Org. techn. Rep. Ser.*, No. 123.

World Health Organization (1963) *Terminology of Malaria and Malaria Eradication*, WHO, Geneva.

World Health Organization (1967) Chemotherapy of malaria, *Wld Hlth Org. techn. Rep. Ser.*, No. 375.

World Health Organization (1969a) Parasitology of malaria, *Wld Hlth Org. techn. Rep. Ser.*, No. 433.

World Health Organization (1969b) *Field Manual for Antilarval Operations in Malaria Eradication Programmes*, WHO, Geneva.

World Health Organization (1971a) Fifteenth Report of the Expert Committee on Malaria, *Wld Hlth Org. techn. Rep. Ser.*, No. 467.

World Health Organization (1971b) *Weekly Epidemiological Record*, **46**, No. 30.

World Health Organization (1972) *Manual of Planning for Malaria Eradication and Control*, Geneva.

World Health Organization (1973a) Information on malaria risks for international travellers, *Wld Hlth Org. Chron.*, **27**, 254, contained in WHO weekly *Epidemiological Record*, **48**, 25–43.

World Health Organization (1973b) Chemotherapy of malaria. Report of a WHO Scientific group, *Wld Hlth Org. techn. Rep. Ser.*, No. 529.

World Health Organization (1973c) Manual on larval operations in malaria programmes, *Wld Hlth Org. Offset Publ. Ser.*, No. 1.

World Health Organization (1974a) Malaria control in countries where time-limited eradication is impracticable at present. Report of a WHO International Conference, *Wld Hlth Org. techn. Rep. Ser.*, No. 537.

World Health Organization (1974b) Sixteenth Report of the Expert Committee on malaria, *Wld Hlth Org. techn. Rep. Ser.*, No. 550.

19

INSECTICIDES FOR USE AGAINST PESTS OF PUBLIC HEALTH IMPORTANCE

J. R. BUSVINE

Modern insecticides have enormously widened the possibilities of eradication of the various diseases carried by arthropods, especially in the tropics. Many arthropod-borne epidemic diseases are readily controlled by these chemicals, and the elimination of such important ones as malaria and urban yellow fever is now being envisaged by WHO. However, the emergence of insecticide-resistant strains of a number of vector species may deprive medicine of this valuable weapon.

Insecticides may be classified according to their mode of attack on the insect as: *stomach poisons, contact poisons,* or *fumigants.* It is also convenient to consider *repellents* in this section. These categories are not entirely exclusive, for some slightly volatile contact poisons may possess fumigant action and others can act as stomach poisons.

Contact poisons have proved most valuable against pests of public health importance. Stomach poisons cannot yet be safely introduced into the blood stream to destroy blood-sucking insects, though some limited success against lice with phenylbutazone taken orally suggests that this possibility exists. At present, however, stomach poisons for public health pests are limited to use against such insects as mosquito larvae, houseflies, and cockroaches.

The gaseous fumigants hydrogen cyanide and methyl bromide are too dangerous to use satisfactorily in human dwellings (which are far from gas-proof), though they find a minor use in treating old furniture in steel vans, to destroy bed bugs. Another minor usage is the disinfestation of lousy garments in a bin or plastic bag by fumigation with ethyl formate. The so-called 'residual fumigant' dichlorvos is a relatively new development. The vapour of this organophosphorus compound, emitted slowly from a dispenser, will destroy delicate insects, such as mosquitoes, in spaces without too much ventilation.

CONTACT POISONS

Types of Contact Insecticides Available

Few natural products, either vegetable or mineral, are now used as contact insecticides, nearly all being replaced by products of the chemical industry. Numerous efficient synthetic insecticides are available, however, many with complex chemical names. Inevitably, such compounds tend to become known by abbreviations (often trade names) and the multiplicity of these may lead to confusion. Recommended common names have been proposed by the British Standards Institution (lists published periodically under B.S. 1831), many of them being taken up by the International Standards Organization. In contrast to proprietary names, the common names are printed without capitals (e.g. heptachlor), except for a few early examples composed entirely of capitals (e.g. DDT).

The most important groups of insecticides, for public health use, are: (1) Pyrethroids; (2) DDT and similar compounds; (3) *gamma* BHC and the chlorinated cyclo-diene insecticides; (4) organophosphorous insecticides; and (5) carbamates.

Pyrethroids. Pyrethrum powder, which has been used as an insecticide for over 100 years, is made from the dried flower heads of the plant *Chrysanthemum cinerariaefolium*. The active principle is a mixture of complex organic esters: for practical purposes these may be described as 'pyrethrins'. After the complex chemical nature of these compounds had been fully determined, some synthetic analogues were eventually prepared from 1950 onward. The first to be commercially available, and widely used, was allethrin. Others have followed (e.g. cyclethrin, furethrin, bioallethrin), and recently an extremely promising new series has been discovered in Britain, the best perhaps being bioresmethrin.

These analogues have chemical and biological properties similar to the natural product and may be conveniently described as pyrethroids All have a rapid paralysing effect on most arthropods, but are more or less innocuous to warm-blooded animals Their insecticidal action can be augmented to different extents (up to about ten times) by non-insecticidal additives known as synergists (e.g. piperonyl butoxide). This can permit economies by reducing the concentration of the active ingredients, which tend to be expensive On the debit side, pyrethroids are chemically rather unstable (especially in light). This prevents them having long residual action, like the chlorinated synthetic insecticides, and restricts their use in the control of insects. They are, in fact, principally employed in circumstances where safety and rapid effect are important. Thus, they are important constituents of the aerosols used for aircraft disinsectization and they are widely used as household sprays against houseflies, cockroaches, etc.

Natural pyrethrins are used much more than the synthetic compounds, of which only allethrin has been manufactured on a large scale (in the United States). Despite its complex manufacture, allethrin is slightly cheaper than natural pyrethrins; but the latter are considerable more toxic to most insects and can be more highly activated by synergists.

DDT. The Swiss discovery of the insecticidal powers of DDT began a new era of insect control, depending on residual action It has been, and still is, extremely widely used, though in recent years it has caused some anxiety on the grounds of persistence of its residues in the environment (see below under Toxic Hazards). Many compounds analogous to DDT have been tested, but none is so effective. Two of them, however,

DDD (or TDE) and methoxychlor, are employed for some purposes because of their extremely low toxicity to mammals [TABLE 52]. DDT and similar compounds are moderately soluble in oils, dissolve easily in fat-solvent organic liquids and are very insoluble in water. They are rather slow in insecticidal action, but their residues are very persistent.

BHC and the Cyclodiene Insecticides. BHC is included in this group because, although it is quite different chemically, its toxicology is rather similar; in particular, resistance to BHC is linked with resistance to the cyclodiene insecticides, and vice versa.

Benzene hexachloride (BHC), or more correctly hexachloro-*cyclo*hexane (HCH), can exist in the form of several stereo-isomers, and it was discovered in 1942 (in Britain) that only one of these—the *gamma* isomer—is insecticidal. Lindane is a refined grade of *gamma* BHC, containing less than 1 per cent. of other isomers. *Gamma* BHC can be used in many ways like DDT; it is more highly insecticidal but less persistent.

The chlorinated cyclodiene insecticides include chlorinated terpenes, from pine oil (e.g. toxaphene) and a whole series of entirely synthetic compounds produced by a chemical reaction known as Diels–Alder condensation (e.g. heptachlor, dieldrin, chlordane). Most of these were developed in the United States from about 1947. Dieldrin has been most widely used against insect vectors of disease on account of its high potency and long residual action. Unfortunately, it is somewhat toxic to mammals and very liable to provoke resistance in arthropods.

Anticholinesterase Insecticides. In the past three decades, numerous anticholinesterase poisons, belonging to the groups organophosphates and carbamates, have been introduced as insecticides. While some of these compounds are dangerous, others have been found with reasonably low toxicity to vertebrates yet with high insecticidal activity. These compounds vary considerably in physical and chemical properties; but, in general, they tend to be less persistent than organochlorine insecticides. Their residual life is therefore shorter and they are more expensive. On the other hand, they are less liable to contaminate the environment.

Organophosphorus Compounds. Following the pioneer work of G. Schrader in Germany, many thousands of organic phosphorus compounds have been made in various research centres. A very large number are insecticidal, but many are unsatisfactory because of dangerous mammalian toxicity or unsuitable chemical or physical properties. Parathion, which was developed early, has been most widely used, but its toxicity curtails its use in medical entomology. In the last two decades, many safer compounds have been marketed. In particular, malathion and difenphos have remarkably low mammalian toxicity [TABLE 52].

Carbamate Insecticides. Carbamic acid esters, toxic to mammals, have been known for many years, but they were not suitable for insecticides. From about 1947, however, a Swiss firm began a search for suitable contact insecticides of this type, which resulted in the commercial production of one or two compounds. Subsequently, a considerable number of insecticidal carbamates has been developed in various countries. One of the most promising for residual action against mosquitoes is propoxur (formerly known as arprocarb).

TABLE 52

Comparison of Insecticidal Potency and Mammalian Toxicity of Some Common Insecticides

Group	Insecticide Common Name	Insecticide Other Names	Contact Fly	Contact Rat	Oral Rat
1	pyrethrin	—	22	1,880	200
	allethrin	—	34	11,200 [1]	920
2	DDT	dicophane	18	2,500	118
	DDD	TDE	20	—	3,400
	methoxychlor	—	24	6,000	6,000
3	*gamma* BHC	*gamma* HCH	1·0	500	88
	chlordane	—	4·0	1,600	457
	dieldrin	—	1·2	60	46
	endrin	—	4·5	15	7·5
	toxaphene	—	30	780	80
4	coumaphos	*Co-Ral*	6·8	860	16
	diazinon	—	6·5	455	76
	dichlorvos	DDVP	1·9	75	56
	difenphos	*Abate*	—	1,930	2,330
	dimenthoate	*Rogor*	1·1	800	250
	fenchlorphos	ronnel	8·2	2,000	1,740
	fenitrothion	*Sumithion*	6·4	3,000 [2]	250
	fenthion	*Baytex*	3·8	320	215
	malathion	—	50	4,100	2,800
	parathion	—	3·2	8	4
	trichlorphon	*Dipterex*	11	2,000	560
5	carbaryl	*Sevin*	245	4,000	400
	dimetilan	—	10	2,000	55
	propoxur	arprocarb	45	2,500	80

Data for houseflies, original data; data for rats, mainly from Martin (1968). The acute LD_{50} (mg./kg.) is the lethal dose in mg. per kg. body weight, which kills 50 per cent. of the insects or animals.

N.B. [1] for rabbits; [2] for mice.

Toxic Hazards from Contact Insecticides

Occasionally, people swallow poisonous doses of pesticides, either accidentally or with suicidal intent. The accidents are liable to happen if concentrated pesticides are decanted into unlabelled bottles, especially if these are in the reach of children. Fatalities from this cause are fortunately very rare; but considerably more important are cases of intoxication among people who regularly handle concentrated pesticides, i.e. those engaged in their manufacture and use. The protection of workers in pesticide factories is a specialized matter, requiring appropriate precautions; but the regular application of pesticides involves many different people (e.g. farmers, sanitary workmen) and is less easily supervised.

Where insect control measures involve the repeated use of insecticides, daily over long periods, there may be a danger from cumulative poisoning. This may result from the slow rate of metabolism, as in the case of dieldrin, or the slow recovery from the biochemical effects, as with parathion. Some idea of the likelihood of cumulative effects arising can be assessed from a knowledge of the dietary levels which animals will tolerate over long periods.

A series of careful measurements have shown that in all the common operations for applying insecticides, the greatest exposure—even from indoor spraying—occurs through the skin and not from the inhalation or swallowing of spray droplets. The potential hazards of insecticides as acute poisons for spraymen can be assessed by comparing the acute oral and acute dermal toxicity of different compounds to animals. Those that go readily through the skin have proved the most dangerous. Thus, dieldrin and fenthion, with dermal LD/oral LD values of about 1·5, have caused poisoning of a certain number of spraymen in antimalarial campaigns who did not take adequate precautions. But DDT, with a ratio of about 20, proved remarkably safe, with no adverse symptoms experienced by the many thousands of spraymen who have applied it regularly to human dwellings.

It is important at this point to distinguish overt chronic intoxication from the accumulation of traces in body tissues which produce no signs or symptoms. Serious risks to the general public from pesticides as used in public health are virtually negligible, except in cases of flagrant carelessness, which would constitute criminal negligence in many countries. On the other hand, it has come to be recognized that the great persistence of organochlorine pesticides has resulted in widely dispersed traces in the environment. Minute traces are found in rainwater, rivers, and drinking water (parts in 10^{12}) and many human foods (parts 10^8); but residues in human fat, and in wild birds and their eggs, for example, are frequently larger, being in the range of 0·1 to 10 parts per million. These facts have caused concern and the situation is being watched by responsible committees in several countries. Their conclusions do not incriminate pesticides as responsible for harm to human health; but cases of death and injury to wildlife have been established. As a result, organochlorine pesticides are being withdrawn from non-essential uses in many countries. This would seem a sensible policy for countries with plentiful food and no insect-borne disease. For tropical countries suffering famine and insect-borne epidemics, the millions of lives undoubtedly saved by DDT may more than balance the intangible hazards mentioned.

The International Agency for Research on Cancer (IARC) has just concluded a multigeneration study of the effects of DDT on mice. A significant increase in the incidence of liver cancer was found in all those treated with DDT even at the lowest level (2 p.p.m.). (World Health Organization, 1974).

Methods of Application

In Powder Form. Perhaps the simplest method of using insecticides, is to mix them with a finely ground inert diluent, such as kaolin, talc, or pyrophyllite. Dusts containing 0·5–1 per cent. pyrethrins, 5–10 per cent. DDT, 0·5 per cent. *gamma* BHC, or 0·5 per cent. dieldrin have been widely used. DDT powder has been successfully used against lice to quell typhus; for DDT-resistant lice, BHC or malathion dust must be used. It is puffed into apertures in the garments of infested people with a hand dusting gun. Treatment is so rapid (no undressing!) that thousands of people can be deloused in a few days. Against plague fleas, DDT, BHC, or dieldrin dusts may be used by blowing them into rat nests and sprinkling in rat runs. Heavily contaminated rats may be killed by the insecticide as well as the fleas.

Lotions and Ointments. Certain human ectoparasites, because of their close association with the body, are controlled by inunctions. Notably, scabies is treated with emulsion concentrates (benzyl benzoate, *gamma* BHC, etc.) applied to the skin surface below the neck in bland emulsion concentrates. Head lice and crab lice are eradicated by lotions (emulsions or spirit solutions) of *gamma* BHC or malathion, applied topically.

Residual Films. Many disease vectors and other troublesome pests, including anopheline and culicine mosquitoes, houseflies, sandflies, and bed bugs, rest on or crawl over wall surfaces, and are therefore vulnerable to residual insecticides. These residues may be applied by simple sprayers, either of the pneumatic knapsack type or the hydraulic bucket-and-stirrup-pump type. Nozzles giving fan-shaped sprays are generally found most convenient. The insecticide may be applied in kerosene solution or as an aqueous emulsion or a suspension. The last mentioned, prepared by simple agitation of a wettable powder, combines the greatest efficiency and cheapness; its only disadvantage is the whitish smears left on dark materials, which may annoy fastidious householders. It is desirable to apply an ample, even deposit, so that walls are usually wetted almost up to the point of run-off (about 2 to 5 litres per 100 m.²). Concentrations are adjusted to leave residues of 1–2 g./m.² of DDT, malathion or propoxur; or 0·25–0·5 g./m.² of dieldrin, *gamma* BHC or diazinon. Residues of DDT and dieldrin are very persistent and may remain active on some surfaces for 8–12 months. The residual life of the other compounds is curtailed by volatility, and is of the order of 2–3 months.

The factors affecting the contamination of insects walking over particulate residues have been very carefully studied. It is known that very fine crystals are most effective and that most of them adhere to the insect's feet when it first alights or takes a few steps. Dried mud is an important surface, because it forms the walls of most dwellings in rural, tropical areas. Particles of insecticide on some varieties of dried mud tend to disappear from the surface *inwards*, owing to adsorption in the micro-capillaries. The ultimate effect on insecticidal action varies with different insecticides. DDT and dieldrin lose activity because they are removed from contact with the insects; but they are chemically stable and may be reactivated by humidity. *Gamma* BHC may actually benefit, since it retains insecticidal action through its vapour and its persistence is increased. Some organophosphorus and carbamate insecticides, however, are chemically less stable and may decompose inside the mud substrate.

Residual deposits on vegetation have been used against a few pests of medical importance, such as tsetse flies and black flies. Owing to the effects of weathering and absorption into the plants, such residues are much less persistent than those inside houses.

Aerosols. Insecticidal aerosols are artificial mists, fogs, or smokes of chemicals used for the rapid destruction of insects in a particular area. They are often used against adult, flying insects, but fine deposits from them may be used against aquatic insect larvae; in neither case is there any appreciable residual action. There are two main types of aerosol treatment: 1. space sprays; and 2. large-scale fogging.

SPACE SPRAYS. Aerosols for relatively small, confined spaces may be produced by hand atomizers (*Flit* guns), but now they are more often emitted from metal dispensers containing insecticide dissolved in liquefied *Freon* (aerosol bombs). Both forms are widely used domestically against household pests. In medical entomology the liquefied gas aerosols are employed for disinsectizing aircraft to prevent insect vectors (possibly carrying pathogens, such as yellow fever virus) from being spread about the world. The original WHO Reference Standard Aerosol for this purpose contains 3 per cent. DDT and 0·4 per cent. pyrethrins. New and improved formulae have been introduced from time to time. All include a pyrethroid (most recently, biomesrethrin) for safety, quick knock-down, and effectiveness against insects resistant to other insecticides. Comparative evaluations are made first by room tests (e.g. British Standard 4172; 1967), and later in actual aircraft. The usual dose is 35 g./100 m.³, dispersed in the cabin, just after passenger embarkation and before take-off (i.e. 'blocks away').

LARGE-SCALE FOGGING. Machines to produce abundant aerosol have been designed on the following principles: 1. Liquid applied to rapidly spinning discs. 2. Opposing jets of liquid and gas (the latter may be compressed air; but in some machines hot engine exhaust or steam is used). 3. Alternatively, ordinary fine-spray nozzles can be employed. For treating extensive areas outdoors, the generator is moved slowly across-wind and the aerosol floats down-wind, for several hundred feet. The output of conventional fogging machines is considerable (say, 2 litres dilute solution or emulsion per minute). Recently, ultra-low-volume (ULV) aerosols have become popular (dispersing about 0·1 litre per minute of concentrated insecticide). Since there is no residual action, treatments must be repeated, usually at weekly intervals.

Aerial Spraying. Spraying from low levels (up to 100 m.) by slow-flying (150–200 mph) aeroplanes, or by helicopters, may be useful for treating large or inaccessible breeding grounds of some pests, such as mosquito larvae in large swamps, or tsetse flies in extensive bush. Urban areas may also be treated to quell certain mosquito-borne epidemics. Most of the spraying systems used for large-scale ground fogging can be adapted to aircraft, including the ULV technique, which shows promise. Sprayers giving coarse droplets produce narrow swaths, with rather irregular coverage. The finer aerosols give more even coverage, but are rather easily displaced by wind. Air spraying can be done satisfactorily only during stable air conditions. In tropical countries, ground heating during the day produces violent air convection, which usually restricts spraying to about an hour either just after sunrise or just before sunset.

Measures against Aquatic Larvae. Two important kinds of insect vector have aquatic larvae: mosquitoes and blackflies, both of which may be controlled in that stage.

MOSQUITOES. The breeding places of mosquitoes vary enormously, from lakes to seepages and from pure mountain streams to brackish swamps or polluted drains. Larval destruction is not difficult, but it is usually intended only to give localized control. Total eradication of indigenous mosquitoes is very difficult, and treatments must be repeated indefinitely at approximately weekly intervals. These difficulties handicap antilarval attacks in any large-scale campaigns against mosquitoes, which have been much more feasible by residual spraying of houses against the adults. However, it is sometimes good policy to attack the larvae; for example, where breeding sites are restricted or close to houses (*Culex fatigans*, *Aëdes aegypti*) or

where resistance has vitiated wall residue treatments. A combined attack against larvae and adults has been used in campaigns against *Aëdes aegypti* in Central America. Kerosene containing insecticide is sprayed on water surfaces and adjacent possible resting places of adults near all houses (perifocal treatment).

Larval treatments against domestic mosquitoes should be chosen in relation to the favoured breeding site. *Aëdes aegypti* breeds in clean water and since domestic drinking vessels are often involved, non-toxic treatments are necessary (e.g. DDT, which is scarcely soluble and, more recently, dilute difenphos, which is harmless). *Culex p. fatigans* tends to breed in polluted water, such as drains. Toxic organophosphorus compounds can be safely used; but they must be unaffected by the polluting matter.

Mosquito larvae breeding in ponds and ditches may be killed by heavy oiling (168 l/ha) by antimalarial oil (with or without a little added insecticide) or by light spraying with kerosene containing high concentration of insecticide (e.g. 5 per cent. DDT), at about 5·6 l/ha. The former treatment also kills weeds in irrigation ditches and seems to have a slightly residual action, the latter saves labour. Both liquids are intended to spread freely across the water surface and must possess good spreading pressure to overcome natural contamination of pools. Larvae breeding among dense standing vegetation, or not rising to the surface (*Mansonia*), may be killed by scattering pellets of insecticide.

BLACKFLIES. Species of *Simulium* breed in clean, rapidly flowing rivers and streams. Good control can be obtained by adding insecticide solution or emulsion to the river and all tributaries at points above the infested region. Recent trials of aerial application have been promising. Concentrations of 0·1–1·0 ppm DDT are appropriate in different conditions, applied for at least 15 minutes; such doses will kill larvae for many miles downstream. This method, systematically applied at about ten-day intervals for a few months, has successfully eradicated *Simulium* from limited areas in Africa.

REPELLENTS

Substances Available

Since ancient times, men have tried to keep noxious insects away from themselves or their dwellings. Primitive measures include smoke from smouldering fires and various odorous substances. In the early years of this century, various essential oils (e.g. citronella) were employed; but from the 1930s onward, various synthetic chemicals were discovered which were more effective and, being nearly odourless, more acceptable for personal use. These synthetic repellents were discovered quite empirically, by testing many thousands of compounds. About 10 per cent. showed high activity, and they belonged to diverse chemical groups, especially esters, amides, imides, ethers, and alcohols. Unfortunately, only a small fraction were safe on the human skin and many of these were ruled out by cost and other criteria. It is somewhat depressing to note that two of the most efficient and widely used modern repellents were discovered, respectively, 15 and 30 years ago. These are *deet* (diethyl *meta*-toluamide) and DMP (di-methyl phthalate). Even these fall short of the perfect repellent, which probably does not exist. Ideally, the application of a few drops should keep off noxious insects for an indefinite period. In practice, modern repellents act mainly by contact, with a little action at a distance, so that only the area treated is completely protected. Furthermore, the protection of treated skin lasts only a few hours and treated garments for a few days. Attempts to find an oral repellent (i.e. a harmless drug which will prevent insect bites) have so far failed.

Use of Repellents

Skin Application. Treatment of exposed skin is used to prevent bites of flying insects such as mosquitoes, blackflies, midges, and stableflies. Both the compounds mentioned can be safely applied to the human skin. The undiluted liquid is sprinkled on the hands and smeared over exposed skin, stockings, and other thin clothing, avoiding lips and eyelids to prevent smarting. Several repellents may damage cellulose plastics, but they are safe on nylon, cotton, or wool. Repellents applied to the skin may be rubbed off, absorbed or leached off by perspiration. The maximum effective time is about three or four hours in a resting subject, but this is much reduced by activity causing sweating.

Application to Nets and Veils. The effective life of a repellent is much prolonged if skin contact is avoided. Biting flies can be kept off the face by a veil worn over the hat. Fairly coarse meshes (up to 1 cm) can be used if impregnated with a repellent such as DMP, and such nets avoid stuffiness and do not greatly impede vision.

Clothing Treatments. Repellents applied to clothing are used to prevent attacks of ticks, chiggers (*Trombicula*), and fleas. DMP, dibutyl phthalate, and benzyl benzoate may be used by simply smearing them over the garments, especially round cuffs, trouser legs, and other openings. The United States Armed Forces impregnate uniforms with a mixture of repellents, giving protection for a week or more.

INSECTICIDE RESISTANCE

The subject of insecticide resistance is too complex to be adequately dealt with here; anyone concerned with prevention of insect-borne disease should read the summaries mentioned in the bibliography. The earliest record of insecticide resistance is nearly fifty years old; but there were very few cases until the big increase in the last decade, involving new synthetic insecticides. The association of resistance with the introduction of these insecticides is almost certainly due to the exceptional selection pressure effected by their very wide use and their residual action. The recrudescence began with DDT-resistant houseflies in 1947 and has continued until nearly 200 species are involved, approximately half of them being of public health importance. These include 35 anophelines, 18 being important malaria vectors and about the same number of culicine mosquitoes (including *Aëdes aegypti* and *Culex fatigans*). Among other important insects may be mentioned houseflies, lice, bed bugs, and fleas (including *Xenopsylla cheopis*).

Resistance has been reported from nearly every country and, since it was growing faster than our ability to cope with it, counter-measures have been co-ordinated by the World Health Organization. The primary need for accurate and comprehensive information necessitated the use of uniform methods of detecting and measuring resistance in all countries. Suitable techniques were devised and were recommended by the World Health Organization, the first tests being for lice and for adult and larval mosquitoes. Subsequently, tests were devised for other arthropods of medical importance, such as fleas, bed bugs, triatomids, sandflies, ticks, etc. The widespread use of such tests, especially for anopheline mosquitoes, has provided a valuable picture of the status of resistance throughout the world. One hopeful sign has been the fact that resistance often does not extend throughout the range of a given species, even when insecticide has been used throughout the area. This suggests that the potentiality for developing resistance may not be universally present in all insect populations.

Basic research, too, has been fostered and co-ordinated. It is known that resistant strains do not arise through tolerance induced by sub-lethal doses; they originate in exceptional individuals which survive insecticide because of defence mechanisms which can be inherited. Persistent selective mortality due to the insecticide eventually causes the resistant form to predominate. True physiological resistance has been observed to involve any of the main groups of insecticide defined earlier. By far the most frequent instances, however, are against one of the two groups of chlorinated insecticides, possible because of their wide use and long residual action. Least common is resistance to the pyrethroids, which is very rarely encountered in the field. Resistance to any compound usually confers resistance to others within the group (though this may depend on varieties of resistance within the main types); it does not confer immunity to the other types of insecticide. However, some insects (housefly, bed bug, louse, and several mosquitoes) have already developed combined resistance to more than one type of poison.

The genetical mechanisms involved in inheritance of resistance have been studied extensively. In several cases elucidated most completely, they have been of normal Mendelian type involving monofactorial inheritance. Studies on the genetics and physiology of resistance, especially in relation to field conditions, have important bearing on its rate of development and its rate of decline on removal of selection pressure when insecticiding is stopped or changed. The last point is very important but the evidence available is not encouraging.

Toxicological and biochemical research on resistance have revealed some of the protective mechanisms involved. Insects resistant to DDT, organophosphorus compounds, or carbamates have been shown to detoxify these poisons by various metabolic pathways. BHC/dieldrin resistance is more mysterious and seems to depend on insensitivity at the site of action. Despite much brilliant research, however, no practical remedy for any case of resistance has been devised. The only solution is to change to a different type of insecticide; but the alternatives are limited. For some 10 years, the World Health Organization coordinated an international search for new types of contact poison, but no outstandingly different compounds were found. Insecticide resistance clearly calls for intensive research of several kinds, for, unless it is overcome, it will gradually drive us back to less efficient control measures.

ALTERNATIVES TO CONTROL BY INSECTICIDES

The problem of insecticide resistance and the growing concern about possible toxic hazards from chemical residues have stimulated scientists to seek alternative methods of controlling insect pests. Among the possibilities which have been envisaged are the following biological methods: (1) control by arthropod parasites or predators; (2) control by pathogenic organisms (see World Health Organization, 1973, on the use of pathogenic viruses for vector control).; (3) replacement of a vector species by a closely related non-vector; and (4) the introduction of strains of the pest species, bearing deleterious genes to cause sterility. Alternative measures involving chemicals could include: (1) use of pheromones (such as sex-attractants) to modify the pests' behaviour; (2) use of insect hormones e.g. the juvenile hormone mimics (insect growth regulation), often called third generation pesticides (World Health Organization, 1974b).; or (3) antibiotics, to disturb the pests' physiology. Combinations of physical and chemical or biological methods include: (1) release of males sterilized by radiation, to prevent breeding of the wild females; (2) use of chemosterilants, in baits, to sterilize both sexes of the wild population; and (3) improved trapping methods, employing pheromones or specially attractive radiation.

Some of these alternatives to conventional pesticides have been discussed in a book by Kilgore and Doutt (1967). Unfortunately, each of these suggestions is fraught with formidable technical difficulties, and it seems most unlikely that, at least in the next decade, any of them will challenge the benefits to health achieved by insecticides. One reason for this is that, whereas the same insecticide treatment can be used against a number of allied species (e.g. mosquitoes), the new methods are highly specific and each pest requires intensive research to determine the feasibility of each proposal. Furthermore, even a successful method is unlikely to be directly profitable, so that funds for the extensive research necessary are unlikely to be forthcoming from industry.

In conclusion, a sound vector-control policy requires a proper balance between expenditure on investigation of resistance, the search for new insecticides, and on the alternative control measure.

REFERENCES AND FURTHER READING

British Standards Institution (1969) *Recommended Common Names for Pesticides*, B.S. 1831, London.
Brown, A. W. A. (1974) The safety of biological agents for arthropod control, *Wld Hlth Org. Chron.*, **28**, 261.
Brown, A. W. A. and Pal, R. (1971) Insecticide resistance in arthropods, *Wld Hlth Org. Monogr. Ser.*, No. 38
Busvine, J. R. (1966) *Insects and Hygiene*, 2nd ed., London.
Kilgore, W. W., and Doutt, R. L. (1967) *Pest Control*, London.
O'Brien, R. D. (1967) *Insecticides*, London.
Symes, C. B., Thomson, R. C. M., and Busvine, J. R. (1962) *Insect Control in Public Health*, Amsterdam.
United Kingdom Department of Education and Science (1969) *Further Review of Certain Organochlorine Pesticides Used in Great Britain*, London, H.M.S.O.
United States Department of Health, Education and Welfare (1969) *Report of the Commission on Pesticides and their Relation to Environmental Health*, Washington, D.C.
World Health Organization (1963) Vector control, *Bull. Wld Hlth Org.*, **29**, Suppl.
World Health Organization (1964) *Equipment for Vector Control*, Geneva.
World Health Organization (1967) *Specification for Pesticides*, 3rd ed., Geneva.
World Health Organization Expert Committee on Insecticides. (1967) 16th Rep. (Safe use of pesticides in public health), *Wld Hlth Org. techn. Rep. Ser.*, No. 356.
(1970) 17th Rep. (Insecticide resistance and vector control), *Wld Hlth Org. techn. Rep. Ser.*, No. 443.
(1971a) 18th Rep. (Application and dispersal of pesticides), *Wld Hlth Org. techn. Rep. Ser.*, No. 465.
(1971b) 19th Rep. (Pesticides) *Wld Hlth Org. techn. Rep. Ser.*, No. 465, No. 474, No. 475.
World Health Organization (1972a) *Vector Control in International Health*, Geneva.
World Health Organization (1972b) Vector surveillance: Developing standard methods, *Wld Hlth Org. Chron.*, **26**, 268.
World Health Organization (1973) Joint FAO/WHO Meeting on Insect Viruses. The use of viruses for the control of insect pests and disease vectors, *Wld Hlth Org. techn. Rep. Ser.*, No. 531.
World Health Organization (1974a) Annual Report I.A.R.C. (1972–1973), *Wld Hlth Org. Chron.*, **28**, 130.
World Health Organization (1974b) The work of WHO in 1973, *Off. Rec. Wld Hlth Org.*, **213**, 51.

20

THE PUBLIC HEALTH ASPECTS OF CERTAIN SKIN DISEASES

L. M. BECHELLI

Many skin diseases constitute a public health problem. This is determined by their prevalence and incidence, duration, human, social and economic implications, the disability they may cause and their mortality rate. Usually, in each disease these factors have a different weight and may be differently combined. For example, ringworm of the scalp (*tinea capitis*) spreads easily and may cause epidemics affecting children, preventing them from attending school, and causing a break in their education. Treatment with griseofulvin is successful, mostly in 6–8 weeks, and therefore the inconveniences caused by the dermatose last only a short period. In contrast to tinea capitis, the pityriasis (tinea) versicolor, is a very common superficial mycosis (in some areas it affects 50 per cent. of the population) but it presents only an aesthetic disadvantage for the patient; its transmission seems to be difficult and the treatment is effective if properly carried out.

Tinea pedis ('foot rot') is a common skin disease and may cause temporary disability, which becomes more frequent under certain conditions. According to Blank, Taplin, and Zaias (1969), it is the commonest cause of disability among American troops in Vietnam: 166 (79 per cent.) out of 209 soldiers stationed in the Mekong Delta had to be hospitalized due to 'foot infections'. In the First World War, it was also very common in British troops in the trenches (static warfare), where it was known as 'trench foot'. It did not, however, occur in the Second World War, as this was a war of movement. Disabilities from skin diseases among American troops in Vietnam engaged in combat have often been the greatest medical cause of non-effectiveness.

Schofield, Parkinson, and Jeffrey (1963) reported that, in Melanesia and Polynesia, patients with tinea imbricata (Tokelau ringworm) experienced severe social disability. The disease was a serious handicap for marriage and patients were discriminated against with regard to employment; employers preferred to engage 'clear skins'. Among the minority of children who can go on to secondary education at a boarding school the disease can also be a handicap.

Let us now consider a deep or systemic mycosis, South American blastomycosis. Its prevalence is relatively very low and it occurs only in certain areas of South America; however, the disease is serious and at times fatal. In addition, treatment with amphotericin B or with sulphonamides is useful, but must be continued for long periods or even indefinitely to prevent relapse. The life of the patient, usually a farm worker, is threatened and seriously affected from both the human and economic viewpoints. Some of the other deep mycoses may also cause multisystem involvement and death if untreated, and even sometimes in spite of treatment. In the case of coc-

cidioidomycosis, to the very serious prognosis of the disseminated and progressive forms should be added its high morbidity in endemic areas. According to Fiese (quoted by Ajello, 1970), 'In the most highly endemic area—Bakersfield, California; Phoenix, Arizona; and El Paso, Texas—nearly 100 per cent. of the population will have been infected in a few years, and about a fifth of them will have had an illness severe enough to cause temporary incapacity and to warrant medical care'.

Onchocerciasis causes human suffering and severe economic damage. Blindness rates of over 10 per cent. or occasionally over 30 per cent. have been found in villages subject to hyperendemic onchocerciasis (Waddy, 1969). (See also CHAPTER 29 on public health ophthalmology, and CHAPTER 17 on arthropod-borne diseases.)

The infections caused by *Staphylococcus pyogenes* and *Streptococcus pyogenes* (pyodermas) are common, may occur in any part of the world, and may spread easily, mainly in children; but the effectiveness of treatment reduced the inconveniences of such dermatoses. They may affect the patient aesthetically when localized in the face (sycosis barbae) or cause limitation in the working capacity (furunculosis, hydrosadenitis, erysipelas), with temporary economic implications.

Regarding leprosy, the seriousness of endemics in relation to other diseases cannot be evaluated only in terms of the total number of patients or the prevalence rates; the duration of the disease, the disabilities that it causes, and the human and social consequences to the leprosy patients and their families must also be taken into account. Patients with disabilities represent a significant loss of man-power for many countries where leprosy is endemic and, as is known, prevalence rates are usually higher in developing countries, which are in particular need of capable men to raise the economic level, the standard of living, and the level of education of the community. To complete the picture of the human and social impact of leprosy, the age-old prejudice against the disease must be added. The discovery of a specific vaccine and/or of very effective drugs would change the outlook for leprosy, already improved to some extent by use of sulphones.

Several skin diseases among the non-communicable dermatoses also deserve the attention of health authorities in a certain number of countries: occupational dermatoses, drug eruptions, dermatoses and skin changes due to physical and chemical agents, precancerous dermatoses and skin cancer, and also hereditary cutaneous disorders. In general, these diseases are of great or almost exclusive concern in countries or areas which have reached a high socio-economic level. Occupational dermatoses are of major importance in these countries, since they account for 50–75 per cent. of all occupational diseases (see also CHAPTER 39 on occupation and health). As indicated by Prieto *et al.* (1968), 'the ever increasing number of industries and the discovery of new chemical products, the expansion of agriculture with mass production techniques, have created a daily increase in the number of possible causes of occupational dermatoses. A particular aspect of this is to be found in iatrogenic skin diseases, caused by various drugs and cosmetics, which also have an occupational facet in factories producing antibiotics, topical medicines, and cosmetics which are liable to provoke these dermatoses.'

These occupational skin diseases, and also precancerous dermatoses and skin cancer, and cutaneous changes due to actinic irradiation, are more liable to appear in individuals of light skin, and at a higher frequency than in dark-skinned persons.

The public health importance of dermatoses is therefore high or low depending on a combination of several factors, and it may vary from one continent to another and often in different areas of the same country. In each country or area, the magnitude of the problem in relation to each disease has to be determined to allow the establishment of a system of priorities in its control.

In the course of years, the discovery of effective therapeutic agents has caused a decrease in importance of some of the communicable dermatoses. The most striking example is yaws, treated by a single injection of penicillin, and controlled in most areas of the world by the World Health Organization and national campaigns.[1] The discovery of griseofulvin and its effect on tinea capitis and other superficial mycoses reduced the inconveniences of these dermatoses. The impact of penicillin on the trend of syphilis is also known.[1] In the case of leishmaniasis, the wise use of insecticides, agricultural development, and chemotherapy have led to the regression of endemic foci. However, due to the exploitation of other regions (deserts and forests) with untouched natural foci, new endemic areas appear.

The skin diseases which have public health importance may be considered in two groups: one comprising the communicable skin diseases and the other, dermatoses which are not transmissible. We shall consider here only some of these diseases, focusing attention on their public health aspects.

In each continent or country, the attention to be given to the above-mentioned diseases and to those that we propose to study should follow a scale of priorities, not only among themselves, but in relation to other diseases. In Africa, where leprosy reaches its maximum degree of endemicity (over 35 per thousand population in some countries, with higher rates in certain foci) it may be fourth or fifth in the scale of priorities, while in other countries, with much lower prevalence rates, it may deserve first priority. Syphilis and venereal diseases were dealt with by special services in several countries before penicillin therapy. After the introduction of antibiotics and the decrease in incidence of these particular diseases, their public health importance was gradually reduced, even though in recent years there has been a recrudescence of the problem. It should be emphasized that in each country the magnitude of each health problem, the resources available, including staff, and other factors (the need for education and other sectors of activities essential for development) should be taken

[1] See CHAPTER 21 on venereal diseases and treponematoses.

into account in determining the priority for the control of certain endemic skin diseases and for the relevant planning. In dealing with skin diseases, an integrated approach—with control activities carried out by general health services—is the long-term goal, which must be achieved gradually and progressively where there are specific services.

COMMUNICABLE SKIN DISEASES

Certain communicable skin diseases tend to be more prevalent or to occur in developing countries (leprosy, yaws) and may also spread in the less developed areas of highly industrialized countries (leprosy). Some diseases (syphilis, venereal diseases), which suffered from the impact of treatment by antibiotics, may spread in any area of the world, usually where there is sexual promiscuity and lack of hygiene and education. There are dermatoses which are located only in certain areas owing to ecological factors (South American blastomycosis, North American blastomycosis and European blastomycosis). In contrast to these deep mycoses, ringworm (tinea corporis, tinea pedis and tinea manuum) is seen both in highly industrialized areas and in developing countries.

Population migration (from poorer areas to industrialized countries), and tourism (when followed by promiscuity) have to be considered in the spread of some communicable skin diseases (venereal diseases, syphilis, leprosy (Browne, 1970), ringworm). Repatriation of people working in certain areas may account for the establishment of certain health problems; among these repatriates, many have leprosy (over 600 repatriates or immigrants in the post-war period in the Netherlands; Leiker, 1970).

The spread of communicable skin diseases varies according to the type of dermatoses and their causative agents. Transmission of ringworm occurs by direct or indirect contact, and the period of communicability lasts as long as lesions are not treated. For others, the transmission occurs presumably by inhalation of contaminated dust or soil. Some dermatoses (e.g. leishmaniasis) are transmitted through bites of infective female sandflies of the *Phlebotomus* species. In leprosy transmission presumably occurs through the skin and, perhaps mainly, via the upper respiratory tract. In others (e.g. candidiasis) transmission occurs by contact with excreta from patients and/or carriers.

In most of the communicable dermatoses, poor hygiene, education and socio-economic conditions play a certain role in their occurrence and maintenance.

Resistance to dermatoses also varies. Adults do not acquire tinea capitis. Most individuals are resistant to leprosy and when some of them acquire it they develop the benign forms of the disease. Individuals of all ages may acquire *Microsporum canis* and *Trichophyton* infections.

The *reservoir* of infection also varies with the disease and may be man, animals (cats, dogs, cattle) or the soil.

The *control* of communicable skin diseases, as does that of any other infectious disease, depends on a knowledge of epidemiology, facilities for diagnosis and availability of therapeutic and/or preventive agents. Funds and trained staff should be available to implement a realistic plan of control, adapted to the country or regional conditions. Very effective therapeutic agents will permit the control of diseases even in unfavourable socio-economic conditions, as happened with yaws following treatment of the patients and their contacts with penicillin.

General measures of prevention would consist of the following:

1. Reduction of the load of infectiousness by the treatment of infected individuals or animals; thus, as for any infectious disease, early diagnosis and early treatment are essential.

2. Avoidance of exposure to infected individuals or animals, and contaminated fomites.

3. Avoidance of infection and/or reinfection by disinfection of infected articles, footwear, combs, head-gear, barber shop tools, and other suspected fomites as in the case of superficial mycoses.

4. Education of patients and their contacts, and of the population exposed.

SUPERFICIAL MYCOSES[1]

In these mycoses the action of fungi, known as dermatophytes, is limited to the superficial layers of the skin, and to the hair and nails. Dermatophytoses (ringworm) may occur at any age and in both sexes; some of them (tinea capitis caused by *Microsporum* and *Trichophyton*) occur almost exclusively in children, while others (tinea pedis and tinea cruris) affect adults.

The skin lesions are caused by the direct action of fungi or by an allergic reaction to them or their derivatives ('ides', dermatophytides), brought from distant primary foci. The fungi may be shown by direct examination or by cultivation, in the former but not in the latter lesions. According to the sites of infection, the dermatophytoses are subdivided into the groups tinea capitis (ringworm of scalp), tinea barbae (ringworm of bearded areas), tinea corporis, tinea cruris (ringworm of inguinocrural region), and tinea unguium (ringworm of the nails). There is a preferential topographical localization according to the genera of fungi: those of the genera *Trichophyton* may affect the scalp, nail, and glabrous skin; *Microsporum*, the scalp and glabrous skin but not the nails; and *Epidermophyton*, the skin and nails, but never the scalp.

The dermatophytes have a worldwide distribution, more common in tropical and semitropical areas; their distribution varies according to countries and within these according to regions, partly because of ecological, epidemiological, and socio-economic factors. The distribution of clinical types also varies. Favus, seen in certain areas of Europe, is rare in the United States and infrequent in Brazil. Tinea barbae occurs in Europe but is rare in the United States and exceptional in Brazil. Tinea imbricata is frequent in Melanesia, Polynesia and Ceylon, but is not seen in Europe and America (except among certain tribes in Goyas and Mato Grosso, Brazil). In France and the United States, *Microsporum audouini* is the most frequent agent of tinea microsporica, while in São Paulo (Brazil) it is very rare, most infection being caused by *Microsporum canis*.

Man and animals (mainly dogs, cats and cattle) are the reservoir of dermatophytes.

<hr>

[1] This and other sections are mainly based on Bechelli and Curban's *Textbook of Dermatology*, 1967.

Individual host susceptibility, environmental factors, socio-economic conditions and virulence of the infecting strain determine the frequency of ringworm in individuals, according to age, sex, and occupation.

Transmission occurs by direct human contact or, in certain dermatophytoses, through contact with an infected animal or carrier. Indirect contact, for example with clothing or seats, also occurs with contaminated materials (hair, skin scales) from infected man and/or animals. Dermatophytoses may be transmitted while affected individuals or animals have untreated lesions, and viable spores are present on contaminated materials.

Tinea Capitis

Excepting favus, ringworm of the scalp is observed almost exclusively in children; in fact, spontaneous healing occurs with puberty. The dermatosis is evidenced by scaling, patchy alopecia and broken hairs at or just above the skin surface and, if untreated, it continues for long periods. With treatment or spontaneous healing the skin and hair resume a normal aspect. The causative agents belong to the genera *Trichophyton* and *Microsporum*, and can be shown by direct examination of hair and scales, and by cultivation. The incubation period is 10–14 days.

Favus (caused by *Trichophyton schoenleini*) is not influenced by age. Hairs are not broken and the mousy odour and the yellowish cup-like crusts or scutulae are characteristic. If untreated the lesions evolve to cicatricial atrophy with consequent permanent alopecia.

Tinea capitis has a worldwide distribution. Tinea capitis caused by *Microsporum audouini* is widespread in the United States, particularly in urban areas. *M. canis* infection occurs in both rural and urban areas. *Trichophyton mentagrophytes* and *T. verrucosum* infections occur in rural areas where the disease exists in cattle, horses, rodents, and wild animals. *Trichophyton tonsurans* infections are epidemic in urban areas in southern and eastern United States, Puerto Rico and Mexico (Benenson, 1970). Favus affects almost exclusively the inhabitants of rural areas, no matter what their age and sex.

Before the advent of griseofulvin the control of tinea capitis presented serious difficulties, because epilation with radiotherapy could be carried out only in certain areas of the world. In other areas, treatment was limited to mechanical epilation of affected hair, topical treatment with tincture of iodine, undecylenic acid, and other drugs; the long duration of treatment acted against its regularity, and satisfactory results could be obtained only in those children who had good surveillance at home. Even with radiotherapy, treatment and surveillance after epilation required great attention. With griseofulvin, tinea captis may be treated more easily and without any eventual inconvenience from irradiation. However, the treatment of great numbers of children is expensive, and many governments are not in a position to offer such an antibiotic to health units; in fact, other diseases may deserve first priority and other problems have to be tackled first.

Besides treating the affected children, the surveillance of contacts is required and they should be examined with Wood's light. During epidemics or in hyperendemic areas, screening of schoolchildren and follow-up surveys should be undertaken. Those affected should be treated and kept away from school.

Griseofulvin by mouth (average of 10 mg. per kg. body weight daily for about a month), local treatment—tincture of iodine (10–20 per cent.), gentian violet (2 per cent.) and other fungicides—daily washing of the scalp, and disinfection of infected articles are recommended. The source of infection should be investigated (an infected person or animal in the household). Education of parents and children is required.

Tinea Corporis (Ringworm of the Body)

The characteristic lesions are well defined, flat, erythematous scaling, oval or ring-shaped, frequently with small vesicles in the centre and/or on the periphery, often progressing peripherally and healing in the central part. Tinea corporis progresses slowly and spontaneous healing is rare. It is widespread throughout the world and is more frequent in children; epidemics may occur among schoolchildren. The incubation period is 10–14 days.

The clinical diagnosis is confirmed by direct examination and cultivation of scales and material obtained by scraping the floor of the vesicles. The infectious agents are fungi of the genera *Microsporum*, *Trichophyton*, and *Epidermophyton*.

Control measures consist of the treatment of the affected individuals and of the sources of infection (man and/or animals). Local treatment gives good result. Infected individuals should be excluded from schools and swimming-pools. Adequate laundering of towels and clothes is required to avoid the spread of the dermatosis or reinfection. Examination of contacts and education of children and adults in the household or in the school (if there is an epidemic) are required.

Tinea Cruris

Tinea cruris is peculiar to adults. The typical lesions, localized in the inguinocrural region and sometimes in the buttocks, are well defined, erythematous scaling with pin-point vesicles on the periphery. They have a chronic evolution, but this chronicity may be interrupted by periods of activity. The infectious agents are fungi of the genera *Trichophyton* and *Epidermophyton*.

Local treatment gives good results but relapse is frequent. Affected individuals and sources of infection should be treated. Proper laundering of underwear and towels is required, and health education is essential.

Tinea Pedis (Ringworm of the Foot)

Ringworm of the foot (athlete's foot) is the most common of the superficial mycoses and is distributed throughout the world. Children are rarely affected. It affects preferentially the plantar region and the spaces between the toes (mainly the last three). Between the toes the main lesion consists of slight scaling, which is not noticed by the affected persons; cracking of the skin is also common. Erythematous-scaling lesions, with vesicles and even bullae (mainly in the acute phase), may be present and, following secondary infection, lymphangitis and adenitis may occur.

Fungi of the genera *Trichophyton* and *Epidermophyton* are the infectious agents, and man is the reservoir. The incubation period is unknown.

With regard to control, treatment of cases and surveillance of contacts is necessary. Local treatment is effective in a great number of cases, but reinfection is frequent. In certain cases

treatment with griseofulvin is required (average of 10 mg. per kg. bodyweight daily for one or two months). Socks and shoes should be disinfected to avoid reinfection; the former should be boiled and the latter placed in a box with formaldehyde for a few hours. The inside of shoes could also be powdered with undecylenic acid and/or its derivates.

Cleaning and disinfection of showers, at home or in the gymnasium, are also recommended.

Tinea Unguium (Ringworm of the Nails)

Caused also by fungi of the genera *Trichophyton* and *Epidermophyton*, tinea of the nails is a common disease. One or more nails of the hands and feet may be affected. They become discoloured, thickened, brittle, with an accumulation of horny material beneath them.

Ringworm of the nails is usually resistant to local treatment. Griseofulvin (250 mg. four times a day) taken for a few months causes the regression of lesions in a high proportion of cases. Relapse and/or reinfection are frequent.

Man is the reservoir and transmission probably occurs by means of the manicuring articles used on an infected person. Disinfection of these articles is required.

CANDIDIASIS

Caused mainly by *Candida* (*Monilia*) *albicans*, candidiasis is a widespread dermatosis, which may be epidemic in nurseries for the newborn. However, its public health importance is limited because it is a sporadic disease and nursery epidemics are limited mainly to thrush.

Clinical manifestations of candidiasis are stomatitis (oral thrush) in children, vulvovaginitis, mainly in adults, intertriginous skin lesions (interdigital, crural and inframammary intertrigo), onychomycosis and paronychia. Generalized candidiasis is rare, as is visceral candidiasis (pulmonary and bronchial lesions, endocarditis, pericarditis, meningitis, ulcers of the gastro-intestinal tract). In contrast to the mucous membrane and skin lesions, the visceral lesions have a reserved prognosis, depending on the organ or system affected.

The clinical diagnosis is confirmed, or made, by the demonstration of *Candida albicans* (direct examination or culture). The yeasts are present in the lesions of candidiasis. However, normal persons may also present them; these would have a saprophytic life and would become pathogenic under the influence of external and/or internal conditioning factors.

Man is the reservoir and transmission occurs by contact with lesions or excretions from patients and carriers. The incubation period is variable, from 2 to 5 days in thrush occurring in infants (Benenson, 1970). Diabetes and the broad-spectrum antibiotics favour the appearance of candidiasis, the former mainly of the genital lesions, vulvovaginitis and balanitis.

Control consists of treating the affected persons: topical application of gentian violet (2 per cent. aqueous solution) or nystatin; in the intertriginous areas, gentian violet solution should be applied and, after this has dried, boric acid 5 per cent in talc. In generalized and/or visceral candidiasis, nystatin (500,000 Units, three or four times a day), cabimicin (50,000 Units three to six times a day); if necessary, intravenous administration should be made of amphotericin B, which, however, is highly toxic. In nurseries, patients with stomatitis should be isolated. Disinfection of excretions and contaminated material is required.

DEEP OR SYSTEMIC MYCOSES

In contrast to the agents of superficial mycosis, fungi of deep mycosis may affect not only the epidermis and dermis but also the hypodermis, bones, joints, viscera, and the central nervous system, producing destructive lesions which leave sequelae when they heal. Thus, grave manifestations may appear, which may cause death.

The distribution of deep mycosis varies according to continents, countries and within these, according to geographical regions. North American blastomycosis is exclusive to the United States, while South American blastomycosis is confined to South America, mainly Brazil. Rhinosporidiosis, first recognized in Argentina, is found in India and Ceylon but is rare in other countries. The distribution of systemic mycoses within a country may vary according to the regions. One example is keloidal blastomycosis (caused by *Loboa loboi*), exclusive to Amazonia; autochthonous cases were not detected in other areas of Brazil. In the United States, coccidioidomycosis (San Joaquin or Valley fever) is endemic from Southern California to West Texas; in Argentina, where it was first described, the disease is endemic only in the northern areas. In Brazil, South American blastomycosis is much more frequent, found almost exclusively in the rural areas. In contrast, sporotrichosis has been reported throughout the world and affects individuals of rural and urban areas alike. The great majority of deep mycoses preferentially affect rural workers.

Sporotrichosis excepted, there is no specific treatment for systemic mycosis; certain progress has been made and many cases benefit from present therapy, but the risk of relapse persists.

The frequency of the deep mycoses is much lower than that of the superficial mycoses. For this reason they will be briefly considered below.

Sporotrichosis

Caused by *Sporotrichum schenkii*, this disease affects the skin, lymphatics and lymph nodes and rarely the viscera. Nodular ascending lymphangitis is characteristic. It has been diagnosed in all continents, though it is relatively uncommon, but epidemics may occur, for example among gold miners in South Africa involving some 3,000 miners (Benenson, 1970).

Soil, vegetation, and wood are the reservoirs of infection. Following pricks from thorns, from slivers of wood or lumber, fungi are introduced into the skin. The incubation period may be a few weeks or months.

As control measures, isolation of patients and surveillance of contacts are unnecessary. Dressings and discharges should be disinfected; patients are treated with potassium iodide in aqueous solution given by mouth; with a dose of 4 g. daily the disease heals in 1 or 2 months. Sodium iodide (10 per cent., 10 ml. intravenously, daily) may also be given. Amphotericin

B may be used for patients with visceral lesions in whom the effect of potassium iodide has not proved satisfactory.

Blastomycosis

European blastomycosis (EB) or cryptococcosis (agent *Cryptococcus neoformans*), North American blastomycosis (NAB) (agent *Blastomyces dermatitidis*) and South American blastomycosis (SAB) or paracoccidioidomycosis (agent *Paracoccidioides brasiliensis*) are serious sporadic diseases, frequently or usually fatal if untreated. They are not directly transmitted from man to man. The reservoir for the last two blastomycoses is probably soil or spore-laden dust, and for cryptococcosis the fungi may be isolated from old pigeon nests and pigeon droppings (in aviaries, on window ledges) and also from the soil. Transmission presumably occurs by inhalation of contaminated soil or spore-laden dust; in addition, in SAB traumatic lesions, mainly of the oral mucosa, are considered by many as a possible way of entry for fungi in the organism. The incubation period is unknown for EB, and not well determined for NAB and SAB (a few weeks to a few months, years?).

Isolation of patients and surveillance of contacts are not required. Contaminated articles and discharges should be disinfected.

Amphotericin B is used for the three blastomycoses[1] and is effective in a certain proportion of cases. However, in view of its high toxicity and side-effects (headaches, vomiting, fever, kidney lesions), it should be used in hospitalized patients under strict clinical and laboratory control. Hydroxystilbamidine isethionate is the alternative drug in the case of NAB. In patients with SAB the use of sulphonamides—sulphadiazine, sulphathiazole, sulphamerazine—introduced by Oliveira Ribeiro in 1939, changed the prognosis of the disease, which before was equivalent to a death sentence. However, the treatment should be continued for years, if not indefinitely, to avoid relapses. In cases of SAB resistant to sulphonamides, amphotericin B should be used.

Coccidioidomycosis

Coccidioidomycosis is caused by *Coccidioides immitis* and starts as a respiratory infection. Its distribution has already been considered. In endemic areas the proportion of reactors to coccidioidin is high, indicating frequent asymptomatic or inapparent infections. The infection shows seasonal variation, and has a higher incidence during the dry and dusty season (July through October in the United States). The reservoir is the soil, and transmission occurs by air-borne spores, inhaled from the dust, soil, and dry vegetation; the infection may also be acquired in laboratories, by the inhalation of spores from culture media. It is not directly transmitted from man to man and, therefore, the isolation of patients and surveillance of contacts are not required. Disinfection of discharges and soiled articles is necessary.

The disease is chronic and fatal if untreated. Amphotericin B is the treatment of choice and has improved the prognosis.

Actinomycosis

Caused by *Actinomyces bovis* (*A. israeli*), *Actinomyces brasiliensis* and by several species of fungi of the genus *Nocardia*, actinomycosis causes thickening and induration of the skin with abscesses and sinuses. It appears in three main forms:

---

[1] Diluted in 5 per cent. glucose in water (the maximum concentration should be 10 mg./100 ml.) and injected slowly intravenously. Start treatment with 1 to 5 mg. and gradually increase the daily dose (by 5 or 10 mg. increments) up to 60–80 mg. (about 1 mg./kg. of body weight); 1–3 g. is the total dosage in a treatment.

cervicofacial, thoracic and abdominal, and podalic actinomycosis.

Man is the reservoir of *Actinomyces bovis*. It grows as a saprophyte in tonsillar crypts, in and around carious teeth. According to Benenson (1970) sample surveys in the United States, Sweden, and other regions demonstrated *A. israeli* microscopically in granules from 40 per cent. of extirpated tonsils; and it has also been isolated in anaerobic culture from as many as 69 per cent. of specimens of saliva or material from carious teeth.

In view of the above, and considering that the disease occurs only sporadically throughout the world, susceptibility to the fungi concerned must be low. Transmission from man to man is rare and therefore isolation of patients and surveillance of contacts are not necessary.

With regard to treatment, penicillin is the drug of choice (up to 15 million units). Tetracycline, chloramphenicol and the sulphonamides are also useful. Combined or alternate treatment may also be proposed. Because of the risk of relapses, treatment should be prolonged for months or years.

Maduromycosis (Mycetoma, Madura Foot)

The foot is mainly affected and the disease is caused by fungi of the genera *Madurella*, *Cephalosporium*, *Monosporium*. The foot becomes enlarged, and the skin thickened with sinuses which eliminate yellow, red, or black grains; there is also destruction and proliferation of bones.

The disease is found in South-East Asia, Africa, and the Americas in tropical and subtropical areas. The fungi, presumably soil or vegetation saprophytes, are introduced into the skin via trauma, in people who go barefoot, or by means of thorns and/or splinters. Direct transmission from man to man does not occur.

To prevent the disease, the use of shoes is necessary and also care in avoiding skin punctures by thorns or splinters. Treatment is similar to that of actinomycosis, also including the administration of dapsone, but the results are not satisfactory.

Chromomycosis

This sporadic disease, caused by *Hormodendrum pedrosoi*, *H. compactum*, *Phialophora verrucosa*, and *P. dermatitidis*, has a worldwide distribution. The area mainly affected is the foot, which presents verrucous plaques and may acquire an elephantiasic aspect. Wood, soil, and/or vegetation are the probable reservoirs. Transmission occurs by the contact of trauma with contaminated material. Direct transmission from man to man has not been reported, thus isolation of patients is unnecessary. The wearing of shoes and avoidance of puncture wounds are the preventive measures to be taken. Besides the electrocoagulation of the lesions, treatment consists of the administration of calciferol (Bopp, 1959) and/or amphotericin B (intravenously or inside the lesions) but there is no specific drug of choice. A new antimycotic agent, 5-fluorocytosine (5-FC), is being tried and initial results seem to be encouraging (Gonzalez Ochoa, 1970).

Histoplasmosis

Caused by *Histoplasma capsulatum*, the primary lesion is usually in the lung but may also occur in the lips, tongue or larynx. The disease is often fatal. It is endemic and common in eastern and central areas of the United States, where 80 per cent. of the people may be infected, as evidenced by reactivity to histoplasmin. It occurs also in some areas of Europe, Africa, and the Far East; it is rare in Brazil.

The fungus has been isolated from mice, dogs, cats, rats, bats, and horses, and may be recovered in the soil in the vicinity of chicken houses, barns, silos, caves, or places where bird manure is abundant. The infection is acquired by inhalation of air-borne spores. 'Characteristically, small groups of men engaged in dusty work such as cleaning out of old chicken houses or silos became ill after an incubation period usually of one or two weeks. The sites of exposure included farm buildings, school houses, a storm cellar, a cave and other locations' (Maxcy-Rosenau, 1965). Thus, preventive measures should consist of reducing exposure to contaminated locations or environment by spraying water or formalin, and the disinfection of contaminated articles and discharges from patients. These are treated with amphotericin B. Contacts living in the same environment should be kept under surveillance.

Rhinosporidiosis

Caused by *Rhinosporidium seeberi*, rhinosporidiosis affects more often the nose, where nodules and tumour masses appear. It is endemic in India, Ceylon, and Malaysia and sporadic in other regions of the world. It appears in persons who come into contact with sand from stagnant rivers. Surgical removal of lesions is the treatment.

LEPROSY

Leprosy is an infectious disease caused by *Myco. leprae*, of chronic course, interrupted in many patients by acute episodes (lepra reaction), determining neural and anaesthetic cutaneous lesions; its evolution is determined by the degree of resistance in the patient, and the disease may evolve either to spontaneous healing or to progressive invasion of the skin, mucosa, eyes, and viscera.

Very often, leprosy has been shown in its ugliest aspects or even presented as a scourge, thus stigmatizing the patient or causing him distress. This also gives a distorted idea of the disease, originating or aggravating the prejudice against it.

The clinical manifestations of leprosy depend essentially on the patient's capacity of resistance—maximum degree of resistance: single skin lesion or in small number and well defined; minimum degree of resistance: numerous lesions, ill defined, spreading in the skin mucosa and nerves, invading viscera, and with progressive evolution leading to blindness and other serious disabilities. It is this degree of resistance to *Myco. leprae* (evidenced by the lepromin reaction) which commands the clinical manifestations, the bacteriological and histological picture, the evolution and prognosis.

The skin lesions may consist of erythema, infiltration, macules, papules, tubercles, nodules, ulcers, and even bullae. A common characteristic of the leprosy skin lesions, no matter what the form of the disease, is *anaesthesia*. The cutaneous lesions of leprosy, apart from recent ones, present impairment of the superficial sensibility and this is one of the most important elements for diagnosis, because anaesthesia is found only in leprosy. Anhidrosis and alopecia also occur frequently and provide further evidence for the diagnosis of leprosy. This may

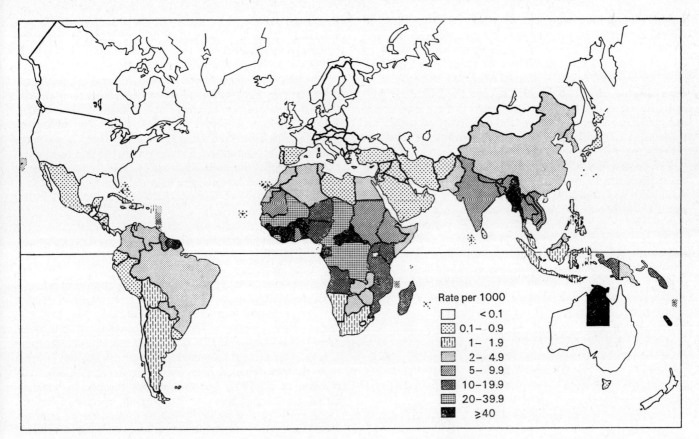

Rate per 1000

	< 0.1
	0.1 – 0.9
	1 – 1.9
	2 – 4.9
	5 – 9.9
	10 – 19.9
	20 – 39.9
	≥ 40

FIG. 74. Distribution of leprosy throughout the world (estimated prevalence). Reproduced with the permission of the *Bulletin of World Health Organization.*

be made on a clinical basis in most patients and may be confirmed in many cases by the bacterial positivity of smears from material collected from skin or mucous lesions.

Classification

According to the Committees of Classification of the International Congresses of Leprology (Havana, 1948; Madrid, 1953), leprosy cases should be classified into two types, tuberculoid and lepromatous, and in two groups, indeterminate and borderline (dimorphous). '*Type* connotes clinically and biologically stereotyped features, characterized by marked stability and mutual incompatibility. *Group* connotes less distinctive or positive characteristics, less stability and less certainty with respect to evolution.'

Lepromatous Type (L). 'A malign type, especially stable,[1] strongly positive on bacteriological examination, presenting more or less infiltrated skin lesions, and negative to lepromin. The peripheral nerve trunks become manifestly involved as the disease progresses, habitually in symmetrical fashion, and often with neural sequelae in advanced stages.'

Tuberculoid Type (T). 'Usually benign, stable; generally negative on bacteriological examination; presenting in most cases erythematous skin lesions which are elevated marginally or more extensively; positive to lepromin.

Sequelae of peripheral nerve trunk involvement may develop in a certain proportion of cases, and this may give rise to serious

and disabling deformity. This frequently appears to occur as a result of extension from or through cutaneous nerve branches, rather than of systemic dissemination, and consequently is often asymmetric and unilateral.'

Indeterminate Group (I). 'A benign form relatively unstable, seldom bacteriologically positive, presenting flat skin lesions which may be hypopigmented or erythematous; the reaction to lepromin negative or positive. Neuritic manifestations, more or less extensive, may develop in cases which have persisted as of this group for long periods. The indeterminate group consists essentially of the "simple macular" cases. These cases may evolve towards the lepromatous type or the tuberculoid type, or may remain unchanged indefinitely.'

Borderline (**Dimorphous**) (B). 'A malign form, very unstable; almost always strongly positive on bacteriological examination; the lepromin reaction generally negative. Such cases may arise from the tuberculoid type as a result of repeated reactions, and sometimes they evolve to the lepromatous type. The nasal mucosa often remains bacteriologically negative even when the skin lesions are strongly positive.' (Madrid, 1953.)

Distribution

The Leprosy Problem in the World. There is a lack of accurate data on the prevalence of leprosy in most countries, primarily because case-finding has not reached the desired level in many of them. Bechelli and Martinez (1966, 1970) have attempted, with many reservations, to provide more realistic figures, using information obtained from several sources and

[1] The word 'stable' implies stability as regards the type, not as regards the severity of the disease.

various criteria for calculating estimated prevalence rates. In all there were, in 1965, 2,831,775 registered patients and 10,786,000 estimated cases; the latter figure could well be an underestimation. The number of treated patients was 1,928,000, some 68 per cent. of the registered cases and 18 per cent. of the estimated cases. About 2097 million lived in areas with prevalence rates of 0·5 per 1,000 or higher; in these areas nearly one million new cases of leprosy could be expected within the subsequent 5 years. The estimated number of disabled patients was 3,872,000.

The geographical distribution of registered, estimated, and treated patients by continents is shown in TABLE 53 and by continents and countries in FIGURE 74. In a further paper Bechelli and Martinez (1970) reported: 'Taking into account on the one hand the estimated number of patients in 1965 and the expected number of cases in the subsequent five years, and on the other hand, deaths and releases from control, it is possible that the total number of cases in 1970 will not greatly depart from the 1965 estimate. In spite of the shortcomings of the data provided it seems that the endemics maintain approximately the same level in most countries.'

TABLE 53

Geographical Distribution of Registered, Estimated and Treated Patients

Con-tinent	LEPROSY PATIENTS				
	No. registered	No. estimated	Treated		
			Number	Per cent. of registered	Per cent. of estimated
Africa	1,712,132a	3,868,000	1,062,527b	62·0	27·5
America	177,813	358,000	95,804c	53·9	26·8
Asia	915,525d	6,475,000e	755,334f	82·5	11·7
Europe	16,624g	52,000	9,973h	60·0	19·2
Oceania	9,681	33,000	4,291i	44·3	13·0
Total	2,831,775	10,786,000	1,927,929	68·1	17·9

[a] No information about 12 countries.
[b] No information about 26 countries.
[c] Information about 16 countries only.
[d] Information about 26 countries only.
[e] No information about Mongolia.
[f] Information about 22 countries only.
[g] No information about Romania.
[h] No information about Romania and U.S.S.R.
[i] No information about New Guinea.

Reproduced with permission of the *WHO Bulletin*.

Epidemiology[1]

Myco. leprae has not yet been cultivated. Substantial progress has been made, however, in attempts to transmit *Myco. leprae* to animals. Local multiplication in the foot-pad of mice was first obtained by Shepard (1960), and its spread in the inoculated animal was reported by Kolesov (1968) and Rees (1968); the latter also reported lepromatoid lesions in mice. The hamster has also been infected. Kirchheimer and Storrs (1971) indicated that an armadillo (*Dasypus novemcintus*) developed lepromatoid infection with *Myco. leprae* approximately 14 months after inoculation of leprosy bacilli, from an untreated case of lepromatous leprosy, into the skin of its abdomen and ear lobes. The hamster has also been infected

[1] Based on Bechelli, (1965, 1966).

and, from reports, it appears that the armadillo would be a susceptible animal. This progress may further epidemiological studies in the future.

Man is the only known reservoir of *Myco. leprae*.

The bacilli eliminated from affected skin and/or mucosa can reach the skin and mucosa of healthy individuals through skin-to-skin contact or by means of the Pflügge droplets. Many leprologists have admitted that the transmission of leprosy might also be indirect. Taking into account that mucosa—due to its structure—offers less resistance than the skin to penetration by bacteria, the nasal mucosa may more frequently be the portal of entry of *Myco. leprae* than the skin.

For the control of leprosy the following epidemiological information is important:

1. Lepromatous and borderline cases are the most infectious. Tuberculoid cases (in reaction) have a certain degree of infectiousness. According to Hanks (1945) one gram of tissue from a leproma could contain as many as seven billion[2] bacilli.

In the Philippines it was found that the risk of contracting leprosy was almost four times as high for those in contact with the lepromatous type as for those in contact with the tuberculoid type (Doull *et al.*, 1942). The risk was almost eight times as high as for persons for whom no history of exposure to either type could be obtained. This was confirmed in a further study (Guinto *et al.*, 1954) but the rate for the non-lepromatous forms was only 1⅓ times that of apparently unexposed persons. Doull *et al.* (quoted by WHO Expert Committee on Leprosy, 1960) have shown that household contact with the tuberculoid type of leprosy does not involve an appreciably higher risk than that to which the general population is normally exposed.

According to the Second Report of the WHO Expert Committee on Leprosy (1960), the continued maintenance of high prevalence rates in hyperendemic areas where tuberculoid type leprosy constitutes as much as 90 per cent. of the total cases may be attributed, at least in part, to the usually undetermined proportion of cases becoming 'open' during periods of reaction.

2. The Third Report of the WHO Expert Committee on Leprosy (1966) emphasized that exposure to known cases cannot be established in an appreciable proportion of leprosy infections, even in young children, partly because of the long incubation period. Undetected cases with inconspicuous lesions may account for some untraceable infections.

3. The majority of individuals are resistant to leprosy, as shown by epidemiological studies (i.e. relatively low percentage of conjugal infection; only some of the children exposed to leprosy acquire it) and by the lepromin reaction (over 80 per cent. of the individuals are lepromin-positive after adolescence).

Lepromin-negative contacts are more likely both to acquire leprosy and to develop it in the lepromatous type, compared with the lepromin-positive contacts. This is generally accepted by leprologists and supported by the findings of Dharmendra and Chatterjee (1955).

4. The attack rate in continuously exposed children aged 3 to 6 years, repeatedly observed for different periods of time, was 36·2 per cent. (Lara, 1961). In the Nauru epidemics, the most important in the world, 30 per cent. of the population (about 1,500 natives) showed signs of leprosy. In the most

[2] Billion = a thousand millions.

endemic countries the rates may exceptionally reach 50 per 1,000 and more.

5. Spontaneous disappearance of certain leprosy lesions is frequent. In Lara and Nolasco's study (1956) 77 per cent. of early childhood cases were free of lesions before adult life. At the Silver Jubilee Children's Clinic, Madras, where 644 non-lepromatous child cases were followed up for periods varying from one to 20 years without any treatment being given to them, spontaneous arrest of the disease was seen in about 65 per cent. of cases—in over 55 per cent. of the maculo-anaesthetic, over 78 per cent. of the minor tuberculoid, and over 88 per cent. of the major tuberculoid cases.[1]

6. Doull *et al.* (1942) have pointed out that the average incidence of lepromatous leprosy is strikingly low at less than 0·5 per 1,000 per year. On the same lines, according to Newell (1966): 'In no survey or study published . . ., even in an epidemic situation, has a lepromatous leprosy point prevalence rate in a population been reported greater than 15 per 1,000 persons . . .'; and 'At no recorded time did the lepromatous rate reach as high as 2 per cent.' This may be evidence that even lepromin-negative individuals may have some resistance against leprosy or against the lepromatous type of the disease.

7. It is known that leprosy has a long incubation period, an average of 3 to 5 years.

8. Leprosy may occur at any age. It seems that the difference in prevalence in the various age-groups would depend chiefly on earlier or later exposure to *Myco. leprae*. In countries where leprosy is highly endemic exposure starts earlier in life and children and young adults have higher leprosy rates (Bechelli and Rotberg, 1949; Doull, 1962; Bechelli, Martinez Dominguez, and Patwary, 1963).

In almost all countries the lepromatous rate is significantly higher in men after puberty.

Leprosy may occur in all races. There is no certain evidence of racial resistance.

9. According to some authors there is no evidence of transmission of susceptibility from parent to child. Some (Beiguelman and Quagliato, 1965) have obtained data which 'strongly suggests an intrafamilial relationship for the lepromin reaction'. Beiguelman, Dall'Aglio, and da Silva (1968) have reported that family concentration of leprosy cases is not random. Beiguelman, in collaboration with Souza-Campos, and Pinto Jr. (1967), also reported that the proportion of strong lepromin reactors after B.C.G. vaccination is significantly lower in the healthy offspring of lepromatous parents as compared to controls of healthy extraction.

Control[2]

The control of leprosy is based on:

1. Health education.
2. Early diagnosis.
3. Early treatment, especially of those who may become infectious, but also of tuberculoid patients in order to prevent deformities.
4. Reduction or elimination of infectiousness of open cases by regular treatment, which should be started as early as possible.

5. Out-patient care and consequent reduction of the number of in-patients to the absolute minimum.
6. Follow-up of those inactive patients who are most liable to relapse and again become infectious.
7. Protection of the susceptible population.
8. Training of medical and auxiliary personnel.
9. Prevention of disabilities and rehabilitation of leprosy cases.
10. Social assistance to the patients and their families.

All these activities have usually been carried out by special services with their own personnel, but a need has gradually arisen for the co-operation of the public health units and the integration of leprosy control activities into the latter.

A public health approach to leprosy control is necessary and has been strongly recommended. At present, leprosy is endemic in developing countries which have to face other public health problems, along with limited resources, and have to carry on educational, socio-economic and other programmes. Full advantage should, however, be taken of these resources to discover and to treat the maximum number of patients—especially the contagious, or those liable to become infectious—to reduce their infectiousness and, in this way, protect the population. Priority should be given to those programmes which contribute most efficiently to reducing the prevalence of leprosy.

The application of present knowledge in the control of leprosy in field projects should be made in a flexible, practical, and economical way, taking into account the characteristics of the endemic, the structure of health services, the availability of resources, and local conditions.

Recognizing the impossibility, in many areas, of overcoming present difficulties, a system of priorities (Bechelli, 1963, 1965; WHO Expert Committee on Leprosy, 1966) should be adopted, based on the limitations of each area and in accordance with local conditions.

Countries with limited budgets, only a few doctors, and facing other serious problems, should first of all treat the lepromatous and other infectious cases and the indeterminate lepromin-negatives.[3] They should keep under surveillance child household contacts, especially those of infectious cases, and try to help patients in the prevention of disabilities. Means and personnel should be concentrated on infectious cases and their contacts, particularly children.

At the other extreme, countries with adequate budgets and good leprosy services, whether or not integrated in the public health service, should diagnose and treat as early as possible *all* patients, maintain surveillance of *all* contacts, prevent disabilities, rehabilitate *all* patients with deformities, and examine systematically certain population groups, in particular children.

The drug currently used for treatment, dapsone, belongs to the sulphone group and is administered orally. Several other drugs have been tried, and some (thiambutosine, long-acting sulphonamides, rifampicin, clofazimine) have been effective to a certain extent. However, the 1970 WHO Expert Committee on Leprosy felt that oral administration of dapsone is still the most practical method of treatment for mass campaigns.

Experience in several centres shows that almost all lepro-

[1] Dr. Dharmendra's communication to WHO, 25 May 1964.
[2] Based on Bechelli 1965 and 1966 (Guide).

[3] In countries in which it is not possible to perform the lepromin test, the indeterminate cases should also receive first priority.

matous patients under very close supervision and regularly treated with sulphone for 10 years no longer show bacilli in skin smears. Among lepromatous cases detected early, about 90 per cent. may become inactive or 'arrested' after 5 years. Theoretically, the existing methods should lead to the control of leprosy, provided that they are thoroughly and correctly applied and that favourable conditions exist in which to do so, including full co-operation of the population and of those concerned. The load of infectiousness should be significantly reduced in a relatively short time. However, dapsone has a slow effect in the serious forms of leprosy. This is its main short-coming.

Because of the length of treatment required in lepromatous cases, a large proportion of patients attend only irregularly. Many drop out or become out-of-control cases. In addition, a high proportion of inactive or 'arrested' cases relapse, mainly those whose treatment was irregular. More than 50 per cent. of these irregularly treated cases may have relapsed at the end of 9 years. Because patients remain infectious for so long, leprosy remains endemic for many decades.

To find out whether dapsone could be used for the *prevention* of leprosy, trials in India and the Philippines have been carried out with partial WHO support. Child contacts of infectious cases, and children living in a sanatorium for leprosy patients, were given either a large dose of dapsone (almost reaching therapeutic levels) or about one-third to two-thirds of this dosage. In both countries, there was a reduction in the number of new cases of about 50 per cent., attributable to the chemo-prophylaxis (WHO Expert Committee on Leprosy, 1970).

Three controlled field trials are currently in progress to investigate the prevention of leprosy by B.C.G. vaccination. The first trial was started in 1960 in Uganda, the second in 1962 in eastern New Guinea, and the third was begun by WHO in Burma in 1964. The findings in the Uganda trial are strikingly different from those so far obtained in Burma and in Karimui, New Guinea, although it is hoped that the value of B.C.G. against leprosy, especially the lepromatous form, will ultimately be clearly determined. For this reason, the WHO Expert Committee on Leprosy (1970) considered it premature to recommend B.C.G. vaccination for the prevention of leprosy. The trials should be extended for at least 10 years; special attention will be paid to the effect of B.C.G. on very young children, particularly the newborn.

The socio-economic, health, and cultural situation is poor or unsatisfactory in most areas where leprosy is endemic. There is usually a shortage of doctors, and many are not interested in working on leprosy control projects. In one area with 500,000 registered cases of leprosy, only five doctors were available for supervision of the paramedical staff. Salaries are not high enough to encourage staff members to devote themselves fully to leprosy work, so doctors prefer to work in other health sectors or to have a private practice. First-rate work is extremely difficult when personnel do not work full-time, or receive inadequate salaries. Leprosy campaigns have been further hampered by the appointment of personnel, even to managerial posts, who lack the necessary technical qualifications. Political instability has also retarded the development of health programmes.

In several countries, leprosy has a low priority in relation to other diseases. Even where it is highly prevalent, the health services may have to deal with other serious diseases which are more widespread and cause more deaths. The health infra-structure is poor in many countries and adequate in only a few. Consequently, the contribution of health units to leprosy control has been limited or unsatisfactory. Not enough time is devoted to the teaching of leprology in most medical schools. Finally, funds are often limited, and the fullest advantage of resources may not be taken because of inadequate planning and programming.

At present, with existing drugs and the prevailing socio-economic and cultural conditions, the prospects of controlling leprosy in a few decades are not bright in most countries. It should be remembered, however, that syphilis has still not been eradicated in the course of half a century, in spite of such drugs as arsenicals, bismuth and, lately, long-acting penicillin. The best solution to the huge leprosy problem is to stimulate and increase research in leprology.

STAPHYLOCOCCAL AND STREPTOCOCCAL SKIN INFECTIONS (PYODERMAS)

In spite of the progress achieved in the therapy of staphyl-ococcal and streptococcal infections, pyodermas continue to be among the most frequent skin diseases. These infections may occur either in the community or in nurseries, medical and surgical wards of hospitals, and may acquire a particular pattern in each circumstance. They have a clinical trait in common: in most of them a pustule is very often one of the skin lesions which leads to the diagnosis of pyodermas. The *Staphylococcus pyogenes* and *Streptococcus pyogenes* infections occur through-out the world and mainly in those areas and layers of the population where personal hygiene does not reach a satisfactory level.

The staphylococcus and the streptococcus may determine inflammatory lesions in the different layers of the skin and in the annexes, thus resulting in skin affections with particular clinical aspects. Only the surface of the skin may be affected, as in *impetigo*, or the epidermis and part of the superficial dermis, as in *ecthyma*. The hair follicle may be affected in its opening (*osteofolliculitis, Bockhardt's impetigo* or *perifolliculitis*), in depth (*folliculitis, sycosis barbae*) and in addition, the sebace-ous glands may also be affected (*furunculosis*). The infection may affect the sweat glands (*periporitis, multiple sweat gland abscesses of infants* and *hydrosadenitis*), the dermis (*cellulitis* and *erysipelas*) or the peri-unguial folds (*paronychia*). *Abscesses* may also occur.

The same organism may therefore produce different clinical manifestations according to the site of infection. This site is conditioned by individual factors. Some patients present only one type of pyoderma while others present two or more forms of the infection. The susceptibility may vary in course of time: on a certain occasion a patient presents furunculosis for weeks or months and, on other occasions, sycosis, hydrosadenitis or another form of pyoderma. The deeper the skin and annexes are affected (furunculosis, abscess, erysipelas, hydrosadenitis), the greater is the possibility of the skin lesion being accom-panied by general symptoms (fever, headaches, and lymph node enlargement). These forms of pyodermas are less frequent than the others. In surgical wards of hospitals, furuncles or stitch abscess, besides the secondary infection of wounds, are the commonest forms of pyodermas.

Most forms of pyodermas are usually uncomplicated. However, impetigo for example may be complicated by glomerulonephritis and, very rarely, by liver abscess and osteomyelitis. Neonatal breast abscess, septicaemia, meningitis, osteomyelitis, brain abscess, and staphylococcal pneumonia may occur in cases of pemphigus neonatorum and exfoliative staphylococcal dermatitis.

In a sensitized organism the blood dissemination of bacterial products or toxins causes scattered lesions (microbides) with few or no bacteria.

The pyodermas are primary skin infections determined by the streptococcus and the staphylococcus. Pyogenic lesions may be observed in certain diseases (acne, tinea pedis, scabiosis, eczema and others), but such lesions are not considered as pyodermas but as secondary infections. Nevertheless, these should be treated and prevented by the same procedures adopted for the pyodermas.

The Infectious Agents

Staphylococcus pyogenes is one of the permanent bacterial flora of normal skin (in the annexes); it is estimated that between 30 to 50 per cent. of healthy individuals carry it on the body surface. It is found with certain frequency in the upper respiratory apparatus: 30 to 40 per cent. and 80 to 90 per cent. in repeated examinations during 10 weeks (Williams, 1946). The streptococcus, on the other hand, is not found among the organisms of the permanent bacterial flora in the normal skin. *Streptococcus pyogenes* is found in the pharynx and nose, less frequently, however, than the staphylococcus (up to 15 per cent. of normal individuals). According to the WHO Expert Committee (1968), surveys made in schools and homes have shown that occasionally as many as 40 to 50 per cent. of children may harbour streptococci at any one time during the school year. These carriers of *Streptococcus pyogenes* usually do not have symptoms of a respiratory disease, but serial determinations of antibody show that some exhibit increasing titres. It follows that a portion of these asymptomatic carriers will have recently acquired the streptococci and therefore have the potential to spread the infection, while the remainder will have been carriers for many weeks and therefore may be considered less dangerous. Streptococci deposited in dust and on objects in the environment may be viable and may cause infections of the skin or of burns.

The pathogenic streptococci and staphylococci which infect the skin or contaminate skin lesions proceed from the upper respiratory tract, through the nose and pharynx and reach the skin by means of droplets or on the fingers of the carriers. Consequently, in the control of the staphylococcal and streptococcal infections it is necessary to prevent transmission by intimate contact. The environmental factors which increase the numbers of such contacts and the duration of carrying the infection will increase opportunities for the spread of the above infections. The role of contaminated articles is not well determined. In nurseries, pathogenic strains colonized in the upper respiratory tract, rectum or circumcision site may be the origin of the skin lesions.

However, as for other infections, the presence of the organism alone is not enough to determine the pyodermas since *susceptibility* to it is also required. Local factors (excoriations, maceration of the skin, traumas, pre-existing dermatosis, lack of hygiene) may play a role as well as internal factors, for instance diabetes. Age may be an important factor and there are some infections which are more common in infants and children (exfoliative dermatitis of the newborn, pemphigus neonatorum, impetigo). Anatomical conditions should also be considered: the horny layer offers resistance to the penetration of bacteria, while the opening of the follicles and the sweat glands offer less resistance.

The *contagiousness* of pyodermas varies. There are certain forms which are very contagious, for instance impetigo. Auto-inoculation may occur and the infection spreads by means of contact of the infected skin with the healthy skin, mainly in intertriginous areas.

The *incubation period* is probably a few days but it may be difficult to determine it.

The *diagnosis* of pyodermas is made on a clinical basis. The simple presence of staphylococci in a lesion may not be the proof that they are causing it, because they may be found in normal skin.

In the *prevention* of pyodermas early diagnosis and early treatment of cases with clinical disease is necessary. This is particularly important for children in families or at schools. Local treatment, in the superficial and crusted lesions, consists in the removal of crusts and exudates with cotton soaked in oil, in the opening of pustules, followed by wet dressings with Alibour's water (diluted 1/10), potassium permanganate (1/4,000 to 1/10,000) or bichloride of mercury (1/2,000) for 15–30 minutes. After this an ointment is applied: yellow oxide of mercury (1 or 2 per cent. in petrolatum), ammoniated mercury, or an ointment with antibiotics (tyrothricin, neomycin, bacitracin, gramicidin). Local treatment is enough when dealing with localized and superficial pyodermas (impetigo, ecthyma, perifolliculitis, periporitis). When the lesions are generalized or there is the possibility of complications, antibiotics or sulphonamides are recommended. It is obligatory to use them when the skin lesions are accompanied by fever, headache, cellulitis, and lymph node enlargement. Septicaemia is efficiently treated or prevented by antibiotics and sulphonamides. After these, vaccinotherapy (mainly anatoxin) can be used, especially for relapsing infections or those which last for a long time. In the case of allergy to penicillin, other antibiotics—erythromycin, cephalosporin, tetracycline, rifampicin—are recommended. 'Hospital' staphylococci may be resistant to several antibiotics and the treatment of the infections they cause may be more difficult. However, there is no sure evidence that these staphylococci are more virulent than the strains prevalent outside hospital. Surgical treatment is indicated for some pyodermas (hydrosadenitis, multiple abscesses of infants) but not for furuncles. Radiotherapy is limited only to special cases (furunculosis, hydrosadenitis) of very painful lesions.

Public health education in modes of transmission and in personal hygiene is necessary to avoid auto-infection or the common use of toilet articles. Contact of infected persons with infants and debilitated persons is to be avoided. Dressings from open lesions should be burned or adequately disposed of. Surveillance of contacts in school or in the family is useful; they should be educated as indicated above, and should report when they present some lesions suspected of being pyodermas.

Aseptic techniques and a high level of staff hygiene are required in nurseries and hospitals. See also the section on hospital cross-infection in CHAPTER 44.

SKIN DISEASES DUE TO ANIMAL PARASITES

Parasitic dermatoses are more frequent in the geographical areas or sectors of the population in which there is poor hygiene and education, or, apparently, during time of war and socio-economic crises. Poor housing, favouring contact and promiscuity, is another important factor in the spread of these diseases. As mentioned earlier, certain types of such skin diseases have a particular geographical distribution in the same country: for instance, in Brazil filariasis is found in the Amazonia region and in limited areas of the north-east, while schistosomiasis dermatitis is found only in the north-east and central-west. Creeping eruption (larva migrans) is more common in the coastal areas; tungiasis and myiasis are seen in rural areas; in contrast, pediculosis capitis and oxyuriasis may occur in any part of the world.

The skin condition is very occasionally caused by a single parasite; usually these are numerous, as in scabies, pediculosis, and creeping eruption. In these dermatoses the lesions are superficial and may be easily treated. However, if untreated secondary infection or eczema may complicate them, and the infected lesions may be the origin—although this happens rarely—of grave internal conditions such as glomerulonephritis in infected scabies.

Scabies

Caused by *Sarcoptes scabiei*, scabies is a widespread disease. Endemic in developing countries or in areas where the standard of living and hygiene is low, the frequency of scabies decreased substantially about 25 years ago. However, in past years its incidence has increased again in many countries, causing epidemics in some areas. Following information received from dermatologists in the United States and 33 other countries, Orkin (1971) indicated that the current epidemic has not yet involved the United States or Canada; scabies is rare in Australia, Hungary, Japan, Romania, Uruguay, and Venezuela, but very common in Argentina, Brazil, Great Britain, France, Germany (East and West), Italy, Mexico, Morocco, Poland, Portugal, and the Soviet Union. According to Orkin, there is no explanation for this recent acceleration of incidence, and cyclic fluctuations of scabies have never been fully understood; changing morality could be a promoting factor, besides poor hygiene. The occurrence of scabies in the sexually active age-group of 16 to 30 years is pointed out by some. Importation of itinerant workers and increased travel could also play a role.

The most important symptom is itching, usually more intense during the night. Pin-point papules or vesicles and tiny linear burrows (with the mites and their eggs) may be seen in the axilla, buttocks, wrists, interdigital spaces, penis and around the mammary areola. In patients with good hygiene a diagnosis of scabies may be very difficult.

The reservoir of infection is man. The disease is very contagious, and transmission occurs by direct and intimate contact, and also by the use of soiled bedclothes or underwear recently contaminated by a patient. In fact, outside the human organism, the larvae usually die in less than 8 hours. As mentioned above, it is frequently acquired during sexual intercourse. Among the persons living with the patient one or several contacts are affected and this epidemiological information is useful in diagnosing scabies.

The incubation period is about a month. Patients stop transmitting the disease usually after one course of treatment. However, most of the clinical manifestations are of an allergic nature and may persist after the destruction of the parasite; this explains the apparent lack of success of treatment in some cases (Borda, 1954). When reinfestation occurs, a single oviparous female is able to cause widespread lesions in the skin due to hypersensitivity. In these cases it is difficult to find the parasite.

Prevention consists in the treatment of patients, examination of contacts and their treatment if infected. All of them should be treated at the same time to avoid a 'ping-pong' scabies. After a warm bath with soap, benzyl benzoate (ointment or solution, 20 to 30 per cent., preferably the latter) is applied all over the body; the medicament is used for three consecutive nights. Usually only one treatment is needed. DDT 5 to 10 per cent. (larvicide) and benzocaine 2 per cent. (ovicide and anaesthetic) may be used in conjunction with the benzyl benzoate. If required, treatment may be repeated after 10 days. Milian and Helmerich's ointments (containing sulphur or its derivatives) are also effective but their odour limits their use. If the scabies is complicated by eczema, the latter should be treated first.

To avoid reinfection, underwear and bedclothes have to be boiled; dust mattress with DDT, 10 per cent. in talc.

Infected children should be prevented from attending school and their closer contacts examined or alerted about the disease. Education of patients, their families, and contacts is necessary.

Pediculosis

Pediculosis is found throughout the world. Three types of pediculosis affect the skin: pediculosis of the scalp caused by *Pediculosis humanus var. capitis*, pediculosis of the body determined by *Pediculus humanus var. corporis*, and pediculosis pubis or phthiriasis whose agent is *Phthirus pubis*.

Pediculosis of the scalp is frequent in persons of low social class but may also occur in individuals with high standards of living. Itching of any part of the scalp, more frequent and intense in the occipital region, is the fundamental symptom. *Pediculus capitis* lives by preference in the occipital region, from where it spreads to other regions of the scalp and occasionally to the interscapular space and proximities. The female's eggs or nits are white and elongated and fixed longitudinally along the hairs by means of a gelatinous substance which becomes solid. Many eggs may be found on the same hair.

Infestation with *Pediculus capitis* is much more frequent in children and women and very rare in the adult male. Epidemics among schoolchildren may occur. Infested persons are the reservoirs of infection. Transmission usually occurs by direct contact with the infested person but may also be indirect through use of clothing, head gear, and other personal belongings of invested individuals. In many cases the parasites are not so numerous and the diagnosis is more difficult. Because of secondary infections, impetigo, folliculitis and also eczema, the real nature of the skin condition may go unnoticed. Thus in all patients with pruritus, pyogenic infection or eczematous dermatitis of the scalp, pediculosis must be remembered and sought for. The lice may also migrate to the eyebrows and eyelashes, axillae and upper parts of the thorax.

Pediculosis of the body is found in the adult. The symptoms are intense itching and linear excoriations revealed by haemorrhagic crusts, localized in the trunk, mainly in the abdomen, interscapular space, buttocks and thighs. Hyperpigmentation may also occur and in this case, with all these manifestations, the disease is known by the name of *maladie des vagabondes*. Secondary infection, impetigo, folliculitis, and furunculosis, occur frequently. Pediculosis of the body is found in individuals of the lower social stratum.

Pediculus corporis does not live on the skin surface like *Pediculus capitis*, but in the folds of clothes where the eggs are deposited and fixed in the threads of tissue. The lice rely on the skin only for food, which they obtain by biting and sucking the host. Exceptionally, they deposit eggs in the hair of the axillae, moustache and even on the scalp.

Pediculosis pubis is evidenced by itching and bluish macules (*maculae cerulae*). Eczematous dermatitis may occur. The parasites are localized in the pubic region and rarely reach the axilla region, moustache, eyebrows, eyelashes, and only very occasionally the hair. As in pediculosis of the scalp, the eggs are deposited on the hairs and transmission occurs by direct contact with infested individuals, particularly during sexual intercourse, but also indirectly through use of toilets.

Control of the three types of pediculosis is undertaken with the treatment of infested individuals, health education of the public concerning hygiene, washing and laundering of clothes to destroy the lice and nits, and examination of contacts, mainly in schools or institutions. Infested individuals and their contacts who are also infested should be treated at the same time. In school epidemics mass treatment may be necessary. The treatment of pediculosis of the scalp consists of washing the scalp with soap followed by application of a solution of DDT 5 per cent. or bichloride of mercury 0·50 per cent. (in conjunction with vinegar and camphorated alcohol in equal parts, 25 per cent. and water) or xylol (two drops in 50 g. of vaseline).

For the treatment of pediculosis of the body, the body itself and personal clothes and bedclothing should be dusted with benzyl benzoate 10 per cent. or DDT 5 per cent. in talc.

Pediculosis pubis is treated by washing with soap and applying DDT 5 per cent. in a solution or 10 per cent. in talc daily for one week. To these agents benzocaine (a larvicide) may be added.

In the three forms of pediculosis when the lice are resistant to DDT, *gamma* benzene hexachloride 1 per cent. dusting powder or 1 per cent. ointment may be used, but not in conjunction with insect repellants or oily liquids applied to the skin.

Larva Migrans or Creeping Disease

This disease is observed in sea-bathers, gardeners, children, or others who are exposed to sandy soil contaminated with dog and/or cat faeces containing hookworms (*Ancylostoma braziliense* and *A. caninum*). Entering through the skin the larva migrates intracutaneously and causes initially a small papule and then a serpiginous threadlike track. It is usually localized in the plantar region but may also be found in the buttocks and trunk. Itching is very intense. Secondary infection may occur.

The disease is treated with thiabendazol by mouth (25 mg./kg. body weight three times a day for three days) or locally with 5 per cent. ointment. If thiabendazol is not available, each larva could be killed by freezing the skin with ethyl chloride spray or with CO_2 snow: both are applied in the oedematous or erythematous extremity of the track in whose vicinity the larva is found.

NON-COMMUNICABLE SKIN DISEASES

Among the non-communicable dermatoses, contact and occupational dermatitis, due to their economic implications, are of great importance in already industrialized countries, and in those countries where industrialization is being developed. Skin cancer and precancerous dermatosis should also be mentioned. The action of sunlight on the skin (lucitis, keratosis senilis, skin cancer) is worth noting: in individuals of the same nationality skin cancer is more frequent where the actinic irradiation is more intense and prolonged (for instance in Australia as compared with the United Kingdom). The pigmentation of the skin plays a role with regard to skin cancer, which is more common in albinos and individuals of light skin, and rare in Negroes. Several dermatoses may potentially evolve into cancer, and require preventive action (senile keratosis, leukoplakia, kraurosis vulvae, radiodermatitis, arsenical keratosis, and certain scars).

Drug eruptions represent another important group of skin affections, sometimes very serious (Stevens-Johnson and Lyell syndromes, giant urticaria) and even fatal; effective control of the use of drugs, taking into account their side-effects, is most important. Sometimes these effects become evident only after large-scale use of a drug.

The hereditary cutaneous disorders (genodermatoses) may be inaesthetic, may cause disability (keratosis palmaris and plantaris, epidermolysis bullosa), death (foetal ichthyosis) and may evolve into cancer (xeroderma pigmentosum). In certain areas they may acquire particular importance. Preventive measures should be taken to decrease the incidence of these dermatoses, following the advice of geneticists, and/or by reducing exposure to mutagenic agents, i.e. ionizing radiation (radiographic and radioscopic examinations, radium and radiotherapy, isotopes).

SKIN DISEASES DUE TO CHEMICAL AGENTS

Chemical agents, organic or inorganic, when in contact with the skin may cause pathological changes; these vary according to the nature, concentration, and physical status of the agent, duration and means of exposure, and also the anatomical, physiological, and immunological conditions of the skin. A diversity of morphological and evolutive aspects of the skin response results from the interaction of the above factors.

Exposure to chemical agents in a concentration which does not affect the skin of most individuals, causes a dermatitis when the exposed person has a specific hypersensitivity to the substances. Into this group fall the majority of cases of contact dermatitis, among which is also included *professional* or *occupational dermatitis*.

Contact dermatitis or *dermatitis venenata*, occurring after exposure of sensitized individuals to certain agents (drug, plant, or commercial products), appears as an eczematous eruption, with erythematous vesicular plaques, sometimes with bullae, accompanied by pruritus. In the majority of cases this is localized in the area of the site exposed to the agent. The site of the dermatitis often suggests the possible causative agent.

Great numbers of agents are known to cause contact dermatitis. They may be present in soaps, cosmetics, scalp dyes or lotions, toothpastes, hand lotions, deodorants, shampoos, dusting powders, lacquer, resinous woods, dyes, leather, volatile oils, formalin, turpentine, cement, plants, and others. Cream bases or vehicles for topical preparations and cosmetics may cause it—and more frequently than is thought (Fisher, Pascher, and Kanof, 1971).

In many areas of the United States, poison ivy is one of the most important causes of dermatitis venenata.

It is not possible to prevent people from using the above articles, and women from using cosmetics; however the public in general should be informed of the possibility of having a skin reaction following the use of certain cosmetics and substances or exposure to certain plants. Moreover, legislation should prevent the word 'harmless' being used on the label of certain products.

When dermatitis venenata appears, the symptomatic treatment consists in the use of wet dressings with boric acid solution (3 per cent.) or potassium permanganate (1/4,000 to 1/10,000) and corticosteroids in creams and eventually by mouth, depending on the seriousness and extent of the process. However, the important measure is the aetiological treatment: based on the anamnesis and on patch tests, the substance which contains the harmful allergen should be detected and the patient recommended to avoid further exposure to it. With the elimination of the allergen the dermatitis heals and does not recur.

The *occupational or professional skin diseases* constitute a very important group because of their human, social, and economic implications. In a broad sense, the group of occupational dermatoses could include not only those caused by allergens and depending on a previous sensitization, but also those related to non-sensitizing agents. Gay Prieto, Jadassohn, Lapière, and Serri (1968) give a list of the most common ones.

1. Occupational stigmata of the skin.
2. Occupational disorders of the sebaceous glands (acne provoked by gases, metals, metaloids, halogens, acids, alkalis, turpentine, lacquers, varnishes, paraffin, lubricants, benzine, gasoline, vaseline, tar, pitch, coal blocks, dyes, vegetable substance, X-rays, etc.). Follicular keratosis.
3. Occupational disorders of the sweat glands (hyperidrosis, anidrosis, bromidrosis).
4. Occupational hair ailments (alopecias).
5. Occupational pigmentation disorders (melanoderma, achromias).
6. Occupational tattoos.

7. Occupational diseases (not accidents) due to cold, heat, electrical current, ionizing rays.
8. Occupational skin infections (erysipeloid, vaccinia milker's nodules, pyodermas, tuberculosis of the skin, etc.).
9. Occupational skin mycosis (ringworm of animal origin in farmworkers, eczema from yeast in bakers, mycosis of the feet in miners, etc.).
10. Cutaneous cancer (the regulations of many institutions consider skin cancer as occupational in workers using tar or asphalt[1] but none considers it occupational in farmworkers, and fishermen. It is far more common in very sunny countries such as those of the Mediterranean basin and the tablelands of South America and Australia).
11. Miscellaneous occupational skin disorders: This group is the largest and most varied and is even more difficult from the diagnostic and therapeutic point of view. The disorders in this group may be due to many different causes, such as eczema in the hands of domestic employees, arising from small, repeated trauma with the use of water, detergents, protective substances, etc.

The most common occupational dermatitis is that caused by cement. Pesticides, used in agricultural work, are also a common cause of dermatitis.

The diagnosis of occupational dermatitis and the detection of the causative agents is based on their clinical aspect, anamnesis, and patch tests. The patient should receive labour compensation and avoid exposure to the harmful agents. Manufacturing processes should be developed to eliminate the allergen from the substances, as in the case of cement. In the manufacture of paints and varnishes, turpentine should be replaced by other products; paraphenylenediamine and ammonium persulphate, used in hair-dressing and causing occupational dermatitis, should be replaced, for instance, by paraphenylenetoludine. Certain agents have to be banned, such as the ammonium persulphate added to flour which causes dermatitis in bakers and pastry cooks. Testing of newly manufactured substances is obligatory to anticipate their eventual action as sensitizers. Workers have to be educated in hygienic precautions and the use of gloves (leather gloves for those working with cement; cotton gloves and over these rubber gloves, when working with detergents, soaps, etc.).

When, in spite of all the measures of prevention, dermatitis and relapses occur, the worker may be advised to take a different job, and such 'changes' may cause serious problems.

In industrialized countries students in medical schools should receive training on the subject. Legislation on occupational dermatitis is required. See also CHAPTER 39 on occupation and health.

DRUG ERUPTIONS

The problem of adverse drug reactions is of interest all over the world. In the United States, recent studies have shown that about 4 per cent. to 6 per cent. of hospital admissions are due to adverse drug reactions and about 10 per cent. to 18 per cent. of hospitalized patients experience a drug reaction before discharge (Friedman, Collen, Harris, Van Brunt, and Davis, 1971). Sometimes, the undesirable effects of a drug become

Pitch, creosote, anthracone oil, tar oils, and soot complete the list.

manifest after it has been in use for many years or after a considerable number of individuals have taken it.

Among the adverse drug reactions those occurring in the skin are an important group. *Drug eruption* or *dermatitis medicamentosa* comprises the skin manifestation caused by ingested, injected, or inhaled drugs. The sudden appearance of the skin lesions after or during use of a drug, their symmetrical widespread distribution and their regression when the administration of the drug is stopped, are factors which favour a diagnosis of drug eruption.

The dermatological manifestations consist of maculopapular lesions, erythematous plaques, papules, nodules, bullae, vegetation, pustules, purpura, and may also mimic certain dermatoses.

Several types of lesions may be produced in the same individual or in different persons by the same drug; the opposite may also occur, as different drugs may produce identical eruption. Certain skin manifestations and the drugs which may produce them are listed below:

Morbilliform or scarlatiniform eruptions: sulphonamides, antibiotics, salicylates, arsenic, digitalis, griseofulvin, isoniazid, tranquillizers.

Erythema multiforme: penicillin, aspirin, antipyrin, salicylate, sulphonamides, quinine, barbiturates.

Vesicular eruptions: antibiotics, meprobamate, anaesthetics, arsenicals, sulphonamides.

Bullous eruptions: iodides, bromides, salicylate, aspirin, arsenic, sulphonamides.

Drug eruption with vegetation and verrucous lesions: bromides, iodides.

Eruptions due to photosensitivity: sulphonamides, griseofulvin, chlorpromazine, tetracycline, reserpine.

Fixed pigmented erythema: barbiturates, phenolphthalein, rarely aspirin, antipyrin, sulphonamides.

Melanosis: arsenic, chloroquine, chlorpromazine.

Acne medicamentosa: bromides, iodides, PAS, and isoniazid.

Urticaria and angioneurotic oedema (*Quincke*): penicillin, atropine, salicylate, aspirin, antihistaminics, tranquillizers, griseofulvin, ACTH.

Exfoliative dermatitis or erythrodermia: arsenic, gold, antibiotics, sulphonamides.

Lupus erythematosus-like eruption: hydrallazine, and hydantoin derivates.

Lichen planus-like eruption: sulphonamides, arsenic, antimalarial drugs, para-aminosalicylic acid, bismuth.

Some of the eruptions (Stevens-Johnson and Lyell syndromes, systemic lupus erythematosus-like eruptions) are very serious.

Treatment consists in the suppression of the harmful drug and symptomatic topical or general treatment (steroids for severe generalized eruption). *Prevention* depends on avoiding the indiscriminate use or prescription of sensitizing drugs, including topical application, and the development of drug monitoring systems, covering large populations. These require the systematic reporting, recording and evaluation of untoward events developing in users of drugs, with or without prescription. A WHO pilot project was set up to investigate the feasibility of establishing an international monitoring system based on case-reports from national centres. WHO consultants considered that, 'an international monitoring system could contribute to health programmes in a number of areas, and, by rapid accumulation and dissemination of information on adverse drug reactions, strengthen and complement the work of national drug monitoring centres. . . . Drug monitoring could assist in producing evidence of a cause-and-effect relationship between a drug and an adverse reaction, give the clinical pharmacologist leads for the elucidation of the mechanisms of adverse reactions and guide the clinician in the selection and use of drugs.' (Royall, 1971).

The number of drug eruptions may be reduced with adequate measures but only to a certain point. For serious diseases the use of drugs with the potentiality to cause eruption cannot be discarded; in such cases, the doctor should weigh the risk of inciting a drug eruption against the risks of the relevant disease.

DERMATOSIS AND SKIN CHANGES CAUSED BY PHYSICAL AGENTS

Mechanical, thermic, actinic, and electrical agents and ionizing radiation may cause skin dermatoses or alterations, whose aspect, histological picture, and evolution vary depending upon the nature of the agent, means and duration of action, and within certain limits upon the conditions of the skin (thickness, colour, anatomical site, and age). For example, with the same exposure to sunlight different individuals present a different skin response according to the thickness, colour, and exposed area of the skin: in blondes or albinos sunlight may produce erythema and bullae while in individuals with dark skin these alterations do not occur or are very mild. The skin pigment offers protection against sunlight and dark-skinned people are better defended against it. As indicated before, skin cancer is very rare among them but frequent in albinos.

Dermatitis or skin conditions produced by exposure to cold (*erythema pernio, dermatitis congelationis*), to heat (burns, *erythema ab igne*), to sunlight (sunburn, photodermatitis, premalignant lesions) and to excessive ionizing radiation (*radiodermatitis*) may and should be avoided or reduced to a minimum by adequate measures of protection or by proper use of ultraviolet lamps and X-ray apparatus.

Among the skin conditions caused by physical agents the commonest are those produced by sunlight. Over-exposure (especially in persons on vacation, not exposed to the sun for a long time) causes sunburn. Continuous, long exposure to actinic radiation (as in the case of sailors, farmers, fishermen) causes premature ageing of the skin and, later, premalignant lesions and then malignant lesions may be a consequence. Sunlight in persons with some genodermatosis such as xeroderma pigmentosum favours the appearance of cancer in a relatively short time. Sunlight may cause photodermatitis when certain agents are applied to the skin: for example, perfumes, eau de cologne, tars and carbanilides, phenols, and halogenated salicylanilides found in cosmetics, deodorant bar soaps, and detergents. Reactions may also occur in individuals taking certain photosensitizing drugs and agents, sulphonamides, tetracyclines, phenothiazines (antihistaminics, tranquillizers, sedatives). There are certain diseases in which sunlight intervenes or participates in their pathogenesis: lupus erythematosus, pellagra, porphyria, hydroa vacciniformis, cheilitis.

With regard to the degenerative action of sunlight it is worth noting the difference in frequency of skin cancer in individuals of the same nationality, which is higher when they live in countries in which the sun's radiation is more intense and prolonged (for instance Australia in contrast to England). According to Schreiber *et al.* (1971) a frequency of 422 skin cancers per 100,000 population, documented by positive biopsy counts, occurred in the area of Southern Arizona served by the city of Tucson. The figure is 20 per cent. above the highest previously reported for any area of the United States, and 34 per cent. above the highest documented rate in the literature. The factors increasing the prevalence of skin cancer in this area 'are metereologic and geographic, producing greater quantity of ultraviolet light. The Tucson area has more sunlight, more clear days . . . and less daytime cloudiness than anywhere in the country.'

Besides avoiding continuous exposure or overexposure to sunshine, individuals prone to skin conditions caused by sunlight should also use protective sunscreening creams (antipyrine 7 per cent.; para-aminobenzoic acid 15 per cent.) Individuals of light skin should take greater care to avoid the carcinogenic action of sunlight.

Ionizing radiation (X-rays, radium, isotopes, thorium) may cause skin changes (radiodermatitis), which deserve special attention because they may be the site of carcinoma. X-ray examinations and radiotherapy should be reduced to the minimum and used only when there is a very precise indication.

PRECANCEROUS DERMATOSES: CARCINOMAS

Some dermatoses favour the development of cancer: xeroderma pigmentosum, senile keratosis, leukoplakia, craurosis vulvae, radiodermatitis, cutaneous horns, arsenical keratosis, seborrheic keratosis, and certain scars. These skin conditions have been called 'precancerous' dermatoses. This does not mean that cancer will develop frequently or in all cases with the above dermatoses, although in xeroderma pigmentosum the development of cancer is the rule. Senile keratosis is histologically considered to be a squamous-cell epithelioma grade one-half; according to MacKee (1942) probably about 25 per cent. of cases terminate in cancer when neglected. The occurrence of squamous-cell carcinoma in leukoplakia (possibly about 30 per cent.; MacKee, 1942) and radiodermatitis is also high, while some of the other 'precancerous' dermatoses are only rarely the site of a carcinoma.

It is important to be able to diagnose those precancerous dermatoses more prone to develop into cancer, in order to treat them prophylactically.

Senile keratosis usually appears in persons over 40, in areas of the skin exposed to actinic radiation. It is more frequent in farmers and sailors and those continuously exposed to sunshine (see Dermatoses Due to Physical Agents). Once diagnosed, the treatment of senile keratosis should not be delayed. When the lesions are very superficial, they can be treated by application of solid carbon dioxide or trichloro-acetic acid (25 to 50 per cent. solution); the latter is removed with alcohol after 1 or 2 minutes. Deeper lesions should be removed by electrocoagulation and curettage. Keratoses of the lip are particularly dangerous and should be destroyed.

Leukoplakia lesions are white, slightly thickened and may appear in the mouth, vulva, and vagina. The irritation caused by decayed teeth, dentures, or from physical and chemical agents, tobacco smoking, and heated pipe stems should be avoided. The lesions which persist, after the suppression of the irritating agents, should be treated with electrodessication or with electrocoagulation.

Radiodermatitis may be avoided by proper technique in the use of X-rays and radium. When the lesion of radiodermatitis presents chronic ulcer and keratosis the affected area should be excised.

Carcinomas of the skin, once diagnosed (with or without histological confirmation) should be treated. Electrocoagulation and curettage afford good results in basal-cell carcinomas as well as surgical excision, X-rays, and radium. For the squamous-cell carcinomas, surgery or radiotherapy is recommended; small tumours could be treated with electrocoagulation and curettage. In countries with all resources, when selecting the method of treatment full consideration should be given to site, duration, speed of growth, and metastasis of the carcinoma.

REFERENCES AND FURTHER READING

Introduction

Ajello, L. (1970) The medical mycological iceberg, in *Proceedings, International Symposium on Mycoses,* Scientific Publication No. 205, p. 3, Pan American Health Organization, Pan American Sanitary Bureau, Regional Office of the World Health Organization, Washington, D.C.

Blank, H., Taplin, D., and Zaias, N. (1969) Cutaneous *Trichophyton mentagrophytes* infections in Vietnam, *Arch. Derm.,* **99,** 135.

Gay Prieto, J., Jadassohn, W., Lapière, S., and Serri, F. (1968) *Public Health Approach to Occupational Dermatoses,* International League of Societies of Dermatology, presented at the 41st Meeting of the WHO Executive Board (unpublished).

Schofield, F. D., Parkinson, A. D., and Jeffrey, D. (1963) Observations on the epidemiology, effects and treatment of *Tinea imbricata, Trans. roy. Soc. trop. Med. Hyg.,* **57,** 214.

Waddy, B. B. (1969) Prospects for the control of onchocerciasis in Africa with special reference to the Volta River Basin, *Bull. Wld Hlth Org.,* **40,** 843.

COMMUNICABLE SKIN DISEASES

Browne, S. G. (1970) Leprosy—an imported disease, *Trans. roy. Soc. trop. Med. Hyg.,* **64,** 223.

Leiker, D. L. (1970) Netherlands. Registration of new leprosy patients, *Int. J. Leprosy,* **38,** 445 (News Item).

Superficial and Deep Mycoses

Bechelli, L. M., and Curban, G. V. (1967) *Compêndio de Dermatologia,* 3rd ed., São Paulo, Brazil, Ch. 18, pp. 335, 368–403.

Benenson, A. S., ed. (1970) *Control of Communicable Diseases in Man,* 11th ed., American Public Health Association, New York. (An official report of the American Public Health Association prepared under the auspices of the Program Area Committee on Communicable Diseases.)

Bopp, C. (1959) *Cromoblastomicose*, Thesis, Porto Alegre, Brazil.

Conant, N. F., Smith, D. T., Baker, R. D., Callaway, J. L., and Martin, D. S. (1954) *Manual of Clinical Mycology*, 2nd ed., Philadelphia.

Gonzalez Ochoa, A. (1970) The prevention and treatment of subcutaneous mycoses, in *Proceedings, International Symposium on Mycoses*, Scientific Publication No. 205, pp. 123–7. Pan American Health Organization, Pan American Sanitary Bureau, Regional Office of the World Health Organization, Washington, D.C.

Maxcy-Rosenau, M. J. (1965) *Preventive Medicine and Public Health*, 9th ed., New York, Ch. 8, pp. 403–5.

Oliveira Ribeiro, D. (1939) Quoted by L. M. Bechelli and G. V. Curban, *Compêndio de Dermatologia*, 1967, 3rd ed., São Paulo, Brazil, Ch. 19, p. 383.

Leprosy

Bechelli, L. M. (1963) Unpublished working paper WP/RC14/TD5 presented for Technical Discussions at the Fourteenth Session of the WHO Western Pacific Regional Committee, Port Moresby.

Bechelli, L. M. (1965) *Leprosy Control*, reported at the First Regional Seminar on Leprosy Control, Manila, Philippines, 21–28 April 1965 (WHO document WPR/163/67) and published in *Acta Leprol. (Genève)*, 1970, Nos. 38–39, pp. 111–27.

Bechelli, L. M. (1966) *A Guide to Leprosy Control*, World Health Organization, Geneva (WHO document PA/66.214).

Bechelli, L. M., and Martinez Dominguez, V. (1966) The leprosy problem in the world, *Bull. Wld Hlth Org.*, **34**, 811.

Bechelli, L. M., and Martinez Dominguez, V. (1970) Further information on the leprosy problem in the world, in *International Leprosy Colloquium, Forschungsinstitut Borstel*, 1970, *Summaries*, p. 94, Abstract No. 58, *Int. J. Leprosy*, 1971, **39**, 601. Original in *Bull. Wld Hlth Org.*, 1972, **46**, 523.

Bechelli, L. M., Martinez Dominguez, V., and Patwary, K. M. (1963) Some epidemiological data collected by the WHO Leprosy Advisory Team in random sample surveys in Nigeria (Katsina), Cameroon and Thailand (Khon Kaen), presented at VIII International Congress of Leprology, Rio de Janeiro, 1963, *Int. J. Leprosy*, **34**, 223.

Bechelli, L. M., and Rotberg, A. (1949) Idade e lepra: estudo dos fatores exposiçao e resistência, *Rev. bras. Leprol.*, **17**, 31.

Beiguelman, B., Dall'Aglio, F. F., and da Silva, E. (1968) Estudo das formas polares de lepra pela analise de pares de irmaos, *Rev. paul. Med.*, **72**, 111.

Beiguelman, B., and Quagliato, R. (1965) Nature and familial character of the lepromin reactions, *Int. J. Leprosy*, **33**, 800.

Beiguelman, B., Souza-Campos, N., and Pinto, W., Jr. (1967) Fatôres genéticos e efeito da calmetizaçao na reaçao de Mitsuda, *Rev. paul. Med.*, **71**, 271.

Dharmendra, and Chatterjee, K. R. (1955) Prognostic value of the lepromin test in contacts of leprosy cases, *Leprosy in India*, **27**, 149.

Doull, J. A. (1962) The epidemiology of leprosy. Present status and problems, *Int. J. Leprosy*, **30**, 48.

Doull, J. A., Guinto, R. S., Rodriquez, J. N., and Bancroft, H. (1942) The incidence of leprosy in Cordova and Talisay, Cebu, P.I., *Int. J. Leprosy*, **10**, 107.

Guinto, R. S., Rodriquez, J. N., Doull, J. A., and de Guia, L. (1954) The trend of leprosy in Cordova and Talisay, Cebu Province, Philippines, *Int. J. Leprosy*, **22**, 409.

Hanks, J. H. (1945) A note on the numbers of leprosy bacilli which may occur in leprous nodules, *Int. J. Leprosy*, **13**, 25.

Kirchheimer, W. F., and Storrs, E. E. (1971) Attempts to establish the armadillo (*Dasypus novemcintus Linn.*) as a model for the study of leprosy, *Int. J. Leprosy*, **39**, 693.

Kolesov, K. A. (1968) The results of experimental infection of mice with material from leprosy patients, *Vestn. Derm. Vener.*, **42**, (10), 55.

Lara, C. B., and Nolasco, J. O. (1956) Self-healing, or abortive, and residual forms of childhood leprosy and their probable significance, *Int. J. Leprosy*, **24**, 245.

Lara, C. B. (1961) Unpublished working paper WPR/Leprosy/24 for the WHO Western Pacific Regional Postgraduate Leprosy Training Course, Manila, Philippines.

Memoria del VI Congreso Internacional de Leprologia (1953) Madrid (Draft Report of Classification Committee), pp. 75–86.

Newell, K. W. (1966) An epidemiologist's view of leprosy, *Bull. Wld Hlth Org.*, **34**, 827.

Rees, R. J. W. (1968) Recent advances in the transmission of human leprosy to mice, *Int. J. Leprosy*, **36**, 584. (Abstract of paper presented at the Ninth International Leprosy Congress, London, 1968.)

Shepard, C. C. (1960) The experimental disease that follows the injection of human leprosy bacilli into foot pads of mice, *J. exp. Med.*, **112**, 445.

World Health Organization (1960) Second Report of the Expert Committee on Leprosy, *Wld Hlth Org. techn. Rep. Ser.*, No. 189.

World Health Organization (1966) Third Report of the Expert Committee on Leprosy, *Wld Hlth Org. techn. Rep. Ser.*, No. 319.

World Health Organization (1970) Fourth Report of the Expert Committee on Leprosy, *Wld Hlth Org. techn. Rep. Ser.*, No. 459.

Staphylococcal and Streptococcal Infections: Pyodermas

Bechelli, L. M., and Curban, G. V. (1967) *Compêndio de Dermatologia*, 3rd ed., São Paulo, Brazil, Ch. 12, pp. 141–61.

Williams, R. E. O. (1946) Skin and nose carriage of bacteriophage types of *Staph. aureus*, *J. Path. Bact.*, **58**, 259.

World Health Organization (1968) Report of the Expert Committee on Streptococcal and Staphylococcal Infections, *Wld Hlth Org. techn. Rep. Ser.*, No. 394.

Skin Diseases Due to Animal Parasites (See also Chapter 22 on the Zoonoses.)

Bechelli, L. M., and Curban, G. V. (1967) *Compêndio de Dermatologia*, 3rd ed., São Paulo, Brazil, Ch. 20, pp. 404–23.

Borda, J. M. (1954) Sarna humana, *Arch. argent. Derm.*, **4**, 101, 255–86.

Orkin, M. (1971) Resurgence of scabies, *J. Amer. med. Ass.*, **217**, 593.

NON-COMMUNICABLE DISEASES

Skin Diseases Due to Chemical Agents

Bechelli, L. M., and Curban, G. V. (1967) *Compêndio de Dermatologia*, 3rd ed., São Paulo, Brazil, Ch. 10, pp. 124–9.

Fisher, A. A., Pascher, F., and Kanof, N. B. (1971) Cream bases for topical agents can cause dermatitis, *J. Amer. med. Ass.*, **217**, 893.

Gay Prieto, J., Jadassohn, W., Lapière, S., and Serri, F. (1968) *Public Health Approach to Occupational Dermatoses*, International League of Societies of Dermatology, presented at the 41st Meeting of the WHO Executive Board (unpublished).

Drug Eruptions

Bechelli, L. M., and Curban, G. V. (1967) *Compêndio de Dermatologia*, 3rd ed., São Paulo, Brazil, Ch. 7, pp. 99–107.

Friedman, G. D., Collen, M. F., Harris, L. E., Van Brunt, E. E., and Davis, L. S. (1971) Experience in monitoring drug reactions in out-patients. The Kaiser-permanente drug monitoring system, *J. Amer. med. Ass.*, **217**, 567.

Royall, B. W. (1971) International aspects of drug monitoring, *Chron. Wld Hlth Org.*, **25**, 445.

Dermatosis and Skin Changes Caused by Physical Agents

Bechelli, L. M., and Curban, G. V. (1967) *Compêndio de Dermatologia*, 3rd ed., São Paulo, Brazil, Ch. 11, pp. 130–40.

Schreiber, M. M., Shapiro, S. I., Berry, C. Z., Dahlen, R. F., and Friedman, R. P. (1971) The incidence of skin cancer in Southern Arizona (Tucson), *Arch. Derm.*, **104**, 124.

Precancerous Dermatoses: Carcinomas

Bechelli, L. M., and Curban, G. V. (1967) *Compêndio de Dermatologia*, 3rd ed., São Paulo, Brazil, Ch. 29, pp. 545–92.

Miller MacKee, G. (1942) Diseases of the skin, in *Preventive Medicine in Modern Practice*, eds. Miller, J. A., Baehr, G., and Corwin, E. H. L., the New York Academy of Medicine, Committee on Public Health Relations, New York.

Montgomery, H., and Doerffel, J. (1967) Bechelli, L. M., and Curban, G. V., *Compêndio de Dermatologia*, 3rd ed., São Paulo, Brazil, Ch. 29, pp. 545–92.

General Works on Skin Diseases

Andrews, G. C., and Domonkos, A. N. (1970) *Diseases of the Skin*, 6th ed., Philadelphia.

Bechelli, L. M., and Curban, G. V. (1967) *Compêndio de Dermatologia*, 3rd ed., São Paulo, Brazil. (In Portuguese.)

Dey, N. (1969) *Skin Diseases in the Tropics*, Calcutta.

Rook, A. J., *et al.*, eds (1969) *Textbook of Dermatology*, Oxford.

21
THE VENEREAL DISEASES AND TREPONEMATOSES

R. R. WILLCOX

INTRODUCTION

In developed countries the venereal diseases now comprise the commonest communicable diseases. Apart from those legally defined, usually syphilis, gonorrhoea, soft sore, lymphogranuloma venereum, and granuloma inguinale, there are a number of other sexually transmitted conditions caused by spirochaetes, bacteria, viruses, protozoa, fungi, and parasites [TABLE 54]. Other organisms are also passed during sexual

TABLE 54

Sexually Transmitted Diseases Affecting Man

	Organism	Disease
Spirochaetes	*T. pallidum*	Syphilis
Bacteria	*Gonococcus*	Gonorrhoea
	Ducrey's bacillus	Chancroid
	Donovania	Granuloma inguinale
Viruses	*Chlamydia*	Non-gonococcal urethritis
		Trachoma; inclusion conjunctivitis
		Lymphogranuloma venereum
	Other viruses	Herpes simplex
		Molluscum contagiosum
		Condylomata acuminata
Protozoa	*T. vaginalis*	Trichomoniasis
Fungi	*C. albicans*	Monilia
	Epidermophyton inguinale	Tinea cruris
Parasites	*Acarus scabiei*	Scabies
	Phthirus pubis	Pediculosis

contact (e.g. mycoplasmas), the roles of which are not yet entirely clear.

THE TREPONEMATOSES

Definition

This group of contact diseases is caused by morphologically similar pathogenic treponemata which include the organisms responsible for venereal and endemic syphilis (*Treponema pallidum*), yaws (*T. pertenue*) and pinta (*T. carateum*). Only venereal syphilis is transmitted sexually. Antibodies are formed in all four conditions, which are indistinguishable by available tests (Willcox and Guthe, 1966).

In addition, *T. cuniculi* is responsible for a naturally occurring treponematosis (cuniculosis; pallidoidosis) in rabbits and another treponeme (*T. Fribourg Blanc*) has been found in the cynocephalus monkey in some yaws areas, which may represent an animal reservoir of the latter condition (Willcox, 1969).

Some have considered the human diseases to be caused by the same organism producing varying clinical patterns in different environments (Hudson, 1958); others that the organisms concerned are closely allied, the spread of each being determined by environmental circumstances. Pinta, yaws and endemic syphilis are the evolutionary forerunners of venereal syphilis (Willcox, 1969).

Venereal Syphilis

Definition. A sexually transmitted disease caused by *T. pallidum*.

Causative Agent. *T. pallidum*, described by Schaudinn and Hoffmann in 1905, is a thin delicate spiral organism entwined with a bundle of 3–4 fibrils which maintains its shape (Willcox, 1964). It has not been successfully cultured *in vitro*, but can be passaged in animals producing infections which are symptomatic in the ape or other primates and in the rabbit, sometimes symptomatic but often asymptomatic in the hamster and guinea-pig, but entirely asymptomatic in the rat and mouse (Turner and Hollander, 1957; Willcox and Guthe, 1966).

Distribution. Venereal syphilis is world-wide except in areas in which the endemic non-venereal treponematoses are rife (Idsøe and Guthe, 1967). In the United States of America there were 106,539 reported cases of primary and secondary syphilis in 1947 (75·6 per 100,000), which number fell to 6,251 (3·8 per 100,000) in 1957, but had risen again to 24,000 cases (11·7 per 100,000) by 1972 (United States Public Health Service, 1973). Because many cases are unreported the actual prevalence in the United States is estimated to exceed 75,000 cases per annum and the total reservoir of untreated syphilis as half a million. In England in 1972, the reported case rate for primary and secondary syphilis was 2·56 per 100,000, a figure which has remained stable in recent years (Department of Health and Social Security, 1973).

Epidemiology. Venereal syphilis is a disease of sexually active adults. Transmission is by means of direct contact with primary and secondary skin and mucous membrane lesions, although in the secondary stage the body fluids are also infective. It may be passed by genital–genital, genito–anal, genito–oral or occasionally oral–oral contact. Indirect transmission by means of eating or drinking vessels or by blood transfusion is rare. Certain population groups are at greater risk than others, owing to differing patterns of sexual behaviour. Homosexual spread accounts for up to 50 per cent. or more of early infections encountered in some cities.

Course of the Disease. *T. pallidum* divides slowly (every

30–33 hours). After an incubation period of 17–28 days (extremes 9–90), a sore (chancre) develops at the site of entry and the local lymph nodes (usually inguinal) are painlessly enlarged. The chancre may be concealed (in the female on the cervix and within the anus in the homosexual male) or it may be absent.

The secondary stage follows within weeks or a few months (usually around six weeks) with generalized signs of the disease which include non-irritant rash, widespread adenitis, mucous patches in the mouth, and condylomata lata by the anus and genitals, by which time serum tests for syphilis have become positive.

Untreated, the secondary lesions heal slowly and the disease becomes latent for many years, even a lifetime. According to the Oslo study (Gjestland, 1955) of a large group of patients with early syphilis left untreated in the period 1891–1910, approximately one in four developed clinical secondary relapse while benign tertiary syphilis (gummata) occurred in about one in six, clinical neurosyphilis (with general paralysis (paresis)), tabes dorsalis—sometimes with optic atrophy—and meningovascular syphilis in 6·5 per cent., and cardiovascular syphilis (with angina pectoris, aortic reflux, and aneurysm) in one in ten patients.

In about one in ten patients syphilis was considered to be the primary cause of death, this being about twice as frequent in males as in females (15·1 versus 8·3 per cent.). Nevertheless, approximately six out of ten infected persons suffer no personal inconvenience from the later effects of the disease either ultimately undergoing apparent spontaneous cure, or remaining in a state of latency until death from some other cause.

Foetal Involvement. *T. pallidum*, as also the cytomegalovirus and the causative organisms of rubella and toxoplasmosis, may be transferred transplacentally to the foetus. This is very likely if the mother has secondary syphilis but uncommon once ten or more years have elapsed. Proved examples of third-generation syphilis are therefore very rare.

Foetal infection may result in miscarriage (four months or later in pregnancy), still birth or a live child which in the early weeks of life develops signs of *early congenital syphilis*. These signs include rash, adenitis, condylomata lata, mucous patches, rhinitis, enlarged liver and spleen, osteitis, and periostitis of lung bones, marasmus, and occasionally meningitis (Nabarro, 1954).

The early signs are followed by a period of latency for years or for a lifetime, but symptomatic *late congenital syphilis* occurs in some cases as gummata (particularly of the nose and palate), neurosyphilis—possibly with optic atrophy—and occasionally cardiovascular syphilis, although this complication is uncommon when the infection is contracted early in life, as it is also in endemic syphilis. In addition, interstitial keratitis and nerve deafness may arise, and dental abnormalities (Hutchinson's teeth and Moon's molars) which, though affecting the second dentition, have arisen from damage to the toothbuds early in the infection (Willcox, 1964).

Diagnosis of Syphilis

1. *Methods.* Diagnosis is confirmed by finding *T. pallidum* by dark-field or by immunofluorescence in material from primary and secondary lesions, and by serum test.

There are two types of serum test, either with lipid or with treponemal antigens (United States Public Health Service, 1969). The latter are more specific and have the greatest value in confirming diagnosis while the former, which may give false-positive results in some other conditions,[1] are best suited for use during post-treatment follow-up and for screening tests.

2. *Test based on lipid antigens.* These include the cardiolipin Wassermann complement-fixation reaction (Kolmer, Maltaner) and the VDRL (Harris). RPR (Rapid Plasma Reagin) and the ART (Automated Reagin test), flocculation or agglutination tests employing cardiolipin antigen. Earlier much-used procedures in which crude extracts of beef heart were used as antigen (e.g. the Kahn), which are less specific especially in the tropics, have now been superseded in most areas.

3. *Test based on treponemal antigens.* The Reiter protein complement-fixation test (using an antigen of the non-pathogenic Reiter strain) may give false-positive and false-negative results. Those using pathogenic *T. pallidum* as antigen—the treponemal immobilization (TPI) test, the fluorescent treponemal antibody-absorption (FTA–ABS) test, and the newer and simpler *Treponema pallidum* haemagglutination (TPHA) test—are specific for disease due to pathogenic treponemes but will not distinguish syphilis from yaws or pinta.

4. *Choice of test.* Tests with cardiolipin antigens usually become positive 1–2 weeks after the appearance of the chancre, are virtually always positive in the secondary stage but may ultimately revert to negative in 30–40 per cent. of cases of late syphilis after some years, even without treatment. Sero-reversal to these tests is to be expected in treated early syphilis. Those with treponemal antigens are also positive in the secondary stage, nearly always remain positive in late syphilis and indeed may do so in 30 per cent. of cases of treated secondary syphilis. The FTA–ABS test becomes positive before those tests with cardiolipin antigens. The TPI test is the last to become reactive.

The best single available test for screening purposes for all of the treponematoses and for assessing the results of therapy is the VDRL or a similar test based on a cardiolipin antigen.

Treatment of Syphilis. Treatment is by means of penicillin, giving 8–15 daily injections of 0·6–1·2 mega units of aqueous procaine penicillin, the duration depending on the stage of the disease. If procaine penicillin with aluminium monostearate (PAM), is used, the World Health Organization (1953) recommends a minimum of 4·8 mega units given in one to eight spaced injections. If benzathine penicillin is used, the United States Public Health Service (1958) recommends single injections of 2·4 mega units for early syphilis. The latter will also abort the disease in the incubation period and is well suited to the treatment of contacts. There are no signs of syphilis becoming resistant to penicillin but the inability to culture the organism makes precise testing impossible (Guthe and Idsøe, 1968b). Erythromycin or tetracyclines are used in persons suspected of being allergic to penicillin.

Treatment given to the infected pregnant female will either prevent infection of the foetus or, if it has already occurred, will cure it *in utero*.

Treponemal forms have been recovered from the lymph nodes, cerebrospinal fluid and aqueous humour of men and

---

[1] Particularly in cases of protein deficiency, leprosy, chronic malaria, trypanosomiasis, certain viral disorders, infectious mononucleosis, liver disease, following smallpox vaccination and in auto-immune conditions (e.g. disseminated lupus erythematosus, Sjögren's syndrome, etc.).

rabbits, even following treatment with effective drugs in accepted dosage. In very few instances have these been proved to be pathogenic *T. pallidum* by infectivity tests. Whether the remainder are *T. pallidum* of lessened virulence or non-pathogenic treponemes from an indigenous or other source is not yet clear (WHO, 1970).

Prevention of Syphilis. Apart from general measures prevention is based on accurate diagnosis of infectious cases and vigorous case-finding of source and spread contacts. Where syphilis represents a public health problem, these should be treated even if they are not found on examination to be clinically or serologically affected (WHO, 1953). Untreated it has been stated that 9–30 per cent. of contacts of infectious cases would otherwise develop the disease.

Serological screening of expectant mothers, blood donors and high-risk groups (prostitutes, 'entertainers', prisoners, seamen, military personnel, etc., including patients with other sexually transmitted diseases), which is extended to food handlers, industrial employees, immigrant labourers, hospital patients, etc., in a number of countries, is a second valuable method of case-finding also leading towards the prevention of later complications. Its value, however, depends on the yield. If very low, the procedure may not be economic and in areas with an endemic treponematosis (e.g. yaws) the results are confused by the high seropositivity rates prevailing in the general population. Its use on expectant mothers is essential for the prevention of congenital syphilis, and the reduction in the prevalence of this condition to a handful of cases in many countries represents one of the triumphs of modern medicine. In the United Kingdom in 1972 seropostivity rates varied from 0·05 to 1·8 per 1,000 in four selected centres involving over 130,000 pregnant women (Department of Health and Social Security, 1973).

Endemic Syphilis

Definition. A non-venereal treponematosis of children caused by *T. pallidum*, the organism responsible for venereal syphilis.

Distribution. Endemic syphilis is found in primitive regions bordering on deserts (Guthe and Willcox, 1954) in Africa (e.g. Niger, Senegal, and around the Sahara in the north and in countries adjacent to the Kalahari desert in Rhodesia (*njovera*) (Willcox, 1950), Botswana and the Transvaal in the south); in the Middle East (*bejel*) (Hudson, 1958) and also occurred in Europe until recently eradicated by a WHO-assisted mass campaign in Bosnia, Yugoslavia (Grin, 1953). Between the wars it was known to be extremely widespread in Eastern Europe and the eastern Mediterranean countries including Greece, Turkey, parts of the Soviet Union and the then Palestine. In past centuries it was rife throughout Europe as the *sibbens* of Scotland, *button scurvy* of Ireland, the *radesyge* of Norway, and occurred under different names in other countries (Guthe and Willcox, 1954; Willcox, 1969).

Epidemiology. In dry climates endemic syphilis is the predominant treponematosis under very poor overcrowded conditions, even in hot regions where the reduced ability to sweat and the colder temperature at night necessitate the wearing of clothes. The majority of cases occur in children who are infected by other children, or from an infection either venereal or asexual in a closely associated adult.

Spread is direct from mouth to mouth during kissing, or indirect by means of the fingers or common eating or drinking vessels. The sharing of pipes, toothpicks, and other unhygienic practices may encourage the same in susceptible adults.

When endemic syphilis is rife, venereal syphilis is not seen in adults as they already have the childhood disease. As living conditions improve children grow up who have not been previously affected. These are now susceptible to the venereal infection, and genital chancres then make their appearance. During the period of transition, asexual infections may be seen in adults if primitive customs persist. The evolution from endemic to venereal syphilis may reverse itself should social conditions deteriorate.

Clinical Course. Primary chancres are rarely seen. The finding of a chancre on the nipple of an uninfected mother suckling her infected child is a strong indication of the presence of the disease. Dark-field positive mucous patches, angular stomatitis, and anogenital condylomata lata are the common early secondary manifestations. All types of serum tests for syphilis are positive. Most patients proceed to latency and in some there is subsequent development of gummatous lesions of skin and bone. Cardiovascular and neurological involvements are also stated to occur, but congenital manifestations are extremely rare due in part to the fact that the early infection is acquired at a younger age than venereal syphilis.

Control. Treatment is by mass campaign. Total mass treatment is recommended when the prevalence of clinically active cases exceeds 3·0 per cent. (Willcox, 1969; WHO, 1960). The doses of penicillin used are similar to those employed in yaws (q.v.) but the dosage is increased by 50 per cent. or more in symptomatic late cases (Willcox, 1964).

Even without active medical measures endemic syphilis tends to wane with improvement of social conditions. Asexual transmission will then tend to persist in adults until unhygienic habits are discarded. It will then be replaced by venereal syphilis.

Yaws

Definition. Synonyms *pian* (French), *framboesia* (German and Dutch), *buba* (Spanish), *bouba* (Portuguese) (Hackett, 1957). A contagious disease caused by *T. pertenue*.

Distribution. Yaws is almost exclusively confined to the humid regions between the Tropics of Capricorn and Cancer. It is found in the northern part of South America and in the Caribbean (including Jamaica and in Haiti, where at one time more than 50 per cent. of the population were affected); in Africa, particularly Central and West Africa; in South-East Asia in Thailand, Indonesia, Malaysia and the States of Indo-China, with scattered pockets in Southern India, Northern Australia and other places, in many of the islands of the Western Pacific (Guthe and Willcox, 1954; Nery-Guimarães, 1970; Willcox, 1964).

It was estimated that two decades ago there were some 50 million cases of yaws throughout the world, of which 25 millions were in Africa. Since then many mass campaigns have been organized by the WHO and the responsible governments, involving many millions of patients and contacts treated. These, together with increased social and technological development, have resulted in marked reduction in prevalence, although in no major territory has complete eradication been achieved.

Epidemiology. Yaws is predominantly a disease of children, particularly those aged 2–10 years. It is found among poor populations, 'at the end of the road', wearing few or no clothes. Transmission is by direct skin-to-skin contact with other children or family members with moist lesions, entry of the organism being assisted by trauma often resulting from walking barefoot in the bush. Flies of the genus *Hippelates* have also been incriminated in its spread.

Yaws is found in moist humid regions and flourishes best at a mean annual isotherm of 80° F. (27° C.) and over, in areas with a heavy rainfall, a poorly draining soil and lush vegetation. A treponeme resembling *T. pertenue* has been found in monkeys in some yaws areas [see p. 281]. The early clinical manifestations become extinct in temperate climates although individual cases are from time to time reported in recently arrived immigrants.

Clinical Course. 1. *Early (contagious) yaws.* A papillomatous initial lesion ('mother yaw', pianoma, framboesioma) develops on exposed parts such as the legs, arms, buttocks or face, after an incubation period of 3–6 weeks (Hackett, 1957; Nery-Guimarães, 1970). This may become ulcerated with a granulomatous centre. After a further 3–6 weeks secondary generalized skin rashes (framboesides) appear from which further papillomata may develop. These are very contagious as *T. pertenue* can readily be demonstrated in them. Antibodies indistinguishable from those of syphilis are found by serum tests with both lipid and treponemal antigens. The secondary lesions usually heal spontaneously after a further 3–6 months but infectious relapses may occur during the ensuing five years, during which time severe osteitis and periostitis may develop and also hyperkeratosis of the palms and soles (crab yaws), the latter being particularly painful and disabling.

2. *Late yaws.* Some patients subsequently develop destructive ulcerative late lesions of skin and bone which may be followed by scarring and contracture. Destruction of the nasal septum or nose and palate results in saddle nose or in gangosa. Other lesions include periostitis, achromia, hyperkeratosis, bursitis, juxta-articular nodes and goundou. The late lesions, too, may heal and relapse.

There are no certain signs of cardiovascular involvement or neuro-yaws, nor of congenital transmission.

Control of Yaws. 1. *Methods used.* Treatment is by means of penicillin but if given only to individual clinical cases is not sufficient to control the disease.

In hyperendemic areas (areas where prevalence of active cases exceeds 10 per cent.) *total mass treatment* is required so as to stamp out not only the clinical cases but also those incubating the disease and latent cases in which infectious relapse might occur later.

In areas of medium prevalence (5–10 per cent. of active cases) *juvenile mass treatment* can be applied, whereby clinical cases and all children are treated, while in areas of low prevalence *selective mass treatment*, involving only clinical cases and all household and obvious contacts, may be used.

The World Health Organization recommends that adults with the active disease receive a single injection of 1·2 mega units of procaine penicillin in oil with aluminium monostearate (PAM), and those under 15 years of age 0·6 mega units. Half of these amounts can be given in latent cases and to contacts.

2. *Principles of mass campaigns* (Willcox, 1964; WHO, 1953; WHO, 1960). The stages of the WHO-assisted mass campaigns may be summarized as follows:

(i) A pilot survey to determine prevalence.

(ii) Examination of the whole population (at least 90 per cent.) by house-to-house visit or by summoning groups to a central place, and application of mass treatment.

(iii) Annual resurveys in which the whole population is again examined when all new clinical cases and their contacts are treated. This process is repeated annually until the prevalence has been reduced to low levels, when the interval between surveys can be extended to every second or third year.

(iv) Subsequent continued surveillance through a strengthened rural health service, and thereafter by means of statistically valid random epidemiological and serological surveys.

Mass treatment with penicillin provides the momentum whereby hyperendemicity can be reduced to hypo-endemicity, or further, within 1–2 years. However, the reduction of clinical cases is not immediately matched by a drop in serological prevalence and serological surveys provide only limited information unless age-profiles are incorporated, when the fall in seropositivity in the younger age-groups indicates a reduction in transmission (Guthe and Idsøe, 1968a).

3. *Results of mass campaigns.* Isolated clinical cases and residual foci may persist. FTA and TPI reactivity in some children usually indicates low-level transmission 10–15 years later. Continued surveillance is therefore required with integration of such activities into the expanding rural health services, as is also a general improvement in hygienic, economic, and environmental standards if the situation is not to regress. Moreover, the danger remains of reintroduction of the infection from outside the area.

With the removal of yaws, also withdrawn is the partial immunity to syphilis which it confers, and the endemic disease will then be replaced by venereal syphilis, e.g. as in Papua and New Guinea (Rhodes and Anderson, 1970) which in turn—if primitive conditions remain—may revert to endemic syphilis, e.g. in Tahiti (Van der Sluis, 1969).

Pinta

Distribution and Epidemiology. First described by Herrejon in 1927 this so-called 'blue stain' disease is endemic in certain rural and jungle areas of Mexico, Venezuela, Argentina, Colombia, Brazil, Peru and Ecuador, and is also present in Guatemala, Haiti, Santo Domingo, Cuba, El Salvador, Honduras, Nicaragua, Panama, Bolivia, Puerto Rico and Guyana (United States Health Service, 1969). It was once estimated that there were 700,000 sufferers from the disease. It is not known for certain outside the Americas. Like yaws, pinta affects peoples of low socio-economic status. Both sexes are equally involved at all ages but most commonly before the age of 20 years. Sufferers from pinta may feel stigmatized and may not be accepted for employment in urban areas.

Causative Agent and Transmission. The causative agent *T. carateum*, recognized in 1938, is indistinguishable from *T. pallidum*, and it evokes antibodies likewise indistinguishable by both types of serum test from those of syphilis.

The disease is contracted early in life by skin-to-skin contact and possibly through flies of the genus *Hippelates*. Patients with pinta rarely contract syphilis or yaws, although syphilitic patients show little resistance to *T. carateum* (Medina, 1967). It has proved difficult to passage the organism in animals, but recently infection has been established in the chimpanzee.

Clinical Course and Treatment. In the experimental infection, the incubation period is 7-20 days after inoculation. The primary lesion is a slowly enlarging salmon-pink papule on the trunk, legs, arms, or face, often surrounded by satellite lesions. After a few months these usually become hypochromic. The genitals are seldom involved and there is generally no enlargement of the lymph nodes. Secondary 'pintides' follow over a period of months or years resembling the primary lesions at first, later turning copper-coloured and then slate blue, and finally becoming depigmented. Hyperkeratosis and juxta-articular nodes have also been described.

The disease is, for practical purposes, confined to the skin and there is no certain evidence of congenitally transmitted pinta or of cardiovascular or neurological involvement. Treatment is similar to that of yaws. Single doses of 1·2 mega units of procaine penicillin with aluminium monostearate (PAM have been used in mass treatment.

SEXUALLY TRANSMITTED DISEASES OTHER THAN SYPHILIS

DISEASES CAUSED BY BACTERIA

Introduction

These include *gonorrhoea*, *soft sore* (*chancroid*) and *granuloma inguinale*. There are also a number of other sexually transmitted bacteria whose significance is not yet clear, e.g. *Haemophilus vaginalis* (which may be associated with vaginitis), *Mimeae*, and *mycoplasmas*, one strain of which has been frequently suggested as a possible cause of *non-gonococcal urethritis*.

Gonorrhoea

Definition. An extremely widespread and common venereal disease caused by the gonococcus, a Gram-negative intracellular diplococcus described by Neisser in 1879.

Distribution. It was estimated a decade or so ago that 60–65 million cases of gonorrhoea occurred throughout the world each year (WHO, 1963). Incidence has since increased markedly in most areas. In the United States, where there is now an estimated annual total of 2½ million cases (Brown, 1971; WHO, 1972a), the reported incidence (which is but a fraction of total incidence), was 284·2 per 100,000 in 1947, fell to 142·8 by 1962 (American Society of Health Association, 1973) but rose to 349·7 by 1972 when it was the most common communicable disease excluding the common cold. In England in 1971, the reported incidence of post-pubertal cases had reached an all-time peak of 121·26 per 100,000 with a fall to 115·28 in 1972 (Department of Health and Social Security, 1973).

Clinical Course. In the male, gonorrhoea causes a purulent urethritis with dysuria although mild and subclinical infections may be encountered. A symptomatic or asymptomatic proctitis occurs in the male homosexual. If untreated, local complications include peri-urethral abscess followed by urethral stricture (and later hypertension), prostatitis and epididymitis. Such complications were once common but are relatively rare in areas with adequate treatment facilities.

In the female adult, the urethra, cervix and rectum are affected but the condition may remain symptomless for long periods if only the cervix and/or rectum are involved. Local complications include abscess of Bartholin's glands and salpingitis, which may occur in about 10 per cent. of cases even in highly developed countries, of whom about one-third become sterile (Willcox, 1964).

In both sexes, systemic complications of acute arthritis and iritis may arise, rarely gross septicaemia with endocarditis. Cases of 'benign' gonococcal septicaemia have been reported, as have oral infections which may be temporary in nature.

Immature girls may be infected sexually or asexually and develop a *vulvo-vaginitis*, and babies born of infected mothers may develop a gonoccocal *ophthalmia neonatorum*.

Epidemiology. Apart from changes in human behaviour, obstacles to control lie in the short incubation period (usually 2–5 days, extremes 1–14), in the frequent asymptomatic infection in the female and male homosexual, in the lack of a suitable screening test without the necessity of initial genital examination, in difficulties in culturing the organism unless considerable care is taken, and in developing resistance of the gonococcus to antibiotics (Willcox, 1970).

Diagnosis. Diagnosis is made by Gram-stained smear and by culture, both methods being essential in the female. A selective medium containing antibiotics (e.g. Thayer-Martin) should be used for the culture. Final identification depends on sugar fermentation tests. The gonococcus ferments dextrose but not maltose. Immunofluorescent techniques are also employed on direct smears but with better results on cultures.

Treatment. Penicillin remains the drug of choice (Willcox, 1968) although there are many alternative antibiotics (new semisynthetic penicillins, numerous tetracyclines, erythromycin, spiramycin, kanamycin, spectinomycin, rifampicin, and others). Sulphamethoxazole with trimethoprim (cotrimoxazole) also gives good results. Many of these drugs, however, are too expensive for mass use in developing countries.

Relative resistance of the gonococcus has developed to penicillin, and also to some other antibiotics, but—apart from streptomycin which is no longer effective and to which resistance is absolute—to a lesser degree. Resistance to penicillin is most marked in the Far East (where single injections of 4·8 million units of aqueous procaine penicillin, which represent the practical limit of what may be given by single injection, will fail in 30 per cent. of cases in some areas (WHO, 1969) and in Africa). It is least marked in the United Kingdom and Northern Europe with Australia, Canada, and the United States in an intermediate position.

Single injection techniques are preferred for epidemiological reasons and injections of 2·4 million units of aqueous procaine penicillin give excellent results in Britain. In high-resistance areas, this or double this amount with added probenecid by mouth may be necessary.

Prevention. Apart from general measures, control lies in accurate diagnosis with delineation of the condition from non-gonococcal urethritis in the male, contact-tracing and treatment of the sexual partners of those affected, screening of high-risk female groups (e.g. those in prisons and remand homes, those undergoing abortion, and other groups in which the yield can be shown to be especially productive), and in the widespread use by all physicians of an effective treatment, the institution of which may result in a reversal of the resistance trend.

Hopes for the future lie in the possibility of more efficient serum tests for screening purposes, in which direction current work is showing some promise, although their value is likely to be limited in populations with a previously high gonorrhoea rate owing to persistent seropositivity. Some research into a vaccine is being undertaken but no field trials have been reported.

Ophthalmia neonatorum can be prevented by the instillation of 1 per cent. silver nitrate into the eyes at birth (available in disposable single-dose plastic packs for use in tropical areas). Other substances are also used (Willcox, 1964). Disadvantages are the induction of a chemical conjunctivitis in some cases and concealment of gonorrhoea in the mother. As the established condition responds well to systemic and local penicillin, ophthalmia prophylaxis is not now used by many physicians in countries in which facilities for post-treatment observation of the child are adequate, but is recommended when this is not the case.

Chancroid (Soft Sore)

Definition. A venereal disease caused by *Haemophilus ducreyi*, discovered by Ducrey in 1889, and characterized by genital ulcers usually painful and multiple, and tender inguinal adenitis, which may progress to unilocular bubo formation with suppuration.

Diagnosis is made by finding the organism by culture, which is difficult, by the Ito-Reenstierna skin test using a vaccine of *H. ducreyi* which is no longer commercially available in Europe, and by the exclusion of other causes of genital sore, e.g. of syphilis by dark-field and serum tests.

Distribution. It is commonest in poorer populations of many parts of the world, especially Africa, the Far and Middle East, Central and South America where in some areas it may be more prevalent than syphilis. It has become rare in countries with high hygienic standards (Willcox, 1964). Only 49 new cases were reported (Department of Health and Social Security, 1973) in England in 1972 while 1,298 cases were reported in the United States (United States Public Health Service, 1973).

Epidemiology. The incubation period is short (usually 3–5 days). Left untreated the genital ulceration may proceed to phagedaena and the burst bubo to ulceration in the groin. The organism is readily inoculable. The infection is many times more common in men than in women, suggesting that the bacillus may be carried asymptomatically in the latter sex.

Control. Improved hygiene and water supply, rendering personal cleanliness easier, is important. The sulphonamides are the drugs of choice when dark-field tests and serum tests have been performed to exclude syphilis. In underdeveloped areas when no such tests have been made, 2·4 million units of procaine penicillin in oil with aluminium monostearate (PAM) should be given in addition or in lieu.

Granuloma Inguinale (Donovanosis)

Definition. A chronic contagious disease characterized by velvety, beefy granulations affecting the genitalia and surrounding skin. Metastatic lesions may occur and malignant change has been reported.

The causative organism is *Donovania granulomatis*, a bipolar staining organism which is found in endothelial and large mononuclear cells. Its properties resemble those of some Gram-negative bacteria.

Distribution. This is an uncommon condition of the poorer classes which is found in the tropics and subtropics of Asia, Africa, and the Americas. In a few areas—e.g. in Southern India (Rajam and Rangiah, 1954) and in Papua and New Guinea (Maddocks, 1967)—it attains high prevalence. In England in 1972, five new cases were reported (Department of Health and Social Security, 1973) and there were 168 cases in the United States in 1972 (United States Public Health Service, 1973).

Epidemiology. The incubation period varies from eight days to a few months. It is more common in males than in females and it has been shown to occur following pederasty with either sex; it is postulated that *Donovania* are essentially faecal organisms which are transferred to the genitalia (Goldberg, 1964). Nevertheless, high rates of conjugal infection have been reported (Rajam and Rangiah, 1954) and straightforward venereal transmission also appears likely.

Control. As for other venereal diseases. For treatment streptomycin or the tetracyclines are the drugs of choice. Resistance to streptomycin may occur. Chloramphenicol, erythromycin, and gentamicin are also used.

DISEASES CAUSED BY VIRUSES AND CHLAMYDIA

Introduction

These include *non-gonococcal urethritis, lymphogranuloma venereum, herpes simplex, condylomata acuminata,* and *molluscum contagiosum.*

Lymphogranuloma venereum and probably many cases of non-gonococcal urethritis are caused by large 'viruses' (*Chlamydia* or *Bedsonia*) which are considered not to be true viruses as they are visible under the light microscope, divide by binary fission, and react to chemotherapy with sulphonamides. A number of other true viruses (e.g. cytomegalovirus) may also be genitally transmitted.

Non-Gonococcal Urethritis

Definition. A urethral discharge in the male resulting from a number of causes other than gonorrhoea.

Aetiology. Once gonorrhoea and physiological discharges (prostatorrhoea, spermatorrhoea, prostaturia) have been excluded, the causes of non-gonococcal urethritis may be classified under five headings: (1) secondary to urethral sores, tumours, and stricture (2) secondary to urinary infections and disease of the urinary tract (including calculus, bilharzia, and urinary tuberculosis); (3) identifiable bacteria (e.g. *Esch. coli*) (4) trichomoniasis; and (5) abacterial urethritis, which is the most common.

The principal contenders as causative organisms of abacterial urethritis are T-strain (tiny culture) mycoplasmas and chlamydia. Inclusion bodies of the latter have been noted in epithelial cells of urethral specimens from those with this condition for many years (Harkness, 1950) and recent work using irradiated synovial (McCoy) tissue culture has given a significant number of positive findings in the urethra of male patients with non-gonococcal urethritis and in the urethra, cervix, and rectum of female sex contacts. These organisms may also be transferred to the child during birth, resulting in a form of ophthalmia neonatorum (Dunlop *et al.*, 1969). The organisms closely resemble those of trachoma and inclusion conjunctivitis and are commonly referred to as TRIC agent. The trachoma agent can therefore be transmitted sexually and may then be transferred from the genitals to the eyes.

Distribution. Non-gonococcal urethritis is world-wide and represents an increasing problem. The condition is frequently diagnosed as 'gonorrhoea' when no tests are taken. It occurs alone or following the treatment of gonorrhoea, when it may indicate a double infection; 62,498 new cases in males were reported in England in 1972, compared with 35,051 post-pubertal infections with gonorrhoea in that sex (Department of Health and Social Security, 1973). Although the virus may undoubtedly be present, to judge from the tests at present available, no clear-cut clinical counterpart can usually be found in the female.

Diagnosis. This is by exclusion of other causes of genital discharge, particularly gonorrhoea and trichomoniasis. Tissue culture techniques for chlamydia are not available except on a limited scale in a few research centres. A promising fluorescent serological typing test is being developed.

Treatment. This is directed at the cause. In abacterial urethritis the old-established tetracyclines given for six days offer a primary clinical cure rate of about 85 per cent. A number of other antibiotics (e.g. erythromycin) can also be used, but penicillin is not usually very effective and ampicillin less so.

Control. Until the course of the disease and the optimum length of the tetracycline course required to eradicate the organism in both sexes have been accurately determined the condition will remain out of control. At present female contacts are examined to exclude gonorrhoea, trichomoniasis, thrush or other identifiable infection in default of more precise tests. General measures of control include establishing a near one-to-one sexual relationship, discrimination regarding sexual associates and the use of the condom.

Reiter's Syndrome

A small proportion (approximately 1·0 per cent.) of male patients with non-gonococcal urethritis and sometimes those with gonorrhoea develop Reiter's syndrome with conjunctivitis and iritis, oral lesions, arthritis, sacroiliitis, subcalcaneal spurs, and occasionally cardiac involvement. The disease tends to be chronic and the response to treatment of rheumatic involvement is slow. It is many times less frequently seen in women. A similar condition may be encountered in both sexes following bacillary dysentery.

Examples of two or more men contracting the disease from a single woman are rare and it seems likely that a constitutional defect exists in those affected, in whom the condition is flared by an infective 'trigger'.

Lymphogranuloma Venereum

Definition. A venereal disease (Favre and Hellerström, 1954; Stannus, 1933) characterized in the male by a fleeting vesiculating primary genital papule followed by inguinal adenitis and multilocular bubo formation (climatic bubo). In the female, genital ulceration, scarring, chronic oedema (esthiomène), rectal stricture, and fistulae may occur following involvement of the pararectal glands.

Aetiology. The causative agent is of the chlamydia group (other agents of this group cause psittacosis, trachoma, non-gonococcal urethritis and enzootic abortion in ewes). It can be cultivated in the chick embryo and by tissue culture.

Epidemiology. The incubation period is 5–21 days. Distribution is world-wide but the disease is more prevalent in tropical or subtropical areas and in Negro or other non-white populations. In 1972, 59 cases were reported in England (Department of Health and Social Security, 1973) usually in immigrants or in association with sea-ports, and 828 cases were notified in the United States (United States Public Health Service, 1973). Men probably cease to be infective when the sore heals but women may remain infective for years.

Diagnosis. This is made by skin (Frei) test using killed cultured virus material and by complement-fixation serum test. Neither is entirely specific (cross-reactions occur with other members of the group) and positivity, once obtained, will persist.

Control. As for other venereal diseases. Treatment is by means of the sulphonamides or tetracyclines.

Herpes Simplex

Definition. A persistent recurrent condition, the commonest cause of a genital sore, which is produced by a true virus, the *herpes virus hominis*.

Epidemiology. There are two types of herpes virus: Type I, which usually affects the mouth and occasionally the genitals, and Type II, which usually affects the genitals but sometimes the mouth, the latter generally following genito-oral contact. They are distinguished by their cultural appearances on the chorio-allantoic membrane of the chick embryo and by serological techniques (e.g. neutralization tests). Infections with one virus do not confer immunity to those of the other.

Serological evidence of Type II virus is seldom found below the age of 14 years and the incidence then rises with age. There is a higher incidence in persons of low socio-economic status (in whom figures of 18–35 per cent. have been reported) than in higher social classes. Much higher seropositivity (80–85 per cent.) has been found in women with invasive cancer of the cervix (Nahmias *et al.*, 1970), suggesting an association between the two disorders.

Clinical Course. The primary infection is not infrequently severe, consisting of a crop of painful vesicles often with a slight but significant tender enlargement of the inguinal lymph nodes. In the female, intense dysuria, sometimes with retention of urine, may occur from urethral lesions and there may be extensive symptomless involvement of the cervix. Fever not infrequently may accompany these signs. Encephalitis and serious generalized infections are rare but very serious complications. Following the primary attack no recurrences may follow, but some patients have recurrent lesions of a much lesser severity at intervals of weeks or months which may persist for years. The foetus may be infected when the mother contracts the condition late in pregnancy and may develop a generalized infection which is usually fatal.

Diagnosis and Treatment. *Diagnosis* is made by virus

culture of the primary or recurrent lesions, by finding of characteristic cells with multinucleate inclusions in the smears (which may be noted during routine cervical cytology), and by serological methods. Complement-fixation tests will be negative at the onset of the primary infection, then within a few weeks antibodies rise to a high titre subsequently falling to a lower one which will persist even through recurrences. Syphilis should be excluded by dark-field and serum test.

Treatment is by means of soothing ointments. The antiviral agent 5 IDU (idoxuridine) may also be applied locally (Hutfield, 1968). Sulphonamides are given if there is secondary infection. There is as yet no known method of preventing recurrences.

Condylomata Acuminata

A common sexually acquired virus infection which results in pink, soft, fleshy papillomata on the genital mucous membranes and around the anus of both sexes, in the vagina and on the cervix uteri. When occurring on the skin they are yellowish-black and hard.

The incubation period varies from a few weeks to some months. The regular consort is often but not always clinically affected (Teokharov, 1969). Electron microscope studies have shown differences between condylomatous viral particles and those of the common skin wart virus. Treatment is by local applications of podophyllin or caustic substances, e.g. trichloroacetic acid, or by cautery. Attention should be paid to co-existing genital discharges.

Molluscum Contagiosum

A chronic condition due to a filterable virus which shows brick-like elementary bodies under the electron microscope. It is manifest by scattered raised shiny red umbilicated papules frequently on or near the genitalia. Spread is by contact frequently during the sexual act (Cobbold and MacDonald, 1970). Treatment is by careful application to the lesions of pure phenol or trichloroacetic acid, or by cautery.

DISEASES CAUSED BY PROTOZOA

The most common sexually transmitted protozoal disease is *trichomoniasis*. Genital ulceration from *amoebiasis* may sometimes be encountered in tropical areas which may, but not necessarily, result from sexual contact.

Trichomoniasis

A ubiquitous condition caused by a flagellated protozoon *T. vaginalis* which contends with candidiasis to be the most common cause of vaginal discharge. It results in a vaginitis in the female and in a urethritis or balanitis in the male, in which the condition is frequently self-limiting. Complications are rare. There were 1,535 male cases and 17,456 female cases reported from the venereal disease clinics in England in 1972 (Department of Health and Social Security, 1973).

Trichomoniasis is extremely prevalent in highly promiscuous women (e.g. prostitutes) and more prevalent in the lower than the upper socio-economic strata (Trussell, 1947). A prevalence of from 1 to 46 per cent. has been found by routine testing in different groups, and of around 40 per cent. of women with gonorrhoea. The reported higher rates in some Negroes probably reflects socio-economic status.

While usually sexually transmitted, spread can occur by indirect contact by means of towels and dirty lavatory seats. Prepubertal girls and post-menopausal women are sometimes infected.

Diagnosis is made by direct microscopy of wet smear, by culture or by suitably stained smear. The organism is frequently identified during routine cervical cytology.

Treatment is by means of metronidazole or nitrimidazine by mouth, except in the first three months of pregnancy when probably the use of one of many available pessaries is best advised. The regular male consort should also be treated, certainly in relapsing cases.

DISEASES CAUSED BY FUNGI

Candidiasis (Moniliasis)

A number of fungi of the *Candida* genus (e.g. *Candida albicans* (*monilia*), *Candida oidium*, and *Candida stellatoidea*) are frequently carried by man, usually in small amounts in the mouth, nose, throat, bowel, vagina, and on the skin.

Under certain conditions (e.g. in the presence of glycosuria, debility of the patient due to intercurrent disease, following the use of systemic or local antibiotics or other chemotherapy, especially immunosuppressive drugs, and possibly also in relation to the use of the contraceptive pill, any of which may alter the local ecology and remove normal competitors), the fungus may overgrow (Catterall, 1971). This results in vulvar soreness and irritation and a vaginal discharge like cream cheese, or in burning and irritation when it occurs in the rectum.

Candidiasis can be a cause of recurrent balanitis in the male partner and occasionally of urethritis. Balanitis may result from infection of the penis (which is common in diabetics) or from allergy to the fungus. *Monilia* is also the cause of a napkin rash and stomatitis in the newborn.

Treatment is local by means of antifungal antibiotics (e.g. nystatin, candicidin or amphotericin B), or other substances of proved worth, locally in the form of pessaries, cream, or paints. Nystatin and amphotericin B, which are not absorbed from the gut, are also used orally in bowel infections and to prevent reinfection of the vagina.

Tinea Cruris

See CHAPTER 20 under dermatomycoses.

Scabies

The itch, caused by *Sarcoptes* (*Acarus*) *scabiei*, is a contact disease which is not infrequently contracted during sexual intercourse. The impregnated female lays her eggs in burrows in the skin commonly around the fingers, wrist, ankles, axillae or genitalia. Papules and vesicles follow on the body, which are characteristically extremely irritant when the patient is warm, particularly at night; secondary infection may result from scratching.

The diagnosis is usually made on clinical grounds but the acarus, just visible to the naked dye, can be recovered from a burrow on the tip of a needle. Treatment is by means of body applications of lotions containing benzyl benzoate or gamma benzene hexachloride.

Pediculosis Pubis

A sexually transmitted infestation with the crab louse (*Phthirus pubis*) which affects the pubic, axillary and body hair including sometimes the beard, eyebrows and eyelashes but never the head hair. The incubation period is believed to be around 30 days (Fisher and Morton, 1970)

The adult motile louse is just visible to the naked eye, and its eggs (nits), which have a convex cap, are best seen with a hand lens and are greyish in colour attached to the hairs. The adult feeds on human blood and its bites cause irritation and a little bleeding.

Treatment is by means of shaving and the application of a lotion or powder containing DDT or gamma benzene hexachloride.

EPIDEMIOLOGICAL ASPECTS OF THE VENEREAL DISEASES

There are many interwoven demographic, social, and medical factors which have led to the present increase in the venereal diseases (Guthe and Willcox, 1971) and these are listed in TABLE 55. The most important are those concerned with alterations in heterosexual and homosexual behaviour and with population mobility, which is facilitating the spread of venereal disease by breaking previously enclosed 'circles' of sexual exposure, and by increasing opportunities of sexual encounter not only internally but also between countries. International population movements today are truly vast. There are an estimated 177 million tourists in the world, of which 126 million are in Europe, where there are also 6 million migrant labourers of both sexes of whom one-third return to their own country each year to be replaced by others (WHO, 1972*b*).

CONTROL OF VENEREAL DISEASE

The basis of venereal disease control is early case-finding and early treatment.

General Measures

These include provision of adequate facilities for free and confidential treatment, effective publicity of whereabouts of clinics at home and overseas (e.g. under the Brussels Agreement by means of the WHO *World Directory of Venereal Disease Treatment Centres in Ports* (WHO, 1964) and health education of the young to acquaint them with the early signs of disease, what they should do if infection is suspected, and how the diseases can be prevented including emphasis on the dangers of promiscuity.

Legislative measures should aim to suppress quackery and the obtaining of antibiotics only on a physician's prescription.

Measures to be Taken by the Patient

These comprise restraint on promiscuous behaviour, discrimination in choice of partner, use of the condom by the male, urination and washing well with soap and water after intercourse. During the Second World War local calomel ointment was employed by the troops to prevent syphilis. Currently, chemical and other foams for the female, which are

TABLE 55
Reasons for Failure of Control of Venereal Disease

Demographic factors	(a) More susceptibles	Increasing population; relatively more young people
	(b) Longer individual sexual span	Longer life; earlier maturity; dispensation of menopause by hormones
	(c) Better contact tracing. More attending clinics	Higher female figures, less unwillingness to attend
Social factors	(a) Breaking of previously closed sexual 'circles' by population movement	Urbanization; industrialization; war and military movement; relatively lower standards of living elsewhere (immigration and migrant labour); increased standards of living at home (more local travel, more cars, more motor bicycles, more tourism, more leisure, more 'club' life, more boredom); technical advancements (more ships, more air travel with larger aircraft)
	(b) Increased promiscuity	*Direct encouragement* from changing attitudes, codes of behaviour and the so-called permissive society, increased emphasis on sex in mass media; more practising promiscuous homosexuals; more premarital intercourse; more money to spend on alcohol, narcotic drugs; broken homes (divorces, illegitimacy); indiscrimination (poorer prospects of contact tracing); *Diminished restraining influence* of religion, parents and family, public opinion, fear of venereal disease (easy treatment), fear of pregnancy (pill and intra-uterine devices), with increased risk of VD from lessened use of the condom (Juhlin and Lidén, 1969)
	(c) Ignorance	Among young persons, teachers, medical students, and doctors
Medical factors	(a) ? Changing pattern of disease	? Milder, ? longer incubation periods, recognition of new clinical syndromes
	(b) No decisive new advance in diagnosis	Too little research. No quick screening test without genital examination, particularly in asymptomatic female, capable of detecting gonorrhoea *before* disease has been passed on
	(c) Increasing failure rates to treatment	Development of resistance of the gonococcus to antibiotics
	(d) Lack of immunizing procedure	Multiple attacks
	(e) Strained facilities	Insufficient money spent on premises, medical and ancillary staff and contact-tracers

also spermicidal, are under evaluation in the United States and elsewhere.

Measures to be Taken by the Physician

Effective Treatment. Prompt and adequate treatment and follow-up to exclude relapse will prevent further community spread.

Contact Tracing. Every effort must be directed towards contact tracing both of source contacts and of secondary contacts after the infection has been acquired. The latter can be induced to attend in about 85 per cent. of cases by patient persuasion, with the use of the 'contact slip'. Source contacts are more difficult to secure and the services of a contact interviewer (venereal diseases social worker in British VD clinics) should be used where available, who will seek out the source where possible and who will often obtain information from the patient regarding secondary contacts over and above those originally stated by the patient to the physician.

When the contacts have been secured the necessary tests should be carried out and, in the case of syphilis, gonorrhoea, and trichomoniasis, the patient treated either for proven disease or epidemiological treatment offered, should the initial tests appear negative. The latter procedure is certainly most desirable for those unable or unlikely later to attend, for known persistent defaulters or highly promiscuous persons and pregnant women.

The social contacts of patients with venereal disease can be regarded as members of a high-risk group, and *cluster testing* has been used in parts of the United States, whereby suspects interviewed as contacts are asked to name their friends, not necessarily sexual associates, who might benefit from a blood test for syphilis. These persons, too, are interviewed and persuaded to have a serological text.

Screening Programmes. Serological screening for syphilis should be obligatory for expectant mothers, blood donors, and hospital patients with neurological and cardiac disease. Attention should also be paid to high-risk groups (e.g. seamen, military, prisoners, prostitutes, and others, depending on yield). This matter is dealt with more fully on page 283.

Screening for gonorrhoea represents greater technical difficulties with varying yields obtained, but should also be applied to high-risk groups [see p. 286].

The control of the venereal diseases is no easy matter, as the effects of social behaviour tend to overcome the effectiveness of medical measures. It depends in the long run on a summation of many efforts, the results from any one of which may seem small.

REFERENCES

Treponematoses

Department of Health and Social Security (1973) *Sexually-Transmitted Diseases*, Report of the Chief Medical Officer for the year 1971, London, H.M.S.O., p. 67.

Gjestland, T. (1955) The Oslo study of untreated syphilis. An epidemiological investigation of the natural course of the syphilitic infection based on a re-study of the Boeck-Bruusgard material, *Acta derm. Venereol.*, **35,** Suppl. 34.

Grin, E. I. (1953) Epidemiology and control of endemic syphilis, *Wld Hlth Org. Monogr. Ser.*, No. 11.

Guthe, T., and Idsøe, O. (1968a) The rise and fall of the treponematoses, II. Endemic treponematoses of childhood, *Brit. J. vener. Dis.*, **44,** 35.

Guthe, T., and Idsøe, O. (1968b) Antibiotic treatment of syphilis, in *Current Problems in Dermatology*, Vol. 2, *Antibiotic Treatment of Venereal Diseases*, Basel, pp. 1–38.

Guthe, T., and Willcox, R. R. (1954) Treponematoses a world problem, *Wld Hlth Org. Chron.*, No. 8, Special Number, 37–114.

Hackett, C. J. (1957) *An International Nomenclature of Yaws Lesions*, World Health Organization, Geneva.

Hudson, E. H. (1958) *Non-Venereal Syphilis. A Sociological and Medical Study of Bejel*, Edinburgh.

Idsøe, O., and Guthe, T. (1967) The rise and fall of the treponematoses, I. Ecological aspects and international trends in venereal syphilis, *Brit. J. vener. Dis.*, **43,** 227.

Medina, R. (1967) Pinta, *Derm. ibero. Latin-Amer.*, (Eng. ed.), **1,** 121.

Nabarro, D. (1954) *Congenital Syphilis*, London.

Nery-Guimarães, F. N. (1970) *Yaws in Diseases of Children in the Subtropics and Tropics*, London, pp. 752–68.

Rhodes, F. A., and Anderson, S. L. J. (1970) An outbreak of treponematosis in the Eastern Highlands of New Guinea, *Papua and New Guinea med. J.*, **13,** 49.

Turner, T. B., and Hollander, D. H. (1957) Biology of the treponematoses, *Wld Hlth Org. Monogr. Ser.*, No. 35.

United States Public Health Service (1968) *Syphilis: a Synopsis*, Public Health Service Publication No. 1660, United States Department of Health, Education and Welfare, Washington D.C.

United States Public Health Service (1969) *Manual of Tests for Syphilis 1969*, United States Department of Health, Education and Welfare, Atlanta, Georgia.

United States Public Health Service (1973) *VD Fact Sheet, 1972* 29th ed., United States Department of Health, Education and Welfare, Atlanta, Georgia.

Van der Sluis, I. (1969) *The Treponematosis of Tahiti*, Amsterdam.

Willcox, R. R. (1950) Njovera: an endemic syphilis of Southern Rhodesia, *Lancet*, **i,** 558.

Willcox, R. R. (1964) *Textbook of Venereal Diseases and Treponematoses*, 2nd ed., London.

Willcox, R. R. (1969) The treponematoses, in *Essays on Tropical Dermatology*, eds. Simons, R. D. G., Ph.D, and Marshall, J., Excerpta Medica Foundation, Amsterdam, pp. 35–47.

Willcox, R. R., and Guthe, T. (1966) *Treponema pallidum*: a bibliographical review of the morphology, culture and survival of *T. pallidum* and associated organisms, *Bull. Wld Hlth Org.*, **35,** Suppl. I.

World Health Organization (1953) Fourth Report of the Expert Committee on Venereal Infections and Treponematoses, *Wld Hlth Org. techn. Rep. Ser.*, No. 63.

World Health Organization (1960) Fifth Report of the Expert Committee on Venereal Infections and Treponematoses, *Wld Hlth Org. techn. Rep. Ser.*, No. 190.

World Health Organization (1970) Treponematoses research. Report of a WHO Study Group, *Wld Hlth Org. techn. Rep. Ser.*, No. 455.

Other Sexually Transmitted Diseases

American Society of Health Association (1973) *Today's VD Control Problem*, New York.

Brown, W. (1971) The national VD problem, in *The VD Crisis*, Amer. Soc. Hyg. Ass. and Pfizer Laboratories, New York.

Catterall, R. D. (1971) Influence of gestogenic contraceptive pills on vaginal candidosis, *Brit. J. vener. Dis.*, **47,** 45.

Cobbold, R. J. C., and MacDonald, A. (1970) Molluscum contagiosum as a sexually-transmitted disease, *Practitioner*, **204**, 416.

Department of Health and Social Security (1971) *Sexually-transmitted Diseases*, Report of Chief Medical Officer for the Year 1970, London, H.M.S.O., pp. 61–70.

Dunlop, E. M. C., Hare, M. J., Darougar, S., Jones, B. R., and Rice, N. S. C. (1969) Detection of *Chlamydia* (*Bedsonia*) in certain infections, II. Clinical study of genital tract, eye, rectum and other sites of recovery of *Chlamydia*, *J. infect. Dis.*, **120**, 463.

Favre, M., and Hellerström, S. (1954) The epidemiology, aetiology and prophylaxis of lymphogranuloma inguinale, *Acta derm. venereol.*, **34**, Suppl. 30.

Fisher, I., and Morton, R. S. (1970) Phthirus pubis infestation, *Brit. J. vener. Dis.*, **46**, 326.

Goldberg, J. (1964) Studies on granuloma inguinale, *Brit. J. vener. Dis.*, **40**, 140.

Guthe, T., and Willcox, R. R. (1971) The international incidence of venereal disease, *Roy. Soc. Hlth J.*, **91**, 122.

Harkness, A. H. (1950) *Non-gonoccocal Urethritis*, Edinburgh.

Hutfield, D. C. (1968) Herpes genitalis, *Brit. J. vener. Dis.*, **44**, 241.

Juhlin, L., and Lidén, S. (1969) Influence of contraceptive gestogen pills on sexual behaviour and the spread of gonorrhoea, *Brit. J. vener. Dis.*, **45**, 321.

Maddocks, I. (1967) Donovanosis in Papua, *Papua and New Guinea med. J.*, **10**, 49.

Nahmias, A. J., Josey, W. E., Naib, Z. M., Luce, C. F., and Guest, B. A. (1970) Antibodies to herpes virus hominis types 1 and 2, II. Women with cervical cancer, *Amer. J. Epidemiol.*, **91**, 547.

Rajam, R. V., and Rangiah, P. N. (1954) Donovanosis, *Wld Hlth Org. Monogr. Ser.*, No. 24.

Stannus, H. S. (1933) *A Sixth Venereal Disease (Lymphogranuloma Venereum)*, London.

Teokharov, B. A. (1969) Non-gonococcal infections of the female genitalia, *Brit. J. vener. Dis.*, **45**, 334.

Trussel, R. E. (1947) *Trichomas Vaginalis and Trichomoniasis*, Springfield, Ill.

United States Public Health Service (1973) *VD Fact Sheet 1972*, 29th ed., Atlanta, Georgia.

Willcox, R. R. (1960) Epidemiological aspects of human trichomoniasis, *Brit. J. vener. Dis.*, **36**, 167.

Willcox, R. R. (1964) *Textbook of Venereal Diseases and Treponematoses*, 2nd ed., London.

Willcox, R. R. (1968) Treatment of gonorrhoea in the male, in *Current Problems in Dermatology*, Vol. 2, *Antiobiotic Treatment of Venereal Diseases*, Basel, pp. 101–40.

Willcox, R. R. (1970) A survey of problems in the antibiotic treatment of gonorrhoea, *Brit. J. vener. Dis.*, **46**, 217.

Willcox, R. R. (1972) A world wide review of venereal disease, *Brit. J. vener. Dis.*, **48**, 163.

World Health Organization (1963) First Report of the Expert Committee on Gonococcal Infections, *Wld Hlth Org. techn. Rep. Ser.*, No. 262.

World Health Organization (1969) *Second Regional Seminar on Venereal Disease Control*, WHO Regional Office for the Western Pacific, Manila, Philippines.

World Health Organization (1972*a*) *Report of WHO and IUVDT International Travelling Seminar to the U.S.A.*, Geneva.

World Health Organization (1972*b*) *Report of WHO Study Group on the Inter-country Spread of Venereal Disease*, Copenhagen.

World Health Organization (1972*c*) *World Directory of Venereal Disease Treatment Centres*, 3rd ed., Geneva.

World Health Organization (1973) Venereal diseases, *Wld Hlth Org. Chron.*, **27**, 418.

World Health Organization (1974) Genital infections in East African women, *Wld Hlth Org. Chron.*, **28**, 264.

World Health Organization Regional Office for Europe (1973) Directory of VD Treatment Centres in the European Region (Euro 1101 (1)), Copenhagen.

22

THE EPIDEMIOLOGY AND CONTROL OF THE ZOONOSES

J. H. STEELE

Introduction

The interrelation of human and animal disease is probably as old as the origin of man, presuming that most of the animals were here before man. All pathogenic micro-organisms are biologically adventuresome in their struggle to survive—they must find a host. The broader the host-range, the easier their survival. As the host-range of animal pathogens expands they become a threat to man's well-being. This is well illustrated by many diseases which at one time were primarily identified with wild life and now have been able to adapt themselves to domestic and pet animals.

The total number of infectious diseases that plague domestic animals is in excess of 400. The 1967 WHO Expert Committee on Zoonoses lists more than 150 diseases which are *common* to man and animals. If one considers the emerging zoonoses (recently identified virus diseases of animals that are closely related to similar entities described in man) the possible size of the reservoir of diseases in the animal kingdom broadens. New disease entities or previously unsuspected human–animal disease relationships are being reported with increasing frequency. Why is this occurring? No one can give a complete answer, but there are many factors at work, the most important being the constant change of host–parasite environment interactions.

Man's success in the control, elimination, and eradication of some of the major communicable disease problems in limited areas of the world has allowed him to redirect his scientific curiosity and pursuits to unresolved problems. Certain of these are periodic epidemic diseases, such as the arthropod-borne encephalitides, epidemic haemorrhagic fever, and fevers of undetermined aetiology (FUA), many of which are known or suspected of having an animal reservoir. The great changes in human and animal ecology which result from the agricultural and industrial development of new territories as well as old ones throughout the world have brought man into contact with animals and disease agents with which he may have had little or no experience. Leptospirosis in Malaya, haemorrhagic fever in Siberia, leishmaniasis in Brazil, enzootic hepatitis in South Africa, and Q fever in Europe are examples of such diseases. Some of these are sporadic diseases that suddenly become epidemic or epizootic in their proportions when susceptible human and domestic animal populations are increased.

It is anticipated that these populations will continue to grow. To develop the food-animal resources needed to provide a standard of living comparable to any of the advanced Western countries will require a three-to-four-fold increase in their numbers. The control of old and new diseases in this population will be a task with which all branches of medicine, public health, and agriculture will be concerned.

Definition and Classification of Zoonoses

The World Health Organization in previous reports defined zoonoses as "Those diseases and infections which are naturally transmitted between vertebrate animals and man' (WHO, 1959). It has been argued that this definition is too wide in that it includes not only infections that man acquires from animals but also: (1) diseases produced by non-infective agents, such as toxins and poisons; and (2) infections that animals acquire from man, that are merely incidental infections of no public health importance. In spite of these drawbacks, the definition has been widely accepted, and the Committee recommends that it should not be modified. However, any list of zoonoses should include only those infections for which there is either proof or strong circumstantial evidence that there is transmission between animals and man.

The Committee agreed that some form of classification of zoonoses is useful, particularly for teaching and the epidemiology evaluation. To meet these demands the following system for the classification of zoonoses has been accepted:

1. *Direct zoonoses* are transmitted from an infected vertebrate host to a susceptible vertebrate host by direct contact, by contact with a fomite, or by a mechanical vector. The agent itself undergoes little or no propagative changes and no essential developmental change during the transmission. Examples are rabies, trichinosis, and brucellosis.

2. *Cyclo-zoonoses* required more than one vertebrate host species, but no invertebrate host, in order to complete the developmental cycle of the agent. Examples are the human taeniases, echinococcosis, and pentastomid infections.

3. *Meta-zoonoses* are transmitted biologically by invertebrate vectors. In the invertebrate the agent multiplies or develops, or both, and there is always an extrinsic incubation (prepatent) period before transmission to another vertebrate host is possible. Examples are numerous, and include arbovirus infections, plague, and schistosomiasis.

4. *Sapro-zoonoses* have both a vertebrate host and a non-animal developmental site or reservoir. Organic matter (including food), soil, and plants are considered to be non-animal. Examples include the various forms of larva migrans and some of the mycoses.

Prevention, Control, and Eradication

The FAO/WHO Expert Committee on Zoonoses recognizes more than 150 zoonoses [see TABLE 55, p. 241]. Prevention, control, and eradication of some of these diseases, particularly where domestic animals are the principal reservoirs, are problems of considerable magnitude in every country. Reservoirs of zoonoses among domesticated animals are the sources of greatest danger for man, since he is in closest contact with such animals. Emphasis should therefore be given to these zoonoses in the development of programmes to combat animal diseases. Notable successes have been achieved when such a procedure has been followed—for example, with bovine tuberculosis, brucellosis, and rabies.

The discharge of governmental responsibilities for zoonoses control requires adequate financial support and close collaboration between different government agencies, particularly the medical and veterinary services. The operation of interministerial (e.g. health and agriculture) committees has proved to be an excellent means of achieving co-operative effort on the zoonoses and has also led to appreciable savings by the pooling of funds, personnel, and equipment. Such formal means of collaboration encourage free and frequent exchange of information on animal and human diseases, joint planning and financing of disease-control campaigns, improved food-hygiene services, and mutual assistance in laboratory and epidemiologic work. Such committees should not, however, remain as paper organizations.

Attention to the zoonoses must be given at all levels of government—local, municipal, provincial, and national. In any area environmental conditions and local customs of the population must be studied carefully before control measures can be instituted. Measures that are successful in economically advanced countries may not be applicable to developing areas without modification.

In planning campaigns against disease, three points are important: prevention, control, and eradication. Prevention is well defined in the lexicons of all nations, and there is little confusion over its meaning. Control is a more ambiguous term that means different things to different officials and workers, depending upon their training, experience, and culture. Definitions of control range from the enactment of regulations or legislation, with little or no attempt at enforcement, to quarantine, restrictions on movement, vaccination, and even destruction of animals and property. In some cases control programmes are enacted with the purpose of complete elimination of a disease, i.e. eradication. (Examples are the elimination of glanders, rinderpest, bovine pleuropneumonia, and fowl plague from Europe and the Americas.) As used in this chapter, the three terms are defined as follows:

Prevention consists of measures to protect man or animals against disease. These may frequently be independent of measures aimed at bringing the disease under control.

Control consists of measures to reduce the prevalence or incidence of disease or infection in animals and man.

Eradication is the total elimination of the aetiologic agent from a region. (The term 'eradication' is used by some authorities to denote elimination of disease and not necessarily of all the infective agents, especially when the chances that the agent will infect a mammalian host are very small.)

Today a nation or state that undertakes campaigns against disease must weigh many factors. Whether to follow a policy of control or one of eradication can be decided only by considering the social organization of a particular country and by weighing the various interests and claims of its economy. Many questions arise in this connexion. Is eradication of a given disease possible? If so, is it economically justifiable? Does a particular policy fit in with the social structure and customs of the country, or would it be a disruptive influence that would be resisted and thus probably fail? Is partial control feasible, or does the situation demand complete eradication and continued freedom from the infective agent or vector?

Eradication of several communicable diseases, such as malaria and smallpox, has become an international goal. National campaigns to eradicate disease include such zoonoses as plague, rabies, bovine tuberculosis, and brucellosis. In certain areas where geographic conditions are favourable and in economically advanced countries some of these diseases have been eradicated. Eradication is possible in selected areas unless animal reservoirs provide inaccessible sanctuaries for infective agents (e.g. the bat and monkey reservoirs for rabies and yellow fever, respectively) and provided the cost is not too great.

The cost factor is often paramount. Economic justification of an eradication campaign, e.g. for bovine tuberculosis or brucellosis, is fairly easy in the early stages, when the returns are greatest for the money invested. When, however, the later stages of the campaign are reached and costs begin to rise for each case revealed great doubts arise. The problem is particularly perplexing if any relaxation of effort means a gradual loss of all ground gained. If one considers the very large costs involved in finally eliminating the extremely small number of residual cases or reservoirs of disease agents, attempts at such a policy are seldom justifiable, particularly in developing countries. But even though eradication may not be practicable, a continuous effort must be made to control the disease so that it does not erupt as an epizootic or continue to take too high a toll in human disease or economic loss.

It is recognized that the goal of eradication has great public appeal, and often gives to disease-control campaigns support that would otherwise not have been forthcoming. However, in cases where it is clear that eradication, if achieved, would be a long and costly process it would be less misleading and perhaps equally effective to label such campaigns 'pre-eradication' or 'suppression'.

Zoonoses as Occupational Hazards and Their Economic Implications

Zoonoses are occupational hazards faced by agricultural, industrial, and laboratory workers and animal handlers. The problems of agricultural workers have been considered by a Joint ILO/WHO Committee on Occupational Health (WHO, 1962). A wide variety of communicable diseases and parasitic infections considered in the present report can be classified as occupational diseases. Some diseases have significantly higher attack rates on workers in the course of their occupations than on the rest of the population. A classic example of this is the occurrence of anthrax in carpet weavers, livestock raisers, and workers with animal hair in the textile industry. Leptospirosis in rice-field workers, brucellosis in agricultural workers, erysipeloid in butchers and fish merchants, tularaemia and trypanosomiasis in hunters, and creeping eruption in plumbers, trench diggers, and others are examples of occupational zoonoses that have been long recognized.

In recent years advances in the control of animal diseases,

changes in agricultural and industrial practices, and changes in the environment have contributed to shifts in the epidemiologic pattern of some of the zoonoses. Thus, brucellosis has in some regions changed from a disease primarily transmitted by the ingestion of milk and milk products contaminated with *Brucella* to one transmitted by contact or inhalation, especially among meat packers and veterinarians; ornithosis has shifted from a disease of owners of pet birds to an occupational disease among workers in poultry-processing plants.

The zoonoses have become, over the years, increasingly identified as occupational hazards. The list includes Q fever in abattoir and rendering-plant workers, jungle yellow fever and tick-borne diseases in woodcutters, salmonellosis in food processers, bovine tuberculosis in farmers, Newcastle disease in poultry raisers and processers, contagious ecthyma (orf) in sheep shearers, and rabies in veterinarians, field naturalists, and dog-control employees.

An important recent addition to the recognized occupational zoonoses is infectious hepatitis transmitted to man from chimpanzees and other subhuman primates. Many hundreds of instances of such transmission have been established by epidemiologic investigation during the last several years. Most of these have involved animal handlers and research biologists working with primate colonies.

The economic impact of zoonoses is extremely difficult to determine accurately, but it is known to be considerable. It includes mortality and acute and chronic debilitating illness of humans, loss of life and impairment of productivity of livestock, and consequent effects on the social fabric and economic development. It is clear that in this connexion developing countries suffer much greater losses than technically advanced countries. This is attributable to the lack of adequately organized public health and veterinary services and to particular social customs prevailing in the predominantly agricultural societies of developing countries. Economic losses caused by brucellosis, bovine tuberculosis, rabies, cysticercosis, and hydatidosis are estimated to be hundreds of millions of dollars annually in Latin American countries alone, quite apart from the human suffering and death caused by these diseases. Worldwide, the economic losses are in billions of dollars.

ANTHRAX

Although the number of reported cases of anthrax, both human and cattle, is relatively low when compared to the other zoonoses, it is felt that these data give a false impression of the true importance of this disease. In a report (Glassman, 1958) it was estimated that about 9,000 human cases are reported annually in the world, although the author believes a truer incidence of disease may be somewhere between 20,000 and 100,000 cases per year. Many thousands of animal cases still occur in some parts of the world, even though good immunizing agents are available. But unfortunately there are vaccines which are neither effective nor safe. The latter occurs when wild strains of *Bacillus anthracis* contaminates live vaccines. It is essential that all animal vaccines be tested continuously, by both the producer and the supervising state authority. When live vaccines are used antibiotics—penicillin, tetracyclines, etc.—should be avoided, as they will neutralize the viable attenuated organisms in the vaccine. Most of the human cases occur

in farmers and animal husbandrymen, but in some areas industrial infections are not uncommon. Epidemiologically the problem can be conveniently divided into its agricultural and industrial aspects.

Agricultural anthrax is most frequently encountered in so-called 'anthrax districts', where the soil is contaminated with the spore form of the *B. anthracis*. Such districts exist on all of the continents, but particularly in Asia, Africa, and parts of southern Europe (Kaplan, 1954). The spores are very resistant to chemical and environmental influence, and can survive for years in certain types of soils and in animal products, such as hides, hair, and wool. When anthrax infection in livestock becomes established in a district there is created a relatively permanent enzootic focus of infection because of the inability of the soil to destroy the spores.

There is considerable evidence to show that anthrax is occasionally carried into some countries by feeds (Van Ness and Stein, 1956), bones and bone meal (Kaplan, 1954), hair and coarse wools, and less frequently hides. Non-infected materials may also become contaminated during transport in vehicles or ships and in warehouses or docks that have previously been seeded with spores. Contamination of agricultural areas may occur through the use of fertilizers or waste materials salvaged from bone-, wool-, and hair-processing plants or by the effluents from tanneries.

Herbivorous animals, especially cattle and sheep, are susceptible to the disease. Horses, deer, buffalo and other wild herbivora, guinea-pigs, rabbits, and mice are also very prone to infection, but swine are less susceptible. Dogs, cats, and most birds are relatively insusceptible, but may be infected artificially. Cold-blooded animals are not affected. The anthrax bacillus can also be spread by flesh-eating birds, animals, and insects from diseased carcasses to healthy animals.

The main sources of infection in agricultural workers are contact with contaminated carcasses, wool, hides, and hair. The ingestion of insufficiently cooked meat derived from infected animals is another source of infection. Inhalation anthrax is rare, but a few cases have been and are still reported among workers handling diseased animal products.

Many factors contribute to the frequency of anthrax among rural people. Despite familiarity on the part of farmers with anthrax in livestock in enzootic districts where the disease recurs periodically, the diagnosis of a single case or group of cases is difficult to recognize because of the lack of striking signs in the hyperacute form of the disease. For economic reasons, farmers are loath to lose the values of hides which are salvaged from dead animals, even where anthrax is recognized as the cause of death. Animals are often slaughtered at the first sign of any illness for meat purposes as well as for their by-products. These practices are highly dangerous and lead to human outbreaks of disease.

Animals that are ill should be placed under the supervision of a veterinarian. If the disease is in the early stages the animal will frequently respond to antibiotic therapy. When animals die of suspected anthrax the attending veterinarian must determine if an autopsy is necessary. Blood smears made directly from the animal immediately after death may provide presumptive evidence of infection, but diagnosis should never be based entirely upon microscopic examination of blood smears. In addition to blood samples, tissues, i.e. spleen and liver, are valuable in establishing a diagnosis. Culture and animal inoculation procedures should always be used for confirmation. *B. anthracis* identification should be confirmed by gamma bacteriophage typing. The carcasses of animals dead from anthrax should be destroyed at the site where the animal died as soon as possible after death. The preferred method is by incineration, followed by deep burial, with lime spread over the area.

Livestock vaccination is the best preventive veterinary medicine in the control of anthrax. Education of the agricultural population about the disease in man and animals is an important practice in control. Naturally, neither meat nor milk from diseased cows should be used by man. When disease outbreaks occur, the animals and premises involved should be quarantined for a period extending 2 weeks beyond the last diagnosed case of anthrax or 2 weeks following effective immunization. The problem of the management and disposal of milk from dairy herds under these conditions can be quite difficult. Fortunately, cattle infected with anthrax do not usually excrete the bacillus in their milk, since milk secretion stops abruptly. Despite the possibility of environmental contamination of milk, there are few reports of milk-transmitted anthrax (Steele and Helvig, 1953).

The recognition or suspicion of anthrax in a carcass in an abattoir calls for drastic measures. Operations should cease until rapid presumptive tests (smears or the Ascoli precipitation test) are made. If these are positive the infected carcasses and all carcasses possibly exposed to contamination should be sterilized, and the contaminated premises should be thoroughly disinfected (with 2 per cent. lye) before operations are resumed. In well-run abattoirs such incidents occur only rarely, because animals ill with anthrax are usually recognized at ante-mortem inspection.

Milk from healthy animals in the herd can be used provided the herd is under veterinary supervision and good sanitary practices are followed. Such milk should be heat treated or pasteurized under special arrangements.

Cutaneous anthrax is by far the most frequent form of disease among industrial workers. Hair, wool, bones, hides, and skins are the usual sources. Although the inhalation form of anthrax (wool sorter's disease) is rare (Morton, 1954), a few cases continue to occur (Plotkin, 1959). Goat hair and skins from areas where anthrax is highly enzootic are the greatest source of human infection. The most dangerous wools are coarse wools from countries where anthrax is a severe and continuing problem. Clipped wool or so-called 'grease' wool is sheared from live animals and is not as often contaminated with *B. anthracis* spores as are 'pulled' wools, since the latter may originate from animals dead of anthrax. Bones have frequently been the cause of industrial anthrax cases in man (Green and Jamieson, 1958).

A fatal case of inhalation anthrax in a person exposed to dust aerosols from a goat-hair processing plant was recently reported in the northern United States. The patient's symptoms were typical of anthrax. Many large Gram-positive bacilli were found in the mediastinal lymph nodes, meninges, and lungs, and *B. anthracis* was recovered from a haemorrhagic mediastinal lymph node (La Force *et al.*, 1969).

Epidemiologic investigation revealed significant surface and aerial contamination with *B. anthracis* at the goat-hair process-ing plant and ample opportunity for aerial spread of the organism.

In the past numerous cases of anthrax in man have been caused from bristles of shaving and some other brushes contaminated with anthrax spores. No animal bristles or hair that have not been sterilized before being embedded in the handle should be used for shaving brushes. In the United Kingdom all goat hair and wool or animal hair has to be imported through Liverpool, where it is disinfected by the 'Duckering' process. The process is carried out mechanically, so that there is no man-handling of the material. The process consists of exposing the material to different disinfecting solutions at a temperature of 81° C.

Control of industrial anthrax has been discussed by numerous authors (Wolff and Heimann, 1951). The problem of decontaminating animal hides is at present still in the process of development. Canada requires by law the decontamination of hides in approved establishments using acid-type disinfectants, such as hydrochloric acid, formic acid, mercuric acid, and sodium bifluoride (Moynihan, 1963). Ethylene oxide fumigation is also effective, but expensive (Sen, 1961). An interesting development is the use of cobalt irradiation for purposes of decontamination (Afagonova, 1963; Turner and Willis, 1959).

An effective human vaccine has been developed and evaluated in the United States (Brachman *et al.*, 1962) for use in high-risk groups. This vaccine is a cell-free, culture filtrate with a high level of protective antigen. Live human vaccines have been developed by other countries, notably Russia, with reported success, where they are used in animal-industry workers.

Wild animal epizootics have been reported world wide from such widely separated regions as the North-West Territories of Canada (Pyper and Willoughby, 1964) and Kruger National Park, South Africa (Pienaar, 1960). The Canadian epizootic caused the death of 281 among 1,300 buffalo who were in the immediate area. Two human cases occurred, one in a biologist who had examined animals bare-handed without any precautions and developed several pustules on the wrists and forearm, and the other in a driver who also handled dead animals. The latter developed a pulmonary disease. Both men recovered with tetracycline therapy. Sporadic cases have continued to occur since the original outbreak. To prevent any further human infections, all men were given tetracycline prophylactically, 250 mg. twice daily. Men in the field were also given protective clothing of overalls, rubber boots, gloves, masks, and goggles.

The source of the outbreak was not clearly identified, but the incidence of disease ended with frost that killed the biting flies.

The Kruger National Park outbreak involved thousands of wild animals and some cattle on farms south of the park. Anthrax was also reported to be rife among buffalo herds in Mozambique, and in Bechuanaland among giraffe, leopards, and hyenas. The immediate cause of the epidemic is unknown. Among the wild animals found dead in Kruger National Park were 771 kudus, 75 waterbucks, 58 buffalo, 41 roan antelope, 28 nyalas, 16 zebras, 13 bushbucks, 10 steenbucks, 7 impalas. Other animals found dead or dying included elephants (3), giraffes (2), wart-hogs (5), leopards (14), lions (2), and a cheetah. All post-mortem diagnoses were based on the examination of blood smears. The South African investigators state that the epidemic was apparently spread by vultures from dead animals, on which they fed, to watering places. The excreta of vultures and other carrion-eating birds is another means of contaminating watering and grazing areas with anthrax spores that pass through their digestive tracts. Blood-sucking insects and tick-eating birds were not considered to be important. On the other hand, carcasses were frequently filled with maggots from which vegetative anthrax bacilli were isolated. Flies and blowflies were considered important disseminators of disease. Contaminated water-holes and forage were considered to be the principal sources of infection. There was no infection among the workers who handled the carcasses or built pyres to burn them. Some natives who attempted to salvage meat became ill, two of whom died.

The cause of morbidity and mortality due to anthrax remains unexplained. Recent studies on this problem by United States investigators suggests that there are probably three toxic factors involved. They are the oedema factor I, protective factor II, and lethal factor III. These factors are thought to act in various combinations and concentrations, resulting in different effects. The mode of actions that lead to death is not known.

BOTULISM

Botulism is a type of food poisoning in man and animals caused by the ingestion of an extremely potent toxin produced by *Clostridium botulinum* during its growth under anaerobic conditions, usually in low-acid foods. Botulism is not an infection but a bacterial poisoning; similar intoxications were called ptomaine poisoning years ago. The poisoning is characterized by headache of varying intensity, and weakness leading to prostration. Vomiting and diarrhoea are not common symptoms. Oculomotor and other paralyses are notable signs. Disturbed vision, difficulty in chewing and swallowing, and respiratory paralysis are seen both in man and animals. The clinical manifestations are caused specifically by the action of the toxin on the central nervous system, rather than the gastro-intestinal tract, where it acts at the synapses at the motor endplates or the myoneural junction. The toxin also affects the parasympathetic nervous system, where it interferes with or inhibits the formation of acetylcholine.

There are seven different types and subtypes of *Cl. botulinum* organisms as characterized by toxin formation. Type A is present in North America, South America, the Far East, and Europe. It is a frequent cause of human illness and may cause disease in animals, especially poultry. Type B is common in North America and Europe, and causes disease in both man and animals. The Type C toxins are almost exclusively associated with animal botulism outbreaks, and are the most common type of poisoning in mink and birds. Subtype Cα is the cause of extensive wild water-fowl epidemics in the United States, South America, Australia, and South Africa. This organism multiplies in decaying vegetation in shallow alkaline waters. Anaerobiosis under these conditions allows the bacteria to multiply and form toxins. These are eventually ingested by water-fowl, who succumb to the poison with a paralysis of the neck muscles called limberneck, which extends to the wings and legs. Subtype Cα is also the cause of botulism in chickens. Subtype Cβ is frequently the cause of forage poisoning in the large domestic animals. This same toxin is apparently the cause

of outbreaks in mink in the United States and Sweden. Type D is reported only from South Africa, but may also be present in other areas. It affects only animals. Type E is found in North America, Europe, and Asia, and is frequently associated with fish and fish products. The organism has been isolated from the intestinal tract of fish in salt and fresh water and marine sediment. Type F is a newly described *Cl. botulinum* affecting man. It was first recognized in 1959 in Denmark, where it produced human illness. The first human cases occurred in the United States in 1966. The organism has been isolated from Columbia River salmon and Pacific marine mud.

A tentative diagnosis of botulism in animals or man can be made by observing the signs and symptoms of the patient. Symptoms usually appear within 12–18 hours or longer after eating the poisoned food, depending on the amount of contaminated food ingested. In the United States and Canada more than half the patients succumb to cardiac or respiratory failure, sometimes within hours, or periods up to 3–7 days, after onset of symptoms. The case fatality rate in Europe is said to be less than 20 per cent. Confirmation of the diagnosis can be made only by isolation and identification of the toxin from the vital organs, blood, or stomach, or gastro-intestinal contents of the victim. Laboratory tests[1] are done by injecting a filtrate of the suspected food, patient's blood, or ingesta into a series of mice or guinea-pigs, some of which receive antitoxin to determine if the suspected toxin can be neutralized. *Cl. botulinum* is widespread in nature, and its isolation does not confirm suspected disease; this is especially true of animal feeds.

The occurrence of botulism in man and animals is sporadic, with groups of cases appearing occasionally in various parts of the world. The organism is commonly found in the soil as previously stated, and may also be present in the intestinal tract of healthy animals. Here it causes no harm, but if the animal should die of other causes the *Cl. botulinum* may multiply and form toxin in the carcass. These carcasses can be poisonous to animals or birds eating them.

Botulism is reported in the United States in man, wild water-fowl, chickens, cattle, and horses. Swine, dogs, and cats are very resistant, and spontaneous cases are very rare. Most human cases of botulism are caused by Type A and B toxins with home-canned low-acid vegetables as the vehicle. In recent years cases of Type E poisoning, associated with canned and smoked fish, have become more common. Meat is seldom involved in cases of human botulism in North America except for products such as liver paste, but in Europe most human cases are associated with the eating of contaminated sausages, meat products, and hams. The largest epidemic of botulism ever reported occurred in the U.S.S.R. in 1933. This was a Type A epidemic caused by the eating of stuffed egg plant. Another major epidemic involving twenty-one cases and twelve deaths was reported in Argentina in 1959 caused by the ingestion of pimentoes contaminated with Type A toxin. Japan has reported a number of unusual Type E epidemics traced to fish salads ('izushi').

Animal botulism is sporadic, although groups of cases are reported in some countries. In the United States forage poisoning is usually caused by Type B *Cl. botulinum*. The organism is

---

[1] The fluorescent antibody technique is now being used to identify the type of toxin that may be circulating in the patient's blood. A blood sample should be taken before antitoxin is given.

found in hay and silage, and other feeds. Botulism in chickens, called limberneck, is said to be caused by the feeding of spoiled canned vegetables. Limberneck of western ducks has previously been described. This disease involves more individuals than any other kind of botulism. Mink are frequently affected, outbreaks occurring every year on mink ranches. The outbreaks follow the feeding of contaminated food, frequently carcasses of animals dead from natural causes, in which toxins have permeated the flesh as previously described. A progressive posterior paralysis is the most common symptom. Other signs include lassitude, squinting, paralysis of the nictitating membrane (medial eyelid) followed by paralysis. The animals then become comatose and death ensues. There are no significant autopsy findings.

Treatment of human intoxications is with polyvalent botulinum antitoxin or the type specific antitoxin. These antitoxins are available from the Center for Disease Control, Atlanta, Georgia, and abroad at State Serum Institutes and Pasteur Institutes.

Botulism may be prevented by adequate processing of foodstuffs. Vegetables which are frequently contaminated include mushrooms, olives, green beans, and other low-acid foods. The home canning of these products is not without danger, and precautions should be taken by the home processer. Government agencies charged with supervision of canned and processed food have done an excellent job in preventing food poisoning, but sporadic cases continue to appear, which emphasizes the importance of constant vigilance.

The control of botulism is in the prevention of the distribution of toxin in low-acid food products. Research carried on over the years has demonstrated that 100° C. for 10 minutes will destroy the toxin. The toxin is also destroyed at 80° C. when the temperature is maintained for 30 minutes. Heat processes are usually designed to destroy the spores and not the toxin. In canning values are set at 116° C. for 10 minutes or 121° C. for 2·78 minutes with a slope (Z valve) of 82° C. (TDT curves). Canning procedures depend on the type of food processed and the size of the container. Processes are calculated on the bases of heat penetration and cooling curves and the thermal death time curve as mentioned above. When large quantities of canned foods are being autoclaved it is important that the temperature in all cans should reach the above levels for the required time. This will vary with the pH of the product. Low pH products require lower temperatures for shorter times. The occasional accidents that occur with canned goods throughout the world are evidence of the lack of proper heating.

BOVINE TUBERCULOSIS

Bovine tuberculosis was one of the first animal diseases that was demonstrated to be communicable to man. The realization that milk could be a vehicle of transmission of tuberculosis stimulated the establishment of public health programmes which resulted in organized efforts to eliminate the disease. Great progress had been made with these programmes in the United States and Canada before 1940, and since 1950 in Europe. Denmark, Finland, Sweden, Norway, and the Netherlands are free of bovine tuberculosis, and Switzerland, Portugal, and Great Britain are rapidly approaching a disease-free status. Considerable progress has also been made in

Eastern Europe. The U.S.S.R. reports that the incidence of bovine tuberculosis is less than a half of 1 per cent. (0·5 per cent.). Poland and Czechoslovakia have made great progress in the past decade, and expect to have eliminated the disease by 1980. Likewise, Yugoslavia has the disease under control. Outside of Europe bovine tuberculosis remains a problem in South America, South Africa, Southern Asia, and parts of Australia. Japan probably has the lowest incidence of bovine tuberculosis in Asia, the incidence being less than a half of 1 per cent. A review in the United States (Steele and Ranney, 1958) stated that only a few proven cases have occurred in the past decade. Even though bovine tuberculosis is rare in man, sporadic cases do occur among individuals who have contact with diseased animals or who have ingested milk from diseased cows. A few such cases are reported even at this late date (1974) in North America and Europe.

Non-specific reactions (i.e those produced in reactors having no visible lesions) to tuberculin tests are a major problem, both in areas where tuberculosis has been virtually eradicated and in those where infection with *Myco. bovis* was relatively rare to begin with. Non-specific reactions to tuberculin vary according to ecologic factors in a given situation. They include: (1) infection with *Myco. paratuberculosis* (Johne's disease); (2) non-progressive infections with *Myco. tuberculosis*, *Myco. avium*, and *Myco. intercellularis*, the organisms causing so-called skin lesions; and (3) various transient sensitizing infections with other myco-bacteria, probably including some soil and water forms. The cause of non-specific sensitivity can be determined only by post-mortem examination of slaughtered reactors and laboratory study of tissues from such animals, including attempted isolation and identification of mycobacteria that might be responsible.

Animals can also become infected from man, and a large number of re-infections of tuberculin-free herds with human- or bovine-type strains have been traced to this source.

Infection of cattle with human strains seldom causes progressive lesions, but often gives rise to a marked tuberculin reaction, frequently temporary in nature, and interferes with the application of the tuberculin test.

As the incidence and prevalence of infection in a population decrease under the influence of an eradication programme, the importance of epidemiologic tracing and of testing procedures increases. If cattle found to be tuberculous by routine meat inspection at the time of slaughter are traced back to the herds of origin the latter can be tested with tuberculin; this is a highly efficient technique for the discovery of infected animals, which can then be eliminated from the herds. Adequate meat inspection services and case-finding programmes can materially reduce the amount of complete area testing that is necessary.

In some parts of the world vaccination of humans against tuberculosis is practised extensively. In cattle experiments have been conducted with vaccines consisting of live cultures of the B.C.G. and vole strains of the tubercle bacillus, and some protection has been achieved under carefully controlled conditions. However, generally speaking, vaccination has no place in the control or eradication of tuberculosis in cattle. Vaccines such such as those composed of B.C.G. or the vole bacillus create a sensitivity to tuberculin that interferes, for varying periods, with control and eradication programmes based on tuberculin testing.

Chemoprophylaxis and Chemotherapy

It is recognized that it is frequently difficult for economically-poor countries to undertake control and eradication programmes based solely on test and slaughter methods. Furthermore, such countries may have great difficulty in obtaining enough calves to replace slaughtered infected cattle. Consequently, many countries have been reluctant to carry out any but the most limited attempts to control bovine tuberculosis; such attempts have frequently been quite ineffective. Recent developments in the chemoprophylaxis and chemotherapy of bovine tuberculosis may offer such countries effective and economical methods for markedly reducing levels of infection; test and slaughter procedures could be introduced subsequently.

Experiments in several countries during the past decade have indicated that chemotherapeutic agents found to be effective against human tuberculosis may also be of value against bovine tuberculosis. An extensive and carefully controlled series of trials recently completed in the Republic of South Africa showed that excellent prophylactic and therapeutic results are achieved by the administration of at least 10 mg./kg. of isoniazid daily for a period of 6–11 months (Kleeberg, 1966). The drug may be given in feed, in water, or in tablet form. Prolonged isoniazid therapy results in a gradual diminution of tuberculin hypersensitivity that is related to the degree of apparent bacteriologic cure.

It was found that some isoniazid resistance had developed in some of the *Myco. bovis* isolated from treated animals, but this did not affect the overall results. The virulence of these strains of *Myco. bovis* in experimental animals was markedly lower than usual; similar observations have been made with mycobacteria isolated from treated human beings. Furthermore, when uninfected cattle were exposed to cattle infected with these strains no evidence of natural transmissibility was found.

BRUCELLOSIS

Brucellosis is one of the most widespread animal diseases that affects man. The number of human infections that occur in the world are estimated in the hundreds of thousands. The highest incidence of human disease is found in southern Europe, North Africa, Central Asia, the Middle East, and Latin America. The U.S.S.R., which formerly had a major problem among agricultural workers, has reduced the incidence 100-fold in the past decade. Goats are the principal source of human infections in these areas. Infection rates among other animals, i.e. cattle, sheep, and swine vary from 1 to 30 per cent. The Scandinavian countries are free of brucellosis, and the disease has almost been eliminated in the United Kingdom, the Netherlands, Germany, and Switzerland. The United States has inaugurated a national brucellosis eradication campaign which is making great strides (Schilf, 1968). By January 1968 nearly all of the states had the disease under control. Individual bovine reactors have declined from 5 to less than 0.1 per cent. in the past 10 years. During the same period the incidence of human infections has dropped precipitously from an estimated 10,709 cases in 1949 (Steele and Emik, 1950) to less than 200 in 1973. Most human disease in North America is attributed to *Brucella abortus* and *Br. suis* from cattle and swine exposure. In Mexico, Argentina, and the Mediterranean region it is *Br. melitensis*, due to goat contact. *Br. melitensis* is also reported to be the most common cause of human infection in the U.S.S.R. Sheep and goats are stated to be the primary source in Russia (Korotich, 1957). Man is usually infected by coming in contact with diseased animals which are discharging brucella. Infected animals which have recently aborted or given birth to young are the greatest hazards to man. The infectious brucella organisms discharged under these conditions may contaminate the environment to such an extent that animals or man not having direct contact with the infected animals may be infected. The transmission of brucella to man by the ingestion or handling of milk and contaminated milk products, meat and meat products is well known. Less known are other foods and water as vehicles of infection. The brucella organism can survive for some period of time in water, and likewise will persist on vegetation. Insects, including flies and ticks, have been found to be harbouring brucella by many investigators, and in some experiments it has been demonstrated that they may transmit infection. The transmission of the disease to laboratory and research workers handling the organism is well known. Since the development of the Strain 19 brucella vaccine for calves, there have been many reports of human illness among veterinarians and livestock handlers who have accidentally inoculated themselves or their assistant (Spink, 1953; Sadusk *et al.*, 1957; Cappucci, 1968).

The control of brucellosis in man and animals is dependent on the removal of infected animals which are shedding the organism. In cattle this is accomplished by the blood-serum agglutination test, which is the standard test. The milk ring test, a modified form of the agglutination test, is used extensively in screening herds for infection. If reactors are found with the ring test the herd is blood tested, and those with a titre of 1:100 or higher are considered positive reactors and are identified as such. Sometimes young animals that have been vaccinated will react. If these animals are not properly identified they are considered infected and are so identified. Vaccination of calves is used in areas where brucellosis-eradication programmes are in progress. In some countries where the disease has been eliminated calfhood vaccination has been dropped.

The pasteurization of all milk and milk products, including cheese, is important in the prevention of human brucellosis. The boiling of milk by rural populations serves the purpose, but in many instances this is done only with fluid milk. Milk that is used for cheese, sour milk, and butter is not boiled, and frequently the brucella organisms will survive the processing and ageing and are ingested by man, with resulting illness. This is especially true of goat-milk products.

The control of brucellosis in goats is more difficult than in cattle. The blood agglutination test is valuable to identify diseased animals, but frequently new infections continue to appear in the herd because of the heavily contaminated area. The best policy is to slaughter the herd and allow the land to remain free of animals for a season. Vaccination of goats with REV 1 has been used in Spain and Mexico with good results. The REV 1 vaccine is now being used on a large scale in Malta, North Africa, Asia, and Peru.

The problem in sheep is very similar to that in goats. Russian veterinarians have reported that vaccination of sheep has drastically reduced the disease but has not eliminated it. Russian public health authorities state that they have immunized more than 5 million rural residents with a modified Strain 19 vaccine in the areas where sheep brucellosis is enzootic with good results, although some individuals suffered systemic reactions comparable to the disease.

Swine brucellosis is found mainly in the United States, Argentina, and Eastern Europe. It has also been reported in Denmark, where hares have been identified as a reservoir (Bendtsen *et al.*, 1954). The disease was eradicated from the swine herds of Denmark on each occasion that it appeared. The first human infection of this type in the British Isles was recently observed in a child on a holiday in Ireland.

Brucellosis is also found in reindeer in the arctic regions. The causal agent is *Br. rangiferi*, a *Br. suis* type IV. This organism can cause disease in man. Another is *Br. canis*, a new species reported as a cause of abortion in dogs in the United States. The first human cases were diagnosed in laboratory workers in 1968 at the New York State Veterinary College. Another new specie is *Br. ovis*, common in sheep in Australia and New Zealand, and more recently has been recognized in the western United States. *Br. ovis* does not affect man or any other species of cattle. *Br. neotomae* is found in rabbits and rodents in some parts of the western United States, but does not cause infection or disease in man or food animals.

Meat inspection is important in the prevention of the spread of the disease to man. The flesh of swine can be a vehicle of infection, while that of cattle, goat, and sheep seldom is. Pigs frequently have a systemic disease, and the *Br. suis* is often found in various organs and muscles. The organisms may survive even pickling. Cattle infections are usually localized in the udder and in pregnant animals in the uterus. Goats and sheep are affected similarly.

The diagnosis of human brucellosis will be increasingly difficult in the future with the widespread use of antibiotics, which arrest the multiplication of the brucella organism and the development of recognizable titres. In these cases only a history of working with diseased animals will provide a clue to a possible diagnosis of brucellosis.

Fortunately, most of the various types of brucella infections in man respond to the broad-spectrum antibiotics, although in some cases it is necessary to continue treatment after the acute disease has subsided, to prevent relapses. The broad-spectrum antibiotic therapy has reduced the seriousness of acute brucellosis, but some cases do not respond to therapy. These cases emphasize the importance of the elimination of animal infections so as to prevent human disease.

The WHO Brucellosis Centre in Moscow has studied the epidemiology of the disease in the USSR and in Mongolia, where it is a disease of great economic importance (World Health Organization, 1974, pp. 27–28).

CAT SCRATCH FEVER

Cat scratch fever or benign inoculation lymphoreticulosis has been identified in many countries, and is presumed to occur throughout the world. The cause of the disease is unknown, although some investigators claim to have isolated a virus which may be related to the psittacosis–lymphogranuloma group. The reservoir and source of infection is believed to be cats, as many patients have had a history of contact with cats before illness, although other animals may have been involved also. No signs of disease have been observed in animals, but it is thought they have an inapparent infection (Steele, 1953). The agent is believed to be widely distributed in nature. The mode of transmission is thought to be from animals to man by scratches, bites, or licks. Minor trauma after insect bites, from thorns and splinters, is a suggested mode of transmission in the frequent instances of no known direct contact with animals.

Published reviews of more than 450 cases disclose that almost 90 per cent. have a history of cat exposure, usually kittens. A review of an epidemic in northern cities of the United States in 1960 reveals that most cases occur during the autumn and early winter months, rising sharply in September and declining after February. Public health officers consider cat scratch fever one of the more common zoonoses they encounter, especially in urban areas.

The first signs of the disease are usually a minor local inflammatory lesion, with swelling, erythema, and slight ulceration or papule formation at the site of scratch wound. The incubation period is thought to be 7–14 days and possibly as short as 2 days. In some cases there is no recollection of a wound or trauma. Subsequent swelling and tenderness of regional lymph nodes proximal to the wound is highly characteristic, with eventual suppuration, the pus being thick, greyish, and bacteriologically sterile. The swelling gradually recedes without treatment in 2 or 3 weeks, but in some instances it persists for months (Daniels and MacMurray, 1954).

Fever is an early symptom occurring particularly in children, who are more often affected, and ranging from 38° to 40° C., being irregular and sometimes undulating. Chills, rash, malaise, and other manifestations of generalized infection have all been described.

There are no recommended control procedures, nor have any vaccines been developed.

A similar infection following a cat bite due to *Pasteurella multocida* is sometimes seen, but it can be differentiated as it progresses by a localized pyogenic reaction which is painful, red, tender, and oedematous. An ascending lymphangitis and lymphadenitis are frequently associated with these infections. In the absence of antibiotic therapy an abscess almost always develops at the site of the bite, which heals slowly. Bryne *et al.* (1956) state that osteomyelitis sometimes follows cat-bite pasteurella infections because of the deep wounds caused by the needle-sharp teeth of the cat, which injure the bone. Other bacterial species may also produce infections following cat bites.

CONTAGIOUS ECTHYMA

Contagious ecthyma, or sore mouth, is an infectious dermatitis of sheep and goats affecting primarily the lips of young animals. It is seen in all parts of the world where sheep and goats are raised, usually in the summer and early autumn. The nature of the lesions warrants its inclusion in pox diseases that affect man and animals.

The disease is caused by the virus which causes vesicles and pustules on the skin of the lips and sometimes the nose and eyes. These vesicles rapidly change to pustules, and finally, thick scabs. The virus is highly resistant to desiccation and is reported to survive for years in scabs that have been held at a moderate temperature. It has been demonstrated that viable virus will survive in scabs that fall off recovered animals. These scabs contaminate the soil and cause infection in new-born animals the following year. Contagious ecthyma seldom causes mortality, except when complications occur due to secondary invasion by the necrosis bacillus (*Spherophorus necrophorus*) or parasitic infestation by the screw worm (*Cochliomyia americana*) larva. It is not uncommon for ewes, suckling infected lambs, to develop lesions on their udders.

Field studies in Texas revealed some years ago that lambs and kids which recovered from this disease were solidly immune thereafter. Later experiments demonstrated that it was possible to immunize them successfully with a technique similar to that used for vaccinating man against smallpox. The vaccine consists of fully virulent material contained in the dried scabs, which is ground and suspended in glycerol and saline solution. This is applied with a stiff bristled brush to a superficially scratched area. A postular lesion develops at the site of the inoculation. This becomes covered with a scab later, which falls off after several weeks.

The disease in man[1] is an occupational problem among shepherds, veterinarians, and others who may handle sick animals, or the viable vaccine. The lesions begin as abrasions. They consist of rather large vesicles that may be multiple in structure. The surrounding skin becomes inflamed and swollen, and may be quite painful. The patient may have some fever, and there may be a moderate swelling of the axillary lymph nodes when the hands or arms are involved. Occasionally there may be lesions on the face or genitalia which may be quite proliferative and distressing. Secondary infections are frequent, and healing is often rather slow. Naturally, such complications result in incapacitation.

Diagnosis in man is usually based on history of occupation and exposure to infected animals, handling of vaccine, or self-inoculation. Confirmation of the diagnosis is established by transmitting the virus from man to a susceptible lamb or kid. The complement fixation test may be of value in the diagnosis.

Treatment is non-specific, except for antibiotics to eliminate secondary bacterial infections, and analgesics to relieve discomfort. Although there are reports that repeated infections are possible, it is thought that an individual who has had the disease, or has been exposed, is usually resistant to further infection.

COWPOX

Pseudocowpox, or milkers nodules, an infection of cows and man is thought to be closely related to contagious ecthyma because of the similarity of the morphology of the viruses.

Other animal-pox diseases affecting man include cowpox, which is relatively rare, except where variola persists. Vaccinia infections transmitted to cows are frequently mistaken for cowpox until differentiated by laboratory procedures. Horse pox or grease, hog pox, camel pox, and simian pox are all diseases that can affect man. These are usually variants or closely related to cowpox. In addition, there are many other pox diseases of animals that do not affect man. These include sheep, goat, mouse, rabbit, fowl, canary, and other pox viruses that are

[1] Known as orf in Australia.

transmitted by insect bites. There is no evidence that animals are a possible reservoir of smallpox, although monkeys are susceptible to variola and vaccinia.

ENCEPHALOMYOCARDITIS

Encephalomyocarditis, or EMC, is a virus disease found in many parts of the world, in a wide range of animals, including primates, mongooses, squirrels, rodents, and swine. It has also been recovered from mosquitoes in Africa and more recently from mosquitoes in Florida. The disease usually occurs only in warm climates, except those cases caused by laboratory accidents. In the United States the naturally occurring disease has been mainly reported in the southern states. It is commonly found in rats and swine, and on a few occasions in squirrels. Rodents do not seem to have any obvious disease signs, whereas swine become quite ill—suffering from depression, loss of appetite, fever, and in some instances, cardiac failure and encephalitis. The disease has become so common in some areas that veterinarians can now diagnose it from the clinical signs. The disease in squirrels causes encephalitic signs which are confused with rabies.

The aetiological agent is a small virus of less than 30 millimicrons. They are quite stable, and can apparently survive in rodent and swine faeces for some time under moderate conditions. The natural transmission among rodents and swine is believed to be by the ingestion of food or water contaminated with animal droppings and urine. The role of squirrels as a reservoir or virus is unknown. Other small animals found in enzootic areas and examined for signs of EMC were uniformly negative.

The clinical features of the diseases in man vary from a mild febrile '3-day fever' to a severe encephalitis from which the patient recovers within a week with no recognizable sequellae. A febrile disease with lymphocytic pleocytosis and some involvement of the central nervous system is the most frequent form in those human cases which have been well studied. Myocarditis, fortunately, is not one of the symptoms observed in man. Severe headache, nuchal rigidity, photophobia, vomiting, and delirium have been seen by some observers. Other cases described include such findings as high fever reaching 40° C. and persisting for 2–3 days accompanied by pharyngitis, stiff neck, and hyperactive deep reflexes. The only notable laboratory finding has been the pleocytosis of from 50 to 500 cells, principally lymphocytes in the spinal fluid. All of the patients recovered with no relapses or sequellae. There are no reported fatalities.

The diagnosis of EMC in man depends on the isolation and dentification of the virus, and the demonstration of specific antibodies. The symptoms and signs of disease in man are not sufficiently diagnostic to differentiate it from other febrile neurologic infections.

Treatment is symptomatic and supportive.

ERYSIPELOID

Erysipeloid is an erysipelas-like infection in man, which is caused by *Erysipelothrix insidiosa* (*rhusiopathiae*), a bacterium, and is world-wide. It is capable of living as a saprophyte, or at least surviving for months in water, soil, pastures, and decaying organic material; also on fish and in the carcasses of meat animals, even after smoking, pickling, or salting. It can also be a pathogen as its name implies, causing disease in domestic and laboratory animals, birds, and man. The bacterium, *Streptococcus pyogenes* Group A, of which there are some forty types, that produces erysipelas in man does not affect animals and can be readily differentiated from erysipeloid infections in man by clinical signs and laboratory tests.

The most frequently encountered form of the disease in man is the localized cutaneous infection, mainly among persons handling swine, turkeys, and fish. Veterinarians sometimes infect themselves when they accidentally puncture their fingers or hands while immunizing swine with virulent live-culture vaccines, or injure themselves while doing necropsies on swine or turkeys. These infections in man apparently provide a good immunity, since reinfections seldom, if ever, occur.

The incubation period in man is from 1 to 5 days. The initial signs at the point of inoculation are redness, swelling, and pain. Sometimes the infection spreads to adjacent parts involving the entire hand and other parts of the body. This is accompanied by twitching, burning, or prickliness. There may be fever as well as swelling and tenderness of the regional lymph nodes and joints. Suppuration does not occur. Most cases are of a moderate nature and recover in 2–3 weeks; rarely some persist longer.

A diffuse or generalized form of disease is occasionally seen. This usually begins as a localized infection which spreads slowly over the body. Sometimes there are eruptions in distant parts that may be the result of re-entry of the organism, or septicaemia. Fever, regional lymphadenopathy, and joint pain accompany the spread. In these cases the patient is depressed and feels that no therapy is of value.

The septicaemic disease is naturally the most serious. All kinds of signs and symptoms are observed, depending upon which organs are affected—lymphadenitis, polyarthritis, and endocarditis. Skin eruptions are usually present and are significant in establishing a diagnosis; confirmation of the disease is by recovery of *E. insidiosa* from the blood. Laboratory mice and pigeons are quite susceptible and are used to isolate the organism.

Morphologically, in smears the bacterium is a slender, Gram-positive, non-motile, non-sporulating rod, 1–2 microns long. On artificial media it is a mixture of short rods and long filaments ranging up to 20 microns in length. The organism is resistant to many disinfectants, including alcohol, formaldehyde, hydrogen peroxide, and phenol. It is, however, readily destroyed by caustic soda and strong chlorinating agents. *E. insidiosa* is quite sensitive to penicillin, less so to the broad-spectrum antibiotics, and is not affected by the sulphonamides. Hence, penicillin is the agent of choice in treatment of both man and animals. Since the advent of penicillin, the complications that were occasionally seen in man are very rare.

Therapy as practised today consists of large doses of penicillin. Antiserum was formerly used, but less so since penicillin has been available and has given such satisfactory results. Other antibiotics are less effective in the following order: tetracycline, chlortetracycline, chloramphenicol, and streptomycin being least efficacious. There is no evidence that the bacterium has developed any resistance to penicillin since it was demonstrated to be effective in 1944.

The disease in animals takes various forms—erysipelas, septicaemia, endocarditis, polyarthritis, and diarrhoea in birds. In swine a variety of signs and symptoms are seen principally in young animals. It is fairly common in the swine-producing areas of North America, Europe, and the U.S.S.R. In young pigs the acute septicaemia is most common, and was formerly frequently fatal. Onset is not characteristic—loss of appetite, depression, and a high body temperature up to 42°–43° C. occur, and an increase in pulse and respiratory rate accompanies the fever. A less severe form of the disease is the cutaneous form, which is called 'diamond skin disease'. The temperature is usually high (40°–42° C.), the appetite depressed, and sometimes the joints are affected. The skin lesions erupt after 18–60 hours. These are light-red patches on the chest, ventral and dorsal surfaces, thighs and shoulders. The number and size vary, but they are usually quadrangular in shape; however, some are rounded. The course of the disease is 8–14 days, and the animals usually recover as the eruptions turn dark red and dry up. A chronic form sometimes occurs, and usually causes enlargement of the joints and a painful arthritis. A vegetative endocarditis may develop in animals that have apparently recovered from the acute disease. This is usually recognized at necropsy, but cardiac insufficiency results in animals being short of breath, coughing, lassitude, and resting on the sternum and elbows, or even sitting on the haunches instead of lying on their side.

Lambs suffer from a non-suppurative polyarthritis. Calves are affected in a similar manner. Infection is usually the result of a wound or navel infection. These animals do not have a localized infection at the wound site or of the skin.

The disease in turkeys is an acute or subacute septicaemia, with males affected more often. It usually occurs in the autumn, about the time birds are ready for market. The first signs are dullness, loss of appetite, and diarrhoea. A red purple swelling of the wattles is suggestive, but this is also seen in other diseases. The case fatality rate is 30–40 per cent. in untreated birds. Treatment consists of penicillin, intramuscularly, at the rate of 5,000 Units/lb. (11,000 Units/kg.). At necropsy multiple diffuse haemorrhages are seen in the muscles and in the viscera. Occasionally, ducks and geese as well as pigeons (squabs) are affected. *E. insidiosa* seldom produces disease in chickens.

The mode of infection is not clearly understood, although wounds are considered the route of entry of the bacterium. It is difficult to reproduce the natural disease under experimental conditions, which suggests that there is great variability in virulence of the agent, and susceptibility of the experimental animals except in the case of mice and pigeons. As stated earlier, the organism is widespread, as demonstrated by finding it in pig pens year after year with no disease occurring, but it is suspected that virulent strains are sometimes introduced in animal feeds, feed supplements, or in new additions to swine herds. Wild birds may be mechanical carriers. Garbage that is fed to swine may carry the infectious agent in meat scraps or viscera.

With the improved immunizing agents available, the disease is being successfully controlled in enzootic areas, where some farms have outbreaks year after year. Also, the extensive use of penicillin in animal medicine has averted outbreaks, and controlled disease when it has occurred. All this in turn has reduced human exposure and disease. Most human infections are now seen as occupational disease among fish handlers and turkey processers, and even here it is rare, as any suspected lesion on the hands is promptly treated with penicillin, and a diagnosis is seldom made.

GLANDERS

Glanders is a highly communicable disease of equidae, but is rare in man. The disease is caused by *Actinobacillus mallei* (synonym—*Pfeifferella mallei*). Three clinical forms occur in animals and man which may be acute or chronic: (1) nasal, in which nodules form and ulcerate in the mucosa of the nasal septum; (2) pulmonary disease is characterized by small nodules in the lungs, which in acute cases consolidate and lead to glanderous pneumonia; and (3) cutaneous or farcy form, in which nodules develop along the course of the lymph vessels and eventually ulcerate. The cutaneous ulcers discharge a thick yellow exudate which is highly infectious. When the disease does occur in man it is usually acute, whereas in animals it is chronic. Bronchopneumonia is the most serious form, and is usually fatal. Laboratory infections cause a pneumonitis similar to virus pneumonia. The organism can be grown readily on artificial media, and can be identified by the FA technique. The FA tests are the same for melioidosis. The same antigen reacts to bacteria causing both diseases.

Diagnosis is by the complement fixation test, agglutination test, mallein reaction, and by bacteriological culture or animal inoculation.

Man and equidae become infected from the discharges of open lesions of the respiratory tract or the skin of diseased individuals. Human infections are usually the result of skin contamination and penetration, and by hand to mucous membranes and through ingestion.

Infections through inhalation are rare, but they do occur among laboratory workers who are handling the organisms or diseased animals. Man is quite resistant. During the Second World War veterinarians who worked with diseased horses and ponies in China and Burma seldom saw or heard of a human case, even though more than one-half of the animals were reactors to the mallein test. Naturally, animals that showed clinical disease were destroyed, and men working around open cases took precautions, such as bathing and removing contaminated clothing.

Glanders is practically unknown in Europe and North America, although it is still observed in Asia, Africa, and South America. The disease is rapidly disappearing from these areas, where mechanization is replacing the horse. Any horses moving in international commerce should be tested for glanders and should not be allowed to enter the country until it has been determined that they are free of disease. In recent years, glanders has been identified in northern India following the importation of horses for military purposes in the 1960s. No human cases have been reported in persons handling or treating these diseased animals (Steele, 1970).

Penicillin, erythromycin, and sulphonamides are recommended as useful therapeutic agents.

Clinical experience with human glanders indicates that the disease can be effectively treated with the sulphonamides and antibiotics with a prolonged regimen.

Melioidosis or Pseudoglanders

Melioidosis, formerly a rare disease in man resembling glanders, is probably more widespread in the world today than glanders. It is caused by *Pseudomonas pseudomallai* (synonym—*Pfeifferella whitmori*), and occurs in South-East Asia from Vietnam to Ceylon. The disease is a military problem in these areas. Melioidosis has also been reported in Australia, New Guinea, Indonesia, Malaysia, Guam, Ecuador, and Aruba. Formerly the natural reservoir was thought to be in rodents. Domestic animals have also been found to be infected. These include equidae, sheep, goats, cattle, swine, dogs, and cats. The first animals in which the disease was described were laboratory animals, i.e. guinea-pigs and rabbits in Malaya. The disease has also been identified in some wild animals, including tree-climbing kangaroos in New Guinea. The transmission of the disease is thought to be by contact with diseased animals and sometimes by the ingestion of contaminated food or water. The isolation of the bacteria from water and soil indicates that it is quite widespread in nature.

The bacillus can remain viable in deep water for as long as 8 weeks, and it is assumed that it can live in mud marshes, rice fields, and stagnant waters for just as long a period. It has been found to remain viable in faeces and urine for 2–4 weeks. This later discovery has raised a question as to the role of infected animals transmitting diseases to man.

The chief clinical features in man as well as animals are septicaemia and granulomatous nodules. These nodules may appear in all parts of the body. Although melioidosis is not a common disease in man, it has a high case fatality rate in those persons having clinical signs of disease.

Up to 1964 over 300 human cases had been recorded in the medical literature since 1912. Almost all were diagnosed *post mortem*, with a case fatality rate exceeding 80 per cent. With improved medical care the case fatality rate has been cut in half. The wide spectrum of clinical signs and the close resemblance of melioidosis to other severe infectious diseases, i.e. cholera, glanders, plague, pyaemia, typhoid fever, and tuberculosis, could account for many unrecognized cases. Recent investigations have revealed that the disease does not always take an acute form and that subclinical or mild unrecognized forms of disease may exist. Since 1964 many additional human cases have been reported in South-East Asia, principally in military personnel and civilians in Vietnam. Fortunately the disease is being treated successfully, and the case fatality rate is much lower than formerly. Exposed persons may not develop the disease for months after their initial contact, hence persons known to be exposed are frequently placed on a prophylactic regime of antibiotics.

LEPTOSPIROSIS

Extensive investigations during the past seventy years have shown that leptospirosis occurs in humans and animals in all parts of the world, and that it is not a single disease but a group of diseases caused by a variety of different serotypes in the genus *Leptospira*. The type species, *L. icterohaemorrhagiae*, was isolated from human cases of leptospirosis in Japan and in Germany in 1915, almost thirty years after Weil's classic clinical description of the disease. After this period many new serotypes were recognized by European and Asian investigators, and knowledge of leptospirae increased considerably. Only in recent years has information been gained regarding the epidemiology, public health importance, and distribution of these diseases in the United States and Europe.

As the search for leptospirae continues, the host range broadens not only among domestic animals but also in a variety of wild mammals. Leptospirosis constitutes a major problem in cattle and swine, and in some areas sheep, goats, and horses become infected. In addition to many rodent carriers, bats, mongooses, bandicoots, jackals, foxes, opossums, racoons, skunks, wild cats, nutria, beaver, armadillo, and even some reptiles (Babudieri, 1958) have been found infected. In these host animals leptospirae become localized in the kidneys and may shed in the urine for long periods. Transmission to man and other animals occurs by direct contact with infectious urine and with tissues of these infected animals or indirectly through contact with contaminated water or other environment. The usual portals of entry are the mucous membranes or abraded skin.

Usually each leptospiral serotype is thought to have a primary animal host, but they may infect other animals, and a so-called primary host for one serotype may become infected with other serotypes or even harbour two types at the same time. Serotype *canicola*[1] is an excellent example of this; found principally in dogs, it has been isolated from cattle, swine, jackals, and hedgehogs, while dogs have been found to harbour at least nine other serotypes.

Although *icterohaemorrhagiae* and *canicola* appear commonly throughout the world, other types have been isolated only in a few areas. For example, serotype *autumnalis*, identified in 1925 in Japan as the cause of autumn fever, is found in eastern Asia and the United States. Here again, the distribution of more than 130 serotypes or subserotypes now recognized broadens as the search continues. In the United Kingdom, where only *icterohaemorrhagiae* and *canicola* had been isolated prior to 1958, *ballum* was found in mice and voles, and an unidentified member of the hebdomadis serogroup in voles. Agglutinins for *bataviae* and *grippotyphosa* appeared in rodent serums, and for *pomona* in pig serums. Similarly, investigations by McKeever *et al.* (1958) yielded serotypes *australis* and *grippotyphosa*, heretofore undetected in the United States, and several new types, including *hyos*, *bakeri*, *atlantae*, *mini* and *georgia*.

The human leptospiral infections compose a multiplicity of separate diseases whose clinical features vary widely and mimic many other diseases (Kalz, 1957). Classic Weil's disease causes hepatic and renal involvement, with marked icterus, uraemia, toxaemia, and haemorrhagic signs, but this is only one clinical form. For clinical differential diagnosis one must consider infectious hepatitis, enteric fever, yellow fever, malaria, brucellosis, influenza, and when meningeal involvement occurs, a number of viral infections, including mumps, meningitis, lymphocytic choriomeningitis, non-paralytic poliomyelitis, and others.

As a result of these varied clinical patterns caused by leptospirae, laboratory confirmation of the diagnosis of leptospirosis is essential. The most desirable and simplest method is isolation of leptospirae by direct culture of blood into a suitable medium (preferably Fletcher's semi-solid) during the febrile stage of illness. Direct culture of urine, tissues, or other body fluids whenever possible is preferred to the indirect method of isolation by animal inoculation, since some laboratory animals may also serve as a natural reservoir of leptospirae. A variety of tests have been developed for the sero-diagnosis of leptospirosis. Probably the most widely used method has been the microscopic agglutination test with living antigens. Several macroscopic agglutination tests have been developed which are performed easily and rapidly. Such a macroscopic slide test has been developed by Galton and her co-workers (1958) which has been found to be extremely valuable for large-volume work. For screening, twelve single leptospiral antigens are combined into four pools of three antigens each. The antigens are prepared from serotypes representative of those known to occur in the United States.

Leptospiral antibodies generally appear from the sixth to the twelfth day of disease and increase rapidly, reaching maximum titres by the third or fourth week. Low agglutinin titres may persist for months or years.

The disease in man is primarily an occupational one, and occurs among miners, sewer-men, fish-cleaners, rat-catchers, swine-herders, abattoir-workers, and veterinarians. It can also be contracted from bathing in water contaminated with urine from domestic animals or rodents and other wild animals. The organism can enter through very slight abrasions, and has been known to affect laboratory workers handling the organism. Prevention and control of animal leptospiroses are similar to the prevention and control of other diseases. The control of the environment in so far as possible by strict sanitary practices, especially the protection of drinking-water, adequate drainage of wet, muddy farm areas, and rodent control are particularly valuable measures. Education of the human population regarding the danger of infection through contact with infected urine or tissue of wild animals will reduce the hazard from these foci. Several vaccines are available for use in cattle and dogs, and while results have been encouraging in the prevention of disease, their role in prevention of infection must be determined to ensure that vaccinated animals are not disseminators of *Leptospira*. Prevention and control of the disease in humans, particularly those exposed in their occupations, depends largely upon improvement of working conditions and protective clothing. The immunization of laboratory workers, veterinarians, and agricultural workers has been studied, but there is little evidence to support the use of vaccines.

Probably one of the most important aspects of control of leptospirosis is the management of the animal shedder who contaminates the environment. There has been little success in developing a practical method for the control of the shedder state of domestic animals with antibiotics. As to wild animals, there is nothing to recommend except reduction of numbers. The contaminated environment can be managed inasmuch as leptospirae are very sensitive to disinfectants, including chlorine and cresol. It goes without saying that all bathing or swimming pools should be disinfected with chlorine. Contaminated barns, pigsties, poultry houses, and laboratory-animal facilities can likewise be disinfected with chlorine or cresol or any other affective agents at hand. Disinfection of large tracts of land, such as rice paddies, with chemicals, i.e. copper sulphate

[1] Nomenclature used is that recommended by the Taxonomic Subcommittee on Leptospira (1963) *Int. Bull. bact. Nomencl.*, **13**, 161–5.

or calcium cyanamide, has been tried, but the results have not been encouraging.

The best protection for those working in contaminated environments is protective clothing. Boots and gloves should be worn by agricultural workers, sewer workers and plumbers, fishermen and hunters, miners, and others that may come in contact with the organism. Human vaccines have been demonstrated to be of value by Torten (1972) in Israel.

Chemoprophylaxis for man by means of penicillin and broad-spectrum antibiotics may be of value when an outbreak or epidemic has started, but the risk of creating sensitivity to penicillin by such programmes must be taken into account. Early serotherapy of Weil's diseases in man using purified antisera of high potency has given excellent results. Specific gamma globulin also appears to be of value in the treatment as well as the prevention of clinical disease. There is some doubt as to the value of penicillin and other antibiotics in the treatment of human leptospirosis. Penicillin seems to be partially efficacious if administered in high doses, 6–12 million Units daily at the beginning of the disease.

WHO has reference centres in Brisbane, Israel, Rome, Tokyo, Amsterdam, London, Moscow and Washington (World Health Organization, 1974, pp. 28–29).

PLAGUE

Plague, caused by the organism *Yersinia pestis*, remains a problem in many parts of the world, even though it has been greatly reduced or eliminated in some areas. WHO expert committees review the problem periodically and set forth principles of control. These principles are sound and are recommended to all authorities concerned with combating plague. Plague is a highly fatal disease with severe toxaemia, manifested by fever, shock, fall in blood pressure, rapid and irregular pulse, restlessness, mental confusion, prostration, delirium, and coma. Bubonic plague is the more common form of the disease. It is characterized by intense pain in the groin and inflammation of the lymph nodes, armpit, or neck, with the appearance of a bubo in the area of the original infection. Secondary invasion of the blood stream leads to localization, which frequently results in terminal pneumonia. This pneumonia may then be the cause of primary pulmonary plague. Sometimes a septicaemic form occurs in which the bubo is not seen or recognized. Tonsillar septicaemic plague is another rare form. Pneumonic and tonsillar plague are transmitted from person to person by contact with patients with primary pneumonic plague or from patients who develop terminal plague pneumonia.

Subclinical upper respiratory infections with virulent *Y. pestis* have recently been observed in persons who have had contact with bubonic plague cases.

The diagnosis may be confirmed by isolation of the organism, animal inoculation, or by the recently developed fluorescent antibody technique.

The bubonic disease is transmitted by the bite of an infected rat flea *Xenopsylla cheopis* or certain other fleas. Fleas may remain infected for days or weeks. The infective fleas are those whose stomachs, proventricules, and oesophagus have become blocked by multiplication of the *Yersinia pestis* at these sites. This prevents the fleas from taking up a blood meal, and results in the blood being regurgitated and returning to the new host upon which the flea is attempting to feed. The blood, in the process of entering the flea and being expelled, becomes grossly contaminated with plague bacilli and carries these bacilli into the host. Fleas that are blocked usually starve to death in a few days. Fleas may also transmit the disease by mechanical means when their proboscides are recently contaminated.

The possibility that the human flea (*Pulex irritans*) may be a vector of infection has caused much concern. A review of past epidemics as well as present-day problems points to this possibility, and emphasizes the need for personal hygiene and insect control, especially among displaced persons.

The natural reservoir of plague is in wild rodents, involving many different species throughout the world. Periodically epizootics affect these populations and result in high mortality. The infection can be transferred to rats living in urban areas, where overlapping with wild rodents occurs. Such events have been rare in recent decades. Sylvatic plague is known to exist in the western United States, but there has not been any urban invasion in more than 20 years, until 1968. In June 1968 a young girl residing in Denver, Colorado, was hospitalized with a high fever and bubo from which *Y. pestis* was later isolated. A dead squirrel (Scimus spp.) found in the same community yielded *Y. pestis* on examination. Subsequent surveys revealed plague to be epizootic in the squirrels. No other animals were infected nor did any other human cases occur. The community is now under surveillance. Sylvatic plague also exists in some regions of South America, but the disease is seldom seen in urban areas. Other foci in the past and present include large areas in central and south Africa, central Asia, Manchuria, Iran, and parts of south-eastern Russia. Recently there have been sporadic cases in Bolivia, 1966; Zaire, 1965; Vietnam, 1967–73; and small epidemics in Nepal, 1967, and Indonesia, 1968. Sporadic cases continue to appear in other enzootic areas where small animals carry the infection. Through the efforts of port quarantine officials and maritime sanitary inspectors the transfer of plague or introduction into new areas is practically unknown today. Nevertheless, plague will continue to be a threat until the disease is eradicated.

Epidemiological studies have revealed that rabbits may act as passive carriers, as may apparently healthy dogs that have contact with infected rodents. A change in the virulence of plague has been noted in many areas. Serologic surveys indicate that latent plague in wild rodents is widespread in natural foci of Africa, Asia, and the Americas. Camels have been shown to be the source of some human infections.

An unusual outbreak occurred on a Navajo Reservation in 1966 when a group of Indians hunting prairie dogs for food became ill. A nine-year-old boy accidentally cut himself with a hunting-knife. Two days later he became very sick with a high fever. At the site of the wound a lesion appeared, and the proximal lymph nodes were affected. The infection was diagnosed as plague. Within a few days five cases occurred, all who had been hunting and skinning prairie dogs, or handling them in cooking preparation.

Plague vaccines have been used since the late nineteenth century, but it has never been possible to measure their effectiveness precisely. There has been continuous research on human immunization, but it is apparent that present-day immunization is not satisfactory, and further investigation is necessary. The killed vaccines available at present offer a reasonable degree of protection if two injections are given, followed by boosters at 6-month intervals. Immunization with plague vaccine, however, is known to reduce the incidence and severity of disease. A single dose of avirulent living plague vaccine has proved of benefit among residents of endemic areas. There is further evidence that the widespread and promiscuous use of antibiotics, particularly at inadequate dosage levels, may lead to the development of streptomycin-resistant strains.

WHO has prepared sets of slides showing various clinical aspects of plague (World Health Organization, 1974, p. 25).

Pseudotuberculosis

Human infections with *Yersinia pseudotuberculosis* are being reported with increasing frequency. Approximately 95 per cent. of such cases are mild mesenteric lymphadenitis and enteritis. The diagnosis is established by isolation of *Yersinia pseudotuberculosis* from the lymph nodes, blood, and stools of patients, by agglutination tests. Except in septicaemic infections, prognosis is excellent when the illness is treated by the administration of streptomycin and tetracycline.

Natural infection with *Yersinia pseudotuberculosis* is widely distributed among many mammals, especially rodents, and birds. Extensive epizootics have been reported in canaries and starlings in the United States and Canada. Sporadic infections in cattle, horses, and dogs are well documented, and cats are frequently infected. In hogs the disease has only rarely been reported. Pseudotuberculosis has been confused with plague in some parts of the world, mainly Alaska and Siberia. The infection may also occur as a hospital-borne infection.

It is generally believed that in most cases transmission of *Yersinia pseudotuberculosis* takes place through the digestive tract and occasionally by the ocular and respiratory routes; there is no evidence that transmission can occur through bites. Contact with infected animals is suspected as the source of human infection in some cases.

Climatic factors and individual metabolic disturbances of the host may contribute to establishment of the disease. Mesenteric lymphadenitis is predominantly a disease of male children, while the septicaemic infection has been observed at all ages in males.

Yersinia pseudotuberculosis may cause mastitis in cows, in which case the milk may serve as a source of human infection.

Enterocolitis

In man, *Yersinia enterocolitica* can cause similar diseases as *Y. pseudotuberculosis*, i.e. lymphadenitis and enteritis. Even rheumatic arthritis has been described. The importance of *Y. enterocolitica* for animals as a cause of disease seems to be limited. In experimental infection even massive doses fail to cause disease. Sporadic cases in chinchilla have been described.

Pasteurella infections

Pasteurella infections have been noted sporadically in man since the early part of the century. These infections are caused by *P. multocida* and *P. haemolytica*. In three cases the same *Pasteurella* found in patients was also isolated from animals with which they had been in contact (a cat, a canary, and a guinea-pig). Since the cat remains an intestinal shedder for a long period and *Pasteurella* contaminate the fur and the anogenital region, it is suspected that transfer to man may occur by the oral route. Faecal and urinary shedding by rats and mice may contaminate food and contribute to the indirect transmission of *Pasteurella*.

Rodent control

Rodent control is an important facet of plague control, as it is of other rodent diseases that are transmissible to man. Plague is by far the most important rodent disease that affects man, although rodents may transmit other zoonoses including bacterial diseases, e.g., leptospirosis, rat bite fever, rickettsial diseases, protozoal diseases, cestode diseases, and viral diseases, e.g. lymphocytic choriomeningitis.

Rodent control today is based on chemicals that destroy or reduce rodent populations so that they are no longer a public health hazard. The brief summary that follows is not conclusive in any sense but summarizes the conclusions of authorities in the field as to what is practical and the hazards that exist in applying these procedures.

Red squill is one of the oldest agents used against rodents, dating back to the middle ages (Siegmund, 1973). It is very effective and acts by producing convulsions with alternate paralysis. It is a potent emetic, and since the rat is incapable of vomiting, red squill is more toxic to rats than other species. However, swine, dogs and cats have occasionally been poisoned despite the unpalatability of squill to these species. Death occurs suddenly as a result of cardiac arrest.

Phosphorus was widely used in the past in food bait preparations employed in the extermination of rodents and rabbits. These preparations were, and to a lesser extent still are, a hazard to domestic animals.

Thallium sulphate is now seldom used as a rodenticide. It has proved to be toxic to all species to which it has been fed and mature animals are more susceptible than young ones.

ANTU (alpha naphthylthiourea). All animals that have been studied have proved to be susceptible to ANTU poisoning. When an animal has a full stomach the poison is absorbed, although in rodents that cannot vomit, absorption occurs regardless of whether the stomach is empty or full.

Sodium fluoroacetate, also known as 1080, is a colourless, odourless, tasteless, water-soluble chemical which is highly toxic to all animals to which it has been fed. It is a very effective poison but also dangerous because of its physical and chemical qualities. Fluoroacetate is toxic in itself, but it is metabolized to fluorocitrate which blocks the tricarboxylic acid cycle—a mechanism necessary for energy production by cells. It produces its effects by two mechanisms: (1) overstimulation of the CNS, resulting in death in convulsions, and (2) alteration of cardiac function which results in myocardial depression, cardiac arrhythmias, ventricular fibrillation and circulatory collapse. Animals that die of 1080 poisoning are dangerous to other animals that may feed on them, hence all rodents or other animals should be collected and buried. It goes without saying that all baits should be identified and those not taken should be picked up so that people and domestic animals do not accidentally ingest them.

Warfarin has potent antiprothrombin activity and is effective in controlling rodent populations that return to the same bait.

Warfarin is safe inasmuch as the animals ingesting it must build up relatively high blood levels before it causes death. Some health authorities have attempted to use it in dog control but with little success as dogs are scavengers that will feed at many sites. Dogs and domestic animals can be poisoned if they are fed large doses maliciously or in contaminated food that is given regularly.

Strychnine is used as a poison in some baits, especially eggs which are commonly used to control skunk populations. It is seldom used as a rodenticide as Warfarin is preferred.

An excellent review of anticoagulant rodenticides in current use is recommended reading (Bentley, 1972). For further information on the effects of various rodenticides and poisons on domestic animals, the Merck Veterinary Manual (Siegmund, 1973) will provide the necessary information. For human poisoning in most countries of the world there are now poison information centres which can provide the latest information on the management of accidental or intentional poisoning.

Q FEVER

Q fever is an inapparent infection of domestic animals. The disease in man is usually inapparent, although many persons develop an acute febrile illness. The causal agent is a rickettsia, *Rickettsia burneti* (synonym—*Coxiella burneti*). Q fever in man is characterized by a sudden onset, fever and chills, headache, malaise, weakness, and severe sweating. The course will vary considerably as to severity and duration. Pneumonia or pneumonitis may occur in acute cases, with a slight cough, chest pain, and little or no upper respiratory involvement. In some aged individuals the disease may be severe, and in rare instances terminate fatally. Since the advent of broad-spectrum antibiotic therapy, e.g. tetracycline and chloramphenicol, the reported fatalities have been negligible.

Laboratory diagnosis is by the complement fixation test and isolation of the rickettsia from the patient. The organism can be readily isolated in guinea-pigs, hamsters, or embryonated hen's eggs. Isolation in the chick embryo can be hazardous to laboratory technicians. The micro-agglutination test has been found to be quite valuable in the hands of experienced technicians. This test remains positive for a long time—often many years after the infection, whereas the complement fixation test usually becomes negative after 6–12 months. For this reason the micro-agglutination test is the preferred laboratory method for epidemiologic survey work. In addition, the capillary agglutination test is a rapid and economical diagnostic test. Recently it has been demonstrated that the indirect fluorescent antibody technique is valuable in diagnosis. The direct FA procedure has been used to detect infected ticks in nature.

The source of the infection for man is primarily infected cattle, sheep, and goats. Q fever infection is common in some wild animals, particularly rodents. Ticks are also known to carry the *R. burneti*. The placental tissues of domestic animals which are grossly contaminated constitute the principal source of infection. The organism can be isolated even when the tissues are diluted 10^{-10}. Dogs can become infected by eating contaminated placentae. In such cases the organism can pass intact through the gut and be spread over a large area by dog faeces.

The rickettsia is quite hardy, and can survive for some weeks in pastures, barns, and barnyards. It is also found in urine and faeces for some time after parturition. The milk of infected animals will often yield organisms for prolonged periods of time. Many outbreaks in labourers have been reported, and in some cases Q fever is legally recognized as an occupational disease.

Man usually becomes infected by inhalation of air-borne rickettsia. Raw milk as well as meat may also carry the agent. Wool, hair, and hides have been identified as sources of human infection.

Q fever has been reported from all continents of the world. Southern Europe, North Africa, Turkey, the U.S.S.R., Australia, and the United States are considered enzootic areas where the disease is found in animals the year round. Eastern and central Europe, the United Kingdom, and Canada are other areas where the disease is enzootic, but to a lesser extent.

Control of the disease is dependent upon limiting it in domestic animals and prevention of contamination of animal products. Vaccination of cattle has been found to be of value in the prevention of infection and shedding of the *R. burneti*, but has not been applied as a means of control. Antibiotic treatment of animals is not practicable. Sanitary measures, i.e. burial of placental tissues, burning of contaminated litter, and removal of manure from the immediate environment, would probably minimize the spread of infectious rickettsiae. As stated earlier, the organism is quite hardy, and can survive for some period of time in bedding, faeces, and animal products.

Pasteurization of all milk and milk products in enzootic areas is recommended. The organism is destroyed by heating to 63° C. for 30 minutes, or to 72° C. for 15 seconds, or by boiling the milk.

Persons exposed to disease, such as laboratory workers, should be immunized. Utilization of vaccine in occupational groups such as veterinarians, animal husbandrymen, and slaughterhouse and rendering-plant workers would be indicated in certain areas of high endemicity.

Areas that are free of Q fever may require that all domestic animals be blood-tested and no infected animals allowed to enter. Outbreaks have occurred on board ship among animals and crew members, and infection has been carried to disease-free islands by imported animals.

RINGWORM

Ringworm is a general term applied to certain mycotic infections of keratinized areas of the body, i.e. hair, skin, and nails. The causative agents are dematophytes, many of which are found in animals and are readily communicable to man. Dogs, cats, cattle, horses, goats, swine, rabbits, rodents, fowl, and many wild animals are affected and may serve as sources of infection for man.

The infection in animals begins by the invasion of the hair or skin by means of thread-like hyphae. Numerous spores arise from the hyphae and serve to spread infection. The initial lesion spreads in a circular manner and gradually becomes larger as more of the skin at the periphery becomes involved. The effect on the hair varies considerably. In some cases the hair becomes dry and encrusted; eventually hairs break off and fall out and a typical ringworm lesion appears on the animal. In other cases the hair does not fall out, and a diagnosis can be made only by examination under an ultra-violet light (3,660 Angström Units) using a Wood's nickel oxide filter or by a microscopic examination of the hair or skin scrapings, or by culture. The ultra-violet-light examination must be used by experienced persons who are familiar with its shortcomings.

Cat and Dog Ringworm

Microsporum canis is the common cause of ringworm in cats and dogs and is readily transmitted to man. It has also been identified in horses and monkeys. Hairless, round lesions are found more frequently around the head and neck. Infected hairs frequently show a green fluorescence under ultra-violet light. The cat is the most frequent source of infection for man, especially when they are kept confined and in large numbers. Dogs are often the source of infection for children. Children are more susceptible to ringworm than adults, but adults are often infected with *M. canis*. Frequently the diagnosis of the human disease is the reason that an animal pet is brought to a veterinarian for examination. In some instances community outbreaks have been traced to infected dogs and cats. In the United States *M. canis* is said to be the cause of 10 per cent. or more of human ringworm involving the exposed parts of the body. Recently *M. audouini*, the most common cause of ringworm of the scalp of children, has been isolated in dogs. The epidemiological significance of this is unknown. *Trichophyton mentagrophytes* and *M. gypseum* are also causes of ringworm in dogs and cats.

Cattle Ringworm

Trichophyton verrucosum causes ringworm in cattle. It is a very common disease among calves and young stock. After an incubation period of 3–4 weeks the affected hair over the infected skin breaks off, and within a few more weeks a sharply circumscribed, thickened patch becomes evident. The lesion expands at the periphery and frequently measures 1–8 cm. in diameter. The head and neck are the first areas affected. Frequently the disease spreads over the entire body. The disease is more commonly seen during the winter months in stabled animals, but may occur at any time in any climate. The fungus is resistant and may survive in stables for months and even years. It may grow as a saprophyte under natural conditions. The disease is also found among other domestic animals.

The infection in man is usually among farmers and members of their families, animal husbandrymen, or those in contact with stabled animals in colder climates. It is a suppurative ringworm frequently affecting the face—'barbers' itch'. Most human infection in the United States occurs in the northern states. The fungus causing ringworm in cattle does not cause infected hairs to fluoresce, and diagnosis must be made by laboratory examination.

Horse Ringworm

Horse ringworm is commonly caused by *T. equinum*. Other causes are *T. verrucosum*, *M. gypseum*, and *M. canis*. *T. equinum* is infrequently transmitted to man. Ringworm in horses is a not uncommon problem. It is transmitted by grooming tools, contaminated saddle blankets and harness, and by animal contact.

Other Animals

The principal dermatophyte isolated from other animals is *T. mentagrophytes*. The disease has a very wide host range from rodents and wild animals to fur farm animals and man. In man *T. mentagrophytes* causes a suppurative ringworm.

T. gallinae of poultry has rarely been reported in humans. *M. nanum*, a disease of swine, has been seen in man on occasions. *T. simii* is found in monkeys, as is *M. distortum*. These latter types have also been found in man. Many of these are found in soil and are considered as geophilic species. Both animals and man are susceptible, and the route of infection can be direct or by contact with diseased animals or persons.

Control

Control of ringworm in animals had been very difficult until the discovery of griseofulvin, a very successful antiringworm drug. Griseofulvin has been found to be very effective experimentally against *M. canis*, *T. verrucosum*, and *T. mentagrophytes* in low levels. The drug is available in the United Kingdom, the United States, and in most of the other countries of the world. It has proved to be very valuable in the treatment and control of animal ringworm, especially in small animals. It may be too expensive to use in cattle and horses, although when these animals are the source of human disease it may be the necessary means. Griseofulvin is also proving to be quite valuable in the treatment of all kinds and forms of ringworm in man.

Naturally, in addition to treating animals and man with ringworm, the environment should be thoroughly cleansed and disinfected. Such items as dog houses, catteries, sleeping baskets, blankets, harnesses, and saddles must all be thoroughly cleansed and disinfected so as to prevent reintroduction of infection [see CHAPTER 20].

SALMONELLOSIS

Salmonellosis in animals has been the subject of many studies since Salmon and Smith in 1885 first described a member of the *Salmonella* group from swine. Early workers classified the salmonellae according to host specificity and pathogenicity into those organisms of human origin that are pathogenic for man and those of animal origin that are non-pathogenic for man. In recent years improved methods of isolation and identification have revealed the widespread distribution of many of the host-adapted and non-host-adapted types of infections of both man and animals. Of the more than 1,300 antigenic types of *Salmonellae* now recognized, few, if any, occur exclusively in one host. Edwards (1958) has observed a distinct correlation between the presence of some types in lower animals and in the human population in a given area. In both man and animals *Salmonella* infection depends largely upon age and general resistance of the individual rather than upon the *Salmonella* type; the young, aged, and debilitated appearing most susceptible.

The incidence of human salmonellosis has increased significantly in many countries in recent years. In the United States the number of reported cases rose from 1,700 in 1956 to 20,865 in 1965. Increases observed in this and other countries must be attributed not only to more efficient bacteriological methods and a greater interest in the problem in general but also to a real increase in numbers of cases. It has been estimated that even in countries with good reporting systems less than 5–10 per cent. of cases are reported.

Any of the *Salmonella* types may produce a variety of clinical manifestations in man, including enteric fever, a mild febrile illness; septicaemia; gastro-enteritis (food poisoning); localized infections (extra-intestinal); and the normal carrier state.

In most countries *Salmonella typhimurium* is the most common serotype and is responsible for 50–60 per cent. of all human cases. The preponderance of the various serotypes affecting man varies from country to country. *S. heidelberg* is important in the United States and the United Kingdom, *S. thompson* in Canada, *S. bovis morbificans* in Australia, and *S. panama* in northern and western Europe.

The role of fowl, swine, cattle, rodents, domestic pets, and many other animals as a source of outbreaks and sporadic cases of salmonellosis in man has long been established. Cold-blooded animals, such as snakes and tortoises, also have been found to carry salmonellae. The studies of Edwards (1958) indicate that domestic fowl and birds probably constitute the largest single animal reservoir of salmonellae. Hinshaw *et al.* (1944) observed cases of gastro-enteritis among attendants on poultry farms caused by contact with acute outbreaks in poultry. Further evidence indicated that transmission of *Salmonella* from human carrier attendants to fowl also occurred. Reports implicating raw, frozen, or dried egg products as sources of *Salmonella* outbreaks appear frequently. Extensive studies on the occurrence of *Salmonella* types in dried egg powder have been reported by numerous investigators. In England public health authorities attribute their increased incidence of human salmonellosis during recent years to dried and liquid egg imports. Recent evidence suggests that *Salmonella* in edible fowl more often results from dissemination during processing than from spread of infection in flocks. The distribution of these organisms was studied in three poultry-processing plants in Florida (Galton *et al.*, 1955). Of 1,244 cultures taken from materials in the plants, 196 (16 per cent.) were positive for *Salmonella*. The highest percentage of positive findings was from edible viscera and the table on which edible viscera were wrapped.

Meat and meat products are the most important sources of *Salmonella* infection in humans in Europe, whereas in North America poultry and poultry products cause more *Salmonella* infections. The danger of meats as a source of large outbreaks of salmonellosis is well illustrated by the Swedish *Salmonella* outbreak of 1953 (Lundbeck *et al.*, 1955), in which nearly 9,000 bacteriologically proved cases were traced to a single slaughterhouse. Where salmonellosis is traced to meat or meat products, insufficient cooking is usually at the root of the problem. Where poultry is incriminated, infection is usually acquired through handling or processing contaminated birds, and infections traced to eggs or egg products are usually the result of undercooking. Salmonellae multiply at temperatures of between 10° and 45° C., and foods that originally were only slightly contaminated can become increasingly dangerous while being processed and stored.

In the United States dried milk has been incriminated as a source of human infection, and salmonellae have been found in such food supplements or additives as dried yeast, soya milk, coconut, cotton-seed protein, cereal powder, and carmine dye.

More and more *Salmonella* serotypes are being isolated from poultry in many parts of the world, although it appears that infection in this species is more common in North America than in Europe.

In cattle *Salmonella dublin* is endemic in many countries and is frequently transmitted to man through infected meat or milk. *Salmonella typhimurium* and other *Salmonella* types have also been found in cattle. Milk-borne outbreaks have been traced to *Salmonella typhimurium* as well as *Salmonella dublin* infection in dairy herds. In the United States recent reports indicate that salmonellosis among dairy and beef cattle is an increasing problem. During a two-year period in one state Ellis (1962) reported forty *Salmonella* isolations from cattle with enteritis. In another state Moore *et al.* (1962) reported the isolation of salmonellae from seventy-eight necropsied cattle during 1960.

Until recently, salmonellosis has apparently been of minor importance in adult cattle. However, in the United States salmonellosis is becoming a recognized problem among dairy and beef cattle, particularly those held for fattening prior to slaughter. In New Zealand and Australia the disease is becoming a common problem. There are few areas in the world that do not have *Salmonella* as a problem in cattle.

The prevalence of *Salmonella* in swine is well known. In a report of 2,788 *Salmonella* cultures derived from animals other than man or fowl Bruner and Moran (1949) found that 76 per cent., including thirty-seven serotypes, came from swine. Many of these cultures were isolated from the enteric lymph nodes of normal animals. Galton and her co-workers (1954) observed a wide difference in the proportion of infected hogs on the farm and in the abattoir. This was attributed to the congested contact of normal and possibly *Salmonella*-infected animals in auction-sale barns, during transportation, and in stockyards, all of which favour the spread of salmonellosis.

Current investigations have shown that subclinical infections of pigs are an important sources of *Salmonella* infection in man. In some countries up to 25 per cent. of swine have been found infected. *Salmonella* carriers harbour the bacteria in the intestinal tract, particularly the caecum, the mesenteric lymph nodes, and, to a much lesser extent, the gall-bladder and portal lymph nodes. Salmonellae are only occasionally found in muscle tissue. Subclinical infections in individual pigs often spread rapidly, involving the entire herd. Conditions under which the animals are subjected to stress, such as transport and confinement in holding pens, promote the spread of *Salmonella* infections.

Recent investigations have clearly shown that contaminated feeds of animal and vegetable origin are the most important sources of salmonellae that infect pigs. Moreover, the contaminated environment and infection of piglets in the first weeks of life are important factors in the spread of infection within the herd. Supplying the animals with *Salmonella*-free feeds seems to control these infections. Pigs can be raised and kept free from salmonellae throughout their lives if they are provided with such feeds in proper hygienic surroundings.

The importance of *Salmonella* infections in sheep has been

underestimated for a long time. These infections play an important economic role in Australia and New Zealand. Although the flock mortality rate is low, a large number of animals remain carriers for a long time; furthermore, the contamination of pastures results in the reinfection of animals.

Outbreaks of severe enteritis in horses with high mortality in foals have been reported with increasing frequency in the United States. Also, subclinical infection is a significant problem in many countries. The appearance of an increasing number of different serotypes in horses has been associated with contaminated feeds.

Practically every species studied has yielded salmonellae. Surveys of dogs have shown incidence rates of from 1 to more than 30 per cent. in different areas. More than fifty serotypes, including the ubiquitous *S. typhimurium*, have been isolated from dogs. Surveys of cats have revealed more than twenty serotypes, the prevalence ranging up to 12 per cent., depending upon the area and conditions under which the animals lived. Chicks, ducklings, pet budgerigars (parakeets), canaries, and exotic species of birds have been incriminated as a source of *Salmonella* infections, especially in children. Recently it has been observed that snakes, lizards, and tortoises play a role in the transmission of salmonellosis to man. The latter, especially, have become popular pets in many countries. The unhygienic conditions under which they are kept in many pet shops and households represent a further health hazard. A number of *Salmonella* infections originating from them have been described recently.

Special attention should be given to the destruction of rodents, flies, and other insects that are often infected in the surroundings of slaughter-houses, food processing plants, and rendering plants.

In connexion with salmonellosis in rodents it should be re-emphasized that salmonellae should in no circumstances be used as rodenticides. Rodents rapidly develop resistance to *Salmonella* serotypes; thus, this method has little practical value. Moreover, it has been shown in different countries that such practices are a public health hazard, because the serotypes used are also dangerous to man.

The role of the human carrier in the contamination of foods in the processing plants must also be considered. Periodic stool-culture examinations of workers in hospitals and food-processing plants should be encouraged when the disease persists. National reporting and surveillance of salmonellosis in man and animals, as well as of salmonellae isolations from human and animal foods, should be established in all countries.

Recent evidence indicates that a high percentage of domestic and imported bone meal, meat meal, fish meal, and similar protein supplements used in animal and poultry feeds are contaminated with salmonellae (Boyer *et al.*, 1962; Pomeroy and Grady, 1961; Watkins *et al.*, 1959). Numerous serotypes have been isolated, and multiple types were obtained frequently from the same sample. Many of these types are those found in poultry, the meat-producing animals, and domestic pets, as well as those commonly recovered from man. Animal feeds, frequently heavily contaminated with salmonellae, cause disease in domestic animals and poultry; they are the main source of infections in animals.

The control of salmonellosis in animals cannot be expected unless careful consideration is given to elimination of sources of contamination through animal feeds. Rigid hygienic control in all food-processing establishments should be maintained [see CHAPTERS 10 and 16]. Further, Savage (1956) has suggested adoption of bacteriological standards for the control of abattoirs and food-processing plants.

TETANUS

Tetanus or lockjaw is one of the oldest clinical entities recorded by physicians. It has been described in man and animals for thousands of years. It is an acute disease induced by the toxin of the tetanus bacillus, *Clostridium tetani*, growing anaerobically at the site of injury. The incubation period is variable, usually 7–10 days and longer. It has been reported as brief as 1 day, and upwards to 35 days. It is characterized by painful muscle contractions, primarily of the voluntary muscles of the head, neck, and trunk; involvement of the facial muscles gives rise to the characteristic appearance of the patient known as 'risus sardonicus' due to retraction of the angles of the mouth. The person affected is frequently unable to speak, and his facial expression is one of fear, pleading for relief. He is helpless yet conscious to suffer the violent muscular seizures which may involve any striated muscle, usually those of the upper body. Opisthotonus with rigid anterior bowing of the abdomen, marked nuchal rigidity, and trismus are often prominent signs. There is also an appearance of marked increase of salivation because the patient cannot readily swallow. Death may occur at the peak of any of the muscular contractions. These painful contractions may last from a few seconds to several minutes, depending on the severity of the disease. Nearly 75 per cent. of all deaths are due to respiratory failure. The diagnosis of tetanus is based on clinical signs and symptoms. In a study of ninety-one clinically diagnosed cases in Minnesota a few years ago the investigators recovered the organism in only 28 per cent. of the cases.

Tetanus is caused by a Gram-positive spore-forming bacillus that is commonly found in soil, street dust, animal and human faeces. The source of contamination is the intestinal canal of domestic animals, especially the horse, and also man, dogs, rats, and even birds. The isolation of *Cl. tetani* from soil and intestinal excretions varies considerably, indicating that the organism is not a normal inhabitant. *Cl. tetani* is highly resistant, and when protected from light and heat remains viable for years. Some strains resist steaming at 100° C. for 40–60 minutes. Five per cent. phenol is said to destroy tetanus spores in 10–12 hours; the addition of 0·5 per cent. hydrochloric acid reduces the time to 2 hours.

Infection in man and all animals is the result of wound contamination, e.g. dirty wounds containing foreign material, particularly soil, animal and human faeces. The organism multiplies at the site of entry and does not migrate. The toxin is thought to be carried either in blood or to the central nervous system via the peripheral nerves by absorption, and that it passes through the nerves centripetally until it reaches the motor cells of the anterior horn of the cord, at which time general symptoms of tetanus appear. The question of animal bites and the possibility of tetanus infection is of concern to all physicians. The biting animal does not normally have *Cl. tetanus* in the mouth or saliva, but contaminates its mouth by feeding habits and anal licking. It is well known that the tetanus spore will live and multiply in dead or anaerobic tissues. The tetanus spore does not germinate in living tissues, probably because of the presence of too much oxygen. It is known that tetanus spores washed free from toxin do not ordinarily produce tetanus when injected into animals, but were taken up by phagocytes and destroyed. Strangely, it has been shown that the injection of washed tetanus spores in a dilute solution of calcium chloride produced tetanus, and that infections regularly occurred in animals receiving inoculated washed spores in areas of the skin in which calcium chloride solution had been injected.

The tetanus organism also enters the body in burned areas. Sometimes trivial or unnoticed wounds provide the entry. Tetanus neonatorum usually occurs through infection of the unhealed umbilicus. The disease may also be a complication of surgery, especially in amputations, where infected or necrotic tissues are favourable sites for the multiplication of the organism.

There is no evidence that the disease can be caused by the ingestion or inhalation of the tetanus bacillus.

The disease is world-wide, in all climates, and affects all age groups, although tetanus neonatorum is seen more frequently in the tropical areas. In the United States less than 300 cases are reported yearly. Most of these are among adults, and with good medical care more than half recover. There is no reason for tetanus to occur in any country where there are public health services, inasmuch as the present-day tetanus immunizations are among the most effective prophylactic disease control measures known. Tetanus toxoid was developed over fifty years ago, and can be manufactured in volume at little cost.

Animal tetanus infections are most frequent in herbivorous animals, especially the horse. Infections in horses are frequently the result of nail wounds in the foot. In cattle it may be a puerperal infection after calving, or it may follow castration, dehorning, and nose ringing of bulls. In swine it usually is seen as a complication of castration wound infections. Carnivorous animals are seldom affected, and birds never have the disease, even though the tetanus bacillus is occasionally found in their intestinal tract. The occurrence of naturally acquired disease seems to correspond with the susceptibility of the animal to tetanus toxin. The amount of toxin per gramme of body-weight to kill a dog is about 600 times greater than that needed to kill a horse,[1] and to kill a chicken requires 350,000 times as much. The brain tissue of chickens and birds seems to have no affinity for the toxin. The brain tissue of all susceptible animals possesses the power of uniting with tetanus toxin *in vitro* and thereby neutralizing it.

Natural immunity occurs in some species, such as birds, that are naturally resistant to infection. The species have no antibodies in their tissues, and the brain tissue does not combine with the toxin. Naturally occurring neutralizing antibodies are found in the blood of cattle, and lesser amounts in sheep and goat blood. These animals are relatively resistant to the disease.

Active immunity follows the administration of tetanus toxoid (anatoxin). This was first used in horses by the French veterinarians Ramon and Lemetayer of the Pasteur Institute. Horses so immunized are resistant to tetanus for at least one year, and

[1] Man and horses are considered to be equally susceptible to tetatus toxin.

if they are exposed at a later date a booster dose will stimulate an increase in antibodies.

The agent of choice in the prevention of tetanus in man is the toxoid. During the Second World War millions of men received the toxoid, usually three doses given 2–3 weeks apart, which proved very successful in preventing tetanus. Today tetanus toxoid should be given to all children in combination with diphtheria toxoid and pertussis vaccine, and booster doses of tetanus toxoid every ten years. Adults who have not previously been immunized should receive two initial doses of toxoid not less than 4 weeks apart, followed by a reinforcing dose 8–12 months later; and thereafter in the absence of injury at intervals of ten years. In case of injury a booster dose of toxoid should be given.

There are a number of factors to consider when a person has an injury in which steps should be taken to prevent tetanus.

1. The patient who has previously been immunized against tetanus should receive a booster or reinforcing dose of 0·5 ml. of tetanus toxoid at the time of injury or as soon as possible thereafter. Toxoid has a great advantage over passive or temporary immunization with tetanus antitoxin, whether human or animal. Naturally, the wound should be cleaned and dead tissue excised. Antibiotic therapy may be considered, and various antibiotics are effective against the vegetative form of the tetanus bacillus, but not spores.

2. The patient who has had no previous immunization against tetanus must receive passive or temporary immunization, provided he is not sensitive to horse serum. The injection of tetanus antitoxin varies considerably. Public health authorities recommend 3,000–5,000 Units of equine tetanus antitoxin provided the patient is seen on the day of injury and there are no compound fractures, gunshot wounds, or other wounds not readily debrided. If delay is greater or complications exist the recommended dose is 6,000–10,000 Units or higher.

Bovine tetanus antitoxin is available for the individual who is sensitive to horse serum. More recently human tetanus antitoxin (immune globulin) has become available. This human tetanus antitoxin, which is hyperimmune gamma globulin, is derived from the serum of persons who have been hyperimmunized against tetanus.

Human tetanus antitoxin has a number of advantages over equine or bovine tetanus antitoxin, including the obvious fact that there is no need to inquire or test for sensitivity. (Properly prepared, human immune globulins do not, as far as is known, transmit serum hepatitis.)

1. Human tetanus antitoxin does not cause any allergic or anaphylactic manifestations that are associated with horse or bovine antitoxin.

2. Human tetanus antitoxin gives protective levels of circulating antibodies for much longer periods of time at much lower dosage than does equine or bovine antitoxin. The currently recommended dose is 500 Units intramuscularly following injury, although more recently the Massachusetts Public Health Laboratories have demonstrated that 250 Units is adequate when given at time of injury. The 500-Unit dose as well as the 250-Unit dose both give protective antibody levels for 3–4 weeks.

3. Human tetanus antitoxin given at the time of injury will not interfere with the primary immune response to the tetanus

toxoid given in another site, and may actually enhance it. Thus, when the second dose of tetanus toxoid is given in 4–6 weeks continuous protection will be provided, as the antibody produced by the toxoid replaces the slowly disappearing passive antibodies.

The increasing availability of human tetanus antitoxin will eventually replace the use of equine or bovine antitoxin and the attendant risks of anaphylaxis and serum sickness.

The availability of human tetanus antitoxin should not decrease the efforts towards active immunization of all persons with toxoid prior to injury, or the initiation of active immunization with toxoid at the time of injury.

There is no reason why any human being should suffer the agonies of tetanus today. With proper immunization with tetanus toxoid in childhood and boosters or reinforcing doses every ten years throughout life the population could be protected.

TOXOPLASMOSIS

The protozoan parasite *Toxoplasma gondii* was discovered in 1908 in north African rodents, and has since been found in a wide variety of wild and domestic animals and birds throughout the world. Infection in humans was not confirmed until 1939 by Wolf. Although many names have been given to toxoplasma organisms isolated from various hosts, biological and serological tests have shown that only the one species exists.

The clinical course of toxoplasmosis in man varies widely from the severe and frequently fatal congenital type in infants to inapparent infections in adults. In animals the clinical and pathological manifestations follow closely those observed in human infections. However, latent infections appear to be more prevalent. Little is known regarding the epidemiology of toxoplasmosis. The widespread distribution of the disease in animals provides many possible sources of infection, but the mode of transmission is unknown. It has been suggested (Siim, 1957) that infection may result from: (1) ingestion or handling raw meat, raw eggs, or raw milk from infected animals; (2) contamination of food by urine or faeces from carrier animals; (3) by droplet infection; or (4) by insect bites. As yet no single animal species has been definitely incriminated as the source of human infection, but there is considerable evidence that cats may be the primary reservoir and dogs, rabbits, farm animals, and birds may serve as reservoirs. Kimball *et al.* (1960) and McCulloch *et al.* (1963) demonstrated a direct relationship between serological reactors to toxoplasmosis and contact with soil or animals. A definite correlation between human and canine infections in the same household has been demonstrated (Cole *et al.*, 1953). Recently, Japanese workers have demonstrated that the infection is widespread in dogs and cats. They found that the infection rate varied between 15 and 30 per cent. Their diagnosis was confirmed by the inoculation of diaphragm samples into mice. Similarly, the geographical distribution of human and game toxoplasmosis has been observed to coincide in certain areas.

Diagnosis of toxoplasmosis must be confirmed by laboratory procedures, since the variable symptoms make a clinical diagnosis difficult. Among the conditions in which the disease should be suspected Siim has included lymphadenopathy, encephalitis, exanthematic diseases, myocarditis, chorioretinitis, and fever of unknown origin. Serological tests are of value in detecting serum antibodies, but isolation of the parasite from the patient by mouse inoculation is necessary for definite confirmation of infection. This can frequently be accomplished by inoculation of a biopsied enlarged lymph node or occasionally by inoculation of peripheral blood during the acute stages of illness.

Of the immunologic tests that have been developed for the diagnosis of toxoplasmosis, the intradermal, complement-fixation, passive haemagglutination, and methylene-blue-dye tests have been widely used. An indirect fluorescent antibody test, agglutination tests with *Toxoplasma* organisms, and latex and bentonite flocculation techniques show promise but require further evaluation.

The methylene-blue-dye test involves the use of living virulent *Toxoplasma* organisms, which must be maintained in mice or in tissue cultures. A human serum containing an 'accessory factor' is also needed, but this may be difficult to obtain and to standardize. Due to the exacting nature of the technique, it can be performed only by skilled personnel in special laboratories.

The complement-fixation test has a lower sensitivity than the dye test and does not detect antibody as early as the latter.

The passive haemagglutination test is a simple, rapid, and inexpensive technique that uses a killed antigen. It is more sensitive than the dye test, and if diagnostic titres ranging from 1:200 to 1:400 are used its specificity is good. If microtechniques are used the test may be employed in sero-epidemiologic studies.

The indirect fluorescent antibody test has a sensitivity similar to that of the methylene-blue-dye test.

Fatal epizootics have been reported in chickens, swine, rabbits, and mink. Spontaneous abortion in sheep and goats is a frequent complication of toxoplasmosis in some parts of the world (see also World Health Organization, 1974, p. 29).

The studies of Eyles (1956) have shown tha tsulphonamides, and pyranethamine will suppress the infection in animals by synergistic action. It is believed that these drugs act only on the proliferative forms of toxoplasma and not on the cysts. This therapy may produce a reversible toxic depression of the bone marrow. As to preventive measures, there are no specific recommendations. General hygienic measures should be followed, such as avoiding intimate contact with sick animals and birds and keeping the premises free from rats and mice. Even though there is evidence that the organism can survive in food products of animal origin, there is no evidence that milk, or eggs are the cause of human disease although raw or undercooked meat has been incriminated as the source of human disease in New York. Nevertheless, every effort should be made to prevent contaminated or diseased foods of animal origin from being used as human food.

TRICHINIASIS

Trichiniasis is a world-wide disease affecting millions of persons, but fortunately only a small number develop an acute infection. The parasite is found in swine, rodents, canidae, and many other species. *Trichinella spiralis* is the causal worm, of which the larva form produces infection and disease in man and animals. Usually the disease is mild and is discovered only in those few cases which are acute. Clinical disease in man is markedly irregular, severity varying with the number or trichinae, organ or tissues invaded, and the general well-being of the host. The overt clinical signs are: (1) gastro-intestinal disturbance, which may cause vomiting and purging; (2) oedema of the upper eyelids and of the legs during the second week of illness; and (3) muscle soreness and pain. Other symptoms may include remittent fever that may reach 40° C. for several days, thirst, profuse sweating, chills, weakness, and prostration. A rapid rise in eosinophils occurs during the second week shortly after the appearance of oedema. Respiratory and neurological symptoms may appear after the second week. Myocardial failure may occur during the second month of illness. Severe or fatal cases are rare.

Diagnosis is confirmed by a rise in the eosinophils and less frequently by biopsy revealing the larvae. Skin, flocculation, and complement-fixation tests aid diagnosis, but these are not conclusive.

The principal reservoir and source of infection for man is swine. Occasionally man may get infected from bear meat, walrus, whale or seal flesh, and dogs and cats where they are used for food. Rats, wild rodents, and some carnivorous animals may serve as a source of infection for swine and other flesh-eating animals.

The cycle of infection begins with the ingestion of flesh that contains encysted larvae. The cyst wall is digested in the stomach, and the liberated larvae congregate on the duodenal and jejunal mucosa. The larvae develop into sexually mature worms within 3–4 days, mate, and then the male dies. The 3–4-mm. female worm penetrates the intestinal mucosa and discharges living larvae by the seventh day. The tiny 0·1-mm. larvae are carried by the lymphatic and portal circulation to the systemic blood stream and on to the various organs and tissues. Those larvae that reach the striated muscle encyst, causing a myositis. When larvae enter other organs and sites they are destroyed by local inflammatory reaction. The diaphragm, tongue, pectoral, and intercostal muscles are the most frequent sites for encystment. Within the muscle the larvae penetrate the muscle fibre and grow to 1 mm. They then coil up and become encysted, in which state they remain viable for years. These encysted larvae are the source of infection for the next host. Some larvae that do not enter the lymphatics pass into the bowel lumen and pass out into the faeces. The adult remains in the intestinal mucosa for 4–5 weeks, producing larvae at a decreasing rate. The total larvae that a female worm produces may exceed a thousand. Following death, the adult worms are digested. They seldom are found in the faeces.

Swine usually become infected by the ingestion of pork scraps or trimmings that contain viable larvae. They also become infected from eating diseased rodents or other animals. Signs of disease are seldom noticed in swine, although they are known to occur, and may be so serious as to cause death. Pig farms where raw garbage is fed and the premises are infested with rats are important sources of diseased swine.

The parasite which causes trichiniasis was formerly widespread in the United States, where one in every six necropsies revealed human infection. Today the incidence according to autopsy surveys is less than 4 per cent., and even lower in persons under the age of 40, where infection is rare. In 1972 less than 100 cases were reported in the United States. The rate of swine infections varies from less than 0·1 per cent. in grain-fed swine to 1 or 2 per cent. in those fed raw garbage. All garbage fed to swine is supposed to be cooked, but there are always exceptions. Canada and England, where all garbage has been cooked for decades, have little human trichiniasis. Recent surveys in Mexico reveal that trichiniasis is a problem. The disease is quite widespread in southern South America, especially Chile and Brazil.

Russia and eastern Europe have found more evidence of disease in nature in recent years. Southern and south-western Europe report a fairly high incidence of disease. Sporadic outbreaks are reported in Western Europe. Epidemics have been reported in the Far East and the Pacific islands. The appearance of the disease in east Africa has caused considerable concern. Apparently wild pigs are the reservoir of the disease.

The most effective control is to forbid the feeding of raw garbage and offal to swine. Cooking of garbage and offal is a formidable task, requiring special equipment and a recording thermometer. Where garbage and offal are fed, the general sanitation must be excellent, otherwise rats and flies are attracted. In Canada, where garbage cooking laws have been in effect for decades, rats have been demonstrated to be the source of infection for swine.

Meat inspection for trichiniasis is impractical, costly, and gives a false sense of security. Even with microscopic examination, it is impossible to thoroughly examine sufficient muscle samples from each carcass. Pork should be thoroughly cooked by the consumer at a temperature and for a time that will ensure the destruction of any cysts. The cysts are destroyed at 66° C., a temperature which provides a good margin. Pork products that are to be consumed raw or partially cooked should be chilled at low temperatures, zero or lower, depending on the time they are held. The cysts are easily destroyed by low temperatures. The freezing of pork and pork products in home freezers or in lockers is thought to have contributed to the decline of human infections in rural areas of the United States [see also CHAPTER 10, and World Health Organization, 1974, pp. 30–31].

Gamma radiation has been used experimentally with good results. There are many problems to be resolved, such as flavour alteration, before it can be used as a public health procedure.

TULARAEMIA

Tularaemia is a highly infectious disease of rabbits and muskrats, and less so of other animals and man. The causal agent is *Francisella tularensis*. The disease in man has a sudden onset with chills, fever, and prostration, with lymphadenopathy. The lymph nodes are swollen, inflamed, and often suppurate. Formerly the pneumonic form had a high fatality rate. This is much lower since the advent of the antibiotics streptomycin, tetracyclines, and chloramphenicol.

Diagnosis is by bacteriological culture, positive agglutination reaction, and animal inoculation.

The sources of human infection are usually diseased animals and infected ticks and flies. All kinds of wild animals are susceptible to infection, and some domestic animals, i.e. sheep and swine, also. A disease of low virulence is seen in some birds. The mode of transmission is by the handling of blood or tissues of diseased animals, which results in the entrance of

TABLE 56

Epidemiological Aspects of Some of the Zoonoses

DISEASE	CAUSATIVE ORGANISM	PRINCIPAL ANIMALS AFFECTED	GEOGRAPHICAL DISTRIBUTION	PROBABLE VECTOR OR MEANS OF SPREAD
1. BACTERIAL DISEASES				
Anthrax	*Bacillus anthracis*	Cattle, sheep, goats, and swine	World-wide	Occupational exposure. Ingestion of contaminated meat. Occasionally airborne or biting insects
Bacterial food infections and intoxications	Various bacteria and their toxins, including: Arizona organisms Salmonellae Staphylococci *Clostridium perfringens* *Clostridium botulinum* (Toxin Types A, B, E, and F) *Bacillus cereus*	Cattle, swine, and fowl	World-wide	Ingestion
Brucellosis	*Brucella abortus* *Brucella suis* *Brucella melitensis* *Brucella canis*	Cattle, sheep, goats, horses, reindeer, and swine	World-wide	Occupational exposure and by ingestion of contaminated milk products and other foods. Occasionally airborne
Colibacillosis	*Escherichia* spp.	Cattle, swine, and domestic fowl	World-wide	Ingestion
Erysipeloid	*Erysipelothrix insidiosa*	Swine, fowl, and fish	World-wide	Occupational contact
Gas gangrene	*Cl. perfringens* and other *Clostridia*	Cattle, sheep	World-wide	Soil
Glanders	*Actinobacillus mallei*	Horses, mules, and asses	Asia, Africa, and South America	Occupational contact
Leptospirosis	*Leptospira* serotypes	Rodents, dogs, swine, cattle, and a variety of wildlife	World-wide	Occupational contact, immersion exposure, and contaminated food
Listeriosis	*Listeria monocytogenes*	Sheep, cattle, chinchilla, swine, goats, and fowl	World-wide	Unknown
Lung abscess	*Bordetella bronchiseptica*	Rodents	World-wide	Contact
Malignant oedema	*Cl. septicum*	Cattle	World-wide	Wound infection
Melioidosis	*Pseudomonas pseudomallei*	Rodents and rabbits	Asia, Australia, Guam, and Philippine Islands	Exposure and ingestion
Pasteurellosis	*Pasteurella multocida*	Mammals and birds	World-wide	Exposure and ingestion
Plague	*Pasteurella pestis*	Rodents	World-wide	Infected fleas and airborne
Pneumonia	*Diplococcus pneumoniae*	Calves (transmitted from man)	Europe and North America	Airborne
Pneumococcal mastitis	*Diplococcus pneumoniae*	Cattle	Northern and Central Europe	Contact
Pseudotuberculosis	*Pasteurella pseudotuberculosis*	Guinea-pigs and other rodents, pigeons, turkeys, and canaries	World-wide	Occupational exposure
Rat bite fever	*Spirillum minus. Streptobacillus moniliformis*	Rodents and wild animals	World-wide	Rodent bites
Relapsing fever, endemic	*Borrelia* spp.	Rodents and wild animals	World-wide	Infected ticks and body lice
Salmonellosis *	*Salmonella* serotypes	Cattle, swine, and fowl	World-wide	Ingestion, airborne, and contact
Staphylococcic disease †	*Staphyllococcus* spp.	Cattle, swine, and fowl	World-wide	Ingestion and contact
Streptococcosis ‡	*Streptococcus* spp.	Cattle and fowl	World-wide	Ingestion and contact
Tetanus	*Clostridium tetani*	Principally herbivorous, but all animals may harbour the agent	World-wide	Wounds
Tuberculosis	*Mycobacterium tuberculosis* var. *bovis* var. *hominis* var. *avium*	Cattle Monkeys Fowl	World-wide	Ingestion, inhalation, and occupational exposure
Tularaemia	*Francisella tularensis*	Rabbits, sheep, and wild rodents	North America, Europe, and Asia	Occupational exposure, handling, ingestion, and bite of infected insects and ticks
Vibriosis	*Vibrio fetus*	Cattle and sheep	Europe, North and South America	Unknown

* Arizona organisms cause similar infections.

† Some strains occur commonly in man and some are common to animals, while others appear in both man and animals.

‡ Group A streptococci have been found in man only. Group B streptococci: common cause of bovine mastitis; other strains cause infection in man; no evidence of interchange. Group C streptococci strains isolated from both human and animal infections. Group D streptococci: found only in animal infections.

TABLE 56 (continued)

DISEASE	CAUSATIVE ORGANISM	PRINCIPAL ANIMALS AFFECTED	GEOGRAPHICAL DISTRIBUTION	PROBABLE VECTOR OR MEANS OF SPREAD
	2. FUNGUS DISEASES				
Actinomycosis	*Actinomyces bovis* §	Cattle, swine, horses, and dogs	World-wide	Endogenous
Aspergillosis	*Aspergillus* spp.	Birds, fowl, and many mammals	World-wide	Contact with organisms in nature
Candidiasis (moniliasis)	*Candida* spp.	Birds, fowl, calves, pigs, rodents, dogs, cats, foals, and other mammals	World-wide	Endogenous
Coccidioidomycosis	*Coccidioides immitis*	Cattle, dogs, wild rodents, sheep, and horses	South-western United States, areas of Mexico, Central and South America	Contact with organisms in nature
Cryptococcosis	*Cryptococcus neoformans*	Cattle, horses, cats, dogs, pigs, and other mammals	World-wide	Contact with organisms in nature
Dermatophilosis	*Dermatophilus congolensis*	Cattle, horses, sheep, deer, and other mammals	World-wide	Not fully understood
Geotrichosis	*Geotrichum candidum*	Cattle	World-wide	Endogenous or exogenous
Histoplasmosis	*Histoplasma capsulatum*	Dogs, cats, cattle, horses, rodents, and other mammals	Probably world-wide	Contact with organisms in nature
Maduromycosis	Several species and genera of fungi	Horses and dogs	World-wide, chiefly tropical areas	Contact with organisms in nature
Nocardiosis	*Nocardia* spp.	Cattle, dogs, and other mammals	World-wide	Contact with organisms in nature
North American blastomycosis	*Blastomyces dermatitidis*	Dogs, horses, and sea lions	North America (occasional human infections in Africa and South America)	Probably contact with organisms in nature
Phycomycosis	Several species and genera of phycomycosis	Cattle, pigs, dogs, and other mammals	Probably world-wide	Contact with organisms in nature
Piedra	*Piedraia hortai*	Lower primates and other mammals	South and Central America, Java, Asia, and Africa	Contact with organisms in nature
	Trichosporon cutaneum	Lower primates and horses	Rare, reported from England and Latin America	Contact with organisms in nature
Rhinosporidiosis	*Rhinosporidium seeberi*	Horses, cattle, and mules	Endemic in India, Ceylon, and areas of western hemisphere. Sporadic in rest of world	Unknown Unknown
Ringworm	*Microsporum* and *Trichophyton* spp.	All mammals and birds	World-wide	Direct contact and fomites; contact with organisms in nature
Sporotrichosis	*Sporotrichium schenckii*	Horses, mules, dogs, cats, rats, mice and swine	World-wide	Contact with organisms in nature
	3. PARASITIC DISEASES				
	a. *Protozoan Diseases*				
Amoebiasis	*Entamoeba histolytica*	Dogs and primates	World-wide	Ingestion
Babesiosis	*Babesia* sp.	Wild and domestic animals	World-wide	Bite of infected ticks
Balantidiasis	*Balantidium coli*	Swine	World-wide	Ingestion
Coccidiosis	*Isospora* spp.	Dogs	World-wide	Ingestion of oocysts
Leishmaniasis: Visceral	*Leishmania donovani*	Dogs, cats, and rodents	South America, Africa, Europe, and Asia	Bite of infected sand flies (*Phlebotomus*)
Oriental sore (cutaneous)	*Leishmania tropica*	Dogs, cats, and gerbils	Asia, Africa, and Europe	Bite of infected sand flies (*Phlebotomus*)
American	*Leishmania braziliensis*	Dogs, cats, and spiny rat	Central and South America	Bite of infected sand flies (*Phlebotomus*)
Pneumocystis infection	*Pneumocystis carinii*	Dogs	World-wide	Unknown
Simian malaria	*Plasmodium knowlesi*	Monkeys	Borneo	*Anopheles* spp.
	Plasmodium malariae	Chimpanzees	Africa	
	Plasmodium cynomolgi	Macaques	Malaya	
	Plasmodium simium	Howler monkeys	South America	
	Plasmodium inui	Macaques	South-east Asia	
	Plasmodium brasilianum	New World monkeys	South America	

§ *Actinomyces bovis* is the cause of actinomycosis in lower animals. It does not cause this disease in man. The agent of actinomyces in man is *Actinomyces israeli*, a different species.

TABLE 56 (*continued*)

DISEASE	CAUSATIVE ORGANISM	PRINCIPAL ANIMALS AFFECTED	GEOGRAPHICAL DISTRIBUTION	PROBABLE VECTOR OR MEANS OF SPREAD
Toxoplasmosis	*Toxoplasma gondii*	Birds and mammals	World-wide	Probably contact and ingestion, although exact route is not known
Trypanosomiasis: African sleeping sickness	*Trypanosoma rhodesiense*	Wild and domestic ruminants	Africa	Bite of infected tsetse fly (*Glossina* spp.)
Chagas' disease	*Trypanosoma cruzi*	Dogs, cats, swine, foxes, bats, rodents, and monkeys	North, Central, and South America	Faecal material of triatomid bug
	Trypanosoma rangeli	Dogs and opossums	Northern part of South America	Faecal material of triatomid bug

b. *Trematode Diseases*

DISEASE	CAUSATIVE ORGANISM	PRINCIPAL ANIMALS AFFECTED	GEOGRAPHICAL DISTRIBUTION	PROBABLE VECTOR OR MEANS OF SPREAD
Amphistomiasis	*Gastrodiscoides hominis*	Swine	Asia	Unknown. Snails (?)
Clonorchiasis	*Clonorchis sinensis*	Dogs, cats, swine, and wild animals	Asia	Ingestion of raw or partially cooked infected fresh-water fish
Fascioliasis	*Fasciola hepatica*	Cattle and sheep	World-wide	Ingestion of contaminated greens
	Fasciola gigantica	Cattle and sheep	World-wide	
Fasciolopsiasis	*Fasciolopsis buski*	Swine and dogs	Asia	Ingestion of raw aquatic plants
Heterophyiasis	*Heterophyes heterophyes* (and other heterophids)	Cats, dogs, foxes, and fish	Nile Delta, Turkey, and the Far East	Eating uncooked fish
Metagonimiasis	*Metagonimus yokogawai*	Cats, dogs, other fish-eating mammals, and fish	Asia, Europe, and Siberia	Eating uncooked fish
Opisthorchiasis	*Opisthorchis felineus*	Cats and dogs	Eastern Europe, Asia, and Siberia	Raw or uncooked fish ingested containing metacercariae
	Opisthorchis viverrine	Dogs, cats, and fish-eating mammals	Thailand and Laos	Eating uncooked fish containing metacercariae
Paragonimiasis	*Paragonimus westermani*	Dogs, cats, and wild animals	Asia and Africa	Ingestion of raw or partially cooked infected crayfish
Schistosomiasis	*Schistosoma japonicum*	Cattle, swine, dogs, and rodents	Asia	Penetration of unbroken skin by cercariae in water
	Schistosoma mansoni	Baboons and rodents	Africa	
Swimmer's itch	*Schistosoma* spp.	Birds and rodents	World-wide	Penetration of unbroken skin by cercariae in fresh and salt water

c. *Cestode Diseases*

DISEASE	CAUSATIVE ORGANISM	PRINCIPAL ANIMALS AFFECTED	GEOGRAPHICAL DISTRIBUTION	PROBABLE VECTOR OR MEANS OF SPREAD
Beef tapeworm	*Taenia saginata*	Cattle	World-wide	Ingestion of measly beef
Dog tapeworm	*Dipylidium caninum*	Dogs and cats	World-wide	Ingestion of dog or cat flea
Fish tapeworm	*Diphyllobothrium latum*	Dogs and fish-eating animals	World-wide	Ingestion of raw or partially cooked infected fish
Hydatidosis	*Echinococcus granulosus*	Dogs, sheep, cattle, swine, and rodents	World-wide	Ingestion of tapeworm eggs
	Echinococcus multilocularis	Foxes, microtine rodents, and dogs	North America, Russia, and Europe	Ingestion of tapeworm eggs
Pork tapeworm and cysticercosis	*Taenia solium* *Cysticercus cellulosae*	Swine	World-wide	Ingestion of measly pork and auto-infection
Dwarf tapeworm	*Hymenolepis nana*	Rodents	World-wide	Ingestion of tapeworm eggs in food, fleas, and mealworms
Mouse or rat tapeworm	*Hymenolepis diminuta*	Rats and mice	World-wide	Ingestion of tapeworm eggs in food, fleas, and mealworms
Sparganosis	*Diphyllobothrium* spp. *Spirometra* spp. (pseudophyllidean tapeworms)	Monkeys, cats, pigs, weasels, rats, chickens, snakes, frogs, and mice	Mostly Far East	Ingestion of Cyclops or poultices from infected animals

d. *Nematode Diseases*

DISEASE	CAUSATIVE ORGANISM	PRINCIPAL ANIMALS AFFECTED	GEOGRAPHICAL DISTRIBUTION	PROBABLE VECTOR OR MEANS OF SPREAD
Capillariasis	*Capillaria hepatica*	Rodents	World-wide	Unknown
Dracunculiosis	*Dracunculus medinensia*	Dogs and racoons	World-wide	Bites of infected Cyclops
Filariasis: Dirofilariasis	*Dirofilaria* spp.	Dogs	World-wide	Bites of infected mosquitoes
Malayan filariasis	*Brugia Malayi*	Dogs and cats	Asia	Mosquito
Tropical eosinophilia	*Brugia* spp.; *Dirofilaria* spp.	Loper primates and mammals	World-wide and Tropical	Bites of infected mosquitoes
Giant kidney worm	*Dioctophyma renale*	Dogs and other carnivores	Europe and North America	Ingestion of infected fish

TABLE 56 (*continued*)

DISEASE	CAUSATIVE ORGANISM	PRINCIPAL ANIMALS AFFECTED	GEOGRAPHICAL DISTRIBUTION	PROBABLE VECTOR OR MEANS OF SPREAD
Gnathostomiasis	*Gnathostoma spinigererum*	Dogs, cats, and wild carnivores	Far East and India	Ingestion of infected fish or amphibians
Larva migrans:				
Ancylostomiasis (cutaneous larva migrans or 'creeping eruption')	*Ancylostoma braziliense*	Dogs and cats	World-wide	Contact with infective larvae which penetrate the skin
Anisakiasis	*Anisakis* spp.	Herring and other marine fish	Europe	Ingestion of raw or partially cooked herring
Parasitic meningoencephalitis	*Angiostrongylus cantonensis*	Rats	Pacific and Orient	Raw prawns and prawn juice, latter used on vegetables; slugs that contaminate raw vegetables and are accidentally ingested
Visceral larva migrans (toxocariosis)	*Toxocara canis*	Dogs	World-wide	Ingestion of dog and cat roundworm eggs
Strongyloidiasis	*Strongyloides stercoralis*	Dogs	World-wide	Contact with infective larvae which penetrate the skin
Thelaziasis	*Thelazia* spp.	Dogs, cats, and sheep	California and Far East	Infected insects
Trichinosis	*Trichinella spiralis*	Swine, rodents, and wild carnivores	World-wide	Ingestion of pork and other flesh containing viable cysts
Trichostrongylosis	*Trichostrongylus colubriformis* and occasionally other species	Domestic and wild herbivorous animals	World-wide	Ingestion of contaminated vegetation

e. Annelid Diseases

DISEASE	CAUSATIVE ORGANISM	PRINCIPAL ANIMALS AFFECTED	GEOGRAPHICAL DISTRIBUTION	PROBABLE VECTOR OR MEANS OF SPREAD
Hurudiniasis	*Limnatis nilotica* and related spp.	Cattle, buffaloes, horses, sheep, dogs, and pigs	Africa, Asia, Europe, and Chile	Direct contact with leech

4. ARTHROPOD DISEASES

DISEASE	CAUSATIVE ORGANISM	PRINCIPAL ANIMALS AFFECTED	GEOGRAPHICAL DISTRIBUTION	PROBABLE VECTOR OR MEANS OF SPREAD
Acariasis (mange)	*Sarcoptes* spp.	Domestic animals	World-wide	Contact with infected individuals or animals and contaminated clothing
Tunga infections	*Tunga penetrans*	Man, dogs, pigs, and other mammals	Western Hemisphere and Africa	Contact with contaminated soil
Myiasis	*Cochliomyia, Cordylobia, Dermatobia, Gastrophilus, Hypoderma, Oestrus,* and other genera	Mammals	World-wide	Invasion of living tissues by fly larvae
Pentastomid infections	*Linguatula* spp. *Armillifer* spp. *Porocephalus* spp. (tongue worms)	Dogs, snakes, and other vertebrates	World-wide	Ingestion of infected animal tissues

5. RICKETTSIAL DISEASES

DISEASE	CAUSATIVE ORGANISM	PRINCIPAL ANIMALS AFFECTED	GEOGRAPHICAL DISTRIBUTION	PROBABLE VECTOR OR MEANS OF SPREAD
Boutonneuse fever	*Rickettsia conori*	Dogs and rodents	Europe and Africa	Bite of infected ticks
Murine typhus	*Rickettsia mooseri*	Rats	North America	Infected rodent fleas
Q fever	*Coxiella burnetii*	Sheep, cattle, goats, fowl, and other mammals	World-wide	Mainly airborne, although milk may be a vehicle and occasionally ticks
Queensland tick typhus	*Rickettsia australis*	Bandicoots and rodents	Australia	Bite of infected tick
Rickettsial pox	*Rickettsia akari*	Mice	Eastern United States and U.S.S.R.	Bite of infected rodent mites
Scrub typhus	*Rickettsia tsutsugamushi*	Rodents	Asia, Australia, and East Indies	Bite of infected larval mites
Spotted fever	*Rickettsia rickettsii*	Rabbits, field mice, and dogs	North and South America	Bite of infected ticks or their crushing on the skin

6. VIRUS DISEASES
a. Arthropod-borne

DISEASE	CAUSATIVE ORGANISM	PRINCIPAL ANIMALS AFFECTED	GEOGRAPHICAL DISTRIBUTION	PROBABLE VECTOR OR MEANS OF SPREAD
Chikungunya	Group A virus		East and South Africa	Mosquito—*Culex* and *Aëdes* spp.
Eastern encephalitis	Group A virus	Wild birds, domestic fowl, horses, mules, and donkeys	Eastern Canada, United States, Mexico, Panama, Trinidad, Colombia, Brazil, and Philippines	Mosquito—*Culiseta melanura* and *Aëdes* sp.
Mayaro	Group A virus		Trinidad, Colombia, and Brazil	Unknown
Middelburg	Group A virus	Sheep	South Africa	Mosquito—*Aëdes* spp.

TABLE 56 (*continued*)

Disease	Causative Organism	Principal Animals Affected	Geographical Distribution	Probable Vector or Means of Spread
Mucambo	Group A virus	Rodents, wild birds, and monkeys	Brazil	Mosquito
O'nyong-nyong	Group A virus		Uganda	Mosquito
Sindbis	Group A virus	Birds	Africa and India	Culicine mosquitoes
Venezuelan-encephalitis	Group A virus	Rodents, wild birds, domestic fowl, horses, mules, and donkeys	Venezuela, Colombia, Brazil, and Trinidad	Mosquito—*Mansonia titillans*
Western encephalitis	Group A virus	Wild birds, domestic fowl, horses, mules, and donkeys	Canada, United States, Mexico, Trinidad, British Guiana, and Argentina	Mosquito—*Culex tarsalis*, *Culiseta melanura*
Bat salivary gland	Group B virus	Bats	Western United States	Unknown. Laboratory infections in man
Central European encephalitis	Group B virus	Cattle, goats (serological evidence only), and wild birds	Central and Eastern Europe from the Baltic to the Balkans	Tick (milk)
Dengue, Type 1	Group B virus		South and South-east Asia, Oceania, and Pacific	Mosquito
Dengue, Type 2	Group B virus	Monkeys and bats (serological evidence only)	Circumglobal in the Tropics	Mosquito—*Aëdes aegypti* and *Aëdes* spp.
Dengue, Type 3	Group B virus		Philippines and Thailand	Mosquito—*Aëdes aegypti* and *Aëdes* spp.
Dengue, Type 4	Group B virus		Philippines	Mosquito—*Aëdes aegypti* and *Aëdes* spp.
Diphasic meningo-encephalitis	Group B virus	Cattle and sheep	U.S.S.R.	Tick (milk)
Ilheus	Group B virus	Wild birds	Northern South America, Trinidad, and Central America	Mosquito
Japanese B encephalitis	Group B virus Group B virus	Wild birds, swine, horses, and cattle	Japan, China, Taiwan, Thailand, Malaya, Burma, India, Guam, Philippines, Australia, and New Guinea	Mosquito—*Culex triaenorhynchus* and *Culex gelidus*
Kunjin	Group B virus	Unknown	Australia	Mosquito
Kyasanur Forest disease	Group B virus	Monkeys and small mammals	Mysore—India	Tick—*Haemophysalis spinigera*
Louping ill	Group B virus	Sheep, goats, and grouse	Great Britain	Tick—*Ixodes ricinus*
Murray Valley encephalitis	Group B virus	Wild birds	Australia and New Guinea	Mosquito—*Culex annulirostris*
Negishi	Group B virus	Rodents	Japan	Ticks suspected
Omsk haemorrhagic fever	Group B virus	Rodents, muskrats, and goats	Omsk, Siberia, U.S.S.R.	Ticks—*Dermacentor pictur*, *Dermacentor marginatus*; goat-milk borne
Powassan	Group B virus	Squirrels	Ontario, Canada	Tick
Russian Spring–Summer encephalitis	Group B virus	Birds, small mammals, and sheep	U.S.S.R.	Tick
St. Louis encephalitis	Group B virus	Wild birds and domestic fowl	United States, Caribbean Islands, and Northern South America	Mosquito—*Culex tarsalis* and *Culex pipiens–quinquefasciatus* complex, *Culex nigripalpus*
Spondweni	Group B virus	Serological evidence in domestic and wild animals	Southern Africa	Mosquito
Wesselsbron	Group B virus	Sheep	East and South Africa	Mosquito—*Aëdes* spp.
West Nile	Group B virus	Wild birds and horses	Africa, Near East, and South Asia	Mosquito—*Culex univittatus* (Egypt) *Culex pipiens*
Yellow fever	Group B virus	Monkeys and marmosets	Tropical Central and South America and Africa	Mosquito—*Aëdes aegypti*, *Haemagogus* sp., *Aëdes leucocelanenus* (S.A.), *Aëdes africanus* (Africa), *Aëdes simpsoni* (Africa)
Zika	Group B virus	Monkeys	Nigeria and Uganda	*Aëdes africanus*
Apeu, Caraparu, Itaqui, Marituba, Murutucu, Oriboca	Group C virus	Rodents and possibly monkeys	Brazil	Mosquito
Madrid, Ossa	Group C virus	Rodents	Panama	Mosquitoes suspected
Restan	Group C virus	Rodents	Trinidad and Surinam	Mosquitoes—*Culex (Melanoconion)*
Bunyamwera	Group Bunyamwera virus		East and South Africa	Mosquito
Germiston	Group Bunyamwera virus		South Africa	Mosquito

TABLE 56 (*continued*)

DISEASE	CAUSATIVE ORGANISMS	PRINCIPAL ANIMALS AFFECTED	GEOGRAPHICAL DISTRIBUTION	PROBABLE VECTOR OR MEANS OF SPREAD
Guaroa	Group Bunyamwera virus		Colombia and Brazil	Mosquito
Ilesha	Group Bunyamwera virus		Nigeria	Mosquito
Wyeomyia complex	Group Bunyamwera virus		Colombia, Brazil, Trinidad, and Panama	Mosquito
Bwamba	Bwamba virus	Monkeys	East, Central, and West Africa	Mosquito—*Aëdes* spp.
California encephalitis virus	Group California virus	Hares and squirrels	Western and Central United States	Mosquito—*Aëdes* spp.
La Crosse virus	Group California virus	Rabbits	Mid-western and Southern United States	Mosquito—*Aëdes* spp.
Tahyna	Group California virus	Domestic animals and hares	Southern United States, Czechoslovakia, and Yugoslavia	Mosquito—*Aëdes* spp.
Catu	Group Guama virus	Rodents and monkeys	Brazil	Mosquito
Guama	Group Guama virus	Rodents	Brazil	Mosquito
Oropouche	Group Simbu virus	Monkeys	Trinidad and Brazil	Mosquito
Argentinian haemorrhagic fever	Tacaribe Group (Junin virus)	Rodents	Argentina	Rodent mite
Bolivian haemorrhagic fever	Tacaribe Group (Machupo virus)	Rodents	Bolivia	Rodent urine
Haemorrhagic uremic syndrome	Tararibe Group virus		Argentina	Unknown
Colorado tick fever	Ungrouped virus	Squirrels, porcupines, and small rodents	Western United States	Tick—*Dermacentor andersoni*
Crimean haemorrhagic fever	Ungrouped virus	Hares	Southern U.S.S.R.	Tick—*Hyaloma marginatum*
Kemerovo	Ungrouped virus	Cattle, horses, and rodents	Siberia	Tick—*Ixodes persulcatus*
Nairobi sheep disease	Ungrouped virus	Sheep	East Africa	Tick
Piry	Ungrouped virus	Rodents and opossum	Brazil	Laboratory infections have occurred
Quaranfil	Ungrouped virus	Wild birds and pigeons	Nile Delta of Egypt	Ticks—*Argus* (*persicargas*) *arboreus*
Rift Valley fever	Ungrouped virus	Sheep, goats, and cattle	Africa	Mosquito—*Aëdes caballua, Aëdes* spp. Contact on autopsy or handling fresh meat
Vesicular stomatitis	Ungrouped virus	Swine, cattle, and horses	North and South America	Contact exposure and insect bites

b. *Not Arthropod-borne*

African Green Monkey disease	Virus	African Green Monkey (*Cercopithecus aethiops*)	Unknown	Contact with infected tissues
Contagious ecthyma	Virus	Sheep and goats	World-wide	Occupational exposure
Cowpox	Virus	Cattle	World-wide, especially where smallpox exists	Contact exposure
Encephalomyocarditis	Virus	Rats, mice, squirrels, swine, monkeys, and baboons	World-wide	Environmental contamination
Foot and mouth disease	Virus	Cattle, swine, and related species	Europe, Asia, Africa, and South America	Contact exposure. Man is quite resistant
Herpes virus-simian (both B virus and T virus)	Virus	Monkeys	World-wide	Bites of monkeys and occupational exposure
Infectious hepatitis (human)	Virus	Sub-human primates	World-wide	Contact exposure
Influenza and para-influenza, including Type A (swine and equine) and Sendai (Type D)	Virus	Swine and rodents	Asia, Europe, and North America	Contact exposure
Lassa fever	Virus	Rats	Nigeria, West Africa	Contact exposure
Lymphocytic choriomeningitis	Virus	Rodents, swine, and dogs	World-wide	Virus contaminates food and environment
Newcastle disease	Virus	Fowl	World-wide	Occupational exposure
Pseudocowpox	Virus	Cattle	World-wide	Occupational exposure
Psittacosis-ornithosis (Bedsonia infections)	Virus	Birds, related virus found in cattle, cats, and sheep	World-wide	Contact and occupational exposure

TABLE 56 (*continued*)

DISEASE	CAUSATIVE ORGANISMS	PRINCIPAL ANIMALS AFFECTED	GEOGRAPHICAL DISTRIBUTION	PROBABLE VECTOR OR MEANS OF SPREAD
Rabies	Virus	Dogs and biting vertebrate animals	World-wide except Australia, New Zealand, Great Britain, Scandinavia, and Japan. A number of smaller islands are also free	Bites of diseased animals
Yaba	Virus	Monkeys	Unknown	Contact
Cat scratch fever	Unknown (virus suspected)	Cats and dogs	World-wide	Wounds and scratches

NOTE: Many proved zoonoses, particularly helminth infections of relatively rare occurrence have been omitted, as well as those diseases caused by fish and reptile toxins.
Prepared by: Veterinary Public Health Section, National Communicable Disease Center, Public Health Service, Atlanta, Georgia. Revised June 1968.

the bacilli via the skin or mucous membranes. The organism can also be ingested in contaminated water or flesh or diseased animals. The organism has been isolated from decaying organic material in stream beds as well as the water. The bite of animals whose mouths are contaminated may rarely cause disease. Laboratory infections are reported.

The disease is rarely spread from man to man. The organism may persist in lesions for a month or longer. Tularaemic papules may harbour virulent organisms for weeks with no clinical illness. Refrigerated rabbits kept frozen were infectious after $3\frac{1}{2}$ years. Lesions occur in rabbit and musk-rat hunters, butchers, and processers.

The disease is common in many areas of North America, especially on the great plains. The highest incidence is during the autumn hunting season, although it can occur throughout the winter. The disease is fairly common in eastern Europe, especially Poland and Russia. It has also been reported in Siberia, China, and Japan. It is unknown in the southern hemisphere.

An attack of tularaemia confirms a solid, lasting immunity. Persons and animals who have had the disease develop agglutinins that persist for long periods. These agglutinins will cross-react with a brucella antigen, or brucella agglutinins will react with a *Francisella tularensis* antigen.

In recent years vaccines have been developed by American and Russian investigators which have proved valuable in protecting against tularaemia. The American vaccine is a phenolized preparation, and is of limited value. The Russian vaccine is a live preparation, and has been used extensively in the endemic areas with success. In most people the live vaccine produced side-effects; newer, improved vaccines have eliminated such reactions. The immunity lasts up to five years.

Other control measures include the education of the public to avoid the handling and dressing of wild cottontail rabbits, and the thorough cooking of wild rabbit meat. Likewise, hunters and farmers should be cautious in handling any sick or strange-acting animals. In areas where ticks are known to be infected, sick sheep, calves, dogs, and birds should not be handled unless necessary, and then only with protective handwear. In these areas people should be warned about the danger of biting insects, such as ticks, flies, and mosquitoes that may carry the tularaemia agent. Likewise, people should be warned about possible contaminated waters where infection prevails among wild animals.

There is little hope that tularaemia can be eliminated or eradicated in nature, hence it is important that knowledge of the disease be widely disseminated, especially as to how it is transmitted, its symptoms in man and animals, diagnosis, treatment, and prevention.

Streptomycin, the tetracyclines, and chloramphenicol have been found to be effective therapeutically.

VIBRIOSIS

Vibriosis or vibrionic abortion was reported first in aborted sheep foetuses, and within a short time the causative agent was isolated from aborted bovine foetuses in Wales. A few years later similar organisms were encountered in bovine abortions in the United States and given the name *Vibrio fetus* by Smith. It is now known to be widely distributed in many areas of the world, and constitutes a major herd breeding problem. Vibriosis, generally considered to be a venereal disease, is characterized usually by a high incidence of infertility, irregular returns to oestrus, and a varying percentage of abortion. The organisms, apparently, are maintained in the testes of the infected bulls indefinitely and transmitted to susceptible cows through venereal contact (Grant, 1955). Cow-to-cow transmission has not been reported.

Laboratory confirmation is essential for a definite diagnosis of *V. fetus* infection, since it cannot be differentiated otherwise with certainty from trichomoniasis, brucellosis, and leptospirosis. Isolation of *V. fetus* from aborted foetuses, placental tissue, vaginal mucus, or semen is the most desirable laboratory procedure. Serological tests on blood serum or vaginal mucus are of limited value for diagnostic purposes.

The disease was thought to be confined to domestic animals until Vinzent in France reported vibrionic abortion and septicaemia in the human female and blood-stream infections were reported in human males. Seven human infections with *V. fetus* and four infections with 'related vibrios' were reported from the United States (King, 1957). These strains were also isolated from blood. All isolations were from males, with the exception of one 'related vibrio' from a three-month-old female infant. More recently, nine additional human infections with *V. fetus* have been reported in the United States by Hinton (1959); Kahler and Huntington (1960); King and Bronsky (1961); Mandel and Ellison (1963); Collins *et al.* (1964); and Bugert and Hagstrom (1964). In man, *V. fetus* infections have been implicated as cause not only in abortion but also in gastro-enteritis, septic arthritis, phlebitis, bacterial endocarditis, and meningitis. The source and mode of transmission of the human infections are unknown. Consumption of contaminated milk and contact with infected cattle has been suspected, but this has not been proved.

Vibrios similar to one of the human strains have been isolated from chickens and are believed to be the cause of avian vibrionic hepatitis (Peckham, 1958).

A new serological test which permits easier diagnosis of *V. fetus* infections in man has been reported by Bokkenheuser. In a New York City survey about 1 per cent. of hospital patients reacted to the *V. fetus* antigen. A higher incidence of antibodies was noted among patients of the lower social economic groups. Among syphilis patients antibodies were found in 7·3 per cent., many times the expected 1 per cent. Bokkenheuser states that this supports the assumption that *V. fetus* is a venereal disease in man as well as cattle. He also points out that over one-half of the fifty-five reported cases that he found in the literature had histories which include direct exposure to cattle. He also states that besides direct transmission from cattle to man, the disease may be transmitted in raw meat and raw milk. He thinks that the true incidence of *V. fetus* infections in man is much greater than indicated by the literature.

REFERENCES AND FURTHER READING

Anthrax

Afagonova, G. S. (1963) The use of gamma rays to disinfect hides contaminated with anthrax bacilli, *Tr. vsesoyuz. Inst. vet. Sanit.*, **22**, 76.
Barlow, H. M., Belton, F. C., and Henderson, D. W. (1956) The use of anthrax antigens to immunize man and monkey, *Lancet*, ii, 476.
Brachman, P. S., *et al.* (1962) Field evaluation of human anthrax vaccine, *Amer. J. publ. Hlth*, **52**, 632.
Glassman, H. N. (1958) Anthrax in man—world incidence, *Publ. Hlth Rep. (Wash.)*, **73**, 22.
Green, D. M., and Jamieson, W. M. (1958) Anthrax and bone-meal fertilizer, *Lancet*, ii, 153.
Kaplan, M. (1954) A brief review of anthrax prevalence and epidemiology outside North America, in *Proceedings of Symposium on Anthrax in Man*, Philadelphia.
LaForce, F. M., Bumford, F. H., Feeley, J. S., Stokes, S. L., and Snow D. B. (1969) Epidemiologic study of a fatal case of inhalation anthrax, *Ann. intern. Med.*, **18**, No. 5, 798.
Lamb, R. (1958) Anthrax and bone-meal fertilizer, *Lancet*, ii, 151.
Lamb, R. (1973) Anthrax, *Brit. Med. J.*, **1**, 157.
Morton, H. E. (1954) Pathogenesis of inhalation anthrax, in *Proceedings of Symposium on Anthrax in Man*, Philadelphia.
Moynihan, W. A. (1963) Anthrax in Canada, *Canad. vet. J.*, **4**, 283.
Pienaar, U. de V. (1960) A second outbreak of anthrax amongst game animals in the Kruger National Park (South Africa), *Koedoe*, No. 4, 1961.
Plotkin, S. (1959) An epidemic of inhalation anthrax, in *Proceedings of CDC Conference for Teachers of Veterinary Public Health and Preventive Medicine and Public Health* (1958), Atlanta, Georgia.
Pyper, J. F., and Willoughby, L. (1964) An anthrax outbreak affecting man and buffalo in the northwest territories, *Canad. Serv. med. J.*, **20**, No. 6, 531.
Sen, S. N. (1961) The sterilization of goat skin with ethylene oxide and some bacteriological studies of the process, *J. appl. Bact.*, **24**, 143.
Shlakhov, E. N. (1957) Anthrax, *J. Micro. Epid. Immun.*, **28**, 748.
Steele, J. H., and Helvig, R. J. (1953) Anthrax in the United States, *Publ. Hlth Rep. (Wash.)*, **68**, 616.
Turner, G. C., and Willis, A. T. (1959) Inactivation of spores of *Bacillus anthracis* by gamma radiation, *Nature (Lond.)*, **183**, 475.
Van Ness, G., and Stein, C. D. (1956) Soils of the United States favorable for anthrax, *J. Amer. vet. med. Ass.*, **128**, 729.
Wolff, A. H., and Heimann, H. (1951) Industrial anthrax in the United States—An epidemiological study, *Amer. J. Hyg.*, **53**, 80.

Botulism

Brandly. C. A., and Jungherr, E. L. (1957) in *Advances in Veterinary Science*, Vol. 3, pp. 482–93, New York.
Foster, E. M., and Sugiyan, H. (1966) Latest developments in research on botulism, *J. of Milk and Food Tech.*, **38**, No. 11, 342.
Lewis, K. H., and Angelotti, R. (1964) *Examination of Foods for Enteropathogenic and Indicator Bacteria*, Public Health Service Publication No. 1142, Washington.
Merson, H. H. (1973) Wound botulism, *N. Eng. J. med.*, **289**, 1105.
Morbidity and Mortality Weekly Report (1966) Vol. 15, No. 42, p. 359, National Communicable Disease Center, Atlanta, Georgia.
Taylor, A., Jnr (1973) Botulism and its control, *Amer. J. nurs.*, **73**, 1380.

Bovine Tuberculosis

Francis, J. (1958) *Tuberculosis in Animals and Man*, London.
Kleeberg, H. H. (1966) Chemotherapy in animal tuberculosis, *Fortschr. Tuberk.-Forsch.*, **15**, 189.
Kleeberg, H. H., Nixon, R. C., and Worthington, R. W. (1966) Studies on chemotherapy in bovine tuberculosis, *J.S. Afr. vet. med. Ass.*, **37**, 219.
Meyr, A. (1957) Progress in the control of bovine tuberculosis in the German Federal Republic, *Rindertuberkulose u. Brucellose*, **6**, 185.
Myers, J. A., and Steele, J. H. (1969) *Bovine Tuberculosis in Man and Animals*, St. Louis, Mo.
Sigurdsson, J. (1945) Studies of the risk of infection with bovine tuberculosis in the rural population, *Acta tuberc. scand.*, Suppl. XV.
Soltys, M. A. (1958) Public health aspects of tuberculosis in domestic animals, *Brit. med. J.*, **2**, 1133.
Steele, J. H. (1959) Epidemiological aspects of tuberculosis control, in *Proc. Symposium on Bovine Tuberculosis*, U.S. Dept. of Agriculture, Washington, D.C.
Steele, J. H., and Ranney, A. F. (1958) Animal tuberculosis, *Amer. Rev. Tuberc.*, **77**, 908.
Wilson, G. S. (1942) *The Pasteurization of Milk*, London.
Wilson, G. S., Blacklock, J. W. S., and Reilly, L. V. (1952) *Non-pulmonary Tuberculosis of Bovine Origin in Great Britain and Northern Ireland*, National Association for the Prevention of Tuberculosis, London.

Brucellosis

Bendtsen, H., Christiansen, M., and Thomsen, A. (1954) Brucella enzootics in swine herds in Denmark, *Nord. Vet.-Med.*, **6**, 11.
Cameron, H. S. (1957) Swine brucellosis, in *Advances in Veterinary Science*, Vol. III, pp. 275–84, New York.
Cappucci, D. (1968) *National Communicable Disease Center Annual Brucellosis Summary, 1967*, Atlanta, Georgia.

Korotich, A. S. (1957) Epidemiological characteristics of brucellosis in the Ukrainian S.S.R., *J. Micro. Epid. Immun.*, **28**, 705.

McCullough, N. B. (1964) Brucellosis, in *Occupational Diseases Acquired From Animals*, pp. 203–13, University of Michigan School of Public Health, Ann Arbor, Michigan.

Renoux, Gerard (1957) Brucellosis in goats and sheep, in *Advances in Veterinary Science*, Vol. III, pp. 242–68, New York.

Sadusk, J. F., Browne, A. S., and Born, J. L. (1957) Brucellosis in man resulting from *Brucella abortus* vaccine, *J. Amer. med. Ass.*, **164**, 1325.

Schilf, E. A. (1968) Progress report on cooperative state federal brucellosis eradication program, U.S. Dept. of Agriculture, Washington, D.C.

Spink, W. W. (1953) Human brucellosis caused by *Brucella abortus*, strain 19, *J. Amer. med. Ass.*, **153**, 1162.

Steele, J. H., and Emik, L. O. (1950) Brucellosis incidence in the U.S., *3rd Inter. Amer. Cong. on Bruc.*, WHO, Washington, D.C.

Thomsen, Axel (1957) The eradication of bovine brucellosis in Scandinavia, in *Advances in Veterinary Science*, Vol. III, pp. 198–235, New York.

Williams, E. (1973) Subclinical brucellosis, *Brit. med. J.*, **2**, 717.

World Health Organization Expert Committee on Brucellosis (1951) First Report, *Wld Hlth Org. techn. Rep. Ser.*, No. 37.

World Health Organization Expert Committee on Brucellosis (1953) Second Report, *Wld Hlth Org. techn. Rep. Ser.*, No. 67.

World Health Organization Expert Committee on Brucellosis (1958) Third Report, *Wld Hlth Org. techn. Rep. Ser.*, No. 148.

World Health Organization Expert Committee on Brucellosis (1963) Fourth Report, *Wld Hlth Org. techn. Rep. Ser.*, No. 289.

World Health Organization Expert Committee on Brucellosis (1971) Fifth Report, *Wld Hlth Org. techn. Rep. Ser.*, No. 464.

World Health Organization (1974) The work of WHO in 1973, *Wld Hlth Org. Off. Rec.*, **213**, 27–28.

Cat Scratch Fever

Byrne, J. J., Boyd, T. F., and Daly, A. K. (1956) Pasteurella infection from cat bites, *Surg. Gynec. Obstet.*, **103**, 57.

Daniels, W., and MacMurray, F. G. (1954) Cat scratch disease, *J. Amer. med. Ass.*, **154**, 1247.

Steele, J. H. (1953) Public health—cat scratch fever, *Vet. Med.*, **48**, 425.

Warwick, W. J., and Good, R. A. (1960) Cat scratch fever in Minnesota. Evidence for its epidemic occurrence, *Amer. J. Dis. Child.*, **100**, 288.

Contagious Ecthyma of Sheep and Goats

Hanson, L. E. (1964) Animal pox viruses and human health, in *Occupational Diseases Acquired from Animals*, pp. 113–14, University of Michigan School of Public Health, Ann Arbor, Michigan.

Hull, T. G. (1963) *Diseases Transmitted from Animals to Man*, 5th ed., Chap. 14, Springfield, Ill.

United States Department of Agriculture (1957) *The Year Book of Agriculture, 1956*, Animal diseases, p. 414, Washington.

Erysipeloid

Merck Veterinary Manual, Fourth Edition (1973) Erysipelothrix infection, pp. 411–18, Rahway, New Jersey.

Shuman, Richard D. (1964) Swine erysipelas, in *Diseases of Swine*, pp. 409–52, Iowa State University Press, Ames, Iowa.

Glanders

Gorelick, Arthur N. (1964) Glanders and melioidosis, in *Occupational Diseases Acquired from Animals*, pp. 228–32, University of Michigan School of Public Health, Ann Arbor, Michigan.

Howe, C., and Miller, W. R. (1947) Human glanders: Report of six cases, *Ann. intern. Med.*, **26**, 93.

Merck Veterinary Manual, Third Edition (1967) Glanders, Rahway, New Jersey.

Leptospirosis

Alston, J. M., and Broom, J. C. (1958) *Leptospirosis in Man and Animals*, Baltimore.

Babudieri, B. (1958) Animal reservoirs of leptospires, *Ann. N.Y. Acad. Sci.*, **70**, 93.

Galton, M. M., Powers, D. K., Hall, A. D., and Cornell, R. G. (1958) A rapid macroscopic-slide screening test for the serodiagnosis of leptospirosis, *Amer. J. vet. Res.*, **19**, 505.

Kalz, G. (1957) The human leptospiroses, *Amer. J. med. Sic.*, **233**, 320.

McKeever, S., Gorman, G. W., Chapman, J. F., Galton, M. M., and Powers, D. K. (1958) Incidence of leptospirosis in wild mammals from southwestern Georgia, with a report of new hosts for six serotypes of leptospires, *Amer. J. trop. Med. Hyg.*, **7**, 646.

Symposium on the Leptospiroses (1953) *Med. Sci. Pub.* 1, Walter Reed Army Medical Center, Washington, D.C.

Van Thiel, P. H. (1948) *The Leptospiroses*, Leiden.

Wolff, J. W. (1954) *The Laboratory Diagnosis of Leptospirosis*, Springfield, Ill.

World Health Organization (1956) Diagnosis and Typing in Leptospirosis. Report of a Study Group, *Wld Hlth Org. techn. Rep. Ser.*, No. 113.

World Health Organization (1967) Current Problems in Leptospirosis Research, *Wld Hlth Org. techn. Rep. Ser.*, No. 380.

World Health Organization (1967) Joint FAO/WHO Expert Committee on Zoonoses, Third Report, *Wld Hlth Org. techn. Rep. Ser.*, No. 378.

World Health Organization (1974) The work of WHO in 1973, *Wld Hlth Org. Off. Rec.*, **213**, 28–29.

Plague

Link, Vernon B. (1955) A history of plague in USA, *Public Health Service Monograph*, No. 26, Washington, D. C.

Morbidity and Mortality Weekly Report (1967) Vol. 16, No. 27, p. 222, National Communicable Disease Center, Atlanta, Georgia.

Pollitzer, R. (1954) Plague, *Wld Hlth Org. Monogr. Ser.*, No. 22.

World Health Organization Expert Committee on Plague (1950) First Report, *Wld Hlth Org. techn. Rep. Ser.*, No. 11.

World Health Organization Expert Committee on Plague (1953) Second Report, *Wld Hlth Org. techn. Rep. Ser.*, No. 74.

World Health Organization Expert Committee on Plague (1959) Third Report, *Wld Hlth Org. techn. Rep. Ser.*, No. 165.

World Health Organization Expert Committee on Plague (1970) Fourth Report, *Wld Hlth Org. techn. Rep., Ser.*, No. 447.

World Health Organization (1973) Plague, *Wld. Hlth Org. Chron.*, **27**, 75.

World Health Organization (1974) A system of plague surveillance, *Wld Hlth Org. Chron.*, **28**, 71.

Q Fever

Enright, J. B. (1951) The role of animals in Q fever, *Vet. Med.*, **46**, 383.

Kaplan, M. M., and Bertagna, P. (1955) The geographical distribution of Q fever, *Bull. Wld Hlth Org.*, No. 13, 829.

Luoto, L., Winn, J. F., and Huebner, R. J. (1952) Q fever studies in Southern California: Vaccination of dairy cattle against Q fever, *Amer. J. Hyg.*, **55**, 190.

Parker, R. R., Bell, E. J., and Stoenner, H. G. (1949) Q fever: a brief survey of the problem, *J. Amer. vet. med. Ass.*, **114**, 55, 124.

Slavin, G. (1952) Q fever: the domestic animal as a source of infection in man, *Vet. Rec.*, **64**, 743.

Stoenner, H. G. (1964) Occupational hazards of Q fever, in *Zoonoses as Occupational Diseases*, pp. 36–53, University of Michigan School of Public Health, Ann Arbor, Michigan.

Syrucek, L., and Raska, K. (1956) Q fever in domestic and wild birds, *Bull. Wld Hlth Org.*, No. 15, 329.

Rodent Control

Bentley, E. W. (1972) A review of anticoagulant rodenticides in current use, *Bull. Wld Hlth Org.*, **47**, No. 3, 275.

Gratz, N. G. (1973) A critical review of currently used single-dose rodenticides, *Bull. Wld Hlth Org.*, **48**, No. 4.

Jackson, W. B. (1973) Biological and behavioural studies of rodents as a basis for control, *Bull. Wld Hlth Org.*, **47**, No. 3.

Mackenzie, R. B. (1973) Public health importance of rodents in South America, *Bull. Wld Hlth Org.*, **47**, No. 2.

Siegmund, O. H., ed. (1973) *Merck Veterinary Manual*, 4th ed., New Jersey.

Wodzichi, I. (1973) Prospects for biological control of rodent populations, *Bull. Wld Hlth Org.*, **48**, No. 4.

World Health Organization (1973) The Unit of Vector Biology and Control has published a bibliography (together with FAO) on rodent pest biology and control for the period 1960–69, the 7000 articles have been taken from the literature of many countries. In 4 parts, Geneva.

World Health Organization (1974) The ecology and control of rodents of public health importance. Report of a WHO scientific group, *Wld Hlth Org. techn. Rep. Ser.*, in the press.

Ringworm

Ainsworth, G. C., and Austwick, P. K. C. (1955) A survey of animal mycoses in Britain: General aspects, *Vet. Rec.*, **67**, 88.

Furcolow, Michael L. (1965), Environmental aspects of histoplasmosis, *Archives of Environmental Health*, Vol. 10, pp. 4–10.

Gentles, J. C., and O'Sullivan, J. G. (1957) Correlation of human and animal ringworm in west of Scotland, *Brit. med. J.*, **2**, 678.

Georg, L. K. (1956) The role of animals as vectors of human fungus diseases, *Trans. N.Y. Acad. Sci.*, **18**, 639.

Kaplan, William (1967), Epidemiology and public health significance of ringworm in animals, *Arch. Derm.*, **96**.

Kaplan, William (1968) Dermatophytosis (ringworm, dermatomycosis), in *Current Veterinary Therapy, III, Small Animal Practice*, ed. Kirk, R. W., Philadelphia.

Rook, A. J., and Frain-Bell, W. (1954) Cattle ringworm, *Brit. med. J.*, **2**, 1198.

Smith, W. W., Menges, R. W., and Georg, Lucille, K. (1957) Ecology of ringworm fungi on commensal rats from rural premises in southwestern Georgia, *Amer. trop. Med. Hyg.*, **6**, 1.

Salmonellosis

Baine, W. B. (1973) Institutional salmonellosis, *J. Infect. Dis.*, **128**, 357.

Boring, John R. (1958) Domestic fish meal as a source of various salmonella types, *Vet. Med.*, **53**, 311.

Boyer, C. I., Jr., Narotsky, S., Bruner, D. W., and Brown, J. A. (1962) Salmonellosis in turkeys and chickens associated with contaminated feed, *Avian Dis.*, **6**, 43.

Bruner, D. W., and Moran, A. B. (1949) *Salmonella* infections in domestic animals, *Cornell Vet.*, **39**, 53.

Edwards, P. R. (1958) Salmonellosis: observations on incidence and control, *Ann. N.Y. Acad. Sci.*, **70**, 598.

Ellis, E. M. (1962) Salmonellosis in cattle, horses and feeds. Presented at the Midwest Interprofessional Seminar on Diseases Common to Man and Animals, Iowa State University, Ames, Iowa.

Galton, M. M., Mackel, D. C., Haire, W. C., and Lewis, A. (1955) Salmonellosis in poultry and poultry processing plants in Florida, *Amer. J. vet. Res.*, **15**, 132.

Galton, M. M., Smith, W. V., McElrath, H. B., and Hardy, A. V. (1954) *Salmonella* in swine, cattle and the environment of abattoirs, *J. infect. Dis.*, **95**, 236.

Hinshaw, W. R., McNeil, E., and Taylor, T. J. (1944) Avian salmonellosis, types of salmonella isolated and their relation to public health, *Amer. J. Hyg.*, **50**, 264.

Kaufmann, A. F., and Feeley, J. C. (1968) Culture survey of *Salmonella* at a broiler-raising plant, *Publ. Hlth Rep. (Wash.)*, **83**, No. 5, 417.

Lundbeck, H., Plazikowski, U., and Silverstolpe, L. (1955) The Swedish *Salmonella* outbreak of 1953, *J. appl. Bact.*, **18**, 535.

Meyer, K. F. (1953) Food poisoning, *New England. J. Med.*, **249**, 765, 804, 843.

Moore, G. R., Rothenbacker, H., Bennett, M. V., and Barnes, R. D. (1962) Bovine salmonellosis, *J. Amer vet. med. Ass.*, **141**, 841.

National Conference on Salmonellosis Proceedings (1964) U.S. Department of Health, Education, and Welfare, Public Health Service, Atlanta, Ga.

Pomeroy, B. S., and Grady, M. K. (1961) *Salmonella* organisms in feed ingredients, in *Proceedings of the 65th Annual Meeting U.S. Livestock Sanitary Association*, p. 449, Minneapolis, Minn.

Report of the Public Health Laboratory Service (1958) The contamination of egg products with *Salmonellae* with particular reference to *S. paratyphi B.*, *Monthly Bull. Minist. Hlth Lab. Serv.*, **17**, 36.

Savage, Sir W. (1956) Problems of *salmonella* food-poisoning, *Brit. med. J.*, **2**, 317.

Walker, John W. (1967) Cooperative State/Federal *Salmonella* control in animal feeds and feed ingredients. Presented to the American Public Health Association, Miami, Florida.

Williams, L. P., and Newell, K. P. (1966) *Salmonella* excretion in joy-riding pigs. Presented to the American Public Health Association, San Francisco, Calif.

Toxoplasmosis

Beverley, J. K. A. (1957) Toxoplasmosis, *Vet. Rec.*, **69**, 337.

Cole, C. R., Prior, J. A., Docton, F. L., Chamberlain, D. M., and Saslaw, S. (1953) Toxoplasmosis: Study of families exposed to their toxoplasma infected pet dogs, *Arch. intern. Med.*, **92**, 308.

Conference on Some Protozoan Diseases of Man and Animals (1956) Anaplasmosis, and toxoplasmosis, *Ann. N.Y. Acad. Sci.*, **64**, 25.

Eyles, D. E. (1956) Newer knowledge of the chemotherapy of toxoplasmosis, *Ann. N.Y. Acad. Sci.*, **64**, 252.

Eyles, D. E., and Frenkel, J. K. (1952) a bibliography of toxoplasmosis and *Toxoplasma gondii*, U.S. Public Health Service Publication, No. 247, Washington, and bibliography of toxoplasmosis and *Toxoplasma gondii*—First supplementum, 1954, Memphis, Tennessee.

Kimball, A. C., Bauer, H., Sheppard, C. G., Held, J. R., and Schuman, L. M. (1960) Studies on toxoplasmosis. III. Toxoplasma antibodies in obstetrical patients correlated with residence, animal contact, and consumption of selected foods, *Amer. J. Hyg.*, **71**, 93.

Manwell, R. D., Coulston, F., Binckley, E. C., and Jones, V. P. (1945) Mammalian and avian toxoplasma, *J. infect. Dis.*, **76**.

Markus, M. B. (1973 Symptoms, prevention and treatment of toxoplasmosis, *S. Afr. med. J.*, **47**, 1588.

Medical Journal of Australia leading article (1973) More about toxoplasmosis, *Med. J. Aust.*, **i**, 126.

McCulloch, W. F., Braun, J. L., Heggen, D. W., and Top, F. H. (1963) Studies on medical and veterinary students skin tested for toxoplasmosis, *Publ. Hlth Rep. (Wash.)*, **78**, 689.

Siim, J. C. (1957) *Toxoplasmosis in Human and Veterinary Medicine:* A survey of present knowledge and future problems, Seminar on Veterinary Public Health, World Health Organization, Warsaw.

Siim, J. C., ed. (1960) *Human Toxoplasmosis*, Report of the Proceedings of the Conference on Clinical Aspects and Diagnostic Problems of Toxoplasmosis in Paediatrics held in Copenhagen, 1956, Copenhagen.

World Health Organization (1969) Report of a WHO meeting, Toxoplasmosis, *Wld Hlth Org. techn. Rep. Ser.*, No. 431.

Trichiniasis

American Medical Association (1952) *Proceedings of the First National Conference on Trichinosis*, Chicago, Ill.

American Medical Association (1954) *Proceedings of the Second National Conference on Trichinosis*, Chicago, Ill.

Gould, Sylvester E. (1945) *Trichinosis*, rev. ed. (1970), Springfield, Ill.

Thornton, Horace (1949) *Textbook of Meat Inspection*, Chicago, Ill.

Timmermann, W. J. (1973) Trichiniasis in U.S.A., 1966–70, *Hlth Serv. Rep.*, **88**, 606.

Tuberculosis

Meyer, J. A., and Steele, J. H. (1969) *Bovine Tuberculosis Control in Man and Animals*, St. Louis, Mo.

Tularaemia

Feldman *et al.* (1973) Tularaemia, *J. Amer. med. Ass.*, **226**, 189.

Jellison, W., and Kohls, G. M. (1955) *Tularemia in sheep and in the industry workers*, Public Health Monograph 28, Public Health Service Publication No. 421, Washington.

Klock, L. E. (1973) Tularaemia epidemic associated with the deerfly, *J. Amer. med. Ass.*, **226**, 149.

Merck Veterinary Manual (1955) Tularemia, Rahway, New Jersey.

Vibriosis

Bokkenheuser, Victor (1968) *Vibrio fetus* infections in humans diagnosed in New York, *Animal Health News*, **2**, 6.

Bugert, W., Jr., and Hagstrom, J. W. C. (1964) *Vibrio fetus* meningoencephalitis, *Arch. Neurol. (Chic.)*, **10**, 196.

Canham, A. S. (1948) *Vibrio foetus* infection in cattle, *J. S. Afr. vet. med. Ass.*, **19**, 103.

Collins, H. S., Blevins, A., and Benter, E. (1964) Protracted bacteremia and meningitis due to *Vibrio fetus*. A case report, *Arch. intern. Med.*, **113**, 361.

Grant, C. A. (1955) Bovine vibriosis: A brief review, *Canad. J. comp. Med.*, **19**, 156.

Hinton, P. F. (1959) Isolation and characterization of an unusual organism in blood culture: *Vibrio fetus*, *Amer. J. med. Technol.*, **25**, 225.

Kahler, R. L., and Huntington, S. (1960) *Vibrio fetus* infection in man, *New Engl. J. Med.*, **262**, 1218.

King, E. O. (1957) Human infections with *Vibrio fetus* and a closely related vibrio, *J. infect. Dis.*, **101**, 119.

King, S., and Bronsky, D. (1961) *Vibrio fetus* isolated from a patient with localized septic arthritis, *J. Amer. med. Ass.*, **175**, 1045.

Mandel, A. D., and Ellison, R. C. (1963) Acute dysentery syndrome caused by *Vibrio fetus*. Report of a case, *J. Amer. med. Ass.*, **185**, 536.

Moynihan, I. W., and Stovell, P. L. (1955) Vibriosis in cattle, *Canad. J. comp. Med.*, **19**, 105.

Peckham, M. C. (1958) Avian vibrionic hepatitis, *Avian Dis.*, **2**, 348.

Zoonoses

Abdussalam, M. (1959) Significance of ecological studies of wild animal reservoirs of zoonoses, *Bull. Wld Hlth Org.*, **21**, 179.

Biester, H. E., and Schwarte, L. H. (1959) *Diseases of Poultry*, 4th ed., Ames, Iowa.

Bruner, D. W., and Gillespie, J. H. (1973) *Hagan's Infectious Diseases of Domestic Animals*, 6th ed., Ithaca.

Hubert, W. T., McCulloch, W. F., and Schurrenberger, P. R. (1974) *Diseases Transmitted from Aninals to Man*, 6th ed., Springfield, Ill.

Lapage, Geoffrey (1956) *Veterinary Parasitology*, Springfield, Ill.

Monath, J. P. (1974) Lassa fever and Marburg virus disease, *Wld Hlth Org. Chron.*, **28**, 212.

Pavlosky, E. N., Petrishcheva, P. A., Zasukhin, D. N., and Olsufiev, N. G., eds. (1955) *Natural Nidi of Human Diseases and Regional Epidemiology*, Leningrad.

Rivers, Thomas M., ed. (1959) *Viral and Rickettsial Infections of Man*, 3rd ed., Philadelphia.

Sanders, M., and Schaeffer, M. (1971) *Viruses Affecting Man and Animals*, St. Louis, Mo.

Schwabe, Calvin W. (1969) *Veterinary Medicine and Human Health*, 2nd ed., Baltimore.

Stableforth, A. W., and Galloway, I. A. (1959) *Infectious Diseases of Animals*, London.

WHO/FAO Joint Expert Committee on Zoonoses (1959) Second Report, *Wld Hlth Org. techn. Rep. Ser.*, No. 169.

WHO/FAO Joint Expert Committee on Zoonoses (1967) Third Report, *Wld Hlth Org. techn. Rep. Ser.*, No. 378.

World Health Organization Expert Committee on Meat Hygiene (1955) First Report, *Wld Hlth Org. techn. Rep. Ser.*, No. 99.

World Health Organization (1973) WHO/FAO programme on comparative virology. (Describes a wide range of animal reference centres for viruses of sera for laboratory use), *Wld Hlth Org. Chron.*, **27**, 10.

World Health Organization (1974*a*) Veterinary public health: a review of the WHO programme; 1 and 2, *Wld Hlth Org. Chron.*, **28**, 103, 178.

World Health Organization (1974*b*) Annual Report of WHO for 1973, *Wld Hlth Org. Off. Rec.*, **213**, 26–31.

23
THE EPIDEMIOLOGY AND CONTROL OF RABIES

J. H. STEELE

EPIDEMIOLOGY

Early Concepts

The epidemiology of rabies has been under review for more than 2,000 years. Rabies was probably known by the ancient civilizations of the Nile, Euphrates, and Hindus river valleys, and they attributed its cause to meteorological conditions, mythological punishment, or ingestion of forbidden substances. The concept of contagion developed from all these causes, which were a consequence of the violation of certain religious or spiritual taboos. The association of bite-wounds and rabies was no doubt known before Hippocrates called attention to the spread of rabies by mad dogs who destroy themselves as well as all they encounter. Aristotle also knew that mad dogs could infect all creatures they bit except man. Why he excluded man is difficult to understand. Pliny, the Roman historian, recognized rabies as a contagious disease of dogs, which was transmitted to man. The innumerable cures cited by Pliny indicate that the disease must have been quite common in the Roman empire.

The *Hippiatrika*, a collection of veterinary writings of Byzantine veterinarians of the ninth and tenth centuries, discusses the disease in detail. Most surprising is the thought that the disease was curable. Among the cures was the excision of the lyssa, the septum linguae at the ventral tip of the tongue. This was also considered a preventive measure (Smithcor, 1957).

That the fable of the 'worm' under the tongue, abetted by Pliny and later 'science' writers, remained more than a myth for a thousand years is attested to by veterinarians of the nineteenth century who described the operation, because sportsmen and hunters demanded the service. Blaine, the author of canine pathology (1817) stated that many educated sportsmen believed that removing the worm under the tongue was essential in the prevention of acute rabies, and that in wormed animals only dumb rabies would occur.

As late as 1874, Fleming, in his work on rabies, stated that the practice was still common, although Blaine had pointed out more than fifty years earlier that surgical cutting of the lyssa was of no value whatever, and might do harm by interfering with the normal movement of the tongue.

That there was both furious and dumb rabies was probably known to medieval physicians and veterinarians; among the first to attempt to differentiate the types was Tuberville (1576). His descriptions of the signs, including the strained howling, are quite interesting, and he stated that the disease killed the animal in 3 or 4 days. He further stated that the disease might last nine months. It is thought that he meant the incubation period, inasmuch as he stated that the animals lived only 3 or 4 days with furious signs and symptoms.

Rabies was known among other domestic animals from the time of Aristotle. The earliest recognition of rabies in wild animals probably occurred at about the same time, although the Roman agriculturists were the first to mention the disease in their essays. Throughout the Middle Ages there are many references to rabid wild animals which destroyed farm animals and invaded cities, but the dog continues to be the source of the disease in so far as one can gather from historical writings.

The earliest appearance of rabies in the Americas was in the eighteenth century when cases were described in both dogs and foxes in the English Colonies. An earlier report, attributed to a priest, states that rabies may have invaded Mexico in the early part of the eighteenth century. The spread of rabies across North America has been reported by explorers, trappers, soldiers, pioneers, scientists, and historians. Reports of the disease in South America were largely confined to the urban areas and sea-ports until the early twentieth century, when bat rabies was first seen in the interior of southern Brazil.

The last hundred years have seen an epizootic explosion of rabies throughout the Americas, with many animal species affected. In the far north, wolves, foxes, and dogs were reported as diseased. In the temperate zones coyotes, foxes, wolves, skunks, and dogs were involved. In tropical America the disease was found mainly in dogs, until the discovery of rabies in bats in the first half of the twentieth century.

Rabies was confirmed as a bite-wound disease by the isolation of the virus from the saliva of diseased animals in the late nineteenth century. This concept was to stand until the mid-twentieth century, when questions were asked about the cycle of rabies virus in nature. Studies of vampire bat rabies raised many questions as to its survival which have not been resolved to this day. It is thought that the disease is transmitted by bite-wounds among the vampire bats, but this is open to question since reports have occurred of non-bite routes of infection among insectivorous bats in the south-western United States. Moreover, the survival of rabies virus in bats and other animals must be reviewed to clarify the possibility of carriers, chronic disease, and latency of disease.

Present-day problems of epidemiology cover a vast biological spectrum that includes many species of mammals—both terrestrial and arboreal—and some arthropods. What the role of various animal hosts may be in maintaining rabies in different geographical areas is a question that is pertinent to any proposed control campaign. If one looks at the Americas, the epidemiological patterns differ between the Arctic tundra, the transitional temperate zones, the deserts, and the tropical areas.

Arctic Disease

The Arctic has an unusual rabies problem of long standing, which was called Arctic dog disease for many decades until

Plummer identified the disease as rabies in 1947 (Plummer, 1947a and b). Since then rabies has been recognized in all of the land and ice-bound areas within the Arctic Circle in both the Eastern and Western Hemispheres. Russian investigators described a disease in foxes which they called 'rabidity', or rabid-like. Other disease names include Arctic nervous disease, polar madness, winter fits, and northern disease. Since Plummer established his observations in 1947, additional reports have revealed that rabies was widespread in Alaska and reached epizootic proportions among wolves, foxes, and dogs in 1945, and continued for a decade (Williams, 1949).

Rausch (1958) has studied the disease in Alaskan wild canidae and believes the disease has been present for many decades, and that the reservoir exists among the Arctic foxes, (*Alopex logopus*), and occasionally is transmitted to wolves, coyotes, and sled dogs by biting animals. The low incidence of human disease is attributed to the heavy protective clothing worn by the Eskimo, although occasional cases have been reported when individuals were bitten on the hands or face.

Russian investigators who studied Arctic fox disease have described the condition as rabies (Kantorovic, 1957; Kantorovic, Konovalov, Buzinov, and Riutova, 1963). Their conclusions are similar to those of other observers, that the disease maintains itself in the Arctic fox (Kantorovic, 1964), and is transmitted to other animals, including polar bears, when the fox is rabid and attacks everything it may encounter. The possibility of the ermine (*Mustela erminae*) or weasel (*Mustela* spp.) as a reservoir has been speculated upon by some scientists, but no evidence has been found to support this hypothesis (Johnson, 1959).

Probably the largest epizootic of rabies in the Arctic is that reported by Danish veterinarians during the last decade (Wamberg, 1960) in western Greenland where more than 1,000 dogs died. The disease was not seen on the coast until 1963 when it appeared in sled dogs. The disease in these dogs was not only a public health threat, but created economic havoc in some districts where more than half the dogs died. The disease is thought to have been present in Greenland for more than a hundred years, but was not proven until 1959 when the first dog and fox tissues were sent to the Communicable Disease Center at Atlanta, Georgia (C.D.C.), and reported to be rabies-positive (Jenkins and Wamberg, 1970). The first proven human case occurred in 1960 in a 4-year old Greenland child (Lassen, 1962).

American and Danish investigators who studied the disease in northern Greenland found that one-third of the dogs or foxes examined yielded rabies virus. The infection rate in foxes was twice that of dogs. Crandall (1966) points out in his study that Negri bodies were seldom present in the material examined. He found that the fluorescent antibody technique and mouse inoculation method for diagnosis were the only acceptable testing procedures. These were equally sensitive. Rausch and Kantorovic, in their original reports, observed that inclusion bodies were rarely found in Arctic animals, although Kantorovic reported in 1964 that cytoplasmic inclusion bodies typical of Negri bodies were found in Arctic foxes for the first time. Crandall is also of the opinion that the Arctic rabies virus is different from the bat and street strains which he compared it with.

The furious disease observed in dogs in the far north was similar to that seen elsewhere, although the incubation period was short, ranging from 4 to 14 days, which may account for the absence of Negri bodies. This short incubation is of special interest inasmuch as others in the Arctic report incubation periods varying from 4 to 5 days to 2 or 3 weeks. Many heads from dogs that died with typical signs of rabies failed to yield rabies virus when examined. Crandall examined thirty heads of sick animals and only sixteen were positive for rabies. The same was true for the foxes examined for rabies; animals with clinical signs of disease did not have virus or Negri bodies in their brains. The possibility that another disease was active in northern Greenland was investigated and the investigators found that the antibodies of canine hepatitis were widespread, whereas canine distemper antibodies were absent. Their conclusion is that canine hepatitis may have been the cause of 'madness' in some dogs. This is difficult to believe unless the encephalitic form of canine hepatitis is common to the Arctic. The authors state that the absence of human disease in persons severely bitten may be explained by canine hepatitis encephalitis. These findings point out the necessity of differential diagnosis when rabies is not confirmed. Similar situations have been reported in other countries where epizootics of distemper, hepatitis and pseudo-rabies (Aujesky's disease) among dogs, and viral encephalitis of cats, squirrels, and other animals have caused serious errors, and confusion. Listeriosis in the fox can also cause encephalitis signs simulating rabies.

The seasonal distribution of rabies appears to be similar to that in the temperature zones, with the highest incidence in late winter and early spring when animals are moving. Density of population and migration also contribute to sudden outbreaks that lead to epizootics.

Crandall concluded that the Arctic fox was probably the reservoir of rabies in Greenland as in Russia, Canada, and Alaska. He supports his premise with the finding of rabies virus in healthy foxes by Kantorovic and, in one instance, by himself. Kantorovic reported in 1964 that he was able to recover virus frequently from apparently healthy Arctic foxes. The percentage of isolations ranged from as high as 75 per cent. during epizootics to a low of 3 per cent. during inter-epizootic periods. The definition of these animals, as to whether they are carriers or are in an incubation period, is important to an epidemiological understanding of the disease. During these studies of the natural foci of rabies in the far north of Russia, Kantorovic examined thousands of murine rodents and fifteen ermines and found no evidence of rabies virus. He concluded that the Arctic fox was the main, if not the only reservoir of rabies in the far north. From the evidence at hand, it appears that the Arctic fox occupies this role in the entire circumpolar area.

The absence of rabies from the Scandinavian peninsula and most of Finland is explained only by the isolation of Norway and Sweden from the Arctic by open water (the Gulf Stream) most of the year. Rabies has been absent from these countries for more than 100 years. Recent studies of sylvatic fur-bearing animals have not revealed any evidence that rabies is present or latent.

Temperate Zone Disease

Rabies in the temperate zones of the Americas has been under observation for at least 200 years or more. The multiple reservoirs, in nature, separate the disease epidemiologically from the Arctic disease. The dog was the principal source of disease for many years but with the successful practice of canine vaccination the dog has declined in importance, and the fox and skunk have become the main source of disease, although it remains to be determined if they are the reservoir. Whether the insectivorous bat is important in maintaining the disease in the North American temperate zone is not clear (Johnson, 1959).

Canada is possibly the only place in the world where the epidemic pattern of the Arctic disease has influenced the pattern in the temperate zones (Moynihan, 1966). Shortly after the confirmation of rabies in the Canadian Arctic, the disease was seen in wildlife in areas to the south and east. Within a few years rabies reached epizootic proportions in Alberta (1952), Ontario (1957), and Quebec and the Maritime Provinces (1964). The disease has been identified in a wide variety of wildlife and domestic animals. Approximately 65 per cent. of reported diagnosed cases are among wildlife, 25 per cent. in domestic food animals and 10 per cent. in dogs. The latter are nearly all attributed to wildlife exposure. Dog rabies is seldom transmitted from dog to dog, but rather from wild animal to dog. The disease in farm animals is likewise always attributed to rabid wild animals, mainly foxes and skunks. Bat rabies has been found in Canada since 1954, and in no instance has been the cause of disease in terrestrial animals, including man. In British Columbia, bat rabies has been identified repeatedly for more than a decade, but no disease has appeared in other animals. It appears that the fox and skunk occupy the all-important niche: reservoir of rabies. Fox rabies is not new in Canada, having been recognized since the eighteenth century; however, skunk rabies is thought to be a new entity, as it appeared only in the present century.

The United States has a very complex epidemiological pattern of disease. The entire country has the problem of sylvatic rabies which varies according to the indigenous population, and is overlain by the bat disease. Urban dogs rabies that has plagued the country for most of the twentieth century is no longer a problem except along the Mexican border. The epidemiological pattern can be said to be much like that of Canada except for the variation in species affected. In the north-east and eastern states fox rabies is the main problem. Likewise, in the south and eastern central states the red and grey fox (*Vulpes fulva* and *Urocyon cinereoargentens*) are the important sources of disease, along with skunks as one goes further west. Attempts have been made by the C.D.C. to determine if the fox is a reservoir, along the lines pursued by Kantorovic, by examining fox in epizootic and pre-epizootic periods to measure virus activity. These studies have shown that the rabies virus increased in amount and virulence until the epizootic crested; thereafter, the concentration would drop sharply, which would be correlated with the short incubation period (Kissling *et al.*, 1955).

A recent observation by Dr. Sikes at the C.D.C. Rabies Laboratory may shed some light on the role of the fox in maintaining rabies virus in nature. He reported on a fox in a challenge study, which developed rabies after challenge when confined for 13 months in a cage. The vaccine used was an inactivated Semple type, which could hardly be considered as a possible cause of disease; hence, the only conclusion is that the diseased animal was exposed before it was captured and confined to the laboratory. If this is so, the fox must be considered as an important reservoir which is activated by time or stress. To set up an experiment to test the hypothesis of long incubation periods in fox is difficult but not impossible. (Hence, it is important that similar findings should be reported by other investigators.) The validity of long incubation periods explaining the inter-epizootic latency of virus should be an important consideration in building an epidemiological hypothesis that explains the natural history of rabies.

Another important observation on rabies in the fox concerns the studies reported by Sikes on the levels of rabies virus necessary to produce disease, and the titres of virus shed by infected animals. The fox is extremely sensitive to rabies when challenged with viruses isolated from salivary glands, or when exposed to aerosol infection in bat caves. Sikes (1962) has presented these data in an earlier report.

An interesting phenomenon reported by Sikes was the relation between the size of the inoculum and the amount of virus recovered in the saliva. Foxes with large inoculum (10^3 mouse LD_{50}) of virus had short incubation periods—less than 18 days, which was usually too short a period for the virus to build up in the salivary gland. Smaller inoculums resulted in longer incubations period—usually 38 days or more, which resulted in almost all the foxes shedding virus in their saliva—some of which titred 10^3 or greater, enough to infect skunks which require a hundred-fold more virus to develop disease. These data support the concept that small doses of viruses are important in keeping rabies alive. This is not only true of rabies but also of many other diseases, otherwise the pathogens would have all died out long ago.

The sharp rise of skunk rabies in some states such as Texas and Tennessee may be explained by the spill-over from foxes to skunks, although there are many areas where skunk rabies appears to have exploded independently of any fox population, i.e. California, Dakota, Minnesota, and Iowa. The skunk is an efficient disseminator of rabies as demonstrated by Sikes, yielding a hundred- to a thousand-fold more virus in their saliva than the fox. The enormous increase of skunks in the Americas has added to the size of the rabies virus reservoir. Conservation authorities, ecologists, and demographers all believe that the skunk and fox as well as many other animals, may be at an all-time modern high. With millions of skunks across the continent, a 1 per cent. infection rate results in a big reservoir, and for the areas where epizootics occur, the number of diseased animals may run into the tens of thousands. Hence, the understanding of their epidemiological niche is most pertinent to the control of the disease.

Johnson (1966) has observed one virus strain from spotted skunks that is unusual in that it ordinarily produces an asymptomatic infection in adult mice inoculated intercerebrally and in those inoculated intermuscularly. Infant mice infected by intercerebral inoculation usually die on day 16 or 17, but some died on day 29. One infant mouse inoculated intercerebrally with original salivary gland virus recovered after having been paralyzed from day 16 to 22. When killed on day 32 F.R.A. test revealed rabies virus.

Johnson (1966) believes that the spotted skunk (*Spilogale putorius*) is probably the true reservoir of rabies in the West, and that this animal should be studied both in laboratory and in nature to determine its role. This is the same animal found on the Great Plains during the last century, which was the cause of much suffering among man and animals. It was recognized as a disseminator of rabies and for that reason was called the 'hydrophobia' cat or 'phobia' cat.

In California, both striped (*Mephitis mephitis*) and spotted (*Spilogale putorius*) skunks are present in equal numbers, but the isolations from striped skunks have exceeded 1,500 during recent years, while only ten were from spotted skunks. Virus isolated from the spotted skunk is different from other isolates in that it has a prolonged incubation period in mice, and the inclusion bodies are different from those seen with other rabies viruses. Subsequent efforts to find other rabies viruses in spotted skunks have yielded only two agents, both unusual in that the virus in the submaxillary salivary gland has a titre of 10–7 when tested in infant mice. Viruses isolated from striped skunks are also different in that only about 60 per cent. produce Negri bodies, while the remaining 40 per cent. were formerly missed as they did *not* produce recognizable inclusion bodies, *nor* did they produce disease in adult mice. The fluorescent antibody test and infant mice inoculation have made it possible to recognize natural strains of low virulence, which may be the reservoir strains that keep the disease alive.

Rabies virus has been isolated from many organs of naturally infected skunks. These include the brain, salivary glands, lungs, pancreas, mammary glands, kidneys, and muscle tissue. The scent gland, spleen, liver, lymph nodes, and intestinal contents, when examined, have not yielded virus to date.

The rabies virus appears to be a Stomatoviridae and the tropism of the virus for respiratory tissues should be expected. Now that the virus has been isolated from lung tissue, this route of infection and excretion must be considered in skunks, foxes, and may be other terrestrial animals as well as bats.

The appearance of bat rabies in the United States is recent. In 1954 the disease was reported in three widely separated states—Florida (Vetners, Hoffert, Scatterday, and Hardy, 1954), Pennsylvania (Witte, 1954), and Texas (Sullivan *et al.*, 1954). Within ten years it had been found in most states, and by 1970 in all the 48 continental states. Bat rabies has not been found in Hawaii, where there is no rabies, nor in Alaska, where bats are rare or unknown.

The discovery of rabies transmission by a non-bite route (Constantine, 1962) is one of the most unusual biological events of recent times. That this experiment can be repeated year after year with highly susceptible animals such as foxes and coyotes during July, when the newborn bats are present in great numbers and put the dams under great stress, is even more unusual. There is considerable evidence that the bats become infected as infants, and most survive the infection. A few develop disease and they are the ones found in late summer and early autumn, paralysed or near death. Those that survive either shed the virus or store it in brown fat (subscapular area) where it remains through the winter. In the spring, when the foetus begins to develop from the previously fertilized ova, stress is added day by day until parturition. It is thought that some animals break down during pregnancy and become rabid. Probably the greatest stress comes with lactation, which results in numerous latent infections, becoming active rabies cases, and these subsequently shed rabies virus. How the virus is secreted is not known, but there may be more than one route.

The urine may be one vehicle inasmuch as fluorescent particles are thought to have been seen in the ureters.

The saliva is known to carry virus and virus has been isolated from upper respiratory tissues. It may be that the virus is shed by the salivary glands and some finds its way to the lungs, while some is shed externally. No one has observed any unusual biting or fighting among colonial or cave bats; hence, this rules out such transmission. Bat milk and mammary glands have been examined for rabies virus by F.R.A. tests, and no evidence of virus has been found. Recently, C.D.C. scientists have recovered the virus from cave air in the south-west United States where millions of newborn bats were developing. After the bats left the cave, no virus could be found as in previous years when sentinel animals were used. The virus is only present in the cave air during July when the young are putting the dams to great stress.

The epidemiology of the colonial bat rabies is unknown. How the free-living bats maintain the virus and transmit it among themselves is *not* known, nor do we have any knowledge if they harbour the virus through the winter. The story of vampire bats transmitting among themselves is also incomplete unless we are to accept the biting and fighting explanation set forth more than sixty years ago by Carini (1911).

The role of insectivorous bats in the maintenance of rabies in any given geographical areas does not seem to be of any significance. The Canadian experience since 1954 is noteworthy. No disease has occurred in terrestrial animals since bat rabies appeared in western Canada. The same situation has been observed in the north-western United States, where bat rabies has been identified in Montana, Idaho, Washington, and Oregon, but no enzootic foci have been established in wildlife or domestic Canidae. The same observations have been noted in other sections of the country, in both rural and urban areas. If the native bats of Canada and the United States were a reservoir of virus for wildlife or domestic farm animals and pets, the evidence would have been forthcoming by now.

The question of rodents as a source of rabies is frequently raised. A survey by Winkler (1966), of the National Communicable Disease Center, revealed that rodents were identified as rabid in less than 0·5 per cent. of the animal tissues examined between 1956–65, and since 1961 the positive findings have dropped more than 43 per cent. [TABLE 57].

TABLE 57

Rabies in Rodents and Other Species, United States,
1956–1965

Years	Rodents	Total Animals	Per cent. Rodents
1956–1960	128	22,972	0·56
1961–1965	71	20,490	0·34
Total	199	43,462	

(Note: In the two periods shown, there is a 10 per cent. decrease in total rabies and a 43 per cent. decrease in rodent rabies in the second half of the decade.)

There has not been a single case of human rabies attributed to a rodent attack for more than twenty years. Experimental observations indicate that most rodents are not particularly susceptible to rabies infection, and even when they are infected, the virus does not usually invade the salivary glands. Hence, the role of rodents, including squirrels, seems to be of no consequence in the epidemiology of the disease.

Recent Spread of Rabies in Europe. Since 1964, rabies has spread into at least six Central European countries: Denmark, Czechoslovakia, Belgium, Luxembourg, Switzerland, and France. Each of these countries had been free from rabies for many years until recently. The disease has apparently spread in concentric circles, emanating from Germany and the area of the former Polish corridor where the disease has been endemic in foxes for many years. According to Steck (1968), the disease spread at the rate of 40 km. per year. This comparatively slow rate is due to the fact that foxes rarely migrate over long distances.

In 1964, rabies was introduced into southern Jutland, Denmark, apparently spreading from the German border. Following an intense fox population reduction programme, in which fox dens were gassed throughout the infected area, the disease was brought under control for approximately two years. It reappeared during 1967 and remains in foxes primarily, although it has also been transmitted to martens, cats, cattle, and deer on several occasions.

In 1965, the disease spread to Austria where it was recognized in foxes in areas adjacent to the German border. Rabies spread into Belgium and Luxembourg in 1966, into Switzerland in 1967, and France in 1968. In each of these countries foxes remain as the primary reservoir of rabies, but they have also transmitted the disease to other species of animals in each of these countries. TABLE 58 presents the incidence of rabies by species for each country for 1968–1969.

TABLE 58
Animal Species Confirmed as Rabid

Central European Countries	Dogs Cats	Foxes	Farm Animals	Deer	Other	Total
Austria . .	15	208	10	28	32	293
Belgium . .	19	509	10	28	167	733
Czechoslovakia .	99	745	18	19	34	915
Denmark . .	4	61	10	2	0	77
France . .	32	226	138	6	6	408
Germany, Fed. Rep. . .	814	5,697	814	618	397	8,340
Poland . .	299	432	73	10	67	881

Apparently the disease has become enzootic in each of these countries as much as it has in wildlife of other developed countries such as the United States and Canada. Intensive selective population reduction programmes of wild animals for short periods of time will probably be used for the control of wildlife rabies in Europe just as they have in the United States.

Telemetry is now being used to track the movements of wild foxes (World Health Organization, 1974).

Tropical Area Disease

Epidemiological concepts of rabies in the tropical and subtropical areas of the Americas have not changed in the past decade. It should be pointed out that urban rabies is a major health problem in most large cities of Latin America. Until these urban epizootics are controlled there is little opportunity to study the epidemic patterns in these regions. The dog has

the same role in urban Latin America as it had in North America twenty-five years ago. Other pet animals, including cats, are also a source of virus in these countries. Sylvatic rabies exists, but little is known about its incidence, distribution, virus characterization, and reservoirs. The vampire bat, as stated earlier, is a reservoir of disease for domestic farm animals, and may be for other animals. The importance of vampire bats (*Desmodus rotundus*)[1] as a source of disease for domestic farm animals cannot be emphasized too strongly. The F.A.O. 1966 survey stated that possibly one million cattle die of vampire bat rabies annually in Latin America between northern Mexico and northern Argentina.

The history of vampire bat rabies in the Americas goes back to 1908 when a paralytic disease of cattle, *mal de caderas*, appeared in epizootic form in southern Brazil. Some of the infected cattle were found to have rabies virus in their brains, but the source of the infection was not known. Later, it was revealed that the ranchers had noted that bats were flying around during the day and fighting one another, and that cattle bitten by these bats often developed the paralytic disease, and died. It was not until 1916 that rabies virus was isolated from a bat caught biting animals during the day. Subsequently, cattle epidemics occurred throughout Brazil and the vampire bat was incriminated as the source of rabies virus. Later, it was discovered that the vampire bat (*Desmodus rotundus*) could transmit the virus for many months as a symptomless carrier. The disease was not known outside mainland South America until 1925 when the virus was found in vampire bats in Trinidad. The Trinidad epizootic is presumed to have spread from mainland South America where the disease was active. The vampire bat disease was confirmed in North America when it was found in Mexico, State of Michoacan, on a ranch where the cattle were dying of *derriengue* or littoral fever, a paralytic disease known in western Mexico since 1910. Rabies virus was isolated from one of the diseased cattle, and thus it was proven that *derriengue* was paralytic rabies transmitted by the vampire bat (Johnson, 1948), in 1945, although the disease had been known for many years.

Since the disease was discovered, it has appeared in all of the countries of Central and South America except Chile and Peru. The vampire bat, except for the hairy legged vampire bat, *Diphylla ecaudata*, has never been seen in the United States, Canada, or the West Indies apart from Trinidad, which is close to mainland South America. The vampire bat is found in Peru and Chile but does not have rabies. An important epizootiological feature of the disease is that the early infections seen in bats thirty to fifty years ago in many of the bats seen were quite vicious, and this suggests that it was the first experience of vampire bats with the disease. Subsequently, the disease has been less vicious in the bats but continues to be deadly to cattle. The infection in vampire bats does not seem to depend on irrational behaviour in order to perpetuate itself, and is now living in balance with its host. How it spreads among vampires remains an unanswered question if viciousness is no longer a common characteristic.

Aside from the vampire bat in the American tropics, there are no important indigenous animals which are reservoirs or disseminators of rabies. The monogose (*Herpestes nyula*) was

---

[1] Other less commonly infected vampire bats are *Diaemus youngi*, and *Diphylla ecaudata*.

introduced into the West Indies in the middle of the nineteenth century by sugar cane planters to destroy snakes and rats. The mongoose has been quite successful in eliminating snakes, as in Puerto Rico, but the rats avoid them except when they are competitive hunters. The mongoose much prefers eggs, poultry, lizards, toads, insects, and fish to rodents, which are taken only of necessity. The story of mongoose rabies in the Americas centres in the West Indies, where it is present in Puerto Rico (Acha, 1967), Cuba, Grenada, and the Dominican Republic. There is no evidence that the mongoose has established itself on the mainlands of the Americas.

The earliest knowledge of rabies in the mongoose came from Eastern Cuba, where it was recognized in the early part of the twentieth century. The discovery of mongoose rabies in Puerto Rico did not occur until the 1950s when Tierkel, Arbona, Rivera, and de Juan (1952) proved that the mongoose was quite susceptible to infection and was a vicious aggressive animal when diseased. Toro (1966) described the normal mongoose as a diurnal hunter who avoids man's habitation and migrates to new hunting areas periodically. It prefers the marginal transitional areas adjacent to agriculturally developed lands. The rabid mongoose has encephalitis, like other terrestrial animals, with the usual changes in behaviour. The rabid animal loses its fear of man and domestic animals, and will seek food and water in the farm yard, or even in urban communities. Sometimes they act 'cute', sitting on their haunches like squirrels. Usually, children are the first to notice the friendly mongoose and, when they approach the animal, they are attacked. Rabid mongooses have been found in homes, barns, warehouses, automobiles, farm machinery, privies, and garden shrubbery; places which they normally avoid. When a rabid mongoose attacks, it bites deeply and does not release the person or animal until it is killed or stunned. Cattle, when they are attacked in the field, are usually bitten on the muzzle or face. The dog that fights with a rabid mongoose usually has face wounds.

The relatively recent appearance of rabies in the mongoose in Puerto Rico and other islands of the West Indies is difficult to understand. Rabies had been present, possibly as early as 1841, according to measures taken to control rabid dogs. The disease was occasionally diagnosed prior to 1934. From 1934 until 1950 the disease was unknown in Puerto Rico, but since that date it has been identified in many species. Why the disease did not become established in mongooses during the enzootic period previous to 1934 is not answerable. Likewise, why mongoose rabies in Cuba has remained in the eastern provinces and has not spread to the western portion of the island has not been explained. The recent epizootic in Grenada is another epidemiological enigma. The Puerto Rico report is only conclusive data that the mongoose is a reservoir host of rabies in the Americas. It should be pointed out that in South Africa and Rhodesia the yellow mongoose is thought to be a reservoir host of rabies (Tierkel, 1959).

There may be other animal reservoirs in tropical America, but there is little or no information about them.

In summing up the epidemiology of rabies in the Americas, there are a number of observations to be considered in developing control programmes:

1. The dog remains the most important vector of disease in urban communities and still accounts for more cases of human disease than any other animal. In rural areas the dog is also an important disseminator of disease except for the United States and Canada.

2. The fox may be the basic reservoir of rabies along with the skunk in certain areas where both animals are indigenous. The long incubation periods and the cyclic changes in virulence of the virus may explain the periodic epizootics between which the virus remains dormant for some generations to regain virulence. The density of population of sylvatic hosts no doubt has an important bearing on the length of the epizootic and inter-epizootic periods. It appears that the relationship may be direct and casual, but more evidence is needed.

3. The skunk of the United States certainly has an important role in maintaining the disease in nature. The data which has been collected in recent years on the variation of virus virulence in these animals is very interesting, and should be studied further in the field and laboratory, in both North and South America.

4. The insect-eating bats of the United States and Canada, as well as other American countries cannot be considered as a basic reservoir of rabies on the evidence gathered to date, but are a cause of disease in man and animals and they will continue to transmit infections; hence, they are important from a health aspect.

5. The vampire bats of tropical America are an important, if not the most important, reservoir of rabies in the Americas. It has been estimated that nearly a million cattle die annually of rabies transmitted by vampire bats in Latin America (Acha, 1966). This disease must be considered among the most serious animal health problems facing Latin America today. The direct economic loss exceeds $100,000,000 annually, and indirect losses including malnutrition approach a quarter of a billion dollars. The disease appears to be increasing. The growing cattle industry provides more hosts for the vampire to feed upon and thus supports larger populations of vampires. The number of people that die from vampire bat bites is unknown, but when one recalls the Trinidad epidemic of the 1920–30s, the public health aspects cannot be forgotten.

Apparently the tropical fruit-eating bats are rarely infected, and do not play a role in the epidemiology of rabies.

6. The mongoose is certainly a reservoir in parts of the West Indies, especially Puerto Rico, and must be treated as such in control programmes. As to other terrestrial animals, including rodents, there is no reason to believe that they are a part of the epizootic or epidemic cycle as we know it today.

CONTROL

Control programmes must be built on epidemiological findings. This has been self-evident in most successful campaigns, and has proved the reason for failure in epidemics in which the pattern was not known. Control efforts must be tailored to the animal and human populations at risk, the socio–economic and cultural structure, the virus characteristics, known reservoirs, and health education of the community; and, most importantly, the availability of safe potent rabies vaccine for both man and animals at a reasonable price.

Vaccines

Investigations as to the possibility of vaccinating dogs against rabies began about a hundred years ago at the Lyons Veterinary College under the guidance of Balard. Pasteur studied with him for a short time before going to Paris. Pasteur was the first to demonstrate that dogs could be successfully immunized against rabies (Pasteur, Chamberland, and Roux, 1884). Pasteur's vaccine was made from spinal cord virus which has been modified or fixed by serial passage in the brains of rabbits, and further attenuated by desiccation at room temperature over potassium hydroxide. Dogs were made resistant to rabies by ten daily subcutaneous injections of the attenuated virus which had been graded as to its virulence by tests in rabbits inoculated intercerebrally. Unfortunately, this procedure was cumbersome, expensive and time-consuming because the dog had to be brought to the laboratory for daily injections, but from these early trials the first successful human vaccine evolved. It was not until Semple (1911) modified Fermi's (1909) phenolized vaccine, that any further thought was given to canine anti-rabies vaccination. The first extensive field trial was carried out in Japan in 1918–20 by Umeno (Umeno and Doi, 1921). During a rabies epizootic in Tokyo, thousands of dogs were vaccinated with a single injection of vaccine made from the brains and cords of rabbits dead of fixed virus disease and inactivated with 1·25 per cent. phenol. They immunized 255,000 dogs during the study, of which 175 (0·08 per cent.) later died of rabies. During the same period, 2,860 non-immunized dogs were diagnosed as being rabid. These observations led to the introduction of phenol-inactivated rabies vaccine for dogs in the United States in 1922 (Eichhorn and Lyon, 1923). Commercial vaccines were in production and rather widely used during the late 1920s. Many communities undertook mass immunization programmes, some of which were successful while others failed. It soon became apparent that the results were inconsistent, and left much to be desired.

As early as 1930 it was suspected that the vaccines were lacking in antigenicity, but this was not proven until Webster (1939) demonstrated in laboratory mice that most of the commercial rabies vaccines used for dogs, as well as those prepared for human use, lacked antigenicity. This came as a shock to the veterinary profession and public health officials, but focused attention on the problem. Habel (1940a) confirmed Webster's findings and developed an assessment test to determine the potency of the vaccine. This is the well-known Habel test. The test involves the use of 48 white mice for each lot of vaccine examined; 30 mice are given six doses of vaccine (0·25 ml/0·5 per cent. brain emulsion) interperitoneally every two days. Fourteen days after the first injection, the mice are divided into small groups of six each, five vaccinated groups and three unvaccinated. Both vaccinated and controls are then challenged with different dilutions of fixed virus. The LD_{50} dose of the virus is that which kills three out of six unvaccinated control mice, and is called the M.L.D. of the virus. The immunity end-point of the vaccinated mice is determined by the largest dose of virus that three out of six mice resist. The protective value is calculated by the ratio between the LD_{50} (M.L.D.) for the vaccinated and control mice. Experimentally, vaccines can be produced that protect against as much as 50,000 M.L.D., but this is difficult to do commercially, although many vaccines are produced with a protective range of 5,000 to 25,000 M.L.D. For the past twenty years all commercial dog inactivated rabies vaccine must protect against at least 1,000 M.L.D.

It is apparent from Habel's studies that many of the strains used for vaccine production were impotent (1940b). Many of these strains were traced to the old Pasteur fixed virus. Further, it was apparent that the strains had changed in the course of propagation, with the use of different animals and methods, and they were no longer useful in vaccine production. Today, government control agencies require that all manufacturers use only potent virus strains in the production of vaccine and that each lot of vaccine be tested for antigenicity.

The handling of vaccine, be it inactivated or live, naturally affects its value. The route of injection is also important: the subcutaneous method has been used widely but it is apparent that intermuscular inoculation results in better protection (Tierkel, Kissling, Eidson, and Habel, 1953) of longer duration.

Attempts to develop other inactivated nervous tissue rabies vaccine using chloroform, ether, or ultra-violet light inactivation were successful experimentally, but failed commercially. Kelser (1928) developed an effective chloroform inactivated vaccine in the late 1920s that proved effective in the Philippines, where it was produced under his supervision, but could not be successfully produced commercially. Later, it was revealed that the conglomerates of nervous tissue insulated and prevented the chloroform from reaching the virus, so it was not attenuated. Ether vaccines failed for the same reason. Today, this could probably be prevented by effective homogenizers, and mechanical agitators. Ultra-violet light successfully inactivates nervous tissue fixed rabies virus, but irradiated vaccines, though proved immunogenic, have had little use in the vaccination of dogs or other animals including man. The principal drawback is that the immunity is often short-lived, so that annual animal revaccination is imperative. Furthermore, the nervous tissue vaccines have sometimes caused post-vaccinal paralysis (Burkhart, Jervis, and Koprowski, 1950). The rate of such accidents may be as high as 1 per 1,000 with phenol-treated nervous tissue vaccines, and higher with ultra-violet-treated nervous tissue.

The advent of the live rabies vaccine began with the adaptation of the Flury strain of rabies virus to day-old chickens and later to the chicken embryo. Johnson isolated the Flury strain from a young girl who died of rabies following an unusual exposure in which there was no evidence of a bite, but a history of the licking of mucous membranes (Johnson, 1965). The virus was passed intercerebrally through 136 transfers of day-old chicks. Later, Koprowski and Cox (1948) propagated the Flury strain virus in chicken embryos. Virus from the 40–50 chicken embryo passage was designated L.E.P. (low egg passage), and found to be avirulent for dogs when injected parenterally. Further experiments with dogs showed that they developed good immunity of long duration (Koprowski and Black, 1950). The successful three-year study of the duration of immunity proved that the live vaccine protected longer than the inactivated vaccines (Tierkel, Kissling, Eidson, and Habel, 1953).

The live L.E.P. canine rabies vaccine has performed admirably since the completion of the C.D.C. study in 1953.

Numerous demonstrations in the United States and abroad have confirmed its safety and efficacy. It has continued to be used in routine veterinary practice and public health organized vaccination campaigns. But, as with all vaccines, there were problems. For example, it was shown that puppies less than 11 weeks of age do not respond as well as older animals (Kaeberle, 1958) and that it may cause encephalitis in puppies under 3 weeks of age. Today, L.E.P. vaccine is not recommended for animals under 3 months of age.

Probably a bigger problem was the shelf-life of live vaccines. Dean and his colleagues (Dean, Evans, and Thompson, 1964) found that many L.E.P. vaccines collected from veterinarians and supply centres were not as potent as when the vaccine was tested at the time of production. The problem was found to be due to poor stabilizers, which are intended to maintain the viability of the vaccine (Peacock, 1966). The importance of stabilizers in protecting the potency of vaccine cannot be stressed too strongly—this will also be true of newly developed tissue culture vaccines.

With the improved L.E.P. vaccines, freed of extraneous tissue debris, it was found that smaller doses of vaccine afforded the same protection as the larger doses of the old 33 per cent. suspensions of infected chicken embryo tissues. The suspension of infected chicken embryo was reduced to 20 per cent. by light centrifugation. These vaccines continued to pass potency tests. Experiments in dogs showed that a 2-ml. dose of the 20 per cent. vaccine was effective. Today this is the standard dose for L.E.P. vaccines.

Dean, Evans, and Thompson (1964) found titres of 33 per cent. vaccine to range from 80,000 mouse LD_{50} (104·85) to 2,000,000 mouse LD_{50} (106·3) and the 20 per cent. to vary less, ranging from 200,000 mouse LD_{50} (105·3) to 630,000 mouse LD_{50} (105·8). Mean values were, however, quite similar for the two vaccines: 500,000 mouse LD_{50} (105·7) for the old 33 per cent. chicken embryo vaccine, and 400,000 mouse LD_{50} (105·6) for the 20 per cent. chicken embryo vaccine. The mean value of the 33 per cent. preparation was seven times the ED_{50}, and the mean value of the 20 per cent. material was six times the ED_{50}. The value of clean vaccines has continued to impress anyone concerned with the problem. Sikes and Larghi (1967) have demonstrated this most conclusively with a purified antigen whose protection index was ten-fold higher than the best tissue vaccines.

The advent of tissue cultures for the study of virus, and the adaptation of rabies virus (Kissling, 1958) to baby hamster kidney has naturally led to the development of both inactivated and live rabies vaccines in a variety of tissue culture systems. These include the Connaught rabid dog strain adapted to hamster kidney, and later to pig kidney, tissue culture (Abelseth, 1964). This strain was named E.R.A. at the sixth passage. The E.R.A. virus strain is pathogenic for mice, guinea-pigs, and hamsters by intercerebral inoculation, but has a very low degree of virulence by the intermuscular route. It is avirulent for domestic animals by the intermuscular route. A single dose is reported to be effective in protecting dogs, cattle, and sheep against rabies, as well as cats, goats, and horses. The challenge resulted in 95 to 100 per cent. mortality in the non-vaccinated controls. Duration of immunity studies have shown good protection for two years in dogs and three years in cattle (Abelseth, 1966).

Kissling reported on the efficacy of rabies vaccine grown on primary hamster kidney tissue culture (Kissling and Reese, 1963). This has led to a development of new tissue culture vaccines with satisfactory concentration of virus.

Ott reported on preliminary trials of a new hamster cell culture rabies vaccine (Ott and Heyke, 1962). One, using C.V.S. mouse origin, fixed rabies virus, is a live virus vaccine. Ott states that hamster kidney cell rabies vaccine can be effective either as an inactivated or as a live attenuated vaccine and that it will reduce post-vaccination tissue reactions to a minimum.

Cabasso and his colleagues have developed a chicken embryo origin tissue culture vaccine (Cabasso, Stebbins, Douglas, and Sharpless, 1965) which has been evaluated in guinea-pigs and dogs. The results indicate that the L.E.P. vaccine prepared in chicken embryo tissue culture will protect dogs in a manner comparable to L.E.P. vaccine produced from chicken embryos. Dogs given a 2-ml. dose of the tissue culture resisted challenge a year later. Dogs have now been given a three-year challenge. Preliminary reports indicate that the dogs resisted challenge (Cabasso, 1966). Other live vaccines used in the trials have also stood up to challenge very well (Sikes, 1969).

Sikes et al. (1971) recently completed a three-year duration of immunity study of eight types of rabies vaccines in 320 pure-bred dogs [TABLE 59]. Results indicated that the four

TABLE 59

Mortality of Beagle Dogs Whose Rabies Immunity was Challenged at 1 Year or 3 Years after Vaccination

Vaccines	Rabies mortality (per cent.)	
	1 year	3 years
I. *Licensed in the United States*		
A. Modified Live		
Low egg passage (L.E.P.)—C.E.O.	0/10 (0)	2/30 (6·7)
L.E.P.—chick fibroblast, tissue culture (T.C.)	0/10 (0)	3/29 (10·3)
L.E.P.—hamster kidney T.C.	1/10 (10)	1/30 (3·3)
High egg passage (H.E.P.)—canine kidney (T.C.)	0/10 (0)	2/29 (6·9)
E.R.A.—porcine kidney T.C.	0/10 (0)	3/30 (10·0)
B. Inactivated		
C.V.S.—hamster kidney T.C. (adjuvanted)	3/10 (30)	12/29 (41·4)
C. Controls, non-vaccinated	10/10 (100)	27/30 (90·0)
II. *Not licensed in the United States*		
A. Inactivated		
Suckling mouse brain (S.M.B.) from Latin America	0/10 (0)	6/29 (20·7)
Purified S.M.B. from C.D.C.	0/10 (0)	0/27 (0)
B. Controls, non-vaccinated	4/10 (40)	27/30 (90·0)

modified live virus (M.L.V.) tissue culture (T.C.) types provided as long-lasting immunity as the L.E.P.–C.E.O. type, following a single injection of these vaccines. On the other hand, the inactivated T.C. vaccine of hamster kidney origin failed to protect the dogs as well as the other vaccines, either for one year or three years, following a single injection of vaccine. A suckling mouse brain vaccine (S.M.B.V.) inactivated with beta propiolacton protected 100 per cent. of the dogs for one year and 80 per cent. for three years. A purified, concentrated S.M.B.V. prepared experimentally at the C.D.C. was the only vaccine that protected all the dogs for one and three years following a single injection of vaccine.

As a result of this study, public health officials now recommend that:

1. Any of the M.L.V. types of rabies vaccines currently licensed in the United States should be used for providing a three-year duration of immunity in adult dogs.

2. If inactivated tissue culture vaccines of the types tested are used, two doses injected 3–4 weeks apart are recommended for primary immunization. Single annual boosters are then recommended with this type of vaccine.

In summary, there is evidence that tissue culture origin vaccines are equal to chicken embryo origin products; however, the duration of immunity must be determined before any final decision is made. The WHO Expert Committee on Rabies, Fifth Report 1966, cautions authorities to reserve judgement until the new tissue culture vaccines have proven themselves by means of laboratory and field tests. Another problem facing many nations is the economics of vaccine production. The cost of vaccine can be high, especially if potency and safety are unknown.

Populations at Risk

Man is the most important population at risk, but other groups must be considered. Man can be protected when exposed, or vaccinated before exposure, when the risk justifies it. With the development of safe potent human vaccines the day may not be distant when health authorities will recommend pre-exposure immunization for everyone.

Dogs are second only to man in importance as a population at risk because of their close relation to man, and their ability to carry disease to man. In any rabies campaign it is very important to have a reasonable estimate of the canine population and of what percentage can be vaccinated by private means and what will remain to be vaccinated at public clinics. In addition, one must know what the stray dog population is. A reasonable estimate of dog population in urban areas is 1 dog to 10 persons. In rural areas the figure may be 1 to 5, and this is subject to many variables, including food such as garbage and slaughter-house waste—indigenous diseases, predators, and poisonous insects and snakes.

Food is naturally a major item; if no one feeds animals, they will not multiply or survive. The availability of food is directly correlated to the economic status of a community. Garbage is the waste food of a community and can feed a sizable canine population. Slaughter-house waste is important in small towns, and these can support hundreds of dogs who are in competition with other scavengers. Disease is also an important limiting factor; distemper and hepatitis are killers in any community. Parasitic diseases, including insect-transmitted infections, are especially important in warm climates. The motor car is another factor limiting dog populations. In American cities it is estimated that 10 to 20 per cent. of the resident dog population is injured or killed by motor vehicles annually. The number of stray dogs killed is probably twice the rate for resident dogs. Predators, poisonous snakes, and insects take their toll

in some places but are of little importance, compared to the above factors, in limiting populations.

On rare occasions other urban animals may be important in rabies control. Cats have been cited as the source of infection in some communities, but they are rarely incriminated independently of dogs. Rabid cats are vicious, dangerous animals. Squirrels have also been associated with rabies epizootics, but in most instances sick squirrels have been found to be suffering from forms of encephalitis other than rabies. Rodents are rarely affected and need seldom be considered in a rabies control campaign, although some persons and societies may want to involve them.

In rural and suburban areas, wildlife is a prime source of rabies and efforts must be undertaken to determine the roles of various species. In the United States the fox is most frequently identified as the source of disease. The skunk likewise can be an urban prowler, especially in sprawling cities which have uninhabited or sparsely occupied areas. Los Angeles is an example of a community where skunk rabies is indigenous. Other wild animals seem to be of little importance as reservoirs, except for stray wildcats or coyotes which enter suburban areas.

The socio–economic cultural structure of a community or country is important in planning any control programme. The socio–economic factors have been discussed under populations at risk but housing should also be mentioned. Poor housing, slums and ghettoes traditionally have large stray dog populations as well as cats and rats in great numbers. Cultural mores and religious taboos are of great significance in many countries, where animals are looked upon as the temporary residence of human souls who are in limbo. Dog wardens and control officers have a difficult role wherever they are, but they are very important in any campaign to control rabies, and need complete support as well as adequate compensation for their efforts.

Problems relating to virus characterization and reservoirs have been discussed under epidemiology, but it is important that they be re-emphasized in this section on control programmes. No programme can succeed if the reservoirs of rabies are not known, or if the virus kinetics are not known. An understanding of the character of the virus can almost determine the course of a control campaign.

In the Americas, bats that carry rabies have different degrees of significance in the temperate and tropical zones. As stated earlier, bat rabies in Canada and the United States is of some concern but is not a major reservoir or cause of disease. However, in the tropical zones, vampire bat rabies is a major problem for which no satisfactory answer is available. Control of vampire bat rabies is probably the biggest challenge facing the animal health authorities today.

Finally, what is the status of health education? What does the population know about rabies? Are they aware of a problem? Do they want to do something about it? Do they believe in vaccination? Will they pay for it? How do they feel about stray animal control? Will they appropriate and collect taxes to support dog pounds or shelters? These and many other questions and answers must be evaluated by any control official. A well-planned health education programme can ensure the success of a rabies control scheme; with no public health education, there will be little community support and most campaigns will be doomed to failure. The opposition to vaccination of any kind is well known, especially in underdeveloped areas where vaccines may not be all they should be.

The prepared community is like the prepared mind—it can accept opportunity when it appears. It is important that the community leaders understand why rabies control is important to them, to their families, to animals, and to prosperity.

REFERENCES

Abelseth, M. K. (1964) An attenuated rabies vaccine for domestic animals produced in tissue culture, *Canad. vet. J.*, **5**, 279.

Abelseth, M. K. (1966) Vaccination of domestic animals with a rabies vaccine produced in tissue culture from the ERA strain, in *Proceedings of the National Rabies Symposium*, N.C.D.C., Atlanta, Ga, p. 53.

Acha, P. (1966) Rabies in the Americas, in *Proceedings of the National Rabies Symposium*, N.C.D.C., Atlanta, Ga, pp. 140–42.

Acha, P. (1967) Personal communication.

British Medical Journal leading article (1974) Rabies vaccination in man, *Brit. med. J.*, **1**, 45.

Burkhart, R. L., Jervis, G. A., and Koprowski, H. (1950) Post-vaccinal paralysis and demyelination in the dog following antirabies vaccination, *Vet. Med.*, **45**, 31.

Cabasso, V. J. (1966) Canine rabies vaccines, in *Proceedings of the National Rabies Symposium*, N.C.D.C., Atlanta, Ga, pp. 45–51.

Cabasso, V. J., Stebbins, M. R., Douglas, A., and Sharpless, G. R. (1965) Tissue culture rabies vaccine (Flury LEP) in dogs, *Amer. J. vet. Res.*, **26**, 24.

Carini, A. (1911) Sur une grande epizootie de rage (vampire bat rabies), *Ann. Inst. Pasteur*, **25**, 843.

Committee of Inquiry on Rabies, Great Britain, Final Report (1970) (The Waterhouse Report), London, H.M.S.O.

Constantine, D. (1962) Rabies transmission by non-bite route, *Publ. Hlth Rep. (Wash.)*, **77**, 287.

Crandall, R. A. (1966) Rabies in Northern Greenland: some observations on the epizootiology and epidemiology, in *Proceedings of the National Rabies Symposium*, N.C.D.C., Atlanta, Ga, pp. 37–42.

Dean, D. J., Evans, W. M., and Thompson, W. R. (1964) Studies on the low egg passage Flury strain of modified live rabies virus produced in embryonating chicken eggs and tissue culture, *Amer. J. vet. Res.*, **25**, 756.

Eichhorn, E., and Lyon, B. M. (1923) Prophylactic vaccination of dogs against rabies, *J. Amer. vet. Med. Ass.*, **61**, 38.

Fermi, C. (1909) *Z. Bakteriol. Parasitenk. Abt.*, Ref. 49, 452; and Ref. 52, 536.

Food and Agriculture Organization (1966) *FAO Survey of Paralytic Rabies in Latin America*, Rome.

Habel, K. (1940a) Factors influencing the efficacy of phenolized rabies vaccines, *Publ. Hlth Rep. (Wash.)*, **55**, 1619.

Habel, K. (1940b) Evaluation of a mouse test for the standardization of the immunizing power of antirabies vaccines, *Publ. Hlth Rep. (Wash.)*, 55:1473.

Jenkins, M., and Wamberg, K. (1960) Rabies discovered in Greenland, *J. Amer. vet. Med. Ass.*, **137**, 183.

Johnson, H. N. (1948) Derriengue; vampire bat rabies in Mexico, *Amer. J. Hyg.*, **47**, 189.

Johnson, H. N. (1959) Rabies in insectivorous bats of North America, in *Proceedings of the Sixth International Congress of Medicine and Malaria*, Vol. 5, pp. 559–67.

Johnson, H. N. (1965) Rabies virus, in *Viral and Rickettsial Infections of Man*, 4th ed., eds. Horsefall, F. L., Jr., and Tamm, I., Philadelphia.

Johnson, H. N. (1966) Sporadic cases of rabies in wildlife: relation to rabies in domestic animals and character of virus, in *Proceedings of the National Rabies Symposium*, N.C.D.C., Atlanta, Ga, pp. 25–30.

Kaeberle, M. L. (1958) Newer tools for the prevention of rabies in domestic animals, *Ann. N. Y. Acad. Sci.*, **70**, 467.

Kantorovic, R. A. (1957) The etiology of madness in polar animals, *Acta virol.*, **1**, 220.

Kantorovic, R. A. (1964) Natural foci of a rabies-like infection in the far North, *J. Hyg. Epidem. (Praha).*, **7**, 100.

Kantorovic, R. A., Konovalov, G. V., Buzinov, I. A., and Riutova, V. P. (1963) Experimental investigations into rage and rabies of polar foxes, natural hosts of the infection, *Acta virol.*, **7**, 554.

Kaplan, H. M. and Koprouski, H. (1973) Laboratory techniques in rabies, 3rd ed., *Wld Hlth Org. monogr. Ser.* No. 23.

Kelser, R. A. (1928) Chloroform-treated rabies vaccine (preliminary report), *Vet. Bull.*, **22**, 95.

Kissling, R. E. (1958) Growth of rabies virus in non-nervous tissue culture, *Proc. Soc. exp. Biol. Med. (N.Y.)*, **98**, 223.

Kissling, R. E., and Reese, D. R. (1963) Antirabies vaccine of tissue culture origin, *J. Immunol.*, **91**, 362.

Kissling, R. E., et al. (1955) Unpublished N.C.D.C. Investigations, Atlanta, Ga.

Koprowski, H., and Black, J. (1950) Studies on chick embryo adapted rabies virus, II. Pathogenicity for dogs and use of egg-adapted strains for vaccination purposes, *J. Immunol.*, **64**, 185.

Koprowski, H., and Cox, H. R. (1948) Studies on chick embryo adapted rabies virus, *J. Immunol.*, **60**, 533.

Lassen, H. C. A. (1962) Paralytic human rabies in Greenland, *Lancet*, **i**, 247.

Moynihan, W. A. (1966) Rabies in Canada, in *Proceedings of the National Rabies Symposium*, N.C.D.C., Atlanta, Gap, p. 134–6.

Ott, G. L., and Heyke, B. (1962) Propagation of rabies virus evaluation of a vaccine, *Vet. Med.*, **57**, 613.

Pasteur, L., Chamberland, C. E., and Roux, M. (1884) Nouvelle communication sur la rage, *C. R. Acad. Sci. (Paris)*, **98**, 457.

Peacock, G. V. (1966) Discussion, canine rabies vaccines, in *Proceedings of the National Rabies Symposium*, N.C.D.C., Atlanta, Ga, pp. 54–5.

Plummer, J. P. G. (1947a) Preliminary note on Arctic dog disease and its relation to rabies, *Canad. J. comp. Med.*, **40**, No. 6, 154.

Plummer, J. P. G. (1947b) Further notes on Arctic dog disease and its relationship to rabies, *Canad. J. comp. Biol.*, **11**, 330.

Rausch, R. (1958) Some observations on rabies in Alaska, with special reference to wild Canidae, *J. Wildl. Mgmt*, **22**, 246.

Semple, A. B. (1972) Rabies and Waterhouse Report, *R. Soc. Hlth J.*, **92**, 303.

Semple, D. (1911) *Science Memorandum*, No. 44, Medical Sanitary Department, Calcutta.

Sikes, R. K. (1962) Pathogenesis of rabies in wildlife, I. Comparative effect of varying doses of rabies virus inoculated into foxes and skunks, *Amer. J. vet. Res.*, **23**, No. 96, 1041.

Sikes, R. K. (1969) Progress in rabies research, *Proc. U.S. Animal Hlth Ass.*, **73**, 302.

Sikes, R. K., and Larghi, O. P. (1967) Purified rabies vaccine: development and comparison of potency and safety with two human rabies vaccines, *J. Immunol.*, **99**, 545.

Smithcor, J. F. (1957) *Evolution of the Veterinary Art*, Kansas City, Missouri, Chs. 1–7, pp. 1–299.

Steck, F. (1968) *Vet. Rec.*, **83**, Suppl. 15.

Sullivan, T. D., et al. (1954) Recovery of rabies virus from colonial bats in Texas, *Publ. Hlth Rep. (Wash.)*, **69**, 766.

Tierkel, E. S. (1959) Rabies, in *Advances in Veterinary Science*, Vol. V, New York, p. 183.

Tierkel, E. S., Arbona, G., Rivera, A., and de Juan, A. (1952) Mongoose rabies in Puerto Rico, *Publ. Hlth Rep. (Wash.)*, **67**, 274–8.

Tierkel, E. S., Kissling, R. E., Eidson, M., and Habel, K. (1953)

A brief survey and progress report of controlled comparative experiments in canine rabies immunization, in Proceedings of the Ninetieth Meeting, *Amer. vet. Med. Ass.*, **443**.

Toro, E. E. (1966) Rabies in Puerto Rico, in *Proceedings of the National Symposium*, N.C.D.C., Atlanta, Ga, pp. 131–3.

Umeno, and Doi (1921) *Kitasato Arch. exp. Med.*, **4**, 89.

Vetners, H. D., Hoffert, W. R., Scatterday, J. E., and Hardy, A. V. (1954) Rabies in bats in Florida, *Amer. J. publ. Hlth*, **44**.

Wamberg, K. (1960) Rabies in Greenland, *Nord. vet. Med.*, **12**, 769.

Webster, L. T. (1939) A mouse test for measuring the immunizing potency of anti-rabies vaccines, *J. exp. Med.*, **70**, 87.

Williams, R. B. (1949) Epizootic of rabies in interior Alaska, 1945–1947, *Canad. J. comp. Med.*, **13**, 136.

Winkler, W. G. (1966) Rodent rabies, in *Proceedings of the National Rabies Symposium*, N.C.D.C., Atlanta, Ga, pp. 34–6.

Witte, E. J. (1954) Bat rabies in Pennsylvania, *Amer. J. publ. Hlth*, **44**, 186.

World Health Organization (1973) Expert Committee on Rabies, Sixth Report, *Wld Hlth Org. techn. Rep., Ser.*, No. 523.

World Health Organization (1974a) New prospects for rabies control, *Wld Hlth Org. Chron.*, **28**, 16.

World Health Organization (1974b) The work of WHO in 1973 (Section on Rabies) *Wld Hlth Org. techn. Rep. Ser.*, No. 213. 26.

FURTHER READING

Nagano, Yasuti, and Davenport, Fred M., eds (1972) *Rabies*, Baltimore, Maryland.

Baer, George, ed. (1974) *Rabies Advances*, New York.

24

THE SPREAD AND CONTROL OF WORM INFECTIONS

T. WILSON

INTRODUCTION

The worms which parasitize man belong to many different genera and species, often with complicated life cycles. They may require special conditions for their survival and transmission, and many of them pass an essential part of their development in some intermediate host or hosts, vertebrate or invertebrate. Although geographical distribution is largely delimited by the climatic requirements of the worm itself or of its hosts, the local standards of environmental sanitation and the habits of the human population can be decisive factors in determining prevalence. In general the less complex the life-cycle and the more direct the route of transmission, the wider the distribution of any particular worm is likely to be.

As with many other parasites, a distinction must be made between worm 'infections' and worm 'diseases'. Many parasitic worms tend to live in harmony with their hosts, and signs and symptoms of disease which can be attributed to the presence of the worm or its products may be relatively rare. Estimates of prevalence are therefore seldom reliable unless based on special surveys designed to reveal infection. There appears to be a general connexion between incidence of disease and average intensity of infection; nevertheless many heavily infected persons may remain free from signs and symptoms, while others, less heavily infected, may suffer severely. Individual reactions to infection obviously play a large part in determining what the end-result will be, and methods of investigating allergy and immunity in relationship to worm infections are still unsatisfactory.

The usual morphological classification of worms does little to explain how worm infections spread in a community, and how they may be controlled. Successful control involves the interruption of transmission, and methods of transmission have little relationship to morphology. Thus, on the one hand, examples of widely different transmission routes may be found among the members of any one zoological group, such as the nematodes; on the other hand, some particular transmission route may be common to the members of several different groups. For a book on preventive medicine a more useful type of classification would seem to be something on the lines of that adopted by Davey and Lightbody (1971). These authors grouped communicable diseases according to route of transmission and epidemiology, and such a system considerably simplifies the discussion of control measures.

Parasitic worms enter the human body in one of three ways. The infective stages may be swallowed; they may penetrate the skin or mucous membranes; or they may be deposited in or on the skin by insect vectors. Routes of exit from the body differ also; in many instances the eggs are passed in the faeces, and these infections tend to be commoner where methods of faeces disposal are unsatisfactory. Man may be the sole host of the adult worm or only one of several hosts; in several instances the normal transmission cycle is from animal to animal, human infection being more or less accidental. Transmission may be direct from man to man, or part of the worm's life-cycle may have to take place outside the body, or in some intermediate host or hosts. All of these factors have to be taken into account when control measures are contemplated. The different routes of transmission arc summarized in TABLE 60.

TABLE 60
The Transmission of Worm Infections

I. TRANSMITTED BY HUMAN EXCRETIONS

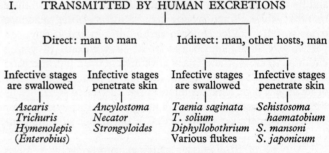

Direct: man to man		Indirect: man, other hosts, man	
Infective stages are swallowed	Infective stages penetrate skin	Infective stages are swallowed	Infective stages penetrate skin
Ascaris	*Ancylostoma*	*Taenia saginata*	*Schistosoma*
Trichuris	*Necator*	*T. solium*	*haematobium*
Hymenolepis	*Strongyloides*	*Diphyllobothrium*	*S. mansoni*
(*Enterobius*)		Various flukes	*S. japonicum*

II. TRANSMITTED BY OTHER ROUTES

Dracunculus
Echinococcus
Trichinella [See Chapter 22]

III. TRANSMITTED BY BITING ARTHROPODS

[See Chapter 17]

Wuchereria bancrofti
Brugia malayi
Loa loa
Onchocerca volvulus

Some worm infections, e.g. schistosomiasis or onchocerciasis, may be responsible for a demonstrable amount of ill health in a community, and specific control measures may be deemed necessary. More often, however, as with most of the intestinal worms, the control of worm infections is incidental to a campaign designed to improve the standard of environmental hygiene, and thus to reduce the prevalence of numerous other diseases which are also spread through contamination of the environment by human excretions. This chapter is concerned mainly with the large group of worm infections spread in this manner, and with two transmitted by some other route. Most of the latter are dealt with elsewhere; arthropod-borne worm infections are described in CHAPTER 17, and trichiniasis in CHAPTER 22.

DIRECT TRANSMISSION BY HUMAN EXCRETIONS

The first worm infections to be considered are those in which man is the only host of the adult worm and transmission is direct from man to man, with or without a brief period of extra-corporeal development. The infective stages may either be swallowed by the victim, or may penetrate his skin.

THE INFECTIVE STAGES OF THE WORMS ARE SWALLOWED

Ascaris lumbricoides, the Large Roundworm

Distribution is world-wide, with the highest incidence in hot, humid climates. The adult worms live in the small intestine, and the eggs are passed in the faeces. Fertile eggs require a period of 14–21 days on moist earth before becoming infective. If then swallowed, the larva contained in the egg emerges and migrates through the intestinal wall to the portal circulation, in which it is carried to the lungs, where it remains and develops for some days. It then makes its way via the alveoli, the bronchi, trachea, and oesophagus, back to the small intestine, where it becomes adult; this whole period of development takes 2–3 months.

Ascariasis is primarily a disease of young children, who infect themselves by crawling around on faeces-contaminated ground, and by the common habit of putting all kinds of things in their mouths; while all age-groups may be infected, the incidence tends to fall in older children and adults. Infection rates are particularly high, approximately 70–80 per cent. in young children, in areas where faeces are stored in open pits and used as fertilizer; the eggs are widely distributed through the agency of fowls and pigs, which commonly have access to such pits, as well as by humans and in dust. The eggs are killed by drying or by high temperature (above 45° C.), but under suitable conditions may remain viable for about a year.

A variety of ill-defined abdominal symptoms have been ascribed to ascaris infection, but a diagnosis usually depends upon the finding of eggs in the stools, or because an adult worm has either been vomited or passed by rectum. Heavy infections, particularly in young children, may occasionally produce respiratory symptoms (ascaris pneumonia) during the migration of larvae through the lungs, or intestinal obstruction may be caused by a mass of adult worms blocking the lumen of the gut.

Trichuris trichiura, the Whipworm

This infection is common throughout the tropics and sub-tropics. The adult worms live in the caecum and large intestine, and the eggs are passed in the faeces. The eggs require a developmental period of several weeks before becoming infective, and this is favoured by high humidity and well-shaded, warm, moist soil. When swallowed, the larvae emerge from the egg and develop into adult worms in the intestine, the slim anterior portion of the worms being threaded into the mucous membrane.

Like ascariasis, trichuriasis is primarily an infection of young children, who acquire both infections in the same manner, and to much the same extent. Heavy infections are reported to be responsible for dysenteric symptoms and rectal prolapse, par-

ticularly in the West Indies, but as a rule a diagnosis is made by the recognition of eggs in the stools.

Hymenolepis nana, the Dwarf Tapeworm

Distribution is wide but patchy, and infection rates are relatively low compared with *Ascaris* and *Trichuris*. The adult worms live in the small intestine, and the eggs are normally passed in the stools and swallowed by another victim. Hatching of eggs in the intestine and auto-infection of the original host is also thought to occur. Again children show the highest incidence of infection. Symptoms are not specific, and diagnosis is by recognition of the eggs (or occasionally segments of the adult worms) in the stools. Although this worm also infects rodents, the human reservoir of infection is probably the important one.

Control

The main control measure against these worm infections, as also against most of those to be described hereafter, consists in the sanitary disposal of human excreta. The principles of sanitation are dealt with in CHAPTER 8, but in many parts of the world the provision of better sanitary facilities is not by itself sufficient to ensure an improvement in standards. Much time and effort may have to be devoted to the study of local habits, to devising a method of disposal which will be acceptable to the people, and then to convincing them that its adoption will be beneficial to them and their children. Apart from the obvious need to use, for example, the type of latrine best suited to the terrain, minor modifications in design may be required to meet local prejudices, and may make all the difference between success and failure. A further point to remember is the need to provide sanitary facilities for people who spend long hours at work outdoors, away from their homes. In countries where human faeces are used as agricultural fertilizer, composting with vegetable refuse or storage for a time in sealed tanks may serve to destroy worm eggs and other pathogens while still preserving their value as manure, but again the farmers concerned will need a lot of convincing that this latter statement is true.

Much can also be done by instructing mothers and children about the importance of personal hygiene in preventing the spread of these worms; in highly endemic areas the mass treatment of young children may be useful, but the effect will be transient unless the chances of re-infection can be reduced as suggested above. *Ascaris* infections can be treated with one of the piperazine salts, with the recently introduced drug tetramisole or its laevorotatory isomer levamisole, with bephenium hydroxynaphthoate, or with thiabendazole. The last two drugs also have an action on *Trichuris* infections. Dichlorophen or niclosamide are effective against *Hymenolepis nana*.

Enterobius vermicularis, the Threadworm

This may conveniently be considered here, although in this infection the eggs are laid by the adult worms on the perianal skin, and are only occasionally found in the stools. Distribution is world-wide, but the infection is said to be commoner in communities with low sanitary standards. The eggs mature in a few hours, and infection is acquired by swallowing the infective eggs; the larvae hatch in the stomach, and the adult worms live in the lumen of the large intestine, whence the females emerge through the anus, especially at night, to lay their eggs on the surrounding skin.

There is little reliable information about the incidence of enterobiasis. It occurs commonly in families and institutions, especially where children are crowded together, but may be found in persons of any age and social status. Infection is transmitted mainly by contaminated fingers and contaminated objects, such as clothes, toilet-seats, chairs, etc.; the eggs may also be present in dust.

The most common clinical feature is perianal irritation, more marked at night, due to the movements of the female worms. The itching can be intense, and the resultant scratching may lead to secondary infection. Diagnosis is made by finding the adult worms or their eggs; the eggs must be looked for by taking cellophane-tape impressions, or swabs, from the perianal skin.

Control

The essential points in the control of enterobiasis are the examination of all members of the family or group, the treatment of all infected persons, usually with viprynium embonate or one of the piperazine salts, and the prevention of further transmission by careful attention to personal hygiene. The hands should always be washed after defaecating and before eating, and infected persons should wash the anal region thoroughly each morning.

THE INFECTIVE STAGES OF THE WORMS PENETRATE THE SKIN

Ancylostoma duodenale and Necator americanus, the Hookworms

Infection with one or other of these worms is widespread throughout the sub-tropics and tropics, with the highest incidence in warm, moist climates. The adult worms live in the small intestine, and the eggs are passed in the faeces. In suitable conditions of temperature and moisture the larvae which hatch from the eggs become infective in a week or ten days, and then enter the body of a fresh victim by penetrating his skin. They are carried in the circulation to the lungs, and pass to the intestine via the trachea and oesophagus. The worms are mature in about five weeks after penetration of the skin.

The epidemiology of hookworm infection is governed by the conditions favouring its transmission, i.e. indiscriminate defaecation on to damp soil, usually with decaying vegetation and in shade, and temperature ranging from 24° to 32° C.; those most liable to be infected will be persons who habitually walk barefoot on, or perhaps handle, the soil containing the infective larvae. Persons of all ages may be infected, but the highest incidence is in adolescents and young adults in endemic areas. Persons whose general health is otherwise good appear to develop an immunity, and the infection remains sub-clinical; the anaemia which is the chief feature of hookworm disease manifests itself predominantly in malnourished children and adults. A combination of malnutrition and heavy worm load may be associated with a severe degree of anaemia, which is typically hypochromic and microcytic; blood loss into the intestine in hookworm disease may be considerable, and has been recorded as up to 150 ml. daily. Occasionally a localized

dermatitis (ground itch) may develop at the place where the larvae have penetrated the skin. Diagnosis of hookworm infection depends upon the finding of the typical eggs in the stools. Differentiation between *A. duodenale* and *N. americanus*, which is sometimes desirable, must be made by examination of the adult worms recovered from the stools after treatment, or of third stage larvae obtained by egg culture.

Strongyloides stercoralis, the Strongylid Threadworm

Infection with *Strongyloides stercoralis* is almost as widespread as hookworm infection, and occurs in much the same areas. The adult worms live in the intestinal mucosa, and the eggs usually hatch in their passage along the intestine, so that larvae are found in the faeces. Outside the body these larvae develop either into free-living adults or into infective larvae which can penetrate the skin of a new host in the same manner as hookworm larvae. Their subsequent migrations within the body are similar to those of the hookworm larvae. The symptoms caused by infection are variable: there may be intermittent diarrhoea and perianal irritation, and in heavy infections intestinal ulceration and damage to the mucosa may occur.

Control

Again the main control measure must be the sanitary disposal of human excreta. Treatment of all infected persons in a community will reduce the reservoir of infection, but this measure is usually applicable only to small communities where the incidence of disease is high. A new drug, phenylene di-isothiocyanate (bitoscanate, *Jonit*) has recently become available which is said to be effective against both species of hookworms; tetrachloroethylene and bephenium hydroxynaphthoate are widely used. Thiabendazole remains the most useful drug against *Strongyloides* infection. Improvement of dietary standards will help to reduce the clinical effects of infection, and some individual protection may be obtained by the wearing of shoes or boots.

INDIRECT TRANSMISSION BY HUMAN EXCRETIONS

In a second group of worm infections transmission is indirect, with part of the parasite's life-cycle taking place in some intermediate host or hosts. The adult worms may be found only in man, or in man and other mammals; the infective stages may be swallowed, as when the intermediate host is an edible animal or vegetable, or may penetrate the skin.

THE INFECTIVE STAGES OF THE WORMS ARE SWALLOWED

Taenia saginata, the Beef Tapeworm

Distribution is world-wide, and infection occurs wherever beef is eaten raw or partially cooked. The adult worms live in the intestine of man only, and gravid segments are passed in the stools. The eggs set free by the rupture of the segments are infective immediately, and under suitable conditions remain viable for about two months. If swallowed by cattle or allied animals, the embryos emerge and pass through the intestinal wall to be carried to the skeletal muscle, where they become small cysts containing the head of the future worm. Man is infected by eating raw or insufficiently cooked meat containing these cysts, cysticercus bovis. The two main factors affecting epidemiology are contamination of cattle pastures or drinking-water by human faeces and the extent to which raw or partially cooked beef is eaten. Cropless birds feeding on sewage have been found to excrete viable eggs, and contamination of pastures by this means is possible, but is probably less important than other sources of contamination. Tapeworm infection in man is usually symptomless, and the diagnosis depends upon the recognition of gravid segments in the faeces; in T. saginata the main uterine branches number 18–30, in T. solium they number 8–12.

Taenia solium, the Pork Tapeworm

The life-history of this worm is similar to that of T. saginata, except that pigs instead of cattle act as the intermediate hosts, and human infection therefore results from eating raw or insufficiently cooked pork containing the cysts, cysticercus cellulosae. One important difference is that the eggs of T. solium can develop to the cysticercus stage if swallowed by man, and localization of these cysts in the brain, eye, or spinal cord may have serious consequences. There is no record of this happening with T. saginata.

Diphyllobothrium latum, the Fish Tapeworm

Infection with this worm occurs most frequently along the Baltic coast and in the neighbourhood of large fresh-water lakes in temperate climates; but may occur wherever infected fish is eaten raw or partially cooked. The adult worm is found in the intestine of man and a number of fish-eating mammals (dog, cat, bear, seal, etc.). The eggs are passed in the faeces and hatch after about two weeks in fresh water, releasing a free-swimming larva which must be swallowed by small crustaceans, Cyclops or Diaptomus. After developing in the body cavity of the crustacean for about six weeks, the larva is infective to fish swallowing the crustacean. In the fish, further development takes place to the form infective to man and the other mammalian hosts of the adult worms. If a small fish containing this infective larva is eaten by a larger fish the larva transfers itself to the muscles of the new host, and most human infections are probably acquired by eating the uncooked flesh of large fish, such as salmon, pike, or perch. Smoking and pickling of the fish are not sufficient to destroy the infective larvae.

Infection with D. latum is usually symptomless, but has occasionally been held responsible for causing a macrocytic anaemia; diagnosis depends upon the recognition of the eggs in the stools, and may be confirmed by the examination of parts of the worm after drug treatment.

Fasciolopsis buski, Clonorchis sinensis, and Paragonimus westermani

These three flukes occur widely, but patchily, in eastern Asia, and P. westermani also occurs in the Pacific islands, Africa, and South America. Although their life-cycles differ in detail, there is sufficient broad similarity to permit their description as a group. The adult worms are found in man and a number of other mammals; the eggs of F. buski, the giant intestinal fluke, and C. sinensis, the Chinese liver fluke, are passed in the stools. The eggs of P. westermani, the Oriental lung fluke, are passed in the sputum, but if this is swallowed will also be found in the stools. The eggs hatch in water, and the larvae enter suitable snails, in which they develop to cercariae. When these leave the snails the free-swimming cercariae of F. buski encyst on the plant on which the snail is feeding, those of C. sinensis penetrate between the scales and into the muscles of fresh-water fish, and those of P. westermani penetrate the flesh of certain crabs and crayfish. The plants commonly involved in the transmission of F. buski are the water caltrop and the water chestnut, which may be cultivated for the market in ponds fertilized with human faeces; the plants are usually eaten raw, the outer leaves being pulled off with the teeth and the inner parts eaten. Fish, crabs, and crayfish may also be reared in ponds, and are frequently eaten raw or pickled, thus allowing the transmission of C. sinensis and P. westermani.

Clinical symptoms and signs of F. buski infection are not distinctive; heavy infections with C. sinensis may produce liver enlargement or cirrhosis, oedema, and diarrhoea; the diagnosis in each instance depends upon the recognition of the characteristic eggs in the stools. P. westermani may cause a chronic bronchitis with brownish-red sputum in which the eggs can be detected.

Control

There are several points in the transmission cycle of all these worms at which the application of control measures might be successful. The sanitary disposal of human faeces would prevent infection of cattle and pigs with T. saginata and T. solium; it would reduce considerably, but not eliminate, the spread of the other worms, which can maintain themselves by means of their other animal hosts; avoidance of indiscriminate spitting would help to reduce the spread of P. westermani. Treatment of infected persons may be of value, particularly the treatment of those with special opportunities for spreading infection, for example farm labourers harbouring T. saginata or T. solium; the drugs dichlorophen and niclosamide have proved effective against the adults of these two worms.

Obviously, however, the adequate cooking of all meat, fish, and shellfish, and the avoidance of possibly infected raw vegetables, would completely prevent the transmission of any of these worms to man. Health education in the endemic areas should stress the importance of this method of control, while at the same time efforts should be made to improve sanitary standards. In countries where much of the slaughtering of cattle and pigs for human consumption is done in central abattoirs, meat inspection may help to prevent the spread of T. saginata and T. solium; and the cysts will be killed by storage of carcasses at — 10° C. for one week.

THE INFECTIVE STAGES OF THE WORMS PENETRATE THE SKIN

Schistosoma haematobium and Schistosoma mansoni

Man is the only important host of the adult worms of these two species of blood flukes. S. haematobium has a widespread distribution in Africa and in parts of the Middle East; a small endemic focus also exists near Bombay in India. S. mansoni has a focal distribution throughout Africa and also in South America and some of the West Indian islands.

The adult worms live in the veins of the human portal system, *S. haematobium* laying its eggs in the vesical plexus and *S. mansoni* in the veins draining the intestinal wall. The eggs pass through the tissues of the bladder and intestine respectively to be excreted in the urine or faeces. For further development to occur, the eggs must reach water within 4–6 weeks, otherwise the contained ciliated larvae, the miracidia, will die. The eggs hatch in water, and the miracidia must penetrate a suitable snail host within a day or two. In its body they develop and multiply through several generations, finally producing the infective forms, the cercariae, in about four weeks. The cercariae leave the snail, enter the water, and can survive up to six days; they penetrate unbroken skin or mucous membrane, and man is infected by contact with, or by drinking, infected water. The cercariae discard their tails during penetration, and pass through the tissues to the circulation, finally reaching the portal veins, where they become adult. This period of development takes about two months.

In endemic areas schistosomiasis is primarily a disease of children and adolescents; adults seem to have developed a considerable degree of immunity, and are often resistant to further infection or at least to its clinical effects. Non-immune adults, however, suffer severely and may have acute toxic and allergic symptoms and high fever within a few weeks of exposure to infection, during the period of development of the worms; the later signs and symptoms are due to pathological changes in the urinary system, the intestine, and the liver, induced by the presence of the worms and their eggs.

Much has yet to be learnt about the vector species of snails and their bionomics. They are aquatic, and normally leave the water only for brief periods, but can survive for months in mud and in cracks in dried-up water-courses. Irrigation canals usually form a suitable habitat, and snails are likely to be especially numerous in eddies and backwaters also frequented by man. They cannot maintain themselves in a water flow faster than about 15 metres per minute, or in water with a salt content above 0·6 per cent. A temperature between 20° and 33° C. is the optimum for the development of the schistosomes in the snails.

Diagnosis of schistosomiasis is made by recognition of the eggs in urine or stools, or perhaps better by diluting these with sterile water, leaving for a few hours, and then examining for the swimming miracidia.

Control

The most permanent and effective control measure would be to prevent human urine and faeces from reaching water in which the vector snails live. This should be the long-term objective, and will require continuous health education combined with the provision of sufficient sanitary latrines in suitable sites and improvements in water supplies. Active control measures consist in making the habitat unsuitable for the snails in various ways, killing the snails with chemicals and mass treatment of all infected persons. The drugs commonly used are one of the antimony compounds or niridazole (Ambilhar). Mass treatment will limit the severity of clinical effects, but by itself does little to control infection. It is becoming clear that the control of schistosomiasis will be achieved eventually only by the use of a variety of control measures, applied in combination over a period of years.

Schistosoma japonicum

This fluke occurs in parts of the Far East, mainly in Japan, China, and the Philippines, and usually with a focal distribution. The adult worms are found in a number of mammals (dog, pig, buffalo, and rodents) as well as in man; they live in the mesenteric veins, and the eggs pass into the bowel and are excreted in the faeces. The developmental cycle is similar to that of *S. mansoni*, but the vector snails are semi-aquatic, and spend part of their time out of the water, in damp, shady places. Because it produces many more eggs, *S. japonicum* is more liable to produce severe clinical effects than the other two schistosomes, and cirrhosis of the liver is a common end-result. In some areas the disease is an occupational one, almost limited to workers in rice-fields. Diagnosis is as for *S. mansoni*.

Control

The human reservoir of infection is more important than the animal reservoir, and transmission could be considerably reduced by improving methods of faeces disposal. Treatment of infected persons with sodium antimony tartrate is also useful; snail control is effective but difficult to carry out, because the snails are not confined to water and may be distributed irregularly in various patches of marshy ground. Intensive cultivation of an area, and the drainage of swampy, uncultivated ground, offers the best hope of permanent snail control and elimination of the disease.

WHO and Schistosomiasis Control

The chemotherapy of schistosomiasis is being studied at the Chemotherapy Centre in Tanga, Tanzania. The work is sponsored by the governments of Tanzania and the United Kingdom, and the World Health Organization. Better molluscicides are being studied, especially the slow-release formulation of niclosamide dissolved in rubber (World Health Organization, 1974, p. 43).

WORM INFECTIONS TRANSMITTED BY OTHER ROUTES

An important group of worm infections is transmitted by biting insects, and these worms are dealt with in Chapter 16; trichiniasis is dealt with in CHAPTER 19. Only two infections under this heading need be considered here, guinea-worm and hydatid disease.

Dracunculus medinensis, the Guinea-worm

This infection occurs patchily in parts of Africa, India, the Middle East, some islands of the West Indies, the Guianas, and Brazil. The gravid female worms are found in the subcutaneous tissues of man and a number of other mammals, the usual sites in man being the ankle and lower leg. A small blister forms over the head of the worm and ruptures to leave an ulcer; on coming into contact with water, the uterus is protruded through this, and larvae are discharged. They can survive in water for two or three weeks awaiting ingestion by a tiny water crustacean, *Cyclops* species, in which they develop in about two weeks to the infective forms. The cyclops then infects man if swallowed in drinking-water, the larvae being liberated in the intestine, and migrating through the tissues for about nine months before becoming mature.

Transmission can occur only when suitable species of cyclops are present in water to which the larvae from the skin can gain access, and that water, including the infected cyclops, is drunk by man. The stagnant water of shallow ponds, tanks, or open step-wells, into which people must wade to fill their water containers, thus supplies ideal conditions for the infection; persons who obtain their drinking-water from small streams or rivers are seldom infected. The greatest incidence is found in young adults. The superficial blister and ulcer are the main clinical features, and secondary bacterial infection of the ulcer is a common complication. Diagnosis may be confirmed by placing a few drops of water on the ulcer and examining for larvae.

Control

Immediate although temporary control may be achieved by chemical treatment of water to kill the cyclops (DDT at 5 parts per million, or copper sulphate 10 to 25 p.p.m.) or by straining or boiling the water. More permanent measures are the provision of protected wells or a piped water supply. Whatever method is adopted, the long incubation period means that infections will continue to appear for about a year after transmission has ceased. Treatment of guinea-worm infections with niridazole has given excellent results.

Echinococcus granulosus

Hydatid disease is a world-wide disease of animals, and human infection is found mainly in the sheep- and cattle-rearing regions of Australia, New Zealand, Africa, and South America. The adult worms live in the intestine of dogs, jackals, wolves, and foxes, and the eggs are passed in the faeces. In the normal transmission cycle these eggs are swallowed by sheep and cattle grazing on contaminated pastures; the eggs hatch in the animal's intestine, and the embryos migrate into the blood stream to be carried to the liver or lungs. In these sites the characteristic hydatid cysts develop, containing enormous numbers of larvae, each one of which is capable of becoming an adult worm if the cyst is eaten by a dog. Human infection with hydatid cyst usually occurs as a result of handling infected dogs, or sheep contaminated by dogs, and occasionally perhaps through the medium of water or raw vegetables contaminated by dog faeces.

Probably many human infections are acquired in childhood, but signs and symptoms may not develop for several years. These vary with the site of the cyst, and differential diagnosis from any other expanding tumour is difficult. An intradermal test with filtered hydatid fluid is a useful aid to diagnosis.

Control

The regular treatment of all dogs (with arecoline hydrobromide) has proved a useful control measure in endemic areas. Transmission can also be reduced by ensuring the destruction of infected offal and meat, by the exclusion of dogs from slaughterhouses, and by deep burial of carcasses. Personal prophylaxis consists in thorough washing of hands after contact with dogs or sheep, and those concerned, including children, should be instructed in the importance of this as a means of safeguarding their own health.

REFERENCES AND FURTHER READING

Beaver, P. C. (1961) Control of soil-transmitted helminths, *Wld Hlth Org. Publ. Hlth Pap.*, No. 10.

Belding, D. L. (1965) *Textbook of Clinical Parasitology*, 3rd ed., New York.

Cowper, S. G. (1971) *A Synopsis of African Bilharziasis*, London.

Craig, C. F., and Faust, E. C. (1971) in *Clinical Parasitology*, 7th ed., ed. Faust, E. C., and Russell, P. F., London.

Davey, T. H., and Lightbody, W. P. H. (1971) *The Control of Disease in the Tropics*, 4th ed., ed. Davey, T. H., and Wilson, T., London.

Davis, A. (1973) *Drug Treatment in Intestinal Helminthiasis*, Geneva.

Faust, E. C., Beaver, P. C., and Jung, R. C. (1962) *Animal Agents and Vectors of Human Disease*, 2nd ed., London.

Hackett, C. J., Buckley, J. J. C., and Murgatroyd, F. (1954) *Manual of Medical Helminthology*, London.

Jeffrey, H. C., and Leach, R. M. (1966) *Atlas of Medical Helminthology and Protozoology*, Edinburgh.

Noble, E. R. and Noble, G. A. (1971) *Parasitology: The Biology of Animal Parasites*, 3rd ed., London.

Watson, J. M. (1960) *Medical Helminthology*, London.

World Health Organization (1973) Schistosomiasis Control: Report of a WHO Expert Committee, *Wld Hlth Org. techn. Rep., Ser.*, No. 515.

World Health Organization (1974) The work of WHO in 1973, *Wld Hlth Org. Off. Rec.*, No. 213, 29.

25

GLOBAL TUBERCULOSIS

G. S. KILPATRICK

Tuberculosis is generally conceded to be the most important communicable disease today. At a conservative estimate there are probably some 15 million cases of infectious tuberculosis in the world at the present time. Every year there are some 2–3 million new cases, while between 1 and 2 million people die of the disease. Not only is the mortality from tuberculosis very considerable but because it is a chronic disease a large amount of human suffering and economic loss result from it. It is also important to realize that more than three-quarters of the cases are in the developing countries of the world.

Tuberculosis has been, and still is, declining in most technically advanced and industrialized countries to such an extent that it is no longer a major public health danger in most of them. Nevertheless, even in these countries, there are some residual problems, and there is little room in them for complacency. In developing countries, however, there is still a very considerable amount of tuberculosis, and because of limited financial and other resources in these countries the approach to the problem must of necessity be different (World Health Organization, 1964). In technically advanced countries the aim as far as tuberculosis is concerned now should be *eradication* of the disease, whereas in the developing countries the first phase should be *control* of the condition. In this chapter the various methods which are available in both circumstances will be described and compared. It is hoped thereby to give a comprehensive and up-to-date appraisal of the global situation as far as tuberculosis is concerned. Specific tools for prevention and cure of the disease are now available, but their use is often inadequately and inefficiently applied. That this is so has been shown by the slow decline of world tuberculosis in

contrast to the very large sums of money and resources expended on it. This has probably been due to lack of national planning, and in particular to unrealistic selection of priorities, together with a failure to reorientate traditional approaches to present knowledge.

Most of what follows deals with the major problem in tuberculosis, namely infectious pulmonary disease. Extra-pulmonary disease, while not of negligible proportions and probably amounting to some 15 per cent. of all cases, is less important from the community point of view. Extra-human sources of infection—usually bovine—are not considered to be as important at present as in the past, because in most parts of the world milk is routinely boiled before consumption, and elsewhere pasteurization of milk with control of bovine infection have already been put into extensive practice. In countries, however, where bovine tuberculosis is still a problem it is also a menace to man, and in these countries complete control of tuberculosis cannot be achieved unless attention is also paid to the reduction or preferably eradication of tuberculosis in cattle.

EPIDEMIOLOGY

Retrospective studies based on reports from industrialized countries have almost invariably shown a decline both in tuberculosis mortality and morbidity since the nineteenth century [see FIG. 75] regardless of the extent and form of the antituberculosis measures taken by the countries concerned (McDonald and Springett, 1954). Before the advent of specific antituberculous drugs and mass B.C.G. vaccination this decline was almost certainly due to improved social conditions.

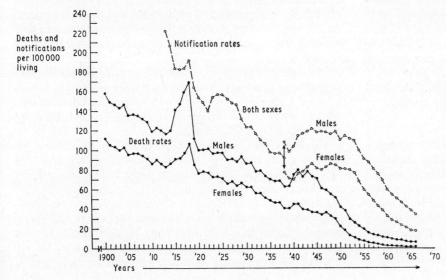

FIG. 75. Annual death rates and notification rates for respiratory tuberculosis in England and Wales (1900–66, all ages).

Since the introduction of specific measures, and particularly as a result of antituberculous chemotherapy, this decline has been accelerated. In general, it has been found that there has been an annual decrease of between 5 and 10 per cent. in both mortality and morbidity in most industrialized countries during the last decade, though there have been considerable variations from country to country.

Since the introduction of specific chemotherapy the indices of mortality and morbidity from tuberculosis are probably not as appropriate as they were, and the tuberculosis mortality rate in particular may give a misleading picture of the importance of the tuberculosis problem in a given country or region. It is known, in general, that if the mortality rate from tuberculosis in a country is high that the figures are so inaccurate as to be practically useless, and where the rate is low that it is a relatively insensitive index. Another source of inaccuracy is the designation as a tuberculous death where tuberculosis is only a minor post-mortem pathological abnormality. It is therefore not possible, or even desirable, to quote figures from various countries. Nevertheless, the mortality rate may still be of some use in countries where accurate records are kept. Notification rates or prevalence studies may give some general idea of the magnitude of the problem in different countries, and a generalization may be made whereby it can be stated that in many developing countries of the world the prevalence of tuberculosis is something of the order of 1 per cent. of the population, whereas in the technically advanced countries the prevalence is less than (and in some instances, very much less than) 1 per 1,000 of the population. The situation in England and Wales has recently been summarized by Springett (1972) and he has made the point that while tuberculosis has substantially declined in the last 25 years that in 1970 there were still 11,280 new notifications and 1,465 deaths were attributed to the condition. Springett (1971) has also pointed out that the mortality for tuberculosis in England and Wales for both sexes in 1945 was 50 per 100,000 of the population, that this had fallen to 4 per 100,000 by 1970 and by extrapolation he estimates that it should be of the order of 0·4 per 100,000 in 1995. In the same way the notification rate in 1945 was 100 per 100,000, 20 per 100,000 in 1970 and an estimated 2 per 100,000 in 1995.

It has been suggested (Styblo and Reil, 1967) that the following three parameters are more likely to give accurate information about tuberculosis either in technically advanced or in developing countries than the more traditional indices. These are: (1) the prevalence of tuberculous infection; (2) the prevalence of 'cases' of tuberculosis; and (3) the prevalence of drug-resistant tuberculosis. These three parameters are closely related, supplement one another, combine information about the past and the present, and may suggest future trends.

Prevalence of Tuberculous Infection

The first of the three parameters enumerated above, namely the prevalence of tuberculous infection, is usually studied in young people. The availability of a standard tuberculin product and of techniques for performing the tuberculin test have made it much easier than it was to estimate the prevalence of infection with *Mycobacterium tuberculosis*. In general, preference should be given to the intracutaneous Mantoux rather than the multiple-puncture Heaf or other test, using a properly administered standard dose of a well-standardized product, making

certain that the reaction is properly read. This is particularly important where comparisons are being made either between groups or between different countries. The use of 5 T.U. Purified Protein Derivative (P.P.D./R.T. 23) with Tween 80 is recommended. This is a purified protein derivative of tuberculin, of which a large batch has been made by the Statens Serum Institut, Copenhagen, under the aegis of the World Health Organization. Tween 80—a detergent—has been added in order to prevent deterioration of the preparation on dilution and storage. The test should be done and read 3 days later; the reading should be made in millimetres according to the largest transverse diameter of induration (or oedema), and not simply as a 'positive' or a 'negative'. Previously, different strengths of the tuberculin test were used, but studies in many parts of the world have demonstrated that nearly all persons infected by *Mycobacterium tuberculosis* will react to a weak dose of tuberculin, while allergies so weak as to be revealed only by a strong test seem to be non-specific, i.e. they represent a cross-reaction to some antigen other than the tubercle bacillus. These infections are often referred to as opportunist, anonymous, non-specific, or unclassified mycobacterial infections, and are thought to be due to such organisms as *Mycobacterium avium*. This non-specific sensitivity is more prevalent in tropical and sub-tropical countries—especially at low altitudes—than in temperate zones.

Sometimes it is necessary to come to an arbitrary decision as to whether a person tested is a 'reactor' or not, when, for instance, it is done before B.C.G. vaccination. In general, it can be stated that a reaction of less than 5 mm. means that the person has probably *not* been infected by *Mycobacterium tuberculosis*; that reactions of greater than 10 mm. probably mean that the person has been so infected, whereas with the reactions of between 5 and 9 mm. they may or may not have been infected, and further careful clinical and laboratory evaluation is required. Using the tuberculin test as a measure of prevalence of tuberculous infection, the World Health Organization (1965) has published a study from fifty-nine different countries or areas where subjects in age group 0–9 years had been investigated, and as can be seen from FIGURE 76, there is a very considerable variation in the prevalence of infection.

In many countries the tuberculin test is not a suitable means of assessing the problem of prevalence of infection, because B.C.G. vaccination has made it impossible to use this sensitive index for determining the ratio of the population infected with virulent mycobacteria. For the future, because allergy and immunity can be dissociated, it should be theoretically possible to produce a non-viable immunizing fraction of *Mycobacterium tuberculosis* that does not sensitize to tuberculin, thus avoiding the loss of the tuberculin test as an epidemiological and diagnostic tool after B.C.G. vaccination.

Finally, it has been suggested that the tuberculin test be used as an indication of success of measures against tuberculosis. Thus the World Health Organization has recommended, on Holm's (1959) suggestion, that the elimination of the disease as a public health problem could not be considered to have been achieved in most instances until the prevalence of natural reactors to tuberculin among children in the 14-year age group had become less than 1 per cent. No country has yet reached this low level of infection, but some are near to it.

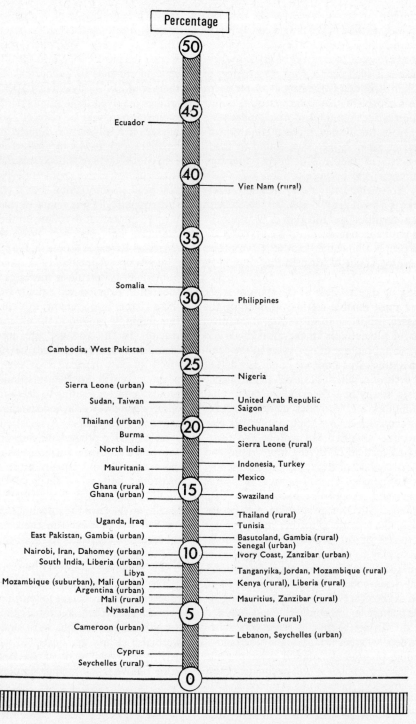

FIG. 76. Estimated prevalence of tuberculosis infection in age group 0–9 years in 59 countries or areas studied.

(*Chron. Wld Hlth Org.* (1965) **19**, No. 8, 313.)

Cases of Tuberculosis

The second of three parameters, namely the prevalence of 'cases' of tuberculosis, presents some problems, and the principal difficulty is the definition of what constitutes a case of tuberculosis. The problem of definition in itself has caused much controversy, especially by those who cannot or will not appreciate the somewhat unpalatable fact that at present there are considerable differences in resources between the technically advanced and the developing countries. In advanced societies a case of tuberculosis will be counted and recorded when notification is made to some central registry. This might result from the finding of tubercle bacilli in the sputum of a patient on direct smear, or only on culture, or because of a radiological abnormality suggestive of tuberculosis, or in the case of non-pulmonary disease, its diagnosis by other means. In developing countries, however, the best and indeed the only satisfactory method of defining a case is one in whom tubercle bacilli are demonstrated in the sputum (Deva-datta *et al.*, 1966). Priority for treatment must be given to these infectious cases, because it is such people who are a danger to the community, and their definition is the best available index of the size of the infector pool in that community. A single direct smear examination of the sputum is of much more relevance than a chest X-ray, as the former, if posititive, immediately defines an infectious case. It has been found in many countries that the majority of people with open pulmonary tuberculosis have symptoms, and because of these symptoms seek investigation and treatment. Individuals are more likely to come forward if there is a good general medical service with which the tuberculosis facilities are integrated. It must be stressed that unless or until adequate facilities are available for the treatment of these people who come because of symptoms —i.e. 'case getting', no programme of 'case finding' should be initiated.

Bacteriological testing by direct smear of the sputum is the simplest, cheapest, and most reliable method of defining the presence of active disease. Initial sputum testing, if positive, provides the diagnosis of tuberculosis in the individual, and therefore the incidence or appearance of new cases in the community. Serial sputum testing gives evidence of efficacy and of the taking of treatment in the individual. The over-all prevalence of sputum-positive cases at any one time indicates the total case load in the community and provides evidence of the quality of tuberculosis control measures. Sputum testing may be done either by the time-honoured but tedious and time-consuming Ziehl–Neelsen method or by the more rapid and equally accurate modern method of fluorescence microscopy. Admittedly there may be included a small number of people who are excreting acid- and alcohol-fast bacilli other than tubercle bacilli, but numerically this proportion will be extremely small. Culture of the sputum is neither necessary nor desirable in the first phase of tuberculosis control, but in affluent societies cultures may be done and the sensitivities of the organisms to the various antituberculous drugs determined.

Radiographs are the least good epidemiological index of disease, partly because of the observer variation in reading X-rays and partly because bacteriological confirmation is required to determine whether a radiological shadow represents active or inactive disease or indeed whether it represents tuberculosis at all. Mass X-ray finding programmes should never precede the development of such basic services as will adequately meet the needs of those seeking help because of symptoms. It is arguable whether mass miniature radiography campaigns are any longer justifiable in countries where there is very little tuberculosis. If X-rays are taken these should be on 70-mm. film, and fluoroscopy should never be employed, partly because of the greater radiation risk from this procedure and partly because of the absence of any permanent record.

Despite the fact that contact examination in tuberculosis case finding and control has been used for many years, there is still considerable controversy about its value. The yield from contact examination varies with the prevalence of infectious disease in the community, and comparisons between different reports cannot be precise because of different definitions. Thus Ferebee and Mount (1962) in the United States reported a yield of active tuberculosis with initial examination of 1·9 per cent. among adult and child household contacts. In Madras (Andrews *et al.*, 1960) there was a yield of 7 per cent.; in Kenya during 1959 (World Health Organization, 1961) 10 per cent. of contacts had abnormal X-rays, while in Korea (Struthers *et al.*, 1961) a yield of 12 per cent. was reported. All these studies involved large numbers of X-rays, and this amount of radiography could be reduced, and not many cases would be missed, if X-raying was limited to tuberculin-positive unvaccinated contacts. In the follow-up study in Madras (Kamat *et al.*, 1966), where B.C.G. was not used, 8 per cent. of initially tuberculin-negative contacts developed tuberculosis during the first year of observation, but a very much smaller percentage subsequently. It was found in that study and by others that it is more important to follow up the initially tuberculin-positive contacts, and especially those with initially large reactions (Medical Research Council, 1963; Ferebee and Mount, 1962). Almeida and Almeida (1964) point out that the likelihood of pulmonary tuberculosis increases steadily with the size of the tuberculin reaction and equally steadily with age. Taking both these factors into account, it is concluded that X-ray examination might be limited to the older age groups and to the strong reactors in the younger age groups. It should also be remembered that some cases of tuberculosis are only recognized at post-mortem, that even in Western Europe some people may still die from tuberculosis and that the commonest avoidable factor leading to death from tuberculosis is failure to observe generally accepted standards of practice (British Thoracic and Tuberculosis Association, 1971).

In general, a progressive case-finding programme for all, i.e. one which gradually increases its efficiency by the adoption of more refined (and usually more expensive) tools, should be instituted only when financially feasible. The primary aim should be to discover those people who are discharging tubercle bacilli, as they are the infectious sources through which transmission is maintained in the community, and the object of tuberculosis control is to break the chain of communication.

Drug-resistant Tuberculosis

The third parameter, the presence of persons excreting tubercle bacilli resistant to antituberculous drugs must now be considered. When antituberculous chemotherapy was first introduced its benefits were undoubted, but its limitations were also clearly demonstrated whereby, when one drug was used, the development of resistance by the organisms to that drug rendered its further employment useless. It has been confirmed in many studies that drug resistance is almost inevitable when one drug is used alone, is always clinically significant, is practically never reversible, and is probably the worst disaster that can befall an individual with tuberculosis today. Not only is the individual's own outlook then less good but he is a further menace to society and may infect other people with his drug-resistant organisms. Patients with tuberculosis who have received no previous treatment and whose pre-treatment cultures yield tubercle bacilli resistant to one or more drugs are described as having primary drug-resistant disease. Acquired or secondary drug resistance is the result of previous inefficient chemotherapy in one individual. The isolation of drug-resistant bacilli from a patient who has never been treated with drugs could have at least two explanations.

First, the patients could have been infected by drug-resistant bacilli from a person who had received inefficient treatment with these drugs, or secondly, the patient's bacterial population could have contained naturally resistant organisms. Evidence in support of the former hypothesis has been produced by several studies, and therefore primary resistance may be assumed to be the direct product of inefficient chemotherapy in another individual.

Knowledge of the prevalence of primary resistant disease is of importance for several reasons. A high or increasing prevalence suggests that drug-resistant strains are being spread from patients whose treatment has been unsatisfactory. This may reflect either current or previous chemotherapeutic regimens. Because patients with primary drug-resistant infections may fail to respond to treatment with standard drugs, the planning of chemotherapy for previously untreated tuberculosis, either in an individual or in a community, should be based on knowledge of the nature of drug resistance in the individual or in the community if it can be determined. Primary resistance in tuberculosis has been investigated in the United Kingdom by the Medical Research Council in two national surveys (Fox et al., 1957; Medical Research Council, 1966). In the first study the prevalence of primary resistance to streptomycin, para-aminosalicylic acid, and isoniazid, alone or in combination, was 4·5 per cent. Only 0·5 per cent. of patients harboured organisms resistant to more than one of these drugs. In the second survey the over-all prevalence of resistant disease was 4·1 per cent., and it was reassuring to find that over the seven-year period there has been no increase in primary resistance. These reports, however, should not lead to complacency, since resistant disease—as with any tuberculous disease—may remain latent for many years. Its prevalence in some other parts of the world is alarmingly high. In Hong Kong (Hong Kong/British Medical Research Council, 1964), for instance, the figure is 20 per cent.

As far as acquired or secondary resistance is concerned, there is a belief that the world total of patients excreting resistant organisms is increasing. In a study carried out in seventeen countries during 1957, Rist and Crofton (1960) demonstrated that from patients who admitted to receiving chemotherapy previously no fewer than 42 per cent. of cultures yielded organisms resistant to one of the first-line drugs. Comparison of the prevalence of acquired resistant disease in different surveys is difficult because of difference in bacteriological techniques and criteria of resistance, but in general, reports from India (Frimodt-Möller, 1962), Africa (Bell and Brown, 1961), Hong Kong (Hong Kong/British Medical Research Council, 1964), and Poland (Zierski, 1964) suggest that at least 50 per cent. of patients first seen in hospitals or clinics with a previous history of chemotherapy are excreting resistant organisms.

Drug-resistant tuberculosis is a measure of the efficacy of past treatment and the extent of future problems. Secondary or acquired resistance in a community declines as treatment improves or clinically infectious cases die; it will increase if treatment is less efficient or if badly treated patients come into a community from other areas. Changes in prevalence of secondary resistance are relatively easy to interpret, as they reflect happenings in the recent past, but changes in primary resistance are less easy to interpret because, for example, one badly treated patient this year may produce a case of primary resistant disease twenty years hence. Drug-resistant tuberculosis is world-wide, and the ultimate solution of the problem depends on the measures of control applied on a global scale. The problem of drug-resistant disease has been particularly relevant in the United Kingdom in recent years because of the immigrant population, who make a large contribution not only to the prevalence of newly notified cases but also to drug-resistant cases in some areas of Britain. This is worthy of some detailed consideration, partly because of its importance in its own right, partly as an example of the application of epidemiological methods to its study, and partly because other countries, especially in Western Europe, may have similar problems either now or in the future.

Tuberculosis in Immigrants in the United Kingdom

One of the residual but quite considerable problems in the United Kingdom today is that of tuberculosis among immigrants. Immigrants from Asian, African, and Caribbean countries have come to the United Kingdom in large numbers since about 1954. The impression that tuberculosis is commoner among immigrants than among the British-born population has been confirmed by various workers, particularly in the Midlands of England (Springett, 1964, in Birmingham; Stevenson, 1962, and Edgar, 1964, in Bradford; Aspin, 1962, in Wolverhampton). Springett found in Birmingham that the highest prevalence of disease was among the Pakistani population, with a notification rate of 18·2/1,000/year in men, compared with British-born subjects, who had a rate of 0·68/1,000/year—a factor of about 20 times. He also found that Indians living in this area had a notification rate of 4·5/1,000/year in men compared with the 0·68/1,000/year previously noted, i.e. a factor of about 6 times. As far as immigrants from Ireland and the West Indies were concerned, the notification rate was between 2 and 4 times that of the British-born population.

A further detailed survey was carried out by the British Tuberculosis Association (1966) in chest clinics throughout England and Wales. This study confirmed that persons born in countries other than the United Kingdom and Ireland contributed a disproportionate share of notified cases. Thus, in the study under review (3 months in 1965), when 3,806 new cases of tuberculosis were notified, 16·5 per cent. occurred in immigrants who formed only 4 per cent. of the total population, and of the total notifications 9·6 per cent. were from India and Pakistan, who formed only 1 per cent. of the total population. It was also found that the Indian and Pakistani patients had a higher proportion of non-respiratory tuberculosis than British-born subjects. The national survey of primary drug resistance (Medical Research Council, 1966) showed that primary drug resistance was more common in the immigrants than in British-born patients, and was commoner in those who had recently arrived in the United Kingdom.

There are three possible explanations for the high prevalence of tuberculosis among the immigrant population. First, it is possible that the immigrants come suffering from tuberculosis; secondly, that they come with latent tuberculosis, which breaks down on arrival in this country, or thirdly, they become infected when they reach this country, possibly from their fellow countrymen with whom they live in close proximity. It is considered that the likeliest explanation is that immigrants bring their disease with them, coming as they do from areas of the world where tuberculosis is common. The problem of tuberculosis among the immigrant population poses difficulties and stretches resources in some parts of the United Kingdom, particularly in the Midlands of England and in London. Until 1962 no health check was required for immigrants coming into the country, but in that year the Commonwealth Immigration Act became law. This gave an immigration officer a right to refuse entry if, on medical advice, the immigrant appeared to be 'suffering from mental disorder or that it was otherwise undesirable for medical reasons that he should be admitted'. Nevertheless, there are administrative difficulties, and it is not practicable to set up examination centres at all possible ports of entry to this country. A better scheme would be to have compulsory medical examinations with a chest X-ray conducted in the immigrant's own country of origin, but this, too, poses both medical and political problems. It would seem reasonable, nevertheless, that some form of screening of immigrants be done, partly to protect the health of the citizens of this country but also in the interest of the immigrants themselves.

Other Methods of Assessment

Emphasis has been laid on the foregoing epidemiological indices, but it should be remembered that there are other methods of obtaining information. Thus by routine reporting of cases to tuberculosis registers fairly accurate information may be obtained, but this is dependent on the quality of the health service in general. Such registers should if possible be built into any scheme of tuberculosis control. The carrying out of either prevalence or of longitudinal surveys should also be done as the occasion arises, and may help to define over-all problems. A prevalence study is useful to determine the size of the problem, though it gives information only at a single point of time. Longitudinal surveys, which are long-term studies of groups, may give information about epidemiological trends, but such studies, though useful, are expensive and time-consuming. The formulation of an efficient tuberculosis control programme under widely varying and rapidly changing conditions rests on the ability to measure the size of the problem. The efficacy of any programme is to be measured not by the number of cases found but by the number effectively treated, by the number successfully followed up, and most of all, by changes in the incidence of the disease. Any national tuberculosis control programme must be on a countrywide and permanent basis, and should be neither sporadic nor patchy. If possible, tuberculosis control should be integrated into the general medical services, and economic considerations demand that such a programme be within the national resources.

In summary, a national tuberculosis control programme must: (1) measure the extent of the problem; (2) adjust its techniques to local conditions; and (3) train personnel for the programmes. This last requirement will include both undergraduate and postgraduate medical instruction, together with paramedical personnel training.

The cost of different programmes must also be taken into account. A computer model has been developed to express the benefits against the cost (Feldstein, 1973).

TREATMENT OF TUBERCULOSIS

Although countries should be actively concerned with programmes aimed at improving the social and economic status of the population, they could make their most effective contribution as far as tuberculosis is concerned by concentrating skills and available resources on the specific aspects of tuberculosis control. Thus attention should be focused on control in those countries where tuberculosis is a serious public health problem and the best use has to be made of limited resources. There can be little doubt that the most important aspect of this is treatment of tuberculosis in the individual, for this is beneficial not only to that individual but also in relation to prevention of the disease in the community. Host factors, such as the type of disease or the patient's immune response, become of decreasing importance as the potency of drug treatment increases. The destruction of the bacilli is done not by the patient but by antituberculous drugs.

While the treatment of tuberculosis has to a large extent become standardized in most countries, there will inevitably be differences in the type of case treated, the type of treatment given, and the duration of that treatment under different conditions. Many of the desiderata are related to finances and to priorities in relation to resources. Thus, undesirable though it may be, and perhaps for some time to come, a two-tier system as far as the treatment of tuberculosis is concerned is inevitable. In the immediately succeeding section general principles of treatment will be considered that should obtain in highly developed industrialized communities with adequate financial and other resources, where the aim is eradication of tuberculosis. These principles should also apply in the developing countries, though their implementation may have to be somewhat modified, as will be described. All forms of tuberculosis respond to chemotherapy, with little need for specialized ancillary methods of treatment and in planning treatment programmes there is no need to make separate provision for the different clinical types of the disease.

TREATMENT OF TUBERCULOSIS IN TECHNICALLY ADVANCED COUNTRIES

The aim of treatment is to find every active or potentially active case of tuberculosis and to bring each case under treatment. This will usually mean long-term chemotherapy, often with initial hospitalization, the provision of free drugs, and social security while the patient is under therapy.

Standard Chemotherapy

It is now fairly generally considered wise to start treatment of fresh cases of tuberculosis with triple drug therapy by means of streptomycin by intramuscular injection together with para-aminosalicylic acid and isoniazid by mouth. It is assumed that in each case, where possible, bacteriological confirmation will be obtained by direct smear, culture, a positive niacin test, and that sensitivity tests will be inaugurated so that precise chemotherapy may be prescribed. If there is a history of inadequate or ineffective therapy in the past drugs other than the standard ones may have to be employed pending the results of sensitivity tests.

While regimens vary somewhat from country to country, it is now fairly well established that the initial therapy should consist of streptomycin, 1 G. in a single dose intramuscularly each day (0·75 G. if over 40 years of age) together with para-aminosalicylic acid in the dose of 10–12 G. in two divided doses and isoniazid in a dose of 300 mg./day, also in two divided doses (Medical Research Council, 1962). This chemotherapy should be continued at least until the sensitivity pattern of the organisms is known, when it is usually possible to dispense with one of the drugs. Usually streptomycin is stopped, and the patient continues on a combination of para-aminosalicylic acid and isoniazid most conveniently given in combined form by cachet. The aim of any antituberculous chemotherapeutic regimen is to render the patient non-infectious, and if possible to eradicate the tubercle bacilli from the body, at the same time preventing the emergence of drug resistance. The use of two antituberculous drugs in combination will prevent the latter, and the continuation of treatment for between 18 months and 2 years will almost invariably ensure the former. In patients suffering from tuberculosis whose organisms are initially sensitive it should be possible to achieve 100 per cent. sputum conversion with virtually no relapse. Physicians must prescribe treatment accurately, must be obsessional in getting their patients to take the prescribed treatment, and there should be an understanding of the importance of impeccable chemotherapy by both parties. Supervised intermittent chemotherapy with twice-weekly streptomycin and high doses of isoniazid (see later) has been recommended in the United Kingdom by Poole and Stradling (1970). That virtually 100 per cent. sputum conversion is possible has been demonstrated in Edinburgh by Ross et al. (1958) and in Birmingham (Thomas et al., 1960). That it has been possible in very many other countries was demonstrated by a report from the International Union against Tuberculosis (1964), where a successful co-operative study in twenty-nine centres was reported. The last few years has seen the introduction of new major chemotherapeutic drugs for tuberculosis, namely rifampicin and ethambutol. Both are powerful and effective though their precise place in chemotherapy has yet to be established. While both are relatively free from serious side-effects, high dosage of ethambutol may lead to ocular toxicity and rifampicin—especially seemingly if given intermittently—may lead to liver damage and thrombocytopenia (Poole et al., 1971; Aquinas et al., 1972). One of the most interesting and exciting possibilities of these drugs is that their introduction may lead eventually to a reduction in the time of treatment required (East African/British Medical Research Council (1972)) and while at present they are expensive, a reduction in time might well offset the high cost.

Treatment of Drug-resistant Tuberculosis

Until recently if a patient was thought or known to have drug resistant tuberculosis the so-called second line or reserve drugs were employed namely, pyrazinamide, ethionamide, cycloserine, thiacetazone, viomycin, and capreomycin. While many of these drugs are very effective antituberculous agents, they are—with the exception of thiacetazone—very considerably more expensive and also very much more toxic. Treatment with these drugs is time-consuming and requires a very considerable amount of persuasion on behalf of the attendant physician and determination on behalf of the patient to take

them for a sufficient length of time. This can, however, be done (British Tuberculosis Association, 1963; Somner and Brace, 1966; Tousek et al., 1967), but it is hoped that with the more general application of good chemotherapy that the number of occasions when second-line therapy will have to be used will become less. With the introduction of rifampicin and ethambutol, however, it seems probable that the management of such cases will be easier and encouraging reports are appearing in the literature (Somner et al., 1971). It is still better to prevent failures than to have to treat them.

Other Considerations and Treatment

There has been a considerable amount of discussion recently whether patients suffering from tuberculosis should be admitted to hospital for any length of time for treatment. The reasons for and against this will be considered more fully in the next section, but it should be remembered that under the conditions of modern technically advanced countries with adequate resources, a 100 per cent. cure rate of tuberculosis should be aimed at, and it has been shown that this can be achieved with good chemotherapy, together with an initial period of hospitalization. It is difficult to recommend that anything less good than this scheme of treatment should be instituted unless or until ambulatory chemotherapy in the technically advanced countries has been shown to be as good as the current schemes. Furthermore, the fact should not be lost sight of that the use of hospital beds for the treatment of tuberculosis shows a 'good return', inasmuch as practically all the patients survive to leave hospital and that the great majority subsequently lead a gainful life. This is more than can be said for the results of hospital treatment of many other conditions. In both the technically advanced and in developing countries hospitalization will inevitably be required for a number of people suffering from tuberculosis, who will include the very sick and those with complications or emergencies, those with concomitant disease, and perhaps those with drug hypersentitivity reactions and the small number who will require surgery.

In summary, tuberculosis therapy in the technically advanced countries must be based on: (1) antituberculous chemotherapy with both main and reserve drugs in adequate supplies to provide a course of chemotherapy of up to 2 years or even longer for every patient; (2) a laboratory service that can undertake numbers of cultures for tubercle bacilli and also sensitivity tests; (3) frequent radiographic examinations; (4) a hospital service with highly equipped thoracic surgical units; and (5) extensive chest clinics. These facilities must be applied in an efficient administrative framework which will include notification of the disease and the collection of other tuberculosis statistics as well as the application of preventive measures. With such facilities, there has been the suggestion that the definition of what constitutes a case suitable for chemotherapy should be broadened. In most centres it is generally agreed that active, inactive, and suspect tuberculosis (Scottish Thoracic Society, 1963; Pamra and Mathur, 1971) should have chemotherapy and also that children with a positive tuberculin reaction under the age of 6 years should be regarded as having active disease and treated. It is important to recognize that in these foregoing groups the chemotherapy that is given should be at least with two drugs, as it constitutes treatment and is in no way a 'prophylactic' measure. While the immediate and short term side-effects of antituberculous chemotherapy have been long recognized it is only now that some of the long-term effects are being documented. One of these is the development of aspergilloma in residual tuberculous cavities (British Thoracic and Tuberculosis Association, 1970) and while this may not be numerically a large problem it is one that may well be more frequently recognized in the future.

Chemoprophylaxis Against Tuberculosis

It has been shown experimentally that guinea-pigs after being treated with isoniazid can receive a challenge dose of virulent tubercle bacilli without developing acute disseminated tuberculosis. It was thought therefore that because isoniazid was cheap, safe, convenient, and an effective killer of tubercle bacilli it could be used not only for the treatment of tuberculosis but also for its prevention. The terms primary and secondary chemoprophylaxis have been suggested, though they have not been universally accepted. Primary chemoprophylaxis in tuberculosis aims at the prevention of infection, secondary prophylaxis at the prevention of disease in people already infected. Isoniazid has been used in both instances usually in the dose of 5–10 mg./kg. body weight for children or a total of 300 mg. for adults given daily in a single dose for a year.

Encouraging results of prophylaxis have recently been reported by Comstock et al. (1967) in Alaska. These favourable results have been reinforced by a more recent report of a 9-year trial of chemoprophylaxis in San Francisco schools (Curry, 1967), in which the results of 2,910 reactors given isoniazid for a year were compared with those in 1,192 reactors whose parents refused this medication for their children. Among those receiving isoniazid, tuberculous lesions developed in only 1 (0·34 per 1,000)—and this in a recent convertor who had not taken the drug regularly—compared with 25 of the untreated group (20·9 per 1,000). The risk, therefore, of developing a tuberculous lesion was many times greater in those not receiving isoniazid. It has been suggested (American Thoracic Society, 1967) that chemoprophylaxis be used more extensively. Thus, patients who may have had inadequate or no drug therapy with a positive tuberculin test and X-ray evidence suggestive of healed adult pulmonary tuberculosis might receive chemoprophylaxis, as might household contacts of active cases with 5 mm. or more of induration to P.P.D., reactors under the age of 20, and known convertors in all age groups. In addition, it might be recommended that chemoprophylaxis be given to any tuberculin-positive patient who has to have corticosteroid therapy, who has to have a gastrectomy, who develops a disease of the reticulo-endothelial system, or has a period of instability of severe diabetes.

Chemoprophylaxis has not been widely adopted, partly because in countries such as the United Kingdom there does not seem to be any impelling need, and partly because there is an understandable reluctance to give only one drug when dealing with tuberculosis. The dividing line between chemoprophylaxis and treatment in tuberculosis is not easy to define, and the most difficult decision to make is whether groups of people (most of whom will be healthy) should be advised to take isoniazid daily for a whole year or more where, even with encouragement and close supervision, the default rate is likely

to be considerable. The risk of drug resistance cannot be discounted, but theoretically in enclosed lesions of low bacterial population this outcome should not be common. Another possible difficulty in recommending isoniazid chemoprophylaxis is the demonstration that this drug can produce neoplasms of the lung and lymph nodes in albino mice. How far, if at all, this finding is relevant to man is not known, but the enormous value of isoniazid as an antituberculous drug should not be lost sight of. Hammond et al. (1967), in a recent study, came to the conclusion that, taken as a whole, their follow-up studies of patients previously treated with isoniazid were reassuring and that they could find no convincing evidence of an increased cancer risk among men, women, or children so treated.

Further work is clearly indicated by means of controlled clinical trials, and cost-comparability studies with B.C.G. should be done in the wealthier countries where eradication rather than control of tuberculosis is the goal. The whole question of chemoprophylaxis is discussed in detail by Ferebee (1970).

TREATMENT OF TUBERCULOSIS IN THE DEVELOPING COUNTRIES

Under the conditions of developing countries, and largely because of financial considerations, ideal treatment as defined in the preceding section may not be possible. Nevertheless, it is clear that as good chemotherapy as possible must be given to all cases of tuberculosis as soon as possible, and the objects of treatment should be the same, namely to render the patient non-infectious and to prevent the emergence of drug-resistant strains of organisms.

Drug Treatment

It should be the aim in developing countries to provide one year of free effective antituberculous chemotherapy for every newly diagnosed case of tuberculosis. The main antituberculous drugs to be used are isoniazid, streptomycin, para-aminosalicylic acid, and thiacetazone. The factors governing their use are efficacy, cost, freedom from toxicity, and the ease of administration. An efficient organization is essential to ensure adequate drug taking and to promote co-operation in relation to local cultural and social settings. While in some of the developing countries standard chemotherapy with isoniazid, streptomycin, and para-aminosalicylic acid may be possible, this is not generally so. Nevertheless, this is the goal to be aimed at, and should be given where possible. From the general principle that active tuberculosis requires two drugs for treatment, the use of isoniazid and para-aminosalicylic acid has been extensively studied (East African/British Medical Research Council, 1960; Fox, 1964). In general, this has been found to be an effective and an acceptable combination of drugs, and provided it is accurately prescribed by the physician and assiduously taken by the patient, a very high rate of bacterial quiescence can be achieved at the end of one year's treatment. Nevertheless, in many developing countries even this regimen may be too expensive, and para-aminosalicylic acid, apart from its expense, does not keep well in tropical countries, is bulky, and is unpleasant to take. Other regimens therefore have been tried, and in particular the efficacy of thiacetazone as a cheap companion drug to isoniazid has been extensively studied. The combination of thiacetazone and isoniazid in one tablet costs only one-tenth of that of the combination of isoniazid and para-aminosalicylic acid.

Many studies have been done, particularly in East Africa, and after testing various dose levels it has been shown that the most effective combination of thiacetazone and isoniazid was a combined tablet in a single daily dose of thiacetazone, 150 mg. and isoniazid, 300 mg. The dosage of the two drugs was shown to be critical, and no advantage arose from a higher dose of isoniazid (East African/British Medical Research Council, 1963, 1966 a and b, 1970; Tuberculosis Chemotherapy Centre, 1966). At the end of one year more than 80 per cent. of patients had bacteriologically quiescent disease. Not only was this combination cheap and effective but in East Africa at least with a level of toxicity similar to that of para-aminosalicylic acid. It was also shown in East Africa that the addition of streptomycin, 1 G. daily for the first two months, substantially improved the results when assessed at the end of one year, but at the same time quite considerably increased the cost of the treatment. Thiacetazone toxicity in several countries has been studied by Miller et al. (1966) and by Ferguson et al. (1971), and there is a suggestion of genuine differences between countries, with Czechoslovakia, Hong Kong, and Pakistan having the highest levels, and Cyprus and India the lowest. The reasons for these differences are not known, but might include racial, dietary, climatic, or reporting differences. It is suggested therefore that before a general scheme of thiacetazone and isoniazid be used a pilot study be made in order to determine acceptability of the drugs. If toxicity is high other regimens may perforce have to be resorted to, and the use of pyrazinamide and ethionamide has been described in Hong Kong by Aquinas (1963).

The above scheme of treatment is largely dependent on the patient taking the drugs in an unsupervised way. An alternative regimen of intermittent chemotherapy has been tested in Southern India with direct supervision (Tuberculosis Chemotherapy Centre, 1964; Nazareth et al., 1966). Studies have been made whereby patients have had 1 G. of streptomycin with isoniazid in a single high dose on two days in the week. The dosage of isoniazid given was equivalent to 14 mg./kg. of body weight with 6 mg. of pyridoxine in order to combat neurotoxicity. This regimen of treatment was found to be effective and acceptable, whereas a regimen of once-weekly streptomycin and isoniazid was found not to be so (Menon, 1965; Tuberculosis Chemotherapy Centre (1970)). It should be remembered that this was done in a suburb of Madras with full and very adequate ancillary services. Whether such treatment could be carried out as efficiently in the rural areas of the developing countries is open to some doubt, as some 80 per cent. of the population in many developing countries live outside the larger towns, though Chaulet et al. (1967) have recommended this regimen in Algeria.

Various other combinations of drugs, dosages, and time schedules have been or are being tried out, including the use in some centres of isoniazid alone as primary treatment of tuberculosis. While this last scheme gives immediately fairly satisfactory results, it is considered by the author that the residual problems of an inevitable proportion of drug-resistant tuberculosis far outweigh any initial benefit that might be obtained. It is probably safer in fact to give efficient (as regards drug combination) but inadequate (as regards time) chemo-

therapy in the hope that the financial situation might improve in the future rather than inefficient chemotherapy in any shape or form. This is particularly important, as second-line drugs are expensive and toxic, and in developing countries should not compete for finances until all newly diagnosed cases are given the best possible treatment with standard chemotherapy. A case can be made for a second year of treatment with isoniazid alone after an initial year of combined chemotherapy (Nazareth et al., 1971). There is probably no place for any collapse method of treatment now and very little place for surgical treatment of pulmonary tuberculosis either in developing countries or elsewhere. Very occasionally surgery will be necessary in some drug-resistant cases and in persistently poor drug takers.

In children in developing countries as elsewhere in the world if a positive tuberculin reaction is discovered under the age of 6 years adequate chemotherapy must be given. If, in developing countries, a mother with active tuberculosis gives birth to a child it is unrealistic and unhelpful to separate the child from its mother, and while the mother is receiving chemotherapy the child should if possible be given isoniazid-resistant B.C.G. together with prophylactic isoniazid by mouth in the hope that infection of the child by the mother will be prevented.

Other Considerations in Treatment

Some further detailed consideration must now be given to the question of hospital versus home treatment. The traditional treatment of pulmonary tuberculosis in Western Europe was a sanatorium regimen with long bedrest, graduated activity, and segregation of the patients from the general population. It has been estimated that the cost of hospital treatment is about fifteen times greater than that for out-patient management. A detailed study has been done in Madras by the Tuberculosis Chemotherapy Centre (1959), where home and hospital management of pulmonary tuberculosis has been compared. Although this report from Madras first appeared in 1959, clinicians have been reluctant to accept the results of this study and the implications therefrom. The results are important and worth quoting in some detail. 193 patients were admitted to a study, of whom 163 were found to have drug-sensitive sputum cultures and allocated at random so that 82 had home treatment and 81 hospital treatment. One year of treatment was given in each group with para-aminosalicylic acid in daily doses of 7·5–10 G. together with isoniazid 150–200 mg. according to weight. The drugs were given together in cachets in two divided doses. In hospital this was supervised and the drugs were shown to have been taken by urine testing in 8 out of 10 cases, whereas at home only 1 in 3 cases when tested gave evidence of having taken their drugs. In 4 out of 10 patients treated at home the diet consisted of less than 50 g. of protein/day, whereas in hospital all had more than this. Thus the patients at home had less rest, less food, and took drugs less regularly than those in hospital, but in contrast the patients at home co-operated better, inasmuch as only 1 absconded, whereas 12 in the hospital group absconded. All the patients suffered from advanced pulmonary tuberculosis and were randomly allocated to the two groups, but by chance the home group had rather more extensive disease, larger cavities, and a more heavily positive sputum than the hospital patients, and therefore the home patients could be said to have been at a considerable apparent disadvantage. At the end of 1 year's treatment 1 patient in the home group had died, whereas 2 in the hospital group had died. Bacterial quiescence at 1 year—defined as negative cultures in the last 3 specimens—showed that 78 per cent. of men at home had quiescent disease and 82 per cent. of men in the hospital group had quiescent disease, but these figures were not statistically significantly different. Analysis of the women was difficult because of greater pre-treatment differences and small absolute numbers. The conclusion reached initially was that one year's treatment at home was no worse for men than treatment in hospital.

These cases have been followed up for 5 years (Dawson et al., 1966), and almost all in the latter 4 years as out-patients. At the end of that time 90 per cent. had bacteriologically quiescent disease—a quite remarkable achievement considering the adverse circumstances under which these people were managed—and there was still no difference between those treated at home and those treated in hospital. It was also found that the incidence of active tuberculosis and of tuberculous infection was no greater in the contacts of patients treated at home than in the contacts of patients treated in hospital, either in the first or over the subsequent years (Andrews et al., 1960; Kamat et al., 1966; Devadatta et al., 1970). The major risk to contacts resulted from exposure to the patient before diagnosis. On the basis of this and other supporting studies, it is recommended that in developing countries all available man-power and resources should be confined to organizing an efficient ambulatory service and not used for building new hospitals or providing more beds for tuberculous patients.

It should be remembered that the home treatment in Madras was very closely supervised by health visitors and a very efficient administration, and it may not be true to say that any home treatment is as good as hospital treatment, but it is almost certainly true that if good home treatment can be given good hospital treatment gives no demonstrable advantage. Having said that as far as developing countries are concerned, many clinicians in technically advanced countries have extrapolated these results and suggest that lessons might be learnt that would be applicable in their own countries. It should be borne in mind, however, that the results in Madras showed evidence of 90 per cent. quiescence at the end of the 5-year period, whereas one would hope for 100 per cent. bacteriological quiescence in patients with initially drug-sensitive organisms in technically advanced countries.

B.C.G. VACCINATION

It is now more than 45 years since B.C.G. (Bacille Calmette-Guérin) was first used in man, but its value as a protective agent is still a matter of controversy for various reasons (Hart, 1967). B.C.G. vaccine is now prepared in many centres from a variety of sub-strains all derived from an attenuated strain of a *Mycobacterium tuberculosis* var. *bovis* originally isolated by Calmette and Guérin at the Institute Pasteur of Lille. All are living vaccines and are issued in liquid or freeze-dried forms. From the technical point of view there is the operational advantage of heat-stable freeze-dried vaccine in hot climates, and also administratively there is an advantage of giving simultaneous B.C.G. and smallpox vaccination. It is recommended that in

general B.C.G. should be given by syringe by the intracutaneous method (World Health Organization, 1966).

Rationale for Using Vaccine

It is known that the consequence of a primary infection with virulent tubercle bacilli in a group of previously uninfected persons is that a small minority develops progressive clinical tuberculosis, but that the great majority is left with enhanced resistance to subsequent infections with virulent tubercle bacilli. Infection of a group of previously uninfected individuals with B.C.G. vaccine, however, does not lead to progressive disease (except in extremely rare circumstances). The aim of B.C.G. vaccination is therefore to replace the natural, potentially harmful, and less predictable primary infection with virulent tubercle bacilli by an artificial and innocuous primary nfection with avirulent bacilli in the hope that this artificial infection will similarly enhance resistance to subsequent infection by virulent tubercle bacilli.

Efficacy of B.C.G. Vaccine

The efficacy of B.C.G. vaccination against tuberculosis in man has been measured in six properly randomized field studies throughout the world. (Aronson et al., 1958; Rosenthal et al., 1961; Palmer et al., 1958; Medical Research Council, 1963; Frimodt-Möller et al., 1964; and Comstock and Palmer, 1966). The efficacy of B.C.G. is usually expressed as a percentage reduction of the attack rate of tuberculosis in the vaccinated group compared with the unvaccinated controls. This figure in the various studies has varied between 14 and 80 per cent. protection [see TABLE 61], and it is because of this quite striking difference that much controversy has centred.

TABLE 61

Results of Six Published Controlled Trials of B.C.G. Vaccination against Tuberculosis

Period of intake	Authors	Population groups	Percentage efficiency B.C.G.
1935–38	Aronson et al. (1958)	North American Indians	80
1937–48	Rosenthal et al. (1961)	Chicago infants	74
1949–51	Palmer et al. (1958)	Puerto Rican children	31
1950	Comstock and Palmer (1966)	Georgia/Alabama	14
1950–52	Medical Research Council (1963)	U.K. schoolchildren	79
1950–55	Frimodt-Möller et al. (1964)	South Indian villagers	69

There are four possible reasons for these discrepant findings: (1) methodological differences; (2) differences in population groups; (3) differences in immunizing potency of the vaccine; and (4) differences in tubercle bacilli in different areas. As far as (1) is concerned there is no evidence that this has contributed to the differences, as all the studies were on a large scale and all involved random allocation. In relation to (2) one of the possible reasons for the differences is the occurrence of natural infection by opportunist mycobacteria, as there is evidence that such infection can affect the efficacy of B.C.G. vaccination.

Thus, in a population exposed to the risk of tuberculous infection it has been found that those with weak degrees of tuberculin sensitivity are at less risk of contracting tuberculosis subsequently than those with no detectable tuberculin sensitivity and also less than those with a strong degree of tuberculin sensitivity. In the last group this is an indication of past infection with virulent tubercle bacilli, whereas those with weak degrees of tuberculin sensitivity are often an indication of past infection with the opportunist mycobacteria. The suggestion has been made that opportunist infections act in a similar way to B.C.G. and provide an innocuous primary infection that enhances resistance to subsequent infection with tubercle bacilli. But the efficiency of this naturally occurring vaccination is less than that of B.C.G. and probably depends on the nature of the mycobacterial infection. It has been shown experimentally (Palmer and Long, 1966) that opportunist infection together with B.C.G. increases the efficiency to that of the B.C.G. alone but no higher. Thus in a population, if a proportion of the group has already acquired a degree of resistance to future virulent infection from past opportunist mycobacterial infection and B.C.G. vaccination is only able to enhance that resistance to a limited extent, the observed efficacy of B.C.G. vaccination will correspond only to this limited enhancement. It will be less than if the same vaccine were used in a population group free from all mycobacterial infection, and thus without any acquired resistance. It has been suggested (Hart, 1967) that this may explain the differences between the Georgia and Alabama groups and that of the United Kingdom, as opportunist mycobacterial infection is much less prevalent in the United Kingdom than in tropical and sub-tropical countries. In the United Kingdom too, 100 TU tuberculin were given and therefore vaccination was given only to 'true' negatives. But this is probably only a partial explanation of the differences, and it is suggested that (3) differences in the potency of the B.C.G. vaccination might well account for a proportion of the differences. As far as (4) is concerned, there is very little evidence of this, though it has been demonstrated that tubercle bacilli found in Southern India are less virulent than those of some other countries.

As far as the duration of protection is concerned, efficacy remains substantial in currently reported follow-up studies, both in North American Indians and in the United Kingdom trials. It has also been shown that B.C.G. is effective irrespective of the age and time of vaccination, and was the same for Chicago infants as for the United Kingdom schoolchildren. It has also been shown that it provides good protection against the most severe forms of the disease, namely miliary and meningeal tuberculosis. As far as revaccination is concerned, there is some suggestion that with vaccine of known potency revaccination is unnecessary, even if the tuberculin test has become negative.

In many countries it is now accepted that 'direct' vaccination be done, i.e. that B.C.G. vaccination be given without prior tuberculin testing. This has been objected to by some, as inevitably, after infancy, some previously infected people will be given B.C.G., but there is no evidence that there is any increased risk of producing progressive clinical disease or for that matter is there any evidence that any additional protection is given by the B.C.G. Direct vaccination has the advantage of avoidance of boredom by the B.C.G. teams in developing countries, and because it saves one visit, produces a lower default rate in subjects.

B.C.G. has not been shown to provide any protection against sarcoidosis or other chest diseases, but it has been shown by Brown et al. (1968) working in Uganda that it does protect children against the early manifestations of leprosy, and therefore has a dual purpose in many developing countries. The order of protection by B.C.G. is approximately 80 per cent. Furthermore, it is of interest to note that the protection given against leprosy to children known to have weak degrees of tuberculin sensitivity was as great as those without, so that local opportunist mycobacterial infections apparently do not protect against leprosy.

Scope of B.C.G. Vaccination

There are two theoretical circumstances where B.C.G. is useless; first, if all members of the community are tuberculin-positive and therefore there would be no scope for protection; secondly, if all members of the community were tuberculin-negative with no likelihood of infection, then there would be no need for any protection. Otherwise the scope of B.C.G. is largely a matter of judgement. Given that B.C.G. offers some degree of protection, its greatest benefit would occur in a community all of whom were tuberculin-negative and all of whom were likely to be infected within the next few years, but this is almost as unlikely as the two extremes envisaged above. The effect of B.C.G. vaccination policy on a community may usefully be expressed in terms of absolute reduction in the annual attack rate of tuberculosis in the whole population which is expected as a result of the vaccination policies. This expected reduction is calculated as a product of three factors: (1) the annual attack rate of tuberculosis and the absence of vaccination among those eligible; (2) the efficacy of the vaccine among those eligible; and (3) the proportion of the whole population which is eligible for vaccination.

In general, one might consider three situations where B.C.G. might be envisaged: (1) In a country with many tuberculin-positive people and a high conversion rate. This is a situation in many developing countries where facilities are limited. B.C.G. in these circumstances would be most effective in newborn children. (2) In a country where there were many tuberculin-positive people with the infection rate falling from previous high levels. This is in fact occurring in many countries where there is good chemotherapy, and B.C.G., in these circumstances, is probably maximally effective at puberty. (3) In countries with a very low infection rate B.C.G. is no longer of real value, and the cost of the scheme and the disadvantages of artificial tuberculin conversion can no longer justify its use (Springett, 1965). At present it would seem, especially in countries with a considerable amount of tuberculosis, that B.C.G. vaccination is a more feasible method of prevention than isoniazid chemoprophylaxis.

In summary, B.C.G. vaccine when given to a subject not previously infected with tubercle bacilli is capable of conferring a substantial degree of protection against subsequent tuberculosis infection. The efficacy of a potent vaccine, i.e. the percentage reduction in the attack rate of tuberculosis in those vaccinated is of the order of 80 per cent. Protection applies to all forms of the disease and remains substantial more than ten years after vaccination. With a potent vaccine the efficacy of B.C.G. in a community in which opportunist mycobacterial infection is widespread is likely to be of the order of between 50 and 60 per cent.

Tuberculosis is a global problem today, but measures are available for its control and subsequent eradication. It is suggested that the gap that exists between the technically advanced and the developing countries could be bridged by international co-operation, and particularly by a maintained medical interest in tuberculosis in the more fortunate countries and a direction of that interest towards other countries' difficulties.

REFERENCES

Epidemiology

Almeida, F. das N., and Almeida, J. M. das N. (1964) Relation between degree of tuberculin sensitivity and prevalence of tuberculosis, *Bull. Wld Hlth Org.*, 30, 519.

British Thoracic and Tuberculosis Association (1971) A survey of tuberculosis mortality in England and Wales in 1968, *Tubercle (Lond.)*, 52, 1.

Devadatta, S., Radhakrishna, S., Fox, W., Mitchison, D. A., Rajagopalan, S., Sivasubramanian, S., and Stott, H. (1966) Comparative value of sputum smear examination and culture examination in assessing the progress of tuberculous patients receiving chemotherapy, *Bull. Wld Hlth Org.*, 34, 573.

Holm, J. (1959) How can elimination of tuberculosis as a public health problem be achieved?, *Amer. Rev. Tuberc.*, 79, 690.

McDonald, J. C., and Springett, V. H. (1954) The decline of tuberculosis mortality in western Europe, *Brit. med. Bull.*, 10, 77.

Springett, V. H. (1971) Tuberculosis control in Britain 1945–1970–1995, *Tubercle (Lond.)*, 52, 136.

Springett, V. H. (1972) Tuberculosis—Epidemiology in England and Wales, *Brit. med. J.*, 1, 422.

Struthers, E. B., Lee, H. K., Ham, S. S., Park, S. O., Park, S. J., Lee, K. Y., Hong, J. K., and Choi, Y. O. (1961) Tuberculosis contacts in Seoul, Korea. An analysis of 3,002 household contacts, 1959, *Amer. Rev. resp. Dis.*, 83, 808.

Stýblo, K., and Reil, I. (1967) Epidemiological parameters of tuberculosis, *Scand. J. resp. Dis.*, 48, 117.

World Health Organization Tuberculosis Chemotherapy Centre, Nairobi (1961) An Investigation of Household Contacts of Open Cases of Pulmonary Tuberculosis amongst the Kikuyu in Kiambu, Kenya, *Bull. Wld Hlth Org.*, 25, 831.

World Health Organization (1965) WHO Assisted Activities in Tuberculosis, *Chron. Wld Hlth Org.*, 19, 313.

World Health Organization Expert Committee on Tuberculosis (1964) Eighth Report, *Wld Hlth Org. techn. Rep. Ser.*, No. 290.

Drug-resistant Tuberculosis

Bell, W. J., and Brown, P. P. (1961) Bacterial resistance in patients with pulmonary tuberculosis presenting for treatment in Ghana, *Brit. J. Dis. Chest*, 55, 192.

Fox W., Wiener, A., Mitchison, D. A., Selkon, J. B., and Sutherland, I. (1957) The prevalence of drug-resistant tubercle bacilli in untreated patients with pulmonary tuberculosis. A national survey, 1955–56, *Tubercle (Lond.)*, 38, 71.

Frimodt-Möller, J. (1962) The tuberculosis situation in India today, *Tubercle (Lond.)*, 43, 88.

Hong Kong Government Tuberculosis Service/British Medical Research Council (1964) Drug-resistance in patients with pulmonary tuberculosis presenting at chest clinics in Hong Kong, *Tubercle (Lond.)*, 45, 77.

Medical Research Council (1966) Primary drug resistance in pulmonary tuberculosis in Great Britain: Second National Survey, 1963, *Tubercle (Lond.)*, 47, 92.

Rist, N., and Crofton, J. (1960) Drug resistance in hospitals and sanatoria, *Bull. int. Un. Tuberc.*, 30, 2.

Zierski, M. (1964) Treatment of patients with cultures resistant to the primary anti-tuberculosis drugs, *Tubercle (Lond.)*, 45, 96.

Tuberculosis in Immigrants

Aspin, J. (1962) Tuberculosis among Indian immigrants to a Midland industrial area, *Brit. med. J.*, 1, 1386.

British Tuberculosis Association (1966) Tuberculosis among immigrants to England and Wales: A national survey, 1965, *Tubercle (Lond.)*, 47, 145.

Edgar, W. (1964) Control of tuberculosis in Pakistani immigrants, *Brit. med. J.*, 2, 1565.

Springett, V. H. (1964) Tuberculosis in immigrants, *Lancet*, i, 1091.

Stevenson, D. K. (1962) Tuberculosis in Pakistanis in Bradford, *Brit. med. J.*, 1, 1382.

Standard Treatment of Tuberculosis

Aquinas, Sister M., Allan, W. G. L., Horsfall, P. A. L., Jenkins, P. K., Hung-Yan, Wong, Girling, David, Tall, Ruth, and Fox, Wallace (1972) Adverse reactions to daily and intermittent rifampicin regimens for pulmonary tuberculosis in Hong Kong, *Brit. med. J.*, 1, 765.

International Union against Tuberculosis (1964) An international investigation of the efficacy of chemotherapy in previously untreated patients with pulmonary tuberculosis, *Bull. int. Un. Tuberc.*, 34, No. 2.

Medical Research Council (1962) Long-term chemotherapy in the treatment of chronic pulmonary tuberculosis with cavitation, *Tubercle (Lond.)*, 43, 201.

Pamra, S. P., and Mathur, G. P. (1971) Effects of chemoprophylaxis on minimal pulmonary tuberculosis lesions of doubtful activity, *Bull. Wld Hlth Org.*, 45, 593.

Poole, Graham, Stradling, Peter, and Worlledge, Sheila (1971) Potentially serious side effects of high-dose twice-weekly rifampicin, *Brit. med. J.*, 3, 343.

Ross, J. D., Horne, N. W., Grant, I. W. B., and Crofton, J. W. (1958) Hospital treatment of pulmonary tuberculosis, *Brit. med. J.*, 1, 237.

Scottish Thoracic Society (1963) A controlled trial of chemotherapy in pulmonary tuberculosis of doubtful activity: five year follow-up, *Tubercle (Lond.)*, 44, 39.

Stradling, Peter, and Poole, Graham W. (1970) Twice-weekly streptomycin plus isoniazid for tuberculosis, *Tubercle (Lond.)*, 51, 44.

Thomas, H. E., Forbes, D. E. P., Luntz, G. R. W. N., Ross, H. J. T., Morrison Smith, J., and Springett, V. H. (1960) 100 per cent. sputum-conversion in newly diagnosed pulmonary tuberculosis, *Lancet*, ii, 1185.

Treatment of Drug-resistant Tuberculosis

British Tuberculosis Association (1963) Ethionamide, pyrazinamide, and cycloserine in the treatment of drug-resistant tuberculosis, *Tubercle (Lond.)*, 44, 195.

Citron, K. (1968) in *Recent Advances in Respiratory Tuberculosis*, ed. Heaf, F. R. G., and Rusby, N. L., 6th ed., London.

Somner, A. R., and Brace, A. A. (1966) Late results of treatment of chronic drug-resistant pulmonary tuberculosis, *Brit. med. J.*, 1, 775.

Somner, A. R., Selkon, J. B., Walton, M., and White, A. B. (1971) Drug resistant pulmonary tuberculosis treated with ethambutol and rifampicin in North East England, *Tubercle* (*Lond.*), **52**, 266.

Tousek, J., Jancik, E., Zelenka, M., and Jancikova-Makova (1967) The results of treatment in patients with cultures resistant to streptomycin, isoniazid and para-amino-salicylic acid, *Tubercle* (*Lond.*), **48**, 27.

Chemoprophylaxis

American Thoracic Society (1967) Chemoprophylaxis for the prevention of tuberculosis, *Amer. Rev. resp. Dis.*, **96**, 558.

Comstock, G. W., Ferebee, S. H., and Hammes, L. M. (1967) A controlled trial of community-wide isoniazid prophylaxis in Alaska, *Amer. Rev. resp. Dis.*, **95**, 935.

Curry, F. J. (1967) Prophylactic effect of isoniazid in young tuberculin reactors, *New Engl. J. Med.*, **277**, 562.

Ferebee, S. H. (1970) Controlled chemoprophylaxis trials in tuberculosis. A General Review, *Advanc. Tuberc. Res.*, **17**, 28.

Ferebee, S. H., and Mount, F. W. (1962) Tuberculosis mortality in a controlled trial of the prophylactic use of isoniazid among household contacts, *Amer. Rev. resp. Dis.*, **85**, 490.

Hammond, E. C., Selikoff, I. J., and Robitzek, E. H. (1967) Isoniazid therapy in relation to later occurrence of cancer in adults and in infants, *Brit. med. J.*, **2**, 792.

Treatment of Tuberculosis in Developing Countries

Andrews, R. H., Devadatta, S., Fox, W., Radhakrishna, S., Ramakrishnan, C. V., and Velu, S. (1960) Prevalence of tuberculosis among close family contacts of tuberculous patients in South India, and influence of segregation of the patient on the early attack rate, *Bull. Wld Hlth Org.*, **23**, 463.

Aquinas, M. (1963) Pyrazinamide and ethionamide in the treatment of pulmonary tuberculosis in Hong Kong, *Tubercle* (*Lond.*), **44**, 76.

Chaulet, P., Larbaoui, D., Grosset, J., and Abderrahim, K. (1967) Intermittent chemotherapy with isoniazid and streptomycin in Algiers, *Tubercle* (*Lond.*), **48**, 128.

Dawson, J. J. Y., Devadatta, S., Fox, W., Radhakrishna, S., Ramakrishnan, C. V., Somasundaram, P. R., Stott, H., Tripathy, S. P., and Velu, S. (1966) A 5-year study of patients with pulmonary tuberculosis in a concurrent comparison of home and sanatorium treatment for one year with isoniazid plus P.A.S., *Bull. Wld Hlth Org.*, **34**, 533.

Devadatta, S., Dawson, J. J. Y., Fox, Wallace, Janardhanam, B., Radhakrishna, S., Ramakrishnan, C. V., and Velu, S. (1970) Attack rate of tuberculosis in a 5-year period among close family contacts of tuberculous patients under domiciliary treatment with isoniazid plus PAS or isoniazid alone, *Bull. Wld Hlth Org.*, **42**, 337.

East African/British Medical Research Council Thiacetazone/Diphenylthiourea Investigation (1960) Comparative trial of isoniazid in combination with thiacetazone or a substituted diphenylthiourea (SU1906) or P.A.S. in the treatment of acute pulmonary tuberculosis in East Africans, *Tubercle* (*Lond.*), **41**, 399.

East African/British Medical Research Council Second Thiacetazone Investigation (1963) Isoniazid with thiacetazone in the treatment of pulmonary tuberculosis in East Africa—Second investigation, *Tubercle* (*Lond.*), **44**, 301.

East African/British Medical Research Council Third Thiacetazone Investigation (1966a) Isoniazid with thiacetazone (thioacetazone) in the treatment of pulmonary tuberculosis in East Africa—Third investigation, *Tubercle* (*Lond.*), **47**, 1.

East African/British Medical Research Council Fourth Thiacetazone Investigation (1966b) Isoniazid with thiacetazone (thioacetazone) in the treatment of pulmonary tuberculosis in East Africa—Fourth investigation, *Tubercle* (*Lond.*), **47**, 315.

East African/British Medical Research Council Fifth Thiacet-azone Investigation—Second Report (1970) Isoniazid with thiacetazone (thioacetazone) in the treatment of pulmonary tuberculosis in East Africa—Second Report of Fifth Investigation, *Tubercle* (*Lond.*), **51**, 353.

East African/British Medical Research Council Controlled Clinical Trial of short-course (6 months) regimens of chemotherapy for treatment of pulmonary tuberculosis (1972) *Lancet*, i, 7760.

Ferguson, G. C., Nunn, A. J., Fox, Wallace, Miller, A. B., Robinson, D. K., and Tall, Ruth (1971) A second international co-operative investigation into thiacetazone side-effects, *Tubercle* (*Lond.*), **52**, 166.

Fox, W. (1964) Realistic chemotherapeutic policies for tuberculosis in the developing countries, *Brit. med. J.*, **1**, 135.

Kamat, S. R., Dawson, J. J. Y., Devadatta, S., Fox, W., Janardhanam, B., Radhakrishna S., Ramakrishnan, C. V., Somasundaram, P. R., Stott, H., and Velu, S. (1966) A controlled study of the influence of segregation of tuberculous patients for one year on the attack rate of tuberculosis in a 5-year period in close family contacts in South India, *Bull. Wld Hlth Org.*, **34**, 517.

Menon, N. K. (1966) Intermittent chemotherapy, *Tuberculosis quart. Rev.*, **17**, 3.

Miller, A. B., Fox, W., and Tall, R. (1966) An international co-operative investigation into thiacetazone (thioacetazone) side-effects, *Tubercle* (*Lond.*), **47**, 33.

Nazareth, O., Devadatta, S., Evans, C., Fox, W., Janardhanam, B., Menon, N. K., Radhakrishna, S., Ramakrishnan, C. V., Stott, H., Tripathy, S. P., and Velu, S. (1966) A 2-year follow-up of patients with quiescent pulmonary tuberculosis following a year of chemotherapy with an intermittent (twice weekly) regimen of isoniazid plus streptomycin or a daily regimen of isoniazid plus P.A.S., *Tubercle* (*Lond.*), **47**, 178.

Nazareth, O., Devadatta, S., Fox, Wallace, Menon, N. K., Radhakrishna, S., Rajappa, D., Ramakrishnan, C. V., Somasundaram, P. R., Stott, H., Subbammal, S., and Velu, S. (1971) Two controlled studies of the efficacy of isoniazid alone in preventing relapse in patients with bacteriologically quiescent pulmonary tuberculosis at the end of one year of chemotherapy, *Bull. Wld Hlth Org.*, **45**, 603.

Tuberculosis Chemotherapy Centre, Madras (1959) A concurrent comparison of home and sanatorium treatment of pulmonary tuberculosis in South India, *Bull. Wld Hlth Org.*, **21**, 51.

Tuberculosis Chemotherapy Centre, Madras (1964) A concurrent comparison of intermittent (twice weekly) isoniazid plus streptomycin and daily isoniazid plus P.A.S. in the domiciliary treatment of pulmonary tuberculosis, *Bull. Wld Hlth Org.*, **31**, 247.

Tuberculosis Chemotherapy Centre, Madras (1966) Isoniazid plus thioacetazone compared with two regimens of isoniazid plus P.A.S. in the domiciliary treatment of pulmonary tuberculosis in South Indian patients, *Bull. Wld Hlth Org.*, **34**, 483.

Tuberculosis Chemotherapy Centre, Madras (1970) A controlled comparison of a twice-weekly and three once-weekly regimens in the initial treatment of pulmonary tuberculosis, *Bull. Wld Hlth Org.*, **43**, 143.

B.C.G. Vaccination

Aronson, J. D., Aronson, C. F., and Taylor, H. C. (1958) A twenty-year appraisal of B.C.G. vaccination in the control of tuberculosis, *Arch. intern. Med.*, **101**, 881.

Brown, J. A. K., Stone, M. M., and Sutherland, I. (1968) B.C.G. vaccination of children against leprosy in Uganda: results at end of second follow-up, *Brit. med. J.*, **1**, 24.

Comstock, G. W., and Palmer, C. E. (1966) Long-term results of B.C.G. vaccination in the Southern United States, *Amer. Rev. resp. Dis.*, **93**, 171.

Frimodt-Möller, J., Thomas J., and Parthasarathy, R. (1964) Observations on the protective effect of B.C.G. vaccination in a South Indian rural population, *Bull. Wld Hlth Org.*, **30**, 545.

Hart, P. D'A. (1967) Efficacy and applicability of mass B.C.G. vaccination in tuberculosis control, *Brit. med. J.*, **1**, 587.

Medical Research Council (1963) B.C.G. and vole bacillus vaccines in the prevention of tuberculosis in adolescence and early adult life, *Brit. med. J.*, **1**, 973.

Palmer, C. E., and Long, M. W. (1966) Effects of infection with atypical mycobacteria on B.C.G. vaccination and tuberculosis, *Amer. Rev. resp. Dis.*, **94**, 553.

Palmer, C. E., Shaw, L. W., and Comstock, G. W. (1958)

Community trials of B.C.G. vaccination, *Amer. Rev. Tuberc.*, **77**, 877.

Rosenthal, S. R., Loewinsohn, E., Graham, M. L., Liveright, D., Thorne, M. G., Johnson, V., and Batson, H. C. (1961) B.C.G. vaccination against tuberculosis in Chicago, *Pediatrics*, **28**, 622.

Springett, V. H. (1965) The value of B.C.G. vaccination, *Tubercle* (*Lond.*), **46**, 76.

World Health Organization Expert Committee on Biological Standardization (1966) Eighteenth Report. *Wld Hlth Org. techn. Rep. Ser.*, No. 329.

FURTHER READING

Barry, V. C. (1964) *Chemotherapy of Tuberculosis*, London.

British Thoracic and Tuberculosis Association (1970) Aspergilloma and residual tuberculous cavities—the results of a resurvey, *Tubercle* (*Lond.*), **51**, 227.

Canetti, G. (1962) The eradication of tuberculosis: theoretical problems and practical solutions, *Tubercle* (*Lond.*), **43**, 301.

Crofton, J. W. (1962) The contribution of treatment to the prevention of tuberculosis, *Bull. int. Un. Tuberc.*, **32**, 643.

East African/British Medical Research Councils (1973) Length of treatment, *Lancet*, **i**, 1331.

Edwards, P. Q., and Edwards, L. B. (1960) Story of the tuberculin test from an epidemiologic viewpoint, *Amer. Rev. resp. Dis.*, **81**. Supplement.

Feldstein, M. S. *et al.* (1973) Resource allocation model for public health planning: A case study of tuberculosis control, *Bull. Wld Hlth Org.*, **48**, Suppl.

Fox, W. (1962) The chemotherapy and epidemiology of tuberculosis. Some findings of general applicability from the Tuberculosis Chemotherapy Centre, Madras, *Lancet*, **ii**, 413 and 473.

Fox, W. (1963) Ambulatory chemotherapy in a developing country: clinical and epidemiological studies, *Advanc. Tuberc. Res.*, **12**, 28.

Fox, Wallace (1971) The scope of the controlled clinical trial, illustrated by studies of pulmonary tuberculosis, *Bull. Wld Hlth Org.*, **45**, 559.

Furcolow, M. L., Shaffer, S. A., and Deuschle, K. W. (1966) Tuberculosis eradication in theory and practice, *Arch. environm. Hlth*, **12**, 287.

Hart, P. D'A. (1967) The place of vaccination in tuberculosis control, *Amer. Rev. resp. Dis.*, **96**, 1.

Heaf, F., and Rusby, N. L., eds (1968) *Recent Advances in Respiratory Tuberculosis*, 6th ed., London.

King, M. (1966) *Medical Care in Developing Countries*, Nairobi.

Miller, F. J. W., Seal, R. M. E., and Taylor, M. D. (1963) *Tuberculosis in Children*, London.

Mitchison, D. A. (1965) Chemotherapy of tuberculosis: a bacteriologist's viewpoint, *Brit. med. J.*, **1**, 1333.

Myers, J. A. (1967) Eighty years after the first glimpse of the tubercle bacillus, *Dis. Chest.*, **51**, 500.

Postgraduate Medical Journal (1971) Tuberculosis in the 1970s, **47**, 691.

Ross, J. D., and Horne, N. W. (1969) *Modern Drug Treatment in Tuberculosis*, 4th ed., London.

World Health Organization (1972) Evaluation of Tuberculosis Control Programmes, *Wld Hlth Org. Chron.*, **26**, 547.

World Health Organization (1973) Tuberculosis control, *Bull. Wld Hlth Org.*, **48**, 448.

World Health Organization (1974) Annual Report of WHO for 1973, *Wld Hlth Org. Off. Rec.*, No. 213, 17–19.

World Health Organization (1974) Ninth report of the Expert Committee on tuberculosis, *Wld Hlth Org. techn. Rep. Ser.*, No. 551.

World Health Organization Regional Office for Europe (1971) Recent reports of meetings on tuberculosis control, Copenhagen.

Study of the effectiveness of the control programmes (Euro 1201).

Integration of Control with the Work of the General Health Services (Euro 1202).

Technical Meeting on Control in Rural Areas (Euro 1203).

Seminar on the Evaluation of the Control Programmes (Euro 1204).

26

ADMINISTRATIVE ASPECTS OF COMMUNICABLE DISEASE CONTROL

ANDREW B. SEMPLE

Communicable disease may be defined as the reaction of a susceptible host to an infectious agent. The precise knowledge of this host parasite relationship forms the basis upon which control measures are based. While many of the principles of control are of a general nature, others are specific and directed at destroying the spread of infection at a particular point in the life history of the parasite.

As the original challenge to public health was the organization of community services for the prevention and control of communicable disease most of the environmental services play their part, and at the same time raise the standard of living so that the public become aware of the value of a hygienic environment.

GENERAL CONTROL MEASURES

It is axiomatic that the prevalence of communicable disease is directly related to environmental standards. Probably the most important factor is population density—where too many people are gathered together in one place—then the path of infection is so facilitated that epidemics readily occur. Examples of this have been seen throughout the ages in armies, in prison camps, and in the slum conditions arising from urbanization. Hence, the control of overcrowding must always be considered as the primary objective, supported by the development of other services. The next is a safe and sufficient supply of water. In developed countries this is largely a civil engineering problem—nevertheless constant vigilance and monitoring is necessary to ensure that the supply is adequately treated and free from harmful chemical agents and the possibility of transmitting pathogenic organisms. Water-borne outbreaks of alimentary disease are explosive in type with large numbers of cases occurring simultaneously which can overwhelm the available treatment services.

Next in order is an efficient system of excreta disposal which is the most effective way to control the alimentary infections such as dysentery, worm infestations, and the more serious epidemic diseases such as cholera. In developed countries a water-borne sewerage system is the rule but other methods may be necessary in special circumstances such as camps, mass gatherings, or in disaster areas. Food control must also be a constant care of the public health service to ensure that the risk from infected food is minimized. Pasteurization of milk and the hygiene of food premises of all types need particular attention, and regular inspection. Such inspection fulfils two purposes, first it ensures that the legal hygiene standards are being maintained; but more important, it gives an oppor-

tunity for the public health inspector to advise and educate both management and staff in food premises.

Other environmental services such as refuse collection all contribute by reducing the reservoirs of infection in the community. In warm climates it may be necessary to maintain some form of insect control. This may be directed against a particular disease vector such as the *Anopheles* mosquito or generally to reduce biting insects because of the public annoyance they cause. Rodent control is also an important local authority service. In particular circumstances general control measures have been developed to deal with recurring events which have been shown to favour outbreaks of infectious diseases, for example, the control measures associated with the annual pilgrimage to Mecca. Pollution in general greatly facilitates the spread of infection and in certain areas control measures against atmospheric pollution will do much to reduce the tendency to chronic respiratory disease.

PERSONAL HEALTH

While the environmental services do much to prevent communicable disease the contribution of the individual cannot be underrated. While the former is provided, the latter must be the result of a definite individual decision which largely depends on training and education. For a food handler to wash his hands after using the lavatory requires not only a washhand basin in the lavatory but also training to make him stop at the basin, and education so that he knows why it is necessary for him to use it. This promotion of good hygienic habits should start in childhood and continue throughout life. In this way the individual gets personal protection and at the same time assists in the prevention of spread of infection to others.

Much of this depends on the level of health education of the community. If individuals practise good personal health habits, then communicable diseases are less likely to spread. Health education is important in many aspects of prevention, it is the main motivating force in many preventive operations such as encouraging parents to bring their children for immunization. Again it is of prime importance in the control of the venereal diseases, and in the prevention of tuberculosis, worm infestations, and certain skin diseases.

Two other personal health factors are involved, namely heredity and nutrition. Certain individuals, and certain races, have a genetically determined susceptibility or resistance to certain diseases. For example, individuals who have the sickle-cell trait have a higher resistance to malaria than those who do not exhibit this abnormal blood picture. In regard to nutrition, although malnutrition *per se* does not render a person more liable to infection, it results in a greater tendency for small doses of infectious agents to gain a foothold and combine with the existing malnutrition to further reduce the individual's low state of health. See CHAPTER 2 for statistics of notifiable infectious disease. See CHAPTER 4 for methods of study of epidemics. For control measures in specific cases, see CHAPTER 10, food hygiene. See CHAPTER 11 for nutrition and epidemic disease, CHAPTER 15 in air-borne infections, CHAPTER 16 in water and food-borne infections, CHAPTER 17 in arthropod disease, CHAPTER 18 in malaria, CHAPTER 19 vector control, CHAPTER 20 in certain skin diseases, CHAPTER 21 in treponematoses, CHAPTER 22 in the zoonoses, CHAPTER 23 in rabies, CHAPTER 24 in worm infections, CHAPTER 25 in tuberculosis, CHAPTER 29 in certain eye diseases, CHAPTER 34 in M.C.H. work (especially in the tropics), CHAPTER 35 in schools, CHAPTER 38 in industry, CHAPTER 44 in hospitals, CHAPTER 49 for health education and communicable diseases, CHAPTER 51 for International aspects of control.

ADMINISTRATIVE CONTROL

Diagnosis

If effective control methods are to be applied it is essential that an accurate diagnosis of the communicable disease should be made as soon as possible. This is not always easy and delay in recognising an early case of smallpox could readily lead to an epidemic. Again, many diseases are most infectious in their early prodromal stages, for example measles and mumps. Here the experienced clinician is invaluable and if doubts exist further consultation should be sought. There are also the many modern diagnostic aids such as the electron microscope, and numerous microbiological procedures, e.g. the fluorescent antibody technique which can determine in many cases the specific antitoxin to be given. However, where the epidemic risk is great, such as with smallpox, it is advisable to take full precautions until the diagnosis is definite. Mass campaigns for treatment of yaws have been most successful [see CHAPTER 21].

Notification

If speedy control action is to be taken by a local authority then it is necessary for a system of prompt notification to operate. In countries with an organized public health service the statutory responsibility is placed upon the medical practitioner. In Britain, current legislation contained in the Health Services and Public Health Act (1968) states that if a medical practitioner becomes aware, or suspects, that a patient he is attending is suffering from a notifiable disease or food poisoning, he must forthwith inform the Medical Officer of Health. With a National Health Service it is assumed that most cases of notifiable disease will be seen by a doctor, but in other countries the responsibility for informing the health authority is also placed on other specified non-medical persons (e.g. head of family, etc.) as the patient may not be seen by a medical practitioner.

The Local Government Act 1972 requires that every local authority shall appoint a 'Proper Officer' for the control of communicable disease and food poisoning and to provide any other medical advice required by the local authority. The National Health Service Reorganisation Act of 1973 requires every Area Health Authority, in consultation with the coterminous local authority, to second a Medical Officer for the above-named duties who will be the 'Proper Officer'.

The Department of Health and Social Security have issued a circular to say that this seconded officer shall bear the title of 'The Medical Officer for Environmental Health' and shall be a specialist community physician on the staff of the Area Health Authority and working under the general direction of the Area Medical Officer. The title of Medical Officer of Health has been abolished as from 1st April 1974.

Notification is the mechanism which brings the control services into action. Regrettably many doctors get the impression that the main purpose of notification is for statistics. This can only be dispelled by good communications and sound and justifiable control measures. Again, notification is sometimes delayed in hospitals as it is feared that the Medical Officer of Health will recommend closing wards which will interfere with the work of the hospital. For this reason, a control of infection committee in a hospital is invaluable. When infection occurs it can be fully discussed by a group of interested individuals with the epidemiologist and the necessary decisions taken on the basis of what is required to prevent further spread with the minimum disturbance to the work of the hospital.

Notification in the way described above is the common practice and a type of notification form is shown in FIGURE 77. The list of notifiable diseases will obviously vary for different geographical areas and may not necessarily be the same for a whole country. This largely depends on the endemic communicable diseases or the diseases which may be imported, and for control, or even occasionally, treatment reasons early warning is desirable.

With certain communicable diseases such as influenza, notification can do little to aid control and in epidemic conditions could prove burdensome, but it is helpful to have a number of medical practitioners who can be called upon for information concerning the numbers and severity of cases occurring in their practices. A daily check on the demand for hospital admissions will also yield valuable information. There must also be an immediate exchange of information between the Medical Officer of Health and the directors of the bacteriological laboratories in his area. If a laboratory finds evidence of a communicable disease in a specimen submitted for examination then epidemiological investigations should be started without delay.

When the infectious disease is of a serious nature then it may involve other areas and even other countries. When this happens the national government health agency should be notified immediately so that accurate information is made available to all likely to be involved.

Isolation

Especially in the case of serious infectious disease efficient isolation is a requirement. This should be provided in a hospital unit specially built for the purpose and with a staff trained to deal with patients suffering from infectious diseases. The degree of isolation will obviously depend on the particular disease; in smallpox for instance it should be as complete as possible. In other diseases a less rigorous isolation will suffice, and home isolation is often satisfactory for minor communicable

NOTIFICATION OF INFECTIOUS DISEASE OR FOOD POISONING

To the Medical Officer of Health for the City of Liverpool

I hereby certify and declare that in my opinion the person named below is suffering from the disease stated.

NAME (in full)	AGE	DISEASE See Note+	DATE OF ONSET
	SEX		

No.

+NOTE When the form is used for a case of food poisoning enter "F.P." (or "F.P. suspected") unless the case is diagnosed as one of specific disease (e.g. dysentery) which is required to be notified as such.

Full address where patient now is:—

If patient is at present in a hospital,
(a) the address in full from which the patient was admitted is:—

(b) in my opinion the disease was/was not contracted in the hospital
(Delete whichever does not apply)

Additional particulars required in cases of certain diseases

Ophthalmia Neonatorum	Date of birth	Name and address of parent or other person in charge of the child
Malaria	Mark "X" where applicable	
	Contracted— (Abroad .... (In this country	If induced— (Therapeutically........ (Accidentally........
Acute Meningitis	Causal organism if known	
Acute Poliomyelitis	Paralytic or non-paralytic (Ring symbol which applies) **P N-P**	(PARALYTIC means that there are or have been signs of weakness and paralysis of muscles either permanent or transient. NON-PARALYTIC means that there have been no such signs)
Acute Encephalitis	Infective or Post-infectious (Ring symbol which applies) **I P-I**	If post-infectious state preceding infection below.
Tuberculosis	Organ or part affected	

Date

Signature of Doctor ....

Address

LIST OF NOTIFIABLE DISEASES

ANTHRAX	MALARIA	SMALLPOX
CHOLERA	MEASLES	TETANUS
DIPHTHERIA	MENINGITIS (ACUTE)	* TUBERCULOSIS
DYSENTERY (AMOEBIC OR BACILLARY)	OPHTHALMIA NEONATORUM	TYPHOID FEVER
	PARATYPHOID FEVER	TYPHUS
ENCEPHALITIS (ACUTE)	PLAGUE	WHOOPING COUGH
INFECTIVE JAUNDICE	POLIOMYELITIS (ACUTE)	YELLOW FEVER
LEPROSY	RELAPSING FEVER	
LEPTOSPIROSIS	SCARLET FEVER	FOOD POISONING

* TUBERCULOSIS is required to be notified in order to check the spread of infection and to bring about the proper management of the individual patient and immediate contacts. A person who should be notified as "suffering from tuberculosis," therefore, is a person who, because of tuberculous infection, may infect others; or a person who is suffering from an active tuberculous lesion which calls for medical treatment or some modification of the patient's normal course of living.

P39596 600 BKS. EST.

FIG. 77. Notification of infectious disease (from 1st April 1974 the title Medical Officer of Health is replaced by Proper Officer for the Control of Communicable Diseases).

diseases. The therapeutic advantages of the isolation hospital must be mentioned as it has a trained and specialist staff versed in modern methods of treatment, which can greatly benefit the patient.

In England and Wales the steps to be taken in the investigation and control of food poisoning are set out in the pamphlet memo/188/Med [see CHAPTER 10].

Carriers

Healthy persons can sometimes harbour in their bodies pathogenic organisms and infect other members of the community. When a carrier of an infectious disease is found it is obvious that he should be treated and the parasite destroyed if possible. Unfortunately, sometimes the carrier state is persistent and then the individual must be trained to avoid as far as possible putting others at risk from his infection and to take

up a suitable job which would not involve risk of spread of the infection.

Disinfection

It is desirable to abolish the infective power of any material on which pathogenic organisms may have lodged. This may be done by using chemical disinfectants, or where possible by collecting the infectious discharges from the patient, e.g. sputum or nasal secretions, and burning them. Bed linen and the like can be boiled and laundered. As far as sick rooms are concerned, thorough domestic cleansing and exposure to the dilutent effect of a current of fresh air normally suffices. Mattresses and blankets can be disinfected by steam.

The detection of carriers has been much facilitated by the use of phage-typing especially by using the vi-antigen. Once a chronic carrier has been detected his name should be entered upon a control register and his employment in the food industry restricted. There are famous examples of persons who have been responsible for numerous outbreaks, e.g. typhoid Mary in U.S.A. Often the gall bladder is the seat of infection and in urinary carriers there may be some abnormality; these carriers may be cured by surgery. The prolonged use of ampicillin may be effective. The treatment of typhoid with chloramphemicol can also result in the production of carriers.

Carriers are important in staphylococcal food posioning, enteric infections and cholera [see CHAPTER 16 and CHAPTER 10] and in the meningococcal infections [see CHAPTER 15].

Techniques are now available for the isolation and control of carriers through the investigation of contamination of sewage at different points in the house where the carrier is shedding the pathogen. Phage typing will confirm the spread of disease to others [see CHAPTER 16].

Prophylaxis

A number of communicable diseases have been brought under efficient control by means of immunization. Polio-myelitis and diphtheria which in the past caused epidemics with death and suffering have now been eradicated from many countries. At present the World Health Organization is sponsoring and largely financing a mass immunization campaign to eradicate smallpox in countries where this disease is endemic. In 1974, smallpox was endemic in only four countries, India, Pakistan, Bangladesh and Ethiopia [see CHAPTER 15]. Mass immunization against many infectious diseases is one of the great success stories of modern medicine.

In malaria a different approach has proved successful. Here the vector has been tackled by using persistent insecticides and at the same time intensive case finding and treatment with antimalarial drugs of all persons found to be harbouring the parasite. Also, in the prevention of communicable disease the standard of environmental hygiene is an important factor.

In dealing with epidemic disease protection of those at risk is especially important. These may be attendants on the sick, contacts, or persons entering an area where the disease is known to be prevalent. If the prophylaxis is a form of active immunization then some time is required for antibodies to develop. For immunization procedures see also CHAPTERS 15, 16, 17, 22, 23, 25 and 34. In some diseases chemoprophylaxis which acts quickly can be given, such as the thiosemicarbazones in the protection of contacts of smallpox; other diseases in which prophylaxis is useful are malaria [see CHAPTER 18], tuberculosis [CHAPTER 25], leprosy [CHAPTER 20], trypanosomiasis [Chapter 17] and onchocerciasis [CHAPTER 17]. Penicillin has also been used to control streptococcal infection and to prevent rheumatic fever (Strasser and Rotta, 1973). Passive immunization which also acts quickly can be given to contacts, e.g. diphtheria antitoxin, or gamma-globulin in measles prophylaxis, in the protection of pregnant women against rubella [see CHAPTER 15] and in the prevention of infective hepatitis, but the protection is short-lived.

Schedules for Immunization

It is important to continue vaccination in developed countries against communicable diseases that have been brought under control e.g. diphtheria, tetanus, poliomyelitis and pertussis and new vaccines against diseases of lesser importance are also being introduced e.g. measles, rubella, mumps. Smallpox has been discontinued in the U.K. but BCG should continue for the time being. Vaccination against typhoid fever is unwarranted in developed countries and there is uncertainty about the value of influenza vaccine. The dosage, number of innoculations, age, should all be reviewed and there should be continuous monitoring against the risks involved.

In developing countries routine immunization should cover tetanus, pertussis, diphtheria, typhoid, measles, smallpox, BCG, poliomyelitis and when indicated, yellow fever. There is little purpose in giving cholera, influenza, rubella or mumps. There is great hope for an effective meningococcal vaccine.

A typical schedule as recommended by Cvjetanović (1973) would be: 1–3 months, DPT and typhoid (a quadruple antigen DPTTy, has proved safe) and BCG, smallpox and when indicated yellow fever and poliomyelitis; 4–8 months, DPT and typhoid and poliomyelitis (trivalent); 9–12 months, poliomyelitis and measles; 5–6 years, DPT plus typhoid and measles [see also CHAPTER 34 for schedules in childhood].

Simultaneous multiple immunization

Efforts are being made to find a one shot method which would immunize a child against all infections at one visit; this is very important because of the difficulty of getting mother and children to attend clinics at frequent intervals, particularly in developing countries. Rubin (1973) in Nigerian children, gave smallpox, measles, yellow fever, diphtheria, pertussis and tetanus at the same time.

Cost effectiveness analysis should always be used in newly developing countries to determine the relative benefits from immunization programmes against the costs, which can often be reduced considerably whilst still maintaining efficacy.

Cvjetanović (1973) has used mathematical models to predict the dynamics of an infection over a long period to serve as a guide in planning control measures.

Evaluation of a programme should be continuous, the following methods should be used in practice.

1. Analysis of the records of vaccination programmes.
2. The use of health statistics to measure morbidity and mortality.
3. Continuing surveillance of the disease.
4. Microbiological surveys of the population.
5. Serological surveys for antibodies etc.
6. Comparison of the incidence of infection in immunized groups with that of a control group of non-immunized persons.

Attack rates in health conscious groups however are always much less than in uncooperative populations, so that the two groups must be comparable in size and make-up.

Contacts

An important aspect of control is the identification and supervision of contacts. First of all it is necessary by careful history-taking from the patient and others to prepare a list of individuals with whom the patient has been in contact during the time he has been infectious. This varies with the disease, some can be passed on in the presymptomatic stage, while others like smallpox or measles are highly infectious when early symptoms are present but before the exanthem has appeared.

Having identified the contacts, they must be questioned to learn whether they have had the disease or not, thus indicating the possibility of immunity or susceptibility. Then they must be seen at regular intervals by a trained observer for a few days longer than the incubation period. Should any signs of infection develop such as pyrexia, then medical advice should be sought immediately. Contacts may also be given some form of prophylaxis as immunization, immunoglobulin or an appropriate chemotherapeutic drug or antibiotic.

In July 1971 routine vaccination in childhood was discontinued in the United Kingdom, and it is considered that should a case of smallpox be imported this disease can be controlled by accurate contact tracing and supervision in the way outlined above.

Epidemiological inquiries are necessary regarding the source of infection and reasons why the outbreak occurred and giving an indication of the control measures which should be undertaken. [See CHAPTER 4 for the methodology.] Time charts and epidemic maps are very useful and will indicate whether an outbreak is e.g. milk-borne or water-borne. The classic investigations of John Snow on cholera, William Budd on typhoid fever and Goldberger on dietetic deficiencies are well known in this field. Phage typing is a useful tool in the search for infection in enteric and staphylococcal infection. Planning control measures can be improved by the use of mathematical models [see CHAPTER 16].

Communications

When there is an outbreak of infectious disease this will have more than local effects and it is essential that other authorities concerned must be informed immediately and kept up to date with subsequent developments. In the United Kingdom it is a legal requirement for the district Medical Officer for Environmental Health to inform the Department of Health and Social Security forthwith when a case of major infectious disease occurs in his area. He should also inform all the medical practitioners and hospitals in his area so that they are alerted to the likelihood of other cases occurring, and inform his health officer colleagues in neighbouring areas. In epidemic situations, misunderstandings and confusion can readily occur and the Medical Officer of Health principally responsible should arrange a daily conference with his medical and health worker colleagues most involved so that aspects of the outbreak can be discussed and everyone has an opportunity to be fully and accurately informed.

Epidemics are news and it may be advisable for the Medical Officer of Health responsible for the control measures to hold a press conference at regular intervals so that he can give an accurate assessment of the situation to the mass media. This should be done on a once daily basis, as frequent interruptions from news-seekers can be distracting and interfere with the work in bringing the epidemic under control. Nevertheless, the need to keep the public informed is an essential part of the handling of the epidemic, if panic and confusion are to be avoided.

Surveillance as a Control Measure

Surveillance of an infectious disease involves the systematic collection of all available information on the occurrence of the disease, including morbidity and mortality data, information from bacteriological and virological laboratories, the results of serological surveys, information on the prevalence of insect vectors, data on the use of vaccines and the results arising therefrom. An important component of a surveillance scheme is the feed-back of collated information to health authorities in the areas concerned.

An epidemiological surveillance unit has been established in the Division of Communicable Diseases at the World Health Organization headquarters at Geneva, and a number of Communicable Disease Surveillance Reports have been produced (Raska, 1966).

Surveillance assumes different forms in different circumstances. Where certain diseases, e.g. diphtheria or poliomyelitis have reached the stage of virtual elimination in some advanced countries, national surveillance programmes are organized to ensure adequate local action if cases of the disease should occur. A special kind of surveillance is called for as a continuing activity after a successful malaria eradication programme in an area.

Sometimes national surveillance programmes are organized for the study of disease of wider prevalence (for example, infectious hepatitis or salmonellosis) for the purpose of defining the paths of spread of these diseases in the community with a view to prevention.

A form of disease surveillance of particular interest to the World Health Organization is the co-ordinated study of the circumstances of incidence of particular diseases that are a problem common to a number of neighbouring states. Collection of information relating to areas transcending national boundaries could lay the foundation for programmes of prevention of such diseases as smallpox or yellow fever over wide areas.

In the worldwide study of incidence of certain diseases a leading part is played by Reference Laboratories for a number of diseases established by the World Health Organization (e.g. the Influenza Reference Laboratory, the Salmonella Reference Laboratory, etc.) to which micro-organisms isolated by laboratories over large areas of the world are forwarded for study and classification. The Reference Laboratories have become centres for epidemic intelligence. They are able to give early warning of any change in type of the prevalent organism. For list of centres see World Health Organization (1974).

The latest surveillance programme relates to poliomyelitis: in which 19 countries participated in 1973.

International Control Measures

The International Health Regulations adopted by the Twenty-second World Health Assembly on 25 July 1969 are the basis for international control measures in force at present by member states of the World Health Organization. They came into force on 1 January 1971. They require notification to the World Health Organization when any area becomes infected with cholera, plague, smallpox, or yellow fever. Provision is also made for the World Health Organization to maintain international surveillance of other communicable diseases such as influenza, salmonellosis, and vector-borne diseases. This international surveillance is a valuable source of information which assists epidemiologists and health departments all over the world to control the spread of disease. The Additional Regulations of 23rd May 1973 adopted by the 26th

World Health Assembly amended the International Health Regulations (1969) with effect from 1st Jan. 1974; this removed any requirement regarding cholera vaccination certificates for International travellers.

The regulations prescribe the measures to be used for dealing with international travel by ships or aircraft to prevent passengers conveying diseases from one country to another. At the same time the regulations are drafted so as to give the maximum protection with the least inconvenience to travellers and the least hindrance to international commerce. Measures are also set out for dealing with ships and aircraft which may be carrying infected persons and for disinfection and disinsection of ships and aircraft. Facilities at ports and airports to help to control the spread of infection are also included, together with instructions relating to the transport of goods. They also prescribe the form and duration of international certificates of vaccination against smallpox, cholera, and yellow fever.

The greatest danger of importation of a disease into a non-infected country comes from air travel, and in Britain the principal threat comes from smallpox. It is therefore necessary to ensure that travellers are aware of this danger and if they feel ill, should consult a doctor. To assist both patient and doctor, a warning card is given to all passengers from areas where certain diseases are known to be present. In instances where travellers are known to be contacts of an infectious disease, they may be kept under supervision as described above in the country of arrival.

The administrative control of infectious diseases requires knowledge of the natural history of these diseases. To further this end there are a number of special centres like the World Influenza Centre in London which conduct research and keep a constant watch on many diseases. There are also great institutes like the Communicable Disease Center in Atlanta devoted to such studies. Finally, the World Health Organization with its many international surveillance and control activities provides up to the minute information on almost every aspect of communicable disease prevalence and sound technical guidance on control measures and especially through its weekly *Epidemiological Record*.

Information on epidemics

WHO has developed an automatic telex reply service for information on communicable disease. It operates 24 hours a day, in English and French.

The code is Telex no. 28150 and ZCZC followed by ENGL for English or FRAN for French or Tel. Geneva 34,60,61 or cable EPIDNATIONS GENEVA.

Special reviews have been issued to provide information on e.g. malaria risks in different parts of the world (see World Health Organization, 1973).

Control in aircraft

The Committee on International Surveillance of Communicable Diseases has stressed the importance of maintaining high standards of drinking water and food in aircraft (see Article 14 of the International Health Regulations). It has also approved the use of resmethrin and bioresmethrin aerosols for aircraft disinfection (World Health Organization, 1974).

REFERENCES AND FURTHER READING

American Public Health Association (1970) *Control of Communicable Diseases in Man*, 11th ed., New York.

Anderson, T. (1971) Whose Responsibility?, *Publ. Hlth (Lond.)*, **85**, 99.

British Medical Journal (1971) International health regulations, **1**, 415.

Burnet, Sir Frank Macfarlane (1970) *Immunicogical Surveillance*, Oxford.

Cruickshank, R., Duguild, J. P. and Marmion, B. P. (1973) *Medical microbiology: a guide to the laboratory diagnosis and control of infections*, 12th ed., Vol. 1, Edinburgh.

Cvjetanović, B. (1973) Immunization programmes, *Wld Hlth Org. Chron.* **27**, 66

Gonzaliz, C. L. (1965) Mass Campaigns and General Health Services, *Wld Hlth Org. Publ. Hlth Pap.*, No. 29.

Notification of communicable diseases (1958). A survey of existing legislation. Geneva.

Pan American Health Organization (1969) *International Movement of Animals*, Washington.

Pan American Health Organization (1971) Proceedings of the conference on the application of vaccines against viral, rickettsial and bacterial diseases of man. Scientific Publication No. 226, Washington.

Raska, K. (1966) Surveillance reports, *Wld Hlth Org. Chron.* **20**, 315.

Roelsgaard, E. (1974) Health regulations and international travel, *Wld Hlth Org. Chron.*, **28**, 265.

Ruben, F. L. et al. (1973) Simultaneous multiple immunization, *Bull Wld Hlth Org.*, **48**, 175.

Strasser, T and Rotta J. (1973) The control of rheumatic fever and rheumatic heart disease: an outline of WHO activities, *Wld Hlth Org. Chron.* **27**, 49.

World Health Organization (1966) Trials of prophylactic agents for the control of communicable disease, *Wld Hlth Org. Monogr. Ser.*, No. 52

World Health Organization (1976) *Airports Designated in Application of the International Sanitary Regulations*, Geneva.

World Health Organization (1968) *Ports designated in Application of the International Sanitary Regulations*, Geneva.

World Health Organization (1970) *Yellow-fever Vaccination Centres for International Travel, Geneva*.

World Health Organization (1971) *International Health Regulations, 1969*, Geneva.

World Health Organization (1971) *Vaccination Certificate Requirements for International Travel*, Geneva.

World Health Organization (1972) *World Directory of Venereal Disease. Treatment Centres at Ports*, 3rd ed., Geneva.

World Health Organization (1973) Information on malaria risks for international travellers, *Wkly epidem. Rec.*, **48**, 25–45.

World Health Organization (1974) Annual Report of the work of WHO for 1973 (Section on surveillance), *Wld Hlth Org. Rec.* No. 213, p. 3–5 and annex. 5 (list of reference centres) p. 297–309.

For more detailed reference to the changes brought about on 1st April 1974 by the reorganization of the National Health Service, see *Management Arrangements in the Reorganized National Health Service* (1972) H.M.S.O., London, and *Report from the Working Party on Collaboration between the NHS and Local Government on its activities to the end of 1972* (1973) H.M.S.O., London.

27

EPIDEMIOLOGY OF CHRONIC DISEASE: THE TOOLS OF PREVENTION

J. A. H. LEE AND J. N. MORRIS

Human life is an uneasy balancing act between biological insults of all kinds, and the basic homeostatic mechanisms of the body. Successful intervention to prevent human disease involves understanding of the disease to be prevented. The depth of knowledge needed for this success is very variable—Jenner knew no virology in 1780 when he invented vaccination; indeed, the subject cannot be said to have been there to know until the twentieth century. Similarly, infant mortality rates were sharply reduced during the early years of this century in developed countries on the basis of the most meagre information about the protection of infant life. In contrast, the modern control of measles by vaccination depended on a long period of steadily deepening knowledge of the nature of the virus, and years of development work to produce the actual vaccine. Until that had been done the spread of measles was uninfluenced by medical action. We know a great deal about the operation of the cigarette as a cause of lung cancer. We know very little about the satisfactions or addiction of the cigarette, and have so far been able to do little about reducing the mortality of this commonest of cancers. Successful prevention depends on the existence of the right body of knowledge—depending on what we know our practical efforts may be very powerful or almost without effect.

Our knowledge of the aetiology of human disease is largely derived from the study of the patients' lives before they became ill. Laboratory studies have made great contributions by their detailed identification and characterization of the agents of disease, but they have provided little information on the situation which determines whether an individual gets or does not get a disease. There are many useful laboratory models of physical states—shock, major infection, etc., and lessons from these can often be transferred quickly to the care of patients. But models of aetiology—exposing animals to carcinogens or to aerosols of bacteria—are difficult to make for a number of reasons. Differences in susceptibility between species are very large, and extrapolation from animals to man difficult; laboratory models are expensive and are seldom designed to realistically imitate the low incidence of human disease. Thus, we can study the effects of limited coronary blood flow very well in the dog, but we cannot cause dogs to develop ischemic heart disease by the routes by which the human disease is produced.

Epidemiologic study may demonstrate a simple association between the occurrence of disease and some antecedent circumstances, and thus enable the disease to be effectively prevented. The recognition of the association between lead consumption and the concentration of a recognizable syndrome in particular population groups (Baker, 1767), or the association between dietary deficiencies and such syndromes as pellagra (Terris, 1964), or goitre (Gillie, 1971) are examples where the knowledge gained led directly to prevention. But a much larger effect may result from the gain in general understanding that these studies provide, and which may be felt even if the immediate prevention of the disease is not possible. Thus, because of the early epidemiological studies and the consequent recognition of the complex ways that lead can be distributed in the community, we are able to pursue the continuing powerful but elusive effects of this useful but toxic metal. The key to the fullest use of epidemiological data is the integration of insights derived from it into the general body of knowledge —the relation of ideas derived from population data with ideas from experimental studies in animals and clinical studies in man. Thus the complex variations in thyroid disease in populations are part of our stock of knowledge about the general physiology of the thyroid gland; the knowledge of the B-vitamin deficiencies part of our general stock of knowledge of carbohydrate metabolism.

The first step in any epidemiologic study is the definition of the people who are affected. This may be a tragically simple matter of counting deaths from lung cancer or mass starvation. But many important and lethal conditions are merely the result of the patient having an extreme level of a variable that is distributed in the population without obvious breaks. For example, blood pressure is continuously distributed in this way. Here the identification of persons with hypertension depends on a division of people by the investigator's decision into two groups—the hypertensive and the normal. This is inevitably only a beginning—the mere division into two groups is a very crude description of a continuously distributed variable. A more refined understanding leads to the evolution of a system of grading or classifying the variable into groups. Only from the experience of people with different levels of blood pressure can we establish the different degrees of risk and make a rational decision as to which levels we will regard as hypertensive for our purposes. People with a mild and unobvious condition—with a slightly raised blood pressure; with a change in the cervix which is not yet a fully invasive carcinoma; infected with poliomyelitis but not clinically ill—may be exceedingly important. In all of these conditions the knowledge for the proper management of the disease in the population and in the individual has been dependent not only on the study of the overtly sick seeking medical attention, but also from a study of the total population.

In practical terms there are two sorts of sick people—the ones with acute disease who were well yesterday, and those who have a long-term disability. Counting each of these is important, for different reasons. For example, it is important to agencies responsible for rehabilitation to know the number of persons who newly become permanently blind each year in a population; it is important to those providing services to know the numbers of blind people in the community. In the conventional terms we need to know the *incidence* of new blind people; we need to know for different purposes the *prevalence* of people who are blind. Both measures are useful; the important thing is to measure the aspect of the disease that is relevant to the purpose in hand. Incidence is usually the useful measure for the acute infections, but the prevalence of influenza may be the relevant statistic to the harrassed manager of a city transport system during an epidemic.

When we consider a sick person, we intuitively consider the number of people who run the risk of getting the disease. A hundred people with a neurological disorder collected in the city of New York means one thing to us; the same number collected from a small island community suggests something quite different. Conventionally, we calculate *rates* relating to the number of sick people (the *numerator*) divided by the number of people at risk (the *denominator*). Equipped with such rates we can make useful comparisons. Thus, in 1967–68 the maternal mortality was 22·5 per 100,000 live births in England and Wales, but 30·5 in France and only 11·5 in Sweden (Metropolitan Life Statistical Bulletin, 1972). Such data raise a whole range of questions about the different societies and the medical services that are part of them. An interesting point is that these rates are in terms of the number of live births, and are not related to the total number of women, or even the total population. Such a selective choice of denominator obviously increases the specificity of the rate greatly (why not total births, what about twins?) Thus the deaths in automobile accidents may be based on total deaths, or separate pedestrians from people inside the vehicles. These can be related to the total population at risk, or to the number of vehicles, or to estimates of the number of miles that they are driven. Each gives a rather different picture of the problem, and their usefulness depends on the needs of the investigator. The recognition of high rates of disease in particular occupations has pinpointed many hazards and sometimes led to effective prevention even without deeper understanding of the relationships between the agent and the target cells, e.g. β-naphthylamine and bladder cancer (Case, 1966 and 1969).

A study of the rates of a disease in different communities may open up a whole new field of human pathology, e.g. the profound but in 1972 still unelucidated relationships between the mineral constituents of drinking-water and the incidence of ischemic heart disease (Crawford *et al.*, 1971; Neri *et al.*, 1971). The effect is large [TABLE 62*a*], but is not found by all communities (Comstock, 1970). The opportunities for the development of large-scale preventive measures—suppose the towns in TABLE 62 could all have the rates of the lowest—are clearly immense. But as well as the potential for direct preventive action, these studies bring a new variable into our ideas on the causation of cardiovascular disease. Vigorous efforts are being made to integrate this finding of the influence of drinking water which was quite unexpected (Crawford and Crawford, 1969; Elwood *et al.*, 1971; Dauncey and Widdowson, 1972) into our general understanding of heart disease. The variation in the incidence of heart attacks in populations with different levels of physical activity at work (Morris *et al.*, 1953; Morris

et al., 1966; Chiang *et al.*, 1968; Paffenbarger *et al.*, 1970) gave us a rather useless lead in terms of prevention [TABLE 62*b* and 62*c*]. The port that gave up its mechanical gear in order to give the longshoremen more exercise would be in several kinds of trouble at once. But the fact is also a major component of our view of the genesis of ischemic heart disease. TABLE 62*d* exemplifies another aspect. Similarly, the map of the variations in the incidence of Burkitt's lymphoma across Africa establishes the conditions which any account of the causation of this disease must meet (Kafuko *et al.*, 1970; Morrow *et al.*, 1971), while providing no useful suggestions about prevention.

TABLE 62
Some Examples of Data on which our View of the Causes of Ischaemic Heart Disease are based

(*a*) *Mean death rates per 100,000 from cardiovascular disease in towns of England and Wales grouped by water calcium, 1958–64*

Calcium (parts per million)	<10	10–39	40–69	70–99	100+
Male	751	721	636	633	546
Female	355	330	306	281	248

From Crawford *et al.* (1971). The independence of sex of the relationship is interesting.

(*b*) *Incidence of ischaemic heart disease in bus conductors and drivers during 5 years by casual systolic blood pressure-level at initial examination*

Quarters of casual systolic blood pressure (mm.Hg)	168–254	150–166	134–148	84–132
Conductors	8·5		3·9*	
Drivers	15		5·6*	
All busmen	13	4·7	5·7	4·1

* For conductors and drivers, first three quarters combined.
From Morris *et al.* (1966). A prospective study, as are *c* and *d*.

(*c*) *Incidence of fatal myocardial infarction per 1,000 per year (age adjusted rates), Health Insurance Plan of Greater New York*

	More active	Less active
Cigarette smokers	1·30	5·18
Not cigarette smokers	0·69	2·57

From Shapiro *et al.* (1969).

(*d*) *Influence of cigarette smoking and blood cholesterol on frequency of heart attacks (Ratios: all men in study as 100)*

	Serum Cholesterol			
	96–193	194–220	221–249	250–534
Cigarette smokers	78	84	118	207
Not cigarette smokers	43	47	57	90

From Kannel (1966)—data from the Framingham study.

A single rate, the incidence of tuberculosis in our town this year, is instructive but again intuitively we recognize that the series of annual rates for a number of years shows us the trend with time of tuberculosis and is much more useful. Routine statistics collected year in year out form the basis of much of our understanding of both progress in the control of old problems—infant mortality, tuberculosis—and of the emergence of new ones—the lung cancer epidemic, or the variety of sudden deaths among the young. Time trends do not always mean what they seem; an increase in death certified to a particular cause may simply mean that physicians have begun to recognize and correctly describe a disease that they previously lumped into a broader category. In many prosperous white populations the incidence of malignant melanoma has been rising steeply in recent years (Lee, 1972), and the incidence now is about 32 per million per year in the white population of the United States (Biometry Branch, 1972). Some of this is undoubtedly due to more frequent pathologic examinations of better quality. One way of critically examining a time trend such as this is to look at the total group, in this case all skin tumors, of which the more refined diagnosis is a part. This trend is also rising, and we are still left wondering whether people are simply becoming more concerned about their cutaneous lumps or because the registries are becoming more efficient. A second strategy is to look at a different variable, subject to different biases from the first. The death rate[1] from malignant melanoma also has risen substantially, which seems to rule out any ideas about the better diagnosis of minor skin lesions being of critical importance in the trend of incidence. Further, the increase in the reported mortality from malignant melanomas is particularly conspicuous in the middle-aged and young—the least likely group to be inadequately certified. This change is large enough to produce an increase in the mortality from all skin cancers combined in people under the age of 65 from 16 per million in the United States white male population in 1950 to 21 per million in 1968, in spite of the improvements in diagnosis and treatment that have occurred. Thus, the analysis of a number of different variables leads us to the reasonably firm conclusion that there has been a real change in the incidence of the malignant melanoma. Similar considerations suggest that the incidence of peptic ulceration is declining in the British population (Meade et al., 1968).

For some reason, when we think about time, we use words that apply to length—a short time, like a short piece of string; never a broad or a shallow time, although the idea seems pleasant. This convention is carried over into scientific work, and studies that collect information about people over long periods of time are spoken of as longitudinal studies. Continuing this simple system, studies of people at the same point in time are spoken of as cross-sectional—when the heights of all the children in a school are recorded on a particular day, a slice has been cut across the stream of time. A group of people who are identified at a particular short period of time—men wounded in a particular period of the Second World War, nuns entering a convent in a particular time period, the group graduating from a school on the same day—can then be followed as time passes. Such a group, defined at the beginning, not supplemented thereafter, is conventionally known as a *cohort*. This is an important idea in the study of the common lethal diseases of developed societies. There are a number of ways in which human diseases are conditioned by long-term features of the patient's life. Ischemic heart disease, for all the suddenness of its presentation, is clearly the result of the long build-up of arterial and coagulation disorder. Lung cancer is a

function of a cigarette habit acquired in adolescence. The incidence of breast cancer in middle life is strongly influenced by the occurrence or non-occurrence of pregnancy in early life Permanent cellular changes may be introduced at a single period of early life—exposure to radiation or an early pregnancy. A habit may be acquired which persists, and exerts a fortunate or disastrous effect over many years. Diseases related to the long-term characteristics of individuals can often best be studied longitudinally. Large differences in the experience at each stage of life of people born at different times can often be demonstrated.

The data of the epidemiologist are derived either from the recorded experience of other people—death certificates, sickness claims, travellers' tales—and/or from the data that he has acquired for the purpose. These approaches complement each other—we know that stomach cancer was common in 1930 because our predecessors made careful records, and we have no access to that aspect of the disease except through these; we know about the interrelationship between smoking and asbestos exposure and lung cancer because of the careful questioning of workers for the purposes of epidemiologic study.

Asking patients about the source of their disease is an epidemiologic method of classic simplicity, but if the factor is both uncommon and powerful this may be all that is needed. Thus the proportion of Pott's patients with epithelioma of the scrotum who were chimney sweeps was clearly too high for the disease to be randomly distributed in the working population (Pott, 1775); equally in a modern example, the association between an epidemic neurological syndrome in humans and animals and the consumption of fish from waters contaminated with mercury from a factory discharge (the Minimata episode) could not have been due to chance (McAlpine and Araki, 1958; Kurland, Faro, and Siedler, 1960). This sort of perceptive questioning is nothing but an extension of the clinical method practiced by every physician. It will not work where the factor is widespread in the community, does not have a high efficiency in producing the disease, or is not its exclusive cause. Then there are numerous people who are clearly exposed to the agent—cigarette smokers, workers in a particular plant—who have not got the disease (lung cancer or bladder cancer), and even some who do get the disease who have never been exposed to the putative agent. Associations of this kind are very common and important, and they can only be disentangled if a method is devised that will demonstrate that those with the disease have a greater experience of the agent than those without. We need an estimate of the exposure in people who did not have the disease—in the conventional terminology a 'control group'.[2] The comparison of histories of some activity, such as cigarette smoking, in patients with the disease, and in people without the disease acting as normal 'controls' is the classical retrospective 'case/control' study. This is a study design which is repeatedly used because it gives answers quickly and cheaply, and has been of great practical importance. Studies of this type have made major contributions to our knowledge of

---

[1] Death rates are the number of deaths from a cause in a period of time as a function of the population at risk; the case-fatality rate relates numbers of deaths to the number of people who had the disease.

[2] This sounds odd in the English language. They do not control anything in the ordinary usage. We do not know how the word came to be used this way. It is apparently derived from the French contre-role, a person acting as a checker in an accounting system. The French themselves call such individuals and groups 'witnesses', which seems much clearer, as they witness to the normal situation.

the aetiology of heart disease, lung cancer, breast cancer, leukemia, and in fact almost all the chronic diseases where we have any knowledge of their aetiology.

The selection of people to act as controls is a subtle and demanding operation. They must be like the patients in age and sex and race, otherwise absurd results will be obtained from the study. But suppose that we carefully match the cases and controls for residence—we have no hope of discovering from our study that the risk is higher in the villages than in the town. Of course we may realize this by simply looking at the distribution. But suppose that the association is subtler. It is possible to match for socio–economic status and neatly obscure a specific factor such as high maize diet by this means. Overmatching of cases and controls is a real possibility.

Another problem of case/control studies is that of observer bias—we see and hear what we expect to see and hear. A factor that the observer or patient expects to be associated with the disease will be reported differently by the patients than by the health controls. If possible, as a means of minimizing the universal human tendency to read into our surroundings our own preconceptions, the person collecting the histories should be unaware which people are patients and which controls; they should be 'blind'. If this cannot be done because, for example, the patients have visible stigmata of their condition, its effects must be searched for. Thus bereaved mothers might remember more closely the events of pregnancy than those with a living child, or the other way round. For at least a sample, the histories should be checked by records made at the time. These effects apply to the patients as well. No alcoholic will give a true account of his consumption, while the non-alcoholic control will search his memory to the last martini in an endeavour to assist the researchers. Bias can get into the conduct of case/control studies in a multitude of unsuspected ways. Helpful colleagues really will select 'typical' cases and thus radically alter the spectrum of the disease observed; or select the articulate and bright, as they give such clear histories. Old men with carcinoma of the prostate give vivid accounts of their sexual life; controls with benign hyperplasia are much more restrained. We do not know if the more dire disease influences the recall, or if we are really seeing a difference in remote lifestyle (Steele *et al.*, 1971).

These difficulties are avoided if the opposite route is employed—data about the factors suspected of causing the disease are collected from a group of healthy people; they are then observed over a period of time, and the occurrence of the disease in the group noted. The incidence can then be related to the distribution of the suspected factor in a situation where the people were put into categories that include them all before anyone became ill. Two examples are shown in TABLE 63. This *prospective* approach is sometimes also termed a cohort study, because clearly cohorts have been set up and followed. Prospective studies have two other major advantages. They enable a direct estimate of the magnitude of the association between the suspected factor and the disease to be made. They also reveal unsuspected further associations between the factor and disease. Thus, for example, it was known from retrospective studies that congenital rubella was associated with hearing and visual defects; it required prospective studies to reveal the full range of the syndrome and to estimate the scale of its effects.

In practice, retrospective and prospective studies are com-

TABLE 63

Two Examples of Prospective Studies

(a) *Average incidence of leukemia by radiation dose estimates in survivors of Hiroshima and Nagasaki, 1950–58*

Estimated dose (rads)	Incidence per million in the time period
0–20	27
21–40	51
41–80	49
81–160	260
161–320	388
321–640	724
641–1,280	1,146
1,281 and over	1,392

Modified from Anderson (1972). In the original the rate is called a prevalence, which is not in terms of the usual definition given here. In general, it is important to check what are the numerator and denominator of rates, rather than relying on the title that they are given.

(b) *Observed and expected deaths between 1930 and 1952 in veterans of the First World War who suffered poisoning with mustard gas, or who underwent amputation of a leg.*

	Cancer of the Lung and Pleura	Other Neoplasms	Other Causes of Death	All Deaths
Mustard Gas 1,267 Men alive 1/1/30				
Observed deaths	29	50	468	547
Expected deaths	14	47	297	357
Amputation 1,114 Men alive 1/1/30				
Observed deaths	13	59	311	383
Expected deaths	16	57	294	366

Modified from Case and Lea (1955). If the data are recorded at the time, it is possible to construct a prospective study years after the events. This is sometimes a powerful technique, as it enables answers to be obtained soon after the question was posed. In this example, the study was done in the 1950s because all the records were there, and the result was the same as if the study had been started in 1918. In contrast with the Hiroshima study there was no distribution of the gas poisoning by dose. The contrast is the numbers of deaths expected on the experience of the general male population over the same period of years; as a check a comparable population of men who were wounded before the date that mustard gas was introduced were also studied. This prospective design shows the total effect of the agent in the difference between the number of deaths observed and expected from all causes—a retrospective case/control study based on mustard gas patients would have missed the large effect on mortality from other causes—in fact, extra deaths due to bronchitis.

plementary. Retrospective studies are cheap and quick, but are susceptible to technical problems and give limited answers. Prospective studies are more costly and may take years to give their answers. One current situation may exemplify the relation between the two types of study. Oral contraceptives are potent steroids, and we do not have the knowledge to be sure that their long-term use is not going to increase the incidence of carcinoma of the cervix or breast cancer—already running at a lifetime level of about 7 per cent. for women in the United States. Prospective studies have been set up, and will provide clear answers in a decade or so. But governments and society need some guidance now, and retrospective studies give the encouraging suggestion that these agents may actually reduce the risk (Vessey *et al.*, 1972). Data from two current studies are shown in TABLE 64.

Several examples have been given of a major component in

TABLE 64

Two examples of Retrospective Studies

(*a*) *Use of oral contraceptives in patients with breast cancer and matched controls*

Time oral contraceptive last used	Breast Cancer		Matched Controls	
	Number of Patients	Percentage	Number of Patients	Percentage
During month before lump noticed	12	13	27	15
More than 1 month before lump noticed	19	21	46	26
Never used	59	66	107	59
Total	90	100	180	100

Modified from Vessey, Doll, and Sutton (1972). There is no indication that within the time scale so far available, the use of oral contraceptives is a factor in the aetiology of breast cancer—if anything, there is some indication that they are protective.

(*b*) *Use of oral contraceptives in patients with preclinical carcinoma of the cervix and a control group. Women aged 25–29.*

Type of Contraception	Percentages	
	Women with preclinical carcinoma of cervix	Controls
Pill	85·8	85·7
Barrier method . . .	26·0	31·5
Intrauterine device . .	12·3	12·2
Other methods . . .	12·5	6·4
All methods	92·2	93·3

Modified from Worth and Boyes (1972). Again, there is no indication that the pill was implicated in the development of these early carcinomas of cervix—found in a screening programme. The percentages do not add to 100 because the women did not restrict themselves to a single type.

our picture of a disease having been derived from epidemiologic study. These tend to be rather unsatisfactory in that they do not connect very obviously to anything else. We do not know why thalidomide is a teratogen for humans but not for mice; why the same dose of radiation is more carcinogenic to elderly people than to the young; indeed, why an elevated blood cholesterol should be associated with ischemic heart disease. The examples from the chronic disease contrast with the neat certainties of our knowledge of the relationship between polio virus and poliomyelitis or the plasmodium and malaria. In infectious processes the agent is foreign and has a life of its own. Its distribution and behaviour and the host's specific response to it determine very largely what happens. Our successful studies of infectious processes have typically depended on the elucidation of a small number of factors. Indeed, we do not know what makes measles a springtime epidemic in temperate climates, or what determines whether an infected and non-immune child will develop apparent rubella or not. But this does not prevent our controlling both these diseases with potent vaccines. The chronic diseases are different. They are the outcome of a number of factors of rather similar importance. Hypertension, deranged blood lipids, diabetes, cigarette smoking, obesity, physical inertia are all factors in the genesis of ischemic heart disease, and none is dominant. The only possible strategy is to conduct studies which include all the known variables, as well as whatever is novel about the particular occasion. This is well recognized for heart diseases, but we still conduct rather elaborate studies of less well-understood diseases in terms of single factors. The practical point is that if only one factor is known in the aetiology of a chronic disease, it is unlikely to account for much of the total determination of that disease, and hence the study should be large enough to describe a rather mild effect. Further, if several factors are known, their distribution should be noted in all future studies.

In sum, epidemiology is the study of the patient in the context of his community, so that the results of the countless natural experiments that we continually perform on ourselves by the way we choose to behave in the environment in which we find ourselves, may be harvested and added to the stock of knowledge of the causation of human disease.

REFERENCES AND FURTHER READING

A wider discussion of some topics is given in Morris's *The Uses of Epidemiology*, 2nd edition, 1964. A valuable survey of current studies is contained in *Epidemiology of Non-Communicable Diseases*, edited by Acheson (1971). Methods are fully discussed in MacMahon and Pugh, *Epidemiology: Principles and Methods*, 1970. The list that follows is not a general reading list, but is provided to enable the student to follow up topics for himself.

Acheson, E. D., ed. (1971) Epidemiology of non-communicable disease, *Brit. med. Bull.*, **27**, 1.
Anderson, R. E. (1972) Leukemia and related disorders, *Hum. Path.*, **2**, 505.
Baker, G. (1767) *An Essay Concerning the Cause of the Endemial Colic of Devonshire*, London. Reprinted Delta Omega, 1964.
Biometry Branch, National Cancer Institute (1972) *Preliminary Report Third National Cancer Survey 1969 Incidence*, Washington, USDHEW.

British Medical Bulletin (1971) Epidemiology of non-communicable disease, vol. 27, no. 1.
Case, R. A. M. (1956) Cohort analysis of cancer mortality in England and Wales 1911–54 by site and sex, *Brit. J. prev. soc. Med.*, **10**, 172.
Case, R. A. M. (1966) Tumours of the urinary tract as an occupational disease in several industries, *Ann. roy. Coll. Surg.*, (*Engl.*), **39**, 213.
Case, R. A. M. (1969) Some environmental carcinogens, *Proc. roy. Soc. Med.*, **62**, 1061.
Case, R. A. M., and Lea, A. J. (1955) Mustard gas poisoning: An investigation in the possibility that poisoning by mustard gas in the 1914–18 war might be a factor in the production of neoplasia, *Brit. J. prev. soc. Med.*, **9**, 62.
Chiang, B. N., Alexander, E. R., Bruce, R. A., and Ting, N. (1968) Physical characteristics and exercise performance of pedicab and upper socioeconomic classes of middle-aged Chinese men, *Amer. Heart J.*, **76**, 760.
Comstock, G. W. (1970) Fatal arteriosclerotic heart disease,

water hardness at home and socioeconomic characteristics, *Amer. J. Epidemiol.*, **94**, 1.

Crawford, M. D., and Crawford, T. (1969) Lead content of bone in a soft and a hard water area, *Lancet*, **i**, 699.

Crawford, M. D., Gardner, M. J., and Morris, N. N. (1971) Cardiovascular disease and the mineral content of drinking water, *Brit. med. Bull.*, **27**, 21.

Dauncey, M. J., and Widdowson, E. M. (1972) Urinary excretion of calcium, magnesium, sodium, and potassium in hard and soft water areas, *Lancet*, **i**, 711.

Elwood, P. C., Bainton, D., Moore, F., Davies, D. F., Wakley, E. J., Langman, M., and Sweetnam, P. (1971) Cardiovascular surveys in areas with different water supplies, *Brit. med .J.*, **2**, 362.

Gillie, R. B. (1971) Endemic goiter, *Sci. Amer.*, **224**, 93.

Kafuko, G. W., and Burkitt, D. P. (1970) Burkitt's lymphoma and malaria, *Int. J. Cancer*, **6**, 1.

Kannel, W. B. (1966) The Framingham heart study: Habits and coronary heart disease, *Publ. Hlth Serv. Publ.*, No. 1515, Washington, USDHEW.

Krugman, S., ed. (1969) International conference on rubella immunization, *Amer. J. Dis. Child.*, **118**, 1.

Kurland, L. T., Faro, S. N., and Siedler, H. (1960) Minimata disease, *Wld Neurol.*, **1**, 370.

Lee, J. A. H. (1973) The trend of mortality from primary malignant tumors of skin, *J. invest. Derm.*, **59**, 445.

MacMahon, B., and Pugh, T. F. (1970) *Epidemiology: Principles and Methods*, Boston, Mass.

McAlpine, D., and Araki, S. (1958) Minimata disease: An unusual neurological disorder caused by contaminated fish, *Lancet*, **ii**, 629.

Meade, T. W., Arie, T. H. D., Brewis, M., Bond, D. J., and Morris, J. N. (1968) Recent history of ischaemic heart disease and duodenal ulcer in doctors, *Brit. med. J.*, **3**, 701.

Metropolitan Life Statistical Bulletin (1972) Maternal mortality —United States, Canada, and Western Europe, *Bull.*, **53**, 2.

Morris, J. N., Heady, J. A., Raffle, P. A. B., Roberts, C. G., and Parks, J. W. (1953) Coronary heart disease and physical activity of work, *Lancet*, **ii**, 1053.

Morris, J. N., Kagan, A., Pattison, D. C., and Gardner, M. J. (1966) Incidence and prediction of ischaemic heart disease in London busmen, *Lancet*, **ii**, 553.

Morrow, R. H., Pike, M. C., Smith, P. G., Ziegler, J. L., and Kisuule, A. (1971) Burkitt's lymphoma: A time-space cluster of cases in Bwamba County of Uganda, *Brit. med. J.*, **2**, 491.

Neri, L. C., Mandel, J. S., and Hewitt, D. (1972) Relation between mortality and water hardness in Canada, *Lancet*, **i**, 931.

Paffenbarger, R. S., Laughlin, M. E., Gima, A. S., and Black, R. A. (1970) Work activity of longshoremen as related to death from coronary heart disease and stroke, *New Engl. J. Med.*, **282**, 1109.

Pickles, W. N. (1939) *Epidemiology in Country Practice*, Bristol.

Pott, P. (1775) Chirurgical Observations. Reproduced in *Percivall Pott's Contribution to Cancer Research* by M. Potter, in *The Biology of Cutaneous Cancer*, ed. Urbach, National Cancer Institute Monograph No. 10, 1963, pp. 1–13, Washington, USDHEW.

Puska, P. (1973) The North Karelia Project: an attempt at community prevention of cardiovascular disease, *Wld Hlth Org. Chron.*, **27**, 55.

Shapiro, S., Weinblatt, E., Frank, C. W., and Sager, R. V. (1969) Incidence of coronary heart disease in a population insured for medical care (HIP), *Amer. J. publ. Hlth*, **59**, Part II, 1.

Steele, R., Lees, R. E., Kraus, A. S., and Rao, C. (1971) Sexual factors in the epidemiology of cancer of the prostate, *J. chron. Dis.*, **24**, 29

Terris, M., ed. (1964) Goldberger on Pellagra, Baton Rouge.

Vessey, M. P., Doll, R., and Sutton, P. M. (1972) Oral contraceptives and breast neoplasia: A retrospective study, *Brit. med. J.*, **3**, 719.

World Health Organization (1974) Cardiovascular diseases: care and prevention. A series of 3 articles. *Wld Hlth Org. Chron.*, **28**, 55, 116, 190.

World Health Organization (1974) The work of WHO in 1973 (section on non-communicable diseases, *Wld Hlth Org. Off. Rec.*, **213**, 58.

World Health Organization Regional Office for the Americas (PAHO) (1973) *Epidemiologic Studies and Clinical Trials in Chronic Diseases*, Washington.

World Health Organization Regional Office for Europe. Reports on chronic heart diseases, Copenhagen.

(1973) *Study on Symptoms and Signs Predicting Acute Myocardial Infarction and Sudden Death, Copenhagen 1972* (Euro 8204(4)).

(1973) *Evaluation of Comprehensive Rehabilitation and Preventive Programmes for Patients after Acute Myocardial Infarction, Prague 1971 and Moscow 1972* (Euro 8206(8)).

(1974) *Working Group on Methodology of Multifactorial Preventive Trials in Ischaemic Heart Disease, Innsbruck 1973* (Euro 8202).

(1974) *Conference on Prevention and Control of Major Cardiovascular Diseases, Brussels 1973* (Euro 8214).

World Health Organization Regional Office for Europe (1973) *The Organization of Comprehensive Cancer Control Programmes, Oslo 1972* (Euro 8102(3)).

Worth, A. J., and Boyes, D. A. (1972) A case control study into the possible effects of birth control pills on pre-clinical carcinoma of the cervix, *J. Obstet. Gynaec. Brit. Cwlth*, **79**, 673.

28

ACCIDENTS AND THEIR PREVENTION

J. P. BULL

A major epidemiological revolution in Western Europe since the Second World War has been the reversal of the roles of infectious diseases and accidents as causes of death. In 1946 deaths in England and Wales due to infectious diseases of all types were twice those due to accidents (28,000 and 14,000 respectively); 5 years later the two were equal and by 1970 deaths from infection were one-fifth of those due to accidents (3,500 and 18,000). Both domestic and road accident deaths had risen during this period, and are each now twice those from infection. The main change has been a reduction of mortality from infection, in particular tuberculosis, but the accident figures rose markedly until 1966. Since then total accident deaths have declined a little; the extent of this is made uncertain by a change of classification since 1967 [FIG. 78]. Nevertheless accidents are the leading cause of deaths of persons aged 1–40 years and are only exceeded by cancer and ischaemic heart disease as a cause of loss of years of working life (Registrar General, 1971).

Though the injuries from different types of accident are often clinically similar, from the epidemiological point of view of causation and prevention, we need to classify accidents by the circumstances in which they occur. Most accidental injuries are related to transport, occupation, or domestic life. A relatively small number fall outside this classification: recreational accidents, falls in the street, and drowning are examples of these. A few types of accident might appear under two heads: for example, injuries to railway employees could appear as 'transport' or 'occupational'. In this study transport accidents involving passengers or employees are included in the 'transport' category. The contribution which the three main groups make to the total deaths from accidents are shown in FIGURE 79. Forty per cent. of accidental deaths in England and Wales occur in and around the home, another 40 per cent. are caused by road transport; and 5 per cent. are occupational. It will be seen that the general rise in total accidental deaths has been due to increases in transport and domestic accidents, whereas occupational deaths have tended to decrease. The marked differences in incidence of these different types of accident at different ages are shown in FIGURE 78 which gives deaths per million population at risk. The total accidental death rate in males is high in infants, and rises again to a peak in the twenties. From 50 years onwards the rate increases rapidly to a maximum at old age. Domestic accidents predominate up to school age; from about 10 to 50 years, road traffic accidents are the main determinant of the total rate, and thereafter domestic accidents again predominate. In childhood and early adult life females follow the same distribution of accident rates, though with a much less prominent peak for road accidents. Their death rate from domestic accidents after 50 years, however, is much higher, and represents an even

greater preponderance of cases, since females of 50 years of age and over outnumber males by one third. Typical circumstances and injuries in the two sexes at different ages will be reviewed in later sections.

Statistical studies in this field necessarily emphasize accidents which cause death, since information about these is much more complete and reliable than it is concerning injuries. All accidental deaths are subject to scrutiny by coroners, and their

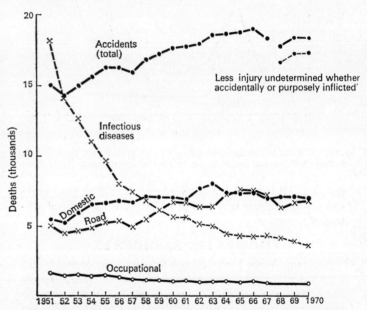

FIG. 78. Deaths due to various types of accidents compared with deaths due to infectious diseases 1951–70. (Data from Registrar General's Statistical Review for England and Wales.)

circumstances are recorded by the Registrar General. Injuries not causing death are much more numerous, but there is no standard system of recording which applies to all types and circumstances of accident. Within the aetiological groups rather more information is available, and will be discussed below. In all groups injuries range from the slight wounds not requiring medical attention and causing only minor and temporary incapacity to those requiring hospital admission and incapacitating for normal employment, and further to those causing permanent disablement or perhaps death. The final severity of the effects of the injury is to a substantial extent determined by the speed and efficiency of treatment. It follows that an epidemiological approach is needed in planning appropriate treatment facilities. Hazardous occurrences and accidents which do not lead to injuries are vastly more numerous again. Information about them is scanty, but is clearly very relevant for prevention. In many such occurrences it seems only by chance that injury does not result. The constituents of this 'chance' merit more attention than they have yet received. From an actuarial aspect it may be adequate to assess the statistical likelihood of injury given certain circumstances, but very often some human action is involved in the escape from injury, just as it is in its causation. In the complex

fabrics usually responsible are of cotton or cellulose, which readily propagate flame. Terylene, nylon and the heavier woollen fabrics are relatively safe, and this accounts in part for boys having fewer serious burns. Nightwear is particularly liable to be ignited, wide-skirted nightdresses being more dangerous than pyjamas. A feature of injuries in children due

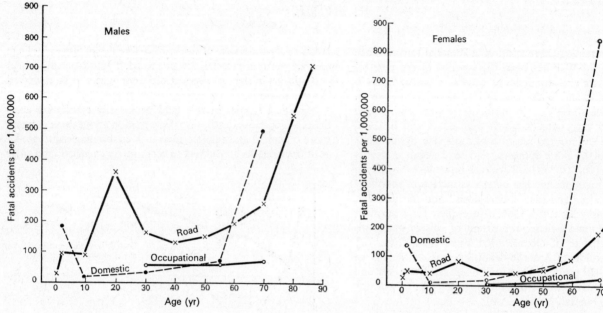

FIG. 79. Fatal accidents per million at risk at different ages, England and Wales, 1970 (except Road Accidents, 1969). Domestic accidents include accidents at home and in residential institutions. (Data from Registrar General's Statistical Review.)

processes of modern life development of skill in preventing and avoiding injury may well be as important as physical protection.

DOMESTIC ACCIDENTS

Accidents in the home, though they account for nearly half the accidental deaths of our community, have received relatively little attention in respect to their causes and prevention. As will be seen from TABLE 65, people at the extremes of life are the most common sufferers. Though much less frequent than previously, death from suffocation and respiratory obstruction by foreign bodies is still prominent in infants. It is the commonest cause of accidental deaths under 1 year in both sexes, and warrants closer investigation of detailed causes, possible underlying disease in some cases, and methods of prevention. When a child learns to walk it encounters a new set of hazards. Many domestic objects and processes which are safe for healthy adults are dangerous for the child, with his poorer co-ordination of movement, less reach and power, less understanding of the hazard, and less capacity to minimize injury. Falls from furniture and elsewhere, scalds from falling into and overturning hot fluids, and injuries from sharp objects affect both sexes about equally in pre-school years (Castle, 1950; Rowntree, 1950). A serious hazard, particularly for young girls, arises from the almost universal use of flammable clothing, both for dresses and nightwear. In India women who wear the cotton sari often receive fatal burns if it catches alight on the open domestic fire. In the United Kingdom the majority of fatal domestic burns are attributable to clothes catching fire. The

to burning is that though many result in death, a great many more cause permanent serious disablement, even after long periods of hospital treatment (Bull et al., 1964).

Deaths from drowning, though often not occurring strictly at home, may be conveniently considered with domestic accidents. They have an even greater importance as a cause of death in boys than have burning accidents in girls. Of 485 accidental deaths from drowning in England and Wales in 1970, nearly half were of children under 15. Accidental falls into open water, such as canals and rivers, account for many of these cases; others result from bathers getting into difficulties. These tragedies do not figure prominently in medical studies, since either death is immediate or complete recovery occurs. In either event the case is seldom admitted to hospital.

Throughout later childhood girls continue to suffer injuries from clothes catching fire, and though commonly able to avoid accidents in normal domestic circumstances, accidental injuries may more easily occur on special occasions, such as parties, when excitement, easily ignited garments, unfamiliar surroundings, and improvised heating increase the hazard.

It is sometimes implied that poisoning is a major hazard of childhood. Mortality statistics do not support this, though numerous cases of non-fatal poisoning do occur which make large demands upon emergency treatment facilities.

Young adults have a relatively low death rate from domestic accidents. In recent years poisoning, usually by household gas or barbiturates, has been the most common cause of these deaths. The deaths from poisoning by household gas have, however, fallen by half since 1967. That this is not due to a reduction in the use of gas is shown by the sales, which have risen by one-third in the same period. The busy housewife often injures herself on sharp tools and objects, and falls causing sprains and sometimes fractures are quite frequent, but seldom in this age-group do they result in death.

The middle-aged adults (45–64 years) have a higher death rate from all the main types of domestic accidents. Deaths from falls and from poisoning show marked increases. Diminished resistance to injury probably plays a part in this higher

come permanently dependent as a result of the injury. An old lady previously able to look after herself and to take a pride in doing so commonly loses this capacity after an injury which even with the best treatment may leave her with stiffness, pain and other disabilities. This situation raises important family and social problems, which are likely to become more prominent in the future as the average age of the population increases (Fisher, 1955) [see also CHAPTER 39].

At all ages people who are subject to attacks of unconscious-

TABLE 65
Domestic Accidents Causing Death (England and Wales, 1970)*

Age-group	Falls	Fires and hot substances	Electric current	Suffocation and respiratory obstruction	Poisons	Other and unspecified	Total	Population (millions)	Rate per million
0–4 years:									
Male . .	32	58	4	215	19	41	369	2·11	175
Female . .	19	59	1	151	10	28	268	2·00	134
5–14 years:									
Male . .	8	16	4	20	5	4	67	3·79	18
Female . .	0	13	3	8	6	2	32	3·60	9
15–44 years:									
Male . .	53	43	21	65	122	21	325	9·77	33
Female . .	16	29	3	17	100	17	182	9·41	19
45–64 years:									
Male . .	146	46	8	39	109	37	385	5·79	66
Female . .	130	68	8	41	129	23	399	6·18	65
65+ years:									
Male . .	848	156	1	29	100	50	1,184	2·38	497
Female . .	2,603	312	4	50	219	83	3,271	3·88	843
All ages:									
Male . .	1,087	319	38	368	355	163	2,330	23·83	98
Female . .	2,768	481	19	267	464	153	4,152	25·08	166

* Includes deaths occurring at home and in residential institutions.

death rate. The injuries themselves may be similar to those in younger persons, but the cumulative effects of previous illnesses and injuries interfere with recovery. All these features become more prominent still in the aged, and the domestic accident death rate rises spectacularly at ages of over 65 years. This, together with the increasing proportion of the aged in the population, is the major cause of the increase of total deaths due to domestic accidents. At ages over 65 years females outnumber males by 5:3, and as will be seen in TABLE 65 deaths of elderly females due to falls alone account for 40 per cent. of domestic accident fatalities. Old people often have poorer sight, hearing, and balance, and their diminished range of movement makes it more difficult to escape injury when an accident occurs; all such factors tend to increase the injury rate, but with respect to the death rate the overriding consideration is that the aged very readily succumb to any disease or injury which requires bed rest. The kind of awkward fall due to the various factors mentioned above can cause several types of fracture. In a year's admissions to the Birmingham Accident Hospital there were among patients 65 years or over 302 patients with Colles' fractures, of whom only 12 were admitted to the main wards and only 1 died. Of 204 patients with fractures of the femur all needed admission and 47 died. Few died directly of their injuries; the average survival was several weeks, and the final cause of death commonly respiratory infection or pulmonary embolism. Another very important aspect of these injuries in the aged is that many of these patients be-

ness have an increased risk of domestic injuries. For example, 14 per cent. of serious domestic burns reviewed by Maisels and Corps (1964) occurred in epileptics. Attacks of collapse or unconsciousness due to cardiovascular accidents are responsible for a further important proportion.

Methods of prevention of domestic accidents follow logically from knowledge of their causes. Improved housing and education in child care will help to reduce infant mortality; increased awareness of the risks to children of burning accidents and of drowning seems necessary. Most parents act as though 'it cannot happen to me'. Practical methods of prevention of burns are now available, fireguards have been carefully designed to give reliable protection (B.S. 2788, B.S. 3140), and guarding of new electric, gas, and oil fires is now compulsory. Work on developing and testing flame-resisting textiles has had considerable success, and fabrics that are acceptable for children's clothing and nightwear, and also of satisfactory low flammability, are now generally available (B.S. 3120, B.S. 3121). Regulations limiting the sale of children's nightdresses to those meeting these specifications are having an encouraging result in a reduction in serious burns from this cause. Another welcome reduction has been in injuries from fireworks. This followed a sustained campaign by surgeons, safety organizations, and government together with co-operation from manufacturers and retailers. Another outstanding example of a practical approach to prevention of burns is the work of Antia in Bombay. On the basis of a survey of the circumstances of these injuries a campaign of instruction was launched in the proper use of pressure stoves, of platforms for cooking fires and care in selection of safer clothing.

The circumstances of drowning accidents need more study. In Norway and also in India investigations have shown that many of these accidents were due to falls into wells. A campaign in Norway to have these properly protected or filled in has been followed by a reduction in this type of accident. In many of our cities derelict canal tow paths are still used as playgrounds, and this not infrequently results in drowning accidents. A more positive approach can be provided by wider opportunities for swimming and life-saving instruction. This should help to reduce the very numerous holiday bathing accidents.

Prevention of accidents in the aged requires that the limitations of old people be recognized by those who look after them, and not least by the aged themselves. Guarding of fires is at least as important as for children, and even more necessary is that obstructions of floors and stairways should be removed. As far as possible stairs should be avoided, and there is scope for special design of rooms, equipment, and homes for the aged to promote the maximum of interest and activity within the limitations of diminished perception and agility [see CHAPTER 39].

TRANSPORT ACCIDENTS

The increase in speed and ease of travel has caused corresponding increases in accidental injuries to a scale which would have appalled previous generations. Transport by air and sea has its own special hazards, but the major contribution to accidental deaths is from motor vehicles on the road. From a few hundred at the beginning of the century the number of deaths in Great Britain from this cause are now 7,500 annually. In a population only about four times as large but with seven times as many vehicles the annual road deaths in the United States are now about 57,000; even more striking are the 19,000 deaths per year in Western Germany, which has a population similar to that of Great Britain and a similar number of vehicles.

Comparative statistics from different countries show that casualties are related to numbers of vehicles and to population. An approximate agreement has been demonstrated between the numbers of casualties and the expression $0{\cdot}0003(NP^2)^{\frac{1}{3}}$ where N is the number of vehicles and P the population (Smeed, 1949). As the number of vehicles per head of population rises, the proportions of the types of accidents change. In the United States, for instance, with one car for every two persons, less than one-fifth of fatal accidents are of pedestrians; in Britain and several western European countries, where there are about four persons per vehicle, pedestrians form about two-fifths of the total casualties. The main trend is that injuries to occupants of vehicles increase in approximate proportion to the increasing number of vehicles. The hazards to certain categories of road user show marked differences in different countries. Risk of death for car occupants is more than twice as high in Germany and Italy as in Great Britain and Sweden. The corresponding figure for the United States is intermediate. In countries with relatively few cars, such as Portugal or Turkey, the hazards to car occupants are also particularly high. Deaths of pedestrians expressed as rates per million at given ages are similar in North America and Britain. They are rather

higher in Germany, but the great excess of road deaths there, as well as in America, is among drivers and passengers of vehicles (Bull, 1969).

TABLE 66 shows the types of fatal road accident in England and Wales. Characteristic peaks of age distribution are found for each type of road user. The deaths among pedestrians are particularly of the very young and the aged. Motor cyclists suffer one-eighth of the fatal accidents, chiefly between the ages of 15 and 25. Deaths of vehicle occupants are becoming increasingly prominent throughout adult life. Pedal cyclists now account for less than one-fourteenth of the fatal casualties. A proportionately similar age distribution of the different types of fatal accident is found in Germany, in spite of the previously mentioned higher total deaths. In contrast to industrial and domestic accidents, road accidents have the highest fatality rate in early adult life. Motor cyclists and car drivers are most often involved; doubtless this is related to the numbers exposed at this age. This peak sustains the role of accidents as the major single cause of mortality from 1 to 40 years in males. Road deaths are relatively uncommon in females. Girls share with boys the fairly high rate due to pedestrian accidents, and elderly women as well as men have high risks as pedestrians. Males, however, continue to have a higher death rate from road accidents than females at all ages. Figures collected by the Economic Commission for Europe confirm that this is true in all western countries (United Nations, 1974).

Head injuries and multiple fractures are the commonest causes of death from road accidents. Similar injuries are found among the survivors, and cause temporary and often permanent disability at an age when there is normally maximum activity and productivity. The detailed causation of these injuries has recently been studied more closely. Experiments, particularly in the United States, have shown the ways in which car occupants are injured by displacement due to the momentum of the body when a vehicle decelerates suddenly on impact. Drivers are thrown against steering-wheel, roof, or windscreen; front-seat passengers against dashboard, screen, and roof, and rear-seat passengers against the back of the front seat. Other injuries are caused by impact against projecting levers and handles, and a characteristic patella fracture results from impact of the knee against the edge of the glove tray. Deformation of the passenger compartment and ejection of occupants are increasingly important as causes of severe injuries in accidents at high speed (Gissane and Bull, 1964). Studies in this country on the circumstances of head injury have been made the basis of the design of protective helmets for motor cyclists and racing drivers, and standard patterns are now available (B.S. 2001 and 2495). Car designers are beginning to make a selling point of safety features, such as special steering-wheel and column, padding of dashboards and antiburst door-locks. The introduction of these features in European cars has been accelerated by recent American legislation. Safety harnesses for car occupants are designed to prevent injuries due to momentum and to ejection, and they have been shown to reduce injuries by about one-half (Lister and Milsom, 1963; Bohlin, 1968). Compulsory fitting of safety harness to new vehicles is now enforced in Great Britain and many other countries. The recent introduction of compulsory wearing of seat belts in Australia is producing very promising reductions of injuries.

Within a given road system prevention of accidents is largely a question of devising and enforcing appropriate rules of behaviour. The problems presented by thousands of vehicles each a ton or more in weight, capable of speeds of 70–120 m.p.h. and each independently controlled, would seem almost insoluble. Add to this that the same roads are used also by pedestrians and cyclists, and it is perhaps the low rather than the high number of accidents which should be the cause of surprise. Important features of the roads themselves, such as surface, lighting, curvature, and line of sight, have been investigated by the Road Research Laboratory. Regulations are

to alertness of other road users. The conditions within which this alertness operates deserve more attention. Propaganda is often directed to the person who breaks the rules. Perhaps more attention should be given to those who keep the rules, but who by doing a little extra may avoid causing injury. Various schemes for training drivers in more expert methods of 'defensive' driving are a welcome development. An elaborate experiment applying many different approaches to the prevention of accidents was made in Slough by co-operation of central and local government, voluntary and research organizations. Many different methods within current legislation were

TABLE 66
Road Accidents Causing Death (England and Wales, 1969)

Age-group	Pedestrians	Pedal cyclists	Motor cyclists	Occupants of other vehicles	Total	Population (millions)	Rate per million
0–4 years:							
Male	146	5	0	28	179	2·11	84·8
Female	69	0	0	20	89	2·00	44·5
5–14 years:							
Male	228	86	1	34	349	3·79	92·1
Female	113	9	2	23	147	3·60	40·8
15–24 years:							
Male	111	45	497	643	1,296	3·64	356·0
Female	45	9	28	211	293	3·52	83·2
25–44 years:							
Male	139	39	93	631	902	6·13	147·1
Female	56	6	12	160	234	5·89	39·7
45–64 years:							
Male	343	111	104	443	1,001	5·79	172·9
Female	209	18	11	207	445	6·18	72·0
65+ years:							
Male	569	82	20	182	853	2·38	35·8
Female	667	9	0	150	826	3·88	21·3
All ages:							
Male	1,536	368	715	1,961	4,580	23·83	192·2
Female	1,159	51	53	771	2,034	25·08	81·1

in force to exclude vehicles which are not roadworthy and these standards need to be under constant revision in the light of experience. Motorways demand new driving methods; on these roads pedestrians and oncoming traffic are excluded, but greater speed increases the risks of being thrown out of vehicles and of multiple vehicles being involved in a single accident. Nevertheless only a relatively small proportion of fatalities occur on motorways even in Germany. In Britain the proportion is less than one-twentieth, most fatalities occurring in built-up areas. While there seems a reasonable prospect of relatively safe fast motor transport between cities, within built-up areas the hazards of intersections and mixed types of traffic suggest the need for exclusion of motor vehicles from shopping centres and stringent speed limitation elsewhere.

There is need for careful assessment of the effectiveness of different measures intended to reduce road accidents. The statistical relation between casualties and numbers of vehicles and population mentioned above should not imply that a given number of accidents is inevitable, but they do suggest a background against which preventive measures can be assessed. The relative value of different types of approach needs to be kept in review; effective prevention may well be more complex than appears at first sight. It is, for instance, common experience that avoidance of accidents and of injury is often due

tested in one area; various forms of publicity were used, extra police advised and warned road users, and, on the engineering side, various minor and major alterations to traffic flow and control were tested. Certain general improvements were found in statistics of casualties, but probably the most important lesson was the limited value of several of the apparently promising preventive procedures and the difficulty of persuading people to change their road behaviour. One of the findings was the advantage of improved street lighting at night, and this has since been separately confirmed in other experiments. More careful tests, preferably of single preventive measures with adequate controls, seem the most promising way to increase the efficiency of road accident prevention. Further details of research in this field are given in the Annual Reports of the Transport and Road Research Laboratory.

Though it is difficult to make precise comparisons, transport by either rail or air appears to be much safer than by road in proportion to the distance travelled. British statistics show about 1·3 deaths of car occupants per 100 million passenger miles as against 0·5 by scheduled air lines and 0·2 by rail. Apart from the 49 rail passengers, 60 railway employees also were killed in crashes and movement accidents in 1970.

The relative safety of air travel in view of its intrinsic dangers is a tribute to the precautionary drill and careful maintenance which is enforced. The major causes of death due to aircraft crashes are deceleration and burning. There is evidence that a greater degree of protection against deceleration forces can be obtained with rear-facing seats. Injuries or death due to rail crashes are very rare in relation to the miles travelled. Improvement might be expected from changes in signalling and control systems; falls on to the line, however, and other accidents due to movement of trains are more common causes of death and injury than train crashes.

INDUSTRIAL ACCIDENTS

In Great Britain about two-fifths of fatal industrial (non-transport) accidents occur in factories and about one-fifth each in the building construction and mining industries. The types of accident are shown in TABLE 67. The main causes are falls,

types of benefit cost £135 million, and this is quite apart from losses of production, disturbance of other work, and costs of treatment. The claim rate is about three times higher in mining than in factories, but the clinical types of injury are in general similar throughout industry. Fractures and other injuries of the limbs are the main causes of lost time. In places under the Factories Act the hand is the commonest site of injury, and studies in light engineering have shown that more than half the injuries and the lost time was attributable to hand injuries. Sepsis was until recently a prominent cause of lost time injury; that the position has now improved may be partly attributable to cleaner methods of working and partly to improved treatment by chemotherapy. Less than 8 per cent. of reportable factory accidents are now attributed to sepsis. Further details of notified accidents, their incidence in different

TABLE 67
Occupational Accidents Causing Death (England and Wales, 1970)

Age-group	Falls	Objects falling, striking or trapping	Machinery and vehicles	Fires and hot substances	Electric current	Suffocation and drowning	Poisoning	Other and unspecified	Total	Estimated working population (millions)	Rate per million
15–44 years:											
Male	113	141	69	18	35	24	15	33	448	7·73	58
Female	2	0	0	2	0	0	1	0	5	4·88	1
45–64 years:											
Male	94	105	45	13	12	12	13	18	312	4·93	63
Female	5	0	0	4	1	1	1	3	15	2·74	5
65+ years:											
Male	18	1	2	0	1	2	1	5	30	0·41	73
Female	6	1	0	0	0	0	0	1	8	0·19	42
All ages:											
Male	225	247	116	31	48	38	29	56	790	13·07	60
Female	13	1	0	6	1	1	2	4	28	7·81	4

and objects falling, striking, or trapping, which between them account for more than half the deaths. Falls are particularly prominent in building construction and more than half the fatal falls are in this industry. In factories falls of persons, machinery accidents, and internal transport each cause about one-fifth of the deaths. In mines falls of ground and haulage accidents are the common causes of fatal accidents. TABLE 67 shows the high rate of fatal accidents in older workers. Not many people over 65 are employed, but the number of accidental deaths is much greater than would be expected from the proportion at work, particularly in view of the fact that many of these men are on the less hazardous jobs. Deaths due to falls account for most of this excess, and they cause more than twice as many deaths as would be expected from the population at risk. It seems probable that this corresponds to the similarly high death rate from falls in domestic accidents and reflects the poorer response of the aged to injury, as well as a somewhat higher liability to such accidents.

As a result of the 1946 Acts in the United Kingdom introducing the present system of National Insurance, an increasing amount of information is becoming available on the numbers and types of claims for industrial injuries. Spells of incapacity due to accidents which qualify for Injury Benefit total about a million per year. Incapacity for longer than six months qualifies for Disablement Benefit, and for this about 15,000 new pensions come into payment annually. Total payments under the two

industries, and method of prevention are given in the Annual Reports of the Chief Inspector of Factories and of H.M. Chief Inspector of Mines.

Very many more injuries occur than cause reportable loss of time. Common minor industrial injuries treated in the larger firms at works surgeries are lacerations, puncture wounds, and bruises, and the great majority again are of the hands. Eye injuries, mostly due to foreign bodies, are common in work involving exposure to coarse dust or other flying particles.

Prevention of industrial accidents has received much attention from government, industry, and voluntary organizations. The Factories Act, 1961, consolidated and strengthened the safety provisions of preceding legislation. Safer design of machinery is prescribed as well as better provision of first-aid treatment of injuries. The Factory Inspectorate and H.M. Inspectors of Mines assist enforcement of these rules and give advice on safe methods of working; most large works also have safety departments. Safe working is ultimately in the interests both of management and men, and Safety Committees, representing both sides of industry have proved of value in obtaining the necessary exchange of information and co-operation in preventive measures.

The current trend towards automation, in substituting machine for manual methods, tends to achieve greater safety as well as greater efficiency. In the design of machine tools, for instance, until recent years technologies have been stretched to their limit, so that the human operator has needed to adapt himself to the machine. Now, with more advanced technology, alternative methods are often available, so that it is possible to choose those which are more appropriate to the abilities of the human operator. However, all new methods need to be studied, since new risks can easily be introduced. It is often possible to alter both old and new processes so as to make them intrinsically safe. The introduction of low-voltage power supplies for portable tools is an example of this. Fatal shocks are virtually impossible at less than 50 volts, and with suitable equipment this can be completely adequate for inspection lamps and hand tools. Other engineering devices for guarding and personal protection are only second and third choices in accident prevention; to make the process intrinsically safe should be the first aim.

Educational campaigns, with special safety weeks and the like, have a useful role so long as the advice is precisely relevant to the industry concerned, and preferably directly based upon studies made in that industry or works. Another aspect of education for safety is the provision of training courses for foremen and for persons in charge of hazardous processes. The pioneer Training Centre in Birmingham organized by the local industrial safety organization and the Factory Inspectorate has shown that this type of training is both welcomed and effective. The emphasis in such training is on safe and good methods of working, the aim being 'safety through skill' rather than the outdated 'safety first'. A recent encouraging example is the marked reduction of accidents on mechanical presses following the introduction of compulsory safety training under the Power Presses Regulations, 1965 [see also CHAPTER 38].

GENERAL FEATURES OF ACCIDENT CAUSATION AND PREVENTION

All life in society entails certain hazards. The more extreme forms have been discussed above as they affect people in domestic, transport, and occupational activities. An attempt to compare their relative importance has been made by Sowby (1965). Taking as an index the number of fatalities per 10^9 hours of exposure, the highest risks seemed to be those self-imposed in, for example, rock climbing (40,000) and riding motor cycles, whether in racing (35,000) or ordinary transport (6,600). On the same basis the highest occupational risk is probably that of air-crew (2,500). Other high occupational risks are in constructional engineering (675), certain railway workers (450), coal miners (400), and fishermen (330) (Schilling, 1966). For comparison, the hazard of accidental death in the general population is calculated as 86, death from cancer as 44, and from cardiovascular disease as 610.

Apart from the specific hazards of home, road, and workshop, certain overriding environmental factors influence the occurrence of accidents. Many years ago the effects of extremes of temperature and humidity were shown to be harmful. For instance, minimum accident rates were found in both male and female factory workers at temperatures about 67·5° F. It is not certain how such factors affect transport and domestic accidents, but there may well be scope here for further investigation. Good lighting has been shown to reduce accidents in factories, docks, and on the roads. Badly lit stairways and passages are known to be a source of accidents in the home (Gray, 1966).

Personal factors in accidents include the obvious increased hazards due to illness and disability. Sudden illness while driving is an occasional cause of traffic accidents (Herner et al., 1966), and collapse causing injury by falling or burning is common in the home. Similarly, impaired attention and judgement due to alcohol is frequently a factor in road accidents. Recent British legislation imposing a maximum possible limit of blood alcohol in drivers has produced a marked reduction in road accidents, particularly at night. During and subsequent to the First World War careful studies showed the harmful effects of excessive hours of work; during the Second World War the effects of fatigue and strain on the performance of skilled tasks, such as piloting aircraft, were investigated. Reduced precision and reliability of response to complex stimuli were found.

When all such definable features have been taken into account there still remains the possibility of certain individuals being more prone to accidents than others. This condition of 'accident proneness', first defined by Farmer (1926), has been demonstrated among factory workers, miners, and vehicle drivers. Conditions must be highly stable with many people doing similar jobs for the demonstration to be convincing, and true accident proneness should not be confused with accident liability, which includes also variations of exposure, health, and age. The results of certain types of psychological tests have been shown to correlate well with accident proneness. Davis (1958) has reviewed the findings in this field, and Häkkinen (1958) has shown in a careful study of bus drivers in Helsinki that accident proneness correlates with particular groups of tests. The correlation, however, is not complete and reliance on the tests for exclusion of applicants could well be unfair in some cases, but may be desirable for responsible and hazardous jobs. Rejection of persons having a large number of accidents may also be unjust in view of the more complex factors in total liability. A better approach is to investigate possible causes in the individual high rates and to try to alter conditions of work and methods of work as appropriate. The studies of Whitfield (1954) among miners showed an interesting difference between the accident proneness of young and older workers. The young accident-prone miners tended to show a failure of perceptual ability which might result in failure of appreciation of a hazard, whereas older workers tended to fail in speed of motor reaction. This would suggest that further training of the younger workers might improve their accident record; probably transfer to intrinsically safer work would be more appropriate for the older men.

Statistical studies show that there are high accident rates in communities where other deaths from violence are common. Whitlock (1971) has demonstrated a correlation in different countries and states between road deaths and murder and other violent crimes. He concludes that an aggressive psychopathy is common to both. In conformity with this, Willett (1964) showed that the drivers convicted of serious motor offences have more than their share of other crime. It is uncertain, however, what proportion of accidents can be attributed to such antisocial attitudes. Possibly only a small proportion of accidents could be prevented by exclusion of drivers with criminal records and whether, indeed, refusal of licences would keep them off the roads is also doubtful.

Prevention of accidents has been summarized as Education,

Engineering, and Enforcement. These three have a role in all groups of accident. Prevention by engineering includes improvement in design of vehicles, roads, machines, methods of working, and domestic buildings and equipment. There must also be proper maintenance so that the safety features continue to operate throughout the life of the equipment. Education has been particularly promising in the prevention of industrial accidents, and more recently of road accidents. It is beginning to be applied to domestic accidents, but needs further development. A recent trend in education in all three main fields of accidents has been an increasing emphasis on positive training rather than exhortation or admonition. Society is likely to continue to be dangerous; its members should integrate safe methods into normal practice which includes pride of performance. Enforcement has also been applied chiefly to transport and to industry. It may take the form of voluntary acceptance of codes of practice in factory or on the road, but these codes usually need to be reinforced at some point by legal sanctions. To only a minor extent has this been applied in the home, where there is naturally an unwillingness to invade domestic privacy. However, it has been possible to act indirectly through introduction of standards of safety in domestic equipment such as electric fires, and further developments on these lines appear promising.

Operational research on methods of accident prevention is highly rewarding. The design of goggles is a recent industrial example. For a long time progress in providing acceptable goggles has been delayed by the assumption that plastics would be unsuitable for protection against hot metal. Simple tests have demonstrated the contrary, so that light goggles with curvature permitting wide range of vision and giving improved protection are now feasible. Studies of the incidence of road accidents by hour of day at different periods of the year suggested that the peak of accidents in the evening was largely determined by lighting. Artificial lighting of experimental stretches of road have now been shown to reduce accidents by up to one-third. It has been widely believed that highly flammable fabrics are a common cause of domestic burning accidents. Simple enumeration and testing of the fabrics involved in accidents has shown the common cellulose materials to be the main culprits; the more highly flammable laces and nets are probably not sufficiently widely used to contribute appreciably to the injuries. Prevention is now therefore directed to replacing or making safe the common textiles used for dresses and nightwear. Social studies on the impact of various measures intended to reduce accidents are also needed. What little has been done in this field suggests that *a priori* theories are often wrong. Much of prevention involves an element of persuasion, and impartial assessment of the degree of success of a campaign is as necessary as it is in commercial advertising (Laner and Sell, 1960).

Though it may be hoped that preventive measures will limit the rate of increase of accidental injuries, in the foreseeable future they will probably demand an increasing proportion of medical attention, and there are now improved methods of treatment which can minimize the ill effects of injuries. Some reorientation of medical services will be required to make such treatment available for accidental injuries whenever they occur.

REFERENCES AND FURTHER READING

Domestic Accidents

Backett, E. M. (1965) Domestic accidents, *Wld Hlth Org. Publ. Hlth Pap.*, No. 26.

British Standards Institution (1957) *The Flammability of Apparel Fabrics in Relation to Domestic Burning Accidents*, London.

Bull, J. P., Jackson, D. M., and Walton, C. (1964) The causes and prevention of domestic burning accidents, *Brit. med. J.*, 2, 1421.

Castle, O. M. (1950) Accidents in the home, *Lancet*, i, 315.

Fisher, A. J. (1955) Injuries in the aged, *Brit. J. prev. soc. Med.*, 9, 73.

Gray, B. (1966) *Home Accidents among Older People*, Royal Society for the Prevention of Accidents, London.

Keswani, M. H., and Antia, N. H. (1971) Prevention of burns—an attempt to educate the masses, in *Research in Burns*, ed. Matter, P., Barclay, T. L., and Konickova, Z., Bern.

Maisels, D. O., and Corps, B. V. M. (1964) Burned epileptics, *Lancet*, i, 1298.

Rowntree, G. (1950) Accidents among children under two years of age in Great Britain, *J. Hyg. (Lond.)*, 48, 323.

World Health Organization (1957) Accidents in childhood, *Wld Hlth Org. techn. Rep. Ser.*, No. 118.

Transport Accidents

Bohlin, N. I. (1968) *Proc. 11th Stapp Car Crash Conference, 1967*, Society of Automotive Engineers, p. 455.

Bull, J. P. (1969) International comparisons of road accident statistics, *Accid. Anal. Prev.*, 1, 293.

Department of Scientific and Industrial Research (1963) *Research on Road Safety*, London, H.M.S.O.

Department of the Environment (1971) *Road Accidents, 1969*, London, H.M.S.O.

Gissane, W., and Bull, J. (1964) A study of motorway (M.1) fatalities, *Brit. med. J.*, 1, 75.

Gissane, W., Bull J., and Roberts, B. (1970) Sequelae of road injuries, *Injury*, 1, 195.

Havard, I. D. J. (1973) Road traffic accidents, *Wld Hlth Org. Chron.*, 27, 83.

Herner, B., Smedby, B., and Ysander, L. (1966) Sudden illness as a cause of motor vehicle accidents, *Brit. J. industr. Med.*, 23, 37.

Lister, R. D., and Milsom, Barbara (1963) Car seat-belts; an analysis of the injuries sustained by car occupants, *Practitioner*, 191, 332.

Norman, L. G. (1960) Medical aspects of road safety, *Lancet*, i, 989, 1039.

Norman, L. G. (1962) Road Traffic Accidents. Epidemiology, Control and Prevention, *Wld Hlth Org. Publ. Hlth Pap.*, No. 12.

Smeed, R. J. (1968) Variations in the pattern of accident rates in different countries and their causes, *Traff. Engng Control*, 10, 364.

Whitlock, F. A. (1971) *Death on the Road. A Study in Social Violence*, London.

Willett, T. C. (1964) *The Criminal on the Road*, London.

United Nations (1974) *Statistics of Road Traffic Accidents in Europe, 1972*, Geneva.

Industrial Accidents

Hunter, D. (1960) *The Diseases of Occupations*, 3rd ed., London.

Department of Employment (1971) *Annual Report of H.M. Chief Inspector of Factories, 1970*, London, H.M.S.O.

Department of Health and Social Security (1973) *Annual Report, 1972*, London, H.M.S.O.

Department of Trade and Industry (1971) *Report of H.M. Chief Inspector of Mines, 1970*, London, H.M.S.O.

Ministry of Power (1967) *Report of H.M. Chief Inspector of Mines, 1966*, London, H.M.S.O.

General Aspects

Davis, D. R. (1958) Accident-proneness, *Med. Press*, **238**, 27.

Farmer, E., and Chambers, E. G. (1926) A psychological study of individual differences in accident rates, *Med. res. Coun. Ind. Fat. Res. Bd*, Report No. 38, London, H.M.S.O.

Häkkinen, S. (1958) *Psychological Tests and Traffic Accident Frequency: Selection of Drivers*, Proceedings of the XII International Congress on Occupational Health, Helsinki, 156 and 529.

Laner, S., and Sell, R. G. (1960) *An Experiment on the Effect of Specifically Designed Safety Posters*, British Iron and, Steel Research Association, OR/HF/15/60.

Pugh, L. G. C. (1968) Isafjordur trawler disaster: Medical aspects, *Brit. med. J.*, **1**, 826.

Registrar General (1971) *Statistical Review of England and Wales for 1969*, London, H.M.S.O.

Schilling, R. S. F. (1966) Trawler fishing: An extreme occupation, *Proc. roy. Soc. Med.*, **59**, 405.

Sowby, F. D. (1965) Radiation and other risks, *Hlth Phys.*, **11**, 879.

Volbov, M. V. (1973) Accidents in the social context, *Wld Hlth Org. Chron.*, **27**, 290.

Whitfield, J. W. (1954) Individual differences in accident susceptibility among coal miners, *Brit. J. industr. Med.* **11**, 126.

World Health Organization Regional Office for Europe (1960) *The Prevention of Accidents in Childhood*. Report on a Seminar, Copenhagen.

World Health Organization Regional Office for Europe, Copenhagen. Reports on Road Traffic Accidents.
(1968) Euro 0147.
(1969) Euro 4113(1).
(1970) Euro 1RC19.
(1972) Euro 5701(2).

29

PUBLIC HEALTH OPHTHALMOLOGY

B. NIŽETIĆ

INTRODUCTION

Objectives and Domain

The science of ophthalmology deals with the processes by means of which the images of external objects are brought to our consciousness (*Encyclopaedia Britannica*). In other words, vision and/or visual impairment (in its different degrees) form the core of ophthalmological interest and activities.

The degree of vision,[1] in most instances, is the functional expression of the eye's[2] health.

As in general health, the health of the eye can be represented as a spectrum or continuum, ranging from complete (optimum) eye health (and full vision) to complete absence of eye health (and the complete absence of vision) or blindness. As applied to *conditions*, the spectrum ranges from asymptomatic stages to conditions serious enough to result in complete anatomical and functional deterioration of the eye. As applied to *persons*, the spectrum ranges from a state of optimum eye health and vision to blindness. It is usually preferable from the operational point of view to use the term *loss of vision* or *visual impairment* instead of employing different variants of the term 'blindness', (economical, legal, social, practical, complete, etc.).

One reason is that we do not have an internationally accepted (by concensus method) definition of blindness. Such a definition in most countries is based partly on medical (measurement) criteria and partly on social-economical and/or cultural grounds. Therefore, an international agreement cannot be expected. The second reason is that the term 'blindness' fits better the concept of the *whole man* in his socio-economic environment, and can be used in the domain of so-called *social ophthalmology* which derives its inspiration from the field of clinical experience and deals with individuals, or more precisely with the social aspects of eye disease in the sick person.

In dealing with problems of *loss of vision* and their causes, two basic approaches are possible. The first is concerned with the spectrum of eye health and vision in the individual, and its traditional domain is that of *clinical ophthalmology*. The second is the community approach to problems related to the promotion of full eye health and particularly to the prevention of disability due to *loss of vision* and *blindness* in the populations at risk—matters entering the domain of *public health ophthalmology*.

With these long-range objectives *public health ophthalmology* endeavours to:

1. Assess the magnitude of the socio-economical impact of this disability on the community.

2. Measure accurately the needs for services for the population, both sick and healthy, in this field.

3. Find and apply the most appropriate solutions, taking into consideration the objective needs, demands (felt-needs) and resources (finances, man-power, and services).

Visual impairment and its most severe stages, represented by economical and total blindness, are becoming of increasingly greater interest and concern to public health authorities in both developing and industrialized areas of the world; this is essentially for two reasons:

1. The rapid progress made in modern technology and the increasing requirements of modern educational systems emphasize the need for full eye health and vision for growing populations.

2. The causes of visual disturbances and blindness vary in space and time, but their economical impact is estimated to be rather significant because of the very high cost to the community represented by:

(i) Direct cost in the form of aid to the blind.

(ii) The cost of medical eye care and rehabilitation.

(iii) Far higher cost of lost productivity from affected individuals, without forgetting the intangible cost of suffering and deprivation.

The Magnitude of the Problem of Loss of Vision and Blindness

In assessing the disability caused by visual impairment we have to consider the differing frameworks in which it occurs.

The loss of vision (including its most severe stages of blindness) may be congenital or may occur at different ages. It may develop suddenly or there may be a gradual progressive loss of the visual function. It may be bilateral or unilateral. Possibly even more important, it may develop as a late consequence of a number of conditions which, if detected in time, may be treated before they affect the vision. Finally, the loss of vision may or may not be curable, and vision may be restored or corrected.

The disability caused by loss of vision is also influenced by social, cultural, educational, and economic factors and by the capacities and personality of the affected individual. From the public health point of view, the basic information necessary for decision-making and setting of priorities in this field includes the prevalence and incidence of persons affected as well as their distribution according to causes of loss of vision and blindness.

The number of blind persons in the whole world has been estimated at 10 to 15 millions (Viswalingham, 1967). This estimate does not include cases with only partial visual impair-

---

[1] 'Vision', here, is used in its full meaning, embracing the visual acuity for distance and nearness, central and peripheral visual field, scotopic and photopic vision, colour vision, depth perception (binocular vision).

[2] 'Eye', here, is used as the expression of the whole visual apparatus (eye globes, annexes).

ment, and therefore the total number of affected people is certainly much higher.

In fact, comparable to an iceberg [Fig. 80], blindness (the complete loss of vision) represents only a small, but visible part of the more general problem of visual loss.

A first compilation of available information on 'blindness' was published by the World Health Organization in 1953 (WHO, 1953). More detailed and more complete information obtained from various sources was published in 1966 (WHO, 1966). In an attempt to complete this information the WHO

estimation of the real situation, and clearly indicate the need to obtain better and more complete information on the subject (WHO, 1972*a*) which would help to add more precision to the assessment of needs.

The fact that a great deal of those in need of eye-health care do not get it at least appropriately, at the present stage, in many areas of the world, represents one of the basic justifications for the community approach in ophthalmology. The analysis of the situation related to the delivery of health care services (organization, financing, man-power) in determined areas

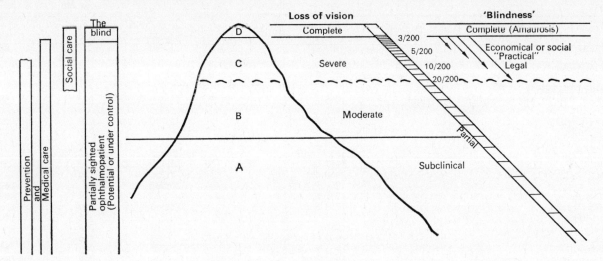

FIG. 80. 'Iceberg' showing the interrelationship between 'blindness', loss of vision, and different aspects of care delivery. (Nižetić, December 1970.)

sent a questionnaire (WHO, 1972*b*) on blindness and its prevention to the national health authorities of all Member States and Associate Members of the WHO in March 1970, but the new up-to-date figures are not yet available.

'Blindness' rates are in general around or below 200 in the United States and in most European countries. In less industrialized countries, and in Africa and Asia, this rate is considerably higher and reaches values above 1,000. It should be noted, however, that relatively high rates may reflect more complete and more accurate information and that in general the quality of available data is better in countries where the average age of the population is higher (WHO, 1972*b*).

A further step in considering the magnitude of the problem related to loss of vision and blindness would be the analysis of available data on *causes underlying visual impairment*.

In general, in approximately one-third of the cases the cause of blindness is unknown or undetermined when it is known, non-infectious causes predominating in the more developed countries, while the ratio between non-infectious and infectious aetiologies is reversed in the less developed countries (Sorsby, 1950). As an example, and taken as a whole with all the reserves made above, 27 per cent. of the total cases of blindness in Africa are attributed to infectious causes, and less than 8 per cent. to non-infectious; in Europe, where less than 39 per cent. of the causes are unknown or undetermined, only 5 per cent. are attributed to infections and 56 per cent. to non-infectious causes.

The figures shown in TABLE 69 certainly represent an under-

helps to define more exactly the magnitude of the local community problem of loss of vision.

The System of Public Health Ophthalmology

At this point the question could be raised as to whether *public health ophthalmology* is to be considered as a special discipline, or body of knowledge, or merely as a particular mental attitude to be adopted by ophthalmologists. We find it useful to consider it as a 'system'.

There are several definitions of a 'system'. Giving some of them will perhaps help an understanding of the text:

1. Any entity, conceptual or physical, which consists of interrelated, interacting, or interdependent parts (Churchman, 1968).
2. A system is a set of parts co-ordinated to accomplish a set of goals.
3. A group of interrelated and interacting elements (Hanika, 1968).
4. A recognizable kind of entity into which are 'input' various types of resources (people, money, techniques).

A 'systems approach' is simply a way of thinking about these total systems and their components. As with every other system, public health ophthalmology is embedded in the larger system of general public health which naturally conditions its performance.

TABLE 68
Number of Blind Persons in Certain Countries and Rate per 100,000 Population

C = Census

E = Estimate

R = Registration

S = Special survey

Country	Year	Definition	Blind population	Rate per 100,000 population	Reference
AFRICA					
Algeria	1946 E		25,000	304	87
Bechuanaland	1954 C		1,880	...	20
Cameroon:					
West Cameroon	1952 S[1]	1			144
North				1,800	
Southern Highlands				400	
Congo, Dem. Rep. of, and former Ruanda-Urundi	1955 S[2]		14,000	118	93
Ethiopia	1962 E		75–90,000	380–450	186
Gambia	1955 E		2,700	983	20
Ghana	1955 E		65,000	959	147
North	1952 S[1]	1		3,000	144
Kenya	1953–55 E	2	65–70,000	1,050–1,150	26
Malawi	1955 E		18,400	724	20
Mauritius	1960 C[3]		250	39	147
Nigeria	1960 E		320,000		147
Eastern Region	1931 C[4]			310	160
Northern Region	1953 E		170,000	1,000	126
Western Region	1931 C[4]			530	160
St. Helena	1956 C		12	258	
Seychelles	1931 C		66	240	
Sierra Leone	1955 E		20,000	952	20
Somalia (Former Italian Somaliland)	1962 E[5,6]		6,000	300	186
South Africa	1957 R				166
Asiatic population			320	75	
Bantu population			26,420	...	
Coloured population			2,058	156	
White population			2,480	84	
Southern Rhodesia	1962 C	3	12,010	332	
African rural areas			9,030	425	
European farming areas			2,190	262	
Urban areas			790	121	
South West Africa	1936 C[7]				
Coloured population			72	176	
White population			13	42	
Tanzania, United Republic of					
Tanganyika	1955 E		50,000	569	20
Zanzibar	1960 R		590	192	147
Togo					
Former British mandated territory	1931 C		827	282	
Former French mandated territory	1937 E		4,000	597	118
Tunisia	1960 S[8]	2	18,000	450	186
Uganda	1955 E		37,500	636	20
United Arab Republic (Egypt)	1960 C[9]	4	75,000	289	186
		5	120,000	462	
Zambia	1961 E	6	10–15,000	500–750	137
AMERICA					
Antigua	1911 C[9]		119	369	160
Argentina	1947 C		14,259	90	
Bahama Is.	1931 C		106	177	
Bermuda	1931 C		25	90	
Bolivia	1900 C		2,126	150	
Brazil	1940 C		60,701	147	
British Guiana	1931 C[10]		524	170	22
British Honduras	1931 C		79	154	
Canada	1965 R[11]	7	24,671	128	101
Cayman Is.	1943 C		17	255	
Chile	1920 C		2,510	78	
Cuba	1943 C		4,629	969	
Dominican Republic	1950 C		2,853	134	
El Salvador	1956 R		660	29	48
Grenada	1911 C[9]		87	130	160

TABLE 68 (continued)

Country	Year	Definition	Blind population	Rate per 100,000 population	Reference
AMERICA (concl.)					
Guadeloupe	1937 R		<100	...	86
Honduras	1935 C		1,040	108	
Jamaica	1955 S[12]		3,123	203	20
Mexico	1940 C[109]		16,884	101	
Netherlands Antilles	1911 C[9]		77	284	160
Nicaragua	1950 E		1,000	100	96
Peru	1940 C		8,972	145	
Puerto Rico	1910 C[9]		1,603	143	160
St. Vincent	1931 C		122	254	
Trinidad and Tobago	1947 C		699	125	
Turks and Caicos Islands	1943 C		26	424	
United States	1960 E[13]	8	385,000	214	83
Uruguay	1908 C[9]		842	81	160
Venezuela	1941 C		4,757	124	
ASIA					
Ceylon	1963 E		50,000	470	3
China:					
Mainland	1947 E		2,000,000	450	102
Taiwan	1930 C[9]		18,510	403	160
Cyprus	1962 E[14]		1,300	224	147
Hong Kong	1963 E		50,000	1,392	3
India	1962 E		2,000,000	460	187
Indonesia (excl. West Irian)	1930 C	9			
Indigenous population			138,983	239	
European population			117	49	
Chinese population			1,254	106	
Other Asiatics			127	111	
Iran	1960 E[15]	2	150,000	750	186
Iraq	1961 E[6]		35–70,000	500–1,000	186
Israel	1961 S	2	5,285	250	186
Japan	1958 E		190,000	208	120
Kuwait	1957 C[9]	10	509	230	186
Malaysia	1963 E		50,000	470	3
Sarawak	1961 E		2,000	260	147
Pakistan	1963 E		400,000	400	3
Philippines	1918 C		8,667	84	
Saudi Arabia	1961 E[16]		180,000	3,000	186
Syria	1958–60 S[6,17]		4,154	95	186
Turkey	1955 C		31,770	132	
Viet Nam					
North Viet Nam					
Tongking	1941 E		30,000	428	91
Yemen	1960 E[6]		180,000	4,000	186
EUROPE					
Austria	1949 E[18]		4,000	66	87
Belgium	1963 R		4,779	51	7
Bulgaria	1945 C[9]		4,000	57	87
Channel Islands					
Guernsey	1911 C[19]		39	87	
Jersey	1911 C[19]		57	110	
Czechoslovakia	1937 E		10,000	61	191
Denmark	1949 E[20]		4,000	100	87
Faroe Islands	1932 R		24	98	141
Finland	1961–62 S[11]	11	3,419	76	176
France	1946 C[21]		42,663	107	
Germany:					
Federal Republic	1962 E		30,000	60	145
Gibraltar	1961 C	12	141	647	
Greece	1951 C		12,987	170	
Hungary	1949 E[22]		10,000	100	87
Iceland	1954 S[11]	13	434	272	14
Ireland	1949 E[23]		7,000	233	87
Isle of Man	1911 C[19]		59	113	
Italy	1963 E[24]		>100,000	>200	63
Malta and Gozo	1960 S[11]	14	638	194	37
Netherlands	1959 E[25]		>6,000	50–60	151
Norway	1948 S[11]	15	3,181	100	81
Poland	1959 E[26]	16	19,000	65	146
Portugal	1960 C[18]		8,225	93	
Rumania	1935 S[27]		13,689	717	17

TABLE 68 (*continued*)

Country	Year	Definition	Blind population	Rate per 100,000 population	Reference
Spain	1953 E	17	16,000	*56*	2
Sweden	1965 E[28]		10,000	*130*	5
Switzerland	1950 C[9]	17	2,864	*60*	162
United Kingdom:					
England and Wales	1963 R	18	96,472	*205*	72
Northern Ireland	1963 R		2,327	*161*	129
Scotland	1964 R	18	10,108	*194*	153
Yugoslavia	1959 E		20,000	*100*	82
OCEANIA					
Australia	1933 C		3,898	*59*	
Fiji Islands	1955 E[29]		4,000	*1,190*	20
New Zealand	1962 R		2,700	*112*	172

TABLE 69
Definitions of Blindness

1. Inability to count fingers at 1 metre.
2. Visual acuity of 3/60 Snellen or less.
3. Totally blind, i.e. those who have to be led.
4. Visual acuity of less than 1/60 Snellen.
5. Partial blindness: visual acuity of 1/60 Snellen or more but less than 3/60 Snellen.
6. Inability to move about in unfamiliar surroundings unaided, such aid including the blind man's stick.
7. Central visual acuity of 6/60 Snellen (20/200) or less in both eyes, even with best correction, or reduction of the field of vision to less than 20 degrees.
8. Central visual acuity of less than 6/60 Snellen (0·1, 20/200) in the better eye or an equally disabling loss of the field of vision.
9. Inability to perceive the movement of fingers close to the eyes.
10. Inability to do any kind of work, industrial or otherwise, for which eyesight is essential.
11. Central visual acuity of 0·1 or less or reduction of the field of vision to less than 30 degrees.
12. Visual acuity of not more than 3/60 Snellen or the presence of gross field defects.
13. Census instructions: all persons who are totally blind, or cannot find their way in places unknown to them before by means of their sight shall be registered as blind.
14. Visual acuity of less than 3/60 Snellen, even with best correction, or inability to find one's way about in unfamiliar places.
15. Inability after the correction of errors of refraction to find one's way about or to count fingers at more than 1 metre.
16. Central visual acuity of 0·05 or less, even with best correction, or reduction of the field of vision to 20 degrees or less.
17. Inability to count fingers at more than 1 metre.
18. Central visual acuity of 3/60 Snellen or less, or between 3/60 and 6/60 Snellen with a gross reduction of the field of vision.
19. Central visual acuity of 3/60 Snellen or less, even with best correction, or reduction of the field of vision to less than 10 degrees.
20. Visual acuity of less than 3/60 Snellen (1/20).
21. Central visual acuity of 6/60 Snellen (20/200) or less in the better eye, even with best correction, or reduction of the field of vision to 20 degrees or less.
22. Visual acuity of less than 1/10 in the better eye, even with best correction.
23. Partial blindness: vision reduced in at least one eye so that the individual cannot count fingers at a distance of 6 metres.
24. Central visual acuity of less than 1/60 Snellen or a field of vision so reduced that the patient can barely go about by himself.
25. Visual acuity in adults of 6/60 Snellen or less and in children of 6/24 Snellen or less. The vision was taken without correction of refractive errors, except in those wearing glasses.
26. Inability to count fingers of an outstretched hand held out from the level of the patient's shoulders, refracting errors being excluded.
27. Inability to count fingers at 2 metres.

28. Central visual acuity of 3/60 Snellen or less in the better eye, even with best correction, or reduction of the field of vision to 20 degrees or less.
29. Partial blindness: visual acuity of more than 3/60 but not exceeding 6/60 Snellen in the better eye, even with best correction.
30. Central visual acuity of less than 3/60 Snellen or reduction of the field of vision to less than 30 degrees.
31. Visual acuity of 6/60 Snellen (20/200) or less.
32. Inability to move about in unfamiliar places, to accomplish work for which eyesight is essential or to count fingers at more than 1 metre, even with the aid of glasses.
33. Visual acuity of less than 3/60 Snellen in each eye.
34. Inability to read ordinary type, even with the aid of glasses, or to carry on ordinary occupations for which eyesight is essential.
35. Inability to find one's way alone.
36. Central visual acuity of less than 0·1, even with best correction, or reduction of the field of vision to less than 10 degrees.
37. Visual acuity of less than 6/60 Snellen (0·1).
38. Central visual acuity of 20/200 or less or reduction of the field of vision to 20 degrees or less.
39. Central visual acuity of 20/200 or less in the better eye or reduction of the field of vision to 20 degrees or less.
40. Central visual acuity of 20/200 or less, even with best correction, or reduction of the field of vision to 20 degrees or less.
41. Light perception only and the recognition of the motion (not the form) of the hand of the examiner at not more than one foot, in either eye.
42. Visual acuity of 6/60 Snellen (20/200) or less in the better eye, even with best correction.
43. Visual acuity too low to permit normal school education in children or normal vocational training or occupation in adults. This corresponds to a visual power of 6/60 Snellen or below.
44. The visual acuity was so low that the children were unable to attend regular public schools due to their visual handicap.
45. Central visual acuity of 20/200 or less in the better eye, even with best correction or reduction of the field of vision to 30 per cent or less or the presence of ocular conditions which do not necessarily involve central visual acuity or peripheral field loss but which constitute a severe visual handicap.
46. Total blindness: absence of light perception in both eyes. Near blindness: the patients are sufficiently handicapped to be unable to look after themselves or find their way about, and visual acuity cannot be brought to 20/200 for either eye.
47. Visual acuity of 20/200 or less in the better eye.
48. Visual acuity not sufficient for the ordinary affairs of life or for the performance of tasks for which eyesight is essential, even with best correction.
49. Central visual acuity of 20/200 or less in the better eye, even with best correction, or impairment of the field of vision or presence of other factors affecting the usefulness of vision to a like degree.
50. Central visual acuity of 20/200 or less.
51. Perception of light, perception of hand movement, or less.
52. Visual acuity of 1/60 Snellen or less in each eye. Persons with tubular fields of vision were not regarded as blind.
53. Inability to count fingers at 1 yard.
54. Visual acuity of 1/60 Snellen or less.

TABLE 69 *continued*

55. Visual acuity of less than 0·04.
56. Visual acuity of 4/60 or less.
57. Blindness: visual acuity of less than 4/60 or considerable reduction of the field of vision. Where the visual acuity could not be measured, blindness was considered to be present when the vision was too poor to allow the patient to move about or to retrieve lost objects other than by touch. Partial sight: visual acuity between 5/60 and 6/18 or presence of conditions where the visual acuity, although reduced, allowed the patient to move about and find lost objects, although small objects could not be seen.
58. Reduction of working capacity by more than two-thirds, with ability to still perform small tasks. Visual acuity of 3/10 in one eye and less than 1/20 in the other eye, or approximately 1/10 in each eye, without central scotoma.
59. Working capacity nil but ability to move about. Visual acuity between 1/10 and 1/20, with or without central scotoma.
60. Total blindness, the patient being always dependent on a third person for the essential activities of life.
61. Visual acuity of 3/60 Snellen or less, even with best correction.
62. Visual acuity of 1/10 or less in both eyes, even with best correction.
63. Central visual acuity of 3/60 Snellen or less or reduction of the field of vision to 20 degrees or less.
64. Visual acuity of 0·2 or less.
65. Central visual acuity of 6/60 Snellen or less with a full field. A reduction of the field of vision raises the degree of central acuity coming within the definition.

FIGURE 81 shows a conceptual systems model for public health ophthalmology. The advantage of this model lies in the fact that it allows us to realize immediately how the problem of *full eye-health promotion* and *prevention of loss of vision* can find the necessary set of solutions only in a truly interdisciplinary approach. In fact, looking at FIGURE 81 we can see that the eye-health situation in a defined population is monitored primarily through the public health administration methods (–A–) (whether or not a formal public health ophthalmological service exists) with the help of investigative techniques, epidemiology, biostatistics (–B–), and health laboratory services (–C–). The system protects the public through:

1. *Preventive programmes* for communicable eye diseases control (–D–), non-communicable eye diseases control (–E–), and control of environmental eye-health hazards (–F–).
2. *Promotive programmes* (–G–) concerned, for example, with nutrition in ophthalmology (g), health education in ophthalmology (gg), prevention of eye accidents (ggg).

The public is composed of four distinct groups each presenting often very specific problems and requiring specialized services, namely for maternal and child health (–I–),[1] school health (–J–), occupational eye health (–K–), geriatric eye health (–L–), which together cover the entire life span of the individual. The public also requires organized medical eye care (–M–), as well as rehabilitative services for the visually impaired and blind (–N–). It is obvious that for the correct execution of all these activities and programmes it is necessary to have the appropriate support of education and training in public health ophthalmology for the supply of necessary manpower at all levels (–O–), and of medical and allied research in this field for new knowledge (–P–). Even if *clinical ophthalmology* does not appear in this model, it is understood that this discipline is an essential part of all the components of the system, for the very simple reason that the eye-health status

---

[1] The body of knowledge belonging to this component of the system is usually labelled as 'paediatric ophthalmology'.

of populations is the sum of the eye-health of their individual members. It becomes obvious, therefore, that public health ophthalmology has to rely a great deal upon the results, trends, and achievements in the field of ophthalmological clinical activities and research.

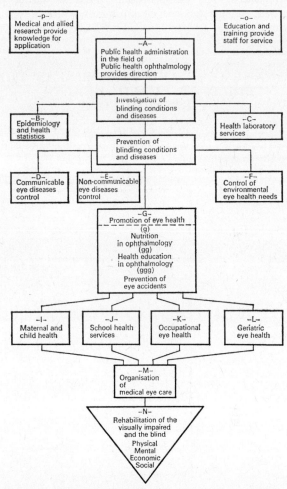

FIG. 81. A systems model of public health ophthalmology illustrating its unity and the interrelationship of its constituent activities.

A considerable amount of data concerning the various components of the P.H.O.-system is scattered throughout the literature, and the utilization of the so-called *systems approach* aims to characterize the nature of this comprehensive structure in such a way that the decision-making process could take place in a logical and coherent fashion and none of the fallacies of narrow-minded thinking would occur.

PUBLIC HEALTH ADMINISTRATION IN THE FIELD OF PUBLIC HEALTH OPHTHALMOLOGY

GENERAL

For the purposes of this chapter the term *public health administration* refers only to the *body of knowledge* necessary at a *collective* (international, national, regional, local) and *personal* level to ensure the proper management, planning, and development of public health ophthalmology activities and programmes, envisaged under the systems approach. It does not refer specifically to administrative and/or institutional settings through which this knowledge has eventually to provide direction for action. The specific patterns of these settings will depend on national and local circumstances, which in turn are functions of larger systems (general public health and general development).

MANAGEMENT AND PLANNING IN THE FIELD OF PUBLIC HEALTH OPHTHALMOLOGY

Without entering into details about the need for modern management and planning methodologies in the field of health,

There are several reasons why eye services are deficient in many parts of the world. Against a background of rapid population growth, migration and urbanization, there has been an increased demand for more and more complex types of health care (WHO, 1971). The competition for allocation of resources (money, man-power or facilities) within the health sector itself makes these resources practically always inadequate. The only rational answer to this situation is that of utilization of careful comprehensive long-term *eye-health planning*.

Continuing and systematic evaluation should be maintained as the programmes develop, because each stage is dependent on the successful implementation of the preceding stage. The need for a multipurpose eye-health planning process is also, in part, a result of the changing patterns of blinding conditions in some areas of the world. *Non-communicable eye diseases and*

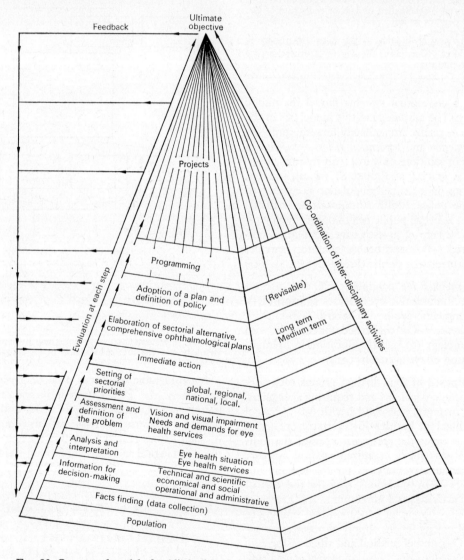

Fig. 82. Conceptual model of public health administrative activities applied to ophthalmology.

it should be pointed out that *loss of vision* and *blindness* constitute an important share of the problem to society; a great deal of those in need of *eye-health care* do not get it at the present stage.

conditions (such as glaucoma, amblyopia, degenerative retinal changes, whether or not of genetic origin), in contrast to the communicable eye diseases, develop and continue over a long period; they have multiple causes, including behavioural factors, and they require long-term care, most of it hospital-based. Plans must therefore take account of, for example, the use of health education, and the contributions to care made by the general practitioner and other community services. *Eye-health planning* should provide a clear and coherent framework for all the myriad decisions, small and large, that affect eye health and eye-health care in the widest sense.

The aim is for the planning process to take care both of the details of the facilities to be provided and of the policies which should govern the correct use of these facilities, without forgetting that planning as such is not a once-for-all commitment but a cyclic process. The careful employment of such a process implies its revision against the background of the problems and the priority objectives of each particular country (Nižetić, 1971*a*).

Eye-Health Information System

The proper deployment of planned ophthalmological public health activities aiming at effective improvement or even the maintenance of the eye-health status of the populations, requires a continuous, comprehensive, and sensitive *eye-health information system*.[1]

Basically, the population-based information which is required concerns data relative to the:

1. Needs.
2. Demands.
3. Resources.

Here, we define the needs as the deficiencies of eye health which might be controlled or eliminated (eradication). The needs might be biological, generally expressed in terms of eye morbidity or blindness (ocular mortality), and also they might be human desires (wishes) and in this case are more the expression of so-called 'demands'.

By 'demands' we define here the effective utilization of ophthalmological facilities.

While the 'assessment' of needs within the planning process reflects almost always and inevitably the viewpoint of one or more professional groups, the demands reflect the subconscious or conscious (but always real in its attitudes) viewpoint of actual or potential beneficiaries. The 'demand' is always dynamic, i.e. fluctuating under the influence of psychological (socio-cultural environment, health education, etc.) and material factors (such as level of life, economical changes, purchasing power, availability, and quality of eye-health services).

By 'resources' is meant the totality of factors on which a country can count to meet the demands.

Among the most important resources are:

1. Financial possibilities—expenditure for eye-health activities analysed according to specific categories and to source of funds.

[1] Among the different definitions of a Health Information System (H.I.S.) the following one given by Glasser (1971) seems to be helpful for the purposes of this chapter: 'A Health Information System is a conglomerate whose function is to collect, analyse, interpret, disseminate measures, indices and messages related to the human conditions as they affect health states, requirements, services and utilization of health systems in defined populations. As a consequence the system must produce reliable indices, methods, and media presentations of sufficient detail and sensitivity to serve the purposes of objective planning, monitoring, and evaluation of health states, programmes and policies in defined populations. It also provides the subjective presentation of the larger health-related issues to the society at large.

2. Man-power—health professionals of different categories, utilized in eye-health activities and indices of utilization.

3. Facilities—buildings, ophthalmic hospital beds, equipment and supplies and indices of utilization.

4. Organization—the organization of eye-health services, with combined functioning of different professionals ('team' concept) and availability of supplies and equipment.

The 'population' from which the data are derived must be carefully defined because it usually varies from study to study. The community may be as small as a neighbourhood or as large as a nation.

All the data concerning needs, demands, and resources should be relevant, complete, accurate, timely and should contain limits of sensitivity (error) on the data itself or on the statistics being produced. They form the core information or so-called *data base* necessary for decision-making at various local, regional, national, and international levels related to the problems of utilization of full eye health on the one hand and loss of vision and blindness on the other.

This data base will allow a first and rough estimate of priority problems on a global (world), regional or national scale, and allow a more objective and scientific approach to the planning process as such.

Data Collection and Sources. In planning the collection of data relevant for public health ophthalmological purposes, the following sources have to be considered:

1. *Blindness statistics:*

(i) *Availability:* as seen previously the existing national registration systems are still rather unsatisfactory in many countries of the world.

(ii) *Population coverage:* in theory, complete for general population.

(iii) *Value and limitations:* when existing, should be routinely available, including diagnostic data.

2. *Ophthalmological data from birth records:*

(i) *Nature of data:* data on congenital eye anomalies.

(ii) *Availability:* may be derived annually from vital registration system of a single country.

(iii) *Population coverage:* in principle, complete for general population.

(iv) *Value and limitations:* in principle, routinely available. Not all congenital eye malformations detected at time of birth.

3. *Notifiable disease statistics:*

(i) *Nature of data:* statistics based on physicians' reports of new cases of notifiable communicable eye diseases.

(ii) *Population coverage:* complete for general population.

(iii) *Value and limitations:* useful in detecting the incidence of certain infectious eye diseases. Reporting spotty, with considerable under-reporting.

4. *Mass diagnostic and screening surveys:*

(i) *Nature of data:* possible by-product of surveys using diagnostic and screening tests for case-finding of specified eye diseases.

(ii) *Availability*: specified population group or for local area on *ad hoc* basis.

(iii) *Population coverage*: unknown degree of completeness.

(iv) *Value and limitations*: identified cases based on fairly good diagnostic information, but findings probably not representative of population under study (for the validity of screening test, see p. 656 and also CHAPTERS 2 and 3).

5. Morbidity surveys of general population:

(i) *Nature of data*: depends upon nature of survey, e.g. household interview survey and eye-health examination survey.

(ii) *Population coverage*: complete for a probability sample.

(iii) *Value and limitation*: household interview surveys yield data on disability (blindness) but diagnostic information not precise; eye-health examinations yield fairly precise diagnostic data but limited to kinds of examination that can be given in the field in each cycle.

6. Epidemiological studies:

(i) *Nature of data*: depends on nature of study. Usually limited to a study of relation between a group of diseases and environmental or social factors.

(ii) *Availability*: *ad hoc* basis for a specified population group or community.

(iii) *Population coverage*: complete.

(iv) *Value and limitations*: usually intense inquiry into the causative factors of eye disease, from which prevalence and sometimes incidence data may be derived. Subject matter and geographical coverage may be limited.

7. Absenteeism data:

(i) *Nature of data*: frequency of absenteeism, for ophthalmological reasons, from work or school.

(ii) *Availability*: may be obtained by special arrangements with school system or industrial concern.

(iii) *Population coverage*: probably complete for school population groups.

(iv) *Value and limitations*: non-specific indicator of disability in a selected population.

8. Social security statistics:

(i) *Nature of data*: data related to eye disability benefit and to hospitalization and eye medical care.

(ii) *Availability*: varies in function from country to country according to the level of administration and population covered by social security.

(iii) *Population coverage*: varies from country to country.

(iv) *Value and limitation*: in many countries there is a complete hospitalization picture and data on those receiving medical eye care for a select but numerically large population group.

9. Hospital in-patient statistics:

(i) *Nature of data*: ophthalmological cases treated in a hospital.

(ii) *Availability*: varies from country to country, but generally not difficult to obtain.

(iii) *Population coverage*: very seldom determinable for individual hospitals.

(iv) *Value and limitations*: population treated in hospitals represents an important segment of the sick population. Diagnostic data presumably of higher quality. Difficult to relate to a defined population from which the hospital cases arise.

10. Hospital out-patient statistics:

(i) *Nature of data*: medical eye care given to patients in clinics and out-patients' services of hospitals.

(ii) *Availability*: generally not available.

(iii) *Population coverage*: not determinable.

(iv) *Value and limitations*: a large volume of eye care is given to ambulatory patients in hospitals. Record system in most instances not well developed; diagnostic data usually poor.

11. Statistics from records of physicians:

(i) *Nature of data*: medical eye care given in physicians' offices.

(ii) *Availability*: not generally available.

(iii) *Value and limitations*: useful information to develop, but physicians' records will range widely in quality and completeness. Problems of identifying new cases and avoiding duplication of counts.

12. Statistics from school eye-health programmes:

(i) *Nature of data*: findings of physical eye examinations of schoolchildren.

(ii) *Availability*: data seldom available.

(iii) *Population coverage*: elementary school population.

(iv) *Value and limitations*: probably of uneven quality and completeness.

13. Statistics on morbidity in Armed Forces:

(i) *Nature of data*:
 (*a*) results of selective service eye examinations;
 (*b*) morbidity and hospitalization figures related to those in Armed Forces.

(ii) *Availability*: easy to obtain in many countries.

(iii) *Population coverage*: military and draftees.

(iv) *Value and limitations*: comprehensive eye morbidity data on select population. Records important source for use in follow-up studies.

14. Eye injury statistics:

(i) *Nature of data*: eye injuries in industry.

(ii) *Availability*: in several countries routinely reported by bureaux of labour statistics.

(iii) *Population coverage*: workers in certain selected large industries in some countries, all workers in industry in certain others.

(iv) *Value and limitations*: useful eye injury data for defined industrial population.

15. Statistics on work-connected eye diseases and injuries:

(i) *Nature of data*: eye illness, eye injury, loss of vision, and blindness arising from occupation.

(ii) *Availability*: varies widely from country to country.

(iii) *Population coverage*: population covered under national laws related to occupational health.

(iv) *Value and limitations*: cases adjudicated by established commission. Presumably well-investigated cases, but determination may be based on different criteria.

Systematic Arrangements of the Data Which Have Been Collected. Such an arrangement is absolutely essential if one is to obtain a picture of the interrelationship among items. The attempt to classify the data means that decisions must be made as to what classification to use.

In the ophthalmological field there are several existing classification and coding systems. Among the most used are:

1. *Standard classification of causes of blindness for international use* (international classification accepted by the General Assembly of the International Association for Prevention of Blindness at New Delhi, on 4 December 1962; published in *Journal of Social Ophthalmology*, 1966).

The purpose of this international standard classification is to achieve a uniform classification of the causes of loss of vision and blindness, so that comparable material can be obtained with some explanation and instructions, followed by an index of diagnostic terms indicating site and type of affection. Finally, a list of some clinical entities causing blindness, supplied with two code numbers, has been added.

2. *Coding system for disorders of the eye (suggested abbreviation C.D.E.)* designed by Schapert-Kimmijser, Colenbrander, and Franken (1968).

This system was devised for the indexing of medical records in ophthalmic departments in 1960, and was completed with alphabetical index in the English language and approved in 1966 by the International Council of Ophthalmology and by the International Federation of Ophthalmological Societies.

3. *Thesaurus for the visual sciences* (Eichhorn, Carroll, and Reinecke), 1969, V.I.C.[1] published by the United States Department of Health, Education and Welfare, Public Health Services, National Institutes of Health.

The thesaurus was designed to satisfy several criteria. First, the need for a highly specific terminology was recognized as a vital prerequisite to a literature retrieval system which must be capable of producing a relevant bibliography in a narrow, specialized area of ophthalmology or the visual sciences. The second requirement was compatibility with *Medical Subject Headings* (MeSH) used by the MEDLARS system of the National Library of Medicine. Lastly, in the V.I.C. system, the thesaurus must serve as an introduction to and link between the two modes of the data base, which includes computer-assisted instruction on selected topics in ophthalmology, as well as literature retrieval.

In addition to MeSH, two other coding systems have been incorporated into the thesaurus. The section designated C13 00 00 00 00 00, Diseases of the Eye, employs the Coding System for Disorders of the Eye, compiled by Schappert-Kimmijser, Colenbrander and Franken (1968). The code

numbers of this system (with a few minor modifications) follow the C13 designation of the V.I.C. system.

The publication contains two forms of thesaurus. The hierarchical structure (VICPRINT) is searchable through the permuted alphabetic index (PERMSORT) in which each term in the thesaurus can be located with its corresponding code number. In the numeric, or hierarchical structure, the level of specificity of the term is indicated by the indentation, as well as by code number. The coding system, consisting of a letter and six pairs of digits, permits seven levels of specificity to be expressed. In many cases, several synonymous terms are listed under the same code number; the non-preferred terms are so indicated by enclosure in parentheses.

The preparation and development of many different classifications was partly necessitated by the lack of an appropriate eye section in the existing *International Classification of Diseases* (I.C.D.) prepared and edited by the WHO.

A ninth revision is actually under preparation by the WHO in which a considerably improved eye section is expected to appear. Different ophthamological groups (Committee on Information of the International Council of Ophthalmology, the American Academy of Ophthalmology and Otolaryngology, and the International Association for the Prevention of Blindness, are collaborating in the preparation of new proposals). It is assumed that the present different classification and coding schemes will be dropped after the improvement of the I.C.D. eye section.

It is useful, perhaps, to mention here that even if they are used largely by physicians and clinical specialists, the different classifications are intended to be used by biostatisticians, not necessarily medically educated. In theory, medical practitioners and specialists are supposed to base their diagnostic recording on recognized nomenclatures which, unfortunately, do not exist. The existing classifications in turn are supposed to be based on such nomenclatures.

The collected data (which can be technical, scientific, economic, social, operational, and administrative) are recorded here following an agreed classification and coding system. Then they are sorted out and tabulated according to the purpose of the study and made ready for analysis, which essentially consists of comparing one set of data with another. It is rare that any given study is undertaken for the sake of the observations themselves. Rather, the objective is to obtain a set of facts which may serve as the basis for prediction about similar situations, that is, the observed material is expected to serve as the *basis for generalization* and the assessment of:

1. The eye-health situation.
2. The situation in eye-health services.

It is therefore extremely important to consider how much the observed sets of data may be expected to vary if additional samples were taken, that is one must consider the *reliability of data* as a basis for generalization.

This requires knowledge of the extent of sampling variations and ways of measuring this.

It should be remembered also that the basic data for the assessment of the eye-health situation depend on diagnoses rather than diseases, and since diagnoses are made by clinicians, the clinical tactics in identifying disease are fundamental elements of the vital statistics branch of ophthalmological

[1] Vision Information Center, the Francis A. Countway Library of Medicine, Howe Laboratory of Ophthalmology, Harward Medical School, Boston, Massachusetts OZ 115. The Vision Information Center is a unit of the national information network of the National Institute of Neurological Diseases and Strokes.

epidemiology. It is beyond the scope of this chapter to go into details of this problem. It is sufficient to state that ophthalmological clinical examination needs to be substantially improved in order to be considered as based on truly scientific measurements and to achieve the desired level of objectivity, precision, consistency, uniformity, and accuracy. To improve the standardization of examination procedures, clinical ophthalmology in fact must continue to develop[1] methods for proving itself more consistent in designating, more uniform in recording, and more reliable in verifying the symptoms and signs that are the main units of clinical measurements. Feinstein's studies and publications in this domain are the most valuable sources for further reading (Feinstein, 1963 to 1968).

The Sectorial Planning Process

The output of an ophthalmological information system, as outlined in previous pages, when analysed with available scientific methods permits more rational decision-making, concerned with:

1. Immediate action, if any.
2. Drawing up short-, medium-, and long-term plans.
3. Conversion of principles and options stated in plans into realistic programmes and projects.
4. Day-to-day monitoring of projects.
5. Continuing appraisal of the progress made towards the attainments of operational targets and final objectives (evaluation).
6. Interdisciplinary aspects (co-ordination) [FIG. 81].

It is beyond any doubt that the available resources (money, equipment, man-power) are always inadequate when compared with ever increasing needs, in both rich and poor countries alike. Therefore, they should be used as efficiently as possible; and because the problems related to eye health and loss of vision are so manifold and complex, the most effective method must be utilized to attack them. Yet, in many instances, criteria of efficiency have not been developed nor has the effectiveness of many ophthalmological programmes been tested.

Comprehensive eye-health planning covers:
1. The planning for eye health of individuals.
2. The planning for eye-health services.
3. The planning for man-power needed to carry out the relevant activities appropriately.

The status of eye health of a defined population cannot be considered as static. The *needs* (expressed also by the ocular mortality (blindness) and morbidity), the *demand* and the *resources* undergo a dynamic variation and the trends are not necessarily positive. A forecast of the possible future situation, on the short, medium, and long term is one of the basic aims of planning.

Long-term comprehensive plans take into consideration the ultimate goal of achieving optimum eye health in the population and preventing totally unnecessary loss of vision, and indicate the broad lines of action necessary to achieve these goals. Medium-term plans should contain more details about precise sub-objectives and the general methodology of work. The public health authorities (with or without the active collaboration of ophthalmologists) adopt one of the alternative

proposed plans, define the policy, taking into consideration the broader context of national resources and priorities, and select fractions of programmes (projects) for implementation under the available budgetary funds. A continuing process of administrative and technical evaluation should provide the necessary feedback for the improvement and revision of activities.

Philosophical and methodological problems connected with planning, programming, and evaluation are elaborated in other parts of this book [see CHAPTERS 3, 41 and 46].

The Ophthalmologist's Role in Eye-health Planning

Comprehensive eye care systems presuppose intra- and extramural activities and a co-ordinated team approach.

Faced with the problem of who has to perform the appropriate planning in this field, we see that there are two possible alternatives:

1. Public health administration, taking the responsibility of sectorial ophthalmological planning, with or without the help of eye specialists.
2. Eye specialists assuming the responsibility of sectorial planning and that of integrating it into general public health planning.

Considering the very specific aspects of loss of vision and related medical processes, the ophthalmologists' active involvement in sectorial planning seems to be highly desirable, even if this entails substantial additions to postgraduate curricula in ophthalmology.

The first step in the planning process as such is a rough estimation of priorities on a global, regional, national, or local scale. As a result of such estimation immediate action is sometimes necessary. These kinds of measures might concern, for example, provision of man-power in understaffed areas, supply of instruments for eye departments or medical action, in cases, for example, of an epidemic of acute keratoconjunctivis in an eye department.

Interdisciplinary Programmes and the Need for Co-ordination

As presented in FIGURE 81 the system of public health ophthalmology requires an interdisciplinary approach in order to move successfully towards the stated objectives, and needs contributions from several professions and technical-administrative units; hence the need for co-ordination. Without such co-ordination, development in this field would be likely to follow the easy course typified by the adoption of a single programme run by one discipline, or by a highly specialized institution.

Such an administrative arrangement might become totally inappropriate when the need arose for larger programmes putting emphasis on comprehensiveness and continuity. Co-ordination might also help to reverse the traditional trend towards a multiplicity of such short-lived projects (especially in the field of research), having little impact and running the risk of duplication or omission. In other words, it is a programme-oriented rather than a unit-oriented development which is required in this field.

The proper co-ordination of public health ophthalmological programmes is a quite complex function which in many instances will require a full-time professional or a specific

---

[1] For activities in this field, see page 389 on trachoma.

administrative unit, whose job will be to obtain a thorough knowledge of the whole programme and to ensure that it is kept comprehensive and continuous.

Whether the leadership of such endeavours will always be the reserve of clinical ophthalmologists, as the most involved specialists, will depend on future trends and curricula in the postgraduate education of this discipline.

The co-ordinator, whoever he is, has to be supported, as needed, by those representing the various disciplines involved in the programme. Co-ordination, to be successful, requires a large degree of co-operation among *all* those involved.

Integration of Some Public Health Ophthalmological Programmes into General Health Services

In providing eye-health care for the population two different approaches are possible. The first is the 'horizontal approach', by which the over-all eye-health problems are tackled on a wide front and on a long-term basis through the creation of a system of permanent institutions (ophthalmological 'infrastructure'). The second, or 'vertical approach' is that through which the solution of a given eye-health problem is sought through the application of specific measures by means of single-purpose machinery. These kinds of activities are well illustrated by effective steps taken against the excessive prevalence of certain endemo-epidemic eye diseases, such as trachoma and seasonal conjunctivitis, which in many areas of the world still constitute a real burden on the population and hamper its economic and social progress.[1] Several trachoma control programmes have shown the need to obtain the best possible knowledge of the local epidemiological behaviour of this disease before launching large-scale operations for its control.

The two approaches 'vertical' and 'horizontal' are not mutually exclusive, for they represent the same effort for eye health and the same final objective. In general, mass campaigns are based on a schedule of successive stages (phases) each of them with well-defined operations and purposes. In the case of communicable eye diseases, the control programmes in their early stage have to be directed, supervised, and executed, either wholly or to a great extent, by a specialized service utilizing health workers exclusive to the task.

In the later stages ('consolidation and maintenance' phases) incorporation into the general health services becomes increasingly important in strengthening epidemiological 'surveillance'.

The culmination of the process whereby a particular eye disease ceases to be the subject of the vertical approach of a special programme or mass campaign and becomes incorporated in the horizontal approach of the general health services and ophthalmological infrastructure, often goes under the term of 'integration of mass campaign into general health services'. This integration usually applies to the peripheral and regional levels of health services, but likewise affects the structural arrangement at the central level, at which the maintenance of an efficient, though somewhat smaller, group of highly skilled specialized personnel is clearly warranted. With the reduction in severity and sometimes also in prevalence and incidence rates of trachoma, the problem of this disease

tends sometimes to be somehow 'forgotten', even in areas where a constant watch is needed to prevent the resurgence of clinical manifestations to the level preceding the mass control measures. The need for a rapid mobilization of resources to cope with any such situation is ample justification for keeping a specialized unit in the national health organization.[2]

INVESTIGATION OF BLINDING CONDITIONS AND DISEASES

EPIDEMIOLOGY AND HEALTH STATISTICS IN OPHTHALMOLOGY

It is largely recognized today that the picture and understanding of a disease process cannot be complete without the description or the thorough study of its behaviour in the population. The term 'epidemiology' can be considered here in two ways. First, it refers to the study of laws governing the frequency and distribution of eye diseases and disability (loss of vision) in population groups and to the factors which influence the occurrence of eye disease in communities. The term is not restricted to communicable eye diseases and does not include communicable eye disease control. Second, epidemiology in large part can be considered also as 'methodology' and this latter interpretation poses also the question of how to bring ophthalmology and epidemiology closer together.

As a matter of fact, epidemiological methods have been rarely applied in ophthalmology. (Surveys in the epidemiological sense[3] have mainly been limited to trachoma, other forms of keratoconjunctivitis and ocular hypertension ('glaucoma').

In general terms, they comprise clinical, laboratory, and field observations where the latter represent the *sine qua non* of the method. Progress in epidemiological inquiry depends to a very large extent indeed on extending methods of standardization in the assessment of symptoms and signs, and on the development of instruments which can be used in field surveys to provide objective measurements.

Substantial progress has been made in this respect in the study of trachoma. The recognition of this disease as a major public health problem has stimulated a multidisciplinary approach. This effort has resulted in substantial improvements towards the basic requirements of any epidemiological study, i.e. towards the basic requirements of any epidemiological study, i.e. definition of the disease, and its various stages, scoring systems, diagnosis and recording, treatment and its evaluation.

For centuries, the centres of trachomatous infections were recognized to be in the Mediterranean basin and in the Orient. Today, the disease is very prevalent in many parts of Africa and Asia, but sporadic cases occur all over the world. Trachoma flourishes in areas that are hot and dry and have a shortage of available water and poor hygienic customs.

It has been estimated that there are actually four to five hundred million cases of trachoma in the world. Together with associated infections, trachoma still represents the main problem of eye pathology in most of the developing countries, and

---

[1] The term 'mass campaign' has become widely accepted for this type of programme.
[2] For further reading see Gonzalez (1965).

[3] That is 'a test applied to a battery of people'. In clinical medicine and ophthalmology the term 'survey' often refers to the concept of a study of a number of cases where a battery of tests are applied to each individual person.

is responsible for visual impairment in many cases which, where complicated by severe sequelae such as entropion and trichiasis and subsequent corneal complications, may lead to more severe loss of vision and blindness. Several studies and surveys have indicated the interrelation of the disease, its degree of endemicity and of severity, with socio-economic factors and with standards of living. Equally, some of these studies have introduced the application of scientific sampling procedures, as well as analysis of different types of experimental errors and biases (by Assaad, Nižetić, Kupka, etc.).

In applying the rules of modern epidemiology, accurate prevalence or incidence rates can be determined for different populations, and it then becomes possible to look for a correlation between disease frequencies and the occurrence of environmental, genetic, demographic, or cultural components of the community. This approach has been called geographical ophthalmology.[1]

The so-called 'descriptive epidemiology' finds its greatest value, in ophthalmology, in the early stages of an investigation when very little is known of suspected environmental factors, and the method is commonly used, in fact, to obtain information that will help to formulate an hypothesis.

Although attractive in theory, the descriptive studies which form the majority of contributions brought by *geographical ophthalmology* are very often fraught with sources of error. Frequently, the cases are not defined, diagnosed, and reported all in the same way in the different geographic areas. The levels of local medical surveillance and sophistication of treatment can influence both blindness and eye morbidity data, and may result in misleading comparisons of prevalence rates.

Disease frequencies, either prevalence or incidence rates, must be based on similarly defined denominator populations that are comparable for the geographic areas under consideration. Limitations are imposed here, since geographic units are usually defined according to local census procedures and may or may not correspond to the geographic area in which it is practical to ascertain numerator cases. The relative accuracy of census records in the comparison populations can also be a source of error.

The second group of epidemiological investigations forms the so-called *analytic epidemiology*. These kinds of studies are specifically designed to examine a particular hypothesis. We can distinguish two types of such analytic investigations, each with its advantages and disadvantages:

1. The *retrospective study* (also called case-control study or case-history study) in which the population is composed of a selected group of cases of a given eye disease and a selected group of controls. An example of this kind of study would be the investigation in which the history of a group of babies with retrolental fibroplasia is compared with the history of a non-diseased control group to determine the relative risk of 'exposure' to such characteristics as prematurity or elevated atmospheric oxygen.

2. The *prospective study* (longitudinal study or cohort investigation) forms part of the general area of analytic epidemiology, and is designed predominantly to test one or more specific

hypotheses. The advantages and difficulties of this method are dealt with in other parts of this book. In ophthalmology there are not many examples of the application of this approach. As an illustration we could mention Linner's longitudinal study of ocular hypertension (Linner, 1969). Departing from the well-known fact that from a clinical point of view it is clearly difficult to differentiate between normal and glaucomatous eyes only by measuring the intra-ocular pressure, Linner, in an attempt to test the influence of borderline pressure of the eyes, longitudinally investigated a group with ocular hypertension for a period of five years. The study population was compared appropriately with a normal control group. As a result of this study, Linner states that there is no exact numeric border between the normal and the pathological pressure of the eye. Single measurements of the intra-ocular pressure are not sufficient for a reliable and early diagnosis of glaucoma, and additional criteria should be found.

The last category of epidemiological investigations is represented by experimental studies, which are technically similar to the longitudinal or cohort approach. The essential difference between the two techniques lies in the fact that in the experimental design the exposure to a suspected factor is controlled through manipulation. In cohort design, on the other hand, the results of a naturally occurring exposure are obtained.

Experimental epidemiology finds common appreciation in therapeutic trials but is not commonly used in the study of causal associations.

Cochrane (1967) has made a critical analysis of screening for glaucoma showing that a raised intra-ocular tension does not always indicate an increased chance of glaucoma.

HEALTH LABORATORY SERVICES IN PUBLIC HEALTH OPHTHALMOLOGY

The laboratory is of great importance in epidemiological investigations. In many communicable eye diseases the aetiological diagnosis can be established only by laboratory examination of appropriate specimens obtained from patients. Furthermore, to gain an adequate understanding of the epidemiology of a certain communicable eye disease, it is essential to determine the incidence of subclinical infection. The type of laboratory support required depends on the nature of the disease to be investigated. Therefore, to ensure optimal results in any epidemiological investigation of communicable eye diseases, close collaboration and adequate communication must exist between the laboratory and the field investigator.

Following extensive trachoma mass treatment campaigns in several areas of the world, the number of so-called 'mild' cases seen in endemic areas is apparently increasing as a consequence of a gradual decrease in the severity of the disease. It is therefore becoming more difficult to establish a diagnosis, more difficult to determine the degree of endemicity in a community, and thus more difficult to determine the degree of risk represented by the disease in individual cases and communities. These diagnostic problems become of critical importance in the evaluation of control measures. An additional difficulty is represented by an apparent trend towards spontaneous disappearance, or at least attentuation of the disease, which may occur even in the absence of specific control measures, perhaps

---

[1] A few years ago, the International Society of Geographical Ophthalmology was constituted. Two conferences have been held so far: the first in Yellowknife (Canada), and the second in Jerusalem (Israel) in August 1971.

as a consequence of general improvements in sanitation and living conditions. The necessary scientific definition of such a trend is also becoming more difficult because of diagnostic problems.

Laboratory techniques could contribute to the solution of these problems. Tarizzo, Nabli, and Labonne's (1968) conclusions confirm that laboratory tests are more likely to be positive when the clinical signs are more pronounced; thus the laboratory tests would be of least assistance in the cases for which they were most needed.

In an individual clinical case, demonstration of the agent, or of the response to its presence, cannot usually provide much more than a confirmation of an already established clinical diagnosis. Tarizzo, Nabli, and Labonne (1968) suggest that if, instead of individual cases, a population group is taken into consideration, the rate of positivity of properly standardized tests may then become a quantitative expression of the density of the causal agent or of the reaction to its presence in a given area or population. Further research in this field will ensure that the best possible use may be made of the diagnostic methods which are available today. It remains, for example, to be proven whether the rate of positivity, by modifications in the endemicity of the disease, is to be accepted as a valid indicator (Tarizzo, Nabli, and Labonne, 1968).

PREVENTION OF BLINDING CONDITIONS AND DISEASES

As in general medicine, ophthalmological prevention started with measures aimed to avoid communicable diseases. The classical example is given by Credé's method to prevent blennorrhoea neonatorum. The modern mass control programmes against trachoma and seasonal conjunctivitis conducted in many areas of the world are another good example of the application of the concept of prevention to community eye health. In many areas of the world, the communicable eye diseases are at present brought under relative control; nutritional deficiencies are identified as an important cause of loss of vision and are becoming preventable.

Nowadays, ophthalmological prevention is becoming increasingly talked about and studied epidemiologically, to include the degenerative, metabolic disease, injuries and other environmental eye-health hazards.

The very concept of prevention has been presented and defined in many different ways. For the purposes of this chapter a few clarifications seem to be necessary.

Some ocular ailments, environmental hazards to eye health, and eye health-related social problems can be *prevented from occurring* (primary prevention). On the other hand, ocular ailments or hazards or social problems are sometimes already present in the individual, family, or community, and in some instances can be *prevented from progressing* (secondary prevention).

In *preventive ophthalmology* it is the individual, sick or well alike, who is the focus of attention. In *public health ophthalmology* or *community ophthalmology*, the focus is on groups of individuals, formed into a community, whose members face common eye-health problems and among whom an organized community effort is essential for the resolution of such problems.

In the planning for and delivery of ophthalmological preventive services, the health administrator has to adopt realistically a pragmatic concept of causality, contrary to the scientist who requires a high degree of plausibility before accepting a causal inference. If all the proofs of causality, which are often missing, were awaited, few programmes of disease control would ever be started.

Preventive programmes in the field of public health ophthalmology contain the mixed elements of *prevention of occurrence*, *prevention of progress*, and *limitation of disability*. Several factors hinder the proper extension of preventive services in ophthalmology. One of them certainly lies in the general clinical attitude of practising ophthalmologists which is strictly related to the type of medical education in the majority of medical schools. Preventive services are further obstructed and retarded by the vast sums of money spent on medical eye care alone, which leaves very reduced funds for prevention. It is usually admitted that if the cost–benefit ratios are to be minimized, the organized eye community services have to be comprehensive. This approach presupposes large financial investments, not always immediately possible even in rich countries, and categorical (ophthalmological) preventive activities often precede an integrated public health action.

COMMUNICABLE EYE DISEASES CONTROL

Acute Bacterial Conjunctivitis and Trachoma

Acute bacterial conjunctivitis can be caused by several infectious agents. The *Morax–Axenfeld diplobacillus* (*Moraxella*) is the most innocuous, *Haemophilus aegyptius* (Koch–Weeks bacillus) the most important and widespread. A Gram-negative diplococcus resembling the gonococcus was in the recent past one of the main causes of conjunctivitis epidemics and of much loss of vision in Africa and the Near East.

Bacterial conjunctivitis infections often occur as seasonal epidemics, in spring and autumn; they may facilitate the onset of trachoma, aggravate its course, and/or prevent it from healing. Secretion and discharges caused by bacterial infections may favour transmission of the trachoma agent. On the other hand, trachomatous conjunctivitis seems to be particularly susceptible to bacterial infections.

In general the magnitude of seasonal epidemics depends on the following factors:

1. The reservoir of bacterial carriers.
2. The abundance of flies during major breeding seasons.
3. The direct influence of climatic conditions on fly breeding, and possibly indirectly on the virulence of the organisms.
4. The lack of personal hygiene of the population.
5. The presence or absence of rational treatment.

The second and third of these factors usually affect the course of the epidemic from May to December, while the first and the fourth exercise a permanent influence.

Seasonal conjunctivitis was and still is in many countries in the world by far the most frequent cause of total blindness. In some North African countries two decades ago, studies have shown that many ulcers occurred in the second half of the season, less often from Koch–Weeks conjunctivitis but frequently from gonoblennorrhoea. Perforations of the eye were relatively frequent, resulting in total or partial adherent leucomata, secondary glaucoma, staphyloma, or phthisis bulbi. Moreover, the bacterial infections have further disastrous effects in that they facilitate the transmission of trachoma, prolong its course and aggravate such complications as pannus and excessive cicatrization of the conjunctiva with its sequelae: entropion, trichiasis, and xerosis.

The unfortunate, widespread co-existence of these infections resulted in a continuous evolution of trachoma throughout life leading, in a very high percentage of cases, to progressive loss of vision.

Wilson (1945) provided circumstantial evidence that the trachoma agent may be transmitted in the infective discharge of conjunctivitis, and it was considered important to check this point in field trials.

Studies carried out in 1952–54 established the fact that in south Morocco the prevalence of both trachoma and seasonal conjunctivitis was high, and that both assumed a grave form resulting in high incidence of impaired vision. In the south eighteen years ago, no solution could be envisaged to this problem. In countries where trachoma and seasonal conjunctivitis are prevalent it is well known that hospital and dispensary services have generally failed to reduce the incidence of communicable eye diseases, although they may have done much to reduce individual suffering and the incidence of blindness.

Because of the insidious onset of trachoma in early childhood and the relative absence of subjective symptoms in the early stages, the children and their parents are unaware of their illness. Usually, only those suffering pain and loss of sight attend hospitals and dispensaries. Persons suffering from conjunctivitis are very often satisfied with the immediate symptomatic relief given by modern treatment and few of them continue the treatment until cured of the underlying trachoma. It is also well known that treatment of a few individual cases cannot change the natural course of an epidemic of conjunctivitis in a community.

As early as 1950, experimental work was conducted in Morocco to find a suitable mass treatment method (Bardon, 1953; Bidart and Racollet, 1953; Ferrand and Parlange, 1951; Ferrand and Soyer, 1953; Gaud, 1949; Gaud and Decour, 1951; Guad, Maurice, Faure, and Lalu, 1950; Pagès, 1938, 1950a, 1950b).

Information on the environmental conditions favouring seasonal conjunctivitis and trachoma infection was available from other countries with similar problems (Wilson, 1945; Maxwell-Lyons, 1953). It has long been recognized that in regions like North Africa and the Middle East, where trachoma and seasonal conjunctivitis co-exist, control measures must be directed against both. In 1952, it was decided that economically feasible mass treatment methods based on this principle could be applied in Morocco, the importance of environmental sanitation and health education being taken into account.

During 1952 and 1953, a joint programme of work was developed for a mass campaign with the participation of the Government of Morocco, the WHO and UNICEF. Within the project area, three experimental sectors were designated: Skoura in 1952, Ouarzazate in 1953, and Goulmima in 1954.

The experimental sectors were used for epidemiological investigations and for the continuous development of simpler, more effective, and more economical methods and schedules of mass treatment.

During the years 1954–58, large-scale clinical trials were carried out in schools in the cities of Marrakesh and Meknès and in the rural areas of Tiznit to determine the effects of a single antibiotic, chlortetracycline, on trachoma, when administered according to different treatment regimens (Reinhards, Weber, and Maxwell-Lyons, 1959). Having established the superiority of the 'intermittent' over the 'continuous' schedule of treatment, further trials were conducted, on a smaller scale, to test the relative efficacy of chlortetracycline and tetracycline; the latter proved slightly better. A study of cure rates in young pre-school children was also carried out to establish a baseline for later assessment of induced drug resistance, if any.

After 1953, the mass treatment campaign was extended and by 1960 covered nearly the whole of the south and also parts of the country north of the Atlas Mountains with a known high prevalence of trachoma. In addition, after 1954, collective treatment was introduced in schools covering an increasing number of children each year; by 1960 treatment was given to all first- and second-grade pupils, and in 1966 treatment was also given to third-grade pupils.

Although the magnitude of the trachoma problem was obvious from the beginning, the shortage of personnel precluded a detailed study of local differences in prevalence, distribution, and gravity of the disease and the role of associated infections, except in the experimental sectors mentioned above. The resulting lack of baseline data on the south as a whole has made difficult the evaluation of the results of the mass campaign (Reinhards, Weber, Nižetić, Kupka, and Maxwell-Lyons, 1968).

Because of these difficulties, large-scale sample surveys have been conducted since 1961 under the auspices of the Moroccan Government, the WHO and UNICEF. These studies used proper sampling techniques and were designed to assess as accurately as possible the changes that had occurred in the level of communicable eye diseases as a result of the introduction of control measures.

They assessed the prevalence, gravity, and frequency of complications of trachoma by ophthalmological examinations, conducted in the home, and the results are compared with data published elsewhere, which were obtained before treatment started in the 1950s in parts of the study area. Additional studies were made of the relations between trachoma and the availability and use of water, and between the prevalence of trachoma in females and their exposure to infection (Kupka, Nižetić, and Reinhards, 1968).

The over-all prevalence of trachoma was unaffected by the mass treatment campaign but a larger proportion of the cases were at stage IV of the disease (healed). In one region, however, the prevalence of active cases (stages I–III) in the younger age-groups had decreased considerably. The occurrence of pannus decreased and while trichiasis decreased in children under 15 years of age, its prevalence increased in adults.

An international group of experts met in 1962 under the auspices of the WHO to review the trachoma problem and make specific recommendations for the organization of anti-trachoma projects. The specific measure to be applied in all these programmes is the specific mass treatment by local application of antibiotic preparations, to be accompanied by training programmes for local personnel, and by health education and environmental sanitation activities whenever possible. The emphasis of the programme and of the criteria for its evaluation, falls on the reduction of the severity of the disease and on avoiding the complications leading to loss of vision, on the utilization of paramedical personnel to facilitate a wider coverage of control activities, on the use of uniform criteria and evaluation of results, and on integration of activities into general health services (WHO, 1962).

Later, in 1970, a field guide with detailed information on principles and procedures in trachoma control activities was prepared by a group of WHO medical officers directly involved in communicable eye diseases control projects (WHO, 1970). Recent work has shown that iododeoxyuridine is an effective chemotherapeutic agent in trachoma (Harris, 1974).

Epidemic Keratoconjunctivitis

Large outbreaks of this disease have been described in Europe, North America, the Far East, and Hawaii, but its occurrence is presumably world-wide. Type 8 adenovirus (occasionally other types) is responsible for this form, which is characterized by an acute unilateral or bilateral inflammation of the conjunctiva, and oedema of lids and peri-orbital tissues, low-grade fever, headache, malaise, tender pre-auricular lymphadenopathy, and opacities of the cornea which become evident within 4 to 14 days. The duration of illness is 2 to 4 weeks and complete recovery is usual, although keratitis with impairment of vision may persist in some patients. Outbreaks among industrial employees in temperate climates commonly involve only a small part of the population at risk. The transmission occurs through direct contact with discharges from the eye of an infected person, or with articles freshly soiled with conjunctival or nasal discharges. In industrial plants, it occurs from trauma to the conjunctiva from dust and dirt with subsequent contamination of the eye in first-aid stations and dispensaries where proper aseptic techniques are not employed. There are reports of cases having originated in eye clinics and physicians' offices.

As far as methods of control and prevention are concerned, education as to personal cleanliness and the danger of using common towels and toilet articles should rank in first place. Use of safety measures, such as goggles in industrial plants and rigid asepsis in ophthalmological procedures in industrial dispensaries, to prevent spread of infection via the hands of attendants or by means of instruments, is to be strengthened.

Epidemic Haemorrhagic Conjunctivitis

Extensive epidemics have been occurring in recent years in Africa, Aisa and Europe from this new disease, caused by a picornavirus (World Health Organization, 1974, pp. 12, 13 and 32).

Protozoal and Metazoan Infections

Protozoal Infections. *Toxoplasmosis*: at present the loss of vision due to manifestations of toxoplasmosis remains mainly in the domain of clinical ophthalmology, because the clinical disease is sporadic though the infection in man is common. The source of human infection is unknown as well as the mode of transmission of post-natal infections. Congenital infection apparently occurs through the placenta of women in the primary stage of infection.

Metazoan Infections. Though the vast majority of infections of the eye, as of other parts of the body, are due to the simplest organisms, a few are caused by multicellular animals, either worms or insect larvae. There are two main types of ocular helminthiasis: that in which a mobile worm (either adult or larva) infects the eye or its adnexa, and that in which the larva is sessile and forms a cyst. Of the former group, *onchocerciasis* is by far the most important, especially from the public health point of view, and of the latter *cysticercosis* most interests the clinical ophthalmologist.

Onchocerciasis: a chonic, non-fatal filarial disease caused by a nematode worm—*Onchocerca volvulus*—producing fibrous nodules in the skin and subcutaneous tissues, particularly of the head and shoulders, pelvic girdle, and lower extremities. The female worm discharges microfilariae which migrate through the skin. From lesions on the head microfilariae frequently reach the eye, producing ocular disturbances and sometimes serious loss of vision. The disease is transmitted by the bite of infected blackflies of the genus *Simulium* and is an excellent example of the interdisciplinary involvement of entomology, helminthology, and ophthalmology. The socio-economic impact of visual loss due to onchocerciasis is likely to be very high, as in certain areas of endemicity the prevalence of this disability has been recorded by various surveys as ranging from 8,000 to 10,000 per 100,000 inhabitants.

The ocular lesions are nearly always irreversible, due to the fact that the diagnosis is almost invariably made at later stages, and the preventive and control measures have to be diverted towards the factors leading to ocular manifestation. This means, in the first place, the destruction of the vector, and, secondly, the reduction of the human parasite reservoir by mass chemotherapy. The first approach is practicable even if extremely expensive. It consists in controlling the vector larvae in rapidly running streams and in artificial waterways by DDT and other insecticides. As for the direct prevention of visual loss from onchocerciasis, practically nothing can be done at present apart from rapid and direct elimination of the human parasite reservoir on a mass scale. The state of present knowledge calls for further research with appropriate and available modern epidemiological methods, aiming to elucidate many still open and controversial issues. These include, among others, studies on the prevalence of subjects with serious loss of vision due to this disease, on the relation of seriously impaired vision and blindness with skin infection in different areas, behavioural studies on subject with and without ocular lesions, and laboratory and epidemiological studies on *Onchocerca volvulus*.

A large-scale oncocerciasis control programme was started in 1974 in the Volta river, financed by UNDP with the participation of FAO. The programme covers nearly 1 million square kilometres in 7 countries. Amongst the 10 million inhabitants, more than 1 million are infected and about 100,000 are economically blind (Fuglsang and Anderson, 1973). WHO has also supported studies on the use of new drugs for chemotherapy by the Organization for Co-ordination and Cooperation in Major Endemic Diseases and the mobile ophthalmology team of the Rural Health Service of the upper Volta (World Health Organization, 1974).

NON-COMMUNICABLE EYE DISEASES

The actual state of knowledge about non-communicable chronic eye diseases from various origins indicates that the means of preventing occurrence are usually not within our grasp. Hence effort has to be expended on *prevention of progression* or minimization of ill-effects (limitation of disability). This is accomplished by organized community health services that provide early and accurate diagnosis, adequate treatment, and also rehabilitation and the meeting of eye health-related social needs.

Early Detection of Potentially Blinding Chronic Eye Conditions

Factors which help to determine the possibilities of a community approach to early detection of potentially blinding chronic eye conditions are represented by the administrative structure of the medical services, the facilities available as regards hospitals and personnel, and the concentration of the population in a defined area or country; ophthalmological practice is then only one factor among such differences as prevail between centres. Furthermore, there are considerable national differences in the attitude to mass screening programmes, and finally, the cost–benefit analysis is everywhere a significant determining factor when it is a question of initiating exploratory investigations into the value of early detection and the techniques to be employed. Consequently, such investigations must clearly be subject to local requirements.

Genetically Determined Conditions

Although a large potential field for early detection, the present state of knowledge is insufficient to allow any widespread activity. Ideally, these abnormalities could be prevented by the development of the twin services of testing for the detection of the heterozygous carrier state, and adequate genetic counselling based upon these results and upon family history. In only three genetically determined conditions, excluding squint with its amblyopia, is early detection of clinical importance. Of these three, two—buphthalmos and retinoblastoma—are genetically determined only occasionally; the third—galactosaemia—appears to be uncommon. Galactosaemia, like phenylketonuria, is one of the few controllable inborn metabolic disorders. Systematic analysis of the urine of neonates is practised in highly developed maternity units, but does not appear to be a routine in most institutions. The occurrence of lens changes in about 75 per cent. of cases— easily recognized from the fairly characteristic early manifestations, simulating a drop of oil in the centre of the lens—may not often be of crucial value in the diagnosis which is readily made on the findings in the urine. Early detection is now less urgent, for early lens changes are likely to be reversible (see also CHAPTER 30).

Hereditary Degenerative Disorders (Abiotrophies)

It seems very likely today that there is no real line of demarcation between congenital hereditary defects and the abiotrophic disorders. The possibility is emerging that some of the so-called senile degenerations of the fundus are also genetically determined. These facts call for increasing endeavour to recognize the *carrier state* where possible. The term *carrier state* is here used in its clinical context: the search for minimal, often non-pathological, anomalies (morphological, serological, or biochemical) which indicate that the individual carries a pathogenic gene. It is interesting that some minor anomalies now recognized as evidence of the carrier state were known to earlier generations of clinicians, and because of their innocuousness were regarded by them as 'physiological variations'.

Evidence of the carrier state is readily available to the ophthalmologist alerted to its existence and significance. In the dominant disorders there is a whole range of incomplete expression in the colobomatous defects (extending from anophthalmos to a minimal iris coloboma), in aniridia, in macular cyst, and possibly also in glaucoma.

Embryopathies

Embryopathy implies a generalized disorder which may or may not include ocular manifestations. It is likely that some purely ocular malformations will ultimately be seen as the result of limited embryopathies. The public health aspect of early detection is as yet of limited significance in embryopathies, as there is nothing to suggest that infective agents, other than the spirochaete, persist to produce damage at more than one pregnancy. In practical terms, this means that early detection in this group has to be restricted to the recognition of mothers at risk and babies at risk.

Amblyopia and Squint

Amblyopia is defined as reduced visual acuity, without any detectable abnormalities, of the optic nerve or retina, as viewed with the opthalmoscope. To the lay public, this is more frequently known as 'lazy eye'.

The incidence of this disability is generally considered to be sufficiently high to present an important public health and economic problem. The necessity of passing increasingly stringent visual tests for employment in industry and for various forms of vehicle licensing makes the problem even more pressing. It is important to distinguish various types of amblyopia when considering possibilities of early detection and treatment.

Von Noorden classifies amblyopia under five headings:

1. Strabismic amblyopia.
2. Amblyopia ex anopsia (or deprivation amblyopia).
3. Anisometric amblyopia.
4. Congenital amblyopia.
5. Ametropic amblyopia.

Since it is generally agreed that amblyopia of the non-organic varieties responds more readily to treatment in direct proportion to the time of its discovery, the problem of early case-finding is crucial. At present, assessment of binocular vision and of amblyopia is entirely subjective. The only objective sign is the onset of squint. Early detection—so greatly dependent upon the subjective features—is thus limited by the age and mental development of the child. It is therefore all the more important to recognize the earliest signs of an actual squint in infants.

In particular, attention should be paid to intermittent squint when reported by parents. Simple tests, such as the cover test and the position of corneal reflexes, should help and they are within the competence of allied health personnel. However, none of these tests is, of course, a measure of amblyopia.

Some conflicting reports exist on the incidence of squint in infancy and childhood. Even if differences between countries are to be excluded, undoubtedly much of the discrepancy is due to lack of uniformity in the criteria used. Adequate data on the incidence of squint, and of amblyopia in *critically observed series*, are needed, as indeed are *systematic studies on the epidemiology of the affection*. As far as treatment is concerned, the simplest procedure is occlusion. This calls for no specialized techniques such as those required in orthoptic treatment or in pleoptics. These specialized facilities are not always available. They appear to have been developed more intensively in Central and Eastern Europe than in the Western and Scandinavian countries. At some centres in Czechoslovakia, Italy, Poland, and the Soviet Union there are residential schools with hospital facilities. Detailed and critical assessment is needed of the results obtained.

The crucial issue in most countries is to get infants with amblyopia and latent or indefinite squint to treatment centres. The medical services for children under school age are nowhere as adequate as the school medical services are, so that apart from diagnostic difficulties, there are variable, but considerable, shortcomings in contact between parents and the treatment centres. Where nursery schools are available on an extensive scale, some of the difficulties in communication can be readily overcome. Elsewhere, there is inevitably much reliance on infant welfare centres, but these are not always able to provide the necessary ophthalmic guidance.

To overcome the lack of contact between parents and ophthalmic treatment centres, propaganda has been used among parents in Sweden and in the Federal Republic of Germany. Even mass screening has been attempted. It would seem that more effective results can be obtained by ensuring that the necessary technical knowledge for early detection is available to general practitioners and allied health personnel who come into professional contact with infants and children.

In a recent report on a Working Group held on this subject in the European Office of the World Health Organization, the following recommendations were made (WHO Regional Office for Europe, 1971):

1. It is desirable that all infant welfare centres, whether well-baby centres or follow-up centres for babies at risk, should be able to tell the groups when they are in danger from squint and amblyopia. While full epidemiological studies are still to come, the risk of squint is definite in the following categories:

(*a*) infants with a family history of squint. It is likely that squint is determined by polygenic inheritance. A history of squint in a sib, in either of the parents or in their first and second degree relatives, is therefore significant;
(*b*) infants with multiple congenital defects;
(*c*) infants with spastic palsy;
(*d*) infants with debilitating disorders.

2. Co-operation of general practitioners needs to be pursued actively. General practitioners should know of the groups at risk and of the danger of delay in treatment.

It should be said that, in some countries, the increasing number of family practitioners and paediatricians who evaluate the visual acuity of their patients as early as possible and refer them for care is encouraging, even if the problem of locating the pre-school child who has undiscovered amblyopia, with or without strabismus, is to be considered as inadequately met on a world-wide basis. The programmes of visual screening in school populations, when they exist, continue to discover those children with visual problems which are still amenable to treatment.

Refraction Anomalies

In all countries, the school medical service can be relied upon to carry out the necessary screening of children at school age. Under school age, the significant error of refraction to be considered is severe myopia. This is a possibility in infants with a history of marked prematurity and may also occur in infants with the same sort of family history as for squint. A recent ophthalmological survey registered a significant increase of myopia in the populations of northern Canada.

Glaucomas

From the prevention and public health point of view, it is especially the so-called *glaucoma simplex* or *chronic simple glaucoma* which has received, in recent years, much attention within the context of prevention of 'blindness'. The other forms of glaucoma—angle-closure glaucoma and secondary glaucoma—tend to produce symptoms at a relatively early stage and thereby come under medical care.

Glaucoma simplex is still a problem which defies solution. Insidious and symptomless in onset, it affects people in middle age. Genetically, it is multifactorial, and the pattern of heredity is therefore not Mendelian, though often familial. It is a major cause of registered 'blindness' in the majority of countries where the communicable eye diseases are kept under control, and because the visual loss does not involve central vision until a later stage, signs of the disease may be present for a long time before the patient notes any symptoms.

Usually it is believed that the raised intra-ocular pressure is responsible for the development of the changes in the disc, and therefore for the progressive loss of vision, although this hypothesis is rejected either in whole or in part by several prominent scientists in this field. The treatment is based entirely on reduction of the intra-ocular pressure to 'safe' levels. During the past twenty years large numbers of people, mostly over the age of 40, have been screened for glaucoma by tonometry, often with very conflicting results, due essentially to the difficulty in interpreting tonometric readings obtained in screening investigations. While the significance of markedly raised tension as evidence of glaucoma is, of course, beyond question, there appears to be growing scepticism as to the value of the borderline readings.

The incidence of false positives may be as high as 90 per cent. when such patients are investigated more completely or kept under prolonged observation. With lack of adequate criteria as to what constitutes normal tension, the high incidence of false positives and a substantial incidence of false negatives (in that some patients, passed as normal, subsequently developed glaucoma) indicate that tonometry, as a diagnostic tool for the detection of early glaucoma, is not sufficiently promising to justify its use for mass screening. On the accumulated evidence now available, the value of tonometry is not very different from that of the provocative tests used in clinical ophthalmology for individual patients suspected of glaucoma.

In view of these disadvantages, the following three possibilities have to be considered as potentially useful for screening purposes:

1. Screening of the visual field.
2. Screening by ophthalmoscopy.
3. Selection by family history.

The normal methods of clinical investigation of the visual field are unsuitable for use in screening, being too tedious and requiring considerable training. The development of the newer type of central field screener—such as Friedman's Visual Field Analyser—has made possible a rapid assessment of the visual field under reasonably standard conditions and also in the hands of less-trained allied health personnel. Such screening is far more specific and sensitive than tonometry, and the incidence of false positives is probably not more than 10 per cent.

It would therefore seem that a first step in the investigation of suspected glaucoma could well be assessment of the central field, much as taking visual acuity is the first step in the routine examination of the eye. Screening of the central field might, in fact, be part of such routine examination, particularly in patients over the age of 40. Further critical studies on the scope and limitations of the available central field screeners are still needed.

Screening for glaucoma by ophthalmoscopy is actually the oldest method and one which, consciously or unconsciously, every ophthalmologist practises in the course of a routine eye test. Even if the routine use of the ophthalmoscope becomes generalized among the general or family practitioners, a very high false-positive rate is to be expected.

The potential value of the selection by family history is based upon the fact that it is possible to show a high prevalence of abnormality among the relatives of patients with glaucoma. This has been shown both for pressure and for fully developed glaucoma, where the familial incidence has been put as high as 38 per cent. Clear simple dominance is not always present, and there is evidence of simple recessive inheritance in some cases. It is, however, likely that the commonest type of inheritance is polygenic rather than monofactorial.

When deciding upon screening activities of any sort, and considering that resources are usually limited, the public health administrator needs information about the actual cost of screening, expressed in terms of time, man-power, and expenditure on materials. In the case of glaucoma, all the screening procedures discussed above are quick and reasonably simple. They have proved acceptable in practice and, although in tonometry there is a theoretical risk of corneal damage, experience in many thousands of measurements has shown that the risk is very small. Field and ophthalmoscopic screening are naturally entirely free from risk, being purely subjective in nature. None of the methods discussed above involves any large expenditure on materials, and Graham (1966), using figures from his own and other surveys, attempted to make a reasonable comparison on the basis of time spent per new case detected. From the results in the detection of unsuspected field defects for a team of ophthalmologist, technician, and secretary, tonometry emerges as clearly the most expensive if the

normal routine of investigation recommended for suspects is followed. The more favourable ratios for field screener and ophthalmoscopy are accounted for, to a large extent, by the simpler nature of the subsequent investigation required. The cost per case detected by tonometry can be reduced if the test is used simply as an indication that the subject requires a visual field test, but it should be remembered that a simple measurement of intra-ocular pressure is an unsatisfactory index for possible field loss.

The second, and even more important problem facing the public health administrator, is that of providing adequate long-term supervision of suspects. Here again, tonometry screening raises the biggest problem, for about 8 per cent. of the population between the ages of 40 and 75 years have pressures which, according to many authors, require long-term supervision. Considering the already overburdened eye clinics and the shortage of ophthalmological man-power in many areas of the world, it is easy to realize the bottleneck which would ensue. At the present time, the available evidence suggests that expansion of facilities, were this possible, to cope with such an influx, is scarcely justified by our limited knowledge of the precise significance of ocular hypertension with normal visual fields. By carrying out visual field screening and ophthalmoscopy, the problem becomes less dramatic, as one cannot deny the desirability of supervision of patients having a definite field defect. The process of eliminating false positives in most cases involves only a single examination, and the number of new cases remaining for long-term surveillance is small, only about 0·3 per cent. for the age-group 40–75. This seems to be more within the bounds of possibility, provided that the initial investigation of suspects can be managed. (See Cochrane (1967) for a critical discussion on screening for glaucoma.)

Diabetic Retinopathy

This retinal disease is recognized as a major and increasing cause of loss of vision in many areas of the world. A number of problems are impeding progress in its clinical and public health management. The protean nature of this disease makes understanding of its natural history difficult. The multiplicity and complexity of body systems affected by diabetes mellitus tax our capacity to integrate with the ophthalmological data, the essential clinical information derived from other specialities. The number of diabetic cases requiring assessment and treatment is already large, and is steadily growing. This represents a challenge to the physician, both in screening and in clinical care. Controlled studies of treatment methods, so necessary for progress in management, usually require an aggregation of suitable patients in a setting appropriate for effective clinical investigation.

Any programme designed to stimulate the multidisciplinary search for solutions should, in particular, emphasize the need for clinicians:

1. To study the epidemiological aspects of the conditions.
2. To examine the possibilities of improving co-operation between ophthalmological and non-ophthalmological public health institutions.
3. In view of the essential need for an effective method of documenting and managing the voluminous data acquired, to consider the possibility of electronic data processing.

Diabetes itself is regarded as genetically determined. Whether the retinopathy is incidental or also genetically determined is not known. Family studies on the incidence of retinopathy in diabetes in both men and women (the latter being especially at risk) would be useful, if it only offers the possibility of establishing criteria for the early diagnosis of progressive retinopathy.

Toxic Disorders

Ocular complications and loss of vision are mainly produced by some pharmacological agent (such as chloroquine and allied preparations, thioridazine (*Melleril*) and ethambutol), while little is known of the ocular toxicity of agents other than medications and addictive drugs, such as tobacco, ethanol, and methanol.

A very large number of newer agents have been reported as producing ocular complications, but the evidence is not always convincing, and the frequency of established complications is apparently low. Further epidemiological data are needed to establish the possible public importance in such instances.

Retinal Detachment

There are very few epidemiologically and preventive-oriented studies on this subject. It is worth mentioning, therefore, the Israel co-operative study (Michaelson and Stein, 1970) on the prevention of retinal detachment, which was begun in 1960 and is still being continued, with the co-operation of heads of eye departments in Israel. Its primary purposes were, first, the assessment of the incidence of retinal detachment in a defined population group during a certain number of years, and the effect on this incidence of a known number of prophylactic measures; second, a study of the natural history of detachment retinopathy. Monthly lists consisting of nominal roles of all cases of preventive treatment and of all cases of idiopathic treatment are centralized for recording from each of the twelve departments. These lists give some general information on the patient, information regarding the situation, shape, and number of the retinal holes, and afford data regarding:

1. The total number of eyes operated on for retinal detachment.

2. The number of second eyes in the total number of eyes operated on for retinal detachment.

3. The number of aphakic myopic eyes in the total number of eyes operated on for retinal detachment.

4. The number of preventively treated eyes.

5. The number of 'second' eyes treated preventively.

6. The number of aphakic myopic eyes treated preventively.

The average incidence of idiopathic retinal detachment between 1962 and 1968 was 8·9 per 100,000 of the population. The percentage of 'second' to 'first' eyes dropped during the years of observation from about 10 to 4·2 per cent. The formula for estimating retinal detachment/retinal hole ratio was discussed and described. It was emphasized that basic to an understanding of the retinal hole/retinal detachment relationship is information regarding the prevalence of retinal holes without detachment in defined eye populations such as myopic, 'second', and aphakic eyes. Such prevalence studies were reported on. A series of tables showing detachment/hole probability ratios were demonstrated, with reference to the shape, position, and size of the holes, and to the general parameter of refraction and of occurrence of retinal detachment in the other eye.

ENVIRONMENTAL EYE-HEALTH HAZARDS

There has so far been no comprehensive study dealing with adverse effects on eye health of the human environment, the latter being defined as 'all physical, chemical, biological, and social processes and influences that, directly or indirectly, have a significant effect on the health and well-being of the human race both individually and as a whole'. Here, we shall briefly mention only some of the physical environmental parameters which have been studied in relation to eye health.

Radiation

In general, radiation, which is harmful to the whole body, is also harmful to the eye, and will similarly induce superficial or deep lesions, depending on its penetration and absorption by the media (Nizetic, 1971b). The common sources of radiation include radio transmitters and diathermy equipment (radio waves, diathermy radiation, and micro-waves), high-temperature furnaces (infra-red rays), the sun (visible rays), welders' electric arc (ultra-violet rays), X-ray tubes operated at 8–25 kV. (grenz rays), X-ray tubes operated at 100–1,000 kV. (ordinary X-rays), radio-active substances, such as radium (gamma rays), and interstellar space (cosmic rays).

Exposure of the whole body to penetrating radiations (X-rays, gamma rays, or neutrons) or the systematic intake of radio-active substances produces so-called radiation sickness. The ocular signs of this condition consist of haemorrhages in the retina. They apparently begin a week or more after the exposure and are local manifestations of the haemorrhagic diathesis. The visual prognosis is the same as for other types of haemorrhagic retinopathy, and depends on the extent and situation of the haemorrhages and the resultant scar formation.

The lesions of the eye ordinarily associated with external radiation (epilation, keratitis, xerosis, and cataract) do not form part of the radiation syndrome, since the dose necessary to cause such lesions, when directly applied to the eye (for example, 500 r. in the case of X-rays), is lethal when applied to the entire body.

Non-ionizing Radiation: Ultra-violet Radiation. Ultra-violet radiation gives rise to keratoconjunctivitis and erythema of the skin. Both occur after a latent period of several hours. The threshold dose is of the order of 2×10^6 ergs/cm.^{2} for the eye (Verhoeff and Bell, 1916), and $4·2 \times 10^4$ ergs/cm.^{2} for the skin (Luckiesh, Holladay, and Taylor, 1936). The sensitivities to various wave-bands, the so-called action spectra, have similar sharp peaks, but in the case of keratitis the peak is at 288 mμ (Cogan and Kinsey, 1946), whereas in the case of erythema it is 294 mμ (Coblenz, Stair, and Hogue, 1932). This difference is no doubt due, in large measure, to the differential scattering effect of the inert layer of keratin overlying the skin. The long-wave limit for both erythema and keratitis is approximately 305 mμ.

The layer of keratin on the skin gives rise to another difference in the reactions of the skin and eye. With chronic exposure, the skin becomes acclimatized through hypertrophy of its keratin layer, while the eye shows no such change in susceptibility with repeated exposure (Cortese, 1930).

Infra-red Radiation. Infra-red radiation has a twofold pathological effect on the eye in doses that do not produce any significant abnormality in the rest of the body. One of these effects is the production of cataract from long exposure to high-temperature furnaces ('glass-blower's' cataract), and the other is the production of focal retinitis ('eclipse blindness') from viewing objects of intense luminosity, such as the sun. The pathogenesis of the former is not well understood, but it seems likely that absorption of heat by the anterior segment of the eye, and particularly by the pigment of the iris, induces metabolic changes that are deleterious to the lens. The lens may be thought to be especially vulnerable, not only because of its proximity to the heavily pigmented layer of the iris, but also because, being avascular, it has no way of dissipating heat readily. The focal retinitis induced by the penetrating infrared and visible rays is a heat burn of the retina attributable to the condensing action of the lens of the eye.

A retinal burn, analogous to 'eclipse blindness', may also result from the explosion of an atomic bomb. One such case was reported as a result of the Hiroshima explosion (Cogan, Martin, Kimura, and Ikui, 1950), and several have subsequently been reported in human beings, monkeys, and rabbits as a result of the Nevada test explosions (Byrnes, Brown, Rose, and Cibis, 1955). This burn may occur at surprisingly great distances (40–50 miles) from the explosion, so long as the pupil is dilated at the time of the flash. The size of the burn varies with the distance. The position of the burn on the retina depends on the direction of gaze at the instant of the explosion. The major portion of the energy reaches the eye and causes the damage before the pupil has had time to contract or before the blink reflex can occur. The relative rarity of retinal burns due to the Hiroshima and Nagasaki explosions, as compared with the test explosions at the Nevada site, is presumably attributable to the fact that the former took place in broad daylight when the pupils were constricted, whereas the latter took place at night when the pupils were dilated.

Micro-wave Radiation. Micro-waves comprise an illdefined portion of the spectrum where radio-waves and infrared radiation overlap. The range of wave-lengths is roughly $10^6 \mu$ to $10^9 \mu$ (1 mm. to 1 m.), and includes those wave-bands used by diathermy equipment and radar installations. Considerable attention has been given to micro-waves, in view of the increased power output of radar equipment. Many instances of known exposure were followed by the development of typical micro-wave lens changes.

Coherent Electromagnetic Radiation. Such radiation is produced by lasers and masers, which are of great interest because of their increasing use for various purposes.

A recent workshop in the United States reaffirmed the belief that the primary hazard from laser radiation is exposure of the eye and that, if radiation levels are kept below those damaging to the eye, no harm will result to other body tissues and organs.

The type of damage inflicted on the human eye by laser beams ranges from a small and insignificant retinal burn in the periphery of the fundus, to severe damage to the macular area, with consequent loss of visual acuity, and finally to massive haemorrhage and extrusion of tissue into the vitreous,

with possible loss of the entire eye. The Q-switched laser, because of its high-power density and short exposure time, represents potentially the greatest hazard. There have been a few bad cases of exposure to Q-switched lasers, but there is no indication at present that such lasers constitute an environmental hazard to large sections of the public. There is the possibility that ranging operations around airports and on military manoeuvres may expose the public inadvertently to Q-switched laser beams. However, this is no more likely at present than exposure of the public to a misfired gun or rocket, or a crashing military aircraft.

While laser beams do not constitute a widespread environmental hazard to the eye at present, there is no assurance that this will not be the case in the future. Lasers may, in the future, be used to beam information over communication channels, whether ground to air, or ship to ship, for airport traffic control, highway surveying alignment, satellite tracking, missile guidance or interception around cities; lasers may also be installed in public places to count traffic, control various contrivances, etc. The number of lasers is increasing rapidly, both in industry and research. They are being constructed by high school students, employed as pointers in lectures and demonstrations, and used to solve illumination problems in art galleries and three-dimensional public displays. It is important that standards and threshold levels for eye damage should be established.

Air Pollution

Partridge, Stebbings, Elsea, and Winkelstein (1966) refer to an outbreak of acute, severe eye irritation in Buffalo, New York, which occurred on 18 September 1963. In a random sample of the residential population of the industrial neighbourhood where the initial complaints arose, the attack rate was 15 per cent. The rate was 48 per cent. for persons exposed out of doors for 10 minutes or more, and only 2 per cent. for those remaining out of doors for less than 10 minutes. A stagnating anticyclone associated with five consecutive nocturnal inversions dominated meteorological conditions in Buffalo for six days before the episode. Twenty-nine equally strong inversions and fifteen instances of five or more consecutive nocturnal inversions had occurred, however, during the previous two years without evidence of illness associated with air pollution. It was hypothesized that on the morning of the episode, a Hewson fumigation brought a concentrated layer of irritating pollutants abruptly to ground level, causing the eye irritation.

PROMOTIVE MEDICINE IN PUBLIC HEALTH OPHTHALMOLOGY

NUTRITION IN OPHTHALMOLOGY

While the nutritional aspects in pathogenesis of ocular diseases and visual disorders are frequent subjects of clinical ophthalmological research, from the public health point of view the most important on a world-wide scale is vitamin A deficiency and consequent xerophthalmia.

This condition is the largest single cause of preventable loss of vision in many developing countries. Severe forms of xerophthalmia are widespread and are important causes of visual impairment in children of pre-school age. The condition is particularly serious in the post-weaning stage in socially and economically deprived areas, and is most frequently associated with protein/energy malnutrition.

The cost of preventive services is only a small fraction of the amount which would be saved by reducing the burden that the visually impaired and the blind inevitably represent to any country's economy.

Signs of vitamin A deficiency are predominantly ocular. They include night blindness, conjunctival xerosis, Bitot's spots, corneal xerosis, and keratomalacia. There is sometimes an investigator-bias in the diagnosis of conjunctival xerosis; Bitot's spots, however, can be used as a reliable indicator of vitamin A deficiency in a great majority of pre-school children.

Several alternative approaches have been considered to provide vitamin A for populations who have serious need for it. These approaches can be grouped into the following categories:

1. *Those intended for specific vulnerable groups within a population.*

These programmes are justified as measures addressed to subgroups of populations at high risk of suffering damage from deficiency of vitamin A. Among these types of programmes is the fortification of special foods and food mixtures designed for specific vulnerable groups, such as weaning foods. Another example of a short-term measure is the administering of massive doses of vitamin A to pre-school children. This method is at present used in India.

2. *Fortification of selected foods with vitamin A.*

A fundamental premise of this approach is that the food to be fortified should be part of the habitual diet of the target population group. In developed countries, the number of possibilities is large because of the large number of components in the daily dietary intake. The limitations of the applicability of these in developing countries are obvious.

3. *Utilization of a universal vehicle.*

This is based on the incorporation of an appropriate amount of vitamin A in a dietary ingredient consumed in relatively constant amounts by all, or practically all the population in all age-groups. This method has been proved effective in many instances with other nutrients. Iodization of salt is perhaps the best example.

HEALTH EDUCATION IN PUBLIC HEALTH OPHTHALMOLOGY

Any successful long-term public health ophthalmological programme has to include carefully studied health educational activities.

This has proved particularly important in several trachoma control programmes carried out in different parts of the world. Work in that field could have no far-reaching effect if the medical and allied health personnel only had knowledge of the communicable eye diseases and the control programmes as such. In this connexion, interest has been shown in some countries in the training of school teachers in eye-health educational matters, and courses on trachomatology have been given both to practising teachers and in teacher training colleges.

In carrying out public health programmes in the field of communicable eye diseases, all types of propaganda could be and have been used, but they must be adapted to local customs: the public must be approached in a language which they can easily understand, and possible local prejudices have to be taken into careful consideration in preparing health educational activities.

ORGANIZATION OF MEDICAL EYE CARE

Medical eye care is offered to the public in:

1. Hospitals (eye departments in general hospitals, autonomous specialized eye hospitals or institutions, eye departments in university and other teaching hospitals).

2. Extended care facilities which are administratively and technically more or less independent of the former institutions.

It is beyond the scope of this chapter to go into details of the different delivery systems when considering extended eye care facilities for specific groups of the population (pre-school and schoolchildren) [see CHAPTER 35], the productive age-group (occupational eye health problems) [see CHAPTER 38]; old age (ophthalmogeriatric problems) [see CHAPTER 39]. It should, however, be mentioned that each of these organizational subsystems has to be closely related to the larger general public health systems of each country. As a consequence, efficient co-ordination with all services involved and careful long-term planning for eye health services clearly become a must. The role of the ophthalmologist in this respect is mentioned earlier in this chapter. It should be pointed out, however, that a substantial amount of research and new knowledge is needed in this field. To meet the requirement of 'comprehensiveness', the systems approach would seem to be the only rational one. White (1971) stated:

> To qualify as a 'system', any arrangement for the provision of personal health services should offer a full range and all levels of patient care for defined populations, have a well-defined organization that is fully accountable, and acceptable records, communications and transportation systems. Requirements for the development of a system include leadership, capital, cash-flow and a clear focus of control and responsibility. Standards would need to be promulgated with respect to organization and staffing, utilization and quality of care. Contractual negotiations between the four parties involved – consumers, physicians, fiscal intermediaries and organizers of services and systems – should encourage diversity, competition, prudent and responsible use of the system and sound quality.

REHABILITATION OF THE VISUALLY IMPAIRED AND THE BLIND

For reasons explained previously in this chapter, there is a certain amount of misunderstanding arising from the term 'blindness'. The difference is not sufficiently stressed between *blindness of man* and *blindness of the organ*, the concepts of which are obviously strongly related, but still different as far as the intervention of society is concerned. When we wish to consider the preventive aspects, we have to turn to activities of primary, secondary, and tertiary prevention of *blindness of the organ* (or more appropriately *unnecessary loss of vision*), and we see that here the greatest burden of direct responsibility lies with the health professionals. *Blindness of man* (where irreversible and in its various degrees) requires more emphasis on social care (educational, economic, and social).

The role of the ophthalmologist, in actively participating with psychologists, educators, economists, and administrators in a team approach to various problems of the blind, is a very important one as far as the assessment of residual visual acuity, or the possibility of recuperation of the latter, etc., are concerned.

EDUCATION AND TRAINING

The comprehensive approach to the delivery of eye-health care to growing populations requires an appropriate quantity and quality of man-power. The necessity of adequate health man-power planning is recognized in most areas of the world (methods to achieve this are described in a recent WHO publication (WHO Regional Office for Europe, 1969)). The relative shortage of highly specialized health personnel, and the necessity of an interdisciplinary approach to the basic problem of prevention of loss of vision, make obvious the need for a structural analysis of the situation and a search for new solutions. One of the proposed solutions is the increasing use of allied health personnel (nurses, ophthalmic assistants, ophthalmic technicians, ophthalmic technologists, orthoptists and pleioptists, as well as the optometrists) working as a team in the delivery of complete eye-health care, under the direction and supervision of the ophthalmologist (Schlossman, 1972).

Many still controversial and, as yet, unsolved problems exist in this field. Before setting out definitively the inter-relationship and responsibilities of different members of such a team, and setting the standards of the educational process for each category, further studies on medical education are mandatory. Methodologically, these studies, to be comparative, should possibly use a universal conceptual model arrived at by systems analysis.

Awareness of the pressing need for man-power studies in ophthalmology is illustrated by the recent appointment of a *Committee on Man-power* by the Canadian Ophthalmological Society, and the organization of the *Joint Commission on Allied Health Personnel in Ophthalmology* (JCAHPO) as the joint effort of six American ophthalmological associations (see *Archives of Ophthalmology*, 1971, Schlossman, 1972).

REFERENCES

Archives of Ophthalmology (1971) Joint Commission on Allied Health Personnel in Ophthalmology, Editorial, *Arch. Ophthal.*, **86**, 611.

Bardon, H. (1953) *Rev. int. Trachome*, **30**, 9.

Bidart, J., and Racollet, R. (1953) *Rev. int. Trachome*, **30**, 36.

Byrnes, V. A., Brown, D. V. L., Rose, H. W., and Cibis, P. A. (1955) *J. Amer. med. Ass.*, **157**, 21.

Churchman, C. W. (1968) *The Systems Approach*, New York.

Coblenz, W. W., Stair, R., and Hogue, J. M. (1932) *J. Res. Nat. Bur. Stand.*, **8**, 541.

Cochrane, A. L. (1967) A medical scientist's view of screening, *Publ. Hlth (Lond.)*, **81**, 207.

Cogan, D. G., and Kinsey, V. E. (1946) *Arch. Ophthal.*, **35**, 670.

Cogan, D. G., Martin, S. F., Kimura, S. J., and Ikui, H. (1950) *Trans. Amer. ophthal. Soc.*, **48**, 62.

Cortese, F. (1930) *Boll. Soc. med-chir. Pavia*, **44**, 555.

Eichhorn, M. M., Carroll, J. M., and Reinecke, R. D., eds. (1969) *Thesaurus for the Visual Sciences*, Vision Information Center, The Francis A. Countway Library of Medicine, Howe Laboratory of Ophthalmology, Boston, Mass.

Ferrand, G., and Parlange, I. A. (1951) *Bull. Soc. Path. exot.*, **44**, 449.

Ferrand, G., and Soyer, R. (1953) *Rev. int. Trachome*, **30**, 18.

Gaud, J. (1949) *Bull. Inst. Hyg. Maroc*, **9**, 139.

Gaud, J., Maurice, A., Faure, P., and Lalu, P. (1950) *Bull. Inst. Hyg. Maroc*, **10**, 55.

Gaud, J., and Decour, H. (1951) *Bull. Inst. Hyg. Maroc*, **11**, 233.

Glasser, J. H. (1971) Health information systems: a crisis or just more of the usual?, *Amer. J. publ. Hlth*, **61**, No. 8, 1524.

Graham, P. A. (1966) *Proc. roy. Soc. Med.*, **59**, 1218.

Hanika, F. de L. (1968) *New Thinking in Management, Journal of Social Ophthalmology*, London.

Kupka, K., Nižetić, B., and Reinhards, J. (1968) *Bull. Wld Hlth Org.*, **39**, 47.

Linner, E. (1969) A longitudinal study of ocular hypertension, *Docum. ophthal.*, **27**, 259.

Luckiesh, M., Holladay, L. L., and Taylor, A. H. (1936) *J. opt. Soc. Amer.*, **20**, 423.

Maxwell-Lyons, F. (1953) *Bull. ophthal. Soc. Egypt*, **46**, 137.

Michaelson, I. C., and Stein, R. (1970) Symposium on Prevention of Retinal Detachment, Israel Ophthalmological Society's meeting, *Amer. J. publ. Hlth*, **69**, No. 5.

Nižetić, B. (1971a) Geographical ophthalmology, semantics and public health action. Paper presented at the 2nd conference of the International Society of Geographical Ophthalmology, Jerusalem.

Nižetić, B. (1971b) *Non-ionizing Radiation and The Eye*, The Hague. (Unpublished WHO working document EURO 4701/11.)

Partridge, R. A., Stebbings, J. H., Elsea, W. R., and Winkelstein, W. (1966) Outbreak of acute eye irritation associated with air pollution, *Publ. Hlth Rep. (Wash.)*, **81**, No. 2, 153.

Pagès, R. (1938) *Epidemiologie du Trachome, Congrès Médical de Tunis*, Vol. I, *Le Trachome*, Tunis, pp. 93–128.

Pagès, R. (1950a) *Maroc med.*, **29**, 106.

Pagès, R. (1950b) *Rev. int. Trachome*, **27**, 91.

Reinhards, J., Weber, A., and Maxwell-Lyons, F. (1959) *Bull. Wld Hlth Org.*, **21**, 665.

Reinhards, J., Weber, A., Nizetic, B., Kupka, K., and Maxwell-Lyons, F. (1968) *Bull. Wld Hlth Org.*, **39**, 497.

Schappert-Kimmijser, J., Colenbrander, A., and Franken, S. (1968) *Coding System for Disorders of the Eye*, Basel.

Schlossman, A. (1972) The role of the Joint Commission on Allied Health Personnel in the USA, in *Proceedings of the Jerusalem Seminar on Prevention of Blindness*, Jerusalem, p. 71

Sorsby, A. (1950) The incidence and causes of blindness, an international survey, *Brit. J. Ophthal.*, Monograph Supplement XIV.

Tarizzo, M. L., Nabli, B., and Labonne, J. (1968) *Bull. Wld Hlth Org.*, **38**, 897.

United States Department of Health, Education, and Welfare (1969) *Thesaurus for the Visual Sciences*, Washington, D.C., p. 31.

Verhoeff, F. H., and Bell, L. (1916) *Proc. Amer. Acad. Arts. Sci.*, **51**, 629.

Viswalingham, A. (1967) Prevention of blindness, *J. Ophthal. soc.*, **38**, 68.

White, K. L. (1971) Personal health services systems, *J. Amer. med. Ass.*, **218**, 1683.

Wilson, R. P. (1945) *Rep. Giza Meml. Ophthal. Lab.* for 1939–1945.

World Health Organization (1953) *Epidemiological and Vital Statistics Report*, **6**, 1.

World Health Organization (1962) Third Report of the Expert Committee on Trachoma, *Wld Hlth Org. techn. Rep. Ser.*, No. 234.

World Health Organization (1966) *Epidemiological and Vital Statistics Report*, **19**, No. 9, 437.

World Health Organization, Regional Office for Europe (1969) *Methods of Estimating Health Manpower*, Report on a Symposium, Copenhagen (Budapest, Oct. 1968, EURO 0289).

World Health Organization (1970) *Methodology for Trachoma Control*, WHO Document VIR/70.3, Geneva.

World Health Organization (1971) Fourteenth Report of the Expert Committee on Health Statistics, *Wld Hlth Org. techn. Rep. Ser.*, No. 472.

World Health Organization, Regional Office for Europe (1971) *Methods for the Early Detection of Potentially Blinding Eye Conditions*. Report on a working group, 1–11 December 1970, Copenhagen.

World Health Organization (1972a) *Press Release* WHA/15, Geneva.

World Health Organization (1972b) *Prevention of Blindness*, Rep. Dir. Gen., WHA 1972, Geneva.

Zammit-Tabona, V. (1969) The WHO programme information retrieval system, *Chron. Wld Hlth Org.*, **23**, No. 7, 295.

Zammit-Tabona, V. (1971) *WHO Programme Information Retrieval System (PIRS)*. Unpublished WHO Document PE/71.2, Geneva.

FURTHER READING

Archives of Ophthalmology (1971) Physicians' assistants, Editorial, *Arch. Ophthal.*, **86**.

Assaad, F. A., and Maxwell-Lyons, F. (1967) Systematic observer variation in trachoma studies, *Bull. Wld Hlth Org.*, **36**, 885.

Bertalanffy, L. von (1972) *General Systems Theory*, New York.

Braunwald, E. (1972) Future shock in academic medicine, *New Engl. J. Med.*, **286**, No. 19.

Buckley, W. (1967) *Sociology and Modern Systems Theory*, Englewood Cliffs, N.Y.

Carlson, C. L., and Athelstan, G. T. (1970) The physician's assistant versions and diversions of a promising concept, *J. Amer. med. Ass.*, **214**, No. 10.

Churchman, C. W. (1968) *The Systems Approach*, New York.

Croft-Long, E. (1971) Medical specialization and world health needs, *J. Amer. med. Ass.*, **217**, No. 12.

De Gennaro, G. (1963) Noziono di oculistica per l'assistenza sanitaria scolastica, *Tip. Osp. Psichiatrico Prov.*, Napoli.

Dowling, M. A. C. (1969) Human resources in tropical health programmes: some aspects of long-term planning and staff training, *Trans. roy. Soc. trop. Med. Hyg.*, **63**, 155.

Emery, F. E., ed. (1970) *Systems Thinking*, London.

Fahs, I. J. (1970) Vision manpower in the United States, *Amer. J. publ. Hlth*, **60**, 1760.

Feinstein, A. (1963) Boolean algebra and clinical taxonomy, I. Analytic synthesis of the general spectrum of a human disease, *New Engl. J. Med.*, **269**, No. 18.

Feinstein, A. (1964a) Scientific methodology in clinical medicine, I. Introduction, principles and concepts, *Ann. intern. Med.*, **61**, 564.

Feinstein, A. (1964b) Scientific methodology in clinical medicine, II. Classification of human disease by clinical behaviour, *Ann. intern. Med.*, **61**, 757.

Feinstein, A. (1964c) Scientific methodology in clinical medicine, III. The evaluation of therapeutic response, *Ann. intern. Med.*, **61**, 944.

Feinstein, A. (1964d) Scientific methodology in clinical medicine, IV. Acquisition of clinical data, *Ann. intern. Med.*, **61**, 1162.

Feinstein, A. (1967) *Clinical Judgement*, New York.

Feinstein, A. (1968a) Clinical epidemiology, I. The populational experiments of nature and of man in human illness, *Ann. intern. Med.*, **69**, No. 4.

Feinstein, A. (1968b) Clinical epidemiology, II. The identification rates of disease, *Ann. intern. Med.*, **69**, No. 5.

Feinstein, A. (1968c) Clinical epidemiology, III. The clinical design of statistics in therapy, *Ann. intern. Med.*, **69**, No. 6.

Fontaine, M. (1969) *Les Cécités de l'enfance*, Paris.

François, J. (1961) *Heredity in Ophthalmology*, St. Louis, Miss.

François, J., ed. (1969) *Occupational and Medicative Hazards in Ophthalmology*, Basel.

Fuerst, H. T., Lichtman, H. S., and James, G. (1965) Hospital epidemiology, *J. Amer. med. Ass.*, **194**, No. 4.

Fuglsang, H., and Anderson, J. (1973) *Lancet*, **ii**, 321.

Gonzalez, C. L. (1965) Mass campaigns and general health services, *Wld Hlth Org. Publ. Hlth. Pap.*, **29**.

Hare, van Court, Jr. (1967) *Systems Analysis: A Diagnostic Approach*, New York.

Keeney, A. H. Moderator (1966) The institute concept in ophthalmology. A symposium, *Surv. Ophthal.*, **11**, No. 1.

Mann, I. (1966) *Culture, Race, Climate and Eye Disease*, Springfield, Ill.

Nižetić, B. (1967) L'Ophtalmologie et la santé publique, *Maroc méd.*, **5071**, 723.

Nižetić, B. (1970) Methodologie scientifique dans l'evaluation des nouveaux traitements, *Voir*, No. 1, Casablanca.

Nižetić, B. (1970) Sur les aspects 'Santé publique' des Problèmes de la Vision et des Maladies oculaires au Maroc, Essai d'une Approche globale devant servir comme base à l'établissement d'un plan d'ensemble dans le domaine de l'ophtalmologie, Unpublished WHO Working Document.

Nižetić, B. (1972) Perspectives in ophthalmology. A public health point of view, *Canad. J. Ophthal.*, **8**, 311.

Nižetić, B. (1973) Public Health Ophthalmology in the European Region, *Public Health in Europe*, **2**, 175.

Perkins, E. S. (1974) Screening for glaucoma, *Health Trends*, **6**, 18.

Prywes, M. (1971) The balance of research, teaching and service in medical education, *Israel J. med. Sci.*, **7**, 1304.

Sartwell, P. E. (1968) Epidemiologic methods in ophthalmology, in *Clinical Methods in Uveitis*, the Fourth Sloan Symposium on Uveitis, p. 3.

Sheldon, A., Baker, F., and McLauglin, C. P., eds. (1970) *Systems and Medical Care*, Boston, Mass.

Singleton, W. T. (1972) Acquisition of evidence about system behaviour, in *Introduction to Ergonomics*, WHO, Geneva, Ch. 12.

Spivey, B. E. (1970) Ophthalmology for medical students' content and comment, *Arch. Ophthal.*, **84**, 368.

Spivey, B. E., and O'Neill (1969) The use of optical scanning as a means of computer in medicine, *J. Amer. med. Ass.*, **208**, No. 4.

Todd, M. C., and Foy, D. F. (1972) Current status of the physicians' assistant and related issues, *J. Amer. med. Ass.*, **220**, No. 13.

White, K. L. (1971) Personal health services systems, Desiderata, *J. Amer. med. Ass.*, **218**, No. 11.

World Health Organization (1973) Prevention of blindness and prevention of xerophthalmia, *Wld Hlth Org. Chron.*, **27**, 21, 28.

World Health Organization (1974) *Field Methods for the Control of Trachoma*, ed. Tarizzo, M. L., Geneva.

World Health Organization (1974) The work of WHO in 1973, *Wld Hlth Org. Off. Rec.* **213**, 12, 13, 32.

30

THE INFLUENCE OF HEREDITY ON HEALTH

J. A. FRASER ROBERTS

With increasing knowledge and with improvement in the conditions of life both mortality and morbidity have been greatly reduced. But the reductions under various headings have not been equal. The progressive conquest of infectious disease and the raising of standards of nutrition have brought about notable falls, but certain diseases and abnormalities do not share in this amelioration, and so assume an ever-growing relative importance as causes of ill health. These include particularly conditions which are genetic or partly genetic, and many about whose causation little or nothing is known. The figures for infant mortality for England and Wales during this century illustrate this very strikingly. They have been analysed by Martin (1949) for the period 1901–47, and data for subsequent years can now be added. Martin groups the causes of death under thirteen headings. Under eleven of these the fall has varied from something substantial to something that can only be called phenomenal. One, namely injury at birth, shows an increase, but this is a subject outside the scope of this chapter. Deaths attributed to congenital malformation have been practically stationary, and there has certainly been no fall. To the nearest whole number the rate has varied in successive quinquennia from 4 to 6 per 1,000 live births, the average figure being a little less than 5. Hence whereas in 1901–5 1 infant death in 32 was attributed to congenital malformation the proportion is now about 1 in 5. The growing relative importance of this cause of infant mortality is shown in TABLE 70.

TABLE 70
Infant Mortality in England and Wales

Period	Rate per 1,000 live births	Proportion attributed to congenital malformation, 1 in:
1901–5	138	32
1906–10	117	24
1911–15	110	29
1916–20	90	22
1921–25	76	18
1926–30	68	14
1931–35	62	11
1936–40	55	9
1941–45	50	8
1946–50	36	8
1951–55	27	6
1956–57	23	5

Figures up to 1941–45 taken from Martin (1949).

Congenital malformations are sometimes, though not very often, wholly genetic. They are much more often partly genetic. But, of course, in many instances their cause is unknown, with little or no indication of genetic determination.

A comparison which comes nearer to an assessment of genetic causation has been made by Carter (1956), who classified causes of death in children coming to post-mortem at The Hospital for Sick Children, Great Ormond Street. The selection of patients is necessarily biased to some extent by various factors, but the changing pattern of mortality emerges very clearly. TABLE 71 shows a comparison of the years 1914 and 1954 respectively.

TABLE 71
Classification of Causes of Death at The Hospital for Sick Children, Great Ormond Street

Year	Percentages			
	Environmental	Unknown	Partly genetic	Wholly genetic
1914	68	15·5	14·5	2
1954	14·5	48	25·5	12

Data from Carter (1956).

In 1914 the environmentally determined group accounted for two-thirds of all deaths, the main conditions being tuberculosis, intestinal infections, and pneumonias. The conditions classified as of unknown causation include certain congenital malformations and the cancers of childhood. The partly genetic group includes such conditions as harelip and cleft palate, infantile pyloric stenosis, and spina bifida.

It is more difficult to make comparisons in terms of morbidity; one particularly notable example, however, is given by Sorsby (1950). A survey of the causes of blindness among school children was made by the Board of Education in 1922 and repeated by him after this not very long interval. During the quarter-century the total rate had been halved, but blindness attributed to congenital and hereditary anomalies (including myopia) showed no reduction. Hence, whereas in 1922 37 per cent. of blindness in the school population was attributed to these causes, by 1950 the figure had risen to 68 per cent. Sorsby emphasizes a finding which is probably true in a number of other fields as well. Over all ages, the relative importance of hereditary and congenital disorders as causes of blindness is much more marked in terms of total years of blindness than it is in terms of case incidence.

It is unnecessary to multiply examples. Over the whole field of medicine it can safely be said that as mortality and morbidity fall the relative importance of hereditary and partly hereditary anomalies (as well as many whose causation is at present unknown) increases in greater or lesser measure, and often in very great measure. To a certain extent advances in therapy produce an absolute as distinct from a relative increase. Caesarean section enables an achondroplastic dwarf woman to bear a living child, and half of these children will be similarly affected. Before the development of adequate treatment nearly all infants with well-marked infantile pyloric stenosis died; now they survive, and a fairly high proportion of their children are also affected. The repair of harelip increases the chances of survival, and, later, of reproduction. Many treatable orthopaedic conditions fall into the same category. These are specific effects, however, and it should be emphasized that there is no justification for generalizing them. There is no evidence, for example, that the decline in infant mortality generally (largely due to the conquest of infection) is preserving weaklings. The infants who previously died of scarlet fever, or tuberculosis, or gastro-enteritis, or bronchopneumonia, would, in all probability, had they survived, have been as fit on the average as anyone else. Susceptibility and resistance (sometimes at least partly genetic) appear to be highly specific. There are no generalized qualities of 'weakness' or of 'strength'.

Apart from the question of reproduction and of some actual increase in incidence, there is also the increased longevity of some of those suffering from congenital and hereditary abnormalities. For example, the proportion of mongols who now live on into adolescence and adult life has materially increased in recent years (Carter, 1958). The extra burden to be borne by the family and the community in this, as in other instances, must be accepted, but it does again emphasize the increasing importance of the contribution of this category of anomalies to morbidity in this community.

GENETIC DISORDERS AND THE PUBLIC HEALTH

Anomalies which are wholly genetic in causation are due to harmful genes which have appeared in the population as the result of mutation. The rates of mutation of these harmful genes are always low. Rates varying from 1 in 10,000 to 1 in 100,000 have been estimated in man, but these must be regarded as outlying values, for only if the rate is relatively high is estimation possible under present conditions. Most mutation rates are undoubtedly much lower. The lowered reproductive fitness of individuals bearing the harmful genes implies a corresponding rate of elimination, applying to all bearers if the gene is dominant, to all affected males with recessive sex linked genes, and to all those possessing the gene in double dose if it is recessive. Hence, in ordinary circumstances simply inherited defects are rare or very rare. But there are very many of them. The importance in numerical terms of a single inherited defect is seldom very great, but in the aggregate their contribution to mortality and morbidity is by no means negligible. Furthermore, there are some exceptions to the general rule that such genes are rare or very rare, and naturally they are important exceptions. Relatively common harmful genes tend to be localized in distribution, and there must always be a reason why they have become common. The usual reason is that the gene in single dose may in certain circumstances confer a positive advantage, which balances the partial, or even total elimination of the homozygotes.

Conditions which are partly genetic may raise rather different problems. If the genetic component is a single gene, then much the same considerations apply, but there are good reasons for supposing, with common diseases and malformations at least, that genetic susceptibilities which in co-operation with other factors result in abnormality are often multifactorial.

This implies a continuous distribution of the underlying genetic susceptibility, although, of course, whether the disease develops or not is an all-or-none phenomenon.

The most immediate and practical problem which arises in connexion with wholly or partly genetically determined disease is the provision of advice on genetic prognosis for those who need it. The proportion of the population who really need genetic advice in regard to marriage and children is relatively small, but those who do need it need it badly, and the provision of facilities for obtaining genetic advice should be a part of any health service. Sometimes the question arises before marriage; one or other partner may suffer from a condition which may be transmitted to children, or there may be something in the family history which, it is feared, may imply an extra risk to offspring. Much more often, however, advice can only be sought after the event, for it is only the birth of an affected child that reveals the potential risk. Then the question is whether or not there is a chance of recurrence in a subsequent child. Knowledge that there is a serious risk of abnormality in children undoubtedly deters some couples from having children, and would deter more if the knowledge were available to them. Naturally, the choice is that of the individual couple, but there is some automatic contribution to the health of the community; some harmful genes are thereby reduced in frequency; others are prevented from coming together in harmful combination. Important though this negative aspect may be, and it is important when the risks are high, it is likely that another consideration is of equal or even greater importance. The welfare of the unborn child is the subject of a rich store of ancient and widespread beliefs. Old wives' tales seldom err on the side of foolish optimism, and so very often indeed couples think that the risk is far greater than it really is, and refrain from parenthood quite unnecessarily. It is probable that the harm done through unnecessary avoidance of parenthood is greater than the harm done by the birth of affected children, when, had the parents known that the risk was high, they would have refrained.

The provision of genetic advice for those who need it involves more, however, than the calculation of chances for offspring or further offspring. Deep emotions are involved; the decision may well be for life. Often there are overt or unconscious feelings of guilt. There may be a sense of loneliness, of being unlike other people. Wise advice from the family doctor and at the health clinic, in addition to specialist genetic advice when necessary on the chances involved, can help to reconcile patients to their misfortune or deprivation. A very important point is reassurance, when this can properly be given, about the chances in regard to marriage and offspring of normal children and other normal relatives.

It is very necessary that the medical adviser should appreciate fully the considerable risks involved in any random pregnancy, the risk that any child will suffer from some serious congenital or hereditary abnormality or other, or that some serious developmental defect will manifest itself during early life. A figure of 1 in 30 is probably not too high. Once the disaster has happened, or if there is something in the family history which points to extra risk, the patient also needs to know the general risk. Such hazards are part of life, and if prospective parents were to be deterred by relatively small risks no one would have a child. Naturally, much depends on the nature of the condition, its severity, whether it is remediable, whether it results in early death or in long years of invalidism. But even with severe conditions a special extra risk does not look very serious to most of those who have been informed of the facts unless it exceeds, say, 1 in 20. Another point is that discussion along these lines helps patients to realize that they are not different from other people. All prospective parents are inevitably running risks, though only a proportion are unlucky.

The second way in which genetic knowledge is relevant to preventive medicine is in regard to diagnosis, and especially early diagnosis. It is, of course, quite wrong to suppose that because a defect is genetic, or partly genetic, it is untreatable; one has only to think of all the orthopaedic conditions amenable to treatment, or harelip, or infantile pyloric stenosis, and many more. And sometimes early diagnosis is very important and may be life-saving. Galactosaemia is a metabolic anomaly due to a recessive gene. The body cannot utilize lactose. Diagnosis is not easy, and early death is a common sequel. Moreover, even should the child survive, irreparable cerebral damage will often have taken place, resulting in mental deficiency. Early diagnosis and the use of milk substitutes can secure normal development. As the condition is recessive, the chance of making an early diagnosis is often confined to a second or later child. But at least the subsequent children of parents who have had an affected child can be watched from birth. Nephrogenic diabetes insipidus provides another example. Early diagnosis is again difficult, early death is common, and again, should the child survive, the profound dehydration often results in cerebral damage and mental deficiency. Prompt recognition and appropriate treatment, with ample fluids, should lead to relatively normal development. This condition is due to a sex linked gene, and in this instance not only is a family history of the condition of value in making an early diagnosis but there is also the immense added advantage that the female carriers of the gene can always, or nearly always, be identified by their failure to produce a normally concentrated urine (Carter and Simpkiss, 1957). Once these women are identified, it is known that the chance that any son will be affected is 1 in 2.

Phenylketonuria is due to a recessive gene. The body is unable to utilize phenylalanine. Toxic products accumulate, and almost always result in cerebral damage so severe as to cause profound mental deficiency. It is now known that feeding on a diet low in phenylalanine may avert much of the cerebral damage, and may sometimes, indeed, ensure relatively normal development. But the treatment, to be effective, must be started very early in life. In the ordinary way a sufficiently early diagnosis is most likely to be made with a second affected child. The incidence of the condition in different parts of the British Isles is believed to vary from about 1 in 10,000 to 1 in 40,000, but the chemical test is so simple that there is a good case for carrying it out on all children soon after birth. This has now become an established practice in a number of countries.

Other examples could be given. Thus, it is often useful to know that a child runs a special risk of congenital dislocation of the hip, or of infantile pyloric stenosis. These conditions are no more than partially hereditary, but there is an appreciable risk for the later sibs or for children of affected persons. It is true, as mentioned earlier, that such conditions tend to be individually rare, but the number in which effective treatment will be developed, especially if a diagnosis is made early, will continue to grow. Provision of the necessary evidence and perhaps ultimately of systematic registration should ensure that it is made as early as possible.

A third way in which genetic knowledge is relevant to preventive medicine is a consequence of the fact that some of those suffering from genetic disorders are exposed to particular hazards. The most notable example is haemolytic disease of the foetus and newborn. Here, of course, it is the genetic constitution of the parents in relation to each other that is important. The institution of early and largely successful treatment has been established for a long time. A very important and striking advance is more recent (Clarke, 1968). There is every hope that sensitization can be prevented in a vast majority of women at risk.

Another example is provided by hereditary porphyria. A particular variety, porphyria variegata, is common in the white and coloured populations of South Africa. It is estimated there are about 8,000 affected persons in that country. The condition is due to a dominant gene, and remarkably enough it seems certain that all these persons have inherited it from a single couple, who married in 1688. Under natural conditions the harm done is not usually very great; some bearers of the gene remain symptomless throughout life, but its presence can always, or almost always, be detected, at least in adults, by a very simple test. It was the introduction of the barbiturates, and above all of barbiturate anaesthetics, that produced a transformation, for barbiturates are liable to produce severe and often fatal reactions. Very large numbers of those at risk have been identified and given cards warning doctors that the dangerous drugs must on no account be given. Furthermore, it is now routine at some South African hospitals to test the faeces for the presence of porphyrin before giving a general anaesthetic (Dean and Barnes, 1955; Dean, 1963).

A similar example is provided by suxamethonium sensitivity (Lehmann, 1956). In about one person in 2,000 in our population the enzyme pseudocholinesterase is absent or defective. Under normal conditions no apparent harm seems to result, but if suxamethonium is given as a muscle relaxant during anaesthesia a dangerous apnoea is liable to occur. The genetics are rather complicated, as it would appear that several different genes, which may well be alleles, are involved. In general, however, the deficiency behaves as a recessive condition.

It is interesting to note that the examples given refer to risks which arise from modern therapeutic advances; in earlier times the genes were at least tolerably harmless. It may well be that the number of such risks will be multiplied in the future.

It is possible that in the future the usefulness of a knowledge of special genetic risks may be greatly extended. This applies particularly to common diseases in whose causation genetic influences play some part. It may be that the knowledge that certain individuals are on the average somewhat more prone than others to develop particular conditions may be of use in the selective application of preventive measures to those who for genetic reasons are especially likely to need them. At present, however, this can only be said with some reservation, the main reason being that the extra measurable genetic risk is usually rather small. Nevertheless, this may be too conservative a view, even in the present state of knowledge. Time and experiment will tell.

Another genetic topic relevant to preventive medicine is the marriage of blood relatives. From the point of view of the community the problem is rather small in our own population, and is continually diminishing, but this is not necessarily so in others. A later section is devoted to this subject.

Agencies which increase the rate of mutation are of great potential importance to the future of the race, and, of course, the question of outstanding interest at present is the hazard of increasing exposure to ionizing radiation. Some reference is made later to this subject also.

Finally, at the risk of being platitudinous, it is highly desirable, to say the least of it, that the genetic element in the aetiology of a very wide variety of diseases should be assessed and understood. Epidemiology (in the wide sense) which ignores genetic differences in susceptibility is at best incomplete, and on occasion might even prove seriously misleading.

THE DOMINANT GENE

Turning to a rather more specific consideration of inherited defects, it is clear that this can be only a rather brief outline. Genetic and partly genetic anomalies are many. Within the space of a single chapter no more can be attempted than some consideration of general principles, illustrated by all too few examples. Moreover, no attempt is made to recapitulate the principles of genetics, or of that part which is human genetics. Knowledge is assumed at the level of the elementary textbooks mentioned at the end of this chapter.

Dominant genes are, strictly speaking, those which produce the same effect whether they are present in single or in double dose. For practical purposes, however, it is convenient to consider under the same head genes which are truly dominant and those which produce a definite effect in the heterozygote, but are sufficiently rare for the marriage of heterozygotes to be ignored. Such genes may or may not be truly dominant; we usually do not know; but the only persons of numerical importance, often the only persons who have been observed, are those with one abnormal gene.

Abnormal dominant genes are very numerous, and, if they are to be transmitted fairly freely from one generation to another, cannot have too serious an effect on reproductive fitness. There seems to be no reason why those with lobster claw or polydactyly should not transmit the defect to their children if they want to; the sufferers are usually just as useful citizens as anyone else, and, indeed, may sometimes compensate specifically for their defect. Hence many dominant genes do not raise problems of any particular importance in regard to the public health. Their possessors not infrequently know the rules of transmission perfectly well. But there are circumstances in which dominant genes do raise problems of importance. This may happen when manifestation is delayed, so that those affected have already had a family before the defect appears. The classical example is Huntington's chorea, with a mean age of onset of about 35 years. In contemplating marriage, not only has the child of an affected person one chance in two of carrying the gene, and so of passing it on to his or her own children, but he or she also has that same chance of developing a long relentlessly progressive disease with increasing dementia. A careful survey by Pleydell (1954) shows that complete ascertainment of affected persons, or rather of the families containing affected persons, would be a very desirable objective. Even

at the present time the condition is not always diagnosed. Furthermore, members of the affected families often do not know about the risks they run. Some said that had they done so, they would never have married.

A second point about dominant genes is that many of them show wide variations in severity of manifestation. Thus, in osteogenesis imperfecta of the so-called mild variety, which is compatible with survival and reproduction, the abnormality ranges from nothing more than blue sclerotics at one extreme to severe crippling and deformity at the other. With conditions like this ascertainment might well be desirable, as well as ensuring that the very mildly affected possessors of the gene know the considerable risks that a child might be severely crippled. In passing, it may be mentioned that it is this variability of expression which is nearly always the explanation of the phenomenon of anticipation, the supposed tendency for severity to increase in later generations. Pedigrees are traced backwards, and so those of early generations who appear in them are those who tended to be more mildly affected and so left descendants.

A further point relates to mutation. With some conditions whose effect on survival or reproduction is serious a relatively high proportion of all instances encountered is due to a recent mutation. Given adequate surveys appropriate advice can be given regarding risks to subsequent children. Thus, with achondroplasia, nearly always due to a dominant gene, sporadic cases, directly due to a mutation, are considerably more numerous than those in which there has been transmission from a parent. If, therefore, a normal couple have an achondroplastic child, they can be assured that the risk to any further child is extremely small. But, of course, when that child grows up and marries, the risk is 1 in 2 that any child of his or hers will be affected.

THE INTERMEDIATE GENE

For practical purposes this category may conveniently be confined to genes which not only produce a greater effect in the homozygote than they do in the heterozygote, but which in addition are sufficiently common to appear with appreciable frequency in the duplex as well as the simplex state. Few such genes are known in man, but of course they are extremely important genes. The outstanding examples are sickling and sickle cell anaemia (as well as some of the other abnormal haemoglobins) and thalassaemia minor and thalassaemia major (Cooley's anaemia). These two genes have become extremely common in some parts of the world. The sickling gene occurs notably all over Africa north of the Zambezi, and the thalassaemia gene notably in Italy and some other parts of the Mediterranean basin. Those with Cooley's anaemia probably never reproduce, and few of those with sickle cell anaemia. Yet the frequency of those with the sickle cell trait is as high (or higher) than 40 per cent. in some parts of Africa, corresponding to an incidence of sickle cell anaemia of nearly 10 per cent. In certain townships in the district of Ferrara about 20 per cent. of the population carry the gene for thalassaemia minor, which, given random mating, corresponds to an incidence of Cooley's anaemia of 1 per cent. It seems certain that with the sickling gene the reason, in part if not wholly, for its extremely high frequency is that the heterozygotes are more resistant than others to malignant tertian malaria. Hence the increased effective fertility of the heterozygotes compensates for the almost total loss of the genes which have come together in pairs in the homozygotes. The corresponding advantage in thalassaemia is not known with certainty, but may well have been resistance to malaria.

Thalassaemia provides the best example up to the present of a scheme for the reduction of a lethal abnormality by enabling those who carry the gene to avoid marrying each other. In parts of Italy where the gene is common, facilities are available for testing the population, so that carriers of the gene, who can always, or nearly always, be recognized, can be registered. Those contemplating marriage can thus find out whether they may both chance to be carriers. It is possible that this scheme will lead to a big reduction in the incidence of Cooley's anaemia. Incidentally, there is little reason to fear that the harm is only being postponed and that the number of carriers will increase. It seems likely that heterozygote advantage has ceased, and that the definite disadvantages attaching to a proportion of those with thalassaemia minor will now gradually reduce the incidence of the gene. It may be that it will not be long before similar measures will be used in Africa to reduce the incidence of sickle cell anaemia.

SEX LINKED GENES

Many sex linked genes are known in man. For numerical reasons (the relatively harmless condition of colour blindness can be ignored), two of these genes are of special importance. They are the gene for haemophilia (or rather the genes for haemophilia and related conditions, all sex linked) and for muscular dystrophy of the classical Duchenne type. The real problem, and the difficult problem, with sex linked genes is the sister of the affected boy. Apart from the chance of mutation, she has one chance in two of being a carrier, with an overall chance of one in four that any son will be affected, or any daughter a carrier. These are high risks, and many people who are aware of them would hesitate before thinking of marriage and children. Once again, as with dominant genes, there is a case for ascertainment and registration so that those who are subject to these chances can be given the facts should they wish.

The frequency of mutation is important with sex linked genes. The rate of elimination is high, through all the affected boys in muscular dystrophy, and through a considerable proportion with haemophilia. Hence about one-third of all haemophiliacs are the first to be affected in their family group, and with muscular dystrophy rather more. The mutation may have occurred in the mother herself; if so, the likelihood of a daughter being a carrier is no greater than for any other woman. Or it may have occurred in the mother's father, or in the mother's mother. So, at the simplest, the likelihood that the sister of the first boy to be affected in the family group is a carrier is $1/2 \times 2/3 = 1/3$. It has been suggested that in haemophilia the mutation rate is much higher in men than in women. If so the chance is little better than $1/2$, but this conclusion cannot be regarded as proved.

Fortunately, with recessive sex-linked genes it is being increasingly found that the carrier state can be detected by suitable observations and tests. With nephrogenic diabetes insipidus, as already mentioned, the carrier women can nearly always, or perhaps always, be detected by their failure to produce a normally concentrated urine. Quite recently it has been found that with muscular dystrophy of the Duchenne type the carrier women can be distinguished with high probability by a raised level of creatine phosphokinase (Wilson, Evans, and Carter, 1965). This also applies to the much rarer and milder sex linked form of the disease. In sex-linked retinitis pigmentosa (which is relatively uncommon compared to the usual recessive variety), and in choroideraemia, the carrier women can be identified by minor and symptomless abnormalities. It is greatly to be hoped that in the future a similar advance will be made with haemophilia.

THE RECESSIVE GENE

Defects due to recessive genes are very numerous, though, as usual, most of them are individually rare. The commonest in our population is that causing fibrocystic disease of the pancreas, which has a frequency of the order of 1 in 2,000 births. Deaf mutism, when hereditary, is nearly always due to recessive genes, and there is good evidence that any one of a number of such genes may (when in double dose) be responsible. Recessive retinitis pigmentosa, much the commonest genetic variety of this disease, has a frequency of perhaps 1 in 4,000. Many recessive conditions are lethal or semi-lethal.

In the very great majority of instances the family history, as far as it can be traced, is negative, and the first indication that a couple happen to carry the same harmful gene is the birth of an affected child. Genetic advice thus relates to subsequent children, and all that can be said is that the chance that any subsequent child will be affected is 1 in 4. Where it is important to be clear is the chances for affected persons themselves, should the condition be compatible with survival and reproduction, as in albinism or retinitis pigmentosa; for the certain carrier, namely, the child of an affected person; for the possible carrier, for example, the normal sib of an affected person. The likelihood of these individuals happening to marry a carrier is small, so the chance of an affected person married to a normal having an affected child is remote, much smaller in fact than the chance of some serious defect or other appearing in any random pregnancy. Marriage to a blood relative may, however, increase the risk considerably. It cannot be stressed too strongly, therefore, that there is no genetic reason why a person suffering from a recessive abnormality should not marry and have children. Nor is there any genetic or nongenetic reason why the sib or any other relative of an affected person should not do so. Parents are always glad to know that their normal children have nothing to worry about in regard to their own children. The lucky parents are those who have had one or more normal children before the birth of the affected child. The unlucky ones are those whose first, or perhaps first and second, children are affected, and who dare not face the 1 in 4 risk which they now know to be present.

There need be no hesitation about encouraging possible carriers, or even affected persons, to marry should they wish to do so. It is true that harmful recessive genes will thus be passed on to children, but everyone is doing this. It is certain that practically everyone must carry at least one such gene; in fact, estimates of the mean numbers per individual (or their equivalent) range from three to eight.

What would be of practical use, if it could be achieved, is preventing the same harmful genes coming together in pairs. As was mentioned above, this is just what is being attempted with Cooley's anaemia in Italy. There is hope that in the future this may be done with some genes now regarded as recessive, for it is found that carriers can sometimes be recognized by suitable tests. With phenylketonuria a phenylalanine tolerance test distinguishes about 90 per cent. of the carriers. This procedure could be applied, even at present, to the normal relatives of affected persons and their proposed marriage partners; but to be really effective the whole population would have to be screened, which is out of the question. If a test could be developed for recognizing the carriers of fibrocystic disease, and if this condition turns out to be always due to the same gene, then complete screening might be worth while, for no less than one person in about twenty must be a carrier. It is true that preventing harmful recessive genes from coming together in pairs would mean a slow increase in gene frequency, but this is a problem for a future so remote that scientific knowledge might be completely revolutionized in the meantime.

The occurrence of recessive defects and the fact that we all carry harmful recessive genes of some kind or other emphasizes the assurance to parents of affected children that they are in no way different from anyone else. They have just been unlucky. Moreover, human families in our community being small, many couples have exclusively normal children in spite of happening to carry the same harmful gene. The chance of all offspring being normal is $(3/4)^n$, where n is the number in the sibship. Thus it is 3/4 for single-child families, 9/16 for two-child families, 27/64 for three-child families, and so on. For every couple who have one or more affected children there is at least one other who might have had, but have been lucky in that the 1 in 4 chance did not come off.

THE MARRIAGE OF BLOOD RELATIVES

Given random mating, the likelihood of identical genes coming together in the child is determined by the frequencies of those genes in the population. The chance is increased when blood relatives marry each other, for a proportion of their genes are necessarily identical, having been received from the same source. The proportion necessarily the same is, for example, 1/8 for first cousins, 1/32 for second cousins, 1/128 for third cousins. The remainder of the genes may be the same or different, with probabilities which are the same as in the marriage of unrelated persons. Clearly, the risk of rare recessive defects appearing is increased in consanguineous marriages, but what is important to the individual couple is not the increase in the relative risk, even should this be considerable, but the amount of the absolute risk. Looked at rather theoretically —almost the only way until fairly recently—the amount of the increased risk has not seemed very large, or of a size that would be a serious deterrent to sensible persons informed of the facts. But, of course, small risks to any given individual may represent serious risks to the community as a whole, and from every point of view the direct test of observing the results of consanguineous marriages is a most desirable goal, though one difficult to achieve.

In recent years some very informative studies have been carried out, including those of Sutter and Tabah (1952), Böök (1957), Schull (1958), and Slatis, Reis, and Hoene (1958). The results show a very considerable measure of general agreement. There is little difference between the outcome of consanguineous and control marriages up to and including birth. That is, the interval to first conception is not longer; there are very few more miscarriages and there is no excess of stillbirths, provided those due to recognizable genetic deformities are excluded. Thus the effect of increased homozygosity does not seem to operate by causing early wastage. From birth onwards, however, the findings are different. Thus Schull (1958), working on Japanese populations, found a death rate at Hiroshima of 116 per 1,000 during the first 8 years of life among the offspring of first cousins, against 56 for second cousins and 55 among the controls. The proportion of major congenital abnormalities was rather less than doubled. Slatis et al. (1958) studied a sample at Chicago. With a lower total death rate the difference in this respect was naturally greater. Of 209 live born children of consanguineous marriages 4 died in the first week and 13 more before the age of 10 years. Of the 167 control children only 1 died in the first week, and only 3 more up to the age of 10. An analysis of quantitative measurements (Morton, 1958) shows very small differences.

A very striking fact is that only a few of the deaths were due to recognized recessive conditions, and the same is true of the congenital malformations not necessarily resulting in death. Multiple congenital defects figure prominently, and these have not hitherto shown any particular indication of being genetic. There are no obvious explanations at present. It may be that a rather small proportion of genetically determined cases have been lost among the remainder. Or it may be that recessive genes with a low frequency of expression are concerned. Or, perhaps, it may be that the effect is more general, that the tendency to homozygosity at a number of loci is unfavourable. Further results must be awaited. It is clear, however, that the extra risks of consanguineous marriage, even if not very great for the individual couple, are quite considerable taken in total from the point of view of the community. It should also be added that small effective breeding populations can give the same result. The problem is not an urgent one in communities like our own, in which the rate of consanguineous marriage is very low, has fallen greatly during the past century, and is continuing to fall. The problem is solving itself. It is doubtful if the first cousin marriage rate in this country now exceeds 3 or 4 per 1,000, and it is lower still in the United States. More distant relationships need cause little concern; genes in common fall off rapidly as relationship becomes more remote. In some other countries, however, in which consanguineous marriages are still relatively frequent, it is clearly of advantage to the health of the community that they should diminish; an outbreeding human population is a healthier population, and this not only because of a falling off in definite known recessively determined defects. It should be mentioned, however, that in communities which have practised close inbreeding for long periods of time there may have been a measure of adaptation which lowers the chances of harmful results.

MULTIFACTORIAL INHERITANCE

Many inherited or partly inherited differences between individuals are due not to single genes, but to the combined action of many genes, each of small effect individually, and additive in their action. The picture we see of variation is then continuous. This is the basis for variations, within normal limits, of stature, for example, in which it is known that the hereditary component is very large, at least in communities in which severe malnutrition is rare. It seems very likely that the bulk of inherited variation in resistance or susceptibility to common diseases has a similar basis. Sometimes it can be seen that disease and normality overlap. This is shown, for example, by the shading of normal intelligence into dullness and then into frank high-grade mental deficiency. It is held by some to be true of level of arterial pressure and benign essential hypertension. More commonly, however, the disease is of an all-or-none character, but the underlying genetic predisposition may still be continuously distributed and due to multifactorial inheritance.

During recent years convincing evidence has been accumulating that the genetic element in the causation of the commoner (and hence the numerically important) congenital malformations is multifactorial. This is not surprising in fact, for it is almost inconceivable that a single gene not always expressed could be responsible when the frequency of the condition exceeds, say, one in 1,000 births. The evidence includes studies on the frequency of the conditions in relatives of various degrees. Sometimes there is a relation between severity and the proportion of affected relatives. It has also been shown that the proportion of affected relatives should fall off more rapidly than the measure of genetic resemblance would imply as we pass from first- to second- and then to third-degree relatives. This has turned out to be so. Finally, when there is a big difference in sex incidence this leads to sex differences in frequencies among relatives which cannot fit a single-gene hypothesis, but fits a multifactorial hypothesis very satisfactorily. This has been demonstrated conclusively for infantile pyloric stenosis by Carter in a number of papers.

MAJOR CHROMOSOME ABNORMALITIES

It is only since 1956 that satisfactory techniques have been available for the examination of human chromosomes. It was then discovered that the diploid number in man is 46, or 23 pairs, and not 48 as had been thought for many years. The next step came early in 1959 with the recognition of abnormalities of human chromosome constitution, and since then new discoveries have been made at an ever-increasing pace.

One important class of chromosome abnormalities involves duplication or loss of the sex chromosomes. About one male in 500 is of constitution XXY. Such individuals suffer from Klinefelter's syndrome. Outwardly they are nearly normal males, but have small testes, with azoospermia, and often gynaecomastia. Often the condition is not apparent before puberty and patients not infrequently come to light because of infertility or gynaecomastia. As is usual with many chromosome anomalies mental deficiency is commoner among them than it is in the general population. Less frequently there may be still more extra X chromosomes, giving the constitutions XXXY and XXXXY. A sex chromosome may be lost, giving an individual with a single unpaired X, of constitution XO. Such persons are outwardly female, but display Turner's syndrome. They are essentially agonadic, with immature external genitalia, and there is a variety of associated anomalies, not, however, always present, including dwarfing, webbed neck, cubitus valgus, and deafness. About one girl in 2,500 suffers from Turner's syndrome. About one woman in 800 or so has three X chromosomes, and in addition to this XXX constitu-

tion, XXXX occasionally occurs, and even XXXXX. Such women are usually outwardly normal, though once again, mental deficiency is unduly common among them. More unusual sex chromosome constitutions include XXYY. It has recently been found that males who have an extra Y chromosome are especially prone to aggressive and anti-social behaviour, often combined with mental backwardness. They appear unduly frequently among inmates of maximum security institutions provided for such subjects.

The hitherto baffling problem of the causation of mongolism (Down's syndrome) was solved in 1959 with the discovery that one of the smallest chromosomes, number 21, is present in triplicate instead of in duplicate. Two other trisomies, which lead to severe malformation and usually to early death, are now well recognized. They are Edwards' syndrome, due to the presence of an extra chromosome of the 16–18 group, and Patau's syndrome, a trisomy in the 13–15 group.

In addition to abnormalities of chromosome number other abnormalities have been reported in increasing numbers. Thus, by the process of translocation, chromosomes of different pairs may exchange segments. This may result in individuals with a normal total number of 46, but having in effect part, or sometimes effectively the whole, of one particular chromosome present in triplicate. A small proportion of Down's syndrome falls into this category, what is practically the whole of an extra 21 being stuck on the end of a 14, a 22, or another 21. The phenomenon is of importance because outwardly normal 'translocation carriers', with 45 chromosomes which in effect represent the genetic material of the normal complement of 46, may transmit abnormality to a fairly high proportion of offspring. Other anomalies of individual chromosomes have been described, including the loss of part of a chromosome and also of chromosomes with one arm represented in duplicate and the other arm missing.

A phenomenon of much importance is mosaicism. Here there are two or more different cell lines. For example, some patients with Klinefelter's syndrome have cells some of which are XXY and some of the normal constitution XY. A number of examples of mosaicism have been described in Down's syndrome.

Finally, it should be mentioned that chromosome abnormalities are far commoner in spontaneously aborted foetuses than in those born alive. It is undoubtedly a mechanism of importance in the determination of foetal loss.

THE GENETIC EFFECTS OF RADIATION

The rate of mutation is increased by radiation, which directly or indirectly produces ionization. If these mutations occur in the cells of the germinal tract the mutant genes are transmitted to future generations. The term mutation may properly be applied to major changes in chromosome structure as well as to point mutations affecting single genes. It will be realized that even in convenient experimental material observation is essentially confined to amounts of radiation which are sufficiently high, on the one hand, to yield measurable counts, and not so high, on the other, as to cause severe disorganization and a high proportion of deaths. Although observations at very low dosages are difficult if not impossible, the nature of the processes involved seems to make it certain that there is no threshold. Any dosage, however small, will induce a corresponding small amount of mutation. Formerly it was supposed that within the ranges most easily studied, the amount of induced mutation seems to be more or less directly proportional to dosage as measured in roentgens. This conclusion now requires modification. With increased dosage the amount of mutation is disproportionately increased. The practical conclusion is important; fairly high dosage applied to relatively few individuals is more harmful than the same total dosage spread over larger numbers; similarly, intensive exposure is more harmful than the same dosage spread over a longer interval.

In this field, as in many others, it is hazardous to assume that what is true of one species is necessarily true for another. For this reason, as well as others, estimates of possible genetic damage have a very wide margin of uncertainty. A useful conception is the doubling dose, namely, the amount of radiation which would double the existing rate of mutation. The usual assumption is a period of exposure of 30 years from birth. Observations on the offspring of those exposed to the atomic bomb in Japan point to a minimum of 10 roentgens. But this is a minimum. The reports of the Medical Research Council

(1956) suggest 30–80 r. and the United Nations Scientific Committee on the Effects of Atomic Radiation (1958) 10–100 r.

It seems clear that at present the peacetime exposure to induced radiation of all kinds is only a very small fraction of these amounts. Much the largest contribution in our community is due to diagnostic radiology. Now that the long-term hazards are better understood, genetic damage due to this cause should be much reduced by avoiding unnecessary X-ray examinations, by improved shielding of the gonads, and by improved instruments with smaller energy requirements.

One practical point may be mentioned. With growing public awareness, parents not infrequently ask whether abnormality in a child might not be due to exposure to radiation. They can be reassured. The likelihood that radiation could be directly responsible in any individual instance is minute.

Much more investigation is needed; in the present state of knowledge many qualifications have to be made; and evidence must be presented at some length if a balanced view is to be given. It is impossible to do this within the limits of a chapter, and the reader is referred to the sources quoted below.

REFERENCES

Böök, J. A. (1957) Genetical investigations in a North Swedish population. The offspring of first-cousin marriages, *Ann. hum. Genet.*, **21**, 191.

Carter, C. O. (1956) Changing patterns in the causes of death at The Hospital for Sick Children, *Gt Ormond Str. J.*, **11**, 65.

Carter, C. O. (1958) A life-table for mongols with the causes of death, *J. ment. def. Res.*, **2**, 64.

Carter, C. O., and Simpkiss, M. J. (1957) The carrier state in sex-linked nephrogenic diabetes insipidus, *Acta genet. (Basel)*, **7**, (1), 111.

Clarke, C. A. (1968) Prevention of Rhesus iso-immunisation, *Lancet*, **ii**, 1.

Dean, G. (1963) *The Porphyrias*, London.

Dean, G., and Barnes, H. D. (1955) The inheritance of porphyria, *Brit. med. J.*, **ii**, 89.

Lehmann, H. (1956) The familial incidence of low pseudo-cholinesterase level, *Lancet*, **ii**, 124.

Martin, W. J. (1949) Infant mortality, *Brit. med. J.*, **i**, 438.

Medical Research Council (1956) The hazards to man of nuclear and allied radiation, London, H.M.S.O.

Morton, N. E. (1958) Empirical risks in consanguineous marriages. Birth weight, gestation time, and measurements of infants, *Amer. J. hum. Genet.*, **10**, 344.

Pleydell, M. J. (1954) Huntington's chorea in Northamptonshire, *Brit. med. J.*, **ii**, 1121.

Schull, W. J. (1958) Empirical risks in consanguineous marriages: sex ratio, malformation, and viability, *Amer. J. hum. Genet.*, **10**, 294.

Slatis, H. M., Reis, R. H., and Hoene, R. E. (1958) Consanguineous marriages in the Chicago region, *Amer. J. hum. Genet.*, **10**, 446.

Sorsby, A. (1950) The causes of blindness in England and Wales, *M.R.C. Memo.* No. 24, London, H.M.S.O.

Sutter, J., and Tabah, L. (1952) Effets de la consanguinité et de l'endogamie. Une enquête en Moribihan et Loir-et-Cher, *Population*, **7**, 249.

United Nations Scientific Committee on the Effects of Atomic Radiation (1958) Report, p. 31, New York.

Wilson, K. M., Evans, K. A., and Carter, C. O. (1965) *Brit. med. J.*, **i**, 750.

FURTHER READING

Roberts, J. A. F. (1973) *An Introduction to Medical Genetics*, 6th ed., London.
An elementary textbook intended for medical students and those studying for postgraduate diplomas.

Neel, J. V., and Schull, W. J. (1954) *Human Heredity*, Chicago.
A more advanced book, useful for research workers. Contains some heavy mathematics.

Stern, C. (1973) *Principles of Human Genetics*, 3rd ed., San Francisco.
An excellent and more extended account, human rather than medical, and with more general background.

Carter, C. O. (1962) *Human Heredity*, London.
A very useful short text.

Sorsby, A. (1960) *Clinical Genetics*, 2nd ed., London.
A useful single volume for looking up individual conditions. Contains some excellent general chapters.

Clarke, C. A. (1964) *Genetics for the Clinician*, 2nd ed., Oxford.
Essentially a stimulating series of essays.

McKusick, V. A. (1968) *Mendelian Inheritance in Man*. Catalogs of autosomal dominant, autosomal recessive and X-linked phenotypes, 2nd ed., Baltimore.
An invaluable book of reference for single gene disorders; a *tour de force*.

Blyth, H., and Carter, C. O. (1969) *A Guide to Genetic Prognosis in Paediatrics*, London.
A very useful practical guide in assessing genetic prognosis.

The following books are also useful for reference:

Brock, D. J. H., and Mayo, O., eds. (1972) *Human Biochemical Genetics*, London.

Cockayne, E. A. (1933) *Inherited Abnormalities of the Skin and its Appendages*, London.

Gates, R. R. (1946) *Human Genetics*, New York.

Harris, H. (1968) *Human Biochemical Genetics*, 2nd ed., London.

Mather, K. (1971) *Biometrical Genetics*, 2nd ed., London.

McConnell, R. B. (1966) *The Genetics of Gastro-intestinal Disorders*, London.

McKusick, V. A. (1961, 1964) *Medical Genetics*, 1958–60, 1961–63, St. Louis.

Penrose, L. S. (1963) *The Biology of Mental Defect*, 3rd ed., London.

Pratt, R. T. C. (1967) *The Genetics of Neurological Disorders*, London.

Race, R. R., and Sanger, S. (1968) *Blood Groups in Man*, 5th ed., Oxford.

Smith, C. (1972) Computer programme to estimate recurrence risks for multifactorial familial disease, *Brit. med. J.*, **1**, 495.

Sorsby, A. (1951) *Genetics in Ophthalmology*, London.

Stevenson, A. C. and Davidson, Clare B. C. (1970) *Genetic Counselling*, London.

World Health Organization. Report of a WHO Scientific Group (1970) Genetic factors in congenital malformations, *Wld Hlth Org. techn. Rep. Ser.*, No. 438.

World Health Organization. Report of a WHO Scientific Group (1971) Methodology for family studies of genetic factors, *Wld Hlth Org. techn. Rep. Ser.*, No. 466.

World Health Organization (1972) Genetic disorders: prevention, treatment and rehabilitation, *Wld Hlth Org. Techn. Rep. Ser.*, No. 497.

World Health Organization (1974a) The work of WHO in 1973, *Wld Hlth Org. Off. Rec.*, **213**, 73.

World Health Organization (1974b) Pharmaeogenetics—the influence of heredity on the response to drugs, *Wld Hlth Org. Chron.*, **28**, 25.

On the genetic hazards of radiation the following are very useful:

Medical Research Council (1960) The hazards to man of nuclear and allied radiations, Second Report, London, H.M.S.O.

Stevenson, A. C. (1958) The genetic hazards of radiation, *Practitioner*, **181**, 559.

World Health Organization Expert Committee on Radiation (1959) First Report. Effect of Radiation on Human Heredity. Investigations of Areas of High Natural Radiation, *Wld Hlth Org. techn. Rep. Ser.*, No. 166.

World Health Organization Expert Committee on Human Genetics (1964) Second Report, Human Genetics and Public Health, *Wld Hlth Org. techn. Rep. Ser.*, No. 282.

World Health Organization Expert Committee on Human Genetics (1969) Third Report, Genetic Counselling, *Wld Hlth Org. techn. Rep. Ser.*, No. 416.

World Health Organization (1973) Methods for the analysis of human chromosome aberrations, ed. Buckton, K. E. and Evans, H. J., Geneva.

3I

MENTAL SUBNORMALITY

A. STOLLER

HISTORICAL BACKGROUND

The modern approach to the mentally subnormal began to develop some 150 years ago following the French Revolution, which led to the re-evaluation of the rights of man and a series of reforms in relation to the treatment of handicapped persons in general. A French physician, Jean Mare Gaspard Itard, obtained world-wide publicity in the early part of the nineteenth century, following his attempt to educate 'the wild boy of Aveyron', who was reported to have been found wandering naked in the woods, subsisting on roots and acorns and only able to utter inarticulate sounds. Although Itard laboured for five years, he was only moderately successful in his task, but his activity caught the imagination of the world as opening up new prospects for the role of education in developing man's intellectual potential. Another French doctor, Eduard Onesimus Séguin, who had studied under Itard, developed the education of subnormals at the Bicêtre Hospital, received official governmental recognition for his methods, and finally published a classical work in 1846 for the total instruction of idiots, involving moral, intellectual, and physiological capacities.

From 1840 on, through the second half of the nineteenth century, there occurred an era of institutional development. Although there were, before this, a few 'asylums' for handicapped persons, including subnormals, attached to churches and hospitals in Europe (including the sections of the Bicêtre and Salpétrière in France), the first distinct institution for 'cretins' was established by Guggenbuhl in the Abendberg, Switzerland, for the purpose of medical care and education. Within twenty-five years many European countries as well as the United States had established institutions for the care of subnormals; relative latecomers were Canada (1876), Italy (1899), Belgium (1892), and Japan (1900). As happened with mental hospitals, early enthusiasms waned with the accumulation of chronic and disturbed cases, and public attitudes became defensive and aggressive to the alienated group in its midst. Subnormals were blamed as being sexually promiscuous, as reducing the quality of human stock because of their high breeding rates, and also as being responsible for a good deal of crime. By the end of the century institutions had become detention centres for undesirable elements in society, and it is not surprising to learn therefore that they had also become the repository for many higher-grade individuals, whose deprived conditions in childhood produced both antisocial behaviour and reduced intellectual capacity. Antipathetic attitudes were stimulated through concepts of eugenics, introduced by Sir Francis Galton in 1865 and reinforced by the publication of family trees, such as the Jukes and the Kallikaks, which seemed to indicate genetic production of large numbers of degenerate individuals. By 1930 sterilization laws had been promulgated in twenty-three States in America, in a Swiss canton, in Denmark, and in Finland. Eugenics, as a general method of controlling the prevalence of mental subnormality, has since been shown to be not valid.

It needs to be appreciated that, in the first half of the nineteenth century, the terms idiocy and cretinism were often used interchangeably, and it was not until after 1850 that the unified concept of idiocy began to break down. Early landmarks were the establishment, around 1850, of the role of lack of iodine in producing cretinism and the description of mongolism by John Langdon Haydon Down in 1866, though this condition was not established as a clinical entity in continental Europe till the early part of the twentieth century. Langdon Down, in line with then current developments in neurology and neuropathology, spoke of three categories of congenital developmental and accidental conditions, with subgroups for each. Coincidentally, classifications were also being developed in relation to educational capacity, and the three categories of idiocy, imbecility, and debile (from the severe to the mildly subnormal) became commonly used.

Special schools began to develop from 1860 onwards, with initial maximal development stemming from German educationalists and then, in rapid succession, in Norway, Switzerland, England, and Italy. It is of interest to note that the United States did not establish its first special class till 1896, in Providence, Rhode Island, and that France, which provided the primary impetus for the education of subnormals through Itard and Séguin, waited until 1909 before its first special schooling was established in Paris.

Stimulus for a major move forward came in the early twentieth century from Alfred Binet and his assistant Theodore Simon, in their formulation of the Binet–Simon Intelligence Test. From 1905 to 1911, when Binet died, three successive versions of statistically evaluated scales of norms of performance for children of various ages were brought out. For the first time a reliable method became available to teachers to enable them to assess mental age, and so become aware of a child's needs and capacities; also, it highlighted the fact that subnormality was not an all-or-none phenomenon, but that there were indeed distinct grades of defect, from profound disturbance through to borderline abnormality. Henry Herbert Goddard in the United States coined the word moron in 1910, adding a new dimension to subnormality in bringing to the notice of educationalists the need for remedial work and special programmes for a large group of persons in the community functioning poorly in the school setting.

The discovery of phenylpyruvic oligophrenia (PKU) by Følling of Norway, in 1934, ushered in a new era of medical interest, in bringing to notice a potentially treatable recessive genetic deficiency; and gradually, with increasing tempo since 1945, more and more biochemical deficiencies have been unearthed. The 1957 determination in the United States by Tijo, an Indonesian, of the exact number of human chromosomes, followed by the 1959 discovery of Lejeune, of France, of trisomy in mongolism, further increased the medical interest, which has now become acute. At the same time research into education by such as O'Connor, Tizard, and Hermelin in the United Kingdom, Kirk in America, and Luria in the U.S.S.R. has opened up new potentials and interests for educational authorities. A third area which has opened up since the 1930s is the area of community care and rehabilitation; Holland, Denmark, Russia, and the United Kingdom have provided outstanding examples of this type of development, but most developed countries have now instituted such programmes in addition to traditional forms of institutional care. Within the last decade international activities have reflected the growing governmental and community interest in this broad field of human welfare, and increasing concern is being shown as to its public health implications. The International Group for the Scientific Study of Mental Deficiency held its first meeting in London in 1960, was officially formed in Copenhagen in 1964, and its first Congress took place in Montpellier in 1967. Groups of parents and laymen have stimulated National Associations for Mental Retardation into forming an international body, the International League of Societies for the Mentally Handicapped. The World Health Organization has established an Expert Committee, publishes regular reports, and has recently produced a revised classification for mental subnormality in its 8th revision of the *International Classification of Diseases*.

DEFINITION AND CLASSIFICATION

Mental subnormality (syn. mental deficiency, oligophrenia, mental retardation, amentia) in a child is recognized by the fact that its intellectual attainments are below that of an average child of the same age. The definition is a pragmatic one, based on the subject's capacity for schooling and for coping with the ordinary skills of everyday life. It must not be regarded as a static condition and possesses no implication of absoluteness or permanence. Improvement in I.Q. has been shown to occur in many subnormals without organic brain damage—possibly due to late maturation. The definition of mental subnormality is therefore descriptive and complex, and the use of intelligence tests may only be seen as a device for sorting out groups of subnormals on the basis of their intellectual functioning, and as a guide for further evaluation of individuals and direction into appropriate social channels. Diminished intellectual functioning, at a point in the life history of an individual, may be due to one, or a combination, of such factors as childhood deprivation, organic cerebral defect, specific metabolic defect, sensory or motor handicap, specific verbal disability, emotional disturbance or socio-cultural handicap.

Standardized intelligence tests sort out those between two and three standard deviations below average intelligence quotient (I.Q. 67–52 approx.) as mildly subnormal; and those more than three standard deviations below average (I.Q. 51 approx. and below) as moderately (I.Q. 51–36 approx.) and severely (I.Q. 35 and below) subnormal. From the latter a

further group of profoundly retarded, idiots, has been distinguished (I.Q. below 20 approx.).

The mildly subnormal are 'educable'—that is, they are able to profit through special schools in Education Departments and will, to large degree, be ultimately absorbed into the general community; while imbeciles, generally those above I.Q. 35, are 'trainable', requiring special programmes for the development of social skills and limited occupational capacity, but still mostly needing supervision all their lives.

Separation into such categories as idiot, imbecile, and feeble-minded, or into severe subnormal (SSN) and educational subnormal (ESN) involves stereotypes. Despite the administrative usefulness of such categorization, each child must still be looked at individually, since there is overlap between trainables and educables, depending especially on emotional stability; also, those educable subnormals who come to need permanent supervision are those with superadded physical or mental disabilities. While these are useful social devices, there is a danger in labelling individuals and a world-wide trend is developing that the education of each retarded person, irrespective of grade, should be based on diagnosis of assets and the fullest development of each of these. It is of interest to note that Britain has recently seen fit to make the Department of Education and Science responsible for the education of every retarded child in the country.

The following table attempts to correlate the terms used in different countries with appropriate I.Q. levels and present-day classification. Since I.Q.s are mere guidelines and do not represent absolutes, WHO figures are used for this purpose; in general, they vary little from what is acceptable in most countries [TABLE 72].

Severe and profound subnormals are found in all social classes, though referrals tend to be greater from inadequately functioning families. Mild subnormals are referred to much lesser degree, constituting less than 50 per cent. of those of I.Q. 52–67 failing to get through school and into a job. Referral is predominantly from lower social classes, except where the mild subnormality is associated with epilepsy, physical handicaps, abnormal EEG, or biochemical or chromosomal aetiologies. Almost no children of higher-social-class parents have children between I.Q. 52 and 85 unless a pathological process is detectable. The non-pathological type of mild subnormality is termed cultural-familial, being thought to be due to an interaction between genetic susceptibility and cultural deprivation.

In the first half of the twentieth century classification was meagre. Tredgold, in 1908, divided cases into two main groups—primary amentia (due to defective germ plasm) and secondary amentia (environmental)—and the few syndromes definitely established were included under these headings. In the light of his appreciation of the cultural origins of milder grades of subnormality, Lewis, in 1933, spoke of pathological and subcultural (physiological) groups.

An attempt at a more comprehensive classification, formulated by Heber in 1959, defined eight categories, the first six being related to causation, of which I–III referred to environmental causes and IV–VI to non-environmental; the final two sections were concerned with those where causation was obscure, VII being those with neurological signs and VIII those without neurological signs.

Category I is a small group, including prenatal infections

TABLE 72

I.Q. level	WHO and Heber classification	Synonyms	Educational capacity
85–68	Borderline (Level 1)	Borderline mental sub-normality (WHO) Borderline mental retardation (Heber) Dull and backward	Educable in normal schools with special attention
67–52	Mild (Level 2)	Mild mental subnorm-ality (WHO) Mild mental retardation (Heber) Educational subnormal —ESN (U.K.) Debile Moron Feeble-minded	Educable in special schools or classes
51–36	Moderate (Level 3)	Moderate mental subnormality (WHO) Moderate mental retardation (Heber) Severe subnormal—SSN (U.K.) Imbecile (high-grade)	Trainable in day training centres and industrial training centres
35–20	Severe (Level 4)	Severe mental subnormality (WHO) Severe mental retardation (Heber) Severe subnormal—SSN (U.K.) Imbecile (low-grade)	Trainable in day training centres. Low industrial potential
Below 20	Profound (Level 5)	Profound mental subnormality (WHO) Profound mental retardation (Heber) Severe subnormal—SSN (U.K.) Idiot	Completely dependent through all ages

such as maternal rubella and congenital toxoplasmosis; the two most important postnatal infections are meningitis and encephalitis, due to various organisms; the pneumococcus and meningococcus are most frequently involved with meningitis and measles with encephalitis.

Category II also comprises a relatively small group, involving most commonly kernicterus, including erythroblastosis foetalis and brain damage associated with retrolental fibroplasia, as well as such rarer conditions as immunization encephalopathy and lead poisoning.

Category III, associated with injuries, is predominantly associated with prenatal obstetric damage (cause often unknown), less frequently with postnatal vascular or other injuries, and occasionally with irradiation encephalopathy.

Category IV, associated with metabolic disorders, includes most commonly phenylketonuria, as well as Hurler's syndrome and other rare neurological degenerations. Cretinism is now quite rare. Over sixty inborn errors of metabolism are now recognized, of which forty-five are associated with mental defect and twenty-five are considered treatable—phenylketonuria, maple syrup disease, Hartnup syndrome, hepatocerebral degeneration, citrullinuria, hyperammonaemia, idiopathic galactosaemia, idiopathic hypoglycaemia, hereditary fructose intolerance, vitamin B_6 dependency, familial cretinism, and renal diabetes insipidus. Although these conditions are numer-

ous, they represent only 3 per cent. of cases of mental subnormality. They are transmitted as autosomal recessives, carriers are clinically healthy, two heterozygote parents are needed to produce the disorder, one-quarter of the children are affected, the gene frequency in the population is 1 in 50, and the child is supported by the mother's enzymes during pregnancy, and is therefore born healthy. Galactosaemia produces obvious evidence of brain damage in the early days of life, PKU at around 4–6 months, Hartnup's disease during school age, and hepatocerebral degeneration usually after adolescence.

Category V, due to tumours, includes most commonly tuberous sclerosis and the Sturge–Weber syndrome, but is probably the smallest group over all.

Category VI, due to unknown prenatal influence, includes the large group of mongolism (Down's syndrome) and other rarer chromosomal defects, dyscranias (malformations of the skull), congenital hydrocephalus, and hereditary syndromes.

Category VII, due to unknown causes and with neurological signs, includes the large group associated with epilepsy, with or without motor disorders, and the rarer neurological degenerations such as Schilder's disease.

Category VIII, due to unknown causes without neurological signs, forms the largest group of subnormals, including cultural-familial retardation, those of unknown cause (idiopathic), and those with major psychotic or personality disorders.

Categories VI, VII, and VIII together make up the main bulk of disorders involved in mental subnormality.

In addition to these eight categories, six supplementary descriptive terms were used: (1) with genetic component; (2) with secondary cranial anomaly; (3) with impairment of special senses; (4) with convulsive disorder; (5) with psychiatric impairment; and (6) with motor dysfunction. The final diagnosis was rounded off with five descriptive categories of levels of intelligence.

This has been used as the basis for the newly introduced WHO Eighth Revision of the *International Classification of Diseases*, as under:

MENTAL RETARDATION (310–315)

310 Borderline mental retardation
Backwardness   Borderline mental deficiency or
Borderline intelligence   subnormality
Deficientia intelligentiae   I.Q. 68–85
311 Mild mental retardation
Feeble-mindedness   Mild mental deficiency or sub-
High-grade defect   normality
Moron   I.Q. 52–67
312 Moderate mental retardation
Imbecile, I.Q. 36–51   Moderate mental deficiency or sub-
    normality
    I.Q. 36–51
313 Severe mental retardation
Imbecile NOS   Severe mental deficiency or sub-
    normality
    I.Q. 20–35
314 Profound mental retardation
Idiocy   I.Q. under 20
Profound mental deficiency
or subnormality
315 Unspecified mental retardation
Mental deficiency or sub-
normality NOS

The following fourth-digit subdivisions may be used with the above categories.

·0 Following infections and intoxications
·1 Following trauma or physical agents
·2 With disorders of metabolism, growth, or nutrition
·3 Associated with gross brain disease (postnatal)
·4 Associated with diseases and conditions due to (unknown) prenatal influence
·5 With chromosomal abnormalities
·6 Associated with prematurity
·7 Following major psychiatric illness
·8 With psycho-social (environmental) deprivation
·9 Other and unspecified.

In Australia and New Zealand it has been decided to separate infection from intoxication (category ·0) and single out mongolism (Down's syndrome) from other chromosomal anomalies.

INCIDENCE AND PREVALENCE

From the public health point of view, we are concerned essentially with subnormals below I.Q. 68, the profoundly and severely subnormal and the educationally subnormal, more so with the former than the latter. Detected profound and severe subnormals, located in hospitals or day training centres, are of the order of 3–4 per 1,000 of children of school age, while estimates of educational subnormals in European countries vary from 10 to 40 per 1,000 of school age, depending on the diagnostic capacity of the school system. Schools are also concerned with the 'dull and backward', or 'slow learners' (I.Q. 70–85), comprising some 5–10 per cent. of the school population, not coming within our definition of subnormality, but calling on medical help for physical handicaps or associated psychiatric disabilities.

There is a distinction between 'administrative' and 'true' prevalence, the former constituting those under care, the latter including additionally those in the community not under care, but in need. As an illustration of this, one might cite the situation in the United States, where it is generally stated that 3 per cent. of the newborn will be diagnosed as mentally subnormal (< I.Q. 70) during their life-time. Of all the newborn, it is estimated that 1 per 1,000 will have an I.Q. less than 20, 4 per 1,000 an I.Q. of 20–50, and 25 per 1,000 of 50–70, based on intelligence tests. The figure of 3 per cent. would, however, be applicable only in regard to later school ages for educational subnormals. In the United States, as in other countries, higher rates of educational subnormality arise from culturally deprived sections of the population; and it has more latterly been estimated that the 'diagnostic' or 'administrative' prevalence is more likely around 1 per cent., which is in line with the accepted figure for most Western communities. The way this figure has been determined illustrates the problems associated with the comparison of prevalences between different countries.

In practice, in the United States only 15 of an estimated educationally subnormal group of 300 children under 6 would be detected; while, of 1,400 educationally subnormal adults over 24, only some 65 would be under care, the rest having gone through the school system undetected or subsequently been absorbed in full employment. Relatively high early death rates would reduce those with I.Q.s <20 from an expected 100 to 50, and those with I.Q.s 20–50 from 400 to 150; while the total number of those with I.Q.s 50–70 would be 700 instead of 2,500.

Denmark, with a population of 4,500,000, registers all known subnormals, and the present register consists of 20,000 persons (approx. 40 per 1,000 of total population), of whom 8,200 live in 35 government institutions, 700 in private institutions, and 11,000 in the community, with 4,550 of the latter using community facilities.

In the United Kingdom there are just under 1·3 beds per 1,000 of total population in institutions and 2·0 subnormals per 1,000 under the care of local authorities. The lower figure than Denmark may be accounted for, in part, by the fact that a proportion of cases are not under direct care. A ten-year plan for the United Kingdom envisages the institutional figure remaining at 1·3 beds per 1,000, which would seem to reflect an irreducible minimum of the accommodation required for severe subnormals. At the same time deficiencies in extra-institutional care are indicated by plans put forward to increase, by 1975, the number of places for subnormals under 16 years of age in Junior Training Centres (16,407 to 23,031 places), in Adult Training Centres for the over-16 age group (11,259 to 27,795 places), and Hostels (947 to 9,907 places). Over-all, considering both institutional and community placements, this will affect 2·5 per 1,000 population, so that it is anticipated that improvements in rehabilitation and job-placement programmes will enable 0·8 subnormals per 1,000 of the population to disappear into the community as integrated working members.

In Holland, at present, the proportion of mentally handicapped persons employed in sheltered industry is 0·7 per 1,000 of total population, but this is below estimated requirements of a probable minimum of 1 place per 1,000. Tizard has estimated that 1·5–2·0 places per 1,000 in training centres and sheltered workshops for adult subnormals in industrial London will be required. A minimum of 1 per 1,000 places is certainly indicated forthwith: planning in the United Kingdom also envisages a minimum of 0·2 per 1,000 hostel places by 1972.

On the basis of the above requirements, which seems to apply to present-day Western communities, and applying the foregoing estimates to a population of 1 million, one would estimate minimal needs as being 1,300 institutional beds, with another 2,000 subnormals under community care. The latter would consist of 500 in Junior Training Centres (0·5 per 1,000), 500 in Adult Training Centres (0·5 per 1,000), and a minimum of 1,000 in Sheltered Workshops (1·0 per 1,000), with 200 of the latter living in hostels (0·2 per 1,000).

Educable subnormals in Education Department special classes constituted 0·8 per cent. of the total school population in the United Kingdom in 1965. A similar figure is quoted for Russia. However, there is a waiting list of 11,000 cases in the United Kingdom, and the figure is at least 1·0 per cent., maybe higher, which comes into line with the more recently quoted United States figures.

In developing countries, of course, a subnormal child may not become manifest because of the lack of pressure from schooling; where schooling exists, however, prevalence rises steadily after school-entrance, and is maximal prior to school-leaving age, or soon after, the latter being due to the pressure of job finding. Kushlik, in his Wessex study in the United Kingdom, found maximum prevalence in the age group 15–19 years. In Victoria, Australia, a survey of mental retardation among children showed that full recognition became manifest at the age of 12–14 years for both males and females. It becomes possible to project backwards from this maximal rate (allowing for death rates which are not considerable after the age of 2 years), and forward (again allowing for death rates in the community). Community absorption is the fate of 90 per cent. of the educationally subnormal group—only 5 per cent. of such adults are institutionalized and another 5 per cent. are in the community as handicapped adults unable to hold down jobs. Profound and severe subnormals, on the other hand, once institutionalized, tend to stay therein; in fact, a study in the United Kingdom has shown that while 30 per cent. of them are in institutions between the ages of 0 and 9, the figure rises to 45 per cent. between the ages of 10 and 19, 70 per cent between 20 and 39, 85 per cent. between 40 and 59, and 100 per cent. of those over the age of 60 years are institutionalized, the institutional prevalence for all ages being 60 per cent. The Wessex study showed rates to be similar in both urban and rural areas.

Over-all rates for profound and severe subnormals show some consistency in surveys, being around 3–4 per 1,000 of population for pre-adult ages; Åkkeson in Sweden produced a figure of 5·8 per 1,000 for all ages. It is interesting to note that mongolism constitutes some 10 per cent. of subnormals below I.Q. 68 and 25 per cent. of moderate and severe subnormals—due to the fact that the majority are in the imbecile range, only 10 per cent. being above I.Q. 50. The prevalence of educational subnormals, on the other hand, shows great inconsistencies in different surveys, due to different criteria used.

Lower grades of subnormals are predominantly associated with organic cerebral pathology, whereas only 25 per cent. of the educationally subnormal show clinical signs of brain damage. The former are now surviving to greater degree, and this is affecting community prevalence. Mongolism, for instance, has quadrupled the survival rate up to the age of 10, since 1929; survival rates have also risen as a result of operative procedures in hydrocephalus, the better treatment of children with low birth weights and the use of antibiotics for such conditions as tuberculous meningitis. Despite increased survival rates, though, the prevalence of institutionalized subnormals has decreased in the United Kingdom since 1938. Diminished length of stay and increased discharges play a part, but it is also contributed to by diminished incidence due to improved obstetrics, control of infections with antibiotics, and the rise in social standards. In the past many with higher I.Q.s than 68 were admitted to institutions because of asocial behaviour, or because of family disturbances; with better diagnosis and improved community facilities these are now tending to be dealt with by other social agencies. Parents are also tending to keep even severely subnormal children at home, with the help of domiciliary services; a recent study in the United Kingdom showed that two-thirds of severe subnormals are being kept in the community, a pattern which is well established in Russia, with its systems of regional community health clinics.

Worries regarding the deterioration of human stock have been answered by the Scottish surveys of 1932 and 1947. Not only are subnormals sub-fertile over-all but mean average intelligence in children born to subnormals tends to rise above that of their parents. Despite a marked brain-drain from Scotland between 1932 and 1947, mean I.Q.s, as measured in 11-year-old schoolchildren, increased from 34·5 to 36·7.

Two United Kingdom studies, one by Cyril Burt in 1925 and another by Gittins in 1952, both showed 7·8 per cent. of delinquents with I.Q. <70, although mean I.Q. for the group as a whole has risen. Nearly 33 per cent. of institutionalized delinquents are seriously illiterate, with low verbal intelligence. Only the educationally subnormal, usually of I.Q. 55–70, become involved in delinquency, and they are generally led into crime by bad companions. This group is more likely to be reconvicted, is especially prone to certain types of crime (e.g. sex crimes), and, because of late maturation, is more likely to be rehabilitatable than other delinquents.

DIAGNOSIS

As already indicated, individuals do not fit readily into classificatory systems, and diagnosis must be in terms of a global assessment of biological, psychological, and sociological aspects; and in each of these particulars one needs to include a listing of assets as well as liabilities. It is, moreover, essential to make a diagnosis as early as possible, in order that counselling of parents and the institution of suitable programmes of management may prevent progressive disability and lay a basis for optimal development.

Physicians are key figures in the detection of those biological factors likely to produce mental subnormality—during pregnancy, at birth, and in the pre-school period. The physician will be especially involved in the diagnosis of severe subnormals, where organic pathological factors predominate. Relatively easily recognizable conditions are mongolism, cranial anomalies, genetic defects, tumours, cerebral palsy, and the sequelae of infectious and neurotropic toxins and traumata. However, many of these develop postnatally or are unrecognized at birth. Mongolism, for instance, is only detected in some 70 per cent. of cases prior to leaving maternity hospital, and such conditions as phenylketonuria develop postnatally and may not be detected till severe brain damage occurs. A study of residents in the Fountain Hospital, London, showed the incidence of cases of unknown aetiology to be 59·0 per cent., and a figure of 63·2 per cent. was obtained for the residential population of the State of Victoria, Australia, with a lower figure for the severe, as compared with moderate and mild, subnormals. If one adds to this figure the 23·0 per cent. of mongols, where the cause of the chromosomal anomaly has still to be established, it becomes apparent that there is much room for research into causation, especially as to this must be added other conditions due to unknown prenatal influence (Heber: Category VI)—prenatal dyscrasia, dyscrasia with malformations, congenital hydrocephalus, meningocele, chromosome anomalies, etc. In the Australian study environmental causes accounted for 18·6 per cent., hereditary causes for 6·0 per cent., while 11·6 per cent. appeared to show a combination of both environmental and hereditary causes. The same picture seemed to hold for admissions to the Fountain Hospital, since a definite cause was obtained in 9·5 per cent., a probable cause in 4·0 per cent., a possible cause in 33·0 per cent., mongolism accounted for 23·0 per cent., and no cause was able to be established for 31·0 per cent. It is interesting to note that almost two-thirds of residential low-grade patients are males, and males also form a high proportion of admissions in this category; it may also be noted that 23 per cent. of admissions have one or more motor, visual, or auditory physical handicaps in addition to the mental subnormality, while 25 per cent. exhibit behaviour problems, such as psychosis or hyperkinesis.

Diagnosis in the first year of life occurs predominantly in the group of I.Q. <35—the lower grades of severe and profound subnormality. There are many helpful developmental schedules which can be used. Severe subnormality is especially associated with muscular atony and lax joints. As many as 40 per cent. of this category have other congenital anomalies in addition to the mental subnormality, and these should always be looked for, otherwise such conditions as congenital cardiac malformations may be missed. At this early stage watch needs to be kept for psychological antecedents of subnormality, such as will occur with maternal deprivation, the battered-child syndrome, and the effects of institutionalization.

In the pre-school period developmental delays in sitting up, walking, vocalization, speech formation, habit control, or muscular co-ordination may bring the subnormality to the attention of the parent or physician, and those of I.Q. 30–50 are now likely to become recognized. Cultural-familial deprivation is beginning also to become a recognizable factor.

In school years the subnormality becomes evident to the educationalist through gross academic failure, withdrawal, negativism, or aggressiveness. The physician is called upon to elucidate the diagnosis of physical and mental handicaps which may occur, to lesser or greater degree, in 20 per cent. of referrals. Failure to make the grade may be due to such handicaps as epilepsy, spasticity, motor inco-ordination, sensory handicaps, or psychiatric disabilities. However, cultural-familial retardation is the commonest aetiological factor in this group.

The global picture of diagnosis should include a general physical examination for congenital anomalies, a neurological assessment (including EEG, special senses, and neuro-muscular co-ordination) and psychological testing for verbal and non-verbal capacities (including observations for attention span, responsiveness to others, trial periods of learning through one or other senses, and play situations through the one-way screen to test motor co-ordination, constructive capacity, and interaction with parents). In addition, help may have to be sought from the specialist paediatrician, psychiatrist, orthopaedist, cytogeneticist, biochemist, ophthalmologist, audiologist, or social worker, to elucidate one or more aspects of the clinical status.

LEGAL AND FORENSIC

Legal provisions for entrance into institutions have involved statutory processes protecting the interests of a minor or dependent adult subnormal. However, since the custodial rigidity of institutions and the tendency for static labels to stick resulted in virtual life-imprisonment for the subnormals admitted, voluntary admissions have come to be preferred to greater degree, but even so, regular assessment seems desirable and needs to be ensured legally. It would also seem reasonable that processes of law ensure that a community provides adequate facilities for the subnormal population.

In many countries it seems to have been appropriate to statutorily establish a central agency to look after the interests of subnormals, taking full cognizance of the special problems involved, and revising out-worn concepts based on static concepts of subnormality and emphasis on institutionalization.

Legislation involves both local communities and public health authorities, and includes a statutory provision for a compulsory register of subnormals.

With respect to areas of guardianship and legal competency, an individual approach to each subnormal problem needs to be ensured, and supervision of the rights of the individual should be the concern of some central governmental agency. Consideration also needs to be given to such matters as voting rights, driving, marriage, and eugenic sterilization. In regard to criminal behaviour, competence to stand trial needs to be determined, and the same range of special adolescent and adult facilities needs to be ensured as for non-criminal subnormals.

INTERNATIONAL ASPECTS

Countries have developed mental retardation programmes in different ways, in accordance with local scientific attitudes and social and political concepts. However, since 1945 a rapprochement in ideation is occurring, and programmes are tending to develop in similar ways. The medical profession would seem to have the important role of initial diagnosis at early ages, the determination of groups-at-risk, and the institution of preventive programmes; however, diagnosis and management, subsequent to school age, is becoming more and more the province of the educationalist, with the medical profession exercising the ancillary role. To illustrate the above, programmes in selected countries will be described.

In both Denmark and Sweden there are Mental Deficiency Acts which allow for a wide spread of integrated programmes at local levels under national planning and control. There are many similarities in these programmes. The Danish programme, which is more recent, will be described. Under the Ministry of Social Affairs, a Directorate of Mental Deficiency Services has been established which supervises programmes in thirteen regional centres and runs a national training school for personnel. Each regional service is run by a team of four leaders of equal status: a business manager, a medical practitioner, a social worker, and an educator. Those treated are persons functioning at a mental subnormality level, as determined by psychological testing and observation. The school age for this group is 7–21 years, the latter figure allowing for late maturation (and this can be extended to 23, in some cases, in Sweden). The special school programme caters for those of I.Q. 45–70 approximately. A wide range of facilities is provided for subnormals: children's homes, foster homes, kindergartens, day schools and boarding schools, special training schools for industrial and occupational training, sheltered workshops, central institutions for care and treatment, and even homes for aged subnormals. Preventive and diagnostic services in Denmark involve free antenatal care, well-baby clinics in the first year, and statutory annual medical examinations from birth to the age of 7, followed by regular annual examination through the School Medical Service. Mothers' Aid Centres, including travelling staff, have been organized on a voluntary basis to provide advice to families with problems, and would constitute another source of detection and help. Sterilization is legal, but has had little effect or prevalence; its main purpose is to help those who would otherwise suffer psycho-socio-economic hardships. The general philosophy is to maintain the subnormal primarily at home, next consider foster care, and institutionalize only as a last resort. The rights of parents are legally protected, and safeguards exist for parents who are not satisfied with a recommendation for placement outside of the home. Pre-school programmes exist for special schools, and there are provisions for regular re-evaluation and shifting from one programme to another. In Denmark 20,000 subnormals are on the central mental deficiency register (0·5 per 1,000), of whom 9,000 (0·25 per 1,000) are in institutional or specialized homes, 9,000 are in family care, and 2,000 are in kindergartens, special schools, and sheltered workshops. There is weighting towards lower-grade subnormals in the registered population. Around 1 per cent. of schoolchildren are receiving education in special schools.

Russia does not operate in terms of I.Q., but has developed its programme of diagnosis on the basis of concepts of neuro-physiology as applied to brain damage; it does not accept psychological intelligence-testing nor concepts of cultural-familial retardation on a genetic basis. Its tests are more neurologically determined, and investigate EEG, motor co-ordination, perceptual defects, conditioning, and concept formation (linguistics). Those of I.Q. <20 are the responsibility of the Health Department, and are cared for by specially trained teachers, defectologists; the rest are looked after by the Education Department. The mild subnormal group seem to filter in much the same sort of way into educational special facilities, and constitute up to 1 per cent. of the school-age population, a figure which is now becoming accepted for most countries. Day and Boarding Special Schools are provided for urban areas and Boarding Schools for rural areas. The Board of Education makes its final decisions in regard to placement through a team consisting of neurophysiologists, defectologists, teachers, and the head of the special school. Before this point is reached a preliminary placement of one year in normal school is undertaken, and 'oligophrenia' is diagnosed only as a last resort; if doubts exist, transfer takes place to diagnostic classes with highly skilled remedial teachers, assisted by a logopaedist and the school paediatrician. The upper limit of schooling for mild subnormals has been shifted from the usual 16–18 years of age, and the curriculum is heavily geared towards vocational training. The Ministry of Social Welfare runs boarding schools for the 'trainable' subnormals, where the key educators are again the defectologists. The latter undergo a five-year programme of training. They are paid 50 per cent. higher stipends than ordinary teachers during training, and their permanent salary is 25 per cent. higher, making them a high-status profession, comparable with physicians. The over-all emphasis is on self-care and work activities leading to pre-vocational training for sheltered industry or return to local regional employment. There are large research institutes, the Institute of Defectology being the major one, employing skills from physiology, paediatrics, psychology, and education. Preventive practices employed include prenatal care as a legal obligation, special attention to the nutrition and health of the expectant mother, and widespread teaching of techniques of resuscitation of the newborn.

These two national programmes illustrate the need for comprehensive integrated programmes for mental subnormality. In the United States, legislation in individual states controls mental subnormality programmes, and emphasis has mainly focused on providing institutional care, which has had relatively low priority; development is now, however, being stimulated by Federal involvement, and research and local community facilities are being encouraged. At the same time, educational authorities are beginning to take a major interest in mild subnormals. The operative figure of 3 per cent. of school population as being subnormal, as already mentioned, is now being scaled down to 1 per cent. Whether other countries are failing to deal with cultural-familial retardation, whether there is a preponderance of these cases in the United States, or whether a statistical artefact has been produced by undue concentration on intelligence testing has yet to be determined. Over-all provisions in the United States are below Scandinavian, and many other European, countries.

Two European countries which have produced solid programmes, though still requiring development in certain areas, are Holland and the United Kingdom. Holland has shown considerable advances in its provisions, first, for institutions and special schools and, more latterly, for reality-based workshop facilities and domiciliary care. It utilizes a combination of governmental and voluntary, mainly religious, agencies. The United Kingdom has produced valuable epidemiological data on needs, and since 1945 has provided many of the insights relating to educability of subnormals. A former concentration on institutions has given way to increased involvement of statutory health regions and public health units of local authorities. Integration is not only developing at the local community level but is also requiring greater functional integration of the Ministries of Health, Education, and Labour.

There is scarcely a developed country in the world which is not moving forward in the field of subnormality through its health and education programmes. A blueprint for a comprehensive service has been recently produced in Eire, and France has reorganized its government programme. Developing countries will be faced with greater problems as their industrial and educational potential increases. Few have gone beyond the stage of extruding a number of severe subnormals into mental hospitals and mild subnormals into prisons. One developing country with which the author is familiar, Thailand, has recently begun to gear its educational facilities to mild subnormals and has instituted a special day training facility of the Department of Health for the care of severe subnormals, but this latter constitutes a mere 300 places for a population of 24 million.

PREVENTION AND MANAGEMENT

Important areas of primary prevention have opened up as a result of the determination of various biological aetiologies. Syphilis has virtually disappeared as a cause of mental subnormality with the advent of antibiotics. The use of iodized salts in iodine-deficient communities has produced the same result with endemic cretinism, while glandular cretinism has responded to hormone therapy. Phenylketonuria, comprising 1 per 10,000 births, is coming under control with early detection and dietary treatment, as is galactosaemia and the other rarer treatable inborn errors of metabolism. Erythroblastosis foetalis is now amenable to the injection of immune antibodies into the mother. Hydrocephaly is responding to surgical treatment in many cases, with the construction of the by-pass between the cerebral ventricles and various areas of the body; premature synostosis of the skull is likewise responding to surgical intervention through craniectomy. Meningitis has now become rare as a cause of subnormality with the modern use of antibiotics, though a small number of patients with tuberculous meningitis, who would formerly have died, are now surviving with varying degrees of brain damage. It is expected that measles encephalopathy will be eliminated as a cause of mental subnormality in the near future, now that a vaccine for this disorder has been perfected; and rubella similarly. Lead poisoning, which was common at the turn of the century, is now rare, its presence in the community having been controlled by legislation.

Genetic counselling may also be usefully employed in the prevention of the rare dominant hereditary conditions, such as acrocephaly, epiloia, and dystrophia myotonica, as well as in the autosomal recessive inborn errors of metabolism and cases of familial translocation mongolism. It is not possible to screen all babies for chromosomal abnormalities, so that one would concentrate on younger mothers of mongoloid infants as being more likely to lead to families with the relatively rare transmissible translocation, and also concentrate on families with multiple cases of subnormality. Guthrie testing, a blood-spot method using a bacterial inhibition technique, is now being applied routinely in many countries for the detection of cases of phenylketonuria, and this test will also locate cases of histidinaemia, maple syrup disease, homocystinuria, tyrosinaemia, and galactosaemia. Biochemical investigation could advisably be undertaken where there are multiple family members in institutions; and paediatricians should also perform screening where there is a progressive failure of mental capacities in children. However, it has to be realized that there is a large group of pathological metabolic disorders, commencing after birth, where causation is unknown and where preventability is not feasible, e.g. amaurotic idiocy, Niemann-Pick disease, Gaucher's disease, gargoylism, glycogenosis (von Gierke's disease), and others. However, somatic foetal cells may now be detected in the amniotic fluid of mothers-at-risk by the 14th to 16th week through amniocentesis and this may be followed by therapeutic termination of pregnancy with parental consent. A wide variety of conditions can be detected by culture of the somatic fibroblast cells, including galactosaemia, maple syrup disease, cystic fibrosis, diabetes mellitus and lipoidoses, such as Niemann-Pick disease, Lesch-Nyhan syndrome and Tay-Sachs disease; thalassaemia, von Gierke's disease and phenylketonuria are not detectable by this means and therefore cannot be diagnosed *in utero*.

Further aspects of primary prevention revolve around improved maternal health and social conditions, the latter tending to decrease nutritional defects and both rates of exposure and susceptibility to infectious diseases. The tendency to complete families earlier could well reduce the incidence of age-dependent disorders, such as mongolism, extra sex chromosomes and hydrocephaly; however, it is necessary ultimately to look into other possible factors in their production, such as genes, viruses, hormones, or irradiation. Evidence has been produced which suggests a link between epidemics of infectious hepatitis and mongolism nine months later. Since the chromosomal abnormality has now been shown to exist in amniotic fluid, amniocentesis may be utilized in high risk cases.

Mention has already been made of the role of genetic counselling in primary prevention, and family planning may also be useful where there is a tendency to obstetric difficulties. Diabetes in the mother is a case in point. Hydramnios, irradiation, drugs (e.g. thalidomide, aminopterin, tridione), and prematurity are all associated with congenital defects. Of those prematures less than 4 lb. at birth, 10 per cent. are reported to be associated with cerebral palsy, sensory defect, or gross deficiency, the rest being normal. The recognition by obstetricians, therefore, of high-risk pregnancies and early and appropriate treatment might well prevent the subsequent development of some cases of cerebral defect. Attention is increasingly being paid to the possible role of infectious conditions during pregnancy, e.g. syphilis, rubella, mumps, vaccinia, smallpox, toxoplasmosis, and infectious hepatitis.

In the postnatal period the control of cerebral infections and lead poisoning has reduced these types of subnormality; however, children are becoming more subject to accidental poisoning with drugs, head injuries through car accidents, the battered-child syndrome, and accidental drownings. There is an area here for increased efforts at primary prevention.

Turning to secondary prevention, it should be realized that since over 50 per cent. of subnormals have no recognizable cause, the best method of attack is early detection, appropriate diagnosis, parent counselling, correction of associated physical disabilities, and appropriate training.

Risk registers are being developed in many places, but risk factors are often ill-defined and screening personnel ill-equipped. It is suggested that specially trained, experienced doctors alone can detect and evaluate cases of minimal cerebral damage, congenital malformations, and neuropsychiatric disorders, which may or may not have been predicted by complicated pregnancy or family background. In fact, emphasis needs to be placed on careful examination of all infants by such experts routinely. Recent work suggests that scoring clusters of adverse factors may be the way to practically determine high risk. This opinion is hardening towards 'prescriptive screening'. Developmental and neurological assessment involves the recognition of visual, auditory, language, motor, intellectual, emotional, and social handicaps. It has been estimated that 70 per cent. of infants with cerebral palsies, 25 per cent. with uncomplicated mental retardation, and most deaf babies can be identified in the first year of life.

A central registry in British Columbia, Canada, has found 40 per cent. of reported severe subnormals to have associated handicaps, and these must be taken into consideration in any programme for training. We have already mentioned the detection and treatment of phenylketonuria, galactosaemia, maple syrup disease, and hypothyroidism, and the need to be on the look-out for lead poisoning. Diagnosis and treatment of subdural haematoma, the excision of temporal lobe foci, and the surgical treatment of hydrocephalus and craniosynostosis can all prevent the development of mental subnormality.

But the prime problem of recognition resides in schooling problems resulting from late maturation, perceptual difficulties, sensory deficits, motor inco-ordination, as well as isolated defects in number concepts, reading, writing, or abstract conceptualization, all of which require specialized teaching. Distractibility and hyperactivity, due to mild brain damage, can result in retardation, and may be helped with amphetamines or phenothiazines, small classes, and improving attention span by limitation of the visual field to the essentials necessary to complete a task. Aphasia, most commonly of the receptive variety, if not recognized early and treated, may lead to retardation or psychotic withdrawal. All of the afore-mentioned problems of schooling may provoke internal frus-trations and aggressive interaction with peers, teachers, and parents, and may prevent development or even encourage regression. Psychiatric services to parents and teachers may be of great help in this regard.

Finally, attention needs to be drawn to the early recognition of the culturally deprived child, who tends to be 1–2 years behind normal by the time schooling begins at around 6 years. Alertness in dealing with the problem of broken families may bring to light children-at-risk, as well as detecting battered-child syndromes and screening of those committed to institu-tions. Institutions, of themselves, tend to create cultural deprivation unless staffing is sufficient to provide adequate mothering.

Tertiary prevention involves attention to associated handi-caps, including psychiatric disability, training for meaningful communications and skills, and encouragement of emotional security. Drugs may be required for such conditions as hyper-activity or epilepsy. Parent counselling can help with the creation of optimal conditions for early development, and parents can be assisted with domiciliary services, temporary institutional placements, and group supports. Institutional placement before the age of 6 is rarely indicated, and there is much to commend development in a normal family milieu during the early formative years. Patterns of custodial care have dominated institutions for many decades, with resultant trends towards therapeutic nihilism, but these are now becom-ing more geared towards treatment, training, education, and rehabilitation. Concepts of large barrack-like units are giving way to small units modelled on the normal home and with adequately trained cottage mothers and fathers. Wherever possible, free communication with the primary family and the community is maintained. The small-group concept applies also to classes, work situations, and recreation.

A variety of facilities are necessary for those subnormals who can be maintained in their homes—day minding centres, day training centres, pre-vocational training workshops, sheltered workshops—and, for those who have no contacts in the com-munity, hostels.

Education for living in the subnormal person, as in the nor-mal, must be geared to the development of full potential. As already indicated, those of I.Q. 50–70 are considered 'educable', capable of absorbing elementary academic skills; while those of I.Q. 35–50 are 'trainable', capable only of developing basic social skills and routine work habits, allowing for some overlap between these two groups. Early activation at home and in pre-school facilities have revolutionized the recognition of potential, and the latter can still be developed through to early adulthood. Since subnormals, especially those who are brain damaged, show rigidity and concreteness of thinking, as well as poor attention and motivation, it is necessary to limit incoming stimuli, introduce more complex experiences gradually, stimu-late motivation through encouragement, and praise and rein-force approaches to single concepts through all sensory modali-ties. Limitation to small aspects of experience enables precise recognition of assets and their encouragement. Operant con-ditioning techniques are being applied to the retarded with

moderate success in habit training; the emphasis is on develop-ing motivation through rewards. Emotional support is essen-tial, and requires close personal attention by teachers in small classes.

Several types of workshop facility are needed for a broad programme of vocational training. The first, which may be termed Pre-vocational Training Workshop, is adjunctive to the Day Training Centre or Special School, and involves training and observation of 14–16-year-olds in the development of in-dustrial and social skills; it is not primarily concerned with productivity though it may have some industrial potential and leads direct to industry or to one of the other units to be des-cribed. The second type of facility, the Activity Centre, is for adult retarded persons who are extremely unlikely to have more than limited industrial potential, but are kept active to prevent deterioration, and are maintained in an institution, hostel, or at home, always in the hope that some may graduate to a more advanced facility. The third type of Workshop, the Adult Training Centre (Transitional Sheltered Workshop), takes those graduating from the Pre-vocational Training Workshops or Activity Centres, or coming direct from an institution, or from the community. Last, there is the Permanent Sheltered Workshop, self-supporting and operating on standard factory lines. The subnormal person must be able to perform as any other worker, even though he may be slower, and pro-duction must be above a prescribed proportion of that of a normal worker. For all those attending workshops it is also necessary to provide adequate social and recreational facilities, as these skills, without practice reinforcement, are just as readily lost as work skills. Communities should plan job oppor-tunities for subnormals. In the Netherlands, for example, industries with more than fifty employees must, by law, em-ploy 2 per cent. of handicapped persons, including the mentally subnormal.

All facilities need to be closely integrated, not only as be-tween the various professions interested in the rehabilitation of the mentally retarded but also as between local and national governmental bodies and the different agencies of government, such as health, social welfare, education, vocational rehabilita-tion, and employment.

CONCLUSION

The public health approach to mental subnormality is providing one of the greatest challenges to present-day medi-cine. Progress is being made in all of the fields of research, prevention, detection, and rehabilitation. The role of the medical profession, in this area of human responsibility, merges with a large number of other professions; and many organs of government are involved other than Departments of Health. However, the medical profession has a primary responsibility to locate families-at-risk, pregnancies-at-risk, and infants-at-risk at as early a stage as possible and institute preventive measures, arrange genetic counselling, and initiate therapeutic follow-up, which may need to extend through life-time. There is need to gear the medical profession as a whole to an understanding of subnormality, arrange adequate maternal and child-health detection programmes, and carry this on through school medical services. The medical profession, except where it is responsible for severe subnormals in institutions, gradually become less involved with age, and adjunctive to educationalists. The degree to which the latter will enter into institutional care, as with the defectologists in Russia, will be determined in time. While one must recognize the different social means for obtaining the same ends, there is needed, most of all, the collection of comparable data for the definition and prevalence of subnormality on an international basis, so that aspects of different social systems can be meaningfully assessed and public health programmes accordingly improved on a world-wide basis.

FURTHER READING

Carter, C. H. (1965) *Medical Aspects of Mental Retardation*, Springfield, Ill.

Clarke, A. D. B., and Clarke, A. M., eds (1965) *Mental Deficiency: The Changing Outlook*, 2nd ed., London.

Craft, M. (1967) A comparative study of facilities for the retarded in the Soviet Union, United States and United Kingdom, in *New Aspects of Mental Health Services*, ed. Freeman. H., and Farndale, S., Chap. 11, Oxford.

Craft, M., and Miles, L. (1967) *Patterns of Care for the Subnormal*, Oxford.

Department of Health and Social Security (1971) *Better Services for the Mentally Handicapped*, London, H.M.S.O.

Eichenwald, H. F., ed. (1968) *Proceedings of the Conference on Prevention of Mental Retardation through Control of Infectious Disease at Cherry Hill, N.J.*, 1966, Bethesda.

Frankenstein, C. (1970) *Impaired Intelligence. Pathology and Rehabilitation*, New York.

Hilliard, L. T., and Kirman, B. H. (1965) *Mental Deficiency*, 2nd ed., London.

Jackson, C. H. (1970) *They Say My Child's Backward: A Guide to the Understanding and Development of Backward Children for Parents, Educationalists, Psychologists and Others*, London.

Kanner, L. (1964) *A History of the Care and Study of the Mentally Retarded*, Springfield, Ill.

Luria, A. R. (1963) *The Mentally Retarded Child*, Oxford.

Morris, Pauline (1969) *Put Away. A Sociological Study of Institutions for the Mentally Retarded*, London.

Oster, J., and Sletved, H. V. (1964) *Report of the International Copenhagen Congress on the Scientific Study of Mental Retardation*, Copenhagen.

President's Panel on Mental Retardation (1962) *Report of the Mission to Denmark and Sweden*, Washington.

President's Panel on Mental Retardation (1962) *Report of the Mission to Russia*, Washington.

Stevens, H. A., and Heber, R., eds (1964) *Mental Retardation*, Chicago.

Tizard, J. (1964) *Community Services for the Mentally Handicapped*, London.

World Health Organization Expert Committee on Mental Health (1968) Organization of services for the mentally retarded, *Wld Hlth Org. techn. Rep. Ser.*, No. 392.

32

THE PROMOTION OF GOOD MENTAL HEALTH

KENNETH SODDY

The concept of mental health, like that of health in general, has proved elusive; but interest in the promotion of good mental health has increased very greatly in many parts of the world during the last two decades. In its development, mental health work has followed a similar path to that taken by public health perhaps two generations earlier. That is, the major emphases have appeared, successively, on: (1) recognition of mental disease and its control by methods of segregation; (2) eradication of aetiological factors by environmental sanitary measures; (3) direct attack on disease processes by refined treatment methods; and (4) more general prophylactic and rehabilitatory measures, together with concern about quality of living.

The constitution of the World Health Organization adopted in 1947 included the statement that 'health is a state of complete physical, mental, and social well-being and not merely the absence of disease or infirmity'. This statement implies that health has a positive, vital quality that not only transcends both resistance to disease and powers of quick recovery, but goes further, to impart zest to life.

A similar positive attitude has become more explicit in mental health thinking in recent years, though it is not new, having been implicit in the intentions of Clifford Beers and his associates when they pioneered the mental hygiene 'movement' in the 1920s and 1930s in the United States and a few other countries.

Since those early days organized mental health work has spread all over the world, stimulated during the 1950s by the World Federation for Mental Health and fostered by the World Health Organization. But whereas Clifford Beers and his fellow pioneers were concerned mainly with the second phase of the historical sequence noted above, the great technical advances of the immediate pre- and post-war periods enabled rapid progress through the third into the fourth phase. Modern interest in this field now concentrates upon the 'positive' aspects of the mental health idea.

In the case of a complex abstraction like mental health it is more useful to develop operational descriptions than to attempt precise definition. A good starting point for discussion is the inclusion of 'mental well-being' in the World Health Organization definition of health, as an equal partner with physical and social well-being; but 'well-being' is by no means the same as 'health'.

The International Preparatory Commission of the Third International Congress of Mental Health in London, 1948, in its publication *Mental Health and World Citizenship*, attempted a definition of mental health which included the following points:

'1. Mental health is a condition which permits the optimal development—physical, intellectual, and emotional—of the individual, so far as this is compatible with that of other individuals.

'2. A good society is one that allows this development to its members while at the same time ensuring its own development and being tolerant towards other societies.'

Before and since this time many definitions have been attempted, none with complete success. More progress has been made through the elucidation of points that contribute towards a more complete understanding of the condition. For example, in his book *The Fear of Freedom*, Fromm introduced the idea of the dependence of mental health upon the satisfaction of tendencies which must be satisfied if the individual is to remain mentally healthy, including growth and the realization of potentialities in common with those of others. Rümke (1955) added the further dimension of the value system—that the individual needs to realize tendencies common to humanity to develop a value system that transcends the individual.

In 1950 the present author developed the concept that a mentally healthy person can meet without strain all normal environmental situations, that absence of strain characterizes his response to life, generally, although he possesses the capacity to meet stressful situations. Additional items of description were that the mentally healthy person's ambitions are within the scope of practical realization; he has a shrewd appreciation of his own strengths and weaknesses; he can be helpful but can also accept aid. He is resilient in failure and level headed in success. He is capable of friendship and of aggressiveness when necessary. His pattern of behaviour has consistency, so that he is 'true to himself', and no one about him will feel that he makes excessive demands on his surroundings; his private beliefs and personal values are a source of strength to him.

Rümke pointed out that the above catalogue of mental health items can apply only to mature people. The factor of development is left out of account. To this justified criticism might be added another, that the description can apply only to those cultures in which such qualities as capacity for adaptation, for friendship, 'legitimate' aggression, and consistency are valued, which is by no means everywhere. For example, the quality of friendship that is prized where Confucius is revered, where there is an emphasis laid on non-attachment, may be very different from that in a Christian society. In an orthodox Buddhist society, aggression can never be 'legitimate'. Or again, in a strictly Hindu society passive submission to fate rules out ambition, and a belief in reincarnation makes qualities such as consistency and trueness to oneself as of little value.

The above examples illustrate the importance of considering mental health from the angle of the community as well as from that of the individual; indeed, it is now generally agreed that not only can no sharp distinction be drawn between the mental health of the individual and that of the community but they are largely interdependent. Some contributors (e.g. Jahoda, 1958) have championed a more 'positive' approach—to seek out and enhance if possible those individual and community factors which contribute to personality strength and harmonious development. Others have concentrated more upon the identification and removal of harmful factors, which is the classical prophylactic approach (see Caplan, 1961); Ackerman in this volume has written about 'positive' mental health as being dynamic rather than static, 'maintained only by continuous striving and the emotional support of others is needed to keep it'.

Our concerns here are to seek to recognize what mental health is, and to find techniques and social practices that can promote it. The most important common ingredient in the studies that have appeared is good interpersonal relationships, and it is clear now, also, that the actual style or conduct of life that results in good human relations is determined largely by community values, aspirations and way of life. Therefore, it is most important to learn more about the relevance of cultural factors, so that mental health work may rest on principles that are valid not only within the confines of a limited social group.

It has been suggested that one of the first conditions for mental health of the individual is a capacity to enter into interpersonal relationships that are appropriate to the community. A second condition might be that the development of the individual should harmonize with the pattern that is characteristic of the society. This is not to suggest that the mature individual must necessarily conform strictly to the pattern of his society, but that during the development period the individual is more likely to be mentally healthy if his pattern of development is acceptable in the community, or rather, in the narrower family setting.

Let us consider further the two points made by the International Preparatory Commission of 1948:

Optimal Development. In a study of middle age Soddy with Kidson (1967) suggested a conceptual analogy to facilitate understanding of individual development. This analogical model represents the individual as a 'chariot' drawn by a large number of 'horses' attached by long elastic traces, each 'horse' representing an aspect of bodily or mental development, e.g. long bones, verbal reasoning, the reproductive system, etc. These 'horses' are of different speeds and strengths, and they run at various speeds at different times of life, e.g. the sex 'horse' runs quickly and strongly around the turn of puberty, but comparatively slowly between the ages of 6 and 11 years. The 'horses' do not always run exactly in the same direction, and this may unsettle the 'chariot', especially during early childhood before the 'driver' (the ego) has learnt how to direct the 'horses'.

The analogy allows for the development of some personalities more rapidly and others more slowly; some reach a higher level of development than others; and the various aspects of personality may develop at different speeds during successive stages of life. Where the 'horses' are not too dissimilar in speed and strength, the passage of the 'chariot' is likely to be smoother

and more stable than when the traction is not well balanced. An outstandingly strong 'horse' pulling off-course may cause a deviation of the whole personality.

But it would be insufficient to consider the traction of the chariot without equally considering the nature of the road, which may be uphill, level, or downhill; rough or smooth; wide and straight or narrow and tortuous; congested or otherwise. School life or learning a new job might be regarded as an uphill period requiring all the strength of the 'horses'; unhappy family life or disappointment and difficulty at work might be a rough 'road'; and a highly demanding or competitive school or community attitude a narrow tortuous route requiring all the skill of the 'driver'.

The Good Society. Expressed in simple terms, among the characteristics of a 'good' society is provision for a wide range of human potentiality and for the satisfaction of all instinctual drives in ways that are acceptable to the community. Would a rather primitive society of simple construction, in which life is strictly regulated according to a narrow pattern of permitted behaviour, be eligible for consideration as a 'good society'? It is commonly believed that people in a simple and rather rigid society live happy, contented, and carefree lives, and on the whole this may be true. Certainly the possibility of making a choice between two or more alternatives and the necessity to bear responsibility are among the more potent causes of anxiety among human beings. There is evidence that where behaviour is regulated by convention, whether this be religious, political, social, or a simple belief that there is only one correct way of doing anything, life tends to be less complicated and people on the whole less anxious than where people are constantly faced with making decisions.

But the crucial question in determining whether a given society is a 'good' society is, perhaps, not so much the happiness or freedom from anxiety of people, but what is the attitude of society to the individual or group that does not conform to the behaviour demanded there? What happens to the mentally retarded or otherwise handicapped person; or to the individual possessed of unusual capacities or drives that are not provided for within the social convention; or to the eccentrics and to people of unusually high ability, in such a society? In other words, the capacity of a society to provide for a wide range of human potentiality and to satisfy the aspirations which the society itself provokes largely determines whether it can be considered to be a society that is conducive to the mental health of its members.

In his study of child-rearing practices, Gorer in 1941 made twelve postulates which have been subsequently elaborated, but of which the last is of particular interest here in its original form: 'In a homogeneous culture the patterns of superordination and subordination, of deference and arrogance will show a certain consistency in all spheres from the family to the religious and political organisations; and consequently the patterns of behaviour demanded in all these institutions will mutually reinforce each other' (see Mead and Wolfenstein, 1955).

To return to the analogy—it may be seen how the way in which the 'chariot' runs over the 'terrain' during childhood, while the 'driver' is gaining control, may facilitate—or otherwise—the individual's development in respect of the community in which he lives. The result of childhood experiences, combined with the inherent qualities of the individual, can have a profound effect upon his or her capacity to live in society.

In *Men in Middle Life* (Soddy with Kidson, 1967) a four-point approach to biographical studies was suggested, with the objective of throwing light on individual career patterns, and personal and group relationships. The suggestion was four series of observations made simultaneously of the developmental pattern of the individual. This notion is theoretical in the present state of knowledge, but the underlying concept is worth application, so that a more fruitful style of inquiry might be set. These four sets of observations are as follows:

1. *Biological*—to show the biological norms—the physiological and psychological capabilities of the individual—as far as possible independently of culture. The observations might show the individual's potential capacity to make adaptive responses to the environment and his ceiling of attainment and learning.

2. *Cultural*—the socio-cultural expectations, norms and stereotypes, and the range of variation considered to be within normal limits in the society to which the individual belongs.

3. *Objective*—the actual levels of attainment and potential of the individual.

4. *Subjective*—the same range of observations as in (3) above, but made by the individual about himself—what he himself believes to be his levels of attainment and potential.

Studies of individuals along these four lines might enable some important further principles of individual and community mental health to be elucidated. The following hypothetical constructs are offered for consideration: (1) a high degree of concurrence between the above four sets of observations is associated positively with optimum mental health; but there may be a degree of concurrence above which tension diminishes, and aspirations and goal-seeking behaviour lessen; (2) wide divergences between biological fact and cultural expectations may cause stresses affecting the whole society; (3) wide divergences between the cultural and the objective data would indicate stress on the individual; complete conformity would tend to enervate the individual; and (4) wide divergences between the subjective series and any or all of the others would probably spell unhappiness and stress for the individual, and possibly a poor state of mental health.

Enough has been written here to illustrate the interdependence of individual and community mental health. To return to the question raised above—ought the society that narrowly controls the behaviour of its members to be considered a 'good' society in the sense used above? The answer must be in the negative, because such a society cannot possibly provide adequately for the wide range of human potential of its members. The effect of a controlling society is to enforce conformity between cultural expectation and objective attainments, (2) and (3) above. The two main possibilities are either that subjective feelings (4) will be at variance with the cultural and objective states, in which case the individual is subjected to frustration and stress; or that the degree of congruence will be so high that individual effort is enervated and potential will not be realized.

MENTAL HEALTH PROBLEMS

At this stage it will be valuable to identify some of the problems which arise among individuals and in communities, when mental health is less than optimal.

The Individual

Most of the signs of deficiency in individual mental health are reflections of inner stress, but their recognition as such naturally varies from society to society. In modern urban, industrial societies generally it may be said that these signs of inner stress do not indicate abnormality in themselves, rather they are exaggerations of normal behavioural phenomena of which everyone may be conscious at times. But when exaggerated beyond a certain degree, which differs by culture, or when in massive combination, these signs of inner stress may indicate failing mental health.

Decided change of established rhythms of life may be significant: e.g. loss of sleep or appetite, dissatisfaction with earlier beliefs, disillusionment with people, or the emergence of new and irrational beliefs. Some changes may be normal and can be expected during times of emotional stress or turmoil and during climacteric periods of life, such as adolescence and the menopause; but when there is apparently nothing to cause the change, it might have a serious significance. In addition, a wide range of anxiety phenomena may appear, e.g. excessive worry over trivial matters, preoccupation with minor physical ailments, such as indigestion or headaches, a sense of tension with no conscious meaning, inability to relax, a succession of physical ailments with no somatic pathological basis, or, in contrast, an unreasonable denial of the reality of illness, difficulty, threat, or danger.

Some common behavioural characteristics operate against harmonious living, e.g. the perfectionist egoist, who must be at the centre of the world, whose possessions are necessarily perfect, who must have things done exactly to his own pattern and cannot bear to be left out. Such an individual always feels that he is in the right, and, in case of dispute, that the other person is invariably in the wrong. Though it may be admitted that the stability and moral evolution of Western society may derive much from people who show mild degrees of perfectionism, such traits may operate against harmonious living in the environment and cause deterioration in interpersonal relationships when excessive, or when they are altering or gaining in strength in individual behaviour. Other common behaviour characteristics may have comparable significance; e.g. excessive shyness or inability to mix; excessive heartiness; lack of discrimination in relationships; miserliness or profligacy; melancholy or euphoria; bursts of terrific energy and inventiveness, or periods of unusual listlessness.

The question of the 'nervous breakdown' raises important social and cultural issues. In modern urban, industrial culture the term 'nervous breakdown' is often used euphemistically for an individual's failure to meet the demands that life is making upon him. When such a breakdown coincides with a period of obvious stress or heavy responsibility, society generally condones the behaviour and provides for it. When a breakdown occurs without obvious justification the attitude of society may be altogether less favourable. Yet from a strictly psychiatric point of view, over-work may be a symptom of a state of excessive and uncontrolled anxiety; and anxiety itself may accumulate when the individual is becoming less and less able to take decisions. A responsibility borne easily in a more balanced frame of mind may be associated with breakdown when the equilibrium is becoming disturbed.

A further range of phenomena has greater morbid significance, though not to a degree that is commonly considered as mental ill health. Here again, normal and near normal traits in excess or in massive combination may not only indicate failing mental health but also may cause disturbances of normal interpersonal relationships, provoking society attitudes that tend to undermine individual mental health. These traits include habitual aggressiveness, irritability, and belligerency; uncooperativeness, hostility, and unfriendliness; and abnormal shiftlessness and dependency. These traits may result from an emotional immaturity that reflects unfavourable reaction patterns dating from early childhood, and are prominent among those who drift into alcoholism or drug addiction; into unstable marriage relationships; and, for obvious reasons, into social problem formation, delinquency, and crime.

Contemporary urban, industrial societies generally regard as constituting more obvious mental disorder such phenomena as delusions, hallucinations, and utterly fantastic ideas; the morbid melancholy that may lead to suicide; the feverish activity of mania that can dissipate the savings of a life-time in a few weeks; utter withdrawal into immobility; and an insane sense of persecution which can lead to dangerous assault, even homicide, and, at least, to excessive litigiousness. These phenomena have in common a glaringly obvious unreality and unreasonableness, and they represent a serious collapse of mental health. Most modern societies also recognize social behaviour problems caused by serious inferiority of intelligence.

The Community

It has been suggested above that it is less useful to think of community mental health than to consider the style of community living that tends to promote the mental health of its members. Certain features of the style of community life may indicate the existence of stresses, interpersonal tensions, and other possible defects in the mental health of individuals. A mentally healthy individual has been described as having a capacity for harmoniousness of human relations, and it follows that a society of mentally healthy individuals is harmonious too. Of course, the harmoniousness of a community is affected by many factors, past and present, among which freedom from outside interference and exposure to outside threat are prominent. For example, it would not be reasonable to expect a community that had been ravaged by war and foreign occupation twice in living memory to display the same kind of harmoniousness and emotional balance which a community that had lived secure and undisturbed for 100 years might show.

It might be expected that a harmonious community would have a deeply rooted way of life which would need little explicit formulation, because its ideals and aspirations would be common to all of its members. Such a community would have a liberal constitution that is permissive rather than restrictive, and a religion and value systems that are enriching, and not merely formal and traditionalist. Community ways of resolving social tensions would be amicable and would

not inflict permanent harm on the weaker party, in a case of dispute.

Among the many possible indications of quality of mental health is the community attitude to minority groups and unpopular minority viewpoints. The questions may be asked whether disapproved minority attitudes are allowed expression and given the test of application to reality, or repressed and perhaps punished; and whether the attitude of the majority to elements that are regarded as antisocial is one of punishment and revenge seeking, or of a desire to treat, to cure, and to reassimilate? Other indications can be found in the class structure of the society—the attitude of all classes to the existing social order and to the distribution of wealth and poverty. Does the social order allow its less-privileged members to aspire to a position of greater social advantage? Are there groups in the community that live generation by generation in a state of protected privilege or superiority; or alternatively, are there community members who are kept permanently in an inferior position as 'second-class citizens'?

This last question is of particular mental health interest. It may be doubted whether any community or section of a community that is in continuous close contact with another community or section which it regards as inferior can escape the adverse consequences of the maintenance of such an attitude. Nor can the section treated as inferior escape evil consequences if they accept the relationship imposed on them.

The chief evil effect is that the maintenance of the oppressive relationship becomes an obsessional preoccupation on the one hand and its consequences a continuous degradation on the other. The very far-reaching question for mental health study here is the psychological motivation of the need to assume and maintain a position of superiority.

Another important indication of mental health in a society is the degree to which citizens themselves are free to study and consider objectively the social institutions of the community, including the prevailing religion, the political structure and the system of government; or to what extent are such studies and possible criticisms openly or tacitly forbidden? Are the social institutions themselves spontaneous or dependent on propaganda; and to what extent do they depend upon authority or tradition for their maintenance?

Community Mental Health Problems

We have suggested that a significant disturbance in individual behaviour, in the absence of an external cause, might indicate the existence of a mental health problem. The same criterion may usefully be applied to the community when there is an unfavourable change in existing patterns of behaviour and in the way of life generally, that cannot be attributed to a known cause.

Let us take for example certain types of change in public behaviour: some increase in rudeness, ill temper, or irritability; or more obvious signs of tension, in the emergence of new political, social, or industrial unrest. A deterioration in the attitude of the majority towards minority viewpoints, and especially in the treatment of minority groups in the absence of an external threat, could be important danger signals.

Sociologists have described a condition of social disorganization that can occur when changes are taking place in a community more quickly than the people can absorb change. This condition is one in which irrational and over-emotional attitudes flourish and unsatisfactory interpersonal relationships are widespread. One effect of social disorganization may be that people become less able to make the best of the resources that they have, often they tend to snatch at random solutions to problems, solutions that may be almost magical in character. There are swings towards magic and authoritarianism in religion and politics, and sometimes there are tendencies for outbursts of public rage to occur against a scape-goat. Thus a public leader may be violently overthrown in an atmosphere of vilification of the overthrown regime. Another important sign of social disorganization is apathy—willingness to give away central values of the culture for the sake of peace.

In the present state of knowledge it is only possible to speculate about the mental health significance of trends in community vital statistics. For example, falling marriage and fertility rates, together with an increasing incidence of divorce, in a society where divorce rates are not artificially held in check, might reflect an unfavourable state of interpersonal relations. A rise in the age at marriage coupled with an increase in the proportion of illegitimate babies born might indicate lack of confidence in that society in its own social institutions and stability.

A more definite indication of morbidity in mental health in a community would be given by the emergence in a society of strongly supported fanatical movements dominated by unreason, especially when accompanied by sharp increases of intolerance and by the claim that all goodness belongs to the movement and all evil to the rest of the world. Moreover, rigid adherence to what passes for good in the community coupled with total intolerance of other ways of life and value systems may indicate a condition of mental health that is as dangerous as the prevalence of recognized evil in the community. Bad crimes have been perpetrated, in all sincerity, in the name of accepted morality.

Since the Second World War there have been signs of social alienation among late teenagers and young people in their early twenties, mainly in industrialized urban areas of countries adversely affected by the war. Obviously such phenomena can appear only in societies where dissident ways of life and self-expression are not repressed, so that their social and mental health significance in different countries is complex and unclear.

This social alienation has taken a number of forms during the 1950s and 1960s, having in common some degree of separate identity formation and of rejection of traditional cultural values. As usually happens when a sub-group acquires a recognizable identity within a community, the behaviour of the young people most deeply involved has been rigid, unadaptable, and self-centred. Their refusal to continue with higher education or technical training, and to accept work, marriage, or child-rearing commitments has had varying effects in different countries, partly according to the reaction of society and affected not least by the climate. (It is not agreeable to live a 'hippy' life in a temperate climate in winter!)

Inevitably socially alienated youth has been caught up in activities which actually or are believed to influence conscious experience—taking various forms of marihuana, L.S.D., cerebral stimulants, tranquillizers, narcotics, and using 'psycheledic' visual and auditory stimulation and rhythmical trance stimulation. Among those with a more active personality pattern, socially disruptive behaviour of an anarchic protesting kind has been seen. As noted above, these tendencies to come out vociferously against actions and attitudes of government or other authority can only be expressed in a country where dissident behaviour is not driven underground.

Among those of less active disposition, perhaps a large majority of affected young people in Great Britain, 'drop-out' has been passive. They have drifted from job to job in casual, unskilled, or routine clerical employment, and from one casual group association to another in their 'pads'. Inevitably they have been exploited by unscrupulous people for their own ends, and their undernutrition and unhygienic conditions threaten public health.

It is too early to estimate the full impact on public mental health of these 'drop out' phenomena. The most serious problem appears to be that of motivation to live in society of those young people who follow a popularized Buddhist philosophy of non-attachment to material values and to other people, with nothing of devout Buddhist striving after spiritual values. It seems most unlikely that anyone who spends several years in the late teens and early twenties in a state of social alienation can adjust later to life in that society. A formidable problem of psychosocial attitude and handling appears to be building up.

Even before the days of sub-cultural alienation, published health statistics gave only doubtful evidence about mental morbidity in the community, and needed much qualification and correction. For example, it is well recognized that the amounts of minor illness in a community and absenteeism from work are closely connected with minor mental health difficulties and thus with public morale and general well-being. Unfortunately even in those countries where medical statistics are comprehensive, medical certification can give little guide to the incidence or prevalence of mental health problems. Comparatively few doctors have been trained in the accurate diagnosis of psychological difficulties, nor do current systems of terminology enable many such diagnoses to be recorded. Diagnoses of the order of influenza, the common cold, peptic ulcer, rheumatism, migraine, fatigue, and overstrain commonly mask an indisposition that relates essentially to an unfavourable emotional attitude of the patient. In addition to the effect of gaps in medical training in the field of psychological medicine, the effect of emotionally-determined public prejudice against mental disorders and maladjustments commonly results in doctors not using terms in public documents that reveal the true state of affairs.

These combined difficulties of terminology and medical training reduce the usefulness of statistics in the field of psychological medicine. The recognized prevalence of mental disorder, mental retardation, and emotional maladjustment depends mainly upon the diagnostic criteria in use in the community, and these, being heavily loaded with social attitude, differ not only in different epochs but also at different ages of people and in social classes. For example, what is permitted in public behaviour varies from generation to generation. Contemporary writings show that it was socially permissible for an eighteenth-century Englishman to shout and jump for joy, to weep when distressed, and to faint when in a moral dilemma. Men were socially permitted to kiss and embrace in public, and women to have the most violent of hysterical fits. The mid-nineteenth-century Englishman had to be much more controlled in his expression of emotionality, although public grief was considered seemly. Women were no longer socially permitted to have violent hysterical fits, but fainting was open to them, and also the pleading of a headache to avoid social embarrassment. In the mid-twentieth century a great deal of public control of emotionality is demanded of both sexes, and even fainting is out of fashion. Even during the last twenty-five years in Great Britain striking changes have occurred in the behaviour phenomena associated with psychotic, severe neurotic, hysterical, and psychosomatic illnesses; for example, crude hysterical paralyses are rare today, and extremes of violence in states of excitement, or of weakness and exhaustion not often seen, as compared with two generations ago.

If to the above considerations be added the fact that different styles of behaviour are demanded of people in different walks of life and at different ages, it will be seen that statistics concerning mental disorder, mental retardation, and emotional disturbances are likely to be unreliable. In those countries, and they are perhaps a majority, in which the certification of psychoses is carried out more for legal than for strictly medical reasons, mental illness statistics may be almost valueless for determining incidence and prevalence. A special difficulty concerning mental retardation statistics in a country with universal compulsory education is that schoolchildren are under the close scrutiny of teachers in a situation in which mental retardation is a serious handicap; but after leaving school, only the most seriously subnormal fail to find simple work where they can escape notice. Comparisons of mental retardation figures among schoolchildren and adults have shown that its presence is recognized perhaps five times as frequently among children of school age as among adults. This is an example of the kind of variation that makes mental disorder statistics hard to interpret in terms of the general population.

It is often hoped to glean mental health data from alcoholism and drug addiction, suicide, crime and delinquency rates, and so on. A common difficulty of all available records within this range is that they depend first of all on compilation by police or other agencies, so that in fact they may not reflect the actual prevalence of the phenomena as closely as the community attitude towards such behaviour, i.e. the degree to which the community will take steps to control and prevent it. In general, it may be summed up that such statistics rarely have value on their own, but if maintained over a number of years in a consistent way, pronounced variations and persistent trends can give valuable information, provided that proper care is taken in interpretation.

Some Principles Governing Mental Health Work

On theoretical grounds it may be anticipated that the degree of success attained by measures designed to improve mental health depends mainly on the quality of active participation of the people concerned. Before mental health work is likely to be acceptable in a given community, people need to know what it is about and to feel that what is aimed at is desirable.

A second condition of success is that the society involved must possess some capacity to assimilate change. In societies in which life is lived in rigid and traditional ways, its influential members scarcely question the practices of the society, and

ordinary people live exactly as tradition demands. Under such circumstances the concept of mental health cannot become an articulate aspiration of ordinary people. Either they live their lives in the correct (i.e. traditional) way or they do not; and if the latter, society will regard them as in error, or even delinquent. It is only when society is showing some tendency to change, some degree of adaptation to new circumstances, that any improvement of mental health can become a realizable aspiration, or indeed, any concept of mental health can be formed.

A third condition of success is that people must be able not only to conceive what mental health may be but also to perceive ways in which the ideal can be approached. In practical terms a proposed mental health programme must appeal to ordinary people as sensible and practicable, and not appear to be merely an idealistic dream.

A fourth condition of success is that people in the community should trust those who are introducing the programme of mental health work. Perhaps it is best introduced by a well-known member of the community, and in any case it is essential that those responsible have a thorough knowledge of and respect for the cultural pattern in which they are working.

The receptiveness of ordinary people to mental health work varies greatly under different conditions and at different times of life, and generally the greatest chance of success lies among people who are conscious of a need for help. It is tactically sound for the mental health worker to seek to define those periods in which people are most receptive to the ideas that are being introduced. One obvious period, for example, would be during the first pregnancy of a young mother, when she may feel that she has been caught up in new experience which is beyond her control. She will be more than usually receptive to skilled help while in that mood. Generally it is sound to introduce mental health work to a new district by centring it on the family, and on children and youth. Other mental health projects tend to develop more soundly from the base of aid given to people in the problems of family life.

THE ORGANIZATION OF
MENTAL HEALTH WORK

It is convenient to discuss mental health projects divided into areas in which there is some unity of concept and practical method; for example: prophylaxis; public education and counselling; definable periods of life; family needs; and social spheres. Each area presents a wide field of opportunity about which we have space for no more than a short comment.

Prophylaxis

It would be logical to base mental health prophylactic measures on eugenic principles, but scientific knowledge about heredity has up to now been insufficient for the formulation of policies. In fact, precise knowledge is currently limited to the inheritance of a few rare somatic diseases and deformities. The various broad psychological characteristics of different people, e.g. introversion or extroversion, over-activity or under-activity, high intelligence or low intelligence, and so on, are complex combinations of many ill-defined genetic factors, and all require interaction with the environment in order to reach full development.

It is a rough approximation that the inheritance of these broad personality traits resembles that of graded polymorphic body characteristics, that is, the offspring inherit the parental average, but because of the complexity of the factors, not reliably and often not recognizably so.

Folk lore and tradition, in the case of most societies, have formulated stringent regulations or taboos about, for example, consanguinity in marriage. These may be regarded as crude prophylactic attempts against the development of mental illness among members of later generations. The length to which such attempts have gone is illustrated in the Korean law which forbade a man and woman bearing the same family name to marry, however far back the common ancestor might be. This law was apparently based on a genetic theory of the causation of mental illness, but it has only curiosity value today because it took only the male, and not the female, line of descent into account.

In societies where marriage is by the partners' own free choice, the influence of inheritance on personality of offspring is obscured also by the likelihood that congeniality of temperament is a decisive factor. This means that not only do the spouses resemble each other in personality, but they will also provide a style of life and family atmosphere in which their children grow up which resembles that of their own families of orientation. Thus environmental influences cannot be disentangled from genetic; and further, decisive evidence is rarely to be found because possession of an extreme temperamental variant is likely to be incompatible with marriage and procreation.

It follows that there is insufficient knowledge to enable a choice of mate to be made with a view either to strengthening family mental health or to avoiding mental illness, with the possible but controversial exception of the case of cyclothymia. Some rare forms of epilepsy, and of structural anomaly and of neurone degeneration are inheritable, but otherwise little is known about the genetics of mental disease. Popular belief inculpates cousin marriages, but though evidence suggests some reduction in fertility, it is inconclusive in relation to mental traits. Nor is there any exact information about the effects of parental ill health, alcoholism, etc., before conception, apart from some evidence that associates some maternal virus infections and excessive hot weather during early pregnancy with foetal brain anomalies. The increase of harmful mutations through parental exposure to ionizing radiation is a modern preoccupation of which due note must be taken, in relation to both men and women during the reproductive period.

Certain psychological and social problems occur in clusters in some families, and tend to follow the association of two or more of various factors, for example low intelligence, excessive excitability, emotional imbalance, and physical ill health. Such clustering may give a false impression of the operation of hereditary factors; whereas the true cause is a vicious circle mechanism. Individual incompetence may result in disadvantageous living conditions with which incompetent individuals cannot cope. Thus, family problems may be perpetuated and recur in successive generations.

A vicious circle giving a false impression of heredity can often be seen, also, when the care of children has been interrupted at formative periods, to the impoverishment of their capacity to form stable, loving interpersonal relations for themselves. In due course their own marriage problems and unsatisfactory emotional ties with their own children may transmit the difficulties to the third generation. In no case is this seen more clearly than in the well-recognized tendency for women born illegitimately themselves to have illegitimate children.

The great dream of eugenics to contribute to the welfare of Mankind by introducing some control of reproduction, on the one hand by encouraging the fitter and, on the other, restricting those who may carry psychosocial disorders, has proved unrealizable. Thus it would be prudent from an eugenic standpoint, for example, for an individual to procreate only at times of physical and mental well-being, to avoid marriage with a member of a family in which psychosocial problems are clustered, not to be pregnant during very hot weather or during an epidemic of rubella, and to be exposed to as little ionizing radiation as possible. Also, it would be eugenically advantageous to reduce fertility among the lowest 10 per cent. on the socio-economic scale of the population, which provide perhaps two-thirds of the known psychosocial problems in the community, and whose birth rate is significantly higher than average. But how to take effective public action in these various respects without unacceptable interference with individual liberty is an unsolved problem.

Two forms of public action, namely, euthanasia and sterilization, have been widely advocated in the past, but their advocacy raises strong, even violent, emotional reactions on moral and humanitarian grounds. They deserve brief discussion from the medical and mental health points of view—without entering into religious and moral considerations.

Because of extreme difficulty in determining which cases have no chance of recovery, there can be very few reliable indications for euthanasia in the fields of mental illness and emotional disorder as distinct from mental subnormality. In some cases of chronic, deteriorated psychosis it may become apparent that the patient's inability to cope with even the simplified life of the mental hospital may be the chief cause of his misery. The compassionate doctor may feel that death would be merciful and might adopt a reserved attitude towards radical life-preserving measures.

Sterilization of the mentally ill or disturbed has been abused from time to time for racist motives, but this does not alter the fact that there are certain individual cases in which sterilization may be beneficial. There are insufficient grounds for action on the basis of the risk of direct transmission of disease. The major issue is the effect of further procreation of children on the health, including the mental health, of the individual, which question needs to be considered in the broader context of the parental functioning of the individual.

The decision is often complicated by sexual guilt of the individual acting as a precipitating factor of the illness, so that sterilization must never be advocated without a thorough study of the psychopathology of each case. This is particularly important whenever sterilization is proposed in order to alleviate a chronic social problem, for example, that of an emotionally disturbed woman who has a succession of illegitimate children whom she abandons or fails to look after properly. It may be felt preferable to offer sterilization as an alternative to some form of social restraint (which it may be difficult to apply). It needs to be borne in mind that sterilization tends to increase rather than decrease the individual's need for psychosocial assistance.

The more radical measure of castration (orchidectomy) offered in some countries, notably Denmark, as a voluntary alternative to imprisonment for persistent serious sexual offenders is still controversial and has no volume of support in the United Kingdom.

Turning now to mental subnormality, euthanasia is commonly advocated in the case of severely retarded newborn babies; but it is essential to be clear about what it is hoped to achieve. The value of euthanasia in this instance is to be found only in the alleviation it may bring to a very severe family problem, there can be no effect on the incidence of mental subnormality in the next generation. The babies affected by the decision have no prospect of procreating children themselves if they live.

The application of euthanasia to subnormal babies is strictly limited to those few babies about whom it is possible to make a firm diagnosis of severe deficiency within a few hours of birth, i.e. those with obvious gross bodily deformity. Even the most experienced diagnostician needs to watch the baby's development for perhaps six months before committing himself to a diagnosis of severe subnormality in the absence of marked physical signs.

Undoubtedly the advocacy of euthanasia for severely subnormal babies is fraught with acute emotional as well as moral problems. Not the least is the parents' reaction to their baby, their shock, grief, and guilt and, in many cases, their psychological need to make atonement for the birth of a handicapped child. The handling of the psychological issues involved requires skill and care.

The voluntary sterilization of the mentally subnormal is an important social issue, but, like euthanasia, its value has to be judged—medically speaking—from the angle of alleviation of social problems rather than from that of eugenics and the reduction of incidence in later generations.

Expressed in the briefest terms, mental subnormality has a three-fold origin:

1. Very rarely as the effect of the direct transmission of a single gene defect.

2. As the lower end of the scale of distribution of mental abilities in the population.

3. As a result of malformation or damage causing impairment of brain development of the foetus or child.

Sterilization of all subnormals in group 1 would involve numbers too small to make any numerical difference; and group 3 into which about one-quarter of all subnormals fall, has no hereditary significance. Group 2 comprises something of the order of 1 per cent. of the whole community. It is a clinical and social impression that perhaps as much as three-quarters of its members are to be found in the families in the lowest socio-economic decile.

It is a crude approximation, therefore, that about half of the cases of mental retardation in the next generation will be found among these bottom decile families, which have a fertility rate significantly above the population average. However, the fertility rate of recognized subnormals is very low and sterilization restricted to this group would have no appreciable effect on prevalence.

Sterilization of the entire bottom decile on the socio-economic scale—obviously impossible on many grounds—might halve the prevalence of mental subnormality in the next generation, but would also deprive the community of some 10 per cent. of its potential children who, though scattered towards the lower end of the intelligence scale, would have been within the range of normality.

Sterilization of subnormals must be judged at a casework and not at an eugenic level. It has two main applications: first, to the not uncommon case of the man or woman who is capable of sustaining a permanent love relationship with a potential spouse but who, in agreement with the other party, is conscious of inability to take responsibility for bringing up children; or in another case, any additional children. Secondly, voluntary sterilization may be appropriate where social restraint is not desirable or not practicable, or where ordinary measures of social supervision fail to prevent the procreation of unwanted children for whom the parents do not take responsibility. Sterilization is never a substitute for measures of social care of subnormals, but it may make a useful contribution to the alleviation of social problems.

In view of the generally negative character of eugenic measures it is a more important contribution to mental health at the present time to ensure that the circumstances in which children are brought up are optimal for their future development. Perhaps the most important single controllable prophylactic mental health factor in the procreation of children is that marriages should be contracted spontaneously on the grounds of congeniality and mutual regard, so that the emotional atmosphere of the home may be stable and satisfying to the children.

Gestation and the Perinatal Period

The period of life surrounding the conception and birth of a child is peculiarly appropriate for mental health work because of the need which parents may feel for help in a situation that is beyond their control. The degree to which there is a felt need for help in this period can be judged from the enormous number of often conflicting ways of bringing up children that are advocated, and the amount of advice that is freely offered on all sides. Fashions come and go quickly in this field.

The need for a helping service has been greatly accentuated during the second half of the twentieth century by advances in medical knowledge about risks and dangers to health of mother and child from the late effects of influences and happenings during pregnancy and the confinement. The scope and importance of preventive mental-health work during this period has been greatly increased. For example: it is now recognized that exposure to rubella infection or ionizing radiation early in pregnancy may result in the birth of a severely damaged child; parental blood incompatibility can be detected and its effects largely controlled; foetal chromosomal abnormalities can be detected early in pregnancy with a reliability of above 90 per cent; very small premature babies can be saved from death by artificial means; and other severely brain-damaged children kept alive.

Wonderful though these spectacular advances in medical techniques have been, they have also increased the need for enlightened counselling help to be available for parents, who may be faced not only with added burdens of anxiety because many of these difficulties can be seen in advance but also with the problem of bringing up a very seriously handicapped child who, a generation before, would not have survived early infancy.

In formulating mental hygiene policies in regard to perinatal work, it needs to be borne in mind that, in modern industrialized countries at least, very little of parental behaviour is determined spontaneously by instinct. During the last 100 years there has been a steady tendency towards artificiality, as knowledge of scientific principles of hygiene and nutrition has increased. Older traditional ways of baby care have given way to more scientifically worked out methods that have resulted in such fashions as scheduled feeding and highly organized schemes of care, of which the Mothercraft system was an outstanding example.

During the last twenty-five years there has been a considerable revolt against artificiality, which has resulted in a widespread return to older practices of feeding more by the demand of the child, and to so-called natural childbirth and rooming-in —i.e. the nursing of the newborn baby in the same room as the mother by day, which has been a popular development of the post-war period in the United States. In the United Kingdom, where a far higher number of confinements take place in the home, such movements have not had the same impact, but here too there has been a general move towards greater spontaneity of parental behaviour.

The interest of mental hygiene in the perinatal period overlaps considerably with that of public health, and for this reason it is important to secure that public health doctors and nurses should be trained to undertake counselling from a mental hygiene point of view. It is particularly important that people who are engaged in this field should understand the principles of social case work, which rely not so much on giving advice to the patient as upon helping the individual to move towards a solution of his own problems, himself. To do this successfully requires an attitude in the counsellor that is different from that of the advice that has traditionally been given in public health clinics. It also requires a willingness to spend a good deal of time in helping an individual to arrive at an appraisal of his own situation and in seeing how to remedy it [see also CHAPTER 34].

Infancy and the Pre-school Period

The interest of mental hygiene in infancy and the pre-school period overlaps with that of the Maternity and Child Welfare Services, and it is important that the latter should be so structured as to take care adequately of the mental health needs of families with young children. The type of problem involved includes the various feeding and habit-training difficulties which are encountered in the first two years of life and the behaviour and psychosomatic difficulties of toddler children, such as temper tantrums, night terrors, undue inhibition, tics, thumb-sucking, nail biting, problems of discipline, asthma, toilet training and so on.

For success in tackling these problems it is usually best to employ a counselling approach, and a counsellor needs to be thoroughly conversant with the social attitudes of the population in which he is working and to understand the ways in which interpersonal relationships in the home are developing. The work will be best based on social case work principles and

it is important to integrate these into the existing Maternity and Child Welfare Services as far as appropriate.

Schoolchildren

Mental health work among schoolchildren can be divided roughly into two broad categories: the first and more general is the need for suitable education to be provided in a positive and constructive way, which is also the concern of the School Psychological Service. The second category includes the more specifically therapeutic needs of the child in emotional difficulties.

It is the function of the School Psychological Service to promote educational measures based on understanding of the psychological needs of children, including appropriate styles of education for children both of superior and of inferior ability, and for the wide range of handicapped children. This involves efficient selection of children for the various types of education that may be available, and study of the individual problems of children who do not fit into the mass programme. Each stage of schooling should be seen by the children to lead on naturally and in an unbroken manner to the next stage.

The system in the United Kingdom of segregating about one-fifth of children aged 11 years plus in a superior stream of education, in 'grammar schools', has been superceded in most parts of the country by 'comprehensive' schools, in intermediate and senior divisions, to cater for pupils between 11 and 19 years of age. These schools may present mental hygiene problems by their size and complexity, the strain they may place upon less adaptable children, and discouragement of the less ambitious. They also do not provide well for the needs of more sparsely populated areas. They involve children in long journeys and in participation in an artificial community life divorced from that of their families.

Children in the lowest five percentiles of ability have been provided for in special classes or schools for educationally subnormal children. Children below a conventional Intelligence Quotient level of 50 have been sent to Junior Training Centres conducted until 1970 by the local health authority, but since that time integrated with the school system by the educational authority. E.S.N. schools provide a somewhat simplified education at a slower pace of learning than the normal. Schools for the severely subnormal concentrate on imparting simple skills in daily group living, and the acquisition of work skills that may keep the individual occupied and to some extent self-supporting.

The more specific mental health needs of schoolchildren cannot be adequately disposed of in a few sentences, but it is very important to reiterate that there should be understanding of children's psychological needs by teachers. Children carry into school with them attitudes developed in their family life, and it is important, too, that there should not be a gulf between home and school. Children with special educational difficulties may need remedial teaching, and particular attention must be paid to the emotional needs of handicapped children, including the handicap of an unfavourable emotional attitude to school. Mental hygiene work needs to be closely integrated with the school medical, nursing and psychological services, for the ascertainment of individual children's needs, for smooth integration with therapeutic services, and for the general supervision of special educational measures [see also CHAPTER 35].

Adolescence and Youth

Much is written and talked today about the needs of youth, and it must be conceded that in a rapidly changing society that is undergoing increasing technological development, the problems of youth are many and varied. The period of greatest difficulty is that just before and after school-leaving age, until the young people have become thoroughly integrated in employment and adult society. Adolescents commonly feel that they do not properly belong either to childhood society or to the adult society around them, and they tend to organize spontaneously in ways which earn the disapproval of society. This problem is common to all urbanized industrial cultures and is the presenting sign of a broad sociological problem briefly discussed above.

Among the cavalcade of teenage and youth phenomena seen successively in the United Kingdom since the early 1950s —teddy boys, beatniks, mods and rockers, hippies, flower children, tribes, and so on—a common factor appears to have been a search by the young for an identity of their own, coupled with varying degrees of protest. But the clarity of definition of these phenomena as social problems has derived as much from adult reactions as from adolescent unrest.

The themes expressed variously by these groups seem to have had in common some degree of refusal to enter into adult society in the way that their seniors expected. Thus, teddy boys appear to have attempted to deny adult sexual responsibility, and beatniks to refuse to take a defined place in society. Mods and rockers, on the other hand, appear to have acted out an intermittent and transient power fantasy in their highly mobile groups in contrast to their static prospects in real life. More recent manifestations have been directed against aggression and have stressed peace, love, and 'togetherness'.

The chief appeal of these various movements has been to the less well-educated or technically trained youth, who are largely not aware of or will not look at the prospects that modern society can offer. It would contribute to a solution if it could be made plainer to the young people how their present stage of life is leading towards the fulfilment of their hopes and aspirations. Adequate technical training for their future needs and opportunities to pursue progressive careers will resolve much of the difficulty over teen-age behaviour. The problem is most intractable in the case of unskilled workers, among whom 'blind alley' occupations form an important part of juvenile employment. The solution to adolescent problems demands the tackling of such practices in industry; but a great deal can be done by a broad programme of youth work, social clubs, and other similar activities. Here mental hygiene overlaps with the general social services of the community, and careful integration is needed [see also CHAPTER 37].

During the second half of the 1960s some social 'drop outs' appeared among teenagers in the higher education group. The origin appears to have been similar to the above, namely, difficulties and uncertainties about gaining university and technical college places. This has led to a passive withdrawal from the 'ratrace', and a search for a separate identity not dependent on winning adult approval.

Among some who succeed in entering university, a more active reaction to the insecurity of the past and uncertainties of the future has been seen. In a number of countries university students are demanding a greater share in their own management. It is not clear yet whether a sense of identity as a student can have the durability that would enable any stable system to be built up on these lines.

Drug dependence is a mental hygiene problem of a different order, which has come into prominence in the later 1960s. During 1967 legislation was introduced to canalize the treatment of 'hard' drug addicts into certain designated hospital clinics. Although this system may have resulted in a tighter control of maintenance prescriptions, it has dispensed with the services of general practitioners, many of whom had a deep knowledge of the needs of the people concerned. It is yet to be seen whether the mental health aspects of this problem are more adequately taken care of by clinics.

The parallel, but not necessarily related problems of 'soft' drug taking—cannabis, amphetamine and their analogues, L.S.D., and so on—remain highly controversial. There is little agreement about how far these drugs create dependency, and opinions vary also about their destructive effect—some authorities maintain that 'soft' drugs do less damage than alcohol or the motor cycle, while others claim that as many as one in seven of 'soft' drug users go on to 'hard' drugs eventually.

Among such conflicting views, the proper organization of mental health work is obscure. There is general agreement that the 'soft' drug problem has much in common with that of youth in search of a distinctive identity, perhaps mainly because the latter are readily identifiable and therefore easily contacted as a potential market. In the author's view a very destructive social role is being played in this area, today, by the mass media of communication—television and radio, newspapers and magazines, the cinema, and the gramophone industry. All of these appear to have been sedulously building up the image and importance of these various teenage groupings, and thereby increasing their vulnerability. These are urgent mental health problems.

Marriage and Family Life

The mental health of the population depends particularly upon harmonious relationships within families, and the promotion of good relationships is an important preoccupation of mental health work. Mental hygiene projects should include broadly based programmes of public education for marriage and family life which need to start in the secondary school, where it is important that school-leavers should be introduced constructively to the prospect of establishing their own families. In a community in which perhaps the majority of teachers have no special, let alone expert, knowledge of human relations in the home or of sociological principles, the first mental health education task lies with the teachers themselves.

Marriage counselling can be helpful in cases of threatening marriage breakdown, provided that the counsellors are suitable people, adequately trained and available early enough in the problem. The success of a marriage counselling service depends largely upon the confidence which it enjoys locally, and in smaller communities the unavoidable use of local people as counsellors has obvious disadvantages, which may not be entirely overcome by making the service totally professionalized and thus more impersonal.

In the 1970s there is a great deal of public anxiety about the state and future of the institution of marriage, the publicizing of matrimonial difficulties, and the rising divorce rate. Anxiety about these matters and the plight of children from 'broken homes' has become a mental health problem of considerable magnitude. There appears to be a wide gap between the beliefs and assumptions of religious, moral, and political leaders, on the one hand, and the realities of interpersonal relationships in the modern so-called 'nuclear' family of Great Britain, on the other. This gap was spectacularly illustrated by the papal encyclical of 1968, which reaffirmed the denial of all so-called artificial methods of contraception to Roman Catholics. One of the great mental health needs of the age is for those who are charged with communication in the fields of theology and morality to arrive at a better level of understanding with those concerned with applied sociology, psychology and anthropology.

Middle Age

Only recently have there been signs of mental health interest in the problems of middle age, although the relatively high morbidity rates of the forties and fifties are a major source of medical concern. Relatively more is known about the problems of women in connexion with the end of the reproductive life, and it is now being increasingly realized that many difficulties previously ascribed to the menopause should be put down to changes in parental identity and role when the children become independent.

The problems of middle-aged men, similarly, are partly the outcome of changing identity and role, both in family life and in the community (Soddy with Kidson, 1967). In family life the middle-aged may commonly be in a pivotal position between the elderly and the rising generation, and to some extent burdened with the problems of both. In their life in the community the middle-aged are expected to provide both management functions and stability. It may be suggested that much of the stereotype of rigidity and incapacity to change and learn new things results from behaviour that is forced upon middle-aged people by their position in the middle. If the middle-aged change their pattern of life it could be seen by other members of the community as a threat to the traditional way of life and the stability of society. There is little objectively known about either the psychology or the physiology of men and women in middle life to suggest that rigidity and difficulty in learning is caused by other than cultural factors.

The difficulties which individuals may find in maintaining their position, with relatively declining abilities in later middle age, including in the case of many the necessity to keep up with or even compete with younger men and women are additional factors to make a middle-aged person rigid and controlling in behaviour. Another common difficulty of individuals in middle life is to keep the self-image truly objective. As discussed above, the subjective range of observations that an individual may make about himself may get seriously out of alignment with the objective. Questions of preparation for retirement and the effect of retirement policies may also loom large in a society in which the employment structure has become rigid.

The practice of a medical check-up in times of health is growing, and although not without some danger of increasing tendencies towards hypochondria, the introduction of a greater degree of sophistication on the mental health side of such assessments would be advantageous.

Old Age

The mental health of old people is the cause of great concern at the present time, particularly in view of the unduly high proportion of senile cases among the admissions to mental hospitals. A constant feature of senility is an increasing disorientation and loss of memory leading to social unreliability, which calls for a certain amount of supervision of old people. In Great Britain, where the size of the independent family group is small, the position of the senile person may be insecure because of lack or non-availability of any relative to exercise the necessary supervision. Often the only possible course is to transfer the old person to a mental hospital, other forms of institutional care not being available. This course is open to criticism on two grounds: first, much simpler measures of supervision of the old person short of deprivation of liberty may suffice; secondly, mental hospitals are not designed for the care and rehabilitation of old people. Many people consider that a grave social injustice is done by the practice of admitting senile patients to mental hospitals for the sole reason that there is nowhere else for them to go.

It is well recognized today that the disorientation to which old people are prone results mainly from the loosening by death or removal of relatives and friends of emotional ties with their present and immediate past, and that it is very important to preserve the symbols of the old person's links, as represented by possessions, furniture, a familiar locality, and so on. To move an old person from his home district, to separate him from his possessions and the company of familiar people cannot be justified from any point of view. This is what much of the current public policy regarding old people is doing.

There are formidable practical difficulties in doing what is right for old people. The ideal may be the provision of small residential communities with a flexible organization that can give the amount of privacy that the old person is used to, with facilities for married couples, and the use of communal feeding arrangements, house cleaning, and nursing provisions as far as the old people need. Such communities are expensive, and the staffing problems are very great.

As noted above, British families are characteristically small —autonomous 'nuclear' units composed of parents and young, dependent children. In this pattern of social organization it is imperative that parents prepare their children to leave the parental home at the latest by the early twenties. It follows that if old people become in need of care themselves it is commonly found that their relationships with their own grown-up children are not intimate enough to bear living together. Moreover, an old person who has brought up children in order to make them independent has usually a strong resistance to becoming dependent in his or her turn. The problem of the old person in a society composed of nuclear families can hardly be solved by stating that it is the duty of the next generation to look after its own old people in the home, and by hoping that such a principle can easily be made effective. This runs so far counter to the spontaneous development of society as to be impractical, and other solutions need to be looked for [see also CHAPTER 39].

Human Relations in Industry

The interest of mental hygiene in industry overlaps with that of occupational health. Mental hygiene is mainly concerned in industry with human relations, including problems of staff/management relations and staff interpersonal relationships. There are also questions of work incentives and congeniality and design of working operations. It has been a modern experience that mental health work in the field of industrial relations is often in danger of being identified by both staff and management with drives towards increased productivity, and thus tends to become politically controversial. For most men in industry and for a large number of women, their industrial life represents a major part of their total life experience, and the protagonists of mental hygiene hold that the principles of human relations need study in that setting just as in other aspects of human living.

In recent years mental health interest has extended to problems of increasing automation and the implications of shorter working hours. Unsolved problems include the satisfying use of the physical energies of the less intelligent when physical energy is less in demand, and the question of the boredom of a stationary occupation mainly concerned with monitoring instruments.

A new problem of wide social significance is that of the second or so-called 'spare-time' job, which shorter working hours are encouraging. In many families with young children the husband has two separate jobs, and the wife a part-time job in addition to running the home and caring for the children.

Experience has shown that mental health work in industry is more acceptable and has a greater chance of success if it starts as a spontaneous movement from within the industrial community itself. Therefore, in principle, specialized mental health workers in industry should be identified with the concern, and should owe loyalty to the group as a whole [see also CHAPTER 38].

General Welfare Measures, including Housing

This, again, is a very wide subject that can only be touched on here. The so-called Welfare State may be still controversial, but some effective form of organization of human welfare by society itself is necessary in a modern industrialized community with a nuclear family structure. The nuclear family can have only limited resources to take care of hardship through illness or accident, or caused by personality factors. It is frequently objected that the Welfare State undermines the independence and self-reliance of people, but it can be argued that welfare measures have been made necessary because the much-prized independence and self-reliance of the majority have reduced the support available for the dependency needs of the minority who cannot stand on their own feet.

The human problems of the increasingly artificial life of big industrial cities cannot be solved completely by general social measures, by securing an adequate standard of living for all people, and by satisfactory housing; but such measures can go a long way to alleviate those problems of interpersonal relationships that are exacerbated by economic insecurity, overcrowding, and lack of privacy. It must be recognized, however, that the people's needs differ very much in these regards among different social classes in the population [see also CHAPTER 5].

THE INSTRUMENTS OF MENTAL HEALTH WORK

The various techniques of mental health work in the community are carried out by a number of specialized agencies, both public and voluntary. A brief description of the main instruments of mental health work follows.

Child Guidance

Child guidance sets out to help children with their emotional and behavioural difficulties, by the use of interdisciplinary team-work of child psychiatrists, educational psychologists, and psychiatric social workers. Child guidance is organized in Great Britain in three main streams: (1) in the hospital services; (2) in the school health services; and (3) in the educational services. The reason for these divisions is largely historical and, in principle, the three streams are supposed to intermingle. In addition to its basic staff, a child guidance clinic should have the consultant services of a paediatrician and such other medical services as may be required. The clinic undertakes the diagnosis and treatment of various mental health problems, behaviour difficulties, psychosomatic illness, social and scholastic difficulties, delinquency, and so on. The clinic normally provides psychological treatment and remedial education for scholastic difficulties. In addition, ideally it should serve as a centre of mental hygiene work in the local community, and forge strong links with the school psychological service. Other natural allies of the child guidance clinic are the maternity and child welfare centre and the school health clinic. Some child guidance clinics also provide consultation services for juvenile courts, remand homes, schools for delinquent children, long stay hostels, orphanages, and other children's institutions.

At its origin in the first decade of this century, child guidance represented an attempt to improve upon the exclusively patient-centred approach which was current in psychiatry at the time, and which, in the sphere of childhood, had resulted in recognition of the existence of mentally defective and 'problem' children. Child guidance employed an ecological approach and was concerned with the child in his natural surroundings.

It is probably fair to say that specialized medical training in child psychiatry has not been adequate for the needs of the growing professional speciality, which has remained weak in its corpus of aetiological and psychopathological knowledge. One result has been dissatisfaction with established child guidance methods and a renewal of the attempt to approach the problem through the family. The establishment of family clinics brings the wheel of development round to its starting point again and leaves the subject still weak in its core of established knowledge and accepted practice.

Maternity and Child Welfare

It has long been realized that child guidance clinics are too cumbrous and too expensive to be applied to the great majority of growing-up problems that arise in ordinary families. There has been a significant movement in recent years for child guidance, maternity and child welfare and school health personnel to participate in each others' services both by clinical co-operation, and by mutual in-service personnel training schemes in the mental health of childhood and the application of mental health principles to work in the community [see also CHAPTER 34].

Mental Health Clinics

Mental health clinics in the community, like child guidance clinics, include out-patient psychiatric departments in general hospitals, specialized psychiatric clinics, and extramural clinics conducted by mental hospitals. It is being increasingly realized that much can be done by early out-patient treatment to take the burden off mental hospitals, in addition to the treatment of cases of neurotic and psychosomatic illness deemed suitable for out-patient psychiatric treatment. There is also an important responsibility for the follow-up and after-care of patients from mental hospitals. More and more, the mental health clinics of the community are providing facilities for social forms of treatment through social clubs and the like, and undertaking mental health educational work in their local districts.

The Psychiatric Hospital and Mental Health

Many writers have drawn attention to the growing role of the psychiatric hospital as a therapeutic community, and to the important effect of this on community attitudes now that mental hospital admission is nearly always informal. Great progress has been made in some parts of the country in reducing the isolation and impersonal character of mental hospitals. In some regions it is planned to do away altogether with old-fashioned and remote mental hospitals and to replace them with psychiatric wings of general hospitals. This is a commendable aim, provided it is always remembered that, unlike the general hospital, the social structure of the psychiatric hospital, its atmosphere and the style of life led by patients while in hospital are themselves essential therapeutic instruments, and need planning and conscious thought, like other medical techniques.

In the days of the Lunacy Act, the diagnosis of a psychiatric illness meant a serious stigma attached not only to the patient but often also to members of his family. The introduction of the principle of voluntary admission by the Mental Treatment Act of 1930 did something to modify the stigma, but did not remove it entirely. Today, much of the success of modern psychiatric treatment depends upon very early diagnosis and quick, informal hospital admission, early discharge home, and on day hospitals, night hospitals, and other forms of part-time in-patient treatment. It is therefore more than ever important that psychiatric diagnoses should not continue to carry with them the traditional stigma of irreversible alienation from society.

Community Mental Health Work

Following changes in the organizational structure of the National Health Service introduced in 1974, the mental health departments that had been established by local health authorities, together with other public health departments, hospital services and general practitioner services, have now been brought into unified administrations by area health authorities.

By this re-organization it is hoped to provide a versatile and comprehensive service of prevention, care and after-care in the field of psychiatric disorders and mental retardation, through the work of teams of general practitioners, community physicians and nurses, specialist psychiatrists, and nurses and in collaboration with psychiatric and general social workers under the administration of local social services departments.

Since 1970 a start has been made by social services departments in the co-ordination of domiciliary care arrangements and the provision of hostels, other social supervision and sheltered employment for adults in need; and of residential nurseries, foster homes and community homes for children.

It is a major aim to reduce to a minimum the number of children and adults in institutional care and the time spent therein. In principle, only those in need of active medical and/or nursing treatment will be hospitalized, in small specialized units within general hospital complexes.

Since 1970, also, the responsibility for junior training centres for severely subnormal children deemed unable to benefit from education in schools for educationally subnormal children has passed to local education authorities which have established schools for the severely subnormal. In 1974 responsibility for senior training centres has passed to the newly created area health authorities [see CHAPTER 35].

Attainment of the long term objective is dependent upon the success of massive training programmes, that have hardly started, in modern casework techniques; and upon a still more massive building programme that in 1974 had not even reached the drawing board stage, nor that of the serious consideration of the financial implications. In the meantime, which may be long drawn out, the specialised hospitals have to carry on, knowing that they are regarded as obsolescent, beset with the staffing problems that are inevitable under such conditions.

Voluntary Effort

Mental health work owes its origin in the early years of the twentieth century to pioneers like Clifford W. Beers in the United States, and Maurice Craig and Evelyn Fox in Great Britain. In 1948 the various public bodies in the field amalgamated to form the National Association for Mental Health which, with its counterparts in Scotland and Northern Ireland, is engaged on broad programmes of public education, professional training, pioneering of new types of project, promotion of legislation, inquiries, advice giving, and support of public and private effort and of local and national governmental programmes. The unique potential contribution of voluntary organizations is that of the possibility of mobilizing citizen support in advance of public opinion and majority support and, therefore, of official action.

More recently there has been a growth in the number of 'self-help' voluntary organizations composed of patients and their relatives, ex-patients, sympathetic professional people, and public-spirited ordinary citizens. The object is radically to increase medical and social aid to sufferers from the disease or disorder which is the focus of their interest. Examples are Alcoholics Anonymous, and the Samaritans, who are available to bring instant aid to those obsessed with thoughts of suicide. A similar self-help organization has been started for neurotics. The interests of children are the concern of the National Society for the Mentally Handicapped Child and the Society for Autistic Children.

These organizations, like for example the British Polio Fellowship and the Spastics Society and many others in cognate fields, have an immense potential for mobilizing support for their particular interest, but have the social disadvantage of sectionalizing effort. There is danger of competition for priority in planning and financial allocation; and the welfare organizations with more general aims may be weakened in their efforts on behalf of much greater numbers who are in need of help but who have not such strong and vocal advocates.

The Institute of Religion and Medicine, which was founded in 1964, set out to bring about closer relationships between clergy, ministers, and doctors in their daily work. The Institute has developed to include all who are vocationally engaged in the broad field of health—physical, mental, and spiritual. It provides opportunities for on-going groups to meet together in local areas for exchange of ideas, study, and mutual professional help. The Institute also organizes conferences and appoints commissions to study and report on important issues of the day.

The World Federation for Mental Health was founded in 1948 to link together and strengthen the work of mental health associations in countries all over the world. It has arranged conferences, commissions, study groups, and seminars, including many in conjunction with the World Health Organization and other United Nations' specialized agencies.

Public Education

Where there is universal literacy, public education is an important way of securing public co-operation. Generally speaking, the best form of public education in the field of mental hygiene can be effected through performing services which the people need. It might be said that the public educational work of the various clinics and counselling departments is about their most important single contribution to society. However, they leave untouched the large majority of the population that does not use their services, including the influential people who shape public opinion and who may control financially the scale of the facilities provided for those who need help.

The mass media are of limited value in public education in this field. It is important in public education in a field in which powerful feelings are involved, not only to be able to foretell but also control the emotional effects produced. As stated above, mental hygiene work is most effective when people feel a need for it, know something about it, and have trust in those who are concerned with it. Thus, the usual mass media of propaganda, such as daily newspapers, radio and television, and public lectures, are not highly effective, and sometimes quite unhelpful in this field. In the case of newspapers of mass circulation the effect of the printed word on the individual reader cannot be controlled, and the whole thing is so impersonal that its results cannot be judged. Exceptions to this do exist in the case of some journals which cater for a known and more defined readership, in which contributors can become figures of trust to the readers. This has applied occasionally to certain regular columnists in daily newspapers, just as it has sometimes been true of radio or television broadcasters when they have built up a quasi-personal relationship with their public.

It is impossible in this chapter to discuss the technique of public education in this field, and it can only be added that, in principle, each effort should be directed towards a known and clearly defined group of recipients and to building up a continuing relationship with them, whether by series of articles, talks, lectures, or discussion groups as appropriate, over a period of several months, using the same contributors or leaders, who themselves are figures of public trust.

Probably more effective work can be done by concentrating upon the education of the leaders of public opinion in a local area and by organizing lecture courses, discussion groups, and particularly working parties and fact-finding commissions in which responsible citizens can engage in a responsible way in the study of this field [see also CHAPTER 49].

SOME SPECIAL PROBLEMS
Children without Families

The proper care of children who are separated from their families, whether temporarily or permanently, is an important mental hygiene preoccupation. It is now recognized that children who are denied the opportunity for normal relationship formation with their mother or a mother figure during the first three years of life are likely to show permanent effects in their character formation, and that some young children who suffer even a short interruption of maternal care develop serious character deformities if no satisfactory alternative arrangements are made. The evidence for this is sufficient to make it imperative that in the public care of children who are separated from their parents, special care be taken to provide for the relationship formation needs of young children.

It will be agreed that it is a biological necessity for all babies and young children to have an opportunity to form an intimate relationship with at least one adult, and that this relationship is best formed with the adult who cares for the baby. The effects of the important training experiences of the toddler period upon character formation are deepest and most salutary if the character training of the child is undertaken by the person with whom the child has the most intimate emotional relationships.

The following are important basic principles of substitute care of children. When a young child is temporarily separated from its mother, great care must be taken to give him the opportunity of forming a special relationship with one adult, which in the case of a child of 12 months or less is the limit of its effective capacity for substitute relationship formation under these conditions. Exposure to several adults may weaken the effectiveness of the child's substitute relationship formation. This point is very important in staffing children's hospitals and short-stay residential nurseries. Another important consideration is that after several weeks in substitute care, the restoration of the infant to his mother may represent a second separation, and the mother may need help with the emotional upsets that may follow. Failure to resolve difficulties that arise after reunion may both harden the child's attitude to loving relationships, and undermine the mother's confidence and patience.

If the separation between child and parents is likely to be long term, provision should be made for the child's formation of satisfactory alternative permanent relationships. The attractive ideal of reconstructing home life has usually proved impracticable. The ideal would be for a married couple to take, say, four children ranging in age and sex like a normal family, and for this synthetic family to function as a unit. In practice, it is very rarely possible to re-create the conditions of life, genuinely. Parenthood normally evolves gradually, and parent–child relationships grow spontaneously. If the couple employed in the substitute home have children of their own there may be problems of jealousy and the necessity to share affection. If the foster-parents have had no children of their own, the fact that the foster-mother has not experienced the discipline of pregnancy and that the ties of instinct with the foster-child may be weak can hardly fail to make the substitute family something very different from the natural family. It is wise to recognize that no re-created home can be the real thing, and to aim with objectivity and realism to set up substitute arrangements that will be the next best thing.

Practical difficulties are such that little more can be done than study the important principles of substitute care, and work in accordance with them as far as possible. It is not reasonable to expect a baby to share an adult with more than one other baby, or a pre-school-age child to share with more than five or six other children; a single sexed and narrow age-group provides the children with limited and often frustrating social experiences; absence of a visible masculine role in the home distorts children's attitudes; and change of staff, however difficult to avoid, inevitably disturbs children's relationship formation. More subtle, but not less important, is the principle that discipline and conduct in the home reflects the quality of the mutual love of parents and children; and where love is not present, the application of a rigid regime and institutional discipline has very different effects upon children's character formation than a normal home environment.

Children in Hospital

Temporary separation of young children from their parents, as when children (or their mothers) are admitted to hospital, is now well recognized as a potential cause of emotional difficulty and relationship disturbance in the case of some children, especially between the ages of 6 months and 3–4 years. To allow mothers to stay in hospital with very young children, and a liberal visiting policy in the case of older children, has been shown to minimize these problems.

Problem Families

The plight of so-called problem families in big cities is a matter of concern in all industrialized countries. Social investigations have shown that there is a clustering of social problems in families in the lowest decile on a socio-economic scale. More than one half of the social situations that require the intervention of a social, medical, or welfare agency occur among the 10 per cent. of the population that lives in the worst or slum districts. The range of problems include poverty, social incompetence, hardship and need, marriage instability, delinquency and crime, drunkenness, unemployment, chronic illness, vagrancy, and so on.

This is a many-sided social problem of considerable significance to mental hygiene. The so-called social problem group owes something to the distribution of intelligence in the population. It may be said that the least intelligent 10 per cent. of the population are the least adequate to deal with the complications of life in a modern industrial city. They are vulnerable and tend to get into social difficulties when conditions are not favourable. They also tend to earn less money and to suffer more interruptions of earning through unemploy-

ment, ill health, and so on. This section of the population has the lowest standard of living and is most subjected to overcrowding and considerable domestic inconvenience. Their vulnerable position is made worse by their comparative inability to overcome social and domestic difficulties and to use their limited resources wisely. Although the unintelligent may form the hard core of the social problem group, other disabilities, such as emotional instability, and some types of neurotic behaviour may drive people into courses of social action which cause them to fall into this group.

One of the great difficulties is that once individuals have succumbed to social difficulties, the cumulative effect of these tends to keep them from rehabilitation. Not only are their domestic conditions the most inconvenient, but the districts in which they live offer the poorest amenities, and they have the greatest need to seek escape and distraction. Helping these people is therefore a many-sided problem. On the one hand, they are in need of social measures to minimize their handicaps and to help them make the best use of their limited facilities. On the other hand, the heart of the problem lies in the poor quality of their interpersonal relationships, their incapacity to conceptualize longer-term objectives and to sustain effort.

The most promising approach is a combination of a policy of rehousing and general social welfare, with carefully planned appropriate forms of education for the children, social care of juveniles just starting work, and practical help in daily living. It is often very difficult to break the vicious circle in which a family may find itself after years of hardship and failure.

Delinquency and Crime

Criminality has many repercussions in the mental health field, and if it cannot be justifiably claimed that all criminality is evidence of mental ill health, yet it can be argued that crime is evidence of an imperfect relationship between the individual and the community; and, further, that a mental health problem is involved in all antisocial and criminal activity. That there may be, and probably is, a moral problem involved as well, does not remove the mental health implications.

There is constant and considerable misunderstanding between those who take a psychological and humanitarian view of delinquency, on the one hand, and those who take a moral or perhaps juridical point of view. Most people agree that unstable and unbalanced people may commit crimes over which they have very little rational control and that when this happens a problem of mental health is involved. Comparatively few people recognize the presence of a mental health problem in a more deliberate, apparently rational and planned crime, especially when a motive of gain is obvious. Such will appear to most people to be more a problem of morality, i.e. of wickedness. From the point of view of mental health, however, the point of interest is the deliberate choice by the individual of a course of action that flouts the interests of others, attempts to profit out of other people's loss, and risks social punishment and degradation. Why should the individual seek to gain personal advantage at the risk of incurring heavy punishment and, almost certainly, at the expense of reputation and the love and respect of his fellows? When put in this light the concern of mental hygiene with criminal behaviour is more apparent. Theoretically, the true prophylaxis against crime and delinquency is the establishment of interpersonal relationships of a quality so excellent that no one values personal gain more highly than care for the interests of others. This ideal may not be fully realizable in practice, but it could be an ultimate aspiration in prophylaxis.

Limited space permits no more than the generalization that there are three main streams of criminal behaviour: the first comes from community sources through social neglect and inequality, and through the urge to gain more advantages felt by some people dissatisfied with their position of social inferiority. The second stream arises out of more personal drives—those of some people whose relationships have been unsatisfying since early childhood and whose need for self-compensation may override all considerations of relationships and morals. The third stream arises out of the character deformity caused by some more severe defect of relationship formation. In some cases the individual is possessed of a deep latent or overt hostility and hateful aggressiveness, with obvious potential consequences—the so-called aggressive psychopath. In other cases the individual is emotionally cold and self-centred, with no loyalties and no feelings of compassion to deter him from criminal activity—the so-called affectionless psychopath.

Therefore, prophylaxis against crime needs to go in two main directions: programmes of social amelioration to remove social injustices that may provoke criminal behaviour among the less compliant of the under-privileged individuals; and the promotion of positive, warm, and stable interpersonal relationships in families and substitute groups in which young children are growing up.

Addictions and Other Behaviour Disorders

Some of the breakdowns in social adjustment that lead to addictions and other behaviour disorders have important mental health implications. Both alcoholism and drug addiction are now generally recognized to be an effect of personality difficulties rather than of the addictive agent itself. The addict has recourse to his drug or to alcohol in order to mask a sense of inadequacy, deaden anxiety, or create an illusory world in which he can gain satisfactions unobtainable in reality. Habit formation comes more from the unbearable qualities of reality to the individual than from the specific effects of the drug, which is one reason why addiction is difficult to cure without effecting a radical change of psychological attitude in the addict.

Alcoholism tends to be linked with homosexuality, directly and indirectly, through the deadening of the sense of guilt and anxiety by alcohol, the reduction of sexual potency among men, and also through the circumstance that daily drinking of alcohol in public places is predominantly for men. The alcoholic who spends every evening in a club or public bar may be using this as a displaced homosexual activity that arouses less sexual guilt.

Since the Second World War the introduction and widespread distribution of new ranges of therapeutic drugs have brought new addiction problems to public notice. Pep pills and tranquillizers, singly, and in combination have had a vogue among teenagers. These practices, together with the use of L.S.D., marihuana, and the like have been mentioned briefly above in connexion with social alienation of youth. So-called 'soft' drug taking is, generally speaking, a problem of group behaviour rather than one of individual personality

disorder. The preventive aim here is to maintain, or re-establish when lost, the feeling of mutual identification between the teenage and the parental generation.

The more chronic problems of alcohol and narcotic drug addiction among adults can be prevented and treated effectively only by dealing with the underlying personality disorders. Problems of 'soft' drug taking demand a wide social programme based on an understanding of the frustrations and anxieties of youth in the modern world. Both problem areas set society a formidable task.

Other forms of behaviour disorder with mental health significance include homosexuality in both sexes; this may be regarded mainly in terms of a developmental failure due to disorders of interpersonal relationship formation during childhood, and its prophylaxis and control lie in the promotion of good intra-family relationships during the childhood period. The forms of behavioural difficulty that have been enumerated earlier in this chapter among the signs of disorder in mental health also have as a common starting-point difficulties in relationship formation [see also CHAPTER 33].

Psychosis

Psychosis represents the extreme form of breakdown in mental health, when the individual is no longer consistently related to the reality situation, but is subjected to irrational and disordered emotional and intellectual processes. Psychosis leads to many forms of aberrant behaviour recognizable by their common quality of unreality.

The role of public health in relation to psychosis is too big a field of discussion for more than a brief mention in this chapter. Public health is concerned with both the securing of early treatment and the after-care and rehabilitation of cases of frank mental disorder; and with securing conditions in society that enable the chronic psychotic to live with a minimum of interference and social difficulty. Although no clear causal connexion has been established between the emotional difficulties of early childhood and the later development of psychoses, the impression of an association is sufficiently strong to justify prophylactic efforts in the direction of preventing early emotional difficulties. Logically, if psychosis is pre-eminently a matter of disorder of the relationship of the individual with external reality, then prophylaxis must look to relationship formation of early childhood.

The profound changes that have taken place during the last twenty-five years in the treatment and management of psychosis and other serious psychiatric illnesses are having important repercussions in the public health world. During this period compulsory admission to psychiatric hospitals has declined to only a small proportion of total admission, which has risen steeply. At the same time the number of patients in mental hospitals—the daily population—has declined, the average length of stay shortened significantly, and the number of re-admissions and re-discharges increased sharply. One inevitable result of these changes is that the ordinary citizen has been brought into closer contact, and personally involved to a greater degree in individual cases of mental illness and treatment. This is creating new problems of attitude towards mental illness and mental health.

Modern active treatment methods, and especially the massive

use of tranquillizers with a view to securing the patient's early return home, have altered the focus of treatment, without a commensurate change in the public concept of treatment provisions, nor as yet in the training and availability of skilled personnel to carry on the treatment process in the patient's home.

It is not widely enough realized that, more and more, the key person in the treatment of psychological illness is becoming the general practitioner who, manifestly, has been ill-equipped up to the present time to bear such a responsibility. This latter covers not only the management of the recovering psychotic after his discharge from mental hospital but also the early detection of signs of psychiatric strain, and the differentiation into those cases which the general practitioner can properly handle himself by psychotherapeutic methods or by some form of physical treatment, and those in need of hospitalization. There is an urgent and pressing need for a realignment of professional training in order to meet these new and growing responsibilities.

One aspect of disordered behaviour that is of special importance to the public health and welfare services is that of suicide. This may be related to psychosis, as in the case of a suicidal depression, and the prophylaxis in this case is that of the psychosis. But attempted and unsuccessful suicide are perhaps more socially disturbing, and these are likely to be more closely related to disturbed emotional relationships. In some ways the attempt at suicide that results from depression is not so dangerous as the more hysterical type of attempt, because of the unmistakable nature of the underlying depressive condition which will put people on guard. Studies of unsuccessful suicide suggest that these cases should be considered mainly as massive and dramatic calls for help by an individual who is facing real or imagined failure in social and personal relationships. The main social danger of attempted suicide is that the individual will be goaded by unresponsiveness in the environment to make even more dramatic gestures, which may be, and frequently are, lethal.

It is in cases of contemplated or attempted suicide of a demonstrative nature that the work of the Samaritans, to which reference has been made above, is most particularly relevant. By telephoning a number the caller is in touch with a skilled social service that can support him while his problems can be worked out constructively.

Needs of Developing Countries

The 1961 International Study Group of the World Federation for Mental Health discussed the introduction of modern psychiatric services into areas in which none had existed previously, and warned against the not uncommon attempt to set up psychiatric hospitals on a European or North American model, without considering how they may fit in with existing medical and social facilities. It is important that administrators be not misled by the likely fact that in a community devoid of medical facilities the problems of mental illness will not be recognized as such; nor should they subscribe to the 'noble savage' or 'child of nature' myth that in simple societies no human suffering is caused by mental illness.

The Study Group recommended a phased approach; first to make a detailed study of the community in order to find out what happens to eccentric, solitary, asocial, and antisocial individuals. Every society has niches into which at least some of its eccentrics, including some of the mentally ill, can be fitted without causing overt problems. It is important that these niches be not invaded and destroyed in the name of 'mental health' without ensuring that something better is provided in their place.

Second: to establish 'shelters' in which those who are so severely disturbed that they are no longer socially competent can receive simple nursing and medical care and social protection, to the extent that can be provided out of existing community resources. Third: to organize a bilateral professional training programme: i.e. concurrently to send promising students of relevant professions to selected training centres abroad, and to invite the same training centres to co-operate in setting up a training centre in the country concerned. In due course the training centre would be taken over by the returned expatriate trainees, but until this happens, programmes of building and social organization should be restricted to whatever is required to support the training programme. Later these could be rapidly expanded according to the design of the returned expatriate trainees.

Long-term overseas training programmes have the disadvantage of detaching—perhaps permanently—the students from their own cultural matrix, and also of familiarizing them with concepts and practices that may be quite untried in the culture in which they are destined to be applied. Training programmes centred in the country chiefly concerned may escape the main difficulties and disadvantages of extrapolation from other cultures.

Population Movements

The twentieth century, even to a greater degree than the nineteenth, has been a time of enormous population movements, both forced by circumstances and voluntarily by planned emigration. In either case the emigrants are faced with serious and complex problems of acculturation: of resolving the old ties of affection or hostility for the former homeland; of learning about the new, its language and customs; of adjusting to its manners and food; of living as a member of a small and sometimes unpopular alien minority; and of seeing their own next generation grow progressively more remote from the old, familiar way of life. These problems, with their counterpart problems in the host community, of intolerance, racist attitudes and prejudice, have nowhere received adequate mental health study.

It is well recognized that processes of acculturation are accompanied by strain which results in heightened incidences of stress disorders and mental illness. Valuable psychiatric studies under the auspices of the International Refugee Organization have resulted in a considerable acquisition of knowledge of how to deal with problems of forced movement. In general these have not been applied sufficiently either to forced or to voluntary migration and have not greatly influenced the preparations made by host countries for the reception of new citizens, nor the information and help available to the immigrants. This is a wide and legitimate field of mental health concern. They have been applied hardly at all to the terrible problems of refugees from war. There is no more expertise available today to deal with the human problems of, for example, the refugees from the India–Pakistan war in Bangladesh (1971) than there has been with the Arab refugees in the Gaza strip during the last quarter of a century. This is a neglected field of international mental health concern of immense importance [see also CHAPTER 40].

Natural Disasters

There is a similar world-wide lack of expertise in dealing with problems of living through natural disasters and epidemics, e.g. earthquakes, floods, tidal waves, cholera, etc. The World Federation for Mental Health has advocated the establishment by United Nations' specialized Agencies of a disaster study centre which could send teams for the immediate study of disaster situations as they occur. The objective would be to help countries set up coping agencies in disaster-prone areas and to have an international reservoir of training and help available when required.

CONCLUSION

Throughout the foregoing section on special problems, the major theme, repeated again and again has been that the way to prophylaxis and prevention lies through the establishment of good interpersonal relationships in family life when children are young. This is a most important principle of the modern, more positive, concept of mental health. It is the duty of society to seek to provide children with experiences that strengthen their reactions to change and development, that inculcate attitudes of acceptance of and satisfaction in adaptation, of stimulation by anxiety, and feelings of security under conditions of threat and danger, not divorced from the reality situation, but leaving the individual free to operate as a wholly integrated person. It is in the establishment of warm and positive patterns of interpersonal relationships with others and of control and constructive utilization of aggressive drives, that the future of humanity will be determined, both in family life and in society at large.

REFERENCES AND FURTHER READING

Books

Bakwin, H., and Bakwin, Ruth M. (1972) *Clinical Management of Behavior Disorders in Children*, 4th ed., Philadelphia.

Bowlby, John (1953) *Child Care and the Growth of Love*, London.

Caplan, G., ed. (1961) *Prevention of Mental Disorder in Children*, London.

Caplan, G. (1964) *Principles of Preventive Psychiatry*, London.

Caplan, G. (1970) *The Theory and Practice of Mental Health Consultation*, London.

Fromm, E. (1956) *The Sane Society*, London.

Funkenstein, D. H. (1959) *The Student and Mental Health*, Cambridge, Mass.

Hargreaves, G. R. (1958) *Psychiatry and the Public Health*, London.

Jahoda, Marie (1958) *Current Concepts of Positive Mental Health*, New York.

Johnson, Mabyl K. (1971) *Mental Health and Mental Illness*, Philadelphia.

Joint Commission on Mental Illness and Health (1961) *Action for Mental Health*, New York.

Jones, Kathleen (1960) *Mental Health and Social Policy, 1845–1959*, London.

Jones, Kathleen (1964) *Mental Hospitals at Work*, London.

Jones, M. (1953) *The Therapeutic Community*, New York.

Levi, L. (1971) *Society, Stress and Disease*, Vol. 1, *The Psychosocial Environment and Psychosomatic Diseases*, London.

Mead, M., ed. (1953) *Cultural Patterns and Technical Change*, Paris.

Mead, M., and Wolfenstein, M. (1955) *Childhood in Contemporary Cultures*, Chicago.

Milbank Memorial Fund (1956) *Elements of a Community Mental Health Program*, New York.

Mills, Enid (1964) *Living with Mental Illness*, London.

Opler, M. K., ed. (1959) *Culture and Mental Health*, New York.

Rees, J. R. (1951) *The Health of the Mind*, London.

Riesman, D., Glazer, N., and Denney, R. (1950) *The Lonely Crowd*, New York.

Soddy, K., ed. (1955) *Mental Health and Infant Development*, Vols. I and II, London.

Soddy, K., ed. (1961) *Identity; Mental Health and Value Systems*, London.

Soddy, K., and Ahrenfeldt, R. H.
Vol. 1. *Mental Health in a Changing World* (1965)
2. *Mental Health and Contemporary Thought* (1967)
3. *Mental Health in the Service of the Community* (1967), London.

Soddy, K., with Kidson, Mary C. (1967) *Men in Middle Life*, London.

Suttie, Ian (1935) *Origins of Love and Hate*, London.

World Federation for Mental Health Conference Reports:
(1954) *Mental Health in Public Affairs*
(1960) *Uprooting and Resettlement*
(1961) Thornton, E. M. *Planning and Action for Mental Health*, London.

Articles and Reports

Berkman, P. L. (1971) Measurement of mental health in a general population, *Amer. J. Epidemiol.*, **94**, 105.

Bowlby, J. (1958) Separation of mother and child, *Lancet*, i, 480.

Bowlby, J. (1958) The nature of the child's tie to his mother, *Int. J. Psycho-Anal.*, **39**, 350.

Clausen, J. A., and Yarrow, Marian R. (1955) The impact of mental illness on the family, *J. Soc. Issues*, **2**, No. 4.

Erikson, E. H. (1950) in *Symposium on the Healthy Personality*, ed. Senn, M. J. E., New York.

Hollingshead, A. B., and Redlich, F. C. (1953) Social stratifications and psychiatric disorders, *Amer. soc. Rev.*, **18**, 163.

Kaiser, A. C., and Cooper, B. (1971) The psychiatric patient, the general practitioner and the out-patient clinic: an operational study and a review, *Psychol. Med.*, **1**, 312.

Rumke, H. C. (1955) Solved and unsolved problems in mental health, *Ment. Hyg. (N.Y.)*, **39**, 178.

World Health Organization Publications

Baker, A., Davies, R. L., and Sivadon, P. (1959) Psychiatric Services and Architecture, *Publ. Hlth Pap.*, No. 1.

Bowlby, J. (1951) Maternal Care and Mental Health, *Monogr. Ser.*, No. 2.

Gastant, H. (1973) *Dictionary of epilepsy* Part 1: Definitions, Geneva.

Lin, Tsung-yi, and Standley, C. C. (1962) The Scope of Epidemiology in Psychiatry, *Publ. Hlth Pap.*, No. 16.

Reid, D. D. (1960) Epidemiological Methods in the Study of Mental Disorders, *Publ. Hlth Pap.*, No. 2.

Various authors (1962) Deprivation of Maternal Care: A Reassessment of its Effects, *Publ. Hlth Pap.*, No. 14.

World Health Organization Expert Committee on Mental Health (1959) Sixth Report, Mental Health Problems of Ageing and the Aged, *Wld Hlth Org. techn. Rep. Ser.*, No. 171.

World Health Organization Expert Committee on Mental Health (1959) Seventh Report, Social Psychiatry and Community Attitudes, *Wld Hlth Org. techn. Rep. Ser.*, No. 177.

World Health Organization Expert Committee on Mental Health (1960) Eighth Report, Epidemiology of Mental Disorder, *Wld Hlth Org. techn. Rep. Ser.*, No. 185.

World Health Organization (1959) Report of a Study Group, Mental Health Problems of Automation, *Wld Hlth Org. techn. Rep. Ser.*, No. 183.

World Health Organization (1969) Report of a WHO Scientific Group. Biochemistry of Mental Disorder, *Wld Hlth Org. techn. Rep. Ser.*, No. 427.

World Health Organization (1970) Report of a WHO Scientific Group. Biological Research in Schizophrenia, *Wld Hlth Org. techn. Rep. Ser.*, No. 450.

World Health Organization (1971) Mental health of adolescents and young persons, *Wld Hlth Org. Publ. Hlth Pap.*, No. 41.

World Health Organization (1973) *The international pilot study of schizophrenia*, Vol. 1., Geneva.

World Health Organization (1974a) The work of WHO in 1973, *Wld Hlth Org. Off. Rec.*, **213**, 67

World Health Organization (1974b) Psychiatry and the general practitioner, *Wld Hlth Org. Chron.*, **28**, 65.

World Health Organization (1974c) The clinical psychologist in the mental health services, *Wld Hlth Org. Chron.*, **28**, 113.

World Health Organization (1974d) Suicide and attempted suicide, *Wld Hlth Org. publ. Hlth Pap.*, No. 58.

World Health Organization Regional Office for Europe (1973) *Report of a Working Group on the Role of the Social Worker in the Psychiatric Services, Nice 1972* (Euro 5438 (1)), Copenhagen.

World Health Organization Regional Office for Europe (1974) *Report of a Working Group on Psychiatry in General Practice* (Euro 5428), Copenhagen.

33

DEPENDENCE AS A PUBLIC HEALTH PROBLEM (ALCOHOL, TOBACCO, AND OTHER DRUGS)

T. H. BEWLEY

INTRODUCTION

Dependence on alcohol, tobacco and other drugs can cause severe health problems. Because of the very widespread use of alcohol and tobacco the amount of ill health caused by socially acceptable drugs still greatly exceeds that caused by misuse of other dependence-producing substances. Treatment of dependence is of limited effectiveness and seldom evaluated adequately. Prevention would be desirable, but is difficult to accomplish. In this chapter some of the problems are spelled out, raising more questions than can as yet be answered.

Alcohol

In the introduction to a review *Alcohol Abuse*, produced by the Office of Health Economics (1970), it was stated:

Alcoholism has been a problem for many hundreds of years, although the word itself is comparatively modern. Like schizophrenia it has, at various times, been described as a sin, a social problem, a disease and an emotional disturbance. Until recently it stood largely outside the field of public health. Alcoholism has been defined in terms of alcohol's adverse effects on the drinker, his family or society; in terms of getting drunk; in terms of the compulsive nature of drinking and, finally, in terms of specific recognizable physical or psychological symptoms. It has been used to describe a symptom of an underlying psychopathological condition or a psychological illness in its own right. This lack of firm definition has been a stumbling block to understanding and progress. Alcoholism is usually a progressive disease. Jellinek (1960) suggested that addiction to alcohol required a very high intake over a period of from three to twenty years. Kessel and Walton (1967) suggested three stages in the development of alcoholism: excessive drinking, the addictive stage, and chronic alcoholism. Excessive drinkers were not alcoholics though they might become so.

Tobacco

Tobacco is known to cause serious health problems. Repetitive use and difficulty in discontinuing smoking indicate the element of dependence present. It has been estimated that in the United Kingdom an adolescent who smokes two cigarettes a day will have a 70 per cent. chance of being a regular smoker for the next forty years (Russell, 1971*a*). Many premature deaths occur each year in England and Wales from diseases brought on by cigarettes. In the report of the Chief Medical Officer (Department of Health and Social Security, 1970), Sir George Godber stated:

In previous reports a very conservative figure of deaths associated with cigarette smoking has been used, but this year an attempt has been made to calculate more closely the total mortality related to cigarette smoking, of which little more than a third is due to lung cancer. On reasonable assumptions about the main groups of such deaths from lung cancer, chronic bronchitis and ischaemic heart disease, some 80,000 premature deaths probably occur in England and Wales each year and for the whole of the United Kingdom the number must approach 100,000. Of course a high proportion of these deaths occurs in older people, but there are enough in the working age-groups up to age 65 to mean that the premature deaths before that age cause each year the loss of 190,000 man years of working life. We cannot estimate the amount of working time lost from illness due to cigarette smoking but it must be responsible at least for the greater part of the 38·6 million days of sickness absence certified as due to bronchitis in 1969.

The World Health Organization has declared itself clearly on this matter of cigarette smoking within the past year. The European and Americas Regional Committees both banned smoking at their meetings in September 1969, and they were followed by the Executive Board in January 1970 and the Assembly and its Committees in May 1970. The benefits to be derived from the abandonment of cigarette smoking are very large and begin soon; it is surely time that every effort was made to help the individual to achieve them. It seems incredible that our country can go on accepting the lavish promotion by advertising and other no less expensive means of a habit that is dangerous to all who indulge in it and offensive to many of those who do not. The benefit to health of abolition of cigarette smoking would be enormous, and economic advantage from the prevention of lost working time and the reduction of the cost of the health care required to relieve the ravages of the habit would certainly add up to many hundreds of millions of pounds each year. This is no harmless indulgence but the biggest single avoidable menace to health in contemporary life in Britain causing, all told, perhaps ten times as many deaths as do road accidents and nearly as many deaths as all the cancers unrelated to smoking put together.

Different methods of control, and prevention of ill health through use, are required for substances which are socially acceptable, such as alcohol and tobacco which, by ingenious casuistry, have been left out of the ambit of the draft protocol on psychotropic substances (United Nations, 1971).[1]

In view of the cumulative evidence of the degree of illness and death it produces, methods to minimize this damage have

[1] 'If the World Health Organization finds:
(*a*) that a substance has the capacity to produce
(i) (1) a state of dependence, and
(2) central nervous system stimulation or depression, resulting in hallucinations or disturbances in motor function or thinking or behaviour or perception or mood, or
(ii) similar abuse and similar ill-effects as a substance in Schedule I, II, III, or IV, and
(*b*) that there is sufficient evidence that the substance is being or is likely to be abused so as to constitute a public health and social problem warranting the placing of the substance under international control, the World Health Organization shall communicate to the Commission an assessment of the substance, including the extent or likelihood of abuse, the degree of seriousness of the public health and social problem, and the degree of usefulness of the substance in medical therapy; together with recommendations on control measures, if any, that would be appropriate in the light of its assessment.'
Tobacco causes a state of dependence and constitutes a public health problem, but as defined in subsection (*a*) (i) (2) it is not psychotoxic and is therefore not liable to control under the protocol.

to be taken into account when considering the use of dependence-producing substances. Already, health education programmes are concerned to dissuade people from smoking, and in this field the principles and measures used apply equally to the socially acceptable and other drugs. There are also associations between the use of alcohol, tobacco and other drugs, and some of the factors leading to use may be similar (Backhouse and James, 1969; Bynner, 1969; Wiener, 1970).

Other Drugs

Sedatives, hypnotics, tranquillizers, stimulants, antidepressants, and analgesics are capable of producing a state of dependence in subjects to whom they are administered repeatedly in sufficient dosage. The use of drugs to produce sedation, oblivion, elation or euphoria is endemic in most parts of the world. These forms are often long established by custom and tradition. They are regulated and stabilized. Their dependence production is low and often they are preparations with minimum risk. Epidemic outbreaks have to be distinguished by such factors as rapid spread, lack of previous social experience, explosive outburst (the introduction of gin in the seventeenth century, the use of amphetamines in Japan, or cannabis smoking by young people in Europe would be examples). With increased communications and travel there have been recent examples of the spread of the use of drugs previously confined to certain areas, for example alcohol from the West to the East and cannabis from the East to the West.

In the first half of the twentieth century the major form of dependence in Europe was alcoholism, and dependence on other drugs was restricted to a small number of health personnel with an equally small number of therapeutic addicts. In the second half of the twentieth century this has changed. There has been a 'recreational' (self-administered for purposes other than medical treatment) use of drugs other than those that are currently socially acceptable (particularly by young people using cannabis, hallucinogens, such as LSD, central stimulants, or opiates). There has been an increase in the number of people therapeutically dependent on such drugs as amphetamines, barbiturates, and analgesics; also there has been an increase in the incidence of non-suicidal self-poisoning (with drugs originally prescribed for other reasons). There was a three-fold increase in admissions to hospital because of poisoning in a period of seven years in England and Wales: 15,900 admissions in 1957, 50,400 in 1964 (Joint Subcommittee of the Standing Medical Advisory Committees, 1968). Finally, there has been an increase in the misuse of drugs in sport (chiefly amphetamines).

DEFINITIONS

The World Health Organization definition of *dependence* is 'a state psychic and sometimes also physical, resulting from the interaction between a living organism and a drug characterized by behavioural and other responses that always include a compulsion to take the drug on a continuous or periodic basis in order to experience its psychic effects and sometimes to avoid the discomfort of its absence. Tolerance may or may not be present. A person may be dependent on more than one drug.' (WHO, 1969.)

The type of dependence, its severity, and the symptoms, if any, that may accompany withdrawal of the drug are characteristic of the type of drug in question. The term 'drug dependence' should be qualified by specifying which of the eight recognized types is referred to:

1. Alcohol-barbiturate type.
2. Amphetamine type.
3. Cannabis type.
4. Cocaine type.
5. Hallucinogen type.
6. Khat type.
7. Opiate type.
8. Volatile solvent type.
(WHO, 1973.)

Dependence upon more than one type of drug may be present, for example concurrent physical dependence on morphine and barbiturate and alcohol, and dependence upon different drugs together, or in succession, is also becoming increasingly common. Such dependence upon drugs may be harmful to the individual or society and is often damaging to both.

Tolerance is defined as 'the phenomenon of dose increase to maintain the drug effect'.

Physical dependence is defined as 'an adaptive state that manifests itself by intense physical disturbances when the administration of the drug is suspended or when its action is affected by the administration of a specific antagonist'.

Psychic dependence is defined as 'a feeling of satisfaction and a psychic drive that requires periodic or continuous administration of the drug to produce pleasure or avoid discomfort. (WHO, 1964, 1965, and 1973).

Drug abuse has been defined as 'persistent or sporadic excessive drug use inconsistent with, or unrelated to, acceptable medical practice'. And the definition of a *drug*, 'any substance that when taken into the living organism may modify one or more of its functions'. In a statement by the American Medical Association Council on Mental Health, the terms 'misuse' and 'abuse' were defined. *Misuse* was applied to the physician's role in establishing a potentially dangerous type of therapy, even though it did not always lead to significant tolerance or physical dependence. *Abuse* was used to describe self-administration of excessive quantities of drugs leading to tolerance, physical and psychological dependence, mental confusion, and other symptoms of abnormal behaviour. The groundwork for drug abuse may often be established by therapeutic misuse by the physician (*Journal of the American Medical Association*, 1965).

Alcoholism has been defined by the World Health Organization (1952): 'Alcoholics are those excessive drinkers whose dependence upon alcohol has attained such a degree that it shows a noticeable mental disturbance or an interference with their bodily and mental health, their inter-personal relations, and their smooth social and economic functioning; or who show the prodromal signs of such developments. They, therefore, require treatment.'

The 'excessive drinkers' of this definition are said to be differentially characterized by '. . . any form of drinking which in its extent goes beyond the traditional and customary "dietary" use, or the ordinary compliance with the social drinking customs of the whole community concerned, irrespective of the aetiological factors leading to such behaviour and irrespective also of the extent to which such aetiological factors are dependent upon heredity, constitution, or acquired physiological and metabolic influences'.

A shorter definition is that given by Mark Keller (1958): *Alcoholism* is a chronic behavioural disorder manifested by repeated drinking of alcoholic beverages in excess of the dietary and social uses of the community and to an extent that interferes with the drinker's health or his social or economic functioning'.

DEPENDENCE ON TOBACCO

In 1604, King James I of England in the *Counterblaste to Tobacco* referred to smoking as 'a branch of the sin of drunkenness, which is the root of all sins', and in 1606 in 'The Copy of a Letter Written by "E.D." Doctor of Physic to a Gentleman by Whom it was Published', E.D. argued that tobacco was 'not safe for youth; it shorteneth life; it breedeth many diseases; it breedeth melancholy; it hurteth the mind; it is ill for the smoker's issue; to conclude: since it is so hurtful and dangerous to youth, I wish that it might have the pernicious nature expressed in the name and that it were as well known by the name of youths' bane as by the name of tobacco'.

As Russell (1971a) has pointed out, King James was right to ally smoking and alcoholism, for it belongs there with dependence on other drugs. E.D. was also correct when he stated that tobacco 'breedeth many diseases' and 'shorteneth life' but it was 350 years before use of the epidemiological method confirmed his statements (Doll and Hill, 1950; Surgeon General, 1964; Royal College of Physicians, 1962, 1971).

As many as three out of four smokers wish to, or have tried to stop their smoking, but less than one in four ever succeeds in becoming a permanent ex-smoker (McKennell and Thomas, 1967). Most smokers only continue smoking because they cannot easily stop. It is easier to become dependent on cigarettes than on alcohol or barbiturates. Most users of alcohol or sleeping tablets are able to limit themselves to intermittent use and to tolerate periods free of the chemical effect. If dependence occurs it is usually in a setting of psychological or social difficulties. Not so with cigarettes, where intermittent or occasional smoking is a rarity (only about 2 per cent. of smokers). Once smoking is tried the most stable, well-adjusted person sooner or later becomes a regular (dependent) user (or misuser). Only about 15 per cent. of those who have more than one cigarette avoid becoming regular smokers (McKennell and Thomas, 1967). In the prevailing social climate it is only the intravenous drugs which have anything like the dependence-producing potential of cigarette smoking, and it may be no coincidence that the absorption of nicotine through the lungs during smoking is about as rapid and efficient as the heroin addict's intravenous injections (Russell, 1971).

Effects of Nicotine

That withdrawal of cigarettes from heavy smokers may cause a subjectively distressed state is widely appreciated. Such symptoms as depression, anxiety, irritability, restlessness, intense craving, and difficulty in concentrating have frequently been described. Some of these withdrawal effects may occur with 'blind' substitution with low nicotine cigarettes (Finnegan,

Larson, and Haag, 1945; Knapp, Bliss, and Wells, 1963). A single study has shown that they can be allayed by injections of nicotine, which are pleasurable to smokers but not to non-smokers (Johnston, 1942). Most people smoke to obtain nicotine and are unsatisfied by nicotine-free cigarettes. Only 9 per cent. of male and 19 per cent. of female cigarette smokers deny that they inhale (Todd, 1969). Smokers unconsciously modify their puff rate to maintain a steady nicotine intake when given high or low nicotine cigarettes (Knapp, Bliss, and Wells, 1963). Intravenous nicotine reduces cigarette consumption significantly compared with a saline control (Lucchesi, 1967). Nicotine is taken up within a few minutes of smoking by receptors in the brain where its action is rapid, complex, and varied. It may act as stimulant or sedative. It shares with other dependence-producing drugs the quality of acting as a primary reinforcer of behaviour in that animals will self-inject it for its own sake. It is in some way intrinsically rewarding (Russell, 1971a).

Apart from the subjective withdrawal symptoms, there is evidence that some smokers exhibit physical withdrawal effects, namely, sleep disturbance, sweating, gastro-intestinal changes, and a fall in pulse rate and blood pressure (Knapp, Bliss, and Wells, 1963). There is little doubt that, in addition to psychological dependence, many cigarette smokers fulfil the criteria of physiological dependence, namely tolerance and physical withdrawal effects (Russell, 1971b).

Starting to smoke

Since dependence leads to difficulty in stopping smoking, prevention by dissuading young people from starting becomes more important. This is difficult since cigarette smoking is seen as a normal adult behaviour, and one that many children aspire to. Children's smoking has recently been reviewed by Bewley, Day, and Ide (1973). They point out that although little is known about how children learn to smoke, the studies reviewed had established, with varying degrees of certainty, some predictors of smoking by school children, which indicated the children most likely to smoke [see also CHAPTER 37].

1. Those whose parents both smoke.
2. Those whose siblings smoke.
3. Those whose friends smoke.
4. Those who are more rebellious and have a greater anticipation of adulthood.
5. Those whose parents are more permissive towards children's smoking.
6. Those who show low academic achievement.
7. Those who live in an urban environment.
8. Those who attend secondary modern schools, particularly of the single sex type.
9. Those whose parents are from social classes IV and V.

EXTENT OF USE

Dependence on the socially acceptable drugs (alcohol and tobacco) is considerably more common than that on illicitly obtained drugs [TABLE 73].

In TABLE 73 a rough estimate of the number of users of different types of drugs in the United Kingdom has been attempted. It is impossible to get accurate figures for all types

TABLE 73

Estimated Prevalence Rates of Misuse of Drugs of Dependence, United Kingdom (1971)

Types of Drug dependence	Rate per 100,000	Comment	References
Cocaine type	<1	Generally associated with opiate dependency	(1) Report to the United Nations on the working of the International Treaties on Narcotic Drugs (1970) Home Office, London (2) Bewley, T. H. (1966) *Bull. Narcot.*, **18**, 1
Morphine type	5–10	Heroin and methadone	(1), (2), and (3) Bransby, C. R. (1971) *Health Trends*, **3**, 15
Hallucinogen type	100–200? 10–20 (?) <1	Have tried Regular users with problems	(2) (4) Report by the Advisory Committee on Drug Dependence (1970), *Amphetamines and LSD*, H.M.S.O., London
Amphetamine type	50–100 100–200 <10	Dependence on prescribed Illicit use Intravenous use	(5) Kiloh, L. G., and Brandon, S. (1962) *Brit. med. J.*, **2**, 40 (2), (4), and (6) *Times*, 20 Dec. 1965 (2)
Barbiturate type	1,000–2,000 100–200 <2	Regular prescription Dependence on prescribed Intravenous use	(7) Adams, B. G. *et al.* (1966) *J. roy. Coll. Gen. Practit.*, **12**, 24 (7) and (8) Johnson, J., and Clift, A. D. (1968) *Brit. med. J.*, **4**, 613 (9) Cahal, D. D.H.S.S. (Personal communication)
Cannabis type	500–1,500 (?) 50–150 (?) <1	Have tried Regular users Medical complications	(2) (10) Cannabis Report by the Advisory Committee on Drug Dependence (1968) (11) Baker, A. A., and Lucas, E. G. (1969) *Lancet*, **i**, 148
Alcohol type	40,000 400 140 35 (men: 25) (women: 10)	Regular users Alcoholism without complications Alcoholism with complications Deaths from alcoholism	(12) Hensman, C., and Zacune, J. (1971) *Drugs, Alcohol and Tobacco*, London (13) World Health Organization (1951) *Wld Hlth Org. techn. Rep. Ser.*, No. 42 (14) Prys Williams, G. (1965) *Chronic Alcoholics*, Rowntree Social Science Trust, London (15) Moss, M., and Davies, E. B. (1967) *A Survey of Alcoholism in an English County*, London (16) Office of Health Economics (1970) *Alcohol Abuse*, London
Tobacco type	58,000 200	Regular users (16+ years) Deaths annually	(17) Todd, G. F. (1969) *Statistics of Smoking in the U.K.*, Tobacco Research Council (18) Report of the Chief Medical Officer (1970) *On the State of the Public Health (1969)*, H.M.S.O., London

TABLE 74

Estimates of the Number of Alcoholics both With and Without Complications, England and Wales, Selected Surveys

Survey	Date	Population	Informants	Area	Rate per 1,000	Number Estimated for 1968*
WHO Expert Committee on Mental Health . . .	1948	Adults 20+	Jellinek formula	England and Wales	11	370,000
College of General Practitioners	1955–56	All	G.P.s	England and Wales	0·2	10,000†
Parr	1956	Adults 15+	G.P.s	England and Wales	1·1	40,000
Prys Williams . . .	1960–63	All	G.P.s, health visitors and probation officers	5 towns	8·5	280,000
Moss and Davies . . .	1961–64	Adults 15+	13 sources	Cambridgeshire	6·2 males 1·4 females	220,000‡
Addiction Research Unit, London	1966	Adults 15+	G.P.s	One London Borough	1·6	—

* The rate per 1,000 found for each survey has been applied to the 1968 England and Wales population.
† Excludes diagnosis of alcoholic psychosis.
‡ An O.H.E. estimate devised by weighting the Cambridgeshire figures according to Parr's regional differentials (Office of Health Economics, 1970).

of drug misuse, and for cannabis and hallucinogen misuse the figures obtained depend on making some rather sweeping assumptions (that one in ten regular cannabis users will be charged with a cannabis offence, and that there will be ten persons who have tried cannabis for each regular user).

Alcohol

Alcoholism rates in the United Kingdom have been variously estimated [TABLE 74].

There are very large variations between rates of dependence on drugs and alcohol between various countries [TABLES 75 and 76].

TABLE 75

Prevalence of Alcoholism, Rates per 100,000 Population Aged 20 Years or More, Selected Countries*

Place	Year	Jellinek method estimate	Independent method estimate
France	1951	5,200	7,300
U.S.A.	1953	4,390	—
Chile	1950, 1953	3,610	4,150
Ontario, Canada	1961	2,460	2,375
Switzerland	1953, 1947	2,100	2,700
Denmark	1948	1,950	1,750
Finland	1951–57	1,120	1,330
England and Wales	1948, 1960–63	1,100	865

* Estimated by both the Jellinek and independent methods. Data originally supplied by the Alcoholism and Drug Addiction Research Foundation, Toronto, Canada (Project No. 23). United States data from Keller, M., and Effron, V. (1955) *Quart. J. Stud. Alcohol.*, **16**, 619.

The separation of two years by a dash indicates that the estimate of prevalence represent averages for the period. Where two years are separated by a comma, the first of these is the year to which the Jellinek estimate applied.

(Source: World Health Organization (1967) *Wld Hlth Org. techn. Rep. Ser.*, No. 363. Office of Health Economics (1970) *Alcohol Abuse*, London.)

Drugs

The patterns of misuse of drugs obtained illicitly have been changing rapidly. In a report for the Council of Europe Public Health Committee on the *Public Health Implications of Recent Developments in Drug Dependence* (1970) it was stated:

In all countries there has been an upsurge in the number of drug dependents which has now attained the dimensions of an epidemic. This concerns mainly hypnotics and some tranquillizers, anti-pyretic analgesics, central stimulants and, recently, cannabis, whereas dependence on opiates seems to be, at present, relatively low. In general, six trends are discernible in drug dependence:

1. A growing incidence in young people;
2. New patterns in drug dependence (e.g. central stimulants, administered intravenously);
3. The rapid increase of the abuse of well-known drugs in other age-groups (hypnotics, anti-pyretic analgesics and central stimulants);
4. A rising frequency of multiple dependence;
5. An increasing number of women dependents;
6. A rapidly increasing problem of alcoholism.

Tobacco

There have been changes in the amounts of tobacco smoked in the United Kingdom in the past decade. Tobacco smoking is now slightly below the peak of the early 60s. In 1968, con-

TABLE 76

Number and Rates per Million of Known Narcotic Addicts, Various Selected Countries,* mid-1960s

Country	No. of addicts (approx.)	Rate per million population	Comments
U.K. (1964) U.K. (1966)	750 1,300	15 25	Mainly heroin
Canada (1965)	3,600	180	Mainly heroin Includes cannabis
Germany (1964)	4,350	80	Mainly synthetics and morphine Includes amphetamines
Japan (1964)	9,400	100	Mainly opium, morphine and heroin
Hong Kong (1965)	10,900	2,900	Mainly heroin
Korea (1964)	15,000	540	Mainly heroin
U.S.A. (1964)	55,900	290	Mainly heroin
Iran (1965)	100,000–200,000 (est.)	6,550	Est. 95 per cent. opium, 5 per cent. heroin
India (1964)	136,000—opium 200,000—cannabis		

(* Note: Only those countries which had a substantially higher number of addicts than the United Kingdom are shown. Many countries reported little or no drug addiction, and for some countries the 1964 United Nations report showed no figures.)

(Source: Summary of Annual Reports of Governments relating to opium and other narcotic drugs (1964); United Nations Commission on Narcotic Drugs (1966); Office of Health Economics (1967), *Drug Addiction*, London.)

sumption per adult male was 8·8 lb. per year while it has been 10·6 lb. per head in 1960. The peak occurred in 1945 when it was 12·5 lb. per head. Although men are smoking less, the over-all consumption in Britain since the mid-50s has been within 10 per cent. of 3·3 lb. per head (*Nature*, 1970; Todd 1969).

The change in smoking habits seems more remarkable than the slow decline in the total amount of tobacco smoked in Britain. Among the public as a whole, the total consumption of cigarettes has been declining since the early 60s and is now 20 per cent. less than the peak of 243 million pounds reached in 1961. Among men, the consumption of cigarettes has fallen from 8·7 lb. per head in 1960 to 7·1 lb. in 1968. There has, however, been a persistent tendency to smoke smaller cigarettes, and sales of cigarettes in Britain have actually increased in the past decade to 121,000 million, more than two-thirds of them tipped. Consumption of cigars has multiplied fourfold in the decade. Although total consumption has declined, the tendency for young people to start smoking early apparently continues. Among 14-year-olds, for example, average consumption among boys rose from 1·9 to 2·4 cigarettes weekly in two years. Among 15-year-olds, girls as well as boys, the incidence of the smoking habit is between four and five times as great among those who have started work than among those who remain at school (*Nature*, 1970; Todd, 1969).

TABLE 77
Reported Misuse of Psycho-active Drugs in 15 European Countries

	Opiates	Hypnotics and Tranquillizers	C.N.S. Stimulants	Cannabis	LSD
Austria	±	+	±	±	±
Belgium	±	+	±	±	−
Czechoslovakia	−	±	±	−	−
Denmark	±	+	++	++	+
Federal Republic of Germany .	±	+	+	++	±+
France	±	+	±	+	±
Greece	±	+	+	++	−
Italy	±	+	+	+	±
Netherlands	±	+	+	++	+
Norway	±	+	±	+	±
Sweden	±	+	++	++	+
Switzerland	±	+	+	+	−
Turkey	±	+	+	++	
United Kingdom . .	++	+	+	++	+
Yugoslavia	±	+	±	+	

± Some misuse reported. + Misuse. ++ Considerable misuse
(Sources: from Council of Europe Report (1970) *Public Health Implications of Recent Developments in Drug Dependence*, Strasbourg; and World Health Organization Regional Office for Europe (1971*b*) *Report on Recent Changes in Drug Abuse in Czechoslovakia, France and Yugoslavia*, Euro 4000/4, Copenhagen.)

EPIDEMIOLOGICAL STUDIES IN ALCOHOLISM

There are two problems in epidemiological studies of alcoholism. Firstly, the concept of alcoholism itself and the difficulty of deriving suitable operational definitions. Keller (1960) considered that clinical definitions based upon either physiologically or psychologically orientated conceptions alone were inadequate, and suggested that the epidemiologist should first identify a drinking pattern with 'undesirable characteristics', and that after that the ill-effects of alcohol upon the subject's health or social or economic status should be demonstrated. The second problem is that many alcoholics deny or conceal their alcoholism. There are three main methods of estimating prevalence:

1. Use of hospital admission rates.
2. The Jellinek formula.
3. General population surveys.

Hospital admission is probably a very poor guide to the extent of the problem and reflects the availability of beds for treating the condition. The increase in the total of admissions for alcoholism and alcoholic psychoses in England and Wales from 1958 to 1971 is shown in FIGURE 83.

Another method of estimating the number of alcoholics is to use the frequency of cirrhosis of the liver as an indirect estimate. Jellinek devised a formula $A = \frac{R(PD)}{K}$ where A is the number of alcoholics, R the ratio of all alcoholics to alcoholics with complications, D the number of deaths from cirrhosis of the liver in a given year, P the percentage of such deaths due to alcoholism, and K the percentage of all alcoholics with com-

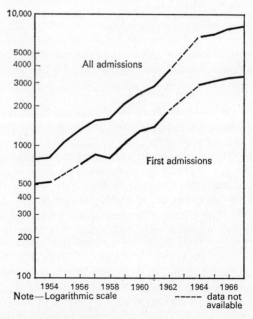

FIG. 83. Alcoholism and alcoholic pyschoses. Mental hospital admissions, England and Wales, 1953–67.

plications, who die from cirrhosis of the liver. The formula has been widely used. The World Health Organization estimate of 350,000 alcoholics in Britain was made by using this formula (WHO, 1951). The formula has been criticized, however, the main criticism being that the constants K, P, and R were changing more rapidly than had been anticipated.

Death from Alcoholism

Deaths from alcoholism and offences of drunkenness in England and Wales, and the consumption of spirits in the United Kingdom between 1875 and 1967 are shown in

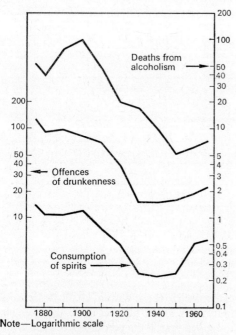

FIG. 84. Deaths from alcoholism and offences of drunkenness (England and Wales) and consumption of spirits (United Kingdom) 1875–1967.
Deaths—rate per million living.
Drunkenness—Offences per 10,000 population over 14.
Consumption—proof gallons *per capita*.

FIGURE 84. Alcoholism death rates per million population living in England and Wales are shown in FIGURE 85.

General Population Surveys

The two main methods of estimation are based on, first, reports from people working in the community who are likely to come into contact with cases of alcoholism and, second, estimates of the prevalence in a random sample of the general population. In a study of psychiatric illnesses in general practice, Shepherd, Cooper, Brown, and Kalton (1966) identified 29 alcoholics out of 14,000 patients, a rate of about 2 per 1,000. The authors thought this was an underestimate, although their numbers were higher than that found by Parr (1957). Reports from probation officers and health visitors (Prys Williams, 1965; Prys Williams and Glatt, 1966) gave a larger number of alcoholics and a rate of 8·5 per 1,000 when early alcoholics were included. This was still below the WHO estimate of 11 per 1,000 based on the Jellinek formula. Probably the most thorough study of this type in England was that carried out by Moss and Davies in Cambridgeshire, who made

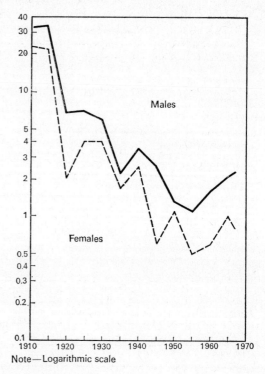

FIG. 85. Alcoholism. Death rates per million living, England and Wales, 1911–67.

an estimate of a rate of 6·2 males and 1·4 females per 1,000 (Moss and Davies, 1967) [FIGURE 86].

Cohort Studies

These have been most widely used in Scandinavia where the special circumstances of a relatively static population and the

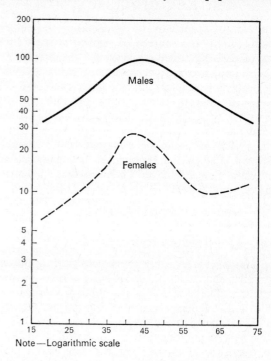

FIG. 86. Alcoholism. Prevalence rates per 10,000 population by age, Cambridgeshire, 1961–64.

systems of public record-keeping facilitated their application. Examples of such studies are those of Fremming (1951), who studied the epidemiology of mental disorder in Bornholm, and Helgason (1964) in Iceland. Fremming selected a cohort of 5,529 persons, born on the island in the period 1883–87, which was traced until 1939. Helgason's cohort consisted of all the Icelanders born during the years 1895–97 and totalled 5,395 probands. They were followed until 1957, by means of data from their personal doctor, various state insurance boards, and hospital and police records. The life expectancy of developing alcoholism for men was found by Fremming to be 3·4 per cent., and for women 0·1 per cent. Helgason obtained life expectancy rates of 6·5 per cent. for men and 0·4 per cent. for women. Only 10 per cent. of Helgason's alcoholic sample were ever admitted to a psychiatric unit.

Field Surveys

Bailey, Haberman, and Alkane (1965) studied Washington Heights, a mixed urban residential area in Manhattan, and the sample consisted of 4,387 families covering 8,082 people. One member of each household was questioned about family drinking habits and the psychiatric, social, and physical ills which might result from alcoholism. The over-all rate of alcoholism was 19 per 1,000. Bailey found a higher prevalence of alcoholism among divorced or separated men (68 per 1,000).

The ratio of male to female admissions for alcoholism in England and Wales is 4·3 to one (Registrar General, 1962). However, the sex ratio changes from a prevalence of 1·8 to one for Negroes in Washington Heights (Bailey, Haberman, and Alkane, 1965) to 30 to one for the expectancy of developing alcoholism on Bornholm (Fremming, 1951).

EPIDEMIOLOGICAL STUDIES IN DRUG DEPENDENCY

In the field of dependency epidemiological studies involve a number of difficulties:

1. The concept of illness. What constitutes illness?
2. The lack of operational definitions.
3. Difficulties of measurement.

If clinical definitions are used they are based on either physiologically or psychologically orientated conceptions and are inadequate for all epidemiological purposes. The epidemiological method may be useful in working out the problem of dependence on a time, persons, and place basis, the exclusions being, for example, that it is rare in the very young age-groups. The prevalance of use or abuse of any drug may vary with high or low prevalence areas. This particularly applies to dependence of the narcotic type. Hawks (1970, 1971) has reviewed the epidemiology of drug dependence in the United Kingdom.

Two community studies are particularly worth noting. The first of these was carried out at Crawley, a new town with a population of 62,000, of whom 41 per cent. were under 20 years of age (de Alarcon and Rathod, 1968). The study covered the age-group 15–20 and employed five screening methods for detecting otherwise unknown heroin use. The methods employed were:

1. Local probation officer reports.
2. Local police reports.
3. The reports of known heroin users.
4. A survey of recent jaundiced in-patients aged 15–25 years.
5. A survey of casualty department records relating to all patients aged between 15–25 years who had been admitted for overdose of hypnotics or stimulants in the previous twelve months.

Classifying all the names obtained by the five screening methods and by direct referral as:

1. Confirmed heroin users;
2. Probable users;
3. Suspects; and
4. Non-users;

revealed that there were 50 confirmed users, 5 probable users, 37 suspects and 6 non-users. What was of particular interest was that only 8 of the 50 confirmed users had been referred through the normal channels, leaving 42 who were first identified through one of the screening methods.

Consideration of the comparative value of the various screening methods showed that the two most productive were the heroin users themselves and the jaundice survey. Heroin users provided first evidence of 46 individuals and the hepatitis survey of 20. These two methods also provided the greatest number of confirmed cases.

Even if the comparison is confined to confirmed cases, only the 50 cases detected by de Alarcon and Rathod contrast with the eight cases of heroin abuse in Crawley known to the Home Office. Had the official figures been used the rate for Crawley would have been 1·4 per 1,000 instead of the 8·5 found.

In a more recent article, de Alarcon (1969) has analysed the spread of heroin abuse in Crawley in greater detail. By establishing the approximate date on which heroin users had their first injection of heroin and the identity of the person who had given them this injection, de Alarcon was able to discern both yearly incidence and source of contagion. This information was obtained from 58 users aged between 15 and 20 from 1962 to 1967 inclusive. By plotting the yearly incidence during this period three stages in the spread of heroin in the town emerged:

1. During 1962–65 a small number of Crawley young people were initiated in other towns.
2. In the first half of 1966 a nucleus of established heroin users, initiated by the former, developed in Crawley.
3. In the second semester of 1966 and first semester of 1967 heroin abuse spread explosively in Crawley.

Two major transmission trees covering 48 cases were traced back to the original initiator; the other included 16 users. Of the total 58 initiations to heroin 46 were carried out by Crawley boys, 7 were initiated in other towns and 5 would not disclose their initiator.

The second study concerned an unidentified provincial town described as being compact and long established with a population of approximately 100,000 (Kosviner et al., 1968). An attempt was made to contact and gain information on all the heroin users living in the town, whether or not they were known to the authorities. The initial approach was made through four known heroin users through whom contact was established with a total of 37 users. While there could be no way of confirming that all heroin users in the town had been contacted the names obtained corresponded very closely with those from official sources. That the subjects were heroin users was confirmed in 22 cases by direct observation of self-injection and in the other cases by hospital notes, general practitioners, or associates.

Of 47 suspected users, 31 were confirmed, 10 were found not to be using heroin and 6 had left town. As was the case in the Crawley study all the authorities approached had under-estimated the extent of the problem—6 users unknown to any of the authorities were identified in the survey.

Associations between Smoking, Drinking, and the Use of Drugs

In a study entitled 'Adults' and Adolescents' Smoking Habits and Attitudes', McKennell and Thomas (1967) showed that smoking is associated with both normal and abnormal drinking. Another study of a hospital out-patient population (Dreker and Fraser, 1968), 'Smoking Habits of Alcoholic Out-patients', showed that 92 per cent. of alcoholics attending as out-patients were smokers and smoked more heavily than the normal population. Two other studies (Bewley and Ben Arie, 1968; Stimson and Ogborne, 1970) showed that most heroin addicts under treatment were smokers (99 per cent. in the second study). Backhouse and James (1969), in a study of delinquent adolescents, showed that 19 per cent. of non-smokers were regular drinkers and 6 per cent. of non-smokers used drugs, while 40 per cent. of smokers were regular drinkers and 21 per cent. of smokers used drugs. The users of heroin and other drug users tended to smoke more heavily and had started at an earlier age [see also CHAPTER 37].

AETIOLOGY OF DEPENDENCE

Possible aetiological factors were discussed in the Eighteenth Report of the WHO Expert Committee on Drug Dependence (WHO, 1970) where some of the many hypotheses to explain the causation of drug dependence of designated types included the following:

1. That such drug dependence may be a manifestation of an underlying character disorder in which immediate gratification is sought in spite of the possibility of long-term adverse consequences and at the price of immediate surrender of adult responsibilities.

2. That it may be a manifestation of delinquent-deviant behaviour in which there is pursuit of personal pleasure in disregard of social convention, so that to some this is primarily a moral problem.

3. That it may be an attempt at self-treatment by persons suffering from: (a) psychic distress either of the normal variety seen, for instance, in adolescence or as a reaction to social and/or economic stress, frustration, or blocked opportunity; or the more persistent problem of depressive illness, chronic anxiety, or other psychiatric disorders; (b) physical distress—hunger, chronic fatigue, or disease; (c) a belief that the drug has special powers to prevent disease or to increase sexual capacity.

4. That it may provide a means of achieving social accep-

tance in a social subculture, particularly for the socially inadequate.

5. That it may be a manifestation of a permanent or reversible metabolic lesion brought about by the repeated use of high doses of drugs.

6. That it may be a part of a rebellion against conventional social values relating to pleasure, tradition, success, and status.

7. That even in the absence of pre-existing psychopathology, it may result from the acquisition of a complex set of instrumental and classically conditioned responses and may, therefore, be a form of learned behaviour.

8. That even in the absence of underlying psychopathology, it may result from socio–cultural pressures leading to heavy use of drug, for example alcohol.

9. That any or all of these factors may play a role in the causation of drug dependence in a given individual.

Since both constitutional and environmental factors determine individual susceptibility to dependence both on alcohol and other drugs it is as important to explore the influence of psychological and cultural factors on individual vulnerability or resistance to dependence (especially for those in contact with a drug subculture or in 'high-risk' groups) as to study the biological and pharmacological effects of dependence-producing drugs.

TREATMENT

Alcoholism

Griffith Edwards (1967) pointed out that previous reviews of the literature and treatment of alcohol dependence largely served to show that claims for the efficacy of specific treatment and treatment regimes had outrun the evidence. Few investigators had attempted any sort of control, and few authors had defined the characteristics of the population they were treating. Few had given a full and clear description of the treatment employed and few had reported outcome in clear-cut terms or had troubled to check the validity of the data. Reports of outcome were often limited to consideration of abstinence alone, and there had been little difference in outcome between patients at special alcoholism clinics and those treated routinely. Edwards ended by pointing out that strict and critical assessment of the literature forced him to the conclusion that the value of any of the wide range of specific treatment methods still had to be incontrovertibly demonstrated—what was effective may well have been the rather non-specific influences of the support, understanding, exhortation, and education. Alcohol dependence is often a chronic relapsing illness and in realistic terms the work of an alcoholism treatment service is largely the long-term care of people more or less frequently in difficulties.

Hospitalization may be necessary at the time alcohol is withdrawn in that there may be withdrawal symptoms which require treatment with sedative drugs. Disulfiram (Antabuse) has been used for over twenty years and patients who continue to take it have a better prognosis than those who stop the drug. Citrated calcium carbamide (Abstem) is another drug which can be used to help some patients who wish to remain abstinent, but have difficulty in doing so. Aversion treatment has also been used but there is still uncertainty as to whether conditioning has anything to offer. Group therapy for alcoholism has been widely used and Alcoholics Anonymous is an enormously valuable supportive organization, although only a minority of patients who are encouraged to join A.A. will in fact do so. Destitute alcoholics may require very long-term or possibly lifetime support, for example in special hostels.

Dependence on Tobacco

Some 18 per cent. of smokers become ex-smokers. This so-called natural discontinuance tends to occur after 30 and increases with age, especially after 60, and the majority of those who give up smoking do not find it difficult. On the other hand, of those who continue to smoke, nearly half would like to stop but are unable to do so. Health, expense, and social pressure are the most important reasons for wishing to stop. There is no evidence that there is any drug or psychological treatment that has any advantage over simple, supportive counselling to guide a patient through withdrawal from tobacco, this to be followed be relearning to function efficiently and contentedly without smoking. There is essentially no specific treatment for those who wish to abandon tobacco.

The medical profession provides a good example of the possibilities and limitations of health education. Physicians, who must be presumed to know more of the hazards and dangers of opiates than comparable non-medical professional groups, nevertheless have significantly higher rates of opiate dependence. In the United States, the incidence of morphine dependence among doctors and nurses is eight times higher than would be expected in the general population. This example illustrates that availability appears to be a more powerful factor than factual knowledge. On the other hand, the smoking habits of doctors have markedly changed, and in some countries the number who are cigarette smokers has been halved, apparently as a result of their professional knowledge of the risks to health.

Drug Dependence

The World Health Organization Expert Committee on Drug Dependence, in their Eighteenth Report (1970), pointed out that the ideal goal of treatment with total abstinence, independence, gainful employment, satisfactory social and personal adjustment, and emotional stability was seldom achieved, though much money had been expended in many countries in the quest for this ideal goal. For this reason, intermediate goals had been formulated which did not insist on abstinence but aimed instead for improvement in the areas of economic stability and employment, social adjustment, and decreased criminality.

Even partially successful treatment with limited aims can be seen as a form of secondary prevention. Treatment can vary from that of complications to special approaches including withdrawal, maintenance, the use of antagonists and the setting up of self-regulating 'therapeutic communities'.

Before discussing various types of treatment it might be helpful to define possible outcomes. These are generally considered to be:

1. Whether or not the patient is continuing to use the drug.
2. Whether the patient is functioning more efficiently, irrespective of whether he is using drugs or not.
3. Whether the patient himself is satisfied with the treatment.

4. Whether the treatment contains or further spreads addiction.

So far, there has been little careful evaluation of any forms of treatment, and disproportionate claims have been made for the efficacy of all methods. It would appear to be true that all types of treatment have had a limited value for a limited number of patients. Finally, since our knowledge of the natural history of different types of dependence on drugs is much poorer than it should be, it is often hard to know whether various treatment methods have improved or worsened the situation. To summarize different treatment approaches: first, there is withdrawal of drugs, in cases where there is physical dependence which may require careful medical supervision. Secondly, some patients who wish to remain totally abstinent and off all drugs will benefit from entering a therapeutic community of the Synanon/Phoenix/Daytop type. However, only a very small percentage of all those dependent on drugs will wish, or be able, to accept this type of programme. For those who are unable to cease using drugs, a less deleterious type of dependence may be substituted by arranging for long-term prescription of drugs. In the United States, the majority of patients in programmes of this type are on long-term methadone maintenance, while in England they may be on methadone or heroin maintenance.

Compulsion

Discussing the role of compulsion in treatment the World Health Organization Expert Committee pointed out that, in principle, compulsion could be used in connexion with problems of drug dependence in three distinct ways:

1. To provide care or treatment that the individual does not desire, or a form of treatment other than that which he prefers.
2. To invoke the principle of quarantine by regarding the individual as a carrier of a communicable disorder that seriously threatens the health of the community ('quarantining a person because he has a dangerous communicable disorder is an acceptable public health practice only if he is afforded such treatment as is reasonably available').
3. To require notification to medical authorities of the disorder of drug dependence, in the same way as notification of other communicable diseases (this, of course, is not compulsory treatment, but rather an obligatory epidemiological procedure).

The Committee reviewed evidence relating to civil commitment for dependence on alcohol and other drugs and reviewed the arguments in favour of, and against, the use of compulsion in connexion with treatment. They considered that the clinical evidence was not sufficient either to support or to refute the case for various forms of compulsory treatment, but noted that, in spite of considerable experience, compulsory detention alone had not been shown to be beneficial.

There is a need for improved evaluation of the effectiveness of various methods (medical, social, legal, educational, and other) of treatment and rehabilitation in different social and cultural settings, with particular emphasis on considering how best to evaluate these adequately.

PREVENTION

Since treatment of drug dependence, alcoholism and cigarette smoking is at present of only limited value, attempts at prevention must be considered seriously. Since one of the factors in the development of dependence of any type is availability of the drug, consideration must be given to control this. A recent report, *Measures for the Prevention and Control of Drug Abuse and Dependence* (which was the Report of a Working Group convened by the Regional Office for Europe of the World Health Organization, 1971*a*), stated in Section 3:

Where alcohol is concerned, taxation policies have been shown in many countries to affect consumption, the incidence of delirium tremens and chronic alcoholism. In Denmark, for example, relatively higher taxes on distilled spirits and lower on beer have led to a change in drinking habits and a decrease in occurrence of the physical sequelae of chronic alcoholism (Nielsen, 1965). There is some evidence from France and

TABLE 78

Average Weekly Spending on Alcoholic Drinks by All Householders in U.K. 1963–69 (new pence)

	1963–65	1965–67	1967–69
Beer and cider . . .	53	62	69½
Wine and spirits . . .	22½	27	33
All alcoholic drinks . .	83	92	104½
Average household income .	£12·42	£26·72	£30·24
All drinks as proportion of total income	3·4%	3·5%	3·5%

(Source: Department of Employment and Productivity (1970), *National Survey of Consumer Expenditure, Representing Households in Great Britain*, London, H.M.S.O.)

Canada (de Lindt and Schmidt, 1968) that *per capita* consumption of alcohol bears a relation to rates of alcoholism. In Finland, where the number of sources for the purchase of alcohol has been recently increased, *per capita* rates of alcohol consumption have similarly altered. In the United Kingdom, a commission studying the alcohol licensing laws has been considering alterations which would permit longer hours for the sale of alcohol. While this might, for example, benefit the tourist industry, the possible social implications of such a change require careful study. If increasing the opportunities for the sale of alcohol can

increase consumption, then any such changes should be looked at not only from the economic standpoint but also from that of their possible effect on the public health.

Bodies promulgating legislation might profitably pay more attention than is usually done to the public health implications manipulating such controls. Health authorities are not usually in a position to advocate the use of revenue controls as a public health measure, while those responsible for taxation do not usually consider the prevention of illness to be one of their functions. Nevertheless, more consideration might be given to the public health consequences of such methods of indirect control, including, for example, taxes on alcohol and tobacco, changes in the times during which alcohol may be consumed, changes in the number of facilities for its sale, controls on sales to minors, or the prohibition of automatic vending machines for cigarettes where it is illegal to sell them to persons under 16.

However, it would appear that in the United Kingdom at present there has been an increase in the amount of alcohol consumed, so that it is possible there will be later increases in rates of alcoholism. Consumer expenditure on alcohol has risen over the past ten years—beer, £563 million in 1960—£1,058 million in 1969 (Department of Employment and Productivity (1970) *National Survey of Consumer Expenditure, Representing Households in Great Britain*). The average weekly spending on alcoholic drinks by all householders in the United Kingdom from 1963 to 1969 is shown in TABLE 78. Spending varied within different income brackets. The greater the income of the households the higher the proportion of money spent on alcoholic beverages. Manual workers spend proportionally more of their income than do people in other occupation. There has also been an increase in the number of drunkenness offences, which again must be a cause for some concern [TABLE 79]. Control of alcohol is provided by controls on price and controls of distribution (and by the breathalyser). Tobacco, too, is controlled by tax and tax limitations on its sale.

Control of Drugs

Some drugs are also controlled by legal measures. The Single Convention of 1961, which came into force in 1964, was the culminating point of efforts at international control which had started in 1909. It aimed to bring under national and international control all narcotic substances. At the national level it provided for:

TABLE 79

Offences of Drunkenness Proved in England and Wales, 1950–1969

Year	Total number of convictions	Number per 10,000 of male population aged 15 years and over	Number per 10,000 of female population aged 15 years and over	Number per 10,000 of total population aged 15 years and over	Variation compared with previous year in number of offences proved	
1950	47,700	26·24	2·83	13·95	+11,984	+33·54%
1961	74,700	41·50	2·51	20·99	+6,585	+9·67%
1962	84,000	45·95	2·54	23·26	+9,298	+12·45%
1963	83,000	45·07	2·51	22·83	−985	−1·17%
1964	76,800	41·31	2·32	20·97	−6,165	−7·43%
1965	73,000	39·17	2·02	19·80	−3,862	−5·03%
1966	70,500	37·50	2·09	19·04	−2,481	−3·40%
1967	75,500	39·94	2·26	20·32	+5,045	+7·16%
1968	79,000	41·69	2·19	21·24	+3,526	+4·67%
1969	80,500	42·27	2·58	21·56	+1,432	+1·81%

(Sources: Home Office (1970*a*) *Offences of Drunkenness 1969*, London, H.M.S.O.; *Drugs, Alcohol and Tobacco in Britain* (1972).)

1. Control of production, manufacture, distribution, and possession of drugs, of internal trade in drugs, and of violation at the international level.

2. Control of the import of an international trade in narcotics.

3. Transmission of estimates and statistical returns to the International Narcotics Board.

4. Provision of information to the United Nations Secretary General.

5. Mutual assistance of states for control purposes.

The main instruments of international control were the regular statistical returns to the International Narcotics Control Board and the estimates for future drug requirements, which make it possible to limit manufacture, import, and export. The Single Convention lays down that the consumption of narcotic drugs is allowed on medical prescription only, and outlaws the non-medical use of narcotic substances (including opium, coca leaves, and cannabis) and their preparations; their possession is permitted to authorized persons only. There is an obligation to supervise constantly all activities related to narcotic drugs and to keep precise records.

A further group of psycho-active drugs (stimulants, sedatives, tranquillizers, and hallucinogens) which have come into use more recently, have shown the need for further measures for international control of such psychotropic substances. This has culminated in a United Nations convention on psychotropic substances signed by twenty countries—subject to ratification and in some cases express reservations (United Nations, 1971). The development of international control of drugs was reviewed by Glatt (1970). An increase in the number of substances to be controlled because of their misuse liability has occurred at a time when greater knowledge, better communications and travel make the implementation of traditional measures more difficult. Study of achievements rather than of aims, and consideration of other methods, besides outright prohibition of use, to curtail and limit consumption might lead to better and more effective controls.

Health Education

Health education in the areas of drugs, alcohol, and tobacco was discussed in a report of a Working Group (WHO, 1971). They pointed out that there was very little reliable information about the effectiveness of health education programmes. The few studies which had been made failed to show any unequivocal benefits. Much health education seemed to be carried out as an act of faith, rather because the ends were seen to be desirable than because their effectiveness was certain and known goals could be achieved. There was a danger that certain groups might be tempted to become self-elected health educators, whose unduly sensational programmes might thus produce an effect which was the reverse of that intended: on the other hand, programmes imposed by remote 'authority' might prove, in practice, to be of limited local value. While changes in behaviour were unlikely to result from appeals to the intellect alone, changes in attitudes and feelings were not easy to produce, and were in any event difficult to measure. There was a very great need for carefully controlled trials of different educational programmes, based on careful organization and planning.

A study of schoolchildren's attitudes to, and knowledge of, dependence-producing drugs (Wright, 1968) showed that the majority of them had knowledge of drug effects, but that much of their knowledge was factually incorrect. Most of them reported that their main source of information was the mass media, particularly television. The effects of school health education have seldom been evaluated. Yet to be of any real value, comparison of 'experimental' (exposed) with 'control' (unexposed) groups of children would seem to be a minimum requirement for effective planning of programmes.

Whether health education programmes dealing specifically with drug abuse are desirable, or whether they should be incorporated in courses of general social education, has been widely discussed, though there has been little attempt to measure the advantages of shortcomings of either approach. It is generally agreed that it is necessary for teachers, youth club leaders, and others dealing with young people to be well-informed about these problems, and that they should themselves receive training in this field before taking part in educational programmes for their pupils.

TABLE 80

United Kingdom

ALCOHOL
£2,000 million spent on alcohol consumption
£900 million taxed revenue
£20 million on advertising alcoholic drinks

(*Alcoholism*)
Hospital admissions 7,000 admissions/year
80,000 arrests for public drunkenness
30,000 arrests for drunken driving
40 per cent. prison population
60 per cent. vagrants } have drinking problems

(*Employment*)
80,000 in brewing and distilling
125,000 licensed premises

TOBACCO
365 million cigarettes smoked daily
£12 million advertising
£1,000 million tax revenue

Mortality
Between 40 and 100 thousand deaths/year as a result of smoking

OTHER DRUGS
Cannabis
3,071 convictions 1968
4,683 convictions 1969
7,520 convictions 1970 (LSD 757 in 1970)

Drug clinics
For opiate dependence 27 to treat 2,881 addicts (London)

Drug prescriptions
37·1 million for sedative and tranquillizing drugs
3·9 million prescriptions for C.N.S. stimulants

(Source: *Drugs, Alcohol and Tobacco in Britain* (1972).)

There are major difficulties in considering how to evaluate the effectiveness of health education campaigns since they are in general minimal when compared with other influences (for example, advertising of alcohol and tobacco), so that it is inherently unlikely that they will produce any but small and transient effects. TABLE 80 gives some idea of the size of this problem [see also CHAPTER 49].

FINAL COMMENT

Dependence-producing substances are a major cause of ill-health. Despite this, adequate information about the size of the problem is lacking. Epidemiological studies are scanty and hard to carry out because of the problem of definition, and society's attitudes to dependence which may favour concealment. Treatment is difficult, and largely entails the long-term case of people more or less frequently in difficulties. Prevention would be desirable, but measures to alter society's attitudes are in their infancy. Research is needed, particularly sociological research, but the meagre findings so far are often platitudes expressed in jargon. As greater success is achieved in treating other illnesses, so the disorders discussed in this chapter will become of greater importance to all those concerned with public health.

The 26th World Health Assembly held in 1973 expressed its concern at the serious public health problem of dependence and stressed the need for WHO to develop programmes in this field. The United Nations Fund for Drug Abuse Control (UNFDAC) works in close liaison with WHO in this field (World Health Organization, 1974).

REFERENCES AND FURTHER READING

Adams, B. G., *et al.* (1966) *J. roy. Coll. gen. Practit.*, **12**, 24.

Advisory Committee on Drug Dependence (1968) *Cannabis, Report by the Advisory Committee on Drug Dependence*, London, H.M.S.O.

Advisory Committee on Drug Dependence (1970) *Amphetamines and L.S.D., Report by the Advisory Committee on Drug Dependence*, London, H.M.S.O.

Alarcon, R. de (1969) *Bull. Narcot.*, **21**, 17.

Alarcon, R. de., and Rathod, N. H. (1968) *Brit. med. J.*, **2**, 549.

Backhouse, C. I., and James, I. P. (1969) The relationship and prevalence of smoking, drinking and drug taking in (delinquent) adolescent boys, *Brit. J. Addict.*, **64**, 75.

Bailey, M. B., Haberman, P. W., and Alkane, H. J. (1965) *Quart. J. Stud. Alcohol.*, **26**, 19.

Baker, A. A., and Lucas, E. G. (1969) *Lancet*, **i**, 148.

Bewley, T. H. (1966) *Bull. Narcot.*, **18**, 1.

Bewley, T. H., and Ben-Arie, O. (1968) Study of 100 consecutive in-patients, *Brit. med. J.*, **1**, 727.

Bewley, B. R., Day, I., and Ide, L. (1973) *Smoking by Children in Great Britain: A Review of the Literature*, Social Science Research Council, London.

Bransby, C. R. (1971) *Health Trends*, **3**, 75.

Bynner, J. M. (1969) *The Young Smoker*, London, H.M.S.O.

Council of Europe (1970) *Public Health Implications of Recent Developments in Drug Dependence*, Public Health Committee Report, Strasbourg.

Department of Employment and Productivity (1970) *National Survey of Consumer Expenditure, Representing Households in Great Britain*, London, H.M.S.O.

Department of Health and Social Security (1970) *On the State of the Public Health, Annual Report of the Chief Medical Officer for the Year 1969*, London, H.M.S.O.

Doll, R., and Hill, A. B. (1950) *Brit. med. J.*, **2**, 739.

Dreker, K. F., and Fraser, J. G. (1968) Smoking habits of alcoholic out-patients, *Int. J. Addict.*, **3**, 65.

'E.D.' in Arber, E., ed. (1895) *Essays of a Prentise, Etc.*, English Reprint Series, London.

Edison, G. R. (1971) The drug abuse pandemic, *J. Amer. med. Ass.*, **216**, 1037.

Edwards, G. (1967) *Hosp. Med.*, **1**, 273.

Finnegan, J. K., Larson, P. S., and Haag, H. B. (1945) *Science*, **102**, 84.

Fremming, K. H. (1951) *The Expectation of Mental Infirmity in a Sample of the Danish Population*, Eugenics Society, London.

General Register Office (1958) *Royal College of General Practitioners Report*, in *Morbidity Statistics from General Practice*, Vol. I, eds. Logan, W. P., and Cushion, A. A., General Register Office, London, H.M.S.O.

Hawks, D. V. (1970) *Bull. Narcot.*, **22**, 15.

Hawks, D. V. (1971) *Int. J. Addict.*, **6**, 135.

Helgason, T. (1964) *Acta psychiat. scand.*, **40**, Suppl. 173, 1.

Hensman, C., and Zacune, J. (1971) *Drugs, Alcohol and Tobacco*, London.

Home Office (1970a) *Offences of Drunkenness 1969*, London, H.M.S.O.

Home Office (1970b) *Report to the United Nations on the Working of the International Treaties on Narcotic Drugs*, London, H.M.S.O.

James I of England (1604) Counterblaste to tobacco, in *Essays of a Prentise Etc.*, ed. Arber, E., English Reprint Series (1895), London.

Jellinek, E. M. (1960) *The Disease Concept of Alcoholism*, New Haven, Conn.

Johnston, L. M. (1942) *Lancet*, **ii**, 242.

Joint Subcommittee of the Standing Medical Advisory Committees (1968) *Hospital Treatment of Acute Poisoning*, Report of Joint Subcommittee of the Standing Medical Advisory Committees, London, H.M.S.O.

Journal of the American Medical Association (1965) *J. Amer. med. Ass.*, **193**, 673.

Keller, M., and Efron, V. (1955) *Quart. J. Stud. Alcohol.*, **16**, 619.

Keller, M. (1958) Alcoholism: nature and extent of the problems, *Ann. Amer. Acad. polit. soc. Sci.*, **315**, 1.

Keller, M. (1960) *Quart. J. Stud. Alcohol*, **21**, 125.

Kessel, N., and Walton, H. (1967) *Alcoholism*, Harmondsworth.

Kiloh, L. G., and Brandon, S. (1962) *Brit. med. J.*, **2**, 40.

Knapp, P. H., Bliss, C. M., and Wells, H. (1963) *Amer. J. Psychiat.*, **119**, 966.

Kosviner, A. M., Mitcheson, M., Myers, K., Ogborne, A., Stimson, G. V., Zacune, J., and Edwards, G. (1968) *Lancet*, **i**, 1189.

Lindt, J. de, and Schmidt, W. (1971) *Addictions*, **18**, No. 2 (1).

Lucchesi, B. R. (1967) *Clin. pharmacol. Ther.*, **8**, 789.

Moss, M., and Davies, E. B. (1967) *A Survey of Alcoholism in an English County*, London.

Nature (1970) *Nature (Lond.)*, **225**, 310.

Nielsen, J. (1965) *Acta psychiat. scand.*, **41**, Suppl. 187, 86.

Office of Health Economics (1967) *Drug Addiction*, London.

Office of Health Economics (1970) *Alcohol Abuse*, London.

Parr, D. (1957) *Brit. J. Addict.*, **54**, 25.

Prys Williams, G. (1965) *Chronic Alcoholics*, Rowntree Social Science Trust, London.

Prys Williams, G., and Glatt, M. M. (1966) *Brit. J. Addict.*, **61**, 257.

Royal College of Physicians (1962) *Smoking and Health*, London.

Royal College of Physicians (1971) *Smoking and Health Now*, London.

Russell, M. A. H. (1971a) Cigarette dependence, 1. Nature and classification, *Brit. med. J.*, **2**, 330.

Russell, M. A. H. (1971b) *Brit. J. med. Psychol.*, **44**, 1.

Shepherd, M., Cooper, B., Brown, A. C., and Kalton, G. (1966) *Psychiatric Illness in General Practice*, London.

Stimson, G. V., and Ogborne, A. (1970) *Bull. Narcot.*, **22**, 13.

Surgeon General (1964) *Report of Advisory Committee to the Surgeon General*, Department of United States Health, Education and Welfare, Washington, D.C.

Todd, G. F., ed. (1969) *Statistics of Smoking in the United Kingdom*, Tobacco Research Council, Research Paper 1, 5th ed., London.

United Nations (1966) *Summary of Annual Reports of Govern-*

ments Relating to Opium and Other Narcotic Drugs 1964, Commission on Narcotic Drugs, Geneva.

United Nations (1971) *Conference for the Adoption of a Protocol on Psychotropic Substances,* Vienna.

Wiener, R. S. P. (1970) *Drugs and School Children,* London.

World Health Organization (1951) Report on the First Session of the Alcoholism Subcommittee, Expert Committee on Mental Health, *Wld Hlth Org. techn. Rep. Ser.,* No. 42.

World Health Organization (1952) Second Report of the Alcoholism Subcommittee, Expert Committee on Mental Health, *Wld Hlth Org. techn. Rep. Ser.,* No. 48.

World Health Organization (1964) Thirteenth Report of the Expert Committee on Drug Dependence, *Wld Hlth Org. techn. Rep. Ser.,* No. 273.

World Health Organization (1965) Fourteenth Report of the Expert Committee on Dependence-producing Drugs, *Wld Hlth Org. techn. Rep. Ser.,* No. 312.

World Health Organization (1966) Fifteenth Report of the Expert Committee on Dependence-producing Drugs, *Wld Hlth Org. techn. Rep. Ser.,* No. 343.

World Health Organization (1967) Fourteenth Report of the Expert Committee on Mental Health, *Wld Hlth Org. techn. Rep. Ser.,* No. 363.

World Health Organization (1969) Sixteenth Report of the Expert Committee on Drug Dependence, *Wld Hlth Org. techn. Rep. Ser.,* No. 407.

World Health Organization (1970) Eighteenth Report of the Expert Committee on Drug Dependence, *Wld Hlth Org. techn. Rep. Ser.,* No. 460.

World Health Organization (1971) The limitation of smoking, *Wld Hlth Org. Chron.,* 25, 242.

World Health Organization (1973) Thirteenth Report of the Expert Committee on Drug Dependence, *Wld Hlth Org. techn. Rep. Ser.,* No. 526.

World Health Organization (1973a) Youth and Drugs, *Wld Hlth Org. techn. Rep. Ser.,* No. 516.

World Health Organization (1973b) Alcohol problems and national health planning in WHO programmes, *Wld Hlth Org. Chron.,* 27, 166.

World Health Organization (1973c) 19th report of the Expert Committee on Drug Dependance, *Wld Hlth Org. techn. Rep. Ser.,* No. 526.

World Health Organization (1974) The work of WHO in 1973, *Wld Hlth Org. Off. Rec.,* 213, 170.

World Health Organization, Regional Office for Europe (1971a) *Measures for the Prevention and Control of Drug Abuse and Dependence,* Report of a Working Group, Copenhagen.

World Health Organization, Regional Office for Europe (1971b) *Report on Recent Changes in Patterns of Drug Abuse in Czechoslovakia, France, and Yugoslavia,* ed. Bewley, T. H., Euro 4000/4, Copenhagen.

World Health Organization (1974a) Twentieth Report of the expert committee on drug dependence, *Wld Hlth Org. techn. Rep. Ser.,* No. 549.

World Health Organization (1974b) Alcohol and drug dependence in 33 countries, *Wld Hlth Org. Offset Publ. Ser.,* No. 6.

World Health Organization (1974c) Evaulation in drug control, *Wld Hlth Org. Chron.,* 28, 283.

Wilmath, S. S., and Goldstein, A. (1974) Therapeutic effectiveness of methadone maintenance programs in the U.S.A., *Wld Hlth Org. Offset Publ. Ser.,* No. 3.

Wright, J. D. (1970). Knowledge and experience of young people regarding drug abuse, *Proc. roy. Soc. Med.,* 63, 725.

34

THE HEALTH OF MOTHER AND CHILD

DERRICK B. JELLIFFE and YNGVE HOFVANDER

Introduction

Problems of maternal and child health (MCH), and ameliorative programmes, vary greatly from one part of the world to another, especially between the extremes of those industrialized affluent countries, with well-developed social services, and many tropical countries with limited resources of all types, including money, trained staff, equipment, and the developmental infrastructure, such as road communications and water supply, on which public health services depend.

Everywhere, but especially in technically less developed countries, pregnant and lactating mothers and young children are biologically, psychologically, and culturally vulnerable. Their nutritional needs are increased physiologically, although, not infrequently, their diets are limited, particularly in protein, because of poverty, lack of knowledge, or custom. They form a substantial segment of the population, and much illness and mortality among this group is preventable, economically and practically.

Biologically, the health of the mother and young child are, to a considerable extent, interdependent. The nutritional stores acquired by the foetus are related to maternal diet in pregnancy, and, subsequently, are of great importance in supplying the needs of the growing infant. In traditional rural circumstances, the young baby's health, nutrition, normal growth and, indeed, even survival, depend on the ability of the mother for successful breast feeding. In all communities, the care, attention, and affection given by the mother to her young offspring, including breast feeding, are of major importance in the psycho-biological development of the infant and, indeed, in subsequent personality development.

Conversely, the health of the mother is dependent in various ways on the cumulative effects of the children she has borne and reared. Early mating, poor maternal diets (often made worse by cultural food restrictions, and by continued hard physical work), and repeated close-spaced reproductive cycles can lead in less well-fed communities to a progressive nutritional drain [see CHAPTER 11] and various forms of 'maternal depletion syndromes', as, for example, with vitamin D and calcium lack (osteomalacia), iron deficiency anaemia, iodine depletion (goitre), or general malnutrition, as evidenced by loss of body weight (due to depletion of stores of subcutaneous fat and body muscle), premature ageing and death. All can be causes of maternal illness or death, especially in pregnancy and childbirth. All, in turn, affect the nutrition of offspring, particularly through foetal stores.

Culturally, pregnancy, labour, and early childhood are well recognized as being hazardous in most societies by special *rites de passage*, especially for childbirth and for weaning. Likewise, unfortunately, many food attitudes, often of a restrictive nature and related to the more nutritious items of the diet, especially protein, are too often directed at mothers, particularly during pregnancy and lactation, and at young children, especially in the first 2 years of life. They can play a considerable role in the aetiology of malnutrition in these vulnerable groups, whose needs, in fact, are increased at these times.

The classical public health 'calendar' divisions in early childhood—that is infant (first year of life) and 'pre-school child' (1–4 years)—are useful statistically and reflect established procedure. However, a more biologically rational categorization is into foetus, 'extero-gestate foetus', and 'transitional'. This emphasizes the dependence—almost complete in all traditional communities—of the young baby in the first 6–9 months of life upon his mother for care and protection, and for nutrition, in the form of human milk and foetal stores.

The term 'transitional' emphasizes the dangerous period characteristic of all mammals, in which the young child moves from being exclusively milk-drinking to gradual omnivorousness ('weaning'), while, at the same time, being in the process of transition immunologically, psychologically, and as regards experience of his environment. It is a period of recognized high-risk, not only nutritionally, but also from accidents and a wide range of microbiological and parasitic infections, varying from region to region, including, for example, whooping cough, ascariasis, and malaria, diarrhoeal disease ('weanling diarrhoea'). In particular, the second year of life brings such severe problems that a special term has been suggested for the 'second year transitional'—the secotrant.

Patterns of MCH

The forms and levels of health problems affecting mothers and young children in any community depend in large measure on four interacting variables—the culture pattern, genetic considerations, geographical–climatic circumstances, and, most important, the 'level of development' of the community.

The culture pattern plainly can affect the forms of physical illness present, as exemplified by the prevalence of tetanus of the newborn where unsanitary practices are customary in dealing with the umbilical cord. Likewise, methods of child-rearing are related to the forms of so-called 'behaviour problems' prevalent.

Genetic diseases vary considerably in different child populations as, for example, the high rate of sickle-cell disease in some communities of African ancestry and of fibrocystic disease in some Caucasian groups. Their importance looms larger as infections and malnutrition become less common.

Geographical–climatic factors play relatively little part in moulding the pattern of maternal and child health, except indirectly, for example, in relation to the easier breeding of

TABLE 81
Changing Pattern of Infant Mortality in the United States 1900–1954

Infant mortality (0–1 Year) . .	1900	1954
Total deaths per 1,000 live births . .	150	26·6

Causes of Death	Percentage of Total	
Infective and parasitic diseases . .	7·9	1·15
Diarrhoea and enteritis . .	24·7	2·97
Pneumonia and influenza . .	14·7	6·93
Congenital malformations . .	6·4	12·54
Certain diseases of early infancy (including prematurity)	34·5	51·14
All other causes	11·8	11·55

(From Williams and Jelliffe, 1972.)

TABLE 82
Infant Mortality Rate, Mortality Rate for the Age-group 1–4 Years, and 'Socio–economic' Development Index

Country	Infant mortality rate per 1000 live births	Mortality rate in children 1–4 yrs old per 1000 children of the same age	Socio-economic development index*
United States of America (1964) .	24·8	1·0	111
England (1964) .	20	0·8	104
Sweden (1963) .	14·2	0·6	103
Australia (1964) .	19·1	1·0	93
Argentina (1963) .	60	3·7	73
Venezuela (1962) .	30	6·0	62
Chile (1962) .	114	7·2	61
Costa Rica (1964) .	75	7·5	50
Panama (1964) .	42·7	8·0	48
Colombia (1964) .	84	13·7	46
Mexico (1964) .	64	12·7	44
El Salvador (1962) .	70	16·0	32
Ecuador (1962) .	39	20·2	31
Guatemala (1962) .	91	26·9	21

* Calculated by United Nations Research Institute for Social Development, Geneva, July 1970.
(From *World Health Organization Technical Report Series* (1971) No. 477; and Joint FAO/WHO Expert Committee on Nutrition, 8th Report.)

certain insect vectors, such as malaria-carrying anopheline mosquitoes.

In fact, the pattern of MCH found in present-day technically less developed countries, situated mainly, but not exclusively, in the tropics and subtropics, is very similar to that of Europe and North America in the last century and earlier [TABLE 81]. The picture is mainly related to 'level of development' [TABLE 82]—a short-hand term to include standards of education, levels of economic prosperity, conditions of environmental sanitation, and the availability of adequate social services, including roads and particularly the availability and use of locally relevant health services, with sufficient outreach to make contact with the majority of the population at risk.

Maternal Ill Health

While child-bearing is a natural process, it has special risks, particularly in less developed regions of the world, where mortality rates can be extremely high [TABLE 83], from such potentially preventable conditions as infections of the birth canal (leading to puerperal sepsis and tetanus), post-partum haemorrhage (often on a background of anaemia), trauma during delivery (including dystocia and ruptured uterus), and, in some areas, severe toxaemias of pregnancy. Thus, in parts of South America the maternal mortality rate has been estimated as over 200 per 100,000 live births as compared with 11·3 per 100,000 live births in Sweden, where such preventable conditions have been very greatly reduced by the improved standard of living, and by antenatal supervision and by the availability of skilled delivery service.

Ill Health in Infancy and the Newborn

The infant mortality rate (IMR) is rightly regarded as an important index of child health, of the effectiveness of health services, and, indeed, of the social progress of a country [FIG. 87]. In developing countries, the IMR is high, often from 50 to 150 per thousand live births, and from 3 to 10 times as great as in industrialized regions of Europe and North America.

Comparisons are made even more meaningful if such data are divided into neonatal mortality (first month of life) and post-neonatal mortality (1–11 months). Difference between less and more developed countries are much greater in the post-neonatal mortality rates, as it is this latter part of infancy in which such 'environmental' conditions as diarrhoea, pneumonia, anaemia, and malaria commence to make their impact. Also, in the latter months of the post-neonatal period, the child under traditional circumstances begins to show early evidence of poor nutrition, as evidenced by flattening of the weight curve, which, in successfully breast-fed babies, is usually excellent in the first 6 months of life. Moreover, in peri-urban communities in developing countries, decline in lactation per-

TABLE 83
Relevant Vital Statistics from some Countries in the Western Hemisphere of Different Levels of Technical and Economic Development

Country	BR	CDR	MMR	IMR	1–4 MR	Percentage total of deaths under 5	Per Capita Income in $ U.S.
United States . . .	21	9·5	0·3	24·8	1·0	6·4	2,707
Canada	23	7·7	0·3	24·7	1·0	9·0	1,691
El Salvador . . .	47	11·7	0·9	65·3	16·0	49·5	235
Equador . . .	46·9	13·1	2·3	89·9	20·0	57·7	174
Jamaica . . .	39·6	7·8	1·7	39·3	4·6	27·9	397
Guatemala . . .	47·3	15·9	2·1	91·6	26·9	48·9	248

BR = birth rate, CDR = crude death rate, MMR = maternal mortality rate, IMR = infant mortality rate, MR = mortality rate.
(From Williams and Jelliffe, 1972.)

formance is often a characteristic and regrettable trend, and is leading to an increasing prevalence of both diarrhoeal disease and of nutritional marasmus in the post-neonatal part of infancy, as mothers attempt unaffordable bottle-feeding in completely unhygienic circumstances.

Neonatal morbidity and mortality in less technologically advanced areas of the world has not been sufficiently studied, especially by autopsy. Nevertheless, it is clear that infections of the newborn (particularly septicaemia and tetanus), birth trauma, and low birth-weight babies (associated with maternal malnutrition and infection) are mainly responsible, as, indeed, they were in Western countries until recent decades. By contrast, in Europe and North America, neonatal mortality has

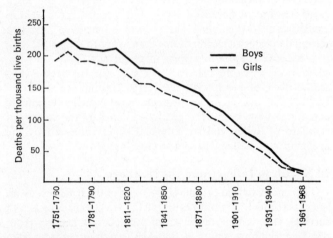

FIG. 87. Infant mortality rates by sex in Sweden from 1751 to 1968. (Reproduced by courtesy of Professor Ragnar Berfenstam, Institute of Preventive Medicine, Uppsala, Sweden.)

fallen considerably, but not proportionately nearly so much as has the death rate in the post-neonatal period. Although infections, damage during the birth process and some forms of low birth weight have been greatly reduced, a core of conditions of less certain aetiology remain, which are less amenable to prevention, such as various congenital abnormalities, premature babies of unknown aetiology and the respiratory distress syndrome.

Ill Health in Pre-School Children

It is in the early so-called pre-school period, especially in the second year, that the major impact of ill health is found in developing countries. Although considerable variations occur, a similar general pattern is to be found widely. The 'Big Three' are everywhere the interacting trio of protein-calorie malnutrition (including kwashiorkor and marasmus), diarrhoeal disease and pneumonia; while the rest of the 'Top Ten' include tuberculosis, intestinal parasites, malaria, whooping cough, measles, anaemia (of various aetiologies), and accidents.

Characteristically, the young child in the populous areas of the Third World grows well for the first 6 months of life, when breast fed. Following this, growth is less adequate during the second semester, and becomes very poor in the second year, partly because of a defective weaning diet, coinciding with a continuous and cumulative barrage of different infections. It is unusual for young children to be suffering from one disease alone, but usually bear an accumulation of several

at the same time. Diagnosis, therefore, in health centres, hospital wards, and at autopsy, is often based on a somewhat arbitrary selection of one of the conditions from which the child is suffering, often reflecting current local medical interest. Usually a background of some degree of protein-calorie malnutrition increases the child's susceptibility to a variety of different infections, such as measles. Rational analysis of causes of death under these circumstances can only be achieved if all the diseases present are recorded, and categorized as being underlying, associated, or primary.

The high prevalence of ill health in this age-group, especially malnutrition, is suggested by attendances at hospitals and health centres, but is fully revealed by community surveys, when it is not uncommon for up to two-thirds of pre-school children to show some degree of malnutrition, as judged anthropometrically.

By contrast, the 1–4 year age group in more technically developed parts of the world is a relatively healthy period with the main causes of death being accidents, particularly poisoning, and malignant diseases, including leukaemia. In developing countries, the death rate among pre-school children may be up to 30–50 times as high as in Europe and North America, with the secotrant especially affected. Forty per cent. or more of the total mortality may occur in children below 5 years of age, compared, for example, with 5 per cent. in countries such as the United Kingdom.

In general, the pattern of ill health in mothers and young children in Western countries has improved greatly because of a dramatic fall in the prevalence of infections and parasitic infestations, of malnutrition and anaemia, and of the complications of poorly supervised pregnancy and childbirth. This has come about as a result of improvement in standards of living and in the application of modern scientific medicine, including health care in pregnancy, childbirth and early childhood, active preventive programmes, such as widespread immunization, and the availability of early treatment.

At the same time, new environmental health problems have emerged, related to urban life-styles, particularly domestic poisoning with medicines and household fluids, and other accidents related to technological innovations, such as road traffic and electrification. The decline of many infections and malnutrition has increased the prominence of, and attention to, less common genetic and metabolic diseases, and to conditions of uncertain aetiology, such as various congenital abnormalities and forms of prematurity. The fall in the infant mortality rate has been mostly concerned with a decline in the prevalence of conditions in the post-neonatal period, while the neonatal mortality has been less affected.

MCH PROGRAMMES

While improvements in community maternal and child health are plainly related to a whole complex of factors usually labelled 'standard of living' and 'level of development', including economics, education, and environmental sanitation, it is also everywhere necessary to devise programmes concerned with the more immediate protection of the health of these vulnerable groups.

Plainly, the form and content of the particular services, and their distribution and staffing, have to be related to local priorities and, in turn, these can only be assessed if based on an analysis of the problems, and the causative factors, in the particular region. Such baseline data should include such *vital statistics* as are available (mortality levels and forms of illness during pregnancy, childbirth, the neonatal period, infancy, and the pre-school age (1–4 years), broken down, when possible, into one year intervals). Biased, but still useful information can be gained from analysis of *attendances at local health services*, and data can be gathered in the course of various special *community surveys* of different degrees of complexity and cost, including cross-sectional and longitudinal studies. Information is needed from all these sources as it is complementary in scope. In many circumstances it may also be possible for information to be collected by the staff of health services, including the 'defined areas' around health centres. This can be most useful and such activities should be built into the training of staff responsible for such services.

Despite great differences in problems in very diverse ecologies in the world, the following ten principles can help to guide a rational development of appropriate MCH services anywhere: (1) adaptation to ecology and needs; (2) with real community participation; (3) within economic constraints; (4) integrated within the general health services; (5) as part of co-operative community development; (6) comprehensive in aim, 'at risk' in focus; (7) with education a primary role; (8) with staff trained to actual function and local need; (9) guided by evaluation; and (10) acceptable within national development planning activities.

In all parts of the world, limited resources of funds and of staff, combined with rapidly rising costs, have led to the realization that there is a need to re-assess priorities, to re-consider the functions of different traditional types of staff and units, to experiment with new forms of service capable of reaching the community, and to consider questions of cost-benefit at all levels. Fortunately, coincidentally with this, national development planners have begun to realize that their task is concerned not only with raising GNP, that is the national income—but also with the 'quality of life' of the population, including the health and nutrition of mothers and children, representing, the 'human resources' of the future. This significant change in attitude is, for example, reflected by the changing goals laid down for the United Nations Second Development Decade commencing in 1970.

MCH services need to be comprehensive in aim, while, at the same time 'at risk' in focus. They should be as comprehensive as possible *physiologically*, that is covering pre-natal and lactating mothers, the newborn infants and weanlings; *geographically*, that is available to all the population including remote rural areas and urban slums; *in range of activity*, that is from health promotion to preventive activities to rehabilitation to treatment; and *in all components of the programme*, that is including hospitals, health centres, other newer units, and, very important, domiciliary activities.

However, within this over-all ultimate aim, 'at risk' districts, families and children need local definition, as requiring special care and supervision, and hence priority attention from limited services and resources. In rural Africa, for example, weaning from the breast or an attack of measles may constitute 'at risk' circumstances in relation to the development of kwashiorkor;

in urban circumstances everywhere low income levels and large numbers of children, especially if closely spaced, clearly indicate families in which mothers and children will be in need of special care and supervision.

MCH services all over the world, but especially in developing countries, must be a major vehicle for family planning advice, and for nutrition education, with emphasis on breast feeding and the best use of weaning multimixes prepared from low-cost locally available foods.

Classical mistakes in the past have been attempts to try to separate the services for sick children and well children, for pregnant women, and for family planning. This may still be practicable [in some Western countries but, in general, the interdependence of all of these activities biologically and also the convenience of the mother and her young children make it necessary to undertake them through one combined set of services. The diagnosis and cure of young children and pregnant women when sick, especially if detected early, constitute as much a 'preventative' aspect of maternal and child health as do more orthodox preventive activities, such as immunization.

However, not only is it desirable for MCH services to be co-ordinated, but, at the same time, they in turn need to be integrated functionally, and preferably physically, within the general health services of a country. Additionally, it is most important that relevant activities, particularly educational in nature, should be undertaken in amicable collaboration with other agencies which may, in some countries, be responsible for extension activities of a parallel nature in the community, including agricultural extension, community development, voluntary agencies, etc.

In all circumstances, but again particularly in less technologically advanced countries, an important role of all aspects of MCH services should be concerned with education of parents and of children, channelling modern scientific knowledge in an understandable and acceptable form to prevent locally important conditions, to detect them early on, and to ensure that the best use is made of available health services.

Health education in the non-didactic modern sense must, then, be a prime function of all levels of all staff in all parts of an MCH programme especially in the home, but also including such traditionally therapeutic enclaves as hospitals.

In all political systems and in countries of all different levels of technical development, rethinking is under way in relation to actual function and to the real needs and resources of the community, rather than to orthodox title and traditionally defined role. This is very much the case, as would be expected in MCH services, dealing as they do with major segments of the population. Many innovative experiments are under way with the use of different varieties of auxiliaries and aides, and of volunteers, both from within the village and also from the educated youth of countries. New roles are in the process of definition for established cadres, including doctors, nurses, and midwives. Many problems need to be overcome including forms of training, interrelationships between different cadres, satisfactory careers for new forms of personnel, and making them acceptable, both to traditional health 'trade unions' and, indeed, to the public, which has often grown to consider a certain service as obligatorily needing a particular type of staff, often a physician.

Components of MCH Services

A large number of systems of MCH services have evolved in various cultural, historical, political, and geographical circumstances in different parts of the world. In all regions, it is necessary to devise a locally appropriate and relevant network which covers comprehensively, as far as possible, the promotive, preventive, and curative health needs of mothers and children in the area concerned, including remoter rural areas and also urban slums, with the constraint of available resources.

Basically, this must include the *early diagnosis and cure of ill health, the supervision of maternal and child health* (especially during more vulnerable periods), *the active prevention of disease*, as by immunization, and *the promotion of good health*, by means of health and nutrition education.

In many countries, this MCH network will be a satellite-system radiating from hospital to health centre to home visiting, with a variety of other units and activities also developed as locally appropriate, including day-care centres, nutrition rehabilitation units (mothercraft centres), etc.

All components of MCH services, as with other aspects of health services, have recently been under reconsideration all over the world. For example, with rising costs, the function and role of the hospital is under review everywhere. In less developed countries, both the paediatric and the maternity wards can very easily become completely overwhelmed with large numbers of patients quite beyond the capacity of the bed space, available staff, and other resources. Under these circumstances the impossibility of administering correct treatment, the high risk of cross-infection, early discharge following inadequate therapy, and the lack of emphasis on health education may make hospitals counter-productive, not only in relation to their high cost compared with the available national health budget, but even to their limited effectiveness in therapy. For example, the present-day mortality rate in kwashiorkor in larger hospitals is still of the order of 20–30 per cent., while many such children die after discharge because of inadequate follow-up, insufficient treatment in hospital and the development of cross-infection that only become manifest after leaving hospital.

The role of hospitals, and especially of paediatric wards, needs re-definition. Adequate screening has to be available to permit those children to be admitted who can benefit most from the usual relative concentration of laboratory and other facilities that is to be found there. This may mean that hospitalization will be principally on short-term basis for children with diagnostic or therapeutic complications that need the special resources available. At the same time, the hospital needs to lay greater emphasis on preventive activities, such as health education and, also, to realize and to assume its role as part of a promotive–preventive–curative network, with real and functional links with other units concerned with delivering health services to communities.

In less developed regions of the world, a major feature of an MCH network will usually be a system of Young Child Clinics (Under Five Clinics), linked with domiciliary activities, at least for 'high risk' families, undertaken by trained health staff, including auxiliaries, together with the use of volunteer personnel, both from the village itself and also from the educated youth of the country.

Coverage

The activities included in the coverage of MCH services can be illustrated in relation to two important components of such services—the Young Child Clinic and the Antenatal Clinic.

Health Supervision. A screening procedure needs to be devised, appropriate to local problems and resources, which will enable the health of pregnant women and young children to be supervised by means of periodic surveillance, both in the homes and at clinics, so that early deviation from normal can be detected and also 'at risk' families or individuals identified and appropriate measures taken including, for example, additional supervision by means of home visiting or extra clinic attendances, by special additional health educational sessions, by relevant therapy, or by the issue of supplementary foods or vitamin and mineral supplements.

The same principles of surveillance and screening also need considering in technically advanced countries for such genetic disorders as phenylketonuria and galactosaemia, using appropriate clinical or biochemical tests from soon after birth.

Serial weighing of young children, using weight charts to record progress, is an important method of assessing growth and of detecting malnutrition at an early stage.

Immunization [See CHAPTER 26]. In all parts of the world, a *continuing* programme of immunization is needed against infectious diseases of local importance in young children. Appropriate schedules need to be devised [TABLES 84, 85, and 86] taking into account the relative costs of both immunization and curative treatment, as well as difficulties in ensuring attendance, and problems of storage and of administration of vaccines in the field.

All over the world, immunization against whooping cough, pertussis, tetanus, poliomyelitis, and smallpox need priority consideration and can be achieved at low cost. In addition, in developing countries the frequency of tuberculosis and the difficulty with its therapy and control by other means make B.C.G. immunization an important, logical, and economical preventive measure. Likewise, the direct effect of measles and its importance in precipitating malnutrition, make immunization a priority, if affordable. Conversely, in technologically advanced countries, immunization against rubella needs to be undertaken by young females, in view of the risk of contracting the infection in a subsequent pregnancy.

TABLE 84

A Combined Compound Immunization Schedule Suitable for Tropical and Subtropical Areas

Age	Proposed schedule
2–6 months	Diphtheria–pertussis–tetanus triple vaccine: 3 doses with 1 month's interval between each dose
6–7 months	Smallpox vaccination
7–10 months	Poliomyelitis vaccine (inactivated): 2 doses with 1 month's interval
15–18 months	Booster dose of triple vaccine: simultaneously third dose of poliomyelitis vaccine
2–4 years	Fourth dose of poliomyelitis vaccine
5–6 years	Booster dose of diphtheria–tetanus vaccine: simultaneously, smallpox revaccination
10–15 years	Booster dose of diphtheria–tetanus vaccine if Schick test positive: no injection of diphtheria prophylactic in Schick pseudo-reactors

(From Stanfield, 1970.)

TABLE 85
A Combined Compound Immunization Schedule Suitable for Tropical and Subtropical Areas

TIME	VACCINE	ROUTE	REMARKS
Antenatal first visit	Tetanus toxoid alum absorbed	IM	1 ml. dose—at least one month apart
7th–8th month of pregnancy	Tetanus toxoid alum absorbed	IM	
Birth	B.C.G.	Intradermal (by Dermojet)	Only feasible in a large maternity unit due to wastage of multidose ampoules
2/12	DPT (triple vaccine) alum adsorbed	IM	Half standard dose has been suggested to minimize reactions
	Poliomyelitis (Sabin) (trivalent)	Oral	Suggested titre for most tropical areas Type 1 $10^{5.3}$ Type 2 $10^{3.4}$ Type 3 $10^{4.7}$
	B.C.G. Vaccinia (smallpox)	Intradermal (by Dermojet) Multiple pressure or Dermojet	Standard skin sites for the county or area should be adhered to
3/12	DPT (triple vaccine alum adsorbed	IM	Read smallpox and B.C.G. vaccinations. Repeat if no lesions visible
	Poliomyelitis (trivalent)	Oral	
4/12	Poliomyelitis (trivalent)		A third monthly dose can be inserted but is probably not necessary if the child can be got back at 9/12 to 1 year
9 months–1 year	DPT (triple vaccine) alum adsorbed	IM	Full dose
	Poliomyelitis (trivalent)	Oral	Combine with measles vaccine
	Measles, live attenuated	Intradermal by Dermojet	Dosage still to be standardized but suggest from 200–1,000 TCD_{50}
School age—5–6 years	DPT (triple vaccine) alum adsorbed	IM	Full dose
	Poliomyelitis (trivalent)	Oral	
	B.C.G.	Intradermal	
	Vaccinia	Multiple pressure or intradermal	
	If child first seen when over 6 months of age and unimmunized		
x/12	DPT alum adsorbed	IM	
	Poliomyelitis (trivalent)	Oral	
	B.C.G.	Dermojet	
	Vaccinia	Multiple pressure or Dermojet)	Standard sites
$\frac{x+1}{12}$	DPT alum adsorbed	IM	Read vaccinia and B.C.G. vaccinations. Repeat if no lesion
	Poliomyelitis (trivalent)	Oral	
	Measles, live attenuated	Intradermal by Dermojet	Use as attraction for second dose. Do not give if child has clear history of measles or is over 3 years of age
$\frac{x+2}{12}$	DPT alum adsorbed	IM	The monthly intervals are not optimal with alum adsorbed DPT but slightly longer intervals might discourage re-attendance
	Poliomyelitis (trivalent)	Oral	

(From Stanfield, 1970.)

Various schedules of immunization have been recommended in different parts of the world. Basically, there is a need to immunize prior to the age at which young children are mainly at risk from the particular condition, but also at a time when the infant's passive immunity is waning and his ability to develop active antibodies has been achieved.

In less developed countries, with difficulties of reaching young children, various adaptive immunization schedules have been developed in an attempt to give as wide as possible a protection against the more important infections with the least number of attendances and with the simplest, speediest methods capable of being undertaken by auxiliary staff.

Health Education. This should be a major concern in all aspects of an MCH programme, and can be undertaken individually, both during a clinic and especially while home visiting, in the form of suggested advice to the mother related to her own problems. In addition, planned activities, usually in the form of group discussion-demonstrations, should be undertaken in all components of MCH services, including hospitals. They are best exemplified in the nutrition rehabilitation centres that have been found to be very effective in recent years in dealing with problems of severe malnutrition in the community. In these, mothers are themselves responsible for preparing and cooking appropriate diets, based on locally available food mixtures, and feeding them to their own malnourished children. In this way, they can see the effect on the child's general appearance, and also in his improved weight, especially if this is recorded serially on a weight chart.

Opportunities for health education are numerous and can range from such sophisticated and costly devices as mechanical film strips with tape recordings played in out-patients while mothers are waiting, to such real-life situations as the develop-

TABLE 86

Revised Schedule for Active Immunization and Tuberculin Testing of Normal Infants and Children in the United States. (Approved by the Committee on Infectious Diseases. American Academy of Pediatrics, October 17, 1971.)

2 months	DTP[1]	TOPV[2]
4 months	DTP	TOPV
6 months	DTP	TOPV
1 year	Measles[3]	Tuberculin Test[4]
1–12 years	Rubella[3]	Mumps[3]
1½ years	DTP	TOPV
4–6 years	DTP	TOPV
14–16 years	Td[5]	and thereafter every 10 years

[1] DTP—diphtheria and tetanus toxoids combined with pertussis vaccine.

[2] TOPV—trivalent oral polio virus vaccine. The above recommendation is suitable for breast-fed as well as bottle-fed infants.

[3] May be given at 1 year as Measles–Rubella or Measles–Mumps–Rubella combined vaccines. Rubella and Mumps for discussion of age of administration.

[4] Frequency of repeated tuberculin tests depends on risk of exposure of the child and on the prevalence of tuberculosis in the population group.

[5] Td—combined tetanus and diphtheria toxoids (adult type) for those over six years of age in contrast to diphtheria and tetanus (DT) containing a larger amount of diphtheria antigen.

Tetanus toxoid at time of injury: For clean, minor wounds, no booster dose is needed by a fully immunized child unless more than 10 years have elapsed since the last dose.

For contaminated wounds, a booster dose should be given if more than 5 years have elapsed since the last dose.

Routine smallpox vaccination is no longer recommended in the United States but is required according to law in many countries, e.g. Sweden.

ment of a low-cost village house and home garden for teaching purposes adjacent to the paediatric unit of a hospital in a developing country.

The main need is to ensure that this philosophy and emphasis permeates all activities, and to be sure that health education receives due emphasis in the training of all staff [see also CHAPTER 49].

Supplementary Foods. Supplements, in the form of appropriate foods, vitamins or minerals, are usually required. However, long-term supplementary feeding programmes need to be considered, most carefully balancing the advantages against various limitations and difficulties.

Modern supplementary feeding programmes for young children need to be based on a carefully thought out, clearly defined policy concerning the purpose, selection, age-group, length of issue, form of packaging and issuing, method of preparation, and assured nutrition education in the preparation of the foods concerned.

In areas where malnutrition in early childhood is common and mainly related to lack of food, at least limited supplementary feeding will be needed for selected children or families for certain periods of time. Thus 'at risk' children who are substantially underweight or following measles, may need food supplementation for the period until they have recovered, or, alternatively, 'at risk' families of large size and low economic level may need food supplementation for longer periods.

Supplementary feeding programmes should not only be selective, but also within the distribution facilities available (including funds for storage and transport, etc.), related to

priority local nutritional deficiencies (as, for example, with regard to any vitamin fortification), culturally and physiologically appropriate—that is to say acceptable to the parents, to their children, digestible and easy to prepare, and without disruptive effect on the local pattern of infant feeding, particularly breast feeding. They should be linked to programmes for the increased local production of foods suitable for the domestic preparation of village level multimixes and for the ingredient foods and for the processing (national and local level) of similar food mixtures ('Incaparina', 'Faffa', etc.).

Supplementary feeding programmes for young children should be primarily an instrument of nutrition education, by demonstration, by home visits, and by all other means. They are more likely to be needed in urban slum areas with impoverished communities within a money economy; their issue free or at low cost through health services can then best be related to the same product which is on sale through regular marketing channels [see CHAPTER 11].

Treatment. Owing to unfortunate historical circumstances, diagnostic-curative activities have tended to develop separately from preventive services in Western countries and, hence, to be regarded as external to MCH services and to the training of their staff. In fact, basic treatment of the major local conditions should form a part of the activities of all components of MCH services, including Young Child Clinics and home visiting, as well as hospital activities.

It is both unnatural and impossible to separate preventive and curative services at any of these levels. Plainly, early treatment has a preventive function, while effective therapy, however simple, of the sick child is the best way to ensure the confidence of parents, and hence their more likely motivation to follow less immediately and obviously beneficial preventive approaches, such as health education and immunization. A major difficulty is in achieving a balance, with sufficient preventive emphasis, in communities where ill health in young children is widespread.

Contraceptive Advice [see CHAPTER 36]. In all communities, but especially in impoverished, poorly nourished groups, family planning needs to be considered not only as a national objective, but also of immediate concern to maternal and child health, both in relation to family size and also to physiologically optimal child spacing. Contraceptive advice, appropriate to the culture, philosophy and practical circumstances of the particular community, should be incorporated into all aspects of MCH services from hospitals, clinics, and domiciliary activities. The opportunities during MCH services are logical, and include the mother's attendances at ante-natal, postnatal, and the Young Child Clinics.

Referral and Co-ordination. Too frequently in the past, isolated components of an MCH network have been developed by governments or by voluntary services. Very frequently, a major need is to ensure a functional relationship between the different existing components, and also to develop new units which will fill the gaps and deficiencies.

Referral and follow-up is very frequently a neglected aspect of MCH service; often, an operative network of services can best be created and developed by means of some form of national MCH advisory committee, with an officer of sufficient seniority at the Ministry of Health, to guide over-all developments, together with, when needed and feasible, local co-ordinating committees for each region and major urban area.

Such a committee should include representatives of groups concerned with paediatrics, obstetrics, nutrition, family planning and health education in the government services, in voluntary agencies (e.g. missions), and in teaching centres, especially universities.

REFERENCES AND FURTHER READING

Bengoa, J. M. (1967) Nutrition rehabilitation centres, *J. trop. Pediat.*, **13**, 169.

Bryant, J. H. (1969) *Health and the Developing World*, Ithaca, New York.

Cameron, M., and Hofvander, Y. (1972) *Manual on Feeding Infants and Young Children in Developing Countries*, Protein Advisory Group of the United Nations.

Cook, R. (1971) Is the hospital the place for the treatment of malnourished children?, *J. trop. Pediat.*, **17**, 15.

King, M., ed. (1966) *Medical Care in Developing Countries*, Nairobi.

Jelliffe, D. B. (1966) The assessment of the nutritional status of the community, *Wld Hlth Org. Monogr. Ser.*, No. 53.

Jelliffe, D. B. (1968) Infant nutrition in the subtropics and tropics, *Wld Hlth Org. Monogr. Ser.*, No. 29.

Jelliffe, D. B. (1969) The secotrant—a possible new age category in early childhood?, *J. Pediat.*, **74**, 808.

Jelliffe, D. B., ed. (1970) *Diseases of Children in the Subtropics and Tropics*, London.

Jelliffe, D. B., and Bennett, F. J. (1962) World-wide care of the mother and newborn child, *Clin. Obstet. Gynec.*, **52**, 64.

Jelliffe, D. B., and Jelliffe, E. F. P., eds. (1971) The uniqueness of human milk, *Amer. J. clin. Nutr.*, **24**, 968.

Jelliffe, D. B., and Jelliffe, E. F. P. eds. (1973) Nutrition programmes for pre-school children, Proceedings of a Conference, Institute of Public Health, Zagreb.

Jelliffe, E. F. P. (1971) A new look at multimixes for the Caribbean, *J. trop. Pediat.*, **17**, 135.

Morley, D. (1963) A medical service for children under five years of age in West Africa, *Trans. roy. Soc. trop. Med. Hyg.*, **57**, 392.

Morley, D. (1968) A health and weight chart for use in developing countries, *Trop. geogr. Med.*, **20**, 101.

Morley, D. (1970) In *Diseases of Children in the Subtropics and Tropics*, ed. Jelliffe, D. B., p. 215, London.

Puffer, R. R. and Serrano, C. V. (1973) *Patterns of Mortality in Childhood*, P.A.H.O. Scientific Publication No. 262, Washington.

Scrimshaw, N. S., Taylor, C. E., and Gordon, J. E. (1968) Interactions of nutrition and infection, *Wld Hlth Org. Monogr. Ser.*, No. 59.

Stanfield, J. P. (1970) In *Diseases of Children in the Subtropics and Tropics*, ed. Jelliffe, D. B., p. 59, London.

Williams, C. D., and Jelliffe, D. B. (1972) *Mother and Child Health, Delivering the Services*, London.

World Health Organization Expert Committee on Maternal and Child Health (1969) The organization and administration of maternal and child health services, *Wld Hlth Org. techn. Rep. Ser.*, No. 428.

World Health Organization (1970) Report of a WHO Expert Committee. The prevention of perinatal mortality and morbidity, *Wld Hlth Org. techn. Rep. Ser.*, No. 457.

World Health Organization (1971) Report on a Seminar. Prevention of perinatal morbodity and mortality, *Wld Hlth Org. publ. Hlth Pap.*, No. 42.

World Health Organization (1974) The work of WHO in 1973, *Hlth Org. Off. Rec.*, **213**, 107.

World Health Statistics Reports. Abortion (1969) Vol. 22, No. 1.

World Health Statistics Reports. Perinatal Mortality (1969) Vol. 22, No. 1.

World Health Statistics Reports, Maternal Mortality (1969) Vol. 22, No. 6.

World Health Statistics Reports. Foetal Mortality (1970) Vol. 23, No. 6.

World Health Organization (1974) Childhood mortality in the Americas, *Wld Hlth Org. Chron.*, **28**, 276.

World Health Organization Regional Office for Europe. Reports of meetings on mother and child health, Copenhagen.

(1970) *Child and Family Psychiatry in Europe 1951–1969* (Euro 0416).

(1972) *Induced Abortion as a Public Health Problem* (Euro 9601).

(1973) *The Role of MCH Services in Family Planning* (Euro 9603).

(1973) *Evaluation of MCH Services in Certain Countries* (Euro 5103(2)).

35

THE HEALTH OF THE SCHOOL CHILD

P. HENDERSON

Introduction

In bringing medicine to the community the provision of health services for children of school age should have a high priority.

A child spends a large part of its life at school exposed to a wide variety of environmental influences, physical, emotional, and social. It is important, therefore, that there should be adequate health supervision of children at school so that early signs of ill health can be detected and the opportunity taken of educating the boys and girls, and their parents, in healthy ways of living.

The requirements of children are basically similar everywhere, and a study of the historical growth and geographical pattern of school health services reveals that they have developed on very similar lines in most parts of the world.

Historical

It was not until the nineteenth century that serious study was given to the health of children at school.

In 1812 James Ware reported on the eyesight of school children in London and of students at Oxford University. In 1840 several doctors were appointed in a number of training colleges in Sweden. In 1866 Herman Cohn investigated the eyesight of over 10,000 children in Breslau; by 1883 he was urging the appointment of school doctors and had the eminent support of Virchow. The first school doctor in Germany was, in fact, appointed that year in Frankfurt-am-Main. Two years later one was appointed in Lausanne. In 1888 the Swedish Government inquired into the physical condition of over 11,000 Swedish children. At about the same time school medical inspection was started in all the Departments of France. In 1895 six school physicians were appointed to supervise the elementary schools in Moscow.

In England, in 1880, Dr. Priestly Smith reported on the prevalence of short sight, and its relation to education, in 2,000 school children and training-college students in Birmingham. In 1882 *Health at School* was published by Dr. Clement Dukes, medical officer to Rugby School; and in 1892 Dr. Francis Warner reported on the medical examination of 50,000 children in schools of various types.

The first publicly appointed school medical officer in England was appointed in London, in 1890; eighty-five had been appointed by 1905, but it was not until 1908 that the school health service was organized on a national basis. The overwhelming evidence, presented in three challenging reports, published at the beginning of the century, that very many children were in poor health or were physically disabled so impressed the Government that the Education (Provision of Meals) Act was passed in 1906, and the Education (Administrative Provisions) Act in 1907.

THE SCHOOL HEALTH SERVICE IN ENGLAND AND WALES

The 1906 Act gave Local Education Authorities the power to provide, or to assist in the provision of, meals for elementary school children who were unable through lack of food to obtain full benefit from education.

The 1907 Act made it a duty for education authorities to arrange for the medical inspection of children in public elementary schools and gave the power to make such arrangements for their treatment as might be sanctioned by the Board of Education. In 1907 a medical branch (renamed Medical Services Branch 1972) was established at the Board of Education (which became the Ministry of Education in 1945 and the Department of Education and Science in 1964). On 1st April 1974 the control of the School Health Service passed into the hands of the Department of Health and Social Security (DHSS) with the reorganization of the National Health Service. The Area Health Boards will be directly responsible for local administration. In 1919, on the establishment of the Ministry of Health, the Chief Medical Officer of the Board of Education was appointed Chief Medical Officer of the new Ministry while remaining Chief Medical Officer of the Board of Education. His successors have, ever since, been Chief Medical Officer of both departments.

In November 1907 the Board of Education issued Circular 576 for the guidance of education authorities:

'The Board desires, therefore, at the outset to emphasise that this new legislation aims not merely at a physical or anthropometric survey or at a record of defects . . . but at the physical improvement, and, as a natural corollary, the mental and moral improvement, of coming generations. . . . One of the objects of the new legislation is to stimulate a sense of duty in matters affecting health in the homes of the people. . . . It is in the home, in fact, that both the seed and the fruit of public health are to be found.'

And that has been the objective of the School Health Service ever since.

The Service expanded with the passing years, and particularly as a result of the legislation that followed the two world wars. Regulations under the Education Act of 1918 made it a duty for Local Education Authorities to provide certain forms of treatment for children in public elementary schools and for the medical inspection of those in secondary schools; it also gave them power to arrange for the treatment of children in secondary schools. The Education Act of 1944 increased further the duties of education authorities.

The Need for a School Health Service

Since all children are entitled to free general practioner, hospital, and specialist advice and treatment through the National Health Service, it might well be asked if there is still need for a special health service for children at school.

This question was considered by the Porritt Committee, that was sponsored by the main British medical organizations including the British Medical Association, the Society of Medical Officers of Health, and the College of General Practitioners, to review the medical services in Great Britain; in its report, published in 1962, it stated: 'The School Health Service performs a special and valuable function which must in our view be continued. Its main functions are to ensure that children who need special educational facilities receive them, and generally to provide for the health and well-being of children at school. . . . It would be a mistake to assume that even were it possible for general practitioners to undertake periodic examination of patients of school age this would do away with the need for a separate School Health Service. The work requires specialized knowledge, and the school child needs to be considered as a person both as regards his school environment and his educational needs. . . . In some circumstances it is possible for family doctors to take part in the School Health Service if they so desire but in many instances we do not think it practical, nor necessarily in the interest of the school child.'

A Report of the British Medical Association on adolescents, published in 1961, contained the statement: '. . . doctors in the School Health Service are in the best position to undertake or suggest preventive measures against the predictable illnesses; they can take the opportunity when examining children at school of talking to them about "ideas of positive health." . . . neither general practitioners nor consultants see very much of their adolescent patients.'

In a report by the Standing Medical Advisory Committee, Ministry of Health, published in 1963, on the Field of Work of the Family Doctor, it was envisaged that even although 'many family doctors still fail to appreciate the value of the public health service and the help that it could give them in the work of their practices yet, in time, it could be expected that they would "participate more fully" ' in the work now done by local authority doctors with a consequent reduction in the number of the latter.

In short, even with a national health service there is continuing need for a preventive health service for children at school.

Purpose, and Field of Work, of the School Health Service

The aim of the Service is to help children at school to achieve the maximum physical and mental health possible for them so that they can obtain full benefit from their education.

The Service provides for the medical examination and supervision of children at school and, in co-operation with the family doctors and the hospital services, helps to arrange for their treatment when this is necessary; it also provides an advisory and counselling service for the boys and girls and for their parents and teachers. It makes recommendations to the local education authority on the special educational requirements of handicapped pupils.

Broadly, the work of the Service in the schools comprises:

1. The medical examination and supervision of children.
2. Finding, investigating, and supervising handicapped children.
3. Health education.
4. The control of infectious diseases (in association with the local health authority).
5. Special inquiries into the health and development (including educational) of school children.

The Service is, essentially, a preventive health service for children at school and is closely geared to the educational service.

STATUTORY BASIS OF THE SERVICE

The Education Act of 1944

This Act, as amended by the Education (Miscellaneous Provisions) Acts of 1948 and 1953, made it a duty for all Local Education Authorities in England and Wales to provide school meals, milk, and medical inspection for pupils in all types of maintained[1] primary and secondary[2] schools, and to provide or secure for them all forms of non-domiciliary medical treatment. The medical inspection and treatment of these children are free of cost to their parents. The establishment of the National Health Service in 1948 enabled education authorities to arrange with Regional Hospital Boards for the free specialist and hospital treatment of children attending maintained schools. Some authorities, however, still prefer to employ and pay the fees of specialists who attend their clinics.

The School Health Service Regulations, 1959

Powers to make these regulations were given to the Minister of Education by the Local Government Act, 1958. The regulations required every Local Education Authority: 1. to provide a School Health Service for pupils at schools and other educational establishments maintained by it; 2. to appoint a Principal School Medical Officer who shall be in charge of the service and responsible to the authority for its efficient conduct; and 3. a Principal School Dental Officer, who shall be in charge of the School Dental Service and responsible to the Principal School Medical Officer for its efficient conduct, and such other medical and dental officers, nurses, and other persons as may be necessary; and 4. to ensure that every nurse (with certain specified exceptions) employed in the School Health Service possesses the qualification of a health visitor.

The Regulations also required that:

1. So far as it is practicable the parent of every day pupil shall be given an opportunity to be present at every medical inspection, and at the first dental inspection, of his child.
2. Medical and dental records in a form approved by the

---

[1] A maintained school is one that has its running costs provided entirely out of public funds. Most of them are owned and wholly provided by Local Education Authorities; the others are owned by voluntary bodies, who provide the premises.
[2] Free milk was withdrawn from pupils in secondary (other than special) schools in 1968, mainly on account of decreasing demand from the pupils.

Minister shall be kept for every pupil attending a maintained school.

The Minister of Education, from powers derived from Section 92 of the Education Act, 1944, required every Local Education Authority to send to him annually a report by their Principal School Medical Officer (including one on the School Dental Service by the Principal School Dental Officer) on the health and well-being of children within the scope of the School Health Service.

The National Health Service Reorganization Act of 1973, that came into force on 1 April 1974, transferred the statutory responsibility of providing school health services from the local education authorities to the Secretary of State for Social Services (including the health services). As from 1 April 1974 all medical, dental and nursing staff formerly employed by the local authorities became employees of either the regional or area health authorities of the National Health Service.

STRUCTURE OF THE SERVICE

In January 1970, about 8 million children, attending over 30,000 maintained and assisted schools, were covered by the service. The whole-time equivalent of about 980 doctors (other than the 250 ophthalmic surgeons and 200 other consultants—whole-time equivalent 75), 1,420 dentists, 3,300 nurses, 470 speech therapists, 170 physiotherapists, and other professional staff, including audiometricians, chiropodists, and orthoptists, were employed. There were over 2,000 school–clinic premises that accommodated about 1,750 minor-ailments treatment clinics, 1,350 dental clinics, 1,500 speech-therapy clinics, 560 ophthalmic clinics, 400 audiology clinics, 394 child guidance clinics, 240 remedial-exercises clinics, 220 orthopaedic clinics, 220 chiropody clinics, 140 ear, nose, and throat clinics, 150 enuretic clincs, and a number of others including asthmatic and cardio-rheumatic clinics.

Of the 3,200 doctors (equivalent whole-time 980) engaged in the Service, only 124 worked in it whole time, 1,780 were also employed in the services of the local health authorities, and about 1,300 were in private practice or were married women working on a sessional basis; of the 9,300 nurses (equivalent whole-time 3,300), 6,679 held the Health Visitor's Certificate, most of whom also worked in the services of the local health authorities.

WORK OF THE SERVICE

In 1970, just under 2 million children were examined at periodic medical inspections, and rather fewer than $1\frac{1}{2}$ million were re-inspected or specially inspected; over 4 million were dentally inspected and just over $1\frac{1}{4}$ million received dental treatment at school dental clinics, but at least as many were treated free by the general dental service of the National Health Service. About 100,000 handicapped children in special schools (and many more in ordinary schools) were supervised by the Service.

School Medical Inspection

About 14 per cent. of children when they first start school are found with defects (other than dental defects) that require treatment, of which from 20–50 per cent. are not being treated despite freely available general practitioner and hospital services. The defects include those of speech, hearing and vision, squint, otitis media, and emotional difficulties, all of which if untreated would retard a child's progress in school. There is thus a very strong case for the medical examination of all children when they first start school.

For more than 50 years the medical examination of all children shortly after first entering school, at least once between the ages of 8 and 12 years, and in their last year at school, has been the basis of the work of the school health service in England and Wales. Children found with defects are re-inspected by the doctor on his next visit to the school. A child can, however, be referred at any time by a parent, teacher, nurse, or doctor for medical inspection either in school or at a school clinic; these special inspections are a very important part of the work of the Service. Also, many children are referred to their own doctors or to hospitals for further examination or treatment.

Selective School Medical Examination

Since a number of years there has been criticism of the large amount of time given by school doctors to the examination of healthy children in the later age groups in England and Wales; in 1970 over a million children in these age groups were medically examined without anything having been found wrong with them (excluding dental disease and infestation with vermin). Many of them were unaccompanied by a parent and the speed of examination was such as not to allow time for discussion of a child's personal problems. In over 50 areas a more selective method of medical examination has been adopted or is being tried. In these areas more time is given to the examination of school entrants; a carefully constructed questionnaire, designed to bring to light conditions that might be missed at a periodic examination, such as emotional difficulties, epileptic seizures out of school hours and enuresis, is sent to all parents of school entrants and of those children in the later age groups who would have had a periodic medical examination under the old system; the cause of a child's absence from school is inquired into, and the doctor and nurse visit the school more frequently. In most areas where the selective method has been adopted children are medically examined on first entering, and shortly before leaving, school; in a few areas the periodic school-leaver examination has been dropped and, instead, every school leaver is interviewed, medical examination being reserved for those who were known to have had some defect or disability at any time in their school life.

Before a selective method of examination is introduced it is essential that it should be explained fully to the teachers and their support enlisted. It is also essential that there should be regular screening tests of the vision of all children, and that all entrants to school should have their hearing tested. The big majority of doctors and teachers with experience of the selective system much prefer it to the periodic one. It does not reduce the number of doctors required for the Service, but it enables them to give more attention to children who are not thriving or who are not making satisfactory progress in school, and to health education. The work of the school doctor is more satisfying, and he no longer experiences the monotony of examining large numbers of healthy children year in year out, to little purpose. Most parents also prefer the selective system; only a small minority are unable, or unwilling, to complete the questionnaire, and in these cases a nurse makes a home visit.

The main argument used against a selective system of examination is that defects are likely to be missed. In the areas where it has been adopted with conviction, and where a check was made on all children some years after it was started, the experience was that significant defects were not missed; indeed, many more, particularly emotional difficulties, were found. No system of clinical examination, however, can guarantee that every child with a defect will be discovered.

Screening Tests of Hearing and Vision

Hearing. Since the most vital period in a child's life for learning to speak is from nine months to three years, and since most children born deaf or who become deaf early in life have some residual hearing, it is now recognized that defective hearing should be diagnosed in infancy or early childhood. Even so, hearing loss is not detected in a number of children till they start school: it is, therefore, essential that every child should have his hearing tested as soon as possible after first entering school. Some doctors doubt the value of screening all children in a number of age-groups because very few are found with hearing loss. Those who hold this view argue that it would be more economical and rewarding if audiometry was reserved for all school entrants and for those children who are liable to have impaired hearing—particularly those with speech defect, otitis media, cerebral palsy, congenital cataract, or who are not making satisfactory educational progress. A puretone audiometer is usually used; this type of instrument was recommended by the Medical Research Council's Committee on the Educational Treatment of Deafness in 1955. Speech audiometry is used in a number of clinics.

Vision. In all areas the vision of school children is tested just before, or at the time of, periodic medical inspection. In some areas vision screening tests are given to all children every two years, and in a few areas annual tests are made. Since about 3 per cent. of children on first starting school at the age of 5 years are found to require treatment for visual defect, the necessity for screening all entrants is becoming generally appreciated. About 13 per cent. of children examined at periodic inspections are found with defective vision.

Hearing and vision screening tests are carried out most often by nurses, occasionally by doctors; but, increasingly, non-professional staff are being trained for this work. Increasing use is made of Keystone and Mavis Vision Screeners.

Clinics

Minor Ailments Treatment Clinics. The number of children treated at school clinics for minor ailments has fallen, due, partly, to diminished prevalence of certain diseases, for example, scabies, impetigo, and chronic otitis media, and, partly, to the facilities provided by the National Health Service. These clinics are, essentially, nurses' clinics; a doctor may attend for a short time daily or, perhaps, only once a week. In some areas provision is made in schools for the treatment of children with simple ailments.

Consultation Clinics. When a doctor at a periodic medical inspection finds he has insufficient time to make a detailed examination of a child he can refer that child to his consultation clinic for further investigation. Parents, nurses, and teachers also send children to them; and there, too, handicapped children are medically examined.

Specialist Clinics. Chief among them are:

1. CHILD GUIDANCE CLINICS. The pattern of provision varies, but, generally, a clinic is part of the School Health Service arrangements and is under the clinical direction of a psychiatrist (who may be employed by the education authority, or his services may be provided free by the Regional Hospital Board), with an educational psychologist and a psychiatric social worker as the other members of the team; a school doctor is often, and a paediatrician sometimes, closely associated with it; occasionally, a lay psychotherapist is an additional member of the team. The educational psychologist usually works also in the School Psychological Service and is an essential link between child and school in the same way as the psychiatric social worker is a link between clinic and child's home. In some areas the child guidance clinic service is provided by the Regional Hospital Board. A few child-guidance clinics undertake the training of local-authority medical officers. There is a serious shortage of psychiatrists, psychologists, and psychiatric social workers. In 1970 over 70,000 children were treated at Child Guidance Clinics. The problem of the maladjusted child was the subject of a special report published in 1955 [see CHAPTER 26].

2. EAR, NOSE, AND THROAT CLINICS. Although there are many fewer children with chronic otorrhoea, 10 per cent. may have acute otitis media at some stage in their childhood: their treatment and supervision are still an important part of the work of aural clinics. Many children are also sent to them for surgical advice on the need for tonsillectomy. Every year just under 200,000 children, aged 5–14 years, undergo tonsillectomy in England and Wales. The investigation of boys and girls with hearing defect, prescribing hearing aids for them, advising on their auditory training, and giving guidance to their parents are now among the chief functions of these clinics.

3. OPHTHALMIC CLINICS. In addition to examining and refracting tens of thousands of children annually, including many with squint, ophthalmologists advise school doctors and local education authorities on blind and partially sighted children. In the Report of the Faculty of Ophthalmologists for 1957–58 it was recommended that school children with distance vision worse than 6/9, on the Snellen chart, in either eye should be referred for examination by an ophthalmologist, and that all school entrants should have their vision tested as soon as possible after starting school.

Children with squint should be found before they start school, but every school child suspected to have a squint should be examined by an ophthalmic surgeon without delay. About 8 per cent. of boys and 0·4 per cent. of girls have defective colour vision: all children should have their colour vision tested at about 10–12 years of age. The Ishihara Confusion Chart Test is commonly used and is a satisfactory test. Children found defective should be referred to an ophthalmologist since there may be pathological conditions of the eyes associated with defective colour vision. Certain industries still insist on a Lantern test for all applicants for employment found defective by the Ishihara Charts.

4. ORTHOPAEDIC CLINICS. In the early days of the Service orthopaedic clinics had to deal with many thousands of children deformed by rickets or tuberculosis. For all practical purposes rickets is non-existent, and tuberculosis of bones and joints is rare. In consequence, more time is now given to children with minor orthopaedic defects.

Increasing attention is being paid to children with postural defects by teachers of physical education, and special remedial classes are held in a number of areas. Much of this work is done in association with the physiotherapists of the orthopaedic clinics.

5. SPEECH THERAPY CLINICS. In England and Wales speech therapists employed by education authorities are on the staff of the Principal School Medical Officer. In 1970 they treated about 90,000 children. There is a serious shortage of therapists due mainly to retirement from the service on early marriage.

School Dental Service

The conditions of a satisfactory school dental service were described in the Report of the Chief Medical Officer of the Ministry of Education for 1962–63. Owing to the national shortage of dentists, the School Dental Service is seriously understaffed and cannot cope with all the children who require treatment. Favourable comment on the work of school dental nurses in New Zealand was made in a Report by a mission from the United Kingdom, published in 1950. The Dentists Act, 1956, provided for the introduction in the United Kingdom of a somewhat similar type of dental ancillary and gave the General Dental Council the duty of arranging an experimental scheme of training and employment so that the value of this type of worker could be assessed. The first training course started in the autumn of 1960, and the students who have since qualified are now working in local authority clinics.

Following the abolition of sweet and sugar rationing in Britain, dental caries increased. A report on the fluoridation of domestic water supplies showed that fluoridation reduced dental caries in children and that there was no risk of mottling of the teeth if the amount did not exceed 1 part per million; the report stressed that there was no scientific evidence that this procedure was injurious to health.

School Nursing Service

The training and work of health visitors, including those in the School Health Service, were reviewed in the Report, published in 1956, of the Working Party appointed in 1953 by the Minister of Health, Minister of Education, and the Secretary of State for Scotland. The Report emphasized that the essential work of a health visitor, in the homes and in the schools, was health education and social advice. Much of the work of a nurse in the School Health Service is concerned with discussing with parents, teachers, and doctors the problems of individual children. Home and school visiting is an essential part of this work. Opinions differ on whether periodic cleanliness inspections of school children should be made by health visitors, or by nurses without the health visitor's qualification, or, indeed, by unqualified, but carefully selected and instructed, women. About 240,000 children (2·5 per cent.) were found verminous in 1970, but this percentage was less than half what it was even ten years ago. Since louse infestation is, usually, very much a family matter, health visitors ought not to detach themselves

completely from this social problem. In a number of schools where all the children have been free from infestation for long periods cleanliness inspections have become more selective: in some, entrants only are inspected; in others, inspections of the older children have been reduced in number or abandoned.

Cleanliness inspections sometimes form part of a general inspection of children by school health visitors; these inspections supplement periodic medical inspections and offer valuable opportunities for nurse–teacher discussion as well as for finding children in need of medical examination or treatment. In 1959, for example, over 3,000 children in Birmingham, and 2,500 in Manchester, were referred by school health visitors to school doctors for further examination and advice.

Much of a school health visitor's work is health education in practical form. An increasing number of teachers, recognizing the health content of this work, now invite health visitors to take a direct part in health education in the schools.

The Medical Examination of Children before Employment

About 100,000 children are employed out of school hours. Although very few are found medically unfit, none the less their medical examination is one of the duties of school doctors. So, too, is the giving of advice to parents and youth employment officers on the suitability or otherwise of certain types of employment for children leaving school.

CONTROL OF INFECTIOUS DISEASES AMONG SCHOOL CHILDREN

Recommendations on the exclusion of children from, and the closure of, schools was given in a Memorandum published by the Departments of Education and Science, and Health and Social Security in 1971. Much of the immunization of school children against diphtheria and vaccination against poliomyelitis, as well as the B.C.G. vaccination of school-leavers, is carried out by school doctors; and, too, they have to investigate school outbreaks of infectious disease, including food poisoning, and tuberculosis; the health of workers in the school meals service and methods employed in the preparation and storage of food in school canteens are also their concern. Advice on the prevention of food poisoning in school canteens was issued in 1954 by the Ministry of Education, and suggestions for the investigation of outbreaks of food poisoning were made in a Memorandum published in 1958 by the Ministry of Health. School canteens come within the scope of the Food Hygiene Regulations, 1955.

SCHOOL MEALS AND MILK

In 1970, 67·9 per cent. of children in maintained and assisted schools had school dinners of whom 12·3 per cent. had them free of charge. Free milk to pupils in secondary schools was discontinued in 1968 since only 58 per cent. of them were taking it. At the beginning of the academic year 1971–72 free milk to pupils in primary schools who were over the age of 7 years was discontinued but it continued to be supplied free to any primary school pupil when recommended by a school medical officer. All children in special schools continued to receive free school milk. Less than one per cent. of school milk was not heat-treated.

THE ASCERTAINMENT AND SUPERVISION OF HANDICAPPED CHILDREN

The Education Act, 1944, lays on Local Education Authorities the general duty of providing sufficient schools in their area for the education of children according to their different ages, abilities, and aptitudes, and the particular duty of seeing that provision is made for the education in special schools or otherwise of those with disability of mind or body. All Local Education Authorities must ascertain which children, aged 2 years and over, in their area require special educational treatment. Education is compulsory from the age of 5 to 15 years for children in ordinary schools, and from 5 to 16 years for those in special schools.

Ten categories of handicapped pupils are defined in the Handicapped Pupils and Special Schools Regulations, 1959, as amended by the 1962 Amending Regulations; blind, partially sighted, deaf, partially hearing, educationally subnormal, epileptic, maladjusted, physically handicapped, speech defective, and delicate.

The Education (Handicapped Children) Act, 1970, that came into force on 1 April 1971, abolished the classification of children who used to be termed 'unsuitable for education at school'; it transferred local responsibility for their education and training from the local health to the local education authorities and central responsibility from the Department of Health and Social Security to the Department of Education and Science. For educational purposes these children are now regarded as educationally subnormal. When the Act came into force there were about 24,000 mentally handicapped boys and girls in 330 training centres, 8,000 in about 100 hospitals for the mentally handicapped, and 750 in separate special care units for those who also had severe physical disabilities or behaviour disorders; others were in private institutions or at home. About 400 special schools have been formed out of the 330 training centres and the 100 hospitals for the mentally handicapped. In the United Kingdom the education of all handicapped children, irrespective of the nature or severity of their handicap, is now the responsibility of the education authorities.

It is the Local Education Authority, not a medical or administrative officer or a teacher, which decides whether a child requires special educational treatment. Before reaching a decision on any child an authority must consider the advice given by a medical officer and any reports or information obtained from teachers or others on the ability and aptitude of the child. A parent has the right of appeal to the Secretary of State for Education and Science against the decision of the Education Authority.

School doctors thus have a vital part in the ascertainment of handicapped children. They have an equally responsible part in the supervision of these children whether they are in special or ordinary schools, in boarding homes, or on home teaching.

Blind and Partially Sighted Children

In January 1970 some 1,100 blind and 1,900 partially sighted children were being educated in special schools. The number of registered blind children, aged 5–16 years, fell from 36·9 per 100,000 children in 1925 to 21·1 in 1950: the reduction was due mainly to the prevention of such diseases as ophthalmia neonatorum, phlyctenular ophthalmia, and interstitial keratitis. In 1948 there was a sudden increase in the number of registrations of blind children under 5 years of age that continued till 1954. This increase was due to retrolental fibroplasia in premature babies. The disease was found to be due to the effect of too much oxygen on the immature eyes of premature babies: when the use of oxygen was restricted the disease virtually disappeared.

There is now one form of certificate (Form B.D.8) covering applicants of any age for registration as blind or partially sighted. The certificate also provides a space for the examining ophthalmologist's recommendation of the appropriate type of school if the applicant is of school age; this provision was made to help education authorities when considering the most suitable form of special educational treatment for a blind or partially sighted child. A copy of Form B.D.8, and the criteria adopted by the Faculty of Ophthalmologists for the guidance of examining ophthalmologists when determining whether a person was blind or partially sighted, were given in Ministry of Health Circular 4/55. Briefly, a person with visual acuity below 3/60 Snellen, or between 3/60 and 6/60 when the field of vision is considerably contracted, is regarded as blind; he may, however, also be regarded as blind if his visual acuity is 6/60 Snellen or better if the field of vision is markedly contracted in the greater part of its extent. A partially sighted child is one with visual acuity of 3/60–6/24 with glasses, and for such a child special education by methods involving vision has to be considered either in a special or an ordinary school.

In 1968 the Secretary of State for Education and Science appointed a Committee to consider the organization of education services for the blind and partially sighted and to make recommendations. The Committee's report was published in 1972 by Her Majesty's Stationery Office.

Children with Defective Hearing

In January 1970, 3,337 deaf and 1,857 partially hearing children attended special or independent schools. Special classes in ordinary schools, in charge of trained teachers of the deaf, for partially hearing children are a relatively recent development in England and Wales; by January 1970 their number had increased to 240 special classes with over 2,200 partially hearing children. These figures reveal the changing attitude to children with defective hearing: as a result of improved methods of diagnosis, early ascertainment and auditory training children who would have been regarded as deaf some years ago are now treated and educated as partially hearing. In addition, a large number of children with defective hearing, many with hearing aids, attend ordinary classes in ordinary schools. The diagnosis of defective hearing in infancy or early childhood, the provision of auditory training, the supply of hearing aids, and the guidance of parents take, or should take, place before the children become the responsibility of the School Health Service. Education authorities have the duty to ascertain children in need of special educational treatment from the age of 2 years. Hospital, Local Health and Education Authority staffs are cooperating increasingly to provide a comprehensive and continuous service for children with defective hearing. In some areas trained teachers of the deaf work in hospital audiology clinics as well as in the special classes for partially hearing children in ordinary schools; and an increasing number (180 by January 1970) visit the other schools in their areas where there are children with defective hearing to observe their progress and advise their teachers. The school doctor has an intimate part in all this work.

A special investigation centre and special school was opened in 1968 by the Manchester Education Authority for children with serious difficulty in communication not entirely due to deafness. This centre works closely with the Department of Audiology and Deaf Education of Manchester University and with Booth Hall Children's Hospital, Manchester. The Report of the Committee on the Possible Place of Finger Spelling and Signing in the Education of Deaf Children was published in 1968.

Educationally Subnormal Children

Before a doctor is employed on the ascertainment of educationally subnormal or ineducable children he must, as required by the Medical Examinations (Subnormal Children) Regulations, 1959, attend an approved course of theoretical and practical instruction and have been present as an observer at the examination of a number of these children. In January 1970 over 50,000 educationally subnormal children were in special schools. This subject is dealt with in more detail in CHAPTER 31.

Epileptic Children

Rather more than 3 per 1,000 children examined at school medical inspections are found to be epileptic. On this basis, there are more than 20,000 epileptic children of school age in England and Wales, about 700 of whom are, at any one time, in seven special schools. As a result of the better control of seizures by modern drugs, and of the increased understanding of the needs of epileptic children by school doctors, teachers, and parents, fewer children are sent to special schools, and for a shorter period, than was expected even ten years ago. The Report of the Sub-committee of the Standing Medical Advisory Committee of the Ministry of Health, on the Medical Care of Epileptics, published in 1956, stressed the need for more diagnostic and treatment centres, and for one or two residential units in the hospital service, for epileptic children with serious behaviour or emotional disturbance. Somewhat similar recommendations were made in the Report of a Study Group of the World Health Organization (1957). The British Epilepsy Association organizes an annual holiday camp for epileptic children. In 1969, 40 boys and girls, aged 5–14 years, died from epilepsy, compared with 111 in 1939.

Maladjusted and Psychotic Children

In addition to the 70,000 children treated at Child Guidance Clinics in 1970 rather more than 10,000 were in special or independent schools or classes or at special boarding homes.

In recent years increasing attention has been given to the needs of psychotic children and by 1970 more than a score of small units had been provided either in, or independent of, mental hospitals. From a survey by Lotter et al., in Middlesex, in 1964, it was suggested that there were probably about 3,000 autistic children in England and Wales. A special school for maladjusted deaf children was opened in 1966 at Stoke Poges, Buckinghamshire.

Physically Handicapped Children

In 1970, about 9,000 physically handicapped children were in special schools. Rickets and tuberculosis of bones and joints are now rare; poliomyelitis appears to have been brought under control and if time proves that this is so then a few years hence a child disabled by the disease will be as uncommon as one with a tuberculous joint is now; acute rheumatism affects many fewer children than it did even twenty years ago (in the 12 areas in England and Wales where juvenile rheumatism is notifiable the notifications are about a tenth of those in 1948). As a consequence of these changes, congenital and hereditary defects are now the chief causes of physical handicap in children, especially cerebral palsy (from 1 to 2 per 1,000 children are affected), spina bifida and muscular dystrophy. In 1963–64 it was reported from a few large areas that there appeared to be a substantial reduction in the number of young children with cerebral palsy but since then there have been no reports of any significant change in incidence elsewhere. Recently, there has been an increase in the number of children surviving with spina bifida; this has been due to highly skilled surgery in the first few hours of life and to excellent nursing. Since 1964, in England and Wales, congenital malformations in newborn babies have been notified to the Registrar General. In 1966 it was estimated that 1,470 children with spina bifida were born alive (1·7 per 1,000), of whom 788 died in the first year. A much smaller number die in later childhood. The number who survive varies according to the quality of treatment they receive. It is still too early to estimate with conviction what percentage of them will require education in special schools for the physically handicapped, but at least half of them would be a prudent estimate in present circumstances.

Local branches of the British Red Cross Society hold a number of annual holiday camps for about 250 physically handicapped boys and girls; most of the children are too severely crippled to attend special schools; instead, they receive education at home. Not more than thirty crippled children attend any one camp; the usual period of stay is ten days.

Speech-defective Children

In 1970 over 90,000 children were treated by speech therapists in speech therapy clinics. There are two special boarding schools, with about 80 places, for children whose speech is so defective that they cannot be educated satisfactorily in a day school; their speech defect is due to injury, disease or developmental defects of the brain, from aphasia or from extensive cleft palate. One of the existing schools is being enlarged to cope with the increasing number of children considered to need residential therapy and education. This school has a residential diagnostic clinic to which children are admitted for a week's intensive investigation and observation. In 1969, the Secretaries of State for Education and Science, Health and Social Security, and Scotland appointed a Committee to inquire into the assessment and treatment of children with speech and language disorders and the role of speech therapy in education and medicine. The Committee's report was published in 1972 by Her Majesty's Stationery Office.

Delicate Children

Just over 7,000 delicate children were in special schools in 1970—several thousands fewer than in 1938 when the school population was about 1½ million less. The reduction in numbers is an indication of the improved health of children. Most of the children in this category are debilitated or have respiratory disease, especially asthma.

There are probably between 3,500 and 4,500 diabetic children in England and Wales; about 100 were in four special boarding homes in 1969; all attended ordinary schools. In 1969, only 10 children, aged 5–14 years, died from diabetes, as compared with 77 in 1939, the year in which the first of these boarding homes was opened. The British Diabetic Association organizes a number of annual holiday camps for diabetic boys and girls. Local Education Authorities can contribute towards the cost of sending children to these camps—and to those held by the British Epilepsy Association and the British Red Cross Society—under Section 53 of the Education Act, 1944.

Home Teaching

In 1970 about 2,000 boys and girls were taught in their homes. They were either children who were too disabled to attend a special school or who were frequently in and out of hospital for treatment and required home tuition in the intervening periods to prevent them falling too far behind in their school work. They were kept under supervision by school doctors.

Assessment Centres for Handicapped Children

Many handicapped children have more than one disability; they pose serious social as well as educational and medical problems. This is particularly the case with severely physically handicapped children and with those with grave difficulty in communication. The Report of the Carnegie United Kingdom Trust, published in 1964, urged the opening of centres where the total needs of handicapped children, particularly in relation to their family circumstances, could be assessed by a group of specialists, and where family counsellors could be trained. The Trust contributed towards the cost of establishing two pilot centres, one in Glasgow and the other in Shrewsbury, that were opened in 1964; both were in local authority, not hospital, premises. Once a handicapped child is found there is continuing need for one agency to be responsible for keeping him under observation right through his childhood and school days and to ensure proper liaison with those responsible for his after care when he leaves school. The School Health Service is well placed to be the responsible agency. The imperfect nature of much of the after care of handicapped young people was stressed in the Report, published in 1963, of the British Council for the Rehabilitation of the Disabled, on The Handicapped School Leaver.

A report issued by the Department of Education and Science in 1970 stated: 'Assessment implies an evaluation of the nature and extent of a child's intellectual, emotional, social, motor and sensory assets and liabilities', and that it was '. . . a continuing process, not a once and for all procedure'.

Health Education

Education for healthy living, in very practical form, is incidental to, but none the less inseparable from, the ordinary day-to-day work of the Service. In some schools doctors and school health visitors are invited to take part in teaching selected groups of pupils and to join parents–teachers associations. But more would be achieved if, from time to time in the various districts, teachers and School Health Service staffs met together to review their work in this field and to consider how each could best help the other. Health education in school is concerned with much more than 'hygiene'; it includes the vitally important, delicate and difficult subject of personal relationships, including sex education. Although an increasing number of schools are accepting the challenge of this wide concept of health education many are still only tackling it in part.

MEDICAL RECORDS AND REPORTS

Standard medical and dental record cards, approved by the Minister of Education, are in use everywhere. One of the objects of having standard cards is that they should be of sufficient uniformity to be of value if a child moves from one area to another. The notes that are issued with the medical cards stress that the medical record is confidential and that if it is kept in a school it should be in a locked drawer or cabinet when not required by the doctor or nurse.

A doctor who examines a child under Section 34 of the Education Act, 1944, to find out if he is suffering from any disability of body or mind must, if requested, give the parent or the Local Education Authority a certificate in prescribed form saying whether the child is suffering from such a disability and, if so, its nature and extent.

THE HYGIENE OF SCHOOL PREMISES

Despite the large school building programme, there are still many old schools that are below the minimum standards prescribed by the Regulations. It is part of the duty of school doctors to report on the hygiene of school premises and on the suitability of classroom furniture. A number of Principal School Medical Officers use their annual reports to bring to public notice the unsatisfactory conditions of certain schools in their area. Some schools have separate medical rooms; in others, suitable accommodation for medical, dental, and nursing examinations is always available, but there are still very many where School Health Service staffs are unable to work either in privacy or quiet.

HEALTH OF CHILDREN TODAY AND FIFTY YEARS AGO

British children are taller and heavier than those of earlier generations; they mature earlier, and few are undernourished. Diseases that once killed or maimed thousands of boys and girls every year have been abolished or controlled. It is seldom that a child is found with defective clothing or footwear, whereas thirty to forty years ago 5–10 per cent. were poorly clad or shod. Then, too, 6 per cent. of children had verminous bodies, but the condition is now rare; the percentage with verminous heads is less than a quarter of what it once was; yet, it is discreditable that over 200,000 are still infested. The death rate per 1,000 children, aged 5–9 years, fell from 9 in 1841–50 to

3·5 in 1901–10, and 0·34 in 1969; for children aged 10–14 years it fell from 5·3 in 1841–50 to 2·1 in 1901–10, and to 0·30 in 1969; less than one per million died from scarlet fever and from whooping cough, none from diphtheria, and 2 from measles in 1969. The expectation of life of a boy or girl at birth was about thirty years more in 1969 than a century earlier.

But, there is still much scope for progress. About 1,000 school children die annually from accidents and other forms of violence—twice as many as die from all the respiratory and infectious diseases together. Many thousands of children are seriously disabled by congenital, hereditary, and developmental defects. And, too, there are puzzling differences in comparable areas in the prevalence of certain defects noted at periodic medical inspections.

THE SCHOOL HEALTH SERVICE IN SCOTLAND AND NORTHERN IRELAND

The pattern of provision in both countries is broadly similar to that in England and Wales, but responsibility for the administration of the service rests with the Central and Local Health Authorities.

SCHOOL HEALTH SERVICES IN OTHER COUNTRIES

Europe

The World Health Organization, acting on the recommendations of one of its Expert Committees, organized at Grenoble, in 1954, a European Conference on School Health Services that was attended by representatives from 22 European countries. Its report was circulated in 1955. A second Conference was held in 1963.

The information given to the 1954 Conference was that in most European countries the pattern of medical examination in primary schools was similar to that in the United Kingdom, but the adequacy of medical inspection in secondary schools varied considerably from country to country. The frequency of periodic medical inspection varied: for example, inspections were carried out annually in Denmark, biennially in Germany, triennially in Austria, and triennially in primary, and biennially in secondary, schools in Sweden; in France, where an annual inspection was the rule, triennial examinations were being experimented with in a few areas. In a number of countries periodic inspections were supplemented by tuberculin testing and chest X-ray examinations.

In most countries there was a serious shortage of dentists; in Norway, however, 200 were employed whole-time in the school dental services, each being responsible for about 1,000 children, and about 300 were also employed in the service part-time.

The Conference considered that although a school health service was mainly a preventive, not a curative, service, it might, none the less, depending on national circumstances, be responsible for some forms of treatment for school children (e.g. treatment of disease of the eyes or skin, of defective speech or posture). It was also thought that work concerned with the mental health of school children was likely to increase. Opinion was unanimous that all persons working or living in schools should have a periodic chest X-ray examination and that school meals service staff should be subject to special supervision.

Administrative arrangements were found to differ considerably: exceptionally (e.g. Finland) the service was administered by a central government department, but, usually, by a municipality, county, canton, or province with, or without, co-ordination on a national basis. In Germany, Iceland, Italy, Monaco, Morocco, Netherlands, and Tunisia the Ministry of Health was the central department responsible for co-ordination, whereas in Belgium, France, Algeria, Greece, Sweden, Switzerland, and Turkey it was the Ministry of Education. In Denmark and Spain both ministries were concerned; in Luxembourg both ministries were combined. In Norway the service was administered by the local authorities, but the Director General was also adviser to the Ministry of Education.

School doctors were employed whole-time or part-time. In 1954 in Denmark there were 50 whole-time and 400 part-time doctors; in the Netherlands all were employed whole-time; in France 682 whole-time doctors did most of the school medical examinations, the remainder being carried out by general practitioners on a sessional basis; in Paris part-time general practitioners were employed who had to pass a special examination with written tests on school health.

The Conference was of the opinion that if a school doctor was full-time and examinations were carried out yearly he could supervise a total of 4,200 children; he should be able to examine four children an hour. It considered that the work of the school health service should include: periodic medical examination of all pupils; the follow-up of children found with defects; advising parents and teachers; the control of infectious disease in school; the sanitary inspection of school premises; the medical supervision of teaching and school meals service staffs; the ascertainment and supervision of handicapped pupils; the medical supervision of children at holiday camps and of those taking part in athletics; and participation in health education in the schools; school doctors should also undertake research. Home and school visiting was an essential part of the work of a school nurse; she was, in fact, a health adviser and should not have more than 1,000–1,5000 school children in her charge. The full co-operation of the teachers was essential; during their training all teachers should receive instruction in the work of the school health service.

The U.S.S.R.

In the U.S.S.R. the children's hospital and polyclinic, which is also a consultation centre, is the standard establishment for preventive and curative medicine. The polyclinic provides all children up to the age of 15 years with all types of medical attention including immunization and vaccination, and home visiting of ill children. The paediatricians employed in polyclinics each have a district with a population of 800–1,000 children. From 1940 to 1965 the number of paediatricians increased from over 19,000 to almost 72,000 and, the number of hospital beds for ill children from about 90,000 to over 350,000. School doctors visit schools to examine and treat school children and to advise on and supervise the hygiene of school premises; they are also concerned with health education. Over 5 million school children go to country pioneer camps in summer.

The United States

The pattern of provision varies greatly from state to state and even in different districts of the same state; in some schools arrangements are comprehensive, in others almost non-existent. A joint report by the American Medical Association and the National Education Association recommended that the duties of a school health service should include: the appraisal of the health of pupils and school staff; the counselling of pupils and parents; encouraging the correction of remedial defects; the ascertainment and supervision of handicapped pupils; the prevention and control of disease; an emergency service for injury or sudden sickness; health education and measures for 'healthful school living' (a 'healthful environment, . . . school day, and the establishment of interpersonal relationships favourable to emotional, social, and physical health'). The provision of medical and dental treatment was not considered to be a function of the school health service, as those unable to afford it could be referred to the appropriate community agency. The teacher–nurse conference was of much value.

The report recommended that all pupils should have a minimum of four medical examinations—on first starting school, in the intermediate grades, at the beginning of adolescence, and before leaving school. Those with serious defects or abnormalities, or who had serious or repeated illnesses, required more frequent examination. It was also recommended that all children should have annual vision screening tests, and three hearing screening tests during the first eight years of school life, with particular attention to the younger children: annual testing of hearing was the goal. All children should be weighed and measured three times every school year.

The joint committee estimated that of every 1,000 pupils, 2 were blind or partially sighted, 15 were deaf or hard of hearing, 15 had speech defects, 10 were crippled, 15 were delicate, 2 were epileptic, and 20 were considerably retarded mentally. These children found it difficult or impossible to benefit fully from the regime of the ordinary school: adjustments or adaptations were required, including particular attention in the regular, or special, classes of ordinary schools, or in day or boarding special schools.

Developing Countries

More than half the world's children live in these countries that are mainly rural and many with poor internal communications. Environmental conditions are, generally, very insanitary. There is much poverty and malnutrition that are made more acute by the rapidly increasing population. Although much progress has been made in the control of serious communicable diseases such as leprosy, malaria, smallpox, and yaws they are still prevalent in some countries, as are tuberculosis, trachoma (the chief cause of blindness in children), and gastro-enteritis; there is much respiratory disease; severe outbreaks of diphtheria and poliomyelitis continue to occur; rheumatic fever and rheumatic heart disease are prevalent; cholera, rabies, and tetanus are causing concern in some districts; worm infestation and scabies are widespread almost everywhere; congenital physical defects are common; there is much preventable blindness; deafness appears to occur in children as frequently

as in developed countries; mental health and social problems are becoming more apparent both in children and young people, and in the latter venereal diseases are on the increase. Mortality rates are high, though falling. In short, as tropical diseases come under control the pattern of disease and disability in children in these countries is seen to be broadly similar to that in children and young people in developed countries.

Everywhere there are serious shortages of doctors, dentists, nurses, health centres, and hospitals, of teachers and schools, of drugs, vaccines, and appliances of all kinds, and of textbooks and other teaching materials.

In general, only about half the children of primary school age are at school, more boys than girls, and many fail to complete the primary school course. Special provision for the health of school children must, perforce, be an integral part of the community health services, particularly the maternity and child health service, and be related to the economic and social circumstances of the country, and to the general educational provision.

The main tasks of a school health service in developing countries are: the control of communicable diseases, including immunization and vaccination; improving the nutrition of children through education in food values as well as school feeding; general health education; the treatment of minor ailments, specially worm infestation; and the detection, treatment, and supervision of handicapped children including their notification to the education authorities.

There is need for improved training in child development and health, and in the disabilities and diseases of childhood and youth, of students in teacher training colleges and of health workers of all types, including midwives and health assistants who do much of the health work in many villages, including schools. The primary responsibility for health education in schools rests with the teachers but the health services can do much to help them both in the schools and through in-service training courses on child and school health. There is need for a close working relationship between departments of health, education, and social welfare both centrally and locally.

THE FUTURE

As a result of changing social circumstances, the work of school health services is becoming more selective: increasing attention is being given to health education and to the investigation and supervision of children who are handicapped or have other defects, or who are not thriving or making satisfactory progress in school, and to advising and helping their parents and teachers.

It is, indeed, a sign of the times, and of the ease of international communication, that the aims of school health services in most countries are almost identical, and that the measures being fashioned to achieve them are of broadly similar form.

FURTHER READING

Reports that Led to the Setting up of the School Health Service in Britain

The Reports of:

The Committee on Children and Their Primary Schools, (1967) London, H.M.S.O.

The Royal Commission on Physical Training in Scotland (1903) London, H.M.S.O.

The Inter-departmental Committee on Physical Deterioration (1904) London, H.M.S.O.

The Inter-departmental Committee on Medical Inspection and Feeding of Children attending Public Elementary Schools (1905) London, H.M.S.O.

General Aspects

Biennial Reports of the Chief Medical Officer, Department of Education and Science, London, H.M.S.O.

British Medical Association (1961) *The Adolescent*, London.

Diagnostic and Assessment Units (1970) Education Survey 9, London, H.M.S.O.

Douglas, J. W. B. (1964) *The Home and the School*, London.

Porritt Committee Report (1962) *A Review of the Medical Services in Great Britain*, London, H.M.S.O.

Pringle, M. L. K. (1965) *Investment in Children*, London.

Pringle, M. L. K., Butler, N. R., and Davie, R. (1966) *Eleven Thousand Seven Year Olds*, London.

Report of the Subcommittee of the Standing Medical Advisory Committee of the Ministry of Health (1963) *The Field of Work of the Family Doctor*, London, H.M.S.O.

UNICEF European Office (1962) *Children in Developing Countries*, Neuilly-sur-Seine.

United Nations Report on Children and Youth (1970)

World Health Organization Expert Committee on School Health Services (1951) First Report, *Wld Hlth Org. techn. Rep. Ser.*, No. 30.

School Health Services in Different Countries are Dealt with in the Following:

Byrd, O. E. (1964) *School Health Administration*, Philadelphia.

Ministry of Health of the U.S.S.R. (1967) *The System of Public Health Services in the U.S.S.R.*, Moscow.

Report of the Joint Committee of the American Medical Association and the National Education Association on School Health Services (1953) Chicago, American Medical Association.

Smiley, J. R. *et al.* (1973) The use of computers in assisting school health programmes in Ontario, *Can. J. Publ. Hlth*, **64**, 141.

World Health Organization Regional Office for Europe (1955) Report of the European Conference on School Health Services, Distributed by WHO Regional Office for Europe, Copenhagen.

Handicapped Pupils

Blakeslee, B. (1963) *The Limb Deficient Child*, Berkeley, California.

British Council for the Rehabilitation of the Disabled (1963) *The Handicapped School Leaver*, London.

Carnegie U.K. Trust (1964) *Handicapped Children and their Families*, Dunfermline.

Goldsmith, S. (1967) *Designing for the Disabled*, London.

Kershaw, J. D. (1967) *Handicapped Children*, London.

Renfrew, C., and Murphy, K. (1964) *The Child Who Does Not Talk*, London.

Report of the Committee on Maladjusted Children (1955) London, H.M.S.O.

Report of the Sub-committee on the Medical Care of Epileptics (1956) London, H.M.S.O.

Speech Therapy Services Report (1972) London, H.M.S.O.

Taylor, I. G. (1964) *Neurological Mechanisms of Hearing and Speech in Children*, Manchester.

The Education of Deaf Children. The Possible Place of Finger Spelling and Signing (1968) London, H.M.S.O.

The Education of Visually Handicapped Chilren (1972) London, H.M.S.O.

West, D. J. (1967) *The Young Offender*, London.

Wing, J K. (1966) *Early Childhood Autism*, London.

Wing. J. K., O'Connor, N., and Lotter, V. (1967) *Brit. med. J.*, **2**, 389.

World Health Organization (1957) Report of a Study Group, Juvenile Epilepsy, *Wld Hlth Org. techn. Rep. Ser.*, No. 130.

Infectious Diseases among School Children, and Food Poisoning

Memorandum on the Control of Infectious Diseases in Schools (1971) Prepared jointly by the Dept. of Education and Science and the Dept. of Health and Social Security.

School Dental Services and Dental Diseases

The Health of the School Child (1956) (Appendix A) for 1954–55, London, H.M.S.O.

Report of United Kingdom Mission (1950) *New Zealand School Dental Nurses*, London, H.M.S.O.

Report of United Kingdom Mission (1953) *The Fluoridation of Domestic Water Supplies in North America as a Means of Controlling Dental Caries*, London, H.M.S.O.

School Nurses

An Inquiry into Health Visiting (1956) London, H.M.S.O.

Medical Records and Reports

Forms 10M, and 11M, London, H.M.S.O.

Schedule (Form 1 H.P.) to the Handicapped Pupils (Certificate) Regulations (1953) London, H.M.S.O.

School Premises

Building Bulletin No. 25 (1965) Secondary School Design (Including Medical Rooms in Schools), London, H.M.S.O.

The Standards for School Premises Regulations (1959) London, H.M.S.O.

36

FAMILY PLANNING AND PUBLIC HEALTH

FRANZ W. ROSA

Introduction

The demographic crisis has been described so widely and so clearly in recent years that it would serve little purpose to repeat again here. The important points from the health viewpoint are the following:

1. With reductions in mortality, excess fertility has become the world's leading health problem. Large family size, in excess of maternal, family, and community resources, is a major obstacle to further improvements in nutrition, growth and development, morbidity, mortality, and well being.

2. In general, the families who are least served by family planning and consequently having the most children, are those whose children are least advantaged developmentally.

3. Little is apparent yet which will prevent areas, which are already over-populated, from facing yet another doubling of their population. Other areas which do not regard themselves as over-populated now, are retarded in achieving health and nutritional coverage as well as other educational, social, and economic progress by rapid population growth rates and high dependency ratios. Even with the most rapidly foreseeable change in present trends, these areas too will reach similar levels of over-population in another generation or so.

4. The economic development which is achieved (in the face of this population growth), associated with industrialization and urbanization, further accentuates the insult on the already strained physical and social human ecology.

5. Despite this critical picture, it is urgent to do what can be done, and to explore how more can be accomplished. Incorporating fertility control with traditional public health concerns for morbidity and mortality control is essential for improving the balance, strength, and results of public health programmes, as well as other community development efforts.

These clear trends should be pertinent to health workers, but many have been slow to become concerned. This has been especially true of government health workers due to lack of motivation to incorporate family planning in their activities. Several studies have shown that governments and their services have lagged behind the population in the desire for family planning. Outmoded laws, religious restrictions, and real or imagined political sensitivities have contributed to this lag. Lack of training in this field has been another factor in the deficient role of health workers. For a description of the world population situation during 1973 see Lorraine (1974). 1974 is World Population Year marked by a conference in Buccharest.

Direct Health Reasons for Family Planning

Analysis of the direct relationships between fertility and family health risks is like 'losing sight of the woods while studying the trees'. However, direct health problems associated with fertility provide significant reasons for family planning as a health measure, regardless of population policy. They have been reviewed extensively elsewhere (IPPF, 1970; Omran, 1971) and here are limited to the following outline:

1. Maternal
   (a) 'Maternal depletion' from a continuous sequence of pregnancy and lactation superimposed on poor diet and heavy labour.
   (b) Other morbidity.
   (c) Emotional consequences of unwanted children.
   (d) Increasing mortality with high parity.
   (e) Unqualified abortion.
2. Infant–child
   (a) Foetal undernutrition, with long-term developmental implications.
   (b) Interruption of breast feeding precipitating protein-calorie malnutrition.
   (c) Consequences of inadequate general infant–child care where the number of children exceeds the family resources.
   (d) Emotional consequences of being unwanted or inadequately cared for.

The majority of all health problems are influenced by the vicious cycle of poverty, malnutrition, high mortality, high fertility, and high dependency ratios. Family planning is one point of attack.

A DECADE OF DEVELOPMENT OF FAMILY PLANNING PROGRAMMES

Although family planning education and services had been provided on a private or voluntary scale previously, the initiation of programmes of family planning is largely a phenomenon of the 1960s. India's family planning programme investment increased from an annual level of 10 million rupees to over a half billion rupees during this decade. China's programme has also been very extensive and apparently successful. Pakistan, Egypt, Turkey, Korea, and Tunisia were other countries to start large programmes in the early sixties. More recently Thailand, Philippines, Indonesia, Ceylon, Iran, and Taiwan have started major programmes. A more complete listing is provided in TABLE 87. Organized family planning activities have been given priority in the highly developed countries as well, as they recognized the health and great social benefits.

TABLE 87

Contraceptive Methods Reported for Official and Voluntary Programmes

	Population in millions 1974[1]	Contraceptive Acceptors (thousands)[2]			
		Pill	IUD	Sterilizations	Other
Afghanistan . . .	18·7	9	4	0	8
Bangladesh and Pakistan .	124·0	7	3,600	1,230	U
Chile	9·4	221	456	55	U
Colombia	23·9	245	267	U	23
Costa Rica . . .	1·9	58	11	0	11
Dominican Republic . .	4·6	31	28	0	18
Egypt	36·7	799	388	0	174
Ghana	9·7	27	12	0	23·7
India	587·0	56	4,370	13,000	7,000
Indonesia . . .	138·0	709	703	0	153
Iran (1971) . . .	32·5	997	50	U	U
Jamaica . . .	2·0	53	13	U	36
Kenya	12·5	85	52	0	13
Korea, South . . .	33·0	934	2,316	193	762
Malaysia, Peninsular . .	9·6	293	5	17	10
Morocco	16·6	62	53	0	10
Nepal (1970) . . .	11·9	25	7	10	37
Philippines . . .	41·4	752	232	0	335
Singapore . . .	2·2	113	11	16	70
Sri Lanka . . .	13·5	143	184	36	44
Taiwan	14·0	295	1,036	2	164
Thailand . . .	38·2	829	423	146	0
Tunisia . . .	5·6	49	91	14	26
Turkey	38·9	41	338	0	0
Venezuela	11·8	78	79	0	8

[1] Projection from *United Nations Demographic Yearbook*, 1971.
[2] Throughout 1972, except where otherwise indicated. From country reports and Nortman, D. (1973).
U Unknown.

TABLE 88

A Decade of Birth Rate Reductions in Selected Areas

Country	Source	Date (unless otherwise indicated)			Principal methods*
		1960	1965	1970	
Barbados . . .	2	33·5	26·1	20·5	L
Bermuda . . .	2	27·2	23·1	18·3 (69)	
Ceylon . . .	2	36·6	33·1	28·4	L P S
Chile . . .	4	35·7	33·2	27·5	L P
Costa Rica . .	2, 1	47·4	42·3	33·8	P L
Egypt . . .	3	44·1		36·8 (69)	P L
El Salvador . .	2	49·5	46·9	39·9	
Fiji . . .	2	39·9	35·9	29·6	L S
Hong Kong . .	2	36·0	28·8	18·9	
India . . .	3	43·0 (61)		38·0 (69)	S L C
Athoor Block . .	4	43·1 (59)	28·1 (68)		
Assam Tea Estates .	4	43·0	26·0 (67)		L
Jamaica . . .	2	42·0	38·9	32·9	
Korea . . .	2	44·7 (1955–65)		29·0	L P S
Malaysia (West) .	2, 1	40·9	36·7	33·0 (69)	P
Malta . . .	1	26·1	17·6	16·3	?
Mauritius . .	2	38·1	36·7	26·0	P L
Pakistan . .	3	48·0 (61)		45·0	L C S
Puerto Rico . .	2	32·3	30·2	25·7	S
Singapore . .	2	38·7	31·1	23·0	P
Taiwan . . .	2, 1	39·5	32·7	28·1	L
Trinidad and Tobago .		39·5	32·8	23·3	

1 UN and WHO Data.
2 IPPF 'Falling Birth Rates and Family Planning' 12/71.
3 Official estimates
4 Special reports
*P Pill.
 L Loop.
 S Sterilization.
 C Conventional (mostly condom).

By the end of the decade it became apparent that the older programmes in Asia and North Africa were reaching a plateau in the number of procedures performed each year, although the cumulative number of couples covered continued to edge upwards. India, after a steady yearly increase in the number of procedures performed over a period of 15 years, showed a levelling off in 1968 and then a drop in the following two years. Pakistan's performance reached a peak in the autumn of 1968 and has since dropped. Taiwan and Korea continued to have a high level of accomplishment but this has been fairly constant for several years.

This levelling off represents both the need for further programme development and a saturation effect. In areas where family planning began years ago, programmes have already reached the most accessible couples who formed a large backlog of potential acceptors. The number of new couples appearing in the population naturally limits a progressive increase in the rate of new acceptors. However, there is still room for programme development since a large number of couples has not been reached, including couples with three or more children.

It is difficult to assess the impact of these programmes on the birth rate. Decreases in birth rates may be the result of coincidental factors such as improvement in education, urbanization, and increasing awareness of population pressure. TABLE 88 shows birth rate reductions that have been recorded or estimated in some representative areas. One can largely say that reductions prior to 1965 would have been seldom due to substantial organized family planning programmes whereas family planning programmes could begin to have impact in some countries after 1965.

At least it is apparent from this data that substantial reductions have taken place in selected areas during the past decade. From the listing it can be seen that a relatively large proportion of the countries where this has occurred are islands. There are two reasons for this, one being that the data are better in these islands (areas with inadequate data are generally excluded from this table), and second, populations began to feel and realize the population pressure due to the distinct delineations of an island population. Furthermore, most of these islands are somewhat more advanced than the continental developing countries.

In some countries it can be seen that the reduction tends to be accelerated after 1965, which could be explained by the introduction of family planning measures. In Mauritius and Fiji, for example, the reduction in birth rate corresponds with what would be estimated from the contraceptive methods which have been provided during these years.

Finally, it is interesting also to observe that extensive birth rate reductions have occurred in areas where no official programme has been provided and in fact where all contraceptive methods have been illegal, such as Malta.

GAINING SUPPORT AND AUTHORITY

Programme support is an initial and continuous requirement. The degree to which family planning programmes have gained support in many countries and at an international level in recent years has been remarkable. This has been brought about by the influence of enlightened leaders, demographers, econo-mists, national planners, and health workers. Deficiencies remain at every level, however, and the continuing provision of information on fertility problems, programme needs, and progress is an essential requirement.

Surveys of public attitudes towards family planning and of problems brought about by excessive fertility have helped to influence leaders. In many areas standard family planning knowledge, attitude, and practice surveys have provided an initial basis for gaining programme support. In other areas, surveys of the induced abortion problems have influenced public authorities. Support of leaders has been gained in several areas by distributing a clear synopsis of the problem.

Another mechanism for gaining adequate programme support has been the establishment of programme authority high enough in the government to have broad and effective influence. This has been accomplished by allowing family planning authorities access to all pertinent agencies, or by providing an inter-agency board or supreme council. Caution must be taken, however, to see that inter-agency councils do not interfere with the effective authority of operational agencies. Separation of authority and operational responsibility is a basic administrative pitfall.

Voluntary and semi-autonomous agencies have in many areas played an important role in mobilizing public support. Their flexibility, latitude, and lack of political restrictions facilitate pioneering in this area. They may be the best authority for programme initiation where governmental encumbrances hinder programme implementation through official channels. However, their goal should always be to mobilize official resources as rapidly as possible, rather than compete, duplicate, or undercut these.

Involvement of community leaders at the local level and mobilization of public support is also an important requirement. To do this, permanent generalized community contacts have many advantages over temporary specialized inputs.

The Family Health Concept as a Basis for Programme Support

Family planning within the context of a health programme that is oriented towards immediate felt needs is likely to be more understandable to the public than family planning presented as a population control programme with economic justifications. The latter may be comprehensible to the economist, the demographer, and the national planner, but it may not be understood by the family, which, from the acceptance viewpoint, is more important. This 'understandability' at the family level is likely to influence political acceptability.

At a World Health Organization African Regional Seminar on the Organization and Administration of MCH Services, held in Brazzaville in November 1969, family planning was introduced into the agenda in response to the interest of the participants. After an extensive and interesting discussion there was harmonious agreement among the representatives of 27 sub-Saharan African countries that family planning was a desirable aspect of health services. There was also a feeling, however, that this should not be tied inflexibly to population questions since the population situation varied from area to area and was in fact likely to be a sensitive subject. Furthermore, they thought that family planning activities could best be developed by national initiative and should not be subject to undue pressures from foreign 'assistance'.

THE ROLE OF HEALTH SERVICES IN FAMILY PLANNING

Reduction of mortality rates and increased survivorship is certainly a prerequisite for receptivity to adoption of family limitation. Health services of course play a leadership role in mortality control, although just as for fertility reduction, broad socio–economic factors and other influences are of much importance. The reduction of mortality rates in fact brings about the need for health programmes to recognize the concurrent need for matching mortality reductions with fertility reductions in order to avoid unhealthful family size and population growth rates.

The health reasons for providing family planning have been outlined in a previous section. These reasons often provide a starting point for introducing the topic to parents. Although studies generally show that economic reasons and 'convenience' overshadow specific health reasons as a motivation for family planning, a broad definition of health, encompassing social well-being, includes all of these motivations as health related.

The rapport health workers establish with families is an advantage in discussing this subject. The time and situation when the patient is in contact with health workers provide further opportunities. Maternity care obviously provides many opportunities and needs for family planning. Counselling is not necessarily given only in separate maternity care programmes but, as with other aspects of maternal health, should be closely related to child health care. The health worker can conveniently introduce the subject when dealing with family nutrition questions, for example. The management of many chronic diseases, such as tuberculosis, calls for family planning. Family planning services should also be available in conjunction with the newly developing field of genetic counselling.

The use of the intra-uterine device, hormonal contraception, and surgical fertility control require health coverage for proper case selection, implementation, follow-up, and management of side-effects.

Health disciplines which contribute to family planning programmes, other than medicine and nursing, include health education and health statistics. The professional skills of the public health educator are closely applicable to the problem of education for fertility management and include improving and supporting the person-to-person education mentioned above, guidance of mass media efforts, the development of sex educational aspects of school health and adult education programmes, strengthening marital counselling, and influencing community leaders and other potential collaborators. The structure established by health programmes to collect data on births, deaths, diseases, health personnel performance, and facilities, serves as a channel for information on family planning programmes. Certain supplementary activities are desirable to evaluate fertility problems, and family planning programme efforts. For this, health programmes are giving increasing recognition to disciplines such as demography and the social sciences. Epidemiology, usually thought of in the context of communicable diseases, is a science of statistical study of influences affecting populations, and can have a closer relation to demography and the study of fertility problems.

Where family planning programmes are not adequately integrated with health programmes there is likely to be friction and opposition. The support of the medical community is highly desirable and its participation for servicing the programme indispensable. At the outset, it is desirable to secure the most prestigious medical support possible for family planning efforts. The medical profession will be involved in advising on the selection of contraceptive methods to be used. Unless medical and health workers are mobilized and supportive to family planning efforts, public support will be deficient. This is true of all levels, from the academic professor of obstetrics to the village midwife.

There are many logistical reasons for integrating programmes for dealing with the priority needs of mothers and children, including family planning. Funding can be pooled, a stronger infrastructure developed, supervision can be strengthened, duplication of facilities can be avoided, and workers can introduce the subject of family planning in relation to many of the reasons for the mother's visit to the clinic. Isolated family planning facilities are likely not to be fully used and workers are often not fully employed, particularly in the rural areas that it is so crucial to cover. In the many areas of the world where mothers can be approached only by female workers, these logistic questions are especially acute, because of the shortages of such workers.

Where funds and personnel are diverted into isolated family planning programmes there is not only the danger that health services will be weakened but also the likelihood that basic infrastructure, which is important for family planning objectives, will be weakened. Where the administration of family planning is carefully balanced with other health services, these programmes should be developed in a way that they will be mutually supportive.

Collaboration with Other Fields

Collaboration with other government departments is essential. Certain agencies can help the family planning organization by printing health education material and arranging for the use of radio, television, and other public information facilities. Social support can be obtained from community developers, agricultural extension agents, and teachers. Aid in programme fulfilment can be sought from the military, the labour ministry, and the department of education.

At an Asian meeting on the 'Administrative Aspects of Family Planning' (ECAFE, 1966) the following contributions from various governmental agencies were identified:

1. Contraceptive supplies (commerce).
2. Public information (communications, information, publications).
3. Social support for small family norm (community development, education, local government).
4. Approach to special groups (labour, social insurance).
5. Evaluation (census, social research).
6. Training (professional education institutions).
7. Research (research facilities).

The co-operation of agencies outside the government can be of great assistance, especially in training personnel and experimenting with new techniques and approaches. However, it is important to be on guard against over-dependence on non-governmental agencies for the actual operation of programmes.

POPULATION CHARACTERISTICS

A factor that certainly affects attitudes towards fertility is the high infant and child mortality remaining in many areas. The average number of children desired ranges widely from two or three in some areas, where the desirability of limiting family size is recognized, to five or six in West Africa. In South Asia about four children are desired but this is conditioned in many areas by the fact that one or two must be boys, and the parents will continue to reproduce until this condition is met. The desire for family limitation is stronger in urban areas where large families are less convenient. Even in rural areas, however, it is observed that the majority of women wish to space pregnancies as well as limit their number.

Amenorrhoea which is associated with prolonged breast feeding and malnutrition is often relied on to delay pregnancy. In some areas taboos on intercourse during the breast feeding period reinforce natural pregnancy spacing. Post-partum amenorrhoea is often found to last a year or more: the number of women who ovulate before resuming menstruation is relatively few, although unfortunately data on the exact number are lacking. Cross-sectional surveys in rural areas in Asia and Africa show that at a given time only half the women in the fertile age range have regular menstrual cycles: the others are either pregnant, have post-partum amenorrhoea or are not menstruating for other reasons. The period of post-partum amenorrhoea is much shorter in urban areas, probably because bottle feeding is, unfortunately, replacing breast feeding.

Beyond post-partum amenorrhoea and abstinence there may be little awareness among uneducated people that birth control is possible. In many cases women depend on useless herbs or on the rhythm method which is ill understood and incorrectly practised. They may resort to hazardous unqualified abortion which is a rapidly growing problem in many areas.

The fertile age range in women is usually considered to be 15–44 years. In tropical countries the onset of ovulation and menstruation is somewhat later than in economically developed countries in the temperate zone. Even with early marriage, pregnancies before age 17 do not constitute a significant proportion of births, although they are a health concern because of increased hazards. About 3 per cent. of couples suffer from primary sterility and an even larger number lack sufficient fertility to need contraception. Because of poor nutrition, chronic infections, and pathology resulting from repeated pregnancies, secondary infertility and early menopause are common. In a few tropical areas fertility appears to be low in all ages, in others it drops off rapidly after age 30.

Given a population structure with a high birth rate and a moderate death rate, the number of women in the fertile age range constitutes about one-fifth of the population. Those who are fertile and exposed constitute about one-seventh of the population. Those women who have had three or more pregnancies constitute a little more than half of these, say one-twelfth of the population. This number represents roughly the group that might be interested in family size limitation, al-though those with less children must also be considered for spacing and for introducing possibilities for eventual limitation of family size. Even among these, only about half will be having ovulation, the remainder either pregnant, post-partum or anovulatory for other reasons.

In such a representative population the number of women entering the fertile range each year is about 1 per cent. of the population, and the number entering the group with three or more pregnancies is about 0·8 per cent. of the population. These figures set long-term margins for the number of new couples to be considered by a family planning programme each year, after the backlog of potential acceptors has been managed.

Representative Population in a Developing Country

1,000	Population
480	Female
200	Age 15–44 Female
140	Potential fertile and exposed (70 ovulating)
80	Three or more pregnancies (40 ovulating)
8	Annual new couples completing desired family size

SOME PROGRAMME POINTS ABOUT BIRTH CONTROL METHODS

These are reviewed in the order of their sophistication and the corresponding requirement for clinical assistance.

Coitus Interruptus. This has undoubtedly made a substantial contribution to fertility control long before family planning supplies were available. It still us an important factor in many areas.

Rhythm Method. This method also has been widely practised both correctly and incorrectly. Even where correctly practised, it has had high failure rates. In areas where prolonged breast feeding is widely practised only a small proportion of the female population is found to have regular cyclical menstruations. Although the rhythm method is usually classified as a 'non-clinical' method, correct practice can actually require more education than more sophisticated methods. Its main disadvantage is that it may interfere with the practice of more reliable methods. On the other hand its acceptability to some families may at least contribute to their acceptance of the concept of family planning, which is certainly an important beginning.

The Condom and Vaginal Agents. Devices that do not require clinical facilities fill a major programme need, despite possible limitations. One of the first steps in any family planning programme should be to ensure that condoms are widely available at low cost, since this does not require waiting for the long-term development of trained manpower and facilities. Vaginal foam tablets have even higher failure rates but it may be desirable to furnish one of the more reliable non-clinical agents to women who want to take the contraceptive responsibility. The rural emphasis is particularly important since condoms are often available only in urban areas, whereas their principal programme advantage is that they can be widely distributed to areas where clinical methods are not available.

In addition to moderate acceptability and reliability, a deficiency of non-clinical methods (also oral contraception) is that they require repeated preventive initiative whereas the IUD and the surgical methods require only a single decision.

Intra-uterine Device. Intra-uterine devices have been

used for contraception in Japan and certain other places since the 1930s but widespread use in family planning programmes developed only in the mid-1960s. At that time a reappraisal was made of the clinical disadvantages of this method (principally complaints of minor bleeding and discomfort) relative to certain distinct programme advantages. This method was thought to be practical for less sophisticated populations not accustomed to practising regular contraception, because only a single decision is required. Continued use is not jeopardized by deficiencies in the availability of supplies. Two other advantages are that the method is easily reversible, and the failure rate of two pregnancies per 100 years of use is much lower than that of traditional contraceptive measures. The device has proved relatively safe. Excessive bleeding and pelvic inflammation have been the most frequent complications. Studies undertaken to date have not shown any carcinogenic influence.

Those women who experience few side-effects from this device regard it as a blessing, but unfortunately a large proportion of women do have some bleeding and discomfort and a smaller proportion expel the IUD spontaneously. Retention rates in Asia have been about 50 per cent. 2 years after insertion [see TABLE 89]. Reinsertion improves retention rates by about 10 per cent. Little headway has been made in overcoming side-effects, and the main progress has depended on extending the availability of this procedure to the proportion of the female population that will accept it. Overcoming the shortage of professional personnel qualified to insert the IUD and to provide adequate follow-up has been a principal need. Some areas have successfully trained paramedical personnel to perform these functions. In Pakistan the Lady Family Planning Visitor—a matriculate with one year of special training—is now filling the gap caused by the shortage of lady doctors. In Punjab State, India, auxiliary nurse–midwives have been trained to handle the procedure. Insertion of IUDs by midwives compared favourably with insertions by physicians in Barbados, Korea, and India.

This method has been a major element in the programmes of Taiwan, Korea, India, and Pakistan during the last few years, with a combined total of over 71,000,000 insertions by 1972.

Hormonal Contraception: 'The Pill'. Oral contraception has become one of the most widely used methods of fertility control in many Western countries during the past decade. Its acceptability in these areas is due to the aesthetics of not needing to employ a device or agent immediately associated with the sexual act, and the negligible failure rate when properly followed. Although oral contraception is now the leading method in the family planning programmes in Egypt, Iran, Malaysia, Mauritius, and Singapore, its effectiveness has been limited by several factors. In the past, price was a consideration but this should no longer be a problem since countries should be able to prepare tablets from basic ingredients that can now be obtained for about U.S.$ 0·10 per cycle. Low acceptance and continuation rates by unsophisticated women are often stated to be objections to the use of the pill in programmes, although experience in several areas shows that illiterate women are able to use it successfully when programmes are carefully developed. In other areas follow-up studies have shown that less than half the acceptors continue for as long as several months, and long-term continuation rates are near to 25 per cent. Continuation rates with the pill (as with

the IUD) are misleading unless there is comprehensive follow-up of acceptors, and, furthermore, they are meaningful only when broken down by months since acceptance. Continuation rates have been improved by the use of 'blank' tablets for the spacing of the cycles so that women can take one tablet daily without interruption, without worrying about calendars or when to start each cycle. Poor acceptance and continuation are due to the ignorance of programme workers as well as to lack of

TABLE 89

Cumulative Retention Rates per 100 IUD Acceptors with Reinsertions

	Months from insertion				
	6	12	18	24	36
Barbados—physicians . .	82	76	70		
nurses . .	87	75	72		
India—Delhi Field Programme	87	78	69	60	
PRAI, Lucknow .	73	63	46		
Korea—National Programme .		71		56	44
Pakistan—Nat. Res. Inst. .	86	79	70	61	
East Pakistan .	82	74	66		
West Pakistan .	68	56	46		
Taiwan—province-wide .	78	69	63		
U.S.A.—CSP Loop D .	87	78	72	67	58

(Sources: Mauldin, P. (1968) *Retention of IUDs: An International Comparison*, Studies in Family Planning No. 18, p. 4, Population Council, New York, .
  Planning Research Action Institute (1967) *A Follow-up of IUD Cases*, PRAI, Lucknow.
  Pakistan Family Planning Council (1968) *Annual Report on the Working of Pakistan's Family Planning Program 1967–68*, Rawalpindi.)

sophistication in the takers, and unless workers are well informed they are likely to discourage use of the pill for a host of misconceived reasons. A most important factor is early follow-up in order that the pill-taking habit may be established and users reassured that side-effects tend to diminish after the first month or two.

All pharmaceutical products, when given to large populations, are likely to affect adversely at least a few persons. The benefits relative to the hazards must always be considered carefully before the desirability of their use may be judged. On the basis of use by millions of women during a decade and under diverse circumstances, oral contraceptives appear to be relatively safe. Intensive studies are continuing on the possible carcinogenic influence of long-term use of these hormones, since high dosages have been carcinogenic in some animal studies. Observed changes in human cervical cytology have been interpreted in various ways, and continue to be discussed. United States data have shown an over-all decrease in deaths from cancers of the cervix, uterus and breast during the past decade, but unfortunately no breakdown in the mortality rates is available as regards women taking the pill and women not taking the pill. Information is more definite for deaths from thrombo-embolism. In 1967 the British Medical Research Council reported an additional thrombo-embolic mortality of 1·3 deaths per annum per 100,000 users under age 35, and 3·4 for users over age 35. This data is supported by a recent analysis which attributes 176 deaths per year to this cause in the United States. Both these figures indicate about one additional death from thrombo-embolism per 40,000 years of oral contraception.

D. M. Potts has illustrated that because of their greater reliability oral contraceptives are one of the safest methods, when over-all mortality from method failure pregancies is considered, as well as deaths due to the method [TABLE 90].

TABLE 90

Method	Occurrences per million years use			
	Pregnancies from method failure	Deaths from these pregnancies at prevailing maternal mortality rates	Deaths from method	Total Deaths
IUD .	48,000	12	?	
Orals .	11,000	3	20	23
Diaphragm .	200,000	52	0	52
Rhythm .	230,000	60	0	60

(Adapted from Peel and Potts, 1969, p. 263.)

In other words, the latter methods, that are regarded as free from mortality risk, are actually associated with more deaths per year of use than the clinical methods, when maternal deaths resulting from method failure are taken into account.

Suppression of lactation is a significant side-effect in areas where infant growth and survival depend on breast feeding. Because of the seriousness of this side-effect and because of negligible fertility in fully lactating non-menstruating women in areas such as India and Pakistan, programme administrators should consider advising women to postpone oral contraception until menstruation is re-established, or, as regards non-menstruating women, to wait at least 6 months after delivery. Optimally, oral contraception and infant feeding supplements should be started at the same time. Elevation of blood pressure occurs in some women taking hormonal contraception.

Oral contraception increases insulin requirements in diabetic women, although many physicians do not consider this an absolute contra-indication to the use of this method. It has also been observed to decrease certain liver functions, but the medical significance of this has not been fully established, particularly in areas with widespread malnutrition.

Oral contraception provides another choice for the many women who will not accept having an intra-uterine device inserted and for many women who try the IUD and find that they cannot tolerate it. Oral contraception as an alternative to condoms may be more acceptable to couples when the male will not take the contraception responsibility or to couples who object to employing an agent or device during the sexual act.

Since successful use of the method is facilitated by close supervision, particularly during the initial stages, and by convenient availability of supplies, the establishment of large numbers of clinical distribution points is important for programme success. It is particularly convenient for private practitioners to prescribe oral contraception but measures must be taken to keep down the cost to the patient. In some areas paramedical personnel and auxiliaries under medical supervision distribute oral contraceptives.

Vasectomy and Tubectomy. Despite predictions that vasectomy would not be widely acceptable, Madras State in India began pioneering this method in its programme in 1959. By 1968, 754,000 operations were reported in that State, a rate of about 12 per 100 married fertile couples. The India family planning programme followed the lead of Madras State and currently it is estimated that 80 per cent. of the eventual birth preventive effect of the programme rests on this procedure. By 1972, a cumulative total of 13,000,000 sterilizations were reported. Pakistan, starting later, has experienced a sudden demand for this method, and reported 559,000 operations performed by November 1968, more than half of which had been done in the previous 6 months. Tubectomy is the leading method of fertility control in Puerto Rico.

The major limitation to these procedures is that they cannot be regarded as reliably reversible, and therefore are likely to be acceptable only to older couples who have already had large numbers of children and are well past the age of peak fertility. However, in these couples this is a reliable and practical procedure, when there are not religious or legal objections.

Induced Abortion. Abortion has been performed as a legal birth control method in countries with a combined population of over 1,200 million. In addition, it is a leading method in many countries where it is illegal. Great increases in illegal abortions are reported from many areas where families are under increasing pressure as a result of large numbers of children surviving, urbanization, and rising aspirations [TABLE 91].

TABLE 91

	Year	Birth Rate	Incidence of Induced Abortions per 100 Live Births	
			Legal	Illegal
Czechoslovakia .	1965	16·4	29	
Hungary . .	1965	13·1	135	
Japan . .	1965	18·6	46	
Poland . .	1964	18·1	32	
United Kingdom .	1965	18·1	0·5	4
United States .	1965	17·9	0·3	25 (1957)
Argentina . .	1964	22		25
Australia . .	1967	19·5		17–35
Colombia . .	1966	41		20

(Source: Adapted from Tables 5 and 6 from Potts, M.: *Induced Abortion: the Experience of Other Nations*, presented at Pakistan International Conference on Family Planning, Dacca, February 1969.)

In at least one country the restriction of previously liberalized abortion has been associated with a marked jump in birth rate. (This restriction in Romania in 1966 was also linked to taxation for childless couples and other pronatalist measures.) The birth rate of 14·3 in 1966 rose to 32·8 in 1968.

Discussion of the legal, moral, and demographic aspects of abortion is beyond the scope of this section. From the medical viewpoint, however, it is important to recognize that legalization is not synonymous with promotion of abortion. Legalization can bring abortion to clinical attention so that supplemental preventive measures can be introduced.

Although abortion is effective in terminating pregnancy it is not efficient in preventing another pregnancy. Unless some preventive method is used, pregnancy soon occurs again. Legalization also leads to the reduction of the number of cases of sepsis and haemorrhage from unqualified illegal abortion. A fall in hospital admissions and declining deaths from induced abortion has been found in Eastern Europe following legalization. The maternal mortality from legal abortion is low, as seen from TABLE 92.

TABLE 92

Country	Year	Abortions	Deaths	Rate per 100,000
Japan . .	1950–53	2,994,000	253	8·5
	1959–65	6,860,000	278	4·1
Czechoslovakia .	1963–67	406,000	10	2·5
Hungary . .	1964–67	739,000	9	1·2
Yugoslavia .	1960–61	177,000	8	4·5
Sweden . .	1960–66	30,600	12	39
Denmark . .	1961–65	21,700	9	41

(Source: Tietze, C., *Legal Abortion in Industrialized Countries*, presented at Pakistan International Conference on Family Planning, Dacca, February 1969.)

The higher mortality in the latter countries is said to be due to a higher proportion of abortions performed on women because of health hazards, and a higher proportion taking place after the sixteenth week of gestation; use of newer methods has proved less hazardous than previous methods. There is a need for further information on the long-term morbidity associated with legal induced abortion.

Programme Needs for Improved Methods and for Employing More Than One Method

Many of the present limitations are due to factors other than deficiencies in existing contraceptive methods. Countries have succeeded in lowering their birth rates, even without the use of modern methods, largely through abortion, coitus interruptus, and postponement of marriage. Nevertheless, it can be seen from the foregoing discussion that all of the presently available methods have certain disadvantages. Therefore, the availability of improved and supplementary contraceptive methods would improve achievement to a certain extent. Research in this direction should be a high international priority. Some improvements might be: a convenient and well tolerated injectable, since injections enjoy wide popularity and can be administered conveniently on a mass basis; a removable implantation that would allow convenient reversal of fertility suppression; the improvement of present sterilization methods to make them conveniently reversible; a safe, convenient hormonal or chemical agent of male contraception; a post-coital oral agent; or a safe chemical agent for legal abortions. Experimentation is proceeding in all of these directions with strong likelihood of improved methods in the future.

It should also be apparent from the preceding presentation that no one method would be ideal for every circumstance, and that it is desirable to provide all of the available methods, since each has a role to play. The provision of alternative methods increases the desirable voluntary aspects of family programmes by allowing families a wider choice. Coercion to employ any particular method is undesirable not only as a matter of principle, but because it is apparent that narrow-minded approaches to improve the performance with any

particular method by limiting the availability of other methods will eventually prove self-defeating.

ORGANIZATION OF FAMILY PLANNING
Central Administrative Functions

The functions of the central administrative unit are similar to and often incorporated with other MCH concerns and include:

1. Serves as the integrated unit at national level for planning, administration, and formulation of policies.
2. Studies needs, evaluates existing programmes for upgrading or improvement of services or centres.
3. Establishes standards, gives operational instructions.
4. Establishes a network of services through the country.
5. Makes mass surveys or large-scale campaigns.
6. Collects data and statistics for tabulation, analysis, evaluation, and use for programme planning purposes.
7. Co-ordinates with other units in Ministries of Health (such as nutrition, nursing, mental health, health education communicable disease, etc.).
8. Co-ordinates with other relevant ministries, e.g. education, welfare, community development.
9. Collaborates with leading professional groups, community leaders.
10. Co-operates and provides guidance to the school health programme if this activity is under the Ministry of Education, or another unit.
11. Stimulates, co-ordinates, and conducts research and evaluation.
12. Is responsible for training and manpower development.
13. Collaborates with teaching institutions (medical school departments of paediatrics and obstetrics, schools of public health, teacher training colleges, nursing and midwifery schools) in service, research, and teaching functions.
14. Establishes uniform service record forms.
15. Establishes performance norms.
16. Advises on and participates in preparation of mass educational media.
17. Stimulates experimentation with new methods and patterns of delivery of family planning education and services.
18. Drafts proposed legislation.
19. Participates in preparation of budgets and receives funds from government and other sources.
20. Gives grants-in-aid to voluntary organizations or financial aid to voluntary organizations or intermediate or local units for new approved projects.
21. Co-operates and provides assistance to private or voluntary organizations.

Peripheral Programme Coverage

One of the serious problems of the delivery of services is that of incomplete coverage of the population requiring care. Among the various reasons accounting for this incomplete coverage are lack of funds; lack of sufficient trained personnel; geographic problems such as unwillingness of professional personnel to work in the more remote rural areas, and inaccessibility of certain populations; lack of acceptance of the health needs of mothers and children as deserving sufficiently high priority for increased support. To deliver services effectively at the peripheral level, planning on a larger geographic basis is essential. At the peripheral level the team needs to have demographic data such as the population to be served (by age-groups), births, deaths, morbidity, etc.

Auxiliary workers, while useful at all levels, are essential for assignment to the more remote rural areas; their training on the job and supervision are essential. The trend is for the basic health centre to provide family planning services, with each health centre having its own subcentres for which it is responsible. The quality and efficiency of services need to be taken into consideration, as well as quantity, in planning for coverage of the population.

Many deliveries are still attended by traditional midwives. Providing training for these indigenous midwives has been a long-standing MCH programme. This work is often not easy and bad performance by the midwives often persists. Nevertheless, a key factor in the success of programmes is the degree to which a programme relationship is promoted with influential local people such as these midwives. This is particularly true for family planning. The traditional midwives are in close contact with the mothers. Where they are not mobilized for the programme they tend to become competitively antagonistic and obstructive to the programme.

The services must be planned and adapted to meet the needs of the people. Where available services are not fully utilized, inquiry must be made to ascertain the reasons. Are the services not provided when the people are free to come? Are the services inappropriate to the needs? Are the people newcomers or so isolated as to be unfamiliar with the use of services?

In order to make these activities effective, the following has to be assured:

1. That there exists an easy system of referral to the next higher health unit.
2. That there is supervision which includes constant in-service training, guidance, and encouragement.
3. That the responsibilities of the workers have to be clearly defined and controlled, and their geographical area specified.
4. That personnel work in a team.
5. That community participation is gained for the services offered.
6. That facilities and equipment are available to perform these activities.

Mobile services are usually considered to supplement the lack of access of fixed clinical facilities. These have been employed both for vasectomy (to a limited extent also for tubectomy) and for loop insertion. They have been successful for vasectomy in India since relatively little individual follow-up is required and unfavourable reactions in the community have not usually been apparent. Mobile clinics for IUD insertion have been less successful, since more individual follow-up is required and, more important, a continuing input is required to prevent adverse rumours over the minor physical side-effects (bleeding and some discomfort). Where widely decentralized clinical facilities have been provided, achievement has been much greater.

The mobile approach can be improved by observing a regular schedule of frequent visits. For example, in Tunisia, after observing some of the above described problems with irregular mobile services for IUD insertions, the Minister of Health directed that all mobile visits would be repeated weekly or at least fortnightly and would appear regularly at a planned time. A second partial solution to the problems of mobility is to co-ordinate with permanent community contacts who can gather cases and answer questions between visits.

Other problems with the mobile approach include lack of roads, problems with vehicle maintenance, inconvenience and travel time demands on staff, climatic problems, and high cost. In general, transport of professionals can be better applied for the supervision and in-service training of local workers, rather than for providing mobile services.

Non-Clinical Coverage

Although we have limited information in many areas, and there is much variation in settings, only a small proportion of the population may be effectively within reach of clinics. Some studies in India show that 75 per cent. of clinic attendance comes from within a radius of 3 kilometres. Rural clinics, including some 5,000 primary health centres and perhaps an equal number of other clinics accessible to rural residents, would then gather 75 per cent. of their attendance from an area of 300,000 square kilometres, which represents only about a tenth of India's total area. The coverage in some other areas is even less.

A first stage programme need is to provide at least the minimum convenient requirements for contraception in all areas and to all people who might be receptive. These can be initially those that do not require delivery by trained personnel nor clinical facilities, and include condoms and vaginal chemicals. Unfortunately, in most family planning programmes this minimum requirement has not yet been fulfilled and in others non-clinical distribution has not even been undertaken. Anticipated poor acceptance and non-use are sometimes cited. These excuses are hardly valid reasons for not pursuing this approach at least to the limits of its acceptability. Even a low degree of acceptance in the predominantly rural countries would contribute more to the programme success than a higher degree of acceptance of more effective methods that depend on clinical facilities which are within reach of only a small urban proportion of the population. In order to provide these at an acceptable price, steps are necessary to remove import licences and taxes, or, better still, to purchase or manufacture and distribute at subsidized prices. An adequate profit incentive for the retailer is desirable to stimulate the programme and a small cost to the purchaser and retailer to facilitate control of wastage.

THE 'MATERNITY-CENTRED' OR POST-PARTUM APPROACH

In any population a large number of women can be found who repeatedly start one pregnancy shortly after completing a previous one. Many of them wish to avoid or postpone further child-bearing but do not know how. The usual mass programme does not contact them promptly after they complete a pregnancy and so it repeatedly finds them 'currently pregnant', and therefore, 'ineligible' for contraceptive services. In fact, it has been determined that without contraception and without lactation, approximately 80 per cent. of fertile women will conceive again within a year following delivery. The action potential becomes obvious. The more time that elapses following pregnancy termination, the greater the likelihood of subsequent pregnancy, and as corollary, less opportunity for contraception.

The antenatal period, the lying-in period, and the post-partum period offer unique opportunities to reach women in a systematic manner. In fact, it has been shown that in an urban setting where most deliveries occur in hospitals most fertile women can be reached within a period of 3 years. The birth (both urban and rural) can be identified by a health worker or registrar, for follow-up of both the mother and child. Additionally, the husbands can also be offered family planning education and services.

The aims of linking maternal and child care and family planning services in any maternity care related activity are:

1. To establish family planning as an important and integral aspect of sound maternal and child health care by initiating, strengthening, and expanding family planning procedures within a maternity service setting.

2. To maximize the extent of effective family planning among the population in need in the surrounding community by focusing on obstetrical and abortion cases via several channels.

3. To promote, support, and upgrade maternal and child health services provided by these hospitals or institutions.

4. To emphasize by demonstration the role of the health and medical community for maternal child health and family planning.

5. To involve other medical and nursing departments, besides that of obstetrics and gynaecology, particularly paediatrics and preventive and social medicine.

6. To participate in teaching programmes of maternal and child health and family planning for medical undergraduates and postgraduates, nurses, midwives, and auxiliaries as well as others coming in contact with the programme.

7. To provide more adequate post-partum follow-up of family planning needs through integration of this concern with child health activities and through home visiting programmes.

8. To promote pertinent co-ordination, supervision, organization, screening, referral, and public education among all pertinent units and levels in the maternity-centred family planning activities.

9. To promote evaluation of the extent and effectiveness of the provision of family planning education and methods through maternity care.

10. To take steps against hazardous unqualified abortion, obstetrical delivery and neonatal care.

11. To promote birth registration and programme follow-up related to this.

12. To increase the provision of needed services by co-ordinating these with wanted services; in other words, to increase the attendance in various maternal and child health activities by providing these in a package which is conveniently available to the family.

Except in the case of post-partum sterilization, there is need for a follow-up beyond the immediate post-partum period. IUD insertion, although it can conveniently be done in the post-partum or post-abortion period, requires follow-up to reassure women about frequent minor side-effects which occur and to provide reinsertion if the IUD is spontaneously expelled. For women who are lactating it is desirable to delay the prescription of hormonal contraception until after supplemental feeding is started for the infant since the oestrogenic component of the pill may reduce the amount of breast milk which is available for the infant and this is of critical importance in developing countries. The mother should be followed closely to advise her that it is necessary to start contraception within 6 months following childbirth, or earlier when post-partum menstruation occurs. As mentioned previously, this follow-up can be provided conveniently in the context of periodic child care.

The principal experience with this approach to date has been under the heading of post-partum programmes in large maternity hospital services. These have been given priority because large numbers of cases could be conveniently reached administratively and evaluated. Support and evaluation have been provided by the Population Council of New York in an international programme which began in 1966. The programme began in 25 hospitals located in 19 cities of 14 countries and has expanded to over 250 hospitals, including multi-hospital networks in Columbia, Honduras, Hong Kong, India, Indonesia, Pakistan, Philippines, Puerto Rico, Thailand, Tunisia, and the United States. During the first 2 years of operation of the 25 original hospitals, 236,000 new acceptors were enrolled representing 11 per cent. of the estimated community target population. A little more than half of the acceptors were women who had been delivered in these hospitals and the remainder were indirect acceptors who had been attracted from the community. The principal dissemination of information outside the hospital was by word of mouth and it is evident that this is quite extensive and highly important for communicating the family planning message. In the seven hospitals in the United States, 45 per cent. of the delivered cases accepted contraception; 21 per cent. accepted in the 18 hospitals outside the United States (Zatuchni, 1970).

There has been less experience with the post-partum approach in smaller maternity units, home delivery services and in rural areas. Several countries have had experience with developing rural maternal child health services and home delivery programmes. Family planning activities are already well advanced in some of these, for example, the role of the rural auxiliary nurse–midwife in India and the lady family planning visitor and village organizer in Pakistan.

To cover the bulk of the population it is essential to extend this activity to small units in rural areas. Furthermore, these areas have been less well served with family planning methods and much more remains to be accomplished here. As rural maternal child health and family planning care becomes a major part of government health programmes further experience and experiment in programme design should be forthcoming. Because the experimental approach is necessary, documentation and evaluation of all aspects of such a programme should have exceptionally high priority.

Recently a study has been done in ten developing countries that seeks to answer the question, 'what would it take of everything—in personnel, physical facilities, training facilities, transport, supplies and equipment, and funding—to bring minimum professional and paraprofessional attention to every pregnant woman before, during, and after delivery, for the double purpose of promoting maternal child health and family planning?' The investigators estimate that the costs are at about 60 cents *per capita* for total programme costs, ranging from U.S.$ 0·32–1·65. These costs are viewed as being relatively low compared to the magnitude of the problem to be solved. Demonstration projects in programme experience in various settings will be necessary to further work out the details and administration to implement and measure these approaches (Taylor and Berelson, 1971).

FAMILY PLANNING PUBLIC EDUCATION

The principal programme method for influencing fertility control behaviour is through education of the family and community leaders.

The observation has been widely confirmed that most changes in knowledge, attitude, and practice result mostly from person-to-person communication. Improvement in maternal and child health practises are usually the result of education by a health worker or indirectly from someone who has been informed by a health worker. Recognizing this requirement, action programmes have generally shifted from an initial phase of providing services to an extension education phase. Covering the population with person-to-person education is a principal MCH/family planning objective.

Education generally requires continuous inputs on appropriate occasions with knowledge of what has gone on before and with plans to follow up actions that are taken. Repeated family visits are especially important for providing the reinforcing educational inputs and follow-up that are essential for successful family planning practice (to reassure against initial side-effects of the pill or the IUD, to provide reinsertion of the IUD where necessary, etc.). The provision of education through a continuity of family care is most advantageous in this respect. At the community level too, continuing inputs are required. This generally cannot be done by transient or mobile workers, but requires workers-in-residence who understand the community and establish rapport with its leaders and opinion leaders.

The rapport that health workers establish in their healing work is an important influence both at the family and at the community level. Family planning education provided in the context of felt health needs is likely to be more understandable and acceptable than 'population education'. There is need to broaden concerns to approach the whole family's needs at each opportune contact. On an international basis the three principal health and educational requirements for optimal child development and human reproduction are nutrition, control of infections, and the management of pregnancies including family planning. These three concerns are mutually interdependent in that nutrition is dependent on avoiding such infections as intestinal parasites and diarrhoea, as well as other infections, the severity of infections is often dependent on the nutritional state, and both the nutritional state and the care that can be provided for infections are related to family size. From the maternal and child health point of view, education on all of these requirements is necessary in order to have optimal success with any of these requirements.

At the most peripheral level in the village in most developing countries, it will usually be necessary for a single agent to cover these priority requirements. Although other educational agents may contribute to various areas of these concerns, it is desirable to approach these comprehensively.

In many areas the most widely distributed agent or worker relative to family planning is the midwife. Most mothers receive some care during delivery although this is often unqualified and hazardous. In these areas concern with upgrading midwifery care, providing education to these agents on the hazards of neonatal tetanus, for example, and mobilizing these agents for family planning education should be an initial consideration for covering the population.

Where education of the family is provided by other agents there should be close co-ordination with health services, so that the necessary health back-stopping can be provided. In family planning, for example, modern methods of contraception must be delivered through trained health persons, and family planning educators from whatever source should work closely together with these health persons. In many cases the best service and education can be provided by a single agent, usually for example, the auxiliary nurse–midwife.

Another channel that is important for family planning education is the school. The back-stopping that health and family planning workers can provide to the teachers and teacher training is the highest priority aspect of school health services.

Maternal and child health education that is provided by workers with very large patient loads with limited training, must be limited to the highest priority and must be specifically oriented towards a most readily available solution in the locality.

TRAINING AND MANPOWER DEVELOPMENT

One of the key problems covering the priorities of family planning is the development and adaptation of workers who can meet the problems at hand and seeing that these are distributed in a way that they cover the population [see also CHAPTER 49].

Principal Points for Orienting Training

1. Workers should be trained to function as a team with close co-operation between doctors, nurses, and other health workers; co-operation between health workers and educators, social workers, and other pertinent workers for family planning; professionals should primarily act as supervisors and administrators of teams of auxiliaries who can cover the population's most pressing needs. There should also be co-ordination between trained workers and indigenous workers, such as the traditional midwife.

2. Workers should be trained to understand community health approaches, how to work with community leaders and how to establish a permanent influential community input.

3. They should become competent in integrating health and family planning approaches to cover the population. They should be well-oriented towards the process of human reproduction and its influence on family and community health. They should be taught the interdependence of nutrition, child care, and management of pregnancy.

4. A most important requirement in this respect is that they become effective public, community and family educators.

5. Orientation should be towards providing a continuity of family care integrating the concerns of development and reproduction so that each may be approached at a most convenient, timely, and effective point, with familiarity of what has proceeded before in the family, and with the follow-up which is so essential for influencing family health practices.

6. They should be oriented and prepared to work where they are needed.

7. They should be taught how to work with the potentially available resources as well as an appreciation of the economy and cost benefits.

Steps in Systematic Development of Family Planning Manpower

1. An analysis and survey of problems in order to adapt the training on a problem basis.

2. Definition of functions for each category of worker.

3. An initial priority for developing teaching staff, co-ordinating all of the essential disciplines.

4. An immediately following priority for providing orientation for key administrators and policy persons at each level, to understand the functions of the family health workers who are to be trained.

5. Assurance that the workers who are to be trained will be employed and utilized.

6. Development of suitable materials and curricula as well as handbooks for reference after training.

7. Provision of opportunities for supervised practical experience.

8. Provision of an opportunity for continuous education and career development through refresher courses, supervision, in-service training, and opportunities for recognition and advancement.

9. Provision for adequate job satisfaction, support, and motivation.

10. Evaluation of training and ongoing requirements.

EVALUATION

Base-line and benchmark assessments of fertility, and knowledge, attitude, and practice of contraceptive methods are basic in programme guidance.

In any evaluation, the results of specific inputs should be measured. To assess programme accomplishment, certain tools are necessary. They should be of a diagnostic nature in order to enhance or complement the programme. If programme procedures are sufficiently elastic, weaknesses can quickly be eliminated and strengths reinforced. Ultimately, the measure of success in attaining goals will be reflected in a declining birth rate.

Ongoing analyses are to be found in monthly compilations of work accomplished, personnel in place, and supplies used. A breakdown is given showing the population served according to age, location, and method. Reports and analyses should flow back to the originating office.

There is a growing body of knowledge accumulating that will influence future programmes substantially. Exchanges of programme experience and the dissemination of information are important to the programme director. Up-to-date information must reach workers at all levels.

Goals and Targets

The goal of the programmes, whether they are operated within or outside the health ministry, is usually stated as an attempt to reduce the natural increase in population for the total well-being of people, including, of course, their health. To accomplish this, a budget with provisions for additional personnel, supplies of material, and clinics are included in the plan. Targets for accomplishment are established, and the need to train workers is recognized. A time-table is established and the necessary forces mobilized.

The goals are stated in various ways as targets; for example, the number of IUDs inserted, sterilizations performed, 'couple years' of protection, and eventual birth preventions. These targets can apply to a country or smaller political subdivision, for a month or a year. This approach can also be used as an administrative tool in analysing programme progress. Other components of target-setting are found in numbers of persons hired, trained, and placed. Also used are quantities of material supplied, numbers of clinics operating, and necessary vehicles provided. Adjustments are made to particular physical and regional characteristics. Urban and rural population distribution, literacy, and several economic factors can influence the target. Accomplishment is dependent upon cultural, ethnic, personal, political, and economic factors.

Most family planning programmes establish targets for performance and/or reduction in birth rates or national growth rates. These targets provide a basis for guiding (or sometimes misguiding) work efforts. They are largely arbitrary, with only superficial relations to estimates of programme potential or fertility control needs. From the standpoint of comparing programmes it is useless to compare achievement with targets because the comparison can suffer either from lack of achievement or lack of reality of the targets. Programme achievement can better be examined in relation to basic population dimensions.

The failure of family planning programmes to achieve targets does not constitute a justification for not supporting present efforts in so far as they can be successful. Nor does this failure in itself justify opinions that alternative approaches such as vaguely proposed 'social engineering', more focus on single-purpose programmes, or, alternatively, more focus on comprehensive health services, would be justified. The only proof comes from testing and observing.

Pilot/Demonstration Activated

In an expanding programme one basis for answering questions about cost-effectiveness is to establish additional inputs on a pilot basis. Many programmes do have pilot and demonstration areas. It is wise to allow these pilot areas to go well beyond the practical scope of immediate programming in order to provide answers to eventual programme development.

It is very difficult to develop controlled cost-benefit experiments under the different conditions of developing countries, and usually pilot areas provide at best empirical experiment for programme guidance. Furthermore, programme development often cannot wait for detailed testing and assessment. Consequently, much programme investment must depend on critical evaluation of ongoing programme experience, and often this provides an even better basis for programme development from the artificial conditions of a pilot programme.

Another important point to stress is that the experience gained in pilot areas should receive administrative attention. Pilot efforts have had an unfortunate tendency in many areas to remain self-contained, rather than means to broader ends.

A limitation of the potential for pilot family planning programmes is that short-term results may not reflect long-term impact. For many approaches, long and broad observations are necessary to fully assess the impact of inputs.

WHAT CAN BE ACCOMPLISHED

One often hears stress on a single facet solution for programmes. Furthermore, there is often a tendency to look for immediate impact. Actually further success in family planning lies in several principal directions which require long-term development. These include:

1. *By further extending current approaches in the programme.* In most family planning programmes there is a wide variation in levels of achievement. Levels may be raised through the delegation of tasks to paramedical workers who can better cover peripheral areas; the development of more facilities; and the improvement of transportation, supervision, and supply.

2. *By introducing additional methods into the programme.* Many programmes suffer, particularly initially, through reliance on ineffective methods of fertility control. The policy acceptance of effective known methods is an important factor in programme progress.

3. *By developing new and more effective methods.* None of the current methods is ideal since disadvantages and drawbacks may be cited for each. The development of easily administered, long-acting, single application, reversible methods would contribute greatly to the improvement of programmes.

4. *By orienting programmes to the provision of contraception during a period of optimum receptivity and need in relation to the maternity cycle.* The post-partum or maternity-centred approach to family planning has demonstrated great potential for making better use of limited resources.

5. *By giving better training to family planning workers.* In-service training is needed where family planning is a new activity, and refresher courses should be given in established programmes to bring workers up-to-date.

6. *By developing stronger public family planning education.* Development of educational programmes, not only through health facilities, but also through schools, the mass media, and all possible information channels is of major importance.

7. *By organizing a comprehensive community programme.* Strong community rapport, the mobilization of opinion leaders and greater cultural acceptance of family planning are necessary to achieve lower norms of family size and wider use of contraceptive methods.

8. *By improving education, socio-economic levels, and general health* and other broad changes such as urbanization will in the long run influence the acceptance of family planning.

9. *By providing better administration of programmes.* Stronger leadership, better management information will improve programmes.

REFERENCES AND FURTHER READING

American Public Health Association (1968) *Family Planning: A Guide for State and Local Agencies*, New York.

Cartwright, Ann (1970) *Parents and Family Planning Services*, London.

Howell, Catherine (1967) *The Use of Mobile Units in Family Planning Programmes*, Working Paper No. 1, International Planned Parenthood Federation, London.

International Planned Parenthood Federation (1970) *The Relationship Between Family Size and Maternal and Child Health*, Working Paper No. 5, London.

International Planned Parenthood Federation (1971) *Falling Birth Rates and Family Planning*, London.

Lorraine, J. A. (1974) The world population situation in 1973, *Lancet*, **i**, 22.

Munroe, Gretel S., and Jones, Gavin W. (1971) *Mobile Units in Family Planning*, Reports on Population/Family Plannning No. 10, Population Council, New York.

Omran, Abdel R. (1971) *The Health Theme in Family Planning*, Monograph 16, Caroline Population Center, Chapel Hill, N.C.

Nortman, D. (1973) *Population and Family Planning Programmes: A Factbook*, Reports on Population/Family Planning No. 2, 5th ed. Population Council, N.Y.

Peel, John, and Potts, Malcolm (1969) *Textbook of Contraceptive Practice*, Cambridge.

Royal Society of Health (1968) *Family Planning*, Report of a Conference on Family Planning for Britain, London.

Taylor, H. C., and Berelson, Bernard (1971) Comprehensive family planning based on maternal/child health services: a feasibility study for a world program, *Studies in Family Planning*, Vol. 2, No. 2, Population Council, N.Y.

United Nations (ECAFE) (1966) *Administrative Aspects of Family Planning*, Asian Population Studies No. 1, United Nations, New York.

United Nations (1971) *Human Fertility and National Development: A Challenge to Science and Technology*, United Nations, New York.

World Health Organization (1969) The organization and administration of Maternal and Child Health Services, *Wld Hlth Org. techn. Rep. Ser.*, No. 428.

World Health Organization (1970) Health Aspects of Family Planning, *Wld Hlth Org. techn. Rep. Ser.*, No. 442.

World Health Organization (1971) Family planning in Health Services, *Wld Hlth Org. techn. Rep Ser.*, No. 476.

World Health Organization (1971) Health Education in Health Aspects of Family Planning, *Wld Hlth Org. techn. Rep. Ser.*, No. 483.

World Health Organization (1971) *Abortion Laws: A Survey of Current World Legislation*, Geneva.

World Health Organization (1973a) WHO research programme in methods of fertility regulation, *Wld Hlth Org. Chron.*, **27**, 356.

World Health Organization (1973b) Advances in methods of fertility regulation. Report of a WHO Scientific Group, *Wld Hlth Org. techn. Rep. Ser.*, No. 527.

World Health Organization (1974) The Work of WHO in 1973, *Wld Hlth Org. Off. Rec.*, **213**, 117.

Wyon, John B., and Gordon, John E. (1971) *The Khanna Study: Population Problems in the Rural Punjab*, Boston, Mass.

Zatuchni, Gerald I. (1970) *Postpartum Family Planning*, New York.

37

HEALTH PROBLEMS OF ADOLESCENTS AND YOUNG ADULTS

ROBERT F. L. LOGAN and JOHN S. A. ASHLEY

For the health policy-makers, adolescents, and young adults—those between the ages of 15 and 25—represent a unique challenge. They form the section of the population which imposes the least burden on current health services, but they are also the group who, given the maximum of persuasive effort, offer the greatest scope for the reduction of its needs for future health services. Although it is clear that effort on younger age groups may produce greater results, young adults can be influenced directly whereas children's behaviour can largely only be modified through their parents or their teachers.

The problem of this age group is thus less that of dealing with present disease but more that of affecting attitudes to causes of future morbidity. In short, this group offers society the best hope of favourably altering the pattern of health care use by the year 2000 when on current experience its members will be moving into the category of maximum preventable risk—action on cigarette smoking, diet, and exercise are obvious examples.

Seeking to change personal habits which lead to physical illness is only one aspect of the problem. Equally, there is a need for example to identify now those situations and factors which may lead to later psychiatric morbidity. Similarly, there is the need to mould attitudes in such a way as to ensure that the best use is made of future medical care, that is at that point in the career of a disease when medical science has the best chance of dealing with it.

Thus the health of young people should be considered not merely in the light of major causes of mortality and in terms of their growth, their nutrition and their mental health, but also more positively by the effectiveness with which they apply their abilities.

In all this, the adolescents and young adults—precisely because of the elongated time-scale—provide the opportunity to make health policy within the wider context of social organization. This indeed is an area where to discuss health, implies in practice, discussing attitudes towards morals, relationships with parents, the effects of rising incomes, education, and many other factors. It is an area, moreover, where fashions of all kinds change so rapidly that generalizations are continually in danger of obsolescence and where the facts about physical development are the relatively firm foundation which inevitably supports more speculative super-structure.

PHYSICAL DEVELOPMENT IN ADOLESCENCE

Puberty occurs earlier each decade and the whole process of growth and maturation has progressively accelerated. Whereas on average 30 years ago adolescent development in girls began at the age of 12, now it starts at 11 when pituitary gonadotrophins first appear in the urine. The typical rapid increase in growth is at its maximum at 12, the menarche is near 13, and by the age of 17 the process is nearly over, 3 months earlier each decade. There is a range of 4 years about the average; but half the 11-year-old girls leaving primary schools show obvious signs of puberty, so it is not without reason that sex education is advocated in such schools.

Throughout the phases of adolescence girls are 1–2 years ahead of the boys in whom the landmarks are less defined. For them puberty begins around 12, maximum growth is about age 14, hair appears on the face by 16 and full physical maturity at age 18 or 19.

With great individual variation in the onset, rate of development, and the attainment of maturity, it is to be expected that many factors must influence the process. Some that have been demonstrated, however, are themselves also puzzling. Douglas, following his cohort of children born in March 1946, showed in 1964 that the more intelligent of them, who were usually at grammar school, reached maturity earlier. Additionally at the age of 15 they were taller and heavier than their secondary school counterparts who had, however, caught up by age 18. He also found that to be early in the birth order lead to a more rapid physical and intellectual development.

These factors were then considered to be secondary to underlying nutritional differences which Tanner (1962) suggested had a marked effect on development. Certainly with adolescents growing faster than at any time since early infancy they need increased protein and a high calorific intake. With boys requiring 3,800 and girls 2,600 Calories per day, their needs are comparable with heavy manual workers or nursing mothers.

Other dietary habits may also be important. For example, despite the absence of signs or symptoms, many young women appear to be anaemic. In a survey in South Wales (Elwood et al., 1964) the mean haemoglobin for females aged 14–15 was 14·0 g./100 ml. and over a quarter of such young women had less than 12·0 g./100 ml.

Adaptation to alterations in their physiology is not the only problem that normal adolescents have to face as they are also developing intellectually, emotionally, and socially. The years round puberty are often crucial educationally, culminating in an abrupt and often traumatic change in environment from the cloistered life of school to the adult community of work or university, associated with an increasing emphasis on self discipline. These changes in themselves form the basis of many fundamental problems for the adolescent but often transcending all of them he or she has to cope with the rapid development of interpersonal relationships and in particular those with the opposite sex.

ADOLESCENT SEXUAL ATTITUDES AND BEHAVIOUR

Although present-day adolescent attitudes to sex are poles apart from those of their parents, in today's 'permissive' society the changes that have occurred in the mores of the young are to a large extent either tolerated or ignored by their elders except when their effects impinge on society. Indeed while both adolescents and adults need more debate on premarital sex, cohabitation, and promiscuity, their effects in terms of illegitimacy and venereal disease are indeed true and pressing public health problems. These problems are to an extent controlled by the better availability of contraceptives, and their continued presence emphasized the need to provide appropriate and universally accessible 'family planning' services. Thus, in 1974, their availability to everyone became a statutory function of the National Health Service.

We have no more up-to-date information on adolescent sexual behaviour than the classical studies of Schofield (1965). He surveyed a representative sample of nearly 1,000 each of boys and girls in English towns, including London. His team of trained interviewers met complete refusals in less than 8 per cent. By age 19 only 8 per cent. of boys and 4 per cent. of girls had no contact with the opposite sex, and there was a steady increase through the six stages of intimacy as they developed in their social experience from age 15. Most of the sample of 2,000 teenagers had 'heavy petting', but by age 19 this had progressed to premarital intercourse in 34 per cent. of the boys and 17 per cent. of the girls [TABLE 93]. There was remarkably little difference in the type of school the adolescents had

TABLE 93

The Sexual Behaviour of Young People: Percentage for Boys and Girls at Each Level of Sexual Activity

Activity in age group	Boys		Girls	
	15–17	17–19	15–17	17–19
No contact with other sex .	22	8	9	4
Kissing only . . .	29	18	31	17
Breast stimulation over clothes . . .	13	11	22	18
Breast stimulation under clothes . . .	12	12	16	17
Genital stimulation .	10	13	9	15
Genital apposition .	3	8	7	13
Sexual intercourse .	11	30	6	16

Schofield, M. (1965) *The Sexual Behaviour of Young People*, London.

attended or in the social class of their families. In four cases out of five the first intercourse for the girl had been with a 'steady' boy-friend, and most of them thought it was because they were in love and were going to marry this boy. It was nearly always unpremeditated and in over half of the cases occurred in the parental home and so the majority of the girls neither took precautions themselves nor insisted upon their boy-friends using any kind of contraception. Indeed, a quarter

of the boys said that they never used any contraception, even though they tended to be intimate with more than one girlfriend. By contrast, at the time of the interview three-quarters of the experienced girls had sexual intercourse with only one person. It would seem that both boys and girls felt that increasing intimacy with a 'steady' partner was a natural and sensible preliminary to marriage, which should be a more mutually considerate and satisfying partnership than it was in the case of their own parents.

Whatever the present day behaviour, without promiscuity veneral disease would vanish, but in England gonorrhoea at least continues to disseminate each year [Table 94]. However latest data show what may be the beginnings of a decrease in incidence in males, although the recent fall has been less in the peak age group for this condition—ages 20–24. For girls the rates are still rising in almost all age groups with the peak at 18–19. Furthermore, new cases with so called non-specific urethritis will outnumber new patients with gonorrhoea. Of all infectious diseases notified, only measles is higher. Also syphylis is not decreasing—indeed it may be starting to rise.

TABLE 94

Gonorrhoea—New Cases Seen in England per 100,000 Population

Age	Males			
	1966	1970	1971	1972
–15	0·9	1·3	2·1	1·8
16–17	75·3	143·2	161·4	144·6
18–19	251·5	503·7	523·9	487·5
20–24	502·3	643·4	683·3	675·7
25+	128·5	156·8	159·3	143·2
All Ages	124·8	164·3	169·3	155·6

Age	Females			
	1966	1970	1971	1972
–15	2·8	7·0	7·0	7·4
16–17	124·1	316·0	348·6	362·9
18–19	220·7	508·3	558·8	575·4
20–24	220·7	332·0	370·1	393·1
25+	22·3	34·0	36·6	36·3
All Ages	40·0	70·0	75·9	77·1

On the State of the Public Health, 1966 *et seq.*, London, H.M.S.O.

ILLEGITIMACY

In 1968 the illegitimate rate at 8·5 per cent. in England and Wales was at its highest since its peak in 1945, when it was over 9 per cent. and since has stayed relatively constant [TABLE 95]. In the late 1950s when illegitimacy was on the increase it started in London and the large cities and spread northwards to Scotland and then outwards (Illesley and Gill, 1968).

Changes in the legitimate birth rate over the last few years have undoubtedly been due to the availability of oral contraception and more recently the Abortion Act. The effect of these innovations has, however, been different in different age groups. Thus although the birth rate for the majority of the child-bearing years started to fall in 1965, due to the appearance of the 'Pill', it was a year later before a similar effect was noticed in the under 20-year-olds. Similarly the effect on illegitimate births was delayed and indeed the rate under age 20 has only just levelled off [TABLE 96].

A short-lived increase in the marriage rates, particularly in the younger age groups, occurred in 1968. This was no doubt due to a combination of factors of which changes in Income Tax benefits and the peak of the bulge reaching the age of 21 that year, are but two quite different contenders as aetiological factors. Whether this increase in marriage or the Abortion Act took us over the hump, in terms of premaritally conceived births, it is impossible to say, but since 1969 there has been a fall in the numbers of such births.

TABLE 95

Illegitimate Births—England and Wales

Year	Percentage illegitimate to total live births
1954	4·7
1959	5·1
1964	7·2
1965	7·7
1966	7·9
1967	8·4
1968	8·5
1969	8·4
1970	8·3
1971	8·4

Registrar General's Statistical Review, Part II, 1954 *et seq.*, London, H.M.S.O.

TABLE 96

Illegitimate Live Births—England and Wales
Rates per 1,000 Unmarried Women

Age	1963	1965	1967	1970	1971
15–19	9·3	11·4	13·5	14·0	14·3
20–24	30·2	32·4	31·6	28·4	28·3
25–29	48·9	52·9	51·4	44·0	45·5
30–34	41·2	44·3	42·9	38·2	40·9
35–39	23·6	26·0	26·5	21·3	21·8
40–44	7·7	7·5	7·8	6·3	6·2
All 15–44	19·1	21·2	22·6	21·5	21·8

Registrar General's Statistical Review, Part II, 1963 *et seq.*, London, H.M.S.O.

Although we are unaware of the number of women seeking abortion for whom there was 'no sufficient grounds to interfere' or who had difficulties in reaching the facilities, not surprisingly most abortions performed are on single girls [TABLE 97]. In 1969 the highest rates were between the ages of 25 and 34, but more recently, they are for those in their early twenties and even younger girls are catching up fast [TABLE 98] with the most marked rise being for those between ages 16 and 19. As with access to the 'Pill', the younger age group are slower in getting abortions than their elder sisters and still seek help later in their pregnancy [TABLE 99].

Whether the major cause in reducing illegitimacy is the 'Pill' or the freer availability of abortions, neither are without their hazards. A rise in thrombo-embolic disease is probably

TABLE 97

Legally Induced Abortions—Cases Resident in England and Wales, 1971 Rates per 1,000 Women

Age	Marital Status		
	Single	Others	All
15–19	12·6	6·0	12·1
20–24	22·1	6·9	13·2
25–34	18·7	9·4	10·4
35–44	3·4	5·8	5·6
45+	0·1	0·3	0·3
All 15–49	14·9	6·3	8·6

Registrar General's Supplement on Abortion, London, H.M.S.O.

TABLE 98

Abortions Notified According to Age of Women Residents of England and Wales

Age	1969	1971	Percentage rise
−16	1,174	2,296	96
16–19	8,059	18,176	126
20–24	12,914	24,465	89
25–29	9,001	17,292	92
30–34	7,981	14,203	77
35–44	9,248	15,892	72
45+	276	451	63
Not stated	1,176	1,795	53
All	49,829	94,570	90

Registrar General's Supplement on Abortion, London H.M.S.O.

TABLE 99

Duration of Pregnancy of Legally Induced Abortions
England and Wales
Proportion Where Stated Duration was Over 13 Weeks

Age	Per Cent.		
	1969	1970	1971
−15	42	37	34
16–19	40	32	28
20–24	34	27	23
25–29	33	28	20
30–34	33	27	19
35–39	32	26	18
40–44	36	29	22
45+	46	32	27
All Ages	35	29	22

Registrar General's Supplement on Abortion, London, H.M.S.O.

attributable to oral contraception—even after withdrawal of products with a high oestrogen content—but the mortality rate is difficult to determine as there is uncertainty as to the number of persons at risk, although estimates in 1968 (Inman and Vessey) indicated that about 17 per cent. of married women over age 20 were 'on the pill'. Notification has revealed a measurable, if small, mortality of legal abortions (11 deaths in 95,000 cases in 1971).

MORTALITY IN YOUNG PEOPLE

Deaths after legal abortion form part of the fifty or so deaths after pregnancy or childbirth each year in women under 25. This number has remained relatively unchanged for 10 years after it was halved during the 1950s. However, the precipitate general fall at that time when today's adolescents were born was largely due to the conquest of tuberculosis. Since the mid 1950s, all cause death rates between the ages of 15 and 24 have been flattening [FIG. 88] although for boys aged 15–19 a minor

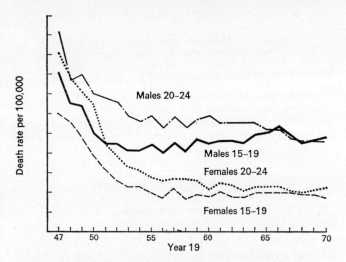

FIG. 88. Death rates per 100,000 living in England and Wales, 1947–70. *Registrar General's Statistical Reviews*, 1947 *et seq.*, Part I, London, H.M.S.O.

peak occurred about 8 years ago. This peak and the subsequent fall since 1966, was almost entirely caused by changes in fashion of youth on the road as reflected in the pattern of deaths from accidents, which are still the principal cause of death in this age group [TABLE 100]. In 1971 total accidents formed almost 60 per cent. of all male deaths between 15 and 25 and over one-third of the female deaths.

The largest component of accident deaths are road deaths and a general fall in the number of these for those aged 15–35 in 1968, was undoubtedly due to increased road safety measures. In particular the revised regulations on drinking and driving, together with the 'breathalizer', which were introduced in October 1967. Consequently this produced a temporary reduction in over-all mortality for boys in the 15–19 age group. More generally, the pattern for road deaths in the young is a complex one [TABLE 101]. In the early 1960s there was great concern about the magnitude of the deaths associated with adolescent male motor cyclists. Indeed at that time, Lee (1963) estimated that a teenage boy had about a 2 per cent. chance each year of being killed or seriously injured on his motor cycle. Since the diminishing interest in this type of vehicle, with fewer on the road each year, the death rates have fallen rapidly and at present are only just about half what they were a decade ago. However, the risk was only transferred to a larger vehicle and deaths in cars and other four-wheeled vehicles continue to rise after a short-lived fall. Young women, on the other hand, have always had lower rates than their brothers and boy-friends but it is a matter of some concern that the death rate, though small is

TABLE 100

Principal Causes of Death in Youth in England and Wales for 1971

Cause of Death	Aged 15–19		Aged 20–24	
	Male	Female	Male	Female
Accidents:				
Road vehicle . . .	708	188	637	151
Drowning . . .	42	5	39	2
Falls . . .	35	7	48	12
Poisoning . . .	22	12	38	15
Other . . .	177	65	220	66
Total accidents . .	984	277	982	246
Suicide	49	26	135	63
Cancer:				
Leukaemia, Hodgkin's, and other blood . .	69	37	84	51
Other . . .	58	53	142	93
Total cancer . .	127	90	226	144
Miscellaneous:				
Pneumonia and influenza	44	32	57	21
Nephritis . . .	13	12	19	10
Congenital abnormalities .	48	30	41	34
Epilepsy . . .	32	14	40	21
Pregnancy, childbirth, and abortion . . .	—	8	—	36
Other Causes . . .	241	48	271	212
Total all causes . .	1,538	631	1,771	787
Total Population (thousands) . .	1,715	1,640	1,874	1,853

Registrar General's Statistical Review, 1971. Part I, London, H.M.S.O.

perceptively rising. High mortality rates from road accidents are mirrored by those for serious injury, and not surprisingly, teenagers have by far the highest rates with 20–24 age group coming second (Rushbrook, 1973).

Apart from accidents, other causes of fatal illness are rare

TABLE 101

Deaths Following Road Accidents—Age 15–24—Rates per Million (Rounded)

	1966	1967	1968	1969	1970	1971
Males						
Car, etc. .	192	188	164	179	201	203
Motor cycle .	202	152	147	138	127	126
Pedal cycle .	12	14	10	13	10	9
Pedestrian .	45	36	29	31	37	36
All road accidents .	451	389	351	360	376	371
Females						
Car, etc. .	56	58	59	60	68	67
Motor cycle .	14	14	13	8	8	13
Pedal cycle .	2	2	2	3	2	1
Pedestrian .	16	16	14	13	18	16
All road accidents .	87	90	87	83	96	97

Registrar General's Statistical Review, 1961 *et seq.*, Part I, London, H.M.S.O.

and so the second cause of death remains cancer which accounts for about one-tenth of all the deaths in both sexes. The largest fraction are deaths due to leukaemia and other haematological cancers. Here the gradual rise in those deaths over the past years has tended to flatten out under age 20 but not after this age, and indeed it still forms almost half the total cancer deaths in young people. Carcinomas in other sites are varied and comparatively rare, although there is now an appreciable number of deaths from neoplasm of the ovary in girls and of the testis in boys. After cancer, the third place is still taken by suicide. The rate for those in their early twenties is now nearly three times that for those in their late teens. Contrary to popular belief, in both age groups there are twice as many 'successful' suicides by males as there are by females.

Surprisingly, despite the present availability and efficacy of antibiotics, there are still 150 or so deaths from pneumonia and influenza a year. The age group also sees the tail end of deaths from congenital diseases.

THE LOW MORBIDITY OF YOUTH

Most of the common crippling diseases are a thing of the past, although it has been estimated that 10,000 males and 9,000 females between the ages of 16 and 29 in Great Britain are appreciably physically handicapped (Harris, 1971). Generally youth makes low demands on medical care services. They have, for instance, low rates of attendance at general practitioners' surgeries and when they go it is largely with minor ailments.

In his suburban London practice, Fry (1968) found that the most common complaint his teenage patients presented was simple respiratory infection and that this accounted for nearly one-third of first consultations. The second reason for consultation was digestive disorders (12 per cent.) followed by minor skin troubles (10 per cent.). This latter group of conditions reaches its peak in adolescence.

In all, 60 per cent. of teenage general practice attendance comes from four causes. The fourth is psychoneurosis (8 per cent. of consultations) although the peak age of psychiatric morbidity is not reached until the fourth decade when the build up of attendances by the chronic and relapsing cases also reaches its maximum. Shepherd et al. (1966) have determined this from attendances at forty-six representative general practices in London [TABLE 102].

TABLE 102

Patient Consulting Rates per 1,000 at Risk for Psychiatric Morbidity

Age	Males	Females
15–24	62	124
25–44	105	195
45–64	111	208
65+	110	149

Shepherd, M. et al. (1966) *Psychiatric Illness in General Practice*, London.

In contrast to the few visits the young pay to doctors, they go to dentists more frequently. This is satisfying as the preservation of young permanent teeth is considered to be of high priority. As there is no general acceptance of fluoridation, as a preventative measure, repair of the damage of pocket money spent on sweets can be the only policy. There is still free treatment for the young and this, combined with a sense of vanity and perhaps a legitimate if uncomfortable reason for absence from work—many factories provide a dental service for this very reason—sends many teenagers to the dental chair [TABLE

TABLE 103

Incidence of Dental Treatment per 1,000 England and Wales, 1967 (Estimated)

Age	Fillings	Extractions	Dentures
15–	377	67	10
18–	385	78	19
21–29	279	70	25

Ministry of Health, 1968 (personal communication).

103]. Nevertheless 1 per cent. of those between 16 and 24 are edentulous (Gray et al., 1970).

ADMISSIONS TO HOSPITAL

It is not surprising that this healthy age group also enjoy low rates of admission to hospital [TABLE 104] and for boys and non-pregnant girls there has been very little change over the last few years. Maternity admissions under the age of 20 however increased by over one-third between 1966 and 1971 and

TABLE 104

Admissions to Non-Psychiatric Hospitals—Rates per 10,000 Population

Age	Males		Females			
			Non-Maternity		Maternity	
	1966	1971	1966	1971	1966	1971
0–4	1,043	1,240	728	875	—	—
5–14	669	658	510	490	1	3
15–19	501	517	500	601	584	743
20–24	503	524	580	686	1,760	1,890
25–34	456	507	620	762	1,268	1,394
35–44	496	558	723	792	326	304
45–64	851	929	775	834	4	3
65–74	1,669	1,639	1,216	1,086	—	—
75+		2,460		1,812		
All ages	768	846	743	830	350	392

Report on the Hospital In-Patient Enquiry, 1966–71, London, H.M.S.O.

it is to be expected that this rate will continue to rise with a goal of 100 per cent. hospital confinement in line with the recent thinking of the Peel Committee (Department of Health and Social Security, 1970). These low admission rates mean that the young only use a small proportion of hospital beds [TABLE 105] and on the whole, less each year. That their use of maternity beds was almost unchanged is of course due to the profound reduction in the length of stay concomitant with the greater introduction of 48-hour confinement and early discharge from hospital.

TABLE 105
Non-Psychiatric Hospital Beds Used Daily per Million Population

Age	Males		Females			
			Non-Maternity		Maternity	
	1966	1971	1966	1971	1966	1971
0–4	3,057	2,603	2,387	2,144	—	—
5–14	1,660	1,171	1,225	902	4	5
15–19	1,544	1,257	1,202	1,160	1,239	1,355
20–24	1,777	1,399	1,326	1,444	3,683	3,408
25–34	1,604	1,604	1,669	1,536	2,710	2,604
35–44	1,868	1,689	2,353	2,024	777	661
45–64	4,440	3,879	3,999	3,316	8	7
65–74	14,245	9,092	14,560	7,219	—	—
75+		2,158		23,569	—	—
All ages	3,701	3,280	4,200	3,835	753	732

Report on the Hospital In-Patient Enquiry, 1966–71, London, H.M.S.O.

The causes of admission to hospital in this age group are reasonably predictable [TABLE 106]. Boys, with their high accident rates are most commonly admitted with head injuries, but the rate after falling is now levelling off. Most head injuries only require observation, so the number of beds used is small. In young men other injuries, half of which are to

condition of nearly 50 per cent. over the boys, is a little less than the 60–70 per cent. shown by Lee in 1961 to have occurred since the 1930s. However, for both males and females, admissions to hospital for appendicitis are falling steadily.

As girls grow up, gynaecological disorders naturally escalate and now completely dominate both admission to hospital and the use of beds. To this must of course be added the rapidly increasing number of admissions for therapeutic abortion. Individual causes are varied but in general these are due to 'irregularities' of menstruation. Curiously there are still many teenage girls having their tonsils removed, but the rate is falling as it did earlier in their younger sisters.

Thus with most adolescent admissions to general hospitals being for 'surgical' causes, young patients in medical wards are rare events as they also are in mental hospitals. Psychiatric admission rates for most older age groups are about double those for teenagers [TABLE 107] in whom first admissions naturally predominate. There is however one readmission to every two first admissions.

Low rates of admission to psychiatric wards may not of course reflect low need for psychiatric care and it may be that the absence of adequate or appropriate services dampens down demand. Certainly many emotional crises are concealed by the label of 'acute poisoning' which already ranks fourth for admitting adolescent girls and young women to a general hospital. In fact, not unlike the 'silent' epidemic of venereal

TABLE 106
Major Causes of Admission to Hospital per 10,000 population

Age 15–19			Age 20–24		
Cause of admission	1969	1971	Cause of admission	1969	1971
Males					
Head injuries	77·3	80·1	Head injuries	59·1	59·5
Fractures and dislocations	57·0	61·2	Fractures and dislocations	48·5	49·2
Soft tissue injuries	50·6	48·2	Soft tissue injuries	41·9	37·7
Appendicitis	48·3	39·4	Appendicitis	33·3	29·9
Diseases of skin	25·2	24·9	Diseases of muscles, bones and joints	25·6	25·6
Diseases of muscles, bones and joints	22·3	27·6	Diseases of teeth	25·6	25·2
Females					
Appendicitis	64·1	58·2	Gynaecological diseases	142·7	155·8
Gynaecological diseases	58·3	63·7	Therapeutic abortion	46·9	68·1
Hypertrophy of Tonsils and adenoids	44·1	37·5	Appendicitis	38·1	32·7
Therapeutic abortion	38·2	72·2	Diseases of teeth	36·2	40·6
Poisoning	35·9	45·6	Poisoning	32·6	40·6
Head injuries	28·0	31·5	Urinary tract diseases	31·8	18·4
Diseases of teeth	21·6	24·3	Benign neoplasms	30·0	21·7
Diseases of muscles, bones and joints	21·3	25·2			
Pregnancy (excluding therapeutic abortion)	626·2	670·3	Pregnancy (excluding therapeutic abortion)	1,694·7	1,821·9

Report on the Hospital In-Patient Enquiry, 1969–71, London, H.M.S.O.

bones, take second and third place. Appendicitis is of course the pre-eminent disease but over age 20, diseases of the teeth (largely extraction of wisdom teeth) are a significant cause of admission. Despite its low incidence, cases of tuberculosis still used an appreciable number of beds in 1971. Indeed, for men between the ages of 20 and 24 at 6·0 beds per 100,000, it rates as high as appendicitis for use of beds.

For young women, trauma is a less significant cause of admission than appendicitis. The present day surplus for this

disease, there has occurred a quiet doubling of the rates of admissions for self-poisoning in the 1960s. This now accounts for up to one-fifth of all emergency medical admissions—second only to myocardial infarction. In Sheffield, females in their teens accounted for one-third, in their twenties another third and outnumbered young men by two to one (Smith, 1972).

At the same time, the development of child psychiatry units has undoubtedly produced more admissions under the age of

TABLE 107

Admission to Psychiatric Units—Rates per 10,000
England and Wales

Age	Males		Females	
	1964	1970	1964	1970
—15	27	46	25	39
15–19	154	200	189	252
20–24	323	378	373	429
25–34	382	438	520	563
35–44	431	435	564	599
45–54	356	409	520	572
55–64	343	339	485	483
65–74	411	414	530	534
75+	644	695	694	745
All ages	279	303	388	414

Department of Health and Social Security (1973) *Health and Personal Social Services Statistics for England*, London, H.M.S.O.

15, but in England and Wales there is still a deficiency of specific facilities for the disturbed adolescent—for example the large shortfall from the thousand or so beds that are currently estimated to be required for these cases (Department of Health and Social Security, 1971*a*). As we catch up on this type of service a further rise can be safely predicted. Is it, however, low health service provision or a degree of unacceptability that has caused the proliferation of self-help organizations by young folk themselves from within their 'alternative' society to cater for their own needs? Are they rejecting the attempts of the therapeutic communities set up by adult organizations?

THE CURRENT EPIDEMIC OF ADDICTION

A new episodic use of psychiatric facilities by youth has been for the treatment of drug dependence. The epidemiology of the taking of 'hard' drugs over the last decade has been as typical as that of the introduction of a new infectious organism into a susceptible population.

Up to the late 1950s addiction to heroin and cocaine was rare and mostly confined to 'professional' addicts in the medical and allied fields. From 1960 to 1967 however, total cases almost quadrupled, with the greatest increase under the age of 35.

In Britain in 1968, two control measures—as recommended in 1965 by the Interdepartmental Committee on Drug Addiction—were instituted. These were compulsory notification of addicts and the restriction of the prescribing of these drugs to specified doctors so that the source of supply could be controlled. The principal effect of the latter regulation was to transfer the burden from general practice to a small number of drug dependency centres, under the direction of licensed psychiatrists, in districts of greatest need principally in London.

In the early months of notification, 38 per cent. of addicts to heroin or methadone were aged under 20 when reported but undoubtedly the presence of a backlog of cases affected the age distribution at this time. Of those receiving hospital treatment up to early 1970, 70 per cent. of males and 68 per cent. of females had first used these drugs in their teens (Bransby, 1971).

Even with more energetic treatment of addiction, the restriction of availability, increased penalties for 'pushers', the epidemic is not yet on the wane. Although the statistics are confusing, most point to an almost stable situation [TABLE 108].

No doubt, as after other epidemics, there will remain a hard core of chronic, often institutionalized, disability as there was from encephalitis lethargica and poliomyelitis, in previous generations.

British youngsters have generally graduated to hard drugs through cannabis or amphetamines and a lesser number have 'taken trips' on LSD or other hallucinogens. A major breakthrough in the control of amphetamine abuse has been the voluntary action taken by increasing numbers of general practitioners to cease to prescribe the drug.

Concerted effort in this direction by general practitioners has enabled the consequent total removal of amphetamines from the shelves of pharmacies in entire towns. It has been by theft from these shelves that youth has found a substantial source of supply of such drugs in recent years. However, this action does not prevent other medicaments being acquired in this way, or taken from family medicine cupboards, and used for experimentation (Hindmarch, 1971). At the same time, most of the issues on the 'soft' drugs are still open.

TABLE 108

Some Recent Statistics on 'Hard' Drug Addiction

	1967	1969	1970	1971	1972
All addicts known during the year†	1,729	2,881	2,661	2,769	2,944
All addicts known at the end of the year†	*	1,466	1,430	1,555	1,619
First notification of addicts—all drugs	*	1,174	762	801	809
Including Heroin addicts aged under 20	*	291	140	*	179
Methadone addicts aged under 20	*	132	94	*	35
Persons found guilty of offences involving 'hard' drugs‡	*	1,082	972	1,253	1,508

* Data not available.
† Heroin, methadone, cocaine, morphine, pethidine.
‡ Opium, heroin, cocaine and other hard drugs controlled under the Dangerous Drugs Act, 1965.
Home Office, 1971, London, and *On the State of the Public Health, 1970*, London, H.M.S.O.

The Wooton Subcommittee (Home Office, 1968), while accepting that cannabis was a potent drug, were unable to assess its total or potential harmfulness and the debate continues unabated—as does the rise in the number of users. If however, the long-term effects of smoking marijuana are still in doubt, those of smoking tobacco certainly are not. As Godber has pointed out (Department of Health and Social Security, 1971*b*), the mortality from smoking-related diseases in Britain is among the highest in the world and thus cigarette smoking is the largest, single, avoidable cause of death today.

The deaths attributable to smoking after an 'incubation period' of some 20 years are of course from lung cancer, bronchitis, and coronary heart disease, and together form at present one-in-eight of all deaths among men aged 35–44, one quarter of those aged 45–64, and one-in-five of those aged 65–

74. Godber comments that 'although few can still be unaware that a danger exists, many do not accept that the hazard is real and applied to them'. As a result Britain is still predominately a smoking community, giving every incentive to children and adolescents to follow the foolish example of their elders.

But what are and have been the cultural, social, or personal pressures acting on the adolescent which encourages him to take up smoking? It was during the First World War that smoking became a national habit for males, and it is the cohort of the teenage boys of that time that appears to be at greatest risk from lung cancer. The Second World War did not increase the numbers of men smoking, only the amount consumed. It did, however, see cigarette smoking become more fashionable in women, who up to then had formed only a small minority. Will the cohort of females born in the twenties form a corresponding lung cancer peak to the men born twenty years earlier? Already an increase is seen in their deaths at all ages.

More recent adolescent attitudes to smoking were revealed by a national survey of a representative sample of 854 adolescents in 1964 (McKennell and Thomas, 1967). They found then that both sexes were taking up smoking at the same rate, but the boys were starting at about age 11 and the girls 2 years later. In consequence, at that time 60 per cent. of boys and close on 40 per cent. of girls by the age of 18 were addicted. Although few adolescents reported enjoying their first cigarette, they took it, usually from a contemporary or slightly older boy or girl, either for reasons of curiosity or to appear more grown-up. They continued to experiment for up to 2 years, finding it difficult to refuse constant offers or to avoid the feeling of being left out or 'different'.

Twenty per cent. of regular adolescent smokers and a further similar proportion of 'triers' were still at school, where any restrictions that existed only seemed to delay the onset of smoking by one year. Outside school, the majority of parents who smoked allowed their children to follow their example and few actually tried to dissuade them, thus adding to the intense social and status pressures put on them by their peers. At the same time half of all smokers said they either wanted to stop or had tried unsuccessfully.

This was in 1964 before any serious efforts began—if not to reduce smoking—to at least lessen encouragement to smoke. The picture since, however, is discouraging. Although tobacco sales have diminished (particularly in the last year) the number of cigarettes sold has only just begun to decrease—largely because untipped brands were replaced by tipped ones (Todd, 1972). There is at least some hope in the young, in that even if the number addicted are not falling, at least they are fairly constant. However, for those that do smoke the latest data seems to indicate that consumption is rising in terms of the number of cigarettes smoked [FIG. 89] but not necessarily the amount of tobacco 'consumed'. What is particularly disappointing is that apparent appreciation of a hazardous habit does not reduce its prevalence, but only results in a transfer to what the consumer hopes is a less risk and any straw is grasped. For example, a report on the tar and nicotine content of different brands (Consumers Association, 1971) only led to a temporary increased demand for those at the head of the league table. For the future, the Royal College of Physicians has made more suggestions (1971) and some have been accepted such as increased non-smoking areas in public transport, but most are based on increased health education which is unlikely to produce a rapid change of mind in a population which seeks the cigarette as a social support if not a pharmacological prop [see also CHAPTER 34].

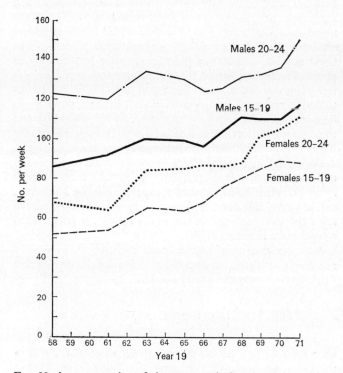

FIG. 89. Average number of cigarettes smoked per week by smokers of manufactured cigarettes. [Todd, G. F., ed. (1972), *Statistics of Smoking in the United Kingdom*, London.]

YOUTH AT LEISURE

At leisure, youth is gregarious by nature and although each succeeding generation has found many different outlets for its exuberance, most of these have been communal in character. Many have also been associated with the 'primitive' cults of music and dancing, but none have so directly impinged on the practice of Public Health as the presently fashionable medium —the outdoor 'Pop Festival'. Attendances have been as high as 200,000 and often extend over several days on open rural sites, devoid of facilities. Fortunately the young are tough and healthy and indeed both the participants as well as the youthful organizers have been, perhaps surprisingly, responsible. With careful, co-operative planning and supervision (valuable guidelines for which are available from the Department of Health and Social Security, 1971c), those mass gatherings that have occurred so far have come and gone, in public health terms at least, reasonably uneventfully; however, the present legal teeth of public health may not be sharp enough to control such situations in the future (Brock, 1971).

Participation in such events seems to satisfy some of the emotional and sensual needs for self-expression. Its attendant publicity presents to the world, however, a false image that today's teenager sheers away from more overtly creative, constructive, or competitive pursuits, and indeed if youth abandons physical exercise in its leisure in the way that older age groups do, we may have lost a major battle against the modern epidemic of coronary heart disease—but hopefully not the war.

With an ever changing kaleidoscope of interests, the general pattern of youthful leisure may already be different from the latest information we have, that for 1966 (Sillitoe, 1969). Then a government social survey of 2,682 persons aged 15 and over living in urban areas, provided data on all kinds of leisure activity. The survey showed that young unmarried adults in towns spent at least a quarter of their leisure time participating in physical recreation (which for this purpose included dancing), but when married it was a great deal less. There was a considerable variety of such recreation and, for example, ten-pin bowling was quite popular at that time. Swimming was one of the chief pursuits as it is indeed at all ages, but was eclipsed for single girls under 22 and boys between 19 and 22 by dancing.

For the future it is disturbing to confirm that the possession of a car in the household reduces, even in the young, the time spent participating in physical recreation. Having access to a car, however, cuts down television viewing which although the most common 'activity' in the whole sample, is relegated to second place in young adults.

Most adolescents of course spend their leisure in socially acceptable activities, but a small but increasing number involve themselves in overt antisocial behaviour.

THE DELINQUENT ADOLESCENT

Crime has more than doubled in the last 10 years and this has been reflected in a similar rise in teenage convictions. It is in the 17–20 age group that the peak of offences occurs [TABLE 109], with the maximum at the age of 17, so that almost half the people before the courts today are under the age of 21.

TABLE 109
Guilty of an Indictable Offence—England and Wales 1972

Age	Males		Females	
	Number	Rate per 100,000	Number	Rate per 100,000
—13	19,278	1,229	1,850	124
14–16	49,784	4,597	5,050	490
17–20	75,059	5,475	8,374	639
21–24	43,700	3,058	5,957	422
25–29	34,547	1,925	5,730	326
30+	71,046	567	19,660	137
All ages	293,414	1,484	46,621	219

Home Office, *Criminal Statistics 1972*, London, H.M.S.O.

That this is admittedly slightly less than a few years ago is probably due to increased 'cautioning' rather than prosecution of young offenders.

It is well known that crime rates are higher in urban than in rural areas and conurbations are even higher with London particularly affected in this respect. Even so there is wide variation within London between neighbourhoods. In six of the 301 census districts in the London Borough of Tower Hamlets 40 per cent. of the boys resident there appeared before the courts before their seventeenth birthday. In contrast, during the same period in a quarter of such districts at most,

only 14 per cent. offended (Power, 1972). There were also wide differences in delinquency rates in apparently similar secondary schools in the Borough with a range of from 4 per cent. of pupils appearing before the Courts while still at school, to ten times this rate. Although nearly half of these first offenders do not appear again, a core of 6 per cent. of them make at least three appearances before they are 17.

While the offences these youngsters commit include most crimes [TABLE 110], stealing is by far the most common reason for a prosecution and there is a constant pattern to these thefts. For boys, cars, and their contents are the prime target account-

TABLE 110
Young Offenders Found Guilty—Age 17–20—England and Wales 1972

Offence	Males	Females
Violence against the person . .	7,312	309
Sexual offences . . .	1,067	5
Burglary and robbery . . .	16,593	477
Theft and unauthorized taking .	35,555	5,817
Handling stolen goods . . .	3,771	568
Fraud	1,678	528
Other indictable offences . .	9,083	670
Total indictable . . .	70,059	8,374
Non-indictable motoring . .	119,773	4,734
Non-indictable other . . .	46,979	4,562
All offences	241,811	17,670

Home Office, *Criminal Statistics, 1972*, London, H.M.S.O.

ing for over 20 per cent. of all indictable offences each year, while for girls, nearly a third of their crime is shop-lifting.

For non-indictable crime, when the mass of motoring offences are excluded, nearly a quarter of that remaining is associated with drink or drunkenness and the rates for such offences have risen 40 per cent. for both boys and girls between 17 and 20 years over the past 5 years, while adult rates have remained low for decades. When convicted, half the young offenders are fined and probation comes a poor second and custodial care third; nevertheless, about 10,000 under the age of 21 are in prisons, borstals, or detention centres today. There is therefore still an increasing need for social services appropriate to this age group to investigate and diagnose the underlying problems which give rise to the symptoms of crime and delinquency.

YOUTH IN ITS ENVIRONMENT

Teenagers at work, particularly the girls, now have the highest inception rates of certified sickness absence [TABLE 111], principally because of all the age groups, their rates have increased more than most in recent years. For young men, in the presence of some unemployment, this trend contrasts sharply with that of those near to retirement—the other group vulnerable to redundancy. In the pre-retirement years not only does the laying off of the 'invalids' increase the general level of health of the survivors but these in their turn cannot afford to be 'off sick' too often and risk the possible consequences. Teenagers, despite the last in, first out, doctrine, perhaps are apparently more complacent but their seemingly increased

TABLE 111

Sickness Absence—Certified Incapacity (Excluding Influenza)
—Great Britain—1970–71 (53 weeks)

Age	Males			Females		
	Spells per 1,000 at Risk	Days per person at Risk	Days per Spell	Spells per 1,000 at Risk	Days per person at Risk	Days per Spell
—19	428	5·9	13·8	537	7·6	14·2
20–24	438	6·8	15·5	483	8·9	18·2
25–29	400	7·4	18·5	411	10·5	25·5
30–34	427	8·9	20·8	487	15·5	31·8
35–39	405	9·9	24·4	457	18·7	40·9
40–44	374	11·5	30·7	448	22·1	49·3
45–49	379	14·3	37·7	401	24·6	61·3
50–54	374	18·3	48·9	428	34·9	81·5
55–59	384	26·0	67·7	359	43·2	120·3
60–64	385	44·6	115·8	N/A	N/A	N/A
All ages	397	15·8	39·8	461	16·9	36·7

On the State of Public Health, 1972, London, H.M.S.O.

proneness to 'illness' is combined with a higher level of resistance and recovery so that the average length of their total incapacity is the lowest of all.

Although inception rates have accelerated over the years, the rise of women aged 20–24 has been lower than in most other young age groups. This has been due to decreasing numbers of married women of this age, in some the rates are particularly high, being not only at work but also eligible for benefit (Whitehead, 1971).

The statistics of absence after industrial accidents, show a parallel pattern to those after illness and suggests that teenagers are the most accident-prone age group. The short duration of their absences of just about one day per year, however, indicates that on the whole the trauma is minor.

There will of course be a considerable contraction of the young work force now that the compulsory school leaving age has been raised from 15 to 16, but it has already been selectively eroded by the ever rising tide towards tertiary education. In 1961, 21 per cent. of children stayed on at school until they were over the age of 16 and 12 per cent. to over 17; now these rates are 35 per cent. and 20 per cent., and it is estimated that by 1985 they will have risen to 63 and 36 per cent. respectively. For every two going on from school to full-time further education in 1961, there were three doing so in 1970—and interestingly more girls than boys. At present, at least one in eleven school leavers transfer to universities or colleges of education [TABLE 112]; in the United Kingdom students now number over 200,000 men and 150,000 women. Just over half of them are under 20 and many of their health problems are of course identical to those of their contemporaries in factories, offices, or department stores. It is, however, also well recognized that they make somewhat greater demands on health care facilities. This is partly because the majority now have access to comprehensive student health services, often on a generous scale. For example, a service with a doctor–student ratio of 1:1500 has been proposed (Mair, 1967). Staffing at such a level enables the worried student to have more than average opportunities for consultation—which he or she undoubtedly takes. It has been observed that a rate of five

attendances per head per year is usual which compares with general practice rates for the traditional heavy users, i.e. infants and the elderly (Gunn, 1970).

Apart from the anticipated stimulation of demand by increased resources, consultation rates are swollen by the effects of stress which may either make minor physical illness intolerable or present itself as minor psychiatric disorders and it has been estimated that 15 per cent. of students go to the university physician for such a reason (Malleson, 1965).

More seriously it has been frequently reported that student suicide rates are about five times those of their contemporaries. There are perhaps four attempts to each successful one and disquietingly, these appear to be rising (Finlay, 1968). On the other hand, students are reported to have minimal venereal disease, less illegitimate pregnancies—with only about 12 per cent. (McChance and Hall, 1972) of unmarried women students on the 'Pill'—although over 40 per cent. are having regular sexual intercourse. Students are also rarely addicted to

TABLE 112

Destination of School Leavers (per cent.)

Destination	Boys		Girls	
	1961–62	1971–72	1961–62	1971–72
	Per cent.	Per cent.	Per cent.	Per cent.
Universities	4·3	7·3	1·8	4·2
Colleges of Education	0·7	1·4	2·5	5·1
Other full time further education	6·8	10·5	10·3	15·0
Employment or other	88·2	80·8	85·4	75·7

Social Trends (1973) London, H.M.S.O.

opiates (Gunn, 1970). The general picture is that adolescents emergent from school are subjected to increased social and mental stress. Quite naturally those entering the hurly-burly of industry and commerce tend to succumb to the former and those translating to the helter-skelter of university or other tertiary education, to the latter.

SUMMARY AND CONCLUSIONS

Freed from the constraints on physical development, youth is taller and physically more fit than ever before. Seizing their educational opportunities, they are more developed intellectually and translate this into more skilled jobs and so are mobile socially upwards. From their good wages, they can afford cars as symbols of strength, power, virility, and success. They feel they are in charge of their own destiny, roaring away from places where they feel cribbed and confined. Most are good drivers and better at speed than their parents, but as risk-taking is a necessary experience for growing-up, their accident risk is higher and more are fatal. Unfortunately the price and tax on alcoholic spirits has not inflated with their wages so new long-term risks, as well as those immediate, are being fostered.

Breaking free from the puritan ethic for work and material competitiveness, youth absents itself from the job more frequently, as well as dropping out from other adult organizations in which it feels it has no say and is not asked to participate. Freed also from the old sex inhibitions and inequalities, coupled with their new ideals of exploring their feelings about themselves and the opposite sex, youth naturally experiments with drugs and sex—but often without love. Thanks to the 'Pill' and abortion on demand, fewer have to get married but despite antibiotics the epidemic of gonorrhoea continues and indeed is out-raced by non-specific urethritis.

The speed of change is too fast and much deprivation, at least in human relationships, still remains so that the youth from a cold home or a hostile school steals a car or its contents and the girl shop-lifts for some compensation. When they cannot externalize their mixed-up emotions in such delinquent behaviour, they may take too many of their tranquillizers prescribed by their family doctor to reduce their stress. This epidemic of self-poisoning in young females is increasing annually at almost fifteen per cent., but few episodes are 'psychiatric' or fatal. The girls concerned just feel that they must stop their personal world for 48 hours.

The impacts from such trauma, youth-made and society fostered, are manifest in the short-term. But the silent and insidious long-term effects may be more important. On the physical side, youth has to sweat less at work, he takes less exercise at leisure and the smoking addiction has spread to girls. All these are pathological omens for future ischaemic heart disease and lung cancer.

Adolescence is the no-man's-land between protected immaturity and the attainment of full physical, mental, and social maturity. Although in biological terms its beginning and duration vary by a few years, society in its wisdom has had to arbitrarily designate its end for administrative, legal, or other practical reasons. The right to drive a car, to drink, to vote, and to marry vary from country to country as does liability to compulsory education, crime, and military service. Youth itself has progressively agitated for a reduction in the age of majority and has now achieved its ambition in Britain. No doubt there are many who have reached the 'age of discretion' at eighteen, but for others it may be 'majority without maturity'. Will the increasing rights that society is giving to these youngsters—and where they feel deprived they still seek them with articulate and sometimes violent protest—lead to secondary consequences? Will, for example, the new sexual freedoms and earlier marriage result in even more divorce? It may take a decade to know.

Adolescence has been described as a process—a series of varied, rapid, and extensive changes—as well as a period of life (World Health Organization, 1965) and that many of the problems of adolescents arise from difficulties in meeting the demands of a highly organized technological society (May et al., 1971).

The present health problems of adolescents illustrate the extent of the medical and social casualties produced by the failure of the process to keep pace with the demands.

REFERENCES

Bransby, E. R. (1971) A study of patients notified by hospitals as addicted to drugs: first report, *Health Trends*, **3**, 75.

Brock, S. H. (1970) Public health and the pop festival, *Community Med.*, **126**, 79.

Consumers Association (1971) Cigarettes, *Which?*, 280.

Department of Health and Social Security (1970) *Domiciliary Midwifery and Maternity Bed Needs*, London, H.M.S.O.

Department of Health and Social Security (1971a) *Hospital Services for the Mentally Ill*, London, H.M.S.O.

Department of Health and Social Security (1971b) *On the State of the Public Health, 1970*, London, H.M.S.O.

Department of Health and Social Security (1971c) *Public Health Guidelines for Large Pop Festivals*, London, H.M.S.O.

Douglas, J. W. B., and Simpson, H. R. (1964) Height in relation to puberty, family size and social class. A longitudinal study, *Milbank mem. Fd Quart.*, **71**, No. 3, 20.

Elwood, P. C., Withey, J. L., and Kirkpatrick, G. S. (1964) Distribution of haemoglobin level in a group of school children and its relation to height, weight and other variables, *Brit. J. prev. Soc. Med.*, **18**, 125.

Finlay, S. E. (1968) Suicides and attempted suicides in Leeds University, *Proc. Brit. Stud. Hlth Ass.*, 37.

Fry, J. (1966) *Profiles of Disease*, Edinburgh; and personal communication.

Gray, P. G., Todd, J. E., Slack, G. L., and Bulman, J. S. (1970) *Adult Dental Health in England and Wales*, SS411, London, H.M.S.O.

Gunn, A. (1970) *The Privileged Adolescent*, Aylesbury.

Harris, A. I. (1971) *Handicapped and Impared in Great Britain*, London, H.M.S.O.

Hindmarch, I. (1971) Age groups at risk, *Drugs and Society*, **1**, 19.

Home Office (1968) *Cannabis*, London, H.M.S.O.

Illsley, R., and Gill, D. G. (1968) Changing trends in illegitimacy, *Soc. Science and Med.*, **2**, 415.

Inman, W. H. W., and Vessey, M. P. (1968) Investigation of deaths from pulmonary, coronary and cerebral thrombosis, and embolism in women of child-bearing age, *Brit. med. J.*, **2**, 193.

Lee, J. A. H. (1961) 'Appendicitis' in young women, *Lancet*, **ii**, 815.

Lee, J. A. H. (1963) Motor cycle accidents to male teenagers: a contemporary epidemic, *Proc. roy. Soc. Med.*, **56**, 365.

McChance, C., and Hall, D. J. (1972) Sexual behaviour and contraceptive practice of unmarried female undergraduates at Aberdeen University, *Brit. med. J.*, **2**, 694.

McKennell, A. C., and Thomas, R. K. (1967) *Adults' and Adolescents' Smoking Habits and Attitudes*, London, H.M.S.O.

Mair, A. (1967) *Student Health Services in Great Britain and Northern Ireland*, Oxford.

Malleson, N. (1965) *A Handbook on British Student Health Services*, London.

May, A. R., Kahn, J. H., and Cronholm, B. (1971) Mental Health of Adolescents and Young Persons, *Wld Hlth Org. Publ. Hlth Pap.*, No. 41, Geneva.

Power, M. J., Benn, R. T., and Morris, J. N. (1972) Neighbourhood, school and juveniles before the courts, *Brit. J. Crim.*, **12**, 111.

Royal College of Physicians (1971) *Smoking and Health Now*, London.

Rushbrook, J. A. (1973) Road accidents and casualties in Great Britain, in *Social Trends, No. 4*, London, H.M.S.O.

Schofield, M. (1965) *The Sexual Behaviour of Young People*, London.

Shepherd, M., Cooper, B., Brown, A. C., and Kalton, G. (1966) *Psychiatric Illness in General Practice*, London.

Smith, A. J. (1972) Self-poisoning with drugs: A worsening situation, *Brit. med. J.*, **4**, 157.

Sillitoe, K. K. (1969) *Planning for Leisure*, SS388, London, H.M.S.O.

Tanner, J. M. (1962) *Growth at Adolescence*, Oxford.

Todd, G. F., ed. (1972) *Statistics of Smoking in the United Kingdom*, Tobacco Research Council Paper No. 1, London.

Whitehead, F. E. (1971) Trends in certified sickness absence, in *Social Trends, No. 2*, London, H.M.S.O.

World Health Organization (1965) Report of an Expert Committee on Health Problems of Adolescence, *Wld Hlth Org. techn. Rep. Ser.*, No. 308, Geneva.

World Health Organization (1973) Youth and drugs: Report of a WHO study group, *Wld Hlth Org. techn. Rep. Ser.*, No. 516.

World Health Organization Regional Office for Europe (1967) *Report of a Symposium on Student Health Services*, Copenhagen.

World Health Organization Regional Office for Europe (1974*a*) *Report of a Symposium on Problems of Deviant Social Behaviour and Delinquency in Young Persons, Bratislava 1973* (Euro 5430III), Copenhagen.

World Health Organization Regional Office for Europe (1974*b*) *Report of a Working Group on Suicide and Attempted Suicide in Young Adults, Zagreb 1973* (Euro 5431III), Copenhagen.

38

OCCUPATION AND HEALTH

R. S. F. SCHILLING

EARLY DEVELOPMENTS

Antiquity and the Middle Ages

The adverse effects that work may have on health have been recognized since the age of antiquity. For instance, early writers referred to the ravages of occupational disease among metal miners in Egypt and Ancient Greece (Rosen, 1943). As the miner of antiquity was a slave or a criminal, there was no incentive to improve his working conditions. Much later, Bernardino Ramazzini (1633–1714), an Italian physician, published the first systematic account of trade diseases (Wright, 1940). Ramazzini conceived it to be the duty of medicine to cultivate this specialty so that workers could earn their living without bodily injury. During his lifetime in the seventeenth and eighteenth centuries, neither his medical colleagues nor the society in which he lived had any strong humanitarian sense to inspire them to heed his words nor at that time was there any economic necessity to protect the life and health of workmen.

Industrial Revolution

The technological inventions of the eighteenth and nineteenth centuries, particularly the use of steam for motive power, laid the foundations of the factory system. This change took place first in the British textile industry and later spread to other industries and into the rest of Europe and North America, and so unsettled family and community life that it became known as the Industrial Revolution. Workers were increasingly exposed to the specific hazards of occupational disease and injury and the adverse effects of excessively long hours of work.

The most serious effects on health which followed the Industrial Revolution were not due to work itself, but were caused by disruption of family life when men moved into the new industrial areas without their families; by overcrowding under insanitary conditions as the factories were built before houses; by malnutrition brought about by the change from peasant to town life; and by poverty from unemployment caused by fluctuations in the economy. It was the poor housing, the overcrowding, and the lack of sanitation of these expanding industrial populations which led to the development of public health services primarily designed to control infectious disease and protect all classes of people living in the new industrial towns.

Government Intervention

In most countries, hazards to health inside workplaces were dealt with separately and by different authorities, such as inspectors of mines and factories. In Britain the public became increasingly concerned about the excessively long hours worked by women and children. The Children's Employment Commissions disclosed almost unbelievable facts about their exploitation, which gave rise to the *first phase* of government activity in occupational health, namely the control by Acts of Parliament of the age of entry of children into workplaces, the restriction of their hours of work, and those of women. The first effective legislation to be enforced by factory inspectors was introduced in 1833. It culminated in the Ten Hour Act of 1847 which restricted the work of women and young persons in factories to 58 hours in the week. The *second phase* was the development of safety laws to deal with the increasing occurrence of fatal and disabling injuries from the new machinery. In Britain the Factory Act of 1844 aimed to prevent this toll of life and limb by making it compulsory to fence all dangerous parts of machinery, and later the Act of 1891 introduced the new principle of making special regulations for particularly dangerous processes. Today, in all industrialized countries, codes of safety for particular processes are one of the most important features of occupational health practice. As the Industrial Revolution proceeded there was a *third phase* of activity aimed at the prevention of occupational disease which had become a problem by reason of the increasing range of new chemicals introduced into factories without consideration of their effects on the worker. Attempts were made to control occupational diseases such as lead and phosphorus poisoning by statutory laws which enforced notification of disease, a higher standard of environmental conditions, and medical surveillance of all workers at risk. These measures were not the first attempts to protect the workman. For centuries the common law practised in many countries, had provided redress by the servant against the negligence of his master. One of the reasons for introducing statutory laws was that the common law by itself was inadequate to protect workers employed in factories and mines.

Employers' Health Services

While the State was taking steps to control hours of work of women and young persons and to prevent the more obvious hazards to health, a few enlightened employers were setting up health and welfare services for the care of their employees. Their motives were almost entirely humanitarian, and there are several outstanding examples of good employers such as the Bradford mill owner who employed a doctor and sent his work children to a health resort when they were 'overdone' (Select Committee, 1832). The first real impetus in Britain for employers to appoint doctors came with the passing of the Workmen's Compensation Act of 1897. The motive, however, was self-protection against claims for compensation, rather than the safeguarding of the health of their employees. The First World War had an important influence on occupational health in many countries. In Britain, the munition famine in 1915 was not made good by excessive hours of work. This led to scientific investigations into the effects of work on health and efficiency, to the study of new toxic problems, and to a rapid growth in industrial medical and nursing services. The motives for this new interest in occupational health were the strongest possible, namely national survival. Interest waned during the economic slump which followed the war. Nevertheless, the more enlightened and wealthy industries continued to provide and to develop their own health services, because the statutory provisions laying down minimum standards of health, safety, and welfare were inadequate. While these services were broadened in their scope, and generally aimed to safeguard employees' health and not merely to protect employers from compensation claims, their achievements were often limited because there was no systematic training of doctors in occupational medicine, and in most countries the practice of occupational hygiene was almost non-existent. Developments in occupational health in other Western European countries and North America followed similar patterns for much the same reasons.

Eastern European Countries

In Eastern Europe there were quite different developments. They began in the Soviet Union after the October Revolution of 1917 when free health services concentrating particularly on prevention were introduced. While in Western Europe and North America occupational health services are provided voluntarily by employers and to a limited extent by Governments, all health services in the Soviet Union are the responsibility of the Ministry of Health and are organized into separate streams of therapeutic and preventive medicine. The former is provided by hospitals, polyclinics, and the medical departments of large plants, and the latter by the sanitary and epidemiological stations (sanepids) in towns, rural areas, and also in large plants. The physicians in the hospitals and polyclinics are responsible for the medical care of people at work and the diagnosis and treatment of occupational diseases, while the staff of the sanepids are responsible for preventive measures including the assessment and control of the environment, both inside and outside the workplace. After the Second World War both Bulgaria and Rumania, which had previously been inactive in this field, followed the Russian method of organizing health services into main streams of therapeutic and preventive medicine, and like the Soviet Union, have placed considerable emphasis on occupational health. Yugoslavia, which had little provision for workers' health and safety before 1945, has also made rapid developments, but in a different way from the other Socialist countries. Therapeutic and preventive services for workers are organized into one health department in large plants and in district centres serving groups of small plants. Thus, Socialist countries have demonstrated the importance they attach to occupational health by the services they have developed and by the large number of research and teaching establishments which they have set up since the 1920s. For example, the Soviet Union has 16 Institutes of Occupational Health sponsored by the Ministry of Health for research and teaching. The Trade Unions also have six institutes to support their technical factory inspectors, who are broadly equivalent in their functions and powers to inspectors in Labour Ministries in Western countries.

Influence of the Second World War

The Second World War and the sustained period of economic expansion which followed this war have had a profound influence on the development of occupational health all over the world. During the war, medical care at the workplace ceased to be a welfare stunt and became important to the war effort. With the Armed Forces taking most of the fit and able men, industry was forced to employ the disabled as well as the fit. As it was necessary to assess ability for work rather than disability, occupational physicians had to get out of their consulting rooms into the workplaces to study the abilities required for different types of work. This encouraged them to take a more active and detailed interest in the working environment. The Armed Forces developed new techniques for selecting personnel. They adapted military equipment to increase fighting efficiency and so gave a boost to ergonomics. The need to get highly trained men who were sick or wounded back into service as soon as possible stimulated developments in the rehabilitation of the injured and sick.

Sustained high employment in the present period of economic expansion has encouraged these developments to continue. The care of the worker has become economically essential and not just a moral or legal obligation. Rapidly developing countries have given a high priority to occupational health, since their national prosperity depends on speedy industrialization in which the worker's health and his environment are especially important.

Factors Influencing Developments

This brief account of developments in occupational health indicates that there are many factors which may influence a nation or an employer to provide for the health of people at work. Both the extent and the quality of service provided will depend on the humanity of a society or of the employer; on national wealth, or on the prosperity of a particular organization; on the social status of the worker, his Trade Union organization, and his representation in Government. Many Governments and employers now recognize the economic advantages and the boost to morale of providing good occupational health services, although it is difficult to measure their benefits in terms of costs saved (Schilling, 1973). These factors in turn influence the importance attached to the training of experts in this field. In the past, when so little was known about the effects of work on health, it was left to a few pioneers to encourage or cajole Governments and industries to improve working conditions by revealing the loss of life and increased sickness and injury caused by disregarding unhealthy conditions of work. Today, in most industrialized countries, there are extensive training programmes for occupational health physicians, nurses, hygienists, factory inspectors, and safety officers [p. 504].

WORK AND HEALTH

In many countries, e.g. as in Britain, occupational health services are separate from the other health services and largely confined to the larger organizations or groups of small firms on the same industrial estate. There are, therefore, many people at work who are not covered by occupational health services and for whom statutory codes of occupational health and safety do not provide adequate cover. For this reason, all those who are responsible for the medical care of people need to be aware of the influence that work may have on health and health on work. Three questions have to be borne in mind. Has the patient's work caused the disease? Has the patient's work exacerbated the illness or injury? Has the patient's illness or incapacity prejudiced ability to work efficiently and safely? The staff of an occupational health service have a major responsibility for dealing with these aspects of medical care, and a good service is organized to do this [p. 501]. But occupational physicians and nurses do not and cannot cover all people at work, many of whom will seek advice in the first place from someone else. Thus, it may be as important for the general practitioner or the doctor in hospital as it is for the works doctor or nurse to consider the influence of work on health and health on work. This demands inquiry into the patient's occupation.

The Occupational History and Occupational Disease

The type of history to be recorded depends on a number of factors. In the general practice or hospital it should include a full description of the patient's present occupation. A comprehensive history covering working life is only needed when the patient's past or present occupation is suspected as being the cause of his illness. In an occupational health service a full occupational history is an essential part of an employee's health record. In studies of the causes of disease in communities or industrial groups, a full occupational history relevant to the particular disease being studied is required. For example, in a disease such as mesothelioma of the pleura and peritoneum which was believed to be due to asbestos, a searching inquiry into all the various types of asbestos and possible sources of exposure during lifetime was required (Newhouse and Thompson, 1965). There are many difficulties in obtaining a history. The job title itself may be misleading or uninformative. A Works Manager in a small factory handling toxic materials may be exposed to risk just as much as one of the operatives. A cooper makes and repairs barrels, which in itself is not a hazardous occupation, but he may be exposed to toxic materials contained in the barrels before repair. For occupational diseases which take many years to develop, the last job may not be the one that provided the cause. The great majority of occupations of men who die of pneumoconiosis in England and Wales are ascribed to the dusty trades, but a substantial number also occur in men employed in what are called 'end-occupations' such as caretaker, clerk, watchman, publican, and store-keeper which are sedentary and require no special skills (Harrington and Schilling, 1973). The patient's pastimes may also be important in elucidating the cause of his complaints. A number of serious illnesses have been attributed to hobbies and do-it-yourself activities. For example, bird fanciers may get a disabling allergic alveolitis from dust from bird droppings. Amateur boat builders and house painters have suffered from asthma as a result of using isocyanates, or lead poisoning from burning off lead paint without taking the necessary precautions. There are numerous examples of housewives becoming sensitized to, or poisoned by, materials used in their work or in the pursuit of their hobbies.

Occupational and pastime diseases often mimic syndromes which are non-occupational in origin and will either be missed or a correct diagnosis will be delayed unless a careful history is taken. A physician should always look at his patient in the light of the type of work he does. It may be important to ask the patient if any workmates are similarly affected. It is often an irrelevant question, but occasionally it provides crucial evidence of the occupational origin of a disease. In essence, this is the epidemiological approach, or being 'group orientated'. This is required by physicians responsible for individual patients as well as those who look after communities. The general practitioner and the hospital doctor do not have the advantages of the occupational physician for whom it is relatively easy to talk to a man's workmates and to examine their working environment. An otorhinologist noticed several men with adenocarcinoma of the nasal sinuses. The rarity of this particular type of tumour prompted inquiry into their occupations. They were found to come from the same area, which was a centre of the furniture-making industry, and all were furniture makers (Acheson, Cowdell, and Hadfield, 1968). A search is now being made for the aetiological agent, which could be certain types of wood dust or glues used in making furniture.

Exacerbation of Non-Occupational Disease

With increasing awareness of the multi-factorial nature of many diseases and the influence that work has on health, it becomes increasingly difficult to classify diseases as strictly occupational or non-occupational. There are, however, several common diseases in which work may be aetiologically important and sufferers from these complaints may need to be advised by their doctor to avoid certain types of work.

Chronic Bronchitis. Certain occupational groups have an increased morbidity and mortality from chronic bronchitis; they have in common hard physical work and exposure to air pollutants both at work and in the home environment. The available evidence suggests that work factors exacerbate rather than cause this disease (Gilson, 1970). Thus, a patient with chronic bronchitis should not be exposed to irritant aerosols nor be employed on heavy work.

Ischaemic Heart Disease. While physical activity at work is protective against ischaemic heart disease, other occupational factors have been identified as having adverse effects. There is an increased risk of angina pectoris and sudden death in men exposed to nitroglycol and nitroglycerine (Lund, Haggendal, and Johnsson, 1968).

Men exposed to carbon disulphide in the manufacture of viscose rayon have death rates from coronary heart disease two-and-a-half times that of men not so exposed (Tiller, Schilling, and Morris, 1968). There is less certain epidemiological evidence that the stress in high-pressure occupations increases the chance of developing myocardial infarction (Russack, 1967). Most patients who have recovered from an acute episode of ischaemic heart disease return to their previous occupation. But where occupational factors are likely to increase the risk of a further attack, the physician should advise them to change or modify their work.

Varicose Veins. These are one of the most common ailments of women in the Western World. They are associated with several factors such as heredity, child-bearing, body weight, and wearing tight corsets. After allowing for these variables, women who stand at their work were found to have a significantly higher prevalence than those who sit or walk. The presence of varicose veins in a shop assistant or waitress should be strong grounds for the physician to recommend early treatment or a change to work which does not involve constant standing (Mekky, Schilling, and Walford, 1969).

Spinal injury and disease may be made worse by heavy lifting; deafness by exposure to excessive noise, chronic skin disease by contact with irritants. These are but a few examples showing the need for inquiry into the patient's occupation. Nevertheless, the physician has to balance the ill against the good effects of work on health before recommending prolonged absence or a change of job. Work provides essentials to living other than an income. To many people it gives a sense of belonging to a group, companionship and recreation.

Illness Jeopardizing the Health and Safety of Others

Airlines and road and rail transport undertakings have their own occupational health services which apply rigorous pre-employment, periodic, and post-sickness medical examinations to their pilots and drivers to protect the travelling public. If they suffer from certain diseases such as myocardial infarction, hypertension, diabetes mellitus, or epilepsy, they will be precluded from this type of work (Raffle, 1970).

Similarly, the major food industries use their occupational health services to protect the public by screening food-handlers for faecal pathogens and infective dermatoses. But there are many workplaces with similar risks but no occupational health service. In these situations, protection of the public may depend on the intervention of the patient's own doctor. A patient who has had one convulsion may demand no action if he is an office clerk, but not if he is a lorry driver. There are other occupations in which certain types of illness or defect may have adverse effects on others. Typical examples are hospital staff who may be a source of infection to vulnerable groups such as children, and the business executive whose diminished responsibility as a result of psychiatric illness, alcoholism, or cerebrovascular disease may have devastating effects on the health of employees as well as on the efficiency of the organization.

CLASSIFICATION OF OCCUPATIONAL DISEASES

Occupational diseases may be classified by their causes as due to: (1) chemical compounds; (2) physical agents; (3) mechanical factors; and (4) infective agents.

Chemical Compounds

Lead, mercury, and silica have been recognized as sources of occupational disease since antiquity; others, such as asbestos, radioactive ores, petroleum products, and a growing range of synthetic or artificially produced compounds have since been added during the present period of increasing industrial activity. Physical state is a major factor in determining the toxic properties of a material. Substances occurring as gases, vapours, and particulate matter are usually more dangerous and difficult to control than liquids.

Some liquids have a local action on skin and mucous membranes. Others are absorbed and act as systemic poisons. Those which have a local action may be classified as primary irritants or as sensitizers which produce allergic reactions. Common primary irritants include inorganic acids and alkalis; salts of metals, such as antimony, chromium, mercury, cadmium, and arsenic; and industrial solvents, such as turpentine, trichloroethylene, and alcohol. Petroleum and coal tar derivatives like pitch, bitumen, and mineral oils are keratogenic and can cause skin cancers.

Many chemical substances such as photographic developers, dyes, oils, resins, and plasticizers, cause sensitization dermatitis. First exposures may be harmless, but if repeated, sensitization develops and subsequent exposure, even to minute quantities, can cause severe dermatitis and reactions to mucous membranes.

Liquids such as nitro and amino derivatives of benzene, phenol, and lead tetraethyl, are readily absorbed through the skin and act as systemic poisons.

Air-borne contaminants occurring as gases, vapours, and particulate matter may be inhaled and produce local effects on the respiratory tract or act as systemic poisons. Those of high solubility, such as ammonia and sulphur dioxide, are absorbed by and act on the upper respiratory passages. Gases of moderate solubility such as chlorine and ozone can damage both the upper respiratory passages and the lungs. Irritants of low solubility such as nitrogen dioxide and phosgene have no effect on the upper respiratory tract but can cause delayed pulmonary oedema with asphyxiation.

Asphyxiants exert their effects by interfering with the oxygen supply to the tissues. The simple asphyxiants, such as carbon dioxide and methane, are physiologically inert gases which act by diluting the atmospheric oxygen below the partial pressure required to maintain an oxygen saturation of the blood sufficient for normal tissue respiration.

Chemical asphyxiants, such as carbon monoxide, hydrogen cyanide, produce their effect by preventing the blood from transporting oxygen from the lungs to the tissues or by interfering with oxygenation in the tissues.

A few compounds such as acetylene and trichloroethylene act primarily as anaesthetics or narcotics without serious systemic effects. Trichloroethylene is widely used as an industrial solvent and its anaesthetic property, which is its most important effect, is a cause of accidents. Cases of addiction also occur since continued exposure to low concentrations creates a pleasant feeling of mild intoxication.

Many substances exert systemic toxic effects on one or more of the organ systems. There are those which cause anaemias and other blood diseases. They include inorganic compounds of lead, derivatives of benzene and its homologues, arsine, and radioactive substances.

There are several compounds which affect the central nervous system, peripheral nerves, or cause behavioural disorders. They include lead, mercury, arsenic, and manganese; trichloroethylene, carbon disulphide, methyl bromide and chloride, and organophosphorus pesticides.

Others act as liver poisons. They include halogenated hydrocarbons such as carbon tetrachloride, chloroform, tetrachlorethane, chlorinated naphthalenes, and methyl chloride, and compounds of selenium, antimony, and phosphorus. There are relatively few substances which attack the kidney. They include compounds of mercury, cadmium, and halogenated hydrocarbons. The renal tract and the bladder are the sites of occupational cancers following exposure to chemicals used in the dyestuff and rubber industry, such as α and β naphthylamines, benzidine, and 4-aminodiphenyl. Virtually any system or organ in the body may be damaged by specific industrial exposures.

Many dusts have a local action on the respiratory tract, and cause disabling and incurable chronic occupational pulmonary diseases. The most important are those due to silica, coal dust, and asbestos. They produce a fibrotic reaction which eventually destroys large areas of lung tissue causing severe breathlessness. Superimposed pulmonary tuberculosis aggravates these dust diseases and makes the prognosis grave.

Metals which act upon the respiratory system include beryllium, cadmium, aluminium, and hard metals such as tungsten carbide and cobalt.

Vegetable dusts from preparing cotton, flax, and soft hemp fibres give rise to byssinosis, characterized by symptoms of chest tightness at the beginning of the working week which may eventually lead to chronic bronchitis and emphysema. Other vegetable dusts like mouldy hay which has become contaminated with mould spores of *Micropolyspora faeni* produce farmer's lung, an allergic alveolitis which can be very disabling.

New occupational pulmonary diseases have been described among those making enzyme washing powders and workers exposed to organic diisocyanate compounds such as toluene diisocyanate used in making paints and lacquers. Occupational cancers of the lung occur among workers exposed to asbestos, bichromates, polycyclic hydrocarbons in gas retort houses, arsenic compounds, and in the mining of radioactive ores and haematite. Cancer of the ethmoid and paranasal sinuses is a hazard among nickel refiners as well as woodworkers.

Physical Agents

Noise. Industrial noise may damage the ears and affect wellbeing by disrupting sleep, causing annoyance, interrupting conversation, and trains of thought. There is no clear evidence that it can cause mental or physical illness apart from injury to the hearing mechanism [see CHAPTER 8].

High and Low Temperatures. Common effects from exposure to high temperatures are:

1. Heat cramps from depletion of sodium chloride lost in the sweat; if replaced with saline drinks the cramps can be prevented.
2. Heat stroke in which sweating suddenly ceases and the body temperature rises in the region of 108°F. If unrelieved, this condition may be fatal.
3. Heat exhaustion which occurs during excessively hot weather in unacclimatized workers. It is caused by peripheral vasodilatation and recovery is rapid after rest.

Exposure to low temperatures occurs among workers in artificially cooled or naturally cold environments. The effects are chilblains, frostbite, and immersion or trench foot, which are prevented by protective clothing and avoiding accidental exposure in cold stores.

Radiation. Non-ionizing sources of radiation include ultraviolet light, laser, and infra-red. Ultra-violet light produced, for example, in electric arc welding can cause conjunctivitis and burning of the skin. Laser is achieved by devices that emit a powerful light over a narrow wavelength band which can be focused to a fine point with very high concentrations of energy. Its industrial applications are expanding. It can cause damage to the eye and produce ionizing radiations.

Infra-red radiation, which is in the lowest range of frequencies on the electromagnetic spectrum, is emitted from hot metal and glass. Workers so exposed, such as glass blowers and furnacemen, may develop cataract and suffer general effects from exposure to heat.

Ionizing radiations include short-wave electromagnetic radiations such as X-rays and gamma rays, and corpuscular radiation emitted from naturally and artificially produced radioactive sources. The most chronic effects are the production of skin cancers which have occurred among radiologists and radiographers, bone tumours among luminizers and lung cancer in miners of radioactive ores. Ionizing radiations can also cause leukaemia, aplastic anaemia, and possibly shortening of the life-span. Acute effects after high exposures include brain damage, nausea and vomiting, diarrhoea, and abdominal pain. [see CHAPTER 12].

High and Low Pressures. Exposures to high or low atmospheric pressures can cause decompression sickness. It occurs typically in workers in compressed air, such as those building tunnels under rivers who are too rapidly decompressed, or when airmen ascend too rapidly to high altitudes. The symptoms are caused by the release of nitrogen within the blood and tissues when the air pressure is reduced. The commonest symptoms are the bends—pains in the joints and bones—the chokes, characterized by dyspnoea and sometimes asphyxia, and the staggers, characterized by vertigo and vomiting. A delayed complication is bone necrosis which can cause persistent pain and ultimately osteoarthritis.

Mechanical Factors

Pneumatic hammers, such as road drills, rotating tools for grinding metals, or mechanical saws, can cause vibration disorders such as Raynaud's phenomenon or dead hand, and damage to joints and soft tissues.

In many industries in which repetitive movements of the hands and forearms are common, such as making boots and shoes, working on an assembly line, or net making, the tendon sheaths and musculotendinous junctions become inflamed causing tyenosynovitis. It affects new employees or regular workers after the introduction of a new process which calls for unusual and repetitive movements.

Cramps or craft palsies also occur in occupations which involve complex and rapid repetitive movements. They occur in writers, telegraphists, and pianists. Co-ordinated movement becomes difficult or impossible. The condition is due to a combination of physical and psychological factors. Neurotic symptoms are common among those affected.

Workers who use hand tools such as picks, hammers, and shovels or who habitually kneel at their work may suffer from 'beat' conditions of the hand, knee, or elbow. Beat hand is a subcutaneous cellulitis which occurs among miners and stokers caused by infection of tissues devitalized by constant bruising. Beat knee or elbow occurs among carpet layers and miners in low seams. It has two forms, a subcutaneous cellulitis and a bursitis.

Infectious Agents

The zoonoses, diseases of vertebrate animals transmissable to man, are the most important sources of occupational diseases due to infections. Examples are anthrax and brucellosis. Brucellosis, or undulant fever, has a worldwide distribution and is caused by *Brucella melitensis*, *Br. abortus*, and *Br. suis*. The disease usually results from direct contact with infected cattle, goats, milk or milk products and occurs among farmers, veterinarians, dairymen, slaughterers, and laboratory workers. There are recurrent bouts of febrile illness and malaise and the illness is often not diagnosed [see CHAPTER 22].

Occupational infections may also be acquired from contaminated water, soil, or air. Leptospirosis or Weil's disease is a risk among miners, sewer workers, slaughterers, and fish gutters. The organism *Leptospira icterohaemorrhagiae* is shed in the urine of infected rats and survives in pools of stagnant water or on moist materials, and so infects man. Tetanus organisms harboured in the intestinal tracts of many animals are passed in their faeces and lie dormant in the soil for long periods. Construction and agricultural workers run the risk of acquiring the disease if tetanus spores contaminate a penetrating wound.

Pulmonary tuberculosis may be contracted by physicians, bacteriologists, and nurses in the course of their work [see CHAPTER 22].

OBJECTIVES OF OCCUPATIONAL HEALTH SERVICES

Prior to the Second World War, occupational health services were mainly confined to large mines and factories doing heavy and hazardous work, and to transport undertakings with responsibilities for public safety. These services were often limited in their scope because at that time, apart from the Soviet Union, there was little formal undergraduate and postgraduate training in occupational health. These services were concerned almost entirely with manual workers and restricted to three main functions—pre-employment medical examinations, provision of treatment for emergencies, and the prevention of accidents and occupational disease.

The new concepts of occupational health which have developed since the pre-war era are epitomized in the following definition of its aims by the Joint Committee of the World Health Organization and the International Labour Office in 1950:

The promotion and maintenance of the highest degree of physical mental and social well-being of workers in all occupations; the prevention among workers of departures from health caused by their working conditions; the protection of workers in their employment from risks resulting from factors adverse to health; the placing and maintenance of the worker in an occupational environment adapted to his physiological and psychological equipment; to summarize: the adaptation of work to man and of each man to his job.

The achievement of these aims depends on having trained and competent staff fulfilling basic functions which will be similar for all working groups. But the type of service provided will depend on needs and resources at local and national levels, the standard of medical care outside the workplace, the type of industry and its size, and the general health of the population and what part of the world they live in; for example, the needs of industries in developing countries in the tropics will be different from those in the temperate climates of Europe or North America.

Placing People in Suitable Work

Pre-employment medical examinations are still used to select the fit and reject the unfit. With increasing shortages of skilled labour and the ethical objections which have been raised to this kind of selection, they have been replaced by preplacement examinations which aim to assess working capacity and, where possible, match such capacity, however limited it may be, with a suitable job.

These examinations can take up so much time that they may prevent an occupational health service from doing other important work. They can be used more selectively by confining them to persons to be employed in occupations which may be potentially dangerous to the employee or others, such as the dusty and chemical trades, radiation work, transport and crane driving, and food-handling. Screening by medical auxiliaries helps to save the physician's time. A current health certificate carried by the worker also avoids the necessity of repeated examinations after each change of job.

Providing a Treatment Service

An efficient treatment service at work for injuries, acute poisonings, and minor ailments is valuable because it prevents complications and assists rehabilitation. It also prevents unnecessary loss of working time by eliminating travelling and waiting in hospitals and dispensaries. Many workers referred to outside agencies with relatively minor complaints are often kept off work quite unnecessarily by doctors and nurses.

A treatment service can also provide valuable epidemiological evidence of hazards and lead to the investigation of causes of serious injuries and of potentially dangerous occurrences which caused only minor injuries. Previously unsuspected occupational risks and their causes may be detected in this way. For example, the repeated attendance for backache by a group of men loading trucks revealed that they were using the wrong methods of work. The records of treatment at one coalfield with unusually thin seams showed a high incidence of beat elbow. By improving treatment and developing special elbow pads, this condition was virtually eliminated (Archibald and Kay, 1966). As well as identifying physical hazards, a treatment service may provide evidence leading to the identification of adverse psychosocial factors in the work environment. It also offers physicians and nurses opportunities for counselling and for the health education of those who attend for treatment and advice.

Identification of Hazards

The most effective way of identifying an occupational hazard is to predict it by toxicity tests in animals or from the chemical formula of a compound. The carcinogenicity of 4-aminodiphenyl was predicted by Walpole, Williams, and Roberts

(1957) because of its similarity in chemical structure to benzidine and other carcinogens. This was confirmed by toxicity tests, with the result that 4-aminodiphenyl was not manufactured in Britain. There are obvious loopholes in any system of identification before human beings are exposed. First, animal tests are not necessarily predictive of such risks; secondly, although toxicity testing is widely practised, and there is an up-to-date index of toxic materials in *Toxicity Bibliography* (1968), it cannot be comprehensive since thousands of new compounds are used by industry every year and manufacturing firms in most countries are not required to get any form of clearance before using new compounds.

The more common method of identifying occupational hazards is through their adverse effects on persons exposed. There are two principle methods of detection.

The first indication that a hazard exists may be an individual worker presenting with symptoms and signs of disease which can be related to a specific exposure at work. It is a method as old as occupational medicine itself and was used by Ramazzini more than 250 years ago to identify hazards such as asthmatic complaints among hemp workers; and by Percivall Pott in the eighteenth century to suggest that soot caused scrotal cancer of chimney sweeps.

New hazards may also be detected by using epidemiology. It may be the only way of discovering occupational risks of such diseases as lung cancer, coronary heart disease, varicose veins, or rheumatic disorders that commonly occur in the general population. Epidemiology may be descriptive or analytical. Descriptive epidemiology is often the first method of inquiry. It deals with the distribution of disease in a population. It reveals the various types of disease measured in terms of the illness, disability, or mortality they cause. It provides clues for analytical epidemiology which is used not only to identify disease but also to determine its causes. There are two main types of investigation, the cohort and the case-control study. The cohort study takes two groups of workers, one exposed and the other unexposed to the suspected agent, and determines how many in each group are affected. It was this method which finally identified and quantified the risk of lung cancer in asbestos workers and later showed that it could be controlled (Doll, 1955; Knox, Doll, Holmes, and Hill, 1968). In the first inquiry eleven asbestos workers died of lung cancer whereas 0·8 deaths would have been expected. After control measures had been introduced a later study of deaths in the same factory revealed that the occupational hazard had been largely eliminated.

The second method, the case-control study, takes two groups of workers matched in all respects except that one group has the disease being investigated (cases) and the other has not (controls), and then compares them for the frequency of the suspected cause. Newhouse and Thompson (1965) took 76 patients who had had mesothelioma of the pleura and peritoneum and 76 other patients from the same hospital without this disease. Occupational and residential histories revealed that 40 (53 per cent.) of the mesothelioma patients had had exposure to asbestos compared with nine (12 per cent.) of the 76 controls.

Many different types of data collected for other purposes are used for identifying occupational hazards, particularly the population census and death registration, records of pensions and sick benefit schemes, and of treatment at the workplace. With the need for more accurate identification of causes of disease and for the better assessment of control measures, epidemiological inquiries are increasingly designed to answer specific questions. Examples are the use of the field survey, and the more sophisticated recording and analysis of sickness absence to provide both epidemiological and personal information.

Control of Hazards

Once hazards have been identified, one of the foremost functions of an occupational health service is their control. The type of preventive measures to be adopted depends on the nature of the harmful substance or agent, its mode of absorption, and how severe the risk is. As a general principle, built-in protection which is an integral part of the process is much to be preferred to a method which depends on continual human implementation or intervention. Safe maintenance needs as much attention as good design.

There are nine main methods of prevention:

1. Elimination by substitution.
2. Total enclosure of the process.
3. Removal of the contaminant at source.
4. Segregation of the process.
5. Limitation of time of exposure.
6. General ventilation.
7. General cleanliness of the workplace.
8. Personal hygiene.
9. Personal protection.

(Schilling and Hall, 1973.)

Substitution of a non-toxic or less toxic material for a poisonous one is the most effective way of eliminating or controlling an occupational disease. Examples are the use of phosphorus sesquisulphide for white phosphorus to prevent phossy jaw in making matches, shot-blasting instead of sand-blasting to prevent silicosis, and finding safer materials than asbestos for insulation.

Total enclosure, which is accompanied by mechanization or automation of the process means that workers, apart from maintenance engineers, are kept out of contact with toxic materials.

Removal at source of toxic aerosols may be achieved by locally applied exhaust ventilation or by wet methods of drilling or grinding.

Segregation of a process limits possible exposure to a specified group of workers. It is important in highly toxic materials and in limiting the effects of noise.

Limitation of time of exposure is a well-established practice among persons exposed to ionizing radiations.

General ventilation of workrooms removes contaminants and maintains safe levels of exposure by adequate dilution. It is important where control by other methods is incomplete or where there is a risk of small leaks of toxic compounds.

General cleanliness or good housekeeping is important for two reasons. It reduces exposure and encourages tidiness and therefore safer methods of working.

Personal hygiene helps to avoid accidental ingestion or skin absorption. Work people should be able to wash exposed skin at the end of a shift and to remove without delay accidental splashes of irritant or toxic materials.

Personal protection by the use of eye-goggles, ear-defenders, respirators, and protective clothing is often required to supplement environmental control measures, particularly where exposures may be high but intermittent, as for cleaners and maintenance workers.

The introduction of such control measures is usually only the beginning of the control programme. An occupational health service has to ensure that prevention is maintained by routine medical surveillance of people at risk, and by environmental monitoring to ensure that hygiene standards are reached. Data from the periodic examination of persons and their exposures also enables dose-response relationships to be deduced, and thus the initiation or reappraisal of hygiene standards to be made.

Health Screening

In addition to screening populations exposed to occupational risks, some occupational health services have applied the same technique to the control of non-occupational disease. In this way they can help to eradicate diseases such as malaria and schistosomiasis in tropical countries and contribute to the control of others such as coronary heart disease and hypertension. In particular, the occupational physician has opportunities for identifying and dealing with mental illness in its mild forms or early stages. Vulnerable groups such as the young, the aged, the disabled, pregnant women, and those with repeated absences from work require special care. They can often be helped by counselling, by rehabilitation, and by modifying their work to remove or reduce harmful influences.

Counselling

Physicians and nurses can perform two different types of counselling. At attendances for routine examinations or treatment, workers can be advised how to deal with health problems and how to prevent recurrence of injuries. Secondly, many go voluntarily to the occupational health service for advice about much broader problems at work or connected with their domestic life. One of the main functions of the occupational physician or nurse is to find the kind of help needed from a wide range of potential counsellors such as their manager, personnel department, general practitioner, or one of the social agencies in the community.

Health Education

An occupational health service has opportunities for both individual and group health education. While much of it is aimed at maintaining health and safety in the job, there is no reason for limiting it so narrowly. The service also has to educate management in its responsibilities for the health and safety of employees and to give effective advice about dealing with environmental hazards and the many individual problems of employees.

Surveillance of Sanitary and Other Amenities

The service has a responsibility to advise management about requirements in respect of toilets, washplaces, and facilities for storing and drying clothes. It also has responsibilities for the routine surveillance of these installations, and other amenities such as kitchens, canteens, day nurseries, and rest homes. Useful advice can also be given on their design, construction, and maintenance.

Environmental Control in the Neighbourhood

While management has an undisputed duty to control environmental hazards in the workplace, there is increasing awareness of the need to avoid various types of pollution affecting the health of neighbouring communities. Occupational health services through physicians and hygienists have opportunities for advising industry on the control of toxic effluents from the workplace, and thus playing a role in the promotion of community health.

Factors Influencing the Type of Service Provided and Its Function

Occupational health services should not be stereotyped, but designed to meet the special needs of the industry concerned, which will depend on its size, the type of work it does, and the people it employs, its location and the standard of medical care provided for the community in which it is situated. Industries in developing countries in the tropics have special problems and needs which have been defined by the Ross Institute of Tropical Hygiene and the TUC Centenary Institute of Occupational Health (1970) as follows:

'(1) The high prevalence of epidemic and endemic communicable diseases such as leprosy, tuberculosis, schistosomiasis, and malaria is a major cause of morbidity and wastage of manpower. The treatment and prevention of these diseases is of paramount importance to industry and often the foremost duty of an occupational health service.

'(2) Public health and social problems arise from industrialization and from the movement of peasant people from rural to urban areas. In addition to communicable diseases there are usually complex problems associated with a rapidly increasing population, malnutrition, and disruption of traditional ways of life. All these interact and have far-reaching effects on community health as well as contributing to mental illness and behavioural disorders such as delinquency, prostitution, and alcoholism. The existence of these public problems calls for joint action by community and occupational health services.

'(3) Hazards of occupational injury and disease tend to be more prevalent in communities unfamiliar with industrial processes and often insufficiently trained and protected against them. An occupational health service has a major responsibility to identify these hazards and to educate and train peasants to become safe and efficient workers. An essential part of any control programme is to deal with the risks of modern agriculture arising from the use of pesticides and new machinery.

'(4) Problems occur of providing medical care for small and widely scattered groups of workers. As most developing countries have an acute shortage of doctors and nurses much of the routine work has to be done by medical auxiliaries who need special training in occupational health.'

WHO co-operates with ILO in international work relating to the health of workers (World Health Organization, 1974).

EDUCATION IN OCCUPATIONAL HEALTH

Everyone who is responsible for patients needs to be aware of the influence that work has on health and that a person's health may seriously affect his or her capacity for work. At work itself, the achievement of good standards of health and safety depends not only on medical and other specialists such as hygienists, engineers, and ergonomists, but also on management and work people without whose co-operation the highly trained experts can do very little. Here, only the education and training programmes of physicians and hygienists are discussed. Much, however, also depends on occupational health nurses and medical auxiliaries specially trained in this field, particularly in developing countries where there is such a great shortage of physicians (Gauvain and Schilling, 1973).

Medical Undergraduates

In the undergraduate curriculum, it is undesirable to over-emphasize any specialty, but in occupational health there are five general educational objectives:

1. To understand the aetiological importance of work in health and disease and the extent to which ill health affects working capacity.

2. To appreciate the therapeutic value of work and to understand the responsibility taken by a physician when advising a change of occupation.

3. To know the epidemiology, pathology, and clinical signs and symptoms of the common occupational diseases, a physician's statutory duties to governmental agencies for notifying accidents and diseases, and to be aware of his responsibility to his patients in ensuring that they receive the social benefits to which they are entitled.

4. To understand the ways of investigating and controlling occupational hazards.

5. To know the aims of occupational health services and their functional relationship with other health services.

Medical Postgraduates

Physicians with direct responsibility for the health of people at work obviously need further training. Many countries now have training programmes coupled with a system of specialist registration. Its aim is to prepare physicians to be directors or senior medical officers in occupational health services and in government departments, and to be consultants or teachers. But there are medical tasks within industry that do not require specialist training; for example many of the services in small plants will continue to be manned by part-time doctors from general practice. In the United Kingdom the training programme for occupational medicine will comprise a three-year period of general professional training which will be broad and suitable for other specialties (Joint Committee on Higher Medical Training, 1972). It will be followed by taking the MRCP (UK) or other equivalent examination in community and occupational medicine, and then by higher specialist training over a period of four years spent working in approved institutes, occupational health departments in industry, and in the services. An academic course in occupational medicine is an important part of this specialist training and its content is markedly similar in different countries. The aims of a course leading to an MSc. offered at the London School of Hygiene and Tropical Medicine, may be summarized as follows:

1. To understand the importance of the effects of work on health and disease and vice versa; to appreciate the general therapeutic value of work and be competent in the resettlement and rehabilitation of patients.

2. To know:

(a) The epidemiology, pathology, clinical signs and symptoms of the relevant occupational diseases.

(b) The statutory duties and responsibilities of the occupational physician, and the assistance available to him from governmental agencies.

(c) The professional responsibilities of an occupational physician including knowledge of the relevant social security provisions.

(d) The importance of the impartiality of his professional conduct and the confidentiality of personal medical information.

3. To know how to identify, assess, and control occupational hazards by observing, measuring, and interpreting the responses of individuals and groups in relation to their total working environment. The teaching and practical experience of statistical, epidemiological, occupational hygiene, and ergonomic methods are essential to this end.

4. (a) To understand the aims and objectives of an occupational health service.

(b) To know how to organize and manage such a service.

(c) To know how to co-ordinate its functions with other health care systems.

5. To develop an understanding of individual and group psychosocial behaviour and its relevance to the relationships at work and their effects on health.

6. To know the sources of supplementary information and advice available to him and to understand the importance of continuing personal professional education in this particular field.

Undergraduates in Other Sciences

In most countries there is usually some formal teaching of occupational health to medical undergraduates but seldom are there any in courses for engineers, chemists, and physicists, although many graduates in these fields are concerned with occupational health hazards in their technical capacities or as directors of enterprises in which they will have over-all responsibility for the health and safety of people at work. The World Health Organization (1971) recommends such instruction in undergraduate courses for engineers and other technical personnel. The subject matter should be similar to that presented to medical undergraduates but with more emphasis on the environmental, safety, administrative, and legal aspects of occupational helath.

Postgraduates in Occupational Hygiene

Throughout the world there is increasing awareness in the larger, more enlightened industries, of the importance of the occupational hygienist who can measure, assess, and advise on the control of the working environment. At present much of this work is carried out unsatisfactorily by engineers, chemists, and physicists who have developed an interest in the subject, through their own experience. Since similar techniques are required for dealing with environmental hazards outside the workplace, the demand for postgraduate training in occupational and environmental hygiene is growing rapidly. The aims of such an MSc. course as that offered at the London School of Hygiene and Tropical Medicine are in many respects similar to those of the occupational medicine course, but with much more emphasis on the measurement and evaluation of chemical, physical, and biological hazards and their control.

REFERENCES

Acheson, E. D., Cowdell, R. H., and Hadfield, M. (1968) Nasal cancer in woodworkers in the furniture industry, *Brit. med. J.*, **2**, 587.

Archibald, R., and Kay, D. E. (1966) A study of beat elbow and related conditions at the colliery, *Occupational Health*, **18**, 118.

Doll, R. (1955) Mortality from lung cancer in asbestos workers, *Brit. J. industr. Med.*, **12**, 81.

Joint Committee on Higher Medical Training (1972) *First Report*, Royal College of Physicians, London.

Gauvain, S., and Schilling, R. S. F. (1973) Education in occupational health, in *Occupational Health Practice*, ed. Schilling, R. S. F., London.

Gilson, J. C. (1970) Occupational bronchitis, *Proc. roy. Soc. Med.*, **63**, 857.

Harrington, J. M., and Schilling, R. S. F. (1973) Man's work and his health, in *Occupational Health Practice*, ed. Schilling, R. S. F., London.

Knox, J. F., Doll, R., Holmes, S., and Hill, I. D. (1968) Mortality from lung cancer and other causes among workers in an asbestos textile factory, *Brit. J. industr. Med.*, **25**, 293.

Lund, R. P., Haggendal, J., and Johnsson, F. (1968) The withdrawal symptoms in workers exposed to nitroglycerine, *Brit. J. industr. Med.*, **25**, 136.

Mekky, S., Schilling, R. S. F., and Walford, J. (1969) Varicose veins in women cotton workers. An epidemiological study in England and Egypt, *Brit. med. J.*, **2**, 591.

Newhouse, M. L., and Thompson, H. (1965) Mesothelioma of plasma and peritoneum following exposure to asbestos in the London area, *Brit. J. industr. Med.*, **22**, 261.

Raffle, P. A. B. (1970) The occupational physician as community physician, *Proc. roy. Soc. Med.*, **63**, 731.

Rosen, Genge (1943) *The History of Miners' Diseases*, New York.

Ross Institute of Tropical Hygiene, and TUC Centenary Institute of Occupational Health (1970) Proceedings of Symposium on Health Problems of Industrial Progress in Developing Countries, *J. trop. Med. Hyg.*, **73**, 731.

Russack, H. I. (1967) Emotional stress and coronary artery disease, *Dis. Chest*, **52**, 1.

Schilling, R. S. F. (1973) Developments in occupational health, in *Occupational Health Practice*, ed. Schilling, R. S. F., London.

Schilling, R. S. F., and Hall, S. A. (1973) Prevention of occupational disease, in *Occupational Health Practice*, ed. Schilling, R. S. F., London.

Select Committee of House of Commons (Gt. Britain) (1832) *Factory Children's Labour*.

Tiller, J., Schilling, R. S. F., and Morris, J. N. (1968) Occupational toxic factors in mortality from coronary heart disease, *Brit. med. J.*, **2**, 407.

Toxicity Bibliography (1968 onwards) National Library of Medicine, Washington, D.C.

Walpole, A. L., Williams, M. H. C., and Roberts, D. C. (1952) The carcinogenic action of 4-aminodiphenyl and 3:2 dimethyl-4-aminodiphenyl, *Brit. J. industr. Med.*, **9**, 255.

World Health Organization (1971) *Report on Symposium on Academic Education and Training in Occupational Health and Hygiene in Ahmedabad*, WHO, New Delhi.

Wright, W. C. (1940) Translation of *De Morbis Artificum* by B. Ramazzini, Chicago, Ill.

FURTHER READING

Hunter, D. (1969) *Diseases of Occupations*, 4th ed., London.

International Labour Office (1971) *International Classification of Radiographs of Pneumoconiosis*, Geneva.

International Labour Office (1971, 1972) *Encyclopaedia of Occupational Health and Safety*, Vols. 1 and 2, Geneva.

Patty, Frank A. (1968, 1967) *Industrial Hygiene and Toxicology*, Vol. 1 (revised), and Vol. 2, New York.

Schilling, R. S. F., ed. (1973) *Occupational Health Practice*, London.

World Health Organization (1963) Occupational Health in Four European Countries, *Chron. Wld Hlth Org.*, **17**, 403 (Jugoslavia and the USSR), 461 (Finland and Sweden).

World Health Organization Regional Office for Europe (1963) *Health Services in Small Factories*, Report of a Joint WHO/ILO Seminar on Health Services in Small Factories, Copenhagen.

World Health Organization Joint ILO/WHO Committee on Occupational Health (1969) Sixth Report. Permissible levels of occupational exposure to airborne toxic substances, *Wld Hlth Org. techn. Rep. Ser.*, No. 415.

World Health Organization (1973a) Environmental and health monitoring in occupational health, *Wld Hlth Org. techn. Rep. Ser.*, No. 535.

World Health Organization (1973b) The role of permissible limits for hazardous airborne substances in the working environment in the prevention of occupational disease, *Bull. Wld Hlth Org.*, **47**, No. 2.

World Health Organization (1974a) The work of WHO in 1973, *Wld Hlth Org. Off. Rec.*, No. 213, 91–93.

World Health Organization (1974b) Biological effects of microwave radiation, *Wld Hlth Org. Chron.*, **28**, 289.

39

COMMUNITY HEALTH PROBLEMS OF AN AGEING POPULATION

W. FERGUSON ANDERSON

Everyman desires to live long but no man would be old.
Swift

Introduction

It is only in recent years that textbooks of public health have included special reference to the problems of an ageing population and a few public health departments have provided means for the medical and psycho-social assessment of older people. The problems, however, have existed for a considerable time, and two decades ago Breslow (1954) drew attention to the excessive restriction of health department services to the young or to those affected by communicable diseases, while Anderson and Cowan (1955) stressed the value of positive ascertainment of disease in the elderly and outlined a possible role for the health department in this respect.

Before the Second World War the problems of maternal and child health were more important, even in those countries with the best medical services and the highest standards of living. Since that time there have been remarkable improvements in the health of mother and child in many countries of the world, particularly in western Europe, North America, Australia, and New Zealand; at the same time in these countries there has been an increase in the percentage of elderly people in the population. Despite many advances in treatment, we have been able to do little to prevent the degenerative diseases of the elderly; this means therefore that the pattern of disease has changed, the chronic diseases of the elderly have become more common, while many of the conditions characteristic of childhood have almost disappeared; or to put it in another way, the child who was saved from death from diphtheria now survives to develop coronary heart disease, diabetes, or chronic bronchitis. In most of the other countries of the world, and particularly those which have the largest populations, e.g. China and India, the greatest problems are still those connected with the health of mother and child; with improving medical services, however, infant and maternal mortality rates are beginning to fall. Drastic efforts are also being made to bring about falls in the birth rate due to the threat of rapidly rising populations; with improving standards of living it is likely that these efforts will bear fruit in the future. All this means, therefore, that eventually nearly all countries of the world will face, to a greater or lesser degree, the problems of an ageing population. As old age has close links with chronic disease, despair, and death, professional workers who care for the aged are exposed to a potential threat to their self-esteem. Those in the public health service have been considerably protected from such harm in their care of mothers and children, and there might thus exist, at least subconsciously, lack of desire to enter the arena of ageing. Rechtschaffen (1959) indicates that there is resistance to working with the aged, and this may stem in part from anxiety aroused in workers by the dependency needs of aged patients; Rudd (1960) states that personnel who care for the ageing, where insecurity is so prevalent, must be secure themselves, and Mullan (1961) suggests that the selection of personnel is crucial, and those with a constructive relationship to self, parents, and other members of the family fare better than those who have not. Interest in the care of the elderly is steadily growing and has brought with it a great flood of research relating to the problems of old age and an increasing usage of new terms. In the *Shorter Oxford English Dictionary*, 3rd ed., 1944, no mention is made of the terms geriatrics and gerontology. In *Websters' New International Dictionary*, 1961, the terms are defined as follows:

Geriatrics (Nascher, 1909): The subdivision of medicine which is concerned with old age and its diseases.
Gerontology (Metchnikoff, 1903): The scientific study of the phenomena of old age.

CONCEPT OF AGEING

Since the nineteenth century the idea of normal and abnormal ageing as distinct processes has gained in popularity. By normal ageing we mean the changes which occur with the passage of time in anatomical structure and physiological function in the absence of disease; and by pathological ageing we mean the increasing occurrence of disease interacting with the processes of normal ageing [FIG. 90]. It is convenient to distinguish five levels of ageing: (1) molecular; (2) cellular; (3) tissue or organ; (4) individual; (5) population.

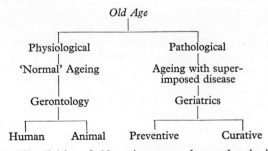

FIG. 90. The division of old age into gerontology and geriatrics.

Molecular Ageing

Recent electron-microscopy studies of the macromolecule of collagen, which is a plastic trihelical polypeptide, have shown that with age there is an increasing production of intra- and intermolecular bridges with associated loss of elasticity. It has been postulated that since the molecular structure of deoxyribonucleic acid is a twin helix, similar structural changes might occur, but there is no experimental proof of this idea.

Cellular Ageing

Cowdry (1952) divided cells into four types: (1) vegetative inter-mitotics; (2) differentiating inter-mitotics; (3) reverting post-mitotics; and (4) fixed post-mitotics.

The vegetative inter-mitotics are the basal cells from which all other cells arise. The differentiating inter-mitotics, e.g. spermatogonia and primitive blood cells, therefore arise from type (1). Both types (1) and (2) are short-lived with environmental influences which promote or inhibit division. The third type of cells, e.g. thyroid cells and capillary endothelium, arise from type (2). Type (3) cells have specialized functions, but are able to revert to a non-specialized form. Type (4) cells, e.g. nerve cells, cardiac and skeletal muscle cells, are cells whose life is fixed and ends in death; they are irreplacable.

There is experimental evidence about ageing in type (3) cells; Court Brown (1967) has shown that human lymphocytes which are reverting post-mitotics can be provoked into cell division in tissue culture and that these cells show a great variation in chromosomal constitution with age, especially in cells derived from the female. Strehler (1971) has reviewed ageing at the cellular level and has stated that antioxidants like the food preservative butylated hydroxytoluene (BHT) increase the longevity of experimental rodents. Vitamin E (another antioxidant) is known to suppress the formation of lipofuscin pigment which occurs in certain tissues such as the rodent uterus in the absence of the antioxidant.

Tissue of Organ Ageing

Many tissues and organs show specific changes in function as they grow old which vary from one individual to the next. Sometimes these alterations can be measured with a fair degree of precision; thus in the case of the human lens, if the range of accommodation is plotted against age in a large number of 'healthy' individuals the values fall within two smooth curves which enclose the normal values for accommodation, and thereby set up standards of 'normality' at the different age-groups. These can be expressed also as mean values. The mean power of accommodation falls steadily with age until the age of 50 years, when it remains stationary; this can be called the normal or physiological ageing of the lens. In India the same process carried out on a random selection of people, obviously not all healthy, shows that these changes in the human lens are reached much earlier, about the age of 40, due to the various additional environmental insults to which the lens is subject in that country [Fig. 91]. Bernstein has devised a 'law' of physiological ageing derived from data on the human eye.

Biological and chronological age are not necessarily the same; furthermore, the biological age of various organs is not uniform throughout the body, because involution may not start at the same time or progress at the same rate in all tissues. Paget named this differential ageing 'errors in the chronometry of life'. On the whole, tissue and organ change follow the same basic pattern, in that there is a progressive loss of cell function, a loss of reserve capacity which may be revealed only under stress, and a slowing of nervous function and failure of sensory discrimination. Goldman (1971) has reviewed in detail decline in organ functioning with age.

Individual Ageing

Ageing in the individual can be defined as a progressive loss of vigour which eventually leads to death; in the past it has been considered that its chief characteristic is a diminished ability to adapt to the environment. This concept of failing homeostasis, however, has recently been challenged by that of homeorhesis, which postulates that ageing is in itself a process of adaptation in which the internal environment is modified to

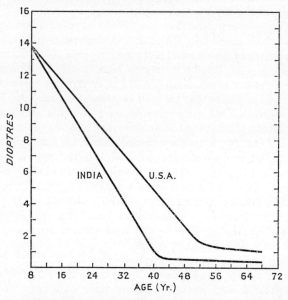

FIG. 91. Mean range of accommodation in dioptres by age in the United States and India (data from Dr. W. Hobson.)

meet the stresses of degeneration as well as external change. There is a great variation in individual ageing, just as there is in tissue and organ ageing, and an individual may reach an advanced chronological age and yet show few of the accepted stigmata of age, and equally, individuals in early middle life may have a biological age greatly in excess of their physical years. In these cases the premature signs of old age are pathological, but it is not easy to say when physiological changes become pathological. Atheromatous changes in the intima of the coronary arteries are considered to be pathological, yet over the age of 60 it is the exception not to find such changes. Usually an old person dies because an organ essential to life has undergone changes which no longer allow it to function adequately.

Nowadays few would agree with Terence that: 'Senectus ipsa morbus est'. The most rewarding attempts to assess old age are those which measure changes in function or overall performance of the individual, e.g. such things as physical capacity, work performance, intellectual ability, and mobility.

Tests of physiological ageing have been described by Bourlière (1969). Le Gros Clark (1956) has used length of working life as a yardstick for measuring the physical changes which characterize old age. Comfort (1969) based a battery of tests to measure human ageing on the work of Hollingsworth and his colleagues (1965) where the highest correlations were for characteristics (hair greying, skin elasticity) which contribute most to the clinical impression of age. Information gained from such tests could measure short-term rates of ageing and give information whether drugs or environmental agents affect ageing rate. Like health and ill health, we cannot separate 'middle age' from 'old age', and one merges gradually into the other. The WHO Seminar on the Health Protection of the Elderly (1963) divided chronological age into three stages: (1) middle-aged persons (46–59); (2) the elderly (60–74); (3) the aged (75 and over). The prevention of human ageing and its control has fascinated mankind for centuries, and claims have been made for a great variety of preparations with little objective evidence of their successful use.

The following facts seem to be based on scientific evidence. Pearl (1931), and later Kallmann, in their twin studies, have demonstrated the essential part played by genetic factors in the ageing process; there is further evidence from pedigree studies (Jarvik *et al.*, 1960). Geill (1963) has described a remarkable example of similarities between two like twins aged 90, from Copenhagen; both were unmarried and were chief stewards in the mercantile marine. They show the same values in most clinical tests, both have myocardial disease, i.e. bundle branch block, but in one it is right-sided, while in the other it is left-sided. Dr. Richard Asher has described a remarkable case of health: 'Fanny aged 90 is doing a hard and responsible job of work as housekeeper and cook to a girls' day school, this she has been doing for 76 consecutive years with only 10 days' illness. Her mother lived to 100, her brother is still alive at 85 and her sisters died at 89 and 86.'

Another interesting finding has been the discovery of an *élite* of elderly people. Birren and his associates (1963) after screening a large group of elderly male volunteers from a Jewish Old Age Home found 27 men aged 65 years and over who had no observed evidence of disease and were supremely healthy. In these optimally healthy men cerebral blood flow and oxygen consumption did not differ from the values obtained in a group of normal young subjects (mean age = 21 years). A similar group (Anderson, 1971) of 80 men and 103 women aged 60–89 years were obtained from those attending the Rutherglen Consultative Health Centre (mean blood pressure: men 152/85, women 157/85).

Bourlière has reviewed a great deal of experimental work on vertebrates and invertebrates showing that increased environmental temperature accelerates the ageing process. Recent experimental work has shown that exposure to ionizing radiation has a similar effect. It has been shown by McKay and his co-workers that rats and trout live longer on a low-calorie diet. Dublin, in an analysis of the statistics of the Metropolitan Life Insurance Company, has shown that overweight causes a decrease in the expectation of life, while Sinclair (1956) has drawn attention to the danger of overfeeding in humans. There is some evidence that a deficiency of unsaturated fatty acids in the diet may predispose to the development of coronary heart disease, but it is far from conclusive. Since we can hardly change our ancestors once we are born, the only hope for prevention in our present state of knowledge seems to be to follow the advice given by Cornaro a hundred years ago and live a life of temperance. As far as human beings are concerned, little is known about the extrinsic factors which may influence the process of ageing, but the following are often quoted: emotional stress, lack of sleep, malnutrition, over-nutrition, excess or lack of physical activity, climatic extremes, abuse of stimulants, effects of chemical agents, chronic diseases, and ionizing radiation. It now seems clear that in many species: (1) longevity is in part genetically determined; (2) increased environmental temperature accelerates the ageing process while lowered temperature slows ageing; (3) exposure to ionizing radiation speeds ageing; (4) a low-calorie diet increases age span; and (5) overweight decreases life expectancy.

Burnett (1970) supports Walford's theory (1969) that the process of ageing is largely mediated by auto-immune processes stating that the progressive weakening of the function of the immunological surveillance is important and may be related to weakness of the thymus-dependent immune system.

Bourlière (1963) has drawn attention to the fact that in France in 1800 the life expectancy for those 80 years of age was 6·7 years for males and 6·8 for females; in 1955 it was not more than 4·0 and 5·9 respectively; in other words, an old person of 80 had fewer years to live than 150 years ago, despite antibiotics and so on. The reason is that this is almost certainly due to a selective process which 150 years ago was extremely rigorous, leaving only the very fit; today many people not so fit are kept going by modern therapy, the so-called medicated survival. The maximum life-span of humans is 100–120 years, the majority die earlier from disease.

Population Ageing

The ageing of human populations is an extremely complex notion. It can happen in three ways:

1. If all the people in one population A become older than those in population B, then the ageing is said to be total.
2. If the proportion of aged persons increases it can be described as ageing at the apex of the population pyramid.
3. If the proportion of young persons decreases it is described as ageing at the base.

It is important, in order to avoid confusion, to keep in mind these definitions.

In this chapter we are specially concerned with the ageing of human populations in different parts of the world, and with the medical, economic, and social problems which result. FIGURE 92 shows population pyramids of a 'young' population and of an 'old' population.

DEMOGRAPHIC TRENDS

Present

In measuring the ageing of human populations for comparative purposes it is convenient to use a single standard. In some countries the retirement age has been used to express this; for example, in the United Kingdom 65 years for men and 60 years for women. Unfortunately, retirement ages vary so much in different countries that no uniformity can result. The statistics published by the United Nations Department of

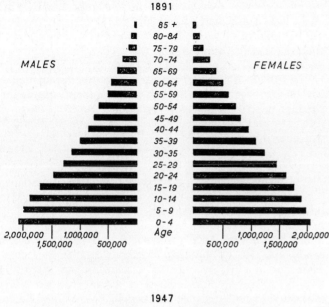

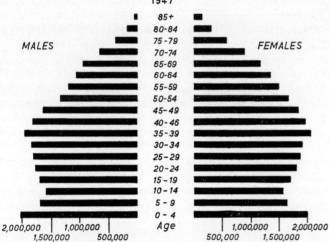

FIG. 92. Population pyramids comparing a 'young' population (Great Britain, 1891) with an 'old' population (Great Britain, 1947).

Economic and Social Affairs (1956) use as an index the percentage of persons above the age of 64 years in relation to the total population, and this measure will be used here.

Populations of the world can be arbitrarily divided into four main groups (Census date 1950 or thereabouts) [FIG. 93].

1. YOUNG POPULATIONS, less than 4 per cent. of persons above the age of 64 years. These include the whole of Africa, Asia, Central and South America, with the exception of the following countries: Japan, Peru, and South Africa (Europeans). Most of the populations of the world fall into this group.

2. MATURE POPULATIONS, where this percentage is between 4 and 7. Peru, Japan, Israel, Finland, Greece, Hungary, South Africa (Europeans), Poland, Portugal, Yugoslavia, and the U.S.S.R.

3. OLD POPULATIONS, where the percentage of old people exceeds 7 but less than 10. Included in this group are the economically advanced countries of Canada, the United States, Australia, and New Zealand. The problem is not as acute in

these countries as in western Europe, because the effect of falling fertility has been offset by the immigration of young people from Europe; moreover, the prospect for the future has been relieved by quite large increases in fertility in Australia and the United States, which have maintained this high level now for several years. Also included in this group are some countries of western Europe where fertility has remained relatively high, e.g. Denmark, Italy, Netherlands, and Spain.

4. VERY OLD POPULATIONS, where the percentage of old people exceeds 10. In this group are the countries of western Europe, where fertility has remained low or where in some cases migration of young people has contributed to the ageing, e.g. Ireland and Sweden. In some countries there were increases in fertility immediately after the war, but these were only temporary. Heading the list in the following order are East Germany (1965) 15·3 per cent., Austria (1968) 13·9 per cent., Sweden (1967) 13·1 per cent., United Kingdom (1970) 12·8 per cent., France (1968) 12·6 per cent., and Norway (1967) 12·4 per cent. The figures for the U.S.S.R. (1961) are 7·9 per cent. and for the United States (1969) 9·4 per cent. The most accurate figure for India is that following the 1961 census giving 3·2 per cent. Another interesting figure is that for Japan (1969), 6·6 per cent., this shows an increase from 1950 due to the fall in birth rate brought about by legalized abortion. Ghana (1960) has increased to 2·9 per cent., being a more accurate figure than previously recorded. The problem is more acute therefore in western Europe than in the United States and the U.S.S.R.

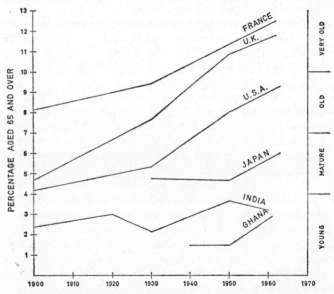

FIG. 93. Percentage of persons aged 65 and above from 1900 onwards in different countries.

The increase in the proportion of old persons has been accompanied by an increase in the percentage of persons of older working age, resulting in an ageing of the labour force; also in these countries the proportion of old women is higher than that of old men. These changes have been balanced by a fall in the proportion of children in almost all the economically developed countries of western Europe.

Past

The populations of western Europe included about 5 per cent. of old people (over 64 years of age) during the middle of the last century, a proportion more than double that found among many populations today. The degree of ageing in France was especially high (6·5 per cent. in 1851) when one realizes that this figure was not achieved by the United States until 1940. At the beginning of the century Sweden (8·5 per cent.), France (8·2 per cent.), and Norway (7·9 per cent.) had already about the same percentages as the United States had fifty years later.

Future

Most countries where the ageing of populations have been acute have made estimations of future population trends, and all have come to similar conclusions, namely, that the ageing process will continue. In the United Kingdom projections for future populations have been prepared by the Royal Commission on Population (1949) for the years 1947–2047 on certain assumptions; at present there is low mortality and fertility; assuming that mortality will continue to decline slowly and that there will be no appreciable migration movement, future trends will depend upon the future levels of fertility. If fertility continues at its present low level the percentage over 64 years of age in 1987 will be 18·3, if there is medium fertility this percentage will be 17·0, and if fertility is high the percentage will be 15·8. The Organization for European Economic Co-operation (1956) made a study of future demographic trends in certain countries of western Europe, the Index of Ageing (percentage of persons above the age of 64 years) obtained from this material for the year 1971 has been calculated for the following countries: Austria (14·4 per cent.), Belgium (14·3 per cent.), France (12·6 per cent.), Ireland (9·0 per cent.), Sweden (13·5 per cent.), United Kingdom (14·4 per cent.).

The most interesting figures are from France, where the ageing process started early and where there has been a recent rise in the birth rate, the forecast shows no change from the figures for 1968, and for Ireland, where a fall is indicated from 11·2 per cent. in 1961 to 9·0 per cent. in 1971 (the 1966 figure remains at 11·2 per cent.); it will be interesting to see how correct are the forecasts.

The latest population projections for the United Kingdom for 1969 to 2001 show an increase of 9 per cent. in the number of retired people. The underlying pattern now is that at age 80 there are roughly two women for every man, at age 85 the ratio has become about three women to each man. Evidence is accumulating of the widening gap between the life expectancy of man as compared with woman. In the United Kingdom in 1901 a male of 80 could expect to live 4·9 more years and in 1966, 5·5 compared with females who in 1901 could anticipate 5·3 more years but in 1966, 6·9 so that in the 65 year interval males had increased life expectancy by 0·6 years and females by 1·6 years.

In Chebotarev and Sachuk's (1964) survey of people 80 years and over in the Ukraine there were seven times as many female centenarians as male. Hamilton and Mestlet (1969) studied subjects in an institution for the mentally retarded in America and found that survival was significantly longer in eunuchs than in intact males; the eunuchs also significantly outlived the intact females. One factor in shortening the length of life of the male animal may well be his male attributes.

The problem of caring for old people in many developed countries is really that of looking after an increasing population of elderly women especially in the 75 and over age group.

In a number of underdeveloped countries the ageing process has already begun, and although accurate forecasting is impossible, the trend is likely to become accelerated in the more distant future; it will depend to a large extent on the degree to which fertility is controlled.

CAUSES OF THE AGEING OF POPULATIONS

The age structure of a population depends upon past trends in fertility, mortality, and migration. These in turn are determined by the reproductive behaviour of couples, by health conditions, and by cultural, economic, and social factors. Reduction in mortality when not accompanied by changes in fertility has had no immediate effect on age structure. There are several examples of this, for example, Formosa and Puerto Rico, where fertility has remained virtually unchanged since 1900 and mortality has decreased considerably, the composition of broad age structures has remained stationary. In all countries of the world where mortality has fallen the most spectacular decreases have occurred in infancy and childhood, and to some extent in young adults. In middle and old age there has been little decline; in fact, in some cases there have been in recent years increases in the death rates for males in the age group 55–64 years. mainly due to coronary heart disease and lung cancer. Grannis (1970) demonstrated in the United States that the ratio of elderly females to males and the ratio of widows to widowers had changed during the past 75 years to the extent expected on the basis of national cigarette consumption by males and the known relation of the degree of cigarette smoking to the premature mortality of males. By 1965 these changes had resulted in a deficit of 1·75 million widowers and an excess of 2·5 million widows. Another way of expressing this is by means of the expectation of life calculated at various ages. In white males, for example, the greatest increase in expectation of life has been in the age group 0–9 years, and has been much less marked in the age group 10–19 years and 20–29 years.

The immediate effect of this was to cause an increase in the numbers of young people. Moreover, these falls in mortality began to be marked only in the present century. It means therefore that the first cohort of persons affected by these changes has now only reached 'middle age'. This is the so-called bulge in the population pyramid; eventually this bulge will move upward into the 'old age' group (over 64 years) and will then contribute materially to the increase in the percentage of 'old persons' (over 64 years) in the population. In economically advanced countries these falls in mortality were later followed by large falls in fertility which caused ageing at the base. A number of detailed studies have been carried out recently on the effect of changes in fertility and mortality on the age structure of populations. These are discussed in detail in Population Studies No. 26, The Ageing of Populations and its Economic and Social Implications (1956), published by the United Nations Department of Economic and Social Affairs.

They all confirm the implication made above, namely, that the decline in mortality has so far been a negligible factor in the increase in the population of old people (over 64 years) in the population, and the main factor responsible has been declining fertility. It is evident that something can be done to control the future ageing of population by attempting to increase fertility. The Royal Commission on Population (1949) in fact recommended that efforts should be made to encourage large families by reducing the financial burden to young couples and to promote family welfare. France raised family allowances for the same reasons, this has already had an effect on the Index of Ageing.

THE PREVENTION AND CONTROL OF THE DISEASES AND DISABILITIES OF THE ELDERLY

In many of the countries of western Europe and in the United States there is a growing awareness of the magnitude and multiplicity of the problems posed by an ageing population in the medical, economic, and social fields. It has been realized that provision for the prevention and control of disease in the elderly cannot be met without adequate knowledge of the relevant facts. Much useful information can be obtained from national mortality and morbidity statistics, but the real needs of the elderly can be determined only by well-planned *ad hoc* surveys. Sheldon (1948) in Wolverhampton was one of the pioneers in this field; he carried out a survey to inquire into the health status of the elderly living in their own homes. Hobson and Pemberton (1955) carried out an important survey in Sheffield. The importance of the Sheffield survey was that in the first place a random sample of the population was taken, i.e. it was not selected, and also a complete clinical examination of the subjects was carried out involving the co-operation of over 200 general practitioners; in addition, many special investigations were carried out, including a complete dietary survey. Brockington and Lempert (1966) assessed the social needs of 77 per cent. of people over 80 living in Stockport and found that 3·9 per cent. of this group were never visited, that much more could be done to help those with defective sight, hearing, and teeth. Recent bereavement, life in the lower social classes, admissions to institutions, and housing in the central and poorer wards of the town militated against survival. Services particularly inadequate were laundry facilities at reduced cost and the smallness of the meals-on-wheels and other services for supplementing the diet. There was no agency concentrating on those old people living alone.

Williamson (1966) found much 'unreported illness' in a survey of old people at home: they did not see fit to bring this to the notice of their own doctors. Such illnesses were those involving the urinary system, the feet, and the presence of anaemia or dementia. High-risk groups selected for special surveillance were: (1) those living alone; (2) those recently bereaved; (3) those with any locomotive deficiency; (4) those showing signs of mental impairment; (5) those recently discharged from a hospital; and (6) those showing a tendency to isolate themselves. Much disability in the elderly has also been reported by Miller (1963) from his examination of women aged 60 years or over and men 65 years or over in his own general practice, and by Richardson (1964). Goldberg (1970) described a field experiment in social work among 300 people aged 70 and over who were clients of a welfare department. Nearly half the applicants were over 80 and nearly half were living in unsuitable housing and two-thirds lived alone. One quarter had serious disease and 15 per cent. suffered from psychiatric disorders. These people were randomly allocated to a special group and a comparison group. Two trained case workers were appointed to take on the social work in this special group while the comparison group remained under the care of the department's welfare officers none of whom had a professional social work training. Those in the special groups received twice the amount of help compared with those in the other group. The trained workers saw more problems and laid more emphasis on case-work and work with relatives. They co-operated more closely with medical and voluntary agencies. It was concluded that closer teamwork between social worker and doctor was essential and many of the minor miseries of old age had not been brought to the notice of the doctors by the clients themselves. These difficulties consisted of foot discomfort, poor sight and hearing, dizziness, urinary symptoms, constipation, and poor sleep. Advice from physicians in geriatric medicine should be available to the social service department concerned with community care.

Numerous cross-sectional studies are now being carried out in different parts of the world with a view to determining the medical, economic, and social needs of old people. Carefully planned and longitudinal studies are in progress, for example, in America, Switzerland, France, Russia, and the Netherlands, to provide the kind of data needed for determining physiological norms and for giving more information on causal relationships. Examples of these are:

1. The Minnesota Longitudinal Study (Brožek *et al.*, 1966) initiated in 1947–48 surveyed 281 business and professional men at that time aged between 45 and 55 years and clinically healthy. In the fifteen-year follow-up it was revealed that the incidence of coronary heart disease was higher among men above median at first examination in relative weight, skinfolds, systolic and diastolic blood pressure, and serum cholesterol concentration, but that only cholesterol concentration was significant.

2. The Duke Study (Busse, 1966) had as a primary objective the effect of ageing upon the nervous system. The sample was composed of volunteers, aged 60 years or over at the beginning of the study, relatively free of disease, functioning at an acceptable level in the community. This study, in operation for more than ten years, has shown that an increase in the severity of cardiovascular disease has little effect on intellectual functioning and on tests of immediate memory, but did produce a significantly extended reaction time; approximately one-third of elderly persons cannot be relied upon to give an accurate assessment of their physical health; a sudden decline in intelligence and an alteration in the E.E.G. suggested the onset of a process of deterioration and approaching death. When studied longitudinally the importance of physical health as a factor in depression became increasingly evident. This longitudinal study provided little support for the disengagement theory. Relatively active elderly subjects were more likely to maintain morale than those who were inactive.

3. In Kiev, Chebotarev and Sachuk (1964) described a mass

medical examination of 27,181 subjects aged 80 years and over and demonstrated that those who survived into old age had started work early in life and left off work at a very late stage. Of the women 91 per cent. were widows, and the great majority of those examined had married and had had large families, usually marrying early and the marriage lasting a long time.

4. Gsell (1967) studying 72 healthy males for 8–10 years found that from the 20th to the 60th year of life body length decreased by 40 mm., vital capacity by 0·3 l., and accommodation of eye by 8–9 dioptres. Other changes were noted, but the author concluded that a 10-year interval was insufficient to produce statistically significant or acceptable age difference in blood pressure.

Haranghy (1965) investigated the physical and mental condition of 23 centenarians, of whom 17 were mobile and clinically healthy. As in the Russian survey, a large number of the centenarians had begun work at a very young age, 10–12 years, and worked hard throughout their lives. This review includes a complete physical examination of these people together with a nutritional survey and a psychiatric analysis.

The use of levodopa has been of immense value in overcoming the disabilities of Parkinsonism bearing in mind the need for starting with small doses and building up the daily intake very slowly (Anderson, 1971).

MORTALITY

Over the age of 50 years the commonest causes of death are heart disease, malignant disease, and respiratory disorders, which in most countries of western Europe are together responsible for about two-thirds of all deaths over the age of 50 years. In the 75 years and over age group in England and Wales heart disease still heads the list of causes, respiratory disease comes next, but vascular disease affecting the central nervous system displaces malignant disease, and this also occurs in women of the 65–74 years age group. One of the great difficulties which arises in a detailed analysis of causes of death in the older age-groups is the question of diagnostic classification. In old age there is rarely one single cause of death; there are several, and it is usually very difficult, even after a post-mortem, to give one primary cause of death; moreover, fashions change. Part of the increase in mortality from coronary heart disease is certainly due to transference of deaths assigned to myocardial disease. A useful measure of health including demographic conditions is the proportion of deaths at 50 years and over to total deaths. More precise measures for comparative purposes are age-specific death rates in quinquennial groups. The death rates per 1,000 for the age group 65–69 years show some remarkable differences in different countries of Europe: the four lowest are Norway (24·4), Holland (28·1), Denmark (28·9), and Sweden (30·3), compared with the United Kingdom (48·0) and Scotland (46·0). Japan (50·0) is also high, while the United States (white) occupies an intermediate position (40·7). In the Scandinavian countries death rates in all the age groups (50–54, 55–59, 60–64, 65–69, 70–74) are about half what they are in Britain Why is this so? Is it due to better health services? Or to healthier ways of living? Or to a healthier environment? Many of the questions can be answered only by more detailed studies,

not only at the national level but also by comparative studies sponsored by such international agencies as the World Health Organization and the United Nations. An analysis of the specific causes of death shows that the higher mortality in Britain can be accounted for by an excess of deaths from 'chronic bronchitis', coronary heart disease, and lung cancer, especially in males, e.g. the recorded mortality rate from chronic bronchitis is 500 times greater, in the age group 65–69 years, in the United Kingdom than it is in Norway. In Scotland the heaviest death rates for respiratory tuberculosis are at ages 65 years and over for males, and among females at ages 75 to 84 years. Death rates for cancer of lung and bronchus have increased among men aged 70 years and over. Some of these differences may be due to differences in fashion of diagnosis or in classification or recording.

MORBIDITY

There is very little objective evidence to indicate whether the health of old people has improved. It has, however, been reported from Sweden that the proportion of invalids in old age has shown a progressive decline over the last three or four

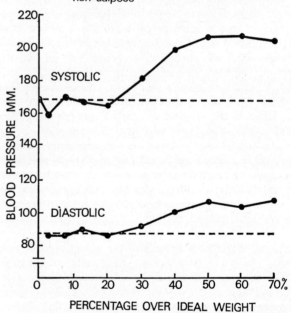

FIG. 94. The systolic and diastolic blood pressure means of 304 women aged 60–79 years in relation to the degree of adiposity. Solid line: mean blood-pressure values for different percentage over ideal weight; broken line: projected mean blood-pressure values for non-adipose.

decades (World Health Organization, 1959). The chronic conditions which produce infirmity and disability become more common in old age, and while it is difficult to prevent the onset of many of these conditions, it is possible to prevent complications and to enable many old people to live at ease with their, often multiple disabilities. Obesity was shown at the Rutherglen Consultative Health Centre (Anderson and Cowan, 1959a) to have a dramatic effect on blood pressure [FIG. 94].

Percentage over ideal weight is estimated from a nomogram

using height and weight. These figures were obtained from healthy fat women as no fit obese men were found. In fact, out of 650 men examined, not one 25 per cent. or more over ideal weight was healthy, and the few obese people reaching old age can be seen [TABLE 113]. Hippocrates describes old men as suffering from 'difficulty of breathing, catarrh accompanied by coughing, strangury, difficult micturition, pains at the joints, kidney disease, apoplexy, cachexia, pruritus, sleeplessness, water discharge from the bowels, eyes and nostrils, dullness of sight, cataract, hardness of hearing'. Times have changed little; recent surveys show that the chief causes of disability in old age are the following: vascular disorders, disorders of the locomotor system, genito-urinary symptoms, respiratory disease, and disorders of the special senses.

TABLE 113
Obesity among Older Patients
Percentage overweight calculated by Anderson's nomogram
(Greene)

Age group years	Under 0–24 per cent.		25–40 per cent.		50 per cent. +		Total	
	Men	Women	Men	Women	Men	Women	Men	Women
55–69	275	205	14	83	2	28	291	316
70–79	272	208	11	37	1	9	284	254
80+	84	59	4	8	—	—	88	67
Total	631	472	29	128	3	37	663	637

Note the small number of men and women in the 50 per cent. overweight column.
From Greene, R., ed. (1951) in *The Practice of Endocrinology*, p. 337, London.

Vascular Disease

Atheromatous arterial disease affects mainly the brain, heart, and legs. The first site is by far the most important cause of disability in the elderly. Both major cerebral infarcts resulting in hemiplegia and multiple minor infarcts which are usually expressed as dementia are very frequent causes of admission to geriatric units for short- or long-stay care. By comparison, ischaemic heart disease, though a major immediate cause of death, is less frequent as a cause of disability. However, its contribution to cardiac failure in the elderly is substantial (Pomerance, 1965a), but in any case modern diuretics have made the management of heart failure much easier than even in the recent past. Peripheral vascular disease is a frequent asymptomatic finding in old age, but comparatively rarely gives rise to symptoms requiring treatment. When it does, modern arterial operations have resulted in the saving of many limbs. There are at present no effective means of preventing arterial disease. It is not known whether reduction of dietary sucrose or animal fat or the long-term administration of clofibrate have any beneficial action whatever. What is clear is that any means that are discovered will necessitate large-scale changes in the habits of the population and will need application in middle rather than later life.

Cardiovascular Disorders

A raised blood pressure can be regarded as almost physiological, at any rate in Europeans, and in healthy older people there is a wide range of acceptable blood pressures (Anderson and Cowan, 1959b); the upper limits for systolic blood pressure in men are 195 mm. Hg (60–69 years), 205 mm. Hg (70–79 years), and 215 mm. Hg (80–89 years), and in women these are 200 mm. Hg, 215 mm. Hg, and 230 mm. Hg respectively. The corresponding diastolic blood pressure upper limits may be taken for men as 100, 104, and 108, and for women as 102, 106, and 110. Blood pressure rises with age, but hypertension, in the sense of a condition producing symptoms or requiring treatment by itself, is not of major importance in the elderly, though it is undoubtedly a risk factor in the development of atheromatous disease and stroke. Pomerance (1965a) found multiplicity of pathological findings in individual hearts was the outstanding feature of cardiac failure in the elderly. The same author (1965b) described senile cardiac amyloidosis at necropsy in 10 per cent. of patients aged over 80 years and in 50 per cent. of those over 90 years. McKeown (1965) analysed the necropsy findings in 1,500 patients aged 70 years or more and described the pathological aspects of the common diseases of old age. Disorders of the cardiovascular system ranked first as a cause of death, while malignancy was almost of equal importance. Pathy (1967) in a clinical study of myocardial infarction noted that only 19 per cent. of 387 patients over 65 years had substernal or epigastric pain. In 81 per cent. the mode of presentation could be divided into fourteen other groups with symptoms of dyspnoea, confusion, giddiness, palpitation, recurrent vomiting, weakness, breathlessness, or sweating, or with syncope, peripheral gangrene, renal failure, stroke, pulmonary embolism, or 'sudden death'. The Sheffield survey showed that nearly one-third of old persons aged 75 years and over had disabling cardiovascular disease.

It was concluded in a Report of the World Health Organization (1963) that there is as yet no effective way of preventing the occurrence of hypertension or ischaemic heart disease.

Cerebrovascular Disease

Strokes occur commonly in older people, and much progress has been made in the understanding of the spatial and perceptive disorders in these patients. Adams (1967) reported a definite improvement in the results of his rehabilitation, comparing his first 710 hemiplegic patients treated between 1948 and 1956 with 729 such patients treated between 1959 and 1963. In his first group 42 per cent. regained independence in walking and self-care; in his second series 59 per cent. reached this stage: while those remaining chronic invalids consisted of 28 per cent. in the first series and 26 per cent. in the second.

Minor attacks of paresis, following cerebral infarction, are common causes of impaired speech or difficulty in walking: partial or complete recovery often occurs spontaneously. Much can be done to help these people by providing adequate housing arrangements, domestic help, and various appliances.

Abnormality in temperature regulation is probably a major aetiological factor in accidental hypothermia in the elderly (MacMillan et al., 1967) and impaired temperature regulation, as well as postural hypotension due to defective baroreceptor reflexes, may be the result of central lesions in the brain (Wollner, 1967).

Disorders of the Locomotor System

Rheumatoid and osteo-arthritis can cause crippling deformities which are a great burden to the housewife, who, let it be noted, does not retire at 65 years. Spondylitis of the spine is a genuine phenomenon of old age, causing great disability. Anderson and colleagues (1966) described osteomalacia in elderly women and felt that this disease might on occasion be due to simple lack of vitamin D arising from defective dietary intake and lack of exposure to sunlight and that the problem of senile osteomalacia might be an extensive one, sufficient to warrant prophylactic vitamin-D therapy in high-risk elderly people. Polymyalgia rheumatica was described by Gatter and McCarthy (1967) as a rheumatic disease of the elderly, and the suggested transition of polymyalgia rheumatica into calssical temporal arteritis by Harrison and Bevan (1967) was of great interest, as cortiscosteroids have been shown to prevent loss of sight associated with temporal arteritis, so that early diagnosis is essential.

Defects of the legs and feet are very common in old people: corns and bunions being most frequently found; sometimes they are associated with varicose veins, peripheral ischaemia, or diabetes. Proper hygiene and care of the feet are essential, including adequate exercise and treatment. The provision of chiropody services is very important. Twenty-six per cent. of all people reporting to the Rutherglen Consultative Health Centre required the attention of the chiropodist.

Respiratory Disease

In the elderly, as in middle life, the two commonest chronic respiratory diseases are chronic bronchitis and bronchogenic carcinoma. The causal role of cigarette smoking is clear in both conditions, while urban atmospheric pollution is undoubtedly of importance in the former, and probably in the latter (Dean, 1966). Cessation of cigarette smoking lessens the risk of bronchial carcinoma (Doll and Hill, 1964), but has little effect on the progress of established chronic bronchitis. Here vaccination against influenza, prophylactic administration of tetracycline or ampicillin throughout the winter and the prompt treatment of acute exacerbations can lessen disability and slow the progression of the disease. Chronic bronchitis is an important cause of premature retirement of men in late middle age, when breathlessness advances to a degree which makes work or getting to work impossible. The provision of sheltered workshops can maintain some of these patients at work. As with arterial disease, it is clear that preventive measures applied earlier in life are necessary to reduce the incidence of chronic bronchitis in old age. The virtually complete failure of all efforts to reduce cigarette smoking makes the prospect for the future very dismal.

The main problem in respiratory tuberculosis in developed countries is now the elderly patient, in whom the diagnosis is of great importance and some difficulty. The risk of infection being transmitted to the younger members of the family must be kept in mind. Many of these elderly men in particular are difficult to reach, as they are people who do not come forward when screening X-ray examination is offered to the public.

Genito-urinary Symptoms

Dysuria, nocturia, frequency, and urgency are a major cause of restricted movement in the elderly, tending to cause social isolation. The most incapacitating genito-urinary symptom, however, is incontinence of urine. It is a frequent cause of admission to hospital and permanent institutional care, and is responsible for much of the heavy work associated with nursing the elderly sick. Two-thirds of the cases of incontinence are due to organic disorders of the central nervous system, usually caused by cerebrovascular disease. This association often results in hospital admission. Incontinence is also due to local disease of the genito-urinary tract, commonly prostatism in men and gynaecological diseases in women. Newman (1969) stressed the importance of depression and felt that urinary incontinence which followed change of environment, e.g. admission to hospital might be prevented by a better understanding of the needs of old people. Psychological disturbances caused by bereavement, resentment, or anger may produce urinary incontinence and drug therapy is also an occasional cause. It is essential that remediable causes of incontinence are recognized and treated and while retraining may be of value the first step must be a correct diagnosis. To look after incontinent elderly people at home requires great devotion on the part of relatives, and it must be supported by good domiciliary services, for example, frequent visits by the district nurse, the supply of necessary appliances, and a domiciliary laundry service.

Disorders of the Special Senses

The sense of taste becomes slightly impaired in the elderly (Hughes, 1969) while few old people have a normal sense of smell (Anand, 1964). Unfortunately, however, the joys of reading and listening to conversation are often denied because of deterioration in vision or hearing. The incidence of deafness found in the Rutherglen series changed from 3 per cent. at 70–74 years, to 8·5 per cent. at 85–89 years, and deafness is often found in patients with late paraphrenia or with depression. A recent random sample of 300 people 65 and over living at home (Caird, 1972) revealed 17 per cent. under 75 and 34 per cent. over 75 had some degree of deafness but only 20 per cent. of those found to be deaf were severely affected. In almost half of all cases the cause was nerve deafness but in a quarter of all deaf people wax in the ears was to blame. The provision of hearing aids can be of great benefit. Impaired sense of smell may result in failure to recognize escaping gas or fire, and is an undoubted cause of accidental household gas poisoning and of increased fire risk. Deterioration of vision is frequent—between the ages of 70 and 80 0·75 per cent. of the population are registered blind and over 80, 3 per cent. (Oxford figures—Caird, Pirie, and Ramsell, 1968). Three main causes predominate—senile macular degeneration, cataract, and glaucoma (Sorsby, 1966). Much can be done by operating on cataract, by the medical and surgical treatment of glaucoma, and even in the case of senile macular degeneration by the provision of visual aids and large print books. Vertigo in old ladies is a frequent cause of accidents, and they should be warned about standing on chairs or in high places.

Psychological Disorders

Psychiatric disturbances in the elderly are often associated with physical disorders or even fear of physical illness; a great deal can be done to reduce periods of disability and certification by early recognition and treatment. The physician has a responsibility to treat the mental disturbance as effectively as the physical disease.

Roth (1964) discussed the prophylaxis, early diagnosis and

treatment of mental illness in later life, basing his work on a survey made in north-east England, and Post (1965) has made a special study of the psychiatry of later life. There is general agreement among psychiatrists that just over 5 per cent. of people over 65 years have organic (senile and arteriosclerotic) psychosis, around 3 per cent. have major functional disorders, 12 per cent. have neurosis or character disorders, and between 5 and 10 per cent. mild mental deterioration. Physicians and psychiatrists have a common interest in the depressions of old age, the delusions and allied states of the elderly, and certain problems of senile and arteriosclerotic psychosis (Roth, 1966). The recognition of emotional disorders, such as depression, is often overlooked in the elderly, and Post (1966) described three symptom complexes which are especially apt to mask the more important depressive disturbances: (1) An increase of long-standing neurotic symptoms which in the elderly is more often due to an intercurrent depressive disorder. (2) Frequency with which depressive illnesses of later life are overlaid with somatic complaints and sensations as well as with hypochondriacal concerns, which are frequently neither bizarre nor obviously delusional. (3) Cognitive impairment with a history of recent decline in various abilities and in memory.

Recent developments in psychogeriatrics (1971) are described with emphasis on the interrelationship between physical and mental disease, the importance of diagnosis and the need for a fully integrated psychogeriatric service.

In a survey of psychiatric outpatient practice in those over 60 years, Straker (1964) pointed out that only 24 per cent. were free of significant associated physical disease, and felt that the best results were often obtained by an initial period of active inpatient treatment. Like many others engaged in this work, he commented on the frequency of late referral to the outpatient clinic. Strachan and Henderson (1965, 1967) drew attention to mental abnormality associated with vitamin B_{12} or folic acid deficiency. This is not commonly found in clinical practice. Shulman (1967) felt that the psychiatrist should be alert to the possibility of vitamin B_{12} deficiency in: (1) patients who had anaemia or a gastrectomy; (2) patients with unexplained fatigue; and (3) those with confusional states or dementia of unknown origin.

The classification of mental disorders which is of value to the physician interested in the elderly is as follows: (1) acute confusional states; (2) dementias; (3) affective disorders; (4) paranoid syndromes; and (5) personality changes. Watch must be kept for the occurrence of mental confusion in the elderly person with an acute illness and for the old man or woman with depression. Suicide is unfortunately not uncommon in the elderly.

The causes of mental illness often have their roots in the general biological phenomenon of ageing, but they are aggravated by loneliness, poverty, or by the awareness of declining vigour and intellect, and may be precipitated by retirement or loss of a near relative. Much can be done to alleviate the mental health problems of the elderly by attending to the various social and economic aspects of their lives.

In the United Kingdom between 1951 and 1960 mental hospital first-admission rates for elderly men increased by between 30 and 40 per cent. and for elderly women by just over 40 per cent. Prevention must be stressed, and social policies concerned with the promotion of mental health in the aged should aim at enabling them to maintain for as long as possible a sense of independence, of having some useful role to perform, and of having meaningful social relationships. One important requirement is the opportunity to go on working for as long as the individual wishes and is able to do so. Another point is the maintenance of physical health. At the Rutherglen Consultative Health Centre, of 663 men and 637 women over the age of 55 years, some 21 per cent. of the men and 25 per cent. of the women were emotionally disturbed, and when these figures were examined in more detail emotional disturbance was found to be commoner in women and increased by a physical illness in both sexes. The factors associated with the emotional disturbance were as follows: an adverse home environment, and this included the state of living alone; physical ill health; bereavement; ill health of a relative; neglectful children; compulsory retirement, and in this series this applied to men only; and financial difficulties. Methods of trying to help the patient were as follows:

1. Reassurance on physical health. The most important method of prevention of mental ill health in the elderly is reassurance on physical health. Adequate time must be made available to establish a good rapport and gain the confidence of the old person.

2. Improving home environment. The mental health of an older person can be assisted by correcting the social circumstances. This does not necessarily mean transfer to a new house or an old person's home. Such steps should be taken only after the most careful appraisal of all the social factors. The presence of good neighbours may be much more important than a modern house. The provision of a well-trained home help, a regular visit by a nurse or voluntary worker, or the pastoral services of a padre may be of great value.

3. Consultation with psychiatrist. Education is urgently required so that the general public and the relatives may understand that while on occasion old people are eccentric, this may pass into an abnormal phase, and where there is doubt a psychiatrist should be consulted. The onset of depression, of a lack of desire to get out of bed or to go on living, these are abnormal findings, and should indicate to the relatives that advice from the patient's own doctor should initially be sought. The modern psychogeriatric unit has much to offer in the way of diagnosis, admission, and cure.

4. Provision of interests. The mental health of old people can be stimulated and mental ill health prevented by the provision of interests. Certainly in men who have been compulsorily retired, a routine of pre-retirement training should be introduced.

The Expert Committee on Mental Health of the World Health Organization (1959) made certain recommendations concerning the mental health problems of ageing: they can be summarized as follows:

1. There should be integrated mental-health services for the elderly, with geriatric guidance centres as their core.

2. The teaching of medical students and nurses should include instruction in the mental-health problems of ageing.

3. Every effort should be made to encourage more favourable community attitudes in relation to the problems of the elderly.

4. They recommended more research and listed a number of important fields for further study; the setting up of institutes of gerontology was recommended.

Nutritional Disorders

McGandy and colleagues (1966) found the total calorie requirements diminished with age and that there is a disproportionate drop in fat intake with age. This may explain the decrease of 15 mg. per 100 ml. in serum cholesterol between the ages of 50 and 70 years. This decrease in total calorie intake was accounted for by decrements in basal metabolism and in energy expended in physical activity. Exton-Smith and Stanton (1965) investigated the diet, clinical condition, and social circumstances of sixty women over the age of 70 years living alone in London. Some diets were ill balanced and provided too little vitamin C, vitamin D, calcium, iron, or protein, and a striking deterioration in health and nutrition was found in the late 70s. These authors made the recommendation that meals designed for the elderly should contain a high proportion of protein with an adequate supply of calcium, iron, and vitamin D presented in such a way that the whole meal is eaten. Vitamin C might require to be provided separately, as food must be kept hot for long periods in a meals-on-wheels service. These authors (Stanton and Exton-Smith, 1970) found that a large number of those women died before they reached their late seventies, about one-quarter developed illnesses which impaired their state of health, physical capacity, and (probably in consequence) nutrient intakes; one-sixth retained health, independence, and dietary intake (the élite). It is not yet known (Watkin, 1968) whether the life-long nutrition pattern of those who reach advanced old age has contributed to their longevity or whether their heredity has not only enabled them to survive but has also, in some manner, characterized their nutrition.

Vitamin C levels are borderline in the elderly, and have been shown to be low in old people in hospital and homes (Kataria *et al.*, 1965; Andrews *et al.*, 1966). Griffiths and his co-workers (1967) found ascorbic acid and thiamine levels low in old people, and Batata and his associates (1967) noted low blood ascorbic acid concentrations in the winter months in new admissions to geriatric departments and low serum folic acid and serum B_{12} but no case of megaloblastic anaemia. Milne and co-workers (1971) measured leucocyte ascorbic acid levels and vitamin C intake in a random sample of men and women 62–94 years. No age difference in leucocyte ascorbic acid levels was found in men but these were significantly lower in older women while the mean value for all women was significantly higher than for all men; both sexes showed higher levels in July to December. Many men over 70 take less than 30 mg. of vitamin C per day and 4·7 per cent. of men and 3 per cent. of women have an intake below 10 mg. daily. These workers have suggested vitamin C supplements for older people especially in the first and fourth quarters of the year.

In the Sheffield survey 'widower's scurvy' was encountered on several occasions, and was in some cases due to sudden bereavement causing intense apathy and depression. Osteomalacia from a simple lack of vitamin D can occur especially in old women and in patients who have had a gastrectomy. The simplest preventive measure is to encourage them to substitute margarine (with added vitamin D) for butter.

Patients who have had partial gastrectomy are at special risk and Williams and colleagues (1969) found clinical and laboratory signs of neurological disease many years after operation. Such patients may have low serum iron or vitamin B_{12} levels and may require permanent replacement therapy especially with parenteral hydroxocobalamin. Folate deficiency can occur in the elderly (Girdwood, 1969) but is usually caused by chronic infection, malignancy, malabsorption, chronic alcoholism, or following anticonvulsant drugs.

Anaemia is common in old people due to gastro-intestinal blood loss (from peptic ulcer, hiatus hernia, or diverticulitis). Salicylate therapy is often a contributing factor. Sideropenia is found in the elderly without anaemia and this may be due to an underlying neoplasm. If no cause is found following iron therapy there is often a reduction of fatigue, lassitude, and irritability with improvement on occasion of the mental faculties. Potassium deficiency can occur in those older people with a marginal potassium intake who suffer an intercurrent infection or require diuretic therapy. This shows itself by muscle weakness, apathy, depression, faecal impaction, or sensitivity to digoxin. The provision of an adequate diet, if necessary by a domiciliary meals service, is of the utmost importance. Brockington and Lempert (1966) felt that a person coming in daily to cook a meal for the older citizen was the best solution to this problem.

The elderly in the community are often at risk nutritionally and those 70 years and over should be visited regularly by someone trained in the dietary problems of old age. The depressed, the recently bereaved, the confused, those with physical disease who depend on others for cooking and those on long-term analgesics are among the people at greatest danger. Doctors should be aware of the risks of diuretic therapy and the need to supplement diet in certain situations, e.g. following serious or long continued illness, surgical operation, accident, or bereavement. It is also most important to ensure that an adequate and appetizing diet is provided in all institutions for the care of the elderly. We should not forget the words of Oliver Wendell Holmes, 'I think as one grows older less food is required, but old people have a right to be epicures, if they can afford it. The pleasures of the palate are among the last gratifications of the senses allowed them.'

Accidents

There has been an increasing occurrence of accidents among the elderly in some countries. Boucher (1966) recorded that 3 per cent. of men aged 65 years or more and 4·8 per cent. of women in this age range died of accidents in 1964. Eighty-two per cent. of fatal accidents in the elderly occur in the old person's own home, and this type of accident increases with age, being particularly high in those aged 80 years or more and those with poor health; 95 per cent. of the fatalities resulted from falls, burns, and scalds, and poisoning by household gas. This is a matter of serious public health concern, since many of them are preventable, particularly those which occur in the home. As people grow older there is an increasing liability to falls, associated with such disabilities as deafness, vertigo, failing vision, degeneration of the posterior columns of the spinal cord, muscular weakness, small unsuspected cerebral thromboses, and fainting spells. Falls are particularly dangerous in the elderly because they are more likely to result in serious injury, e.g. fracture of the femur due to osteoporosis. An accident of this nature can be a most serious event in the life of an old person because it often results in a prolonged stay in bed which may precipitate senile decay.

Stairs may be a special menace, especially in those who suffer from weakness, dyspnoea, stiff joints, or those who have had a stroke. Special housing for the elderly is very important from this point of view. An adequate environment for a healthy old person may become a most inadequate one with even a minor deterioration in health. A minor defect in environment, such as steps that are too steep, may render an old person housebound.

The doctor or nurse can often do much to prevent accidents by giving the necessary advice on such things as the right kind of accommodation, adaptation of kitchen appliances, adequate lighting in dark corners, guards for heating appliances, non-skid rugs, hand-rails on stairs or ramps to avoid steps, and guide ropes for blind persons.

From this short account of the chief disorders and disabilities of the elderly it is clear that a great deal can be done to prevent and control them, particularly by education in healthy ways of living, by early detection of disease, and by providing a whole range of domiciliary and institutional services for the care of the elderly [see also CHAPTER 28].

HEALTH EDUCATION

This is most effective when begun in childhood, but the following problems can be tackled by education directed towards middle-aged and elderly persons: accident prevention, care of the bowels, abuse of drugs, the hygiene of healthy living, mental health, diet and nutrition, retirement and the proper use of leisure, and the better use of medical and welfare services. Health education should be a special task of the family doctor, the public health nurse (health visitor), and the social worker; it should be organized, however, by the appropriate medical authorities, especially by the Medical Officer of Health. In countries where general practitioners work at health centres, health education for the elderly should be organized from these at community level.

An example of one activity is that of the Metropolitan Life Insurance Company of New York, which has undertaken an advertising campaign in a number of periodicals under the heading, 'Cancer's Seven Warning Signals', they are as follows:

1. Any sore that does not heal.
2. A lump or thickening in the breast or elsewhere.
3. Unusual bleeding or discharge.
4. Any change in a wart or mole.
5. Persistent indigestion or difficulty in swallowing.
6. Persistent hoarseness or cough.
7. Any change in normal bowel habits.

Readers are advised that should one of these signals appear, no time should be lost in seeing the doctor.

A great deal of further study is required in order to evaluate the ultimate effect of such methods. The special methods and techniques of health education are described in CHAPTER 49.

ROUTINE HEALTH EXAMINATIONS

The aim of routine health examinations is the early detection of physical, mental, and social deviations from health; the application of health education, and to provide opportunity for defining with greater precision the term 'health' in old age. Such examinations should, if possible, be carried out before retirement and be part of a pre-retirement counselling programme. The techniques of multiphasic screening may be of value in the early detection of such diseases as tuberculosis, potential diabetes, anaemia, glaucoma, hypertension, and some forms of cancer. It is the detection of early, previously undiagnosed, conditions which is so important from the public health point of view. The 'iceberg' phenomenon of unreported illness is now well known. The World Health Organization Advisory Group on the Public Health Aspects of the Ageing of the Population which met in Oslo in 1958 suggested that at least two health examinations should be carried out during middle age, namely, soon after the age of 40 and 6 months prior to retirement (World Health Organization Regional Office for Europe, 1959). Another appropriate time might be following bereavement, as this period is fraught with danger for the individual left alone.

Cancer

Early detection has come to play a key-role, so much so that in the United States a presidential committee investigating the cancer problem stated 'each premature death from cancer is a personal tragedy; each preventable death is a national reproach; each year more and more such deaths are occurring for the pace of science is bringing more within our reach, but the pace of application allows them to slip through our grasp'.

Two main categories of cancer exist; the first when found early is often curable by relatively simple procedures. The second in sites such as pancreas, stomach, and kidney are not readily accessible to early detection, but as new techniques develop the position may change. Cancer found at a late stage typically involves extensive procedures, which are too often palliative.

In view of the great increase of lung cancer in recent years, one of the greatest needs is an accurate method of detecting the early stages.

Raven (1971) suggests that populations should be divided into high and low risk groups, the former including women descended from mothers or grandmothers with breast carcinoma; offspring of patients with gastric, colonic, and rectal carcinoma. Also in this group are patients with pernicious anaemia who are at risk of gastric carcinoma and patients with familial adenosis of the colon and rectum or with total chronic ulcerative colitis who are at greater risk of colonic or rectal carcinoma.

Precancerous Lesions. A precancerous lesion is one which as long as it is present gives an increased risk of developing cancer. In these groups can be included rectal polyps, leukoplakia, senile keratoses, pigmented naevi, moles, and thyroid adenomas. Hitchcock and Aust (1954) found rectal polypi in 10 per cent. of routine examinations at the University of Minnesota Clinic.

The removal of such lesions by surgical and other procedures is an important way of preventing cancer.

Screening Methods. The routine examination of large numbers of 'healthy individuals' by physicians is time-consuming and costly, and opinion is divided on the wisdom of such methods, especially as the majority of doctors are not convinced of health surveillance. Continuing evaluation of cancer detection is needed, but figures strongly supporting screening have been given by Day (1967) in comparing five-year survival period of two periodic examination programmes with the national average of the United States [TABLE 114], and also by quoting the potential effect of cancer detection on cancer mortality statistics [TABLE 115]. See also CHAPTER 50 for a more detailed discussion.

Cytology. The realization that exfoliated cancer cells can be recognized under the microscope was first developed as a practical test for early cancer detection by Papanicolaou in 1928.

The vaginal smear is the only procedure which has been developed on a wide scale. The use of this method is limited by the number of slides which a trained technician can examine in one day—this has been estimated as between twenty-five and thirty. A microfluorimetric scanner has been devised to detect cancer cells automatically; there are clearly great possibilities for this type of investigation. There is a great need for a critical evaluation of cytological examinations in the detection of early cancer and of mammography screening for breast cancer.

Routine X-ray Screening. Although this method is of value in detecting tuberculosis, its value in detecting lung cancer is very limited.

In Los Angeles experience with nearly 2 million chest X-rays revealed 0·2 per cent. of cases of lung cancer (Guiss, 1955). Of the cases discovered, half were inoperable, and only 14 per cent. were alive three years later.

TABLE 114

Comparison of Five-year Survival:* Two Periodic Examination Programmes against National Average of the United States

Selected sites	National average	Strang Clinic (1954–56), Day (1963)		Gilbersten and Wangensteen (1963)	
		Result	Improvement	Result	Improvement
Breast	50	70	20	84	34
Colon and rectum	32	73	41	67	35
Uterine cervix	53	88	35	80	27
Uterine corpus	78	95	17	100	22

* All figures are given in percentages.

[From Day, E. (1963) Early detection of cancer as a control measure, *Ca.* (*A Cancer Journal for Clinicians*), **13**, 2; and Gilbertson, V. A., and Wangansteen, O. H. (1963) *Surg. Gynec. Obstet.*, **116**, 413.]

Certain specialized points can be made; the heavy consumer of alcohol should know of his risk of cancer of the upper alimentary tract, especially when he smokes heavily as well. Many surveys have established a clear, quantitative relationship between numbers of cigarettes smoked and incidence of lung cancer. If present smoking habits continue, it has been forecast that there will be some 50,000 deaths from the disease each year in England and Wales in the 1980s. If cigarette smoking were to cease there might in 20 years time be no more than 5,000 annual deaths from the disease (*Smoking and Health Now*, 1971). Nutritional deficiencies suspected to relate to cancer of the upper alimentary tract, cancer of the stomach, and cancer of the liver are associated with deep-rooted socio-economic problems. It is obvious that a recommendation to raise a population's intake of protein, fat, and vitamin-rich food cannot be easily accomplished. Nevertheless, attempts to improve the staple diet by making it richer in protein and by increasing the consumption of vitamin-rich fruit and vegetables can be made.

Preventive methods in various sites are: cancer of the oral cavity can be detected early by a regular examination of the

TABLE 115

Potential Effect of Cancer Detection on Cancer Mortality Based on United States Statistics, 1966

Selected sites	Deaths	Percentage preventable	Salvage
Cervix	10,000	100	10,000
Skin *	4,400	75	3,300
Colon and rectum	43,000	65	27,950
Breast	27,000	50	13,500
Prostate	16,000	50	8,000
Head and neck†	10,000	50	5,000
Endometrium	4,000	50	2,000
Lung	50,000	10	5,000
Stomach	18,000	10	1,800
Urinary organs	14,000	10	1,400
Ovary	9,000	10	900
Total	206,000	38·8	78,850

* Includes melanoma.
† Includes buccal cavity, pharynx, larynx, and thyroid.

mouth and throat, and abolition of betel chewing would lower the incidence if this measure could be instituted. Cytodiagnosis is being developed for cancer of the oesophagus and stomach, and here the risk of malignant change in association with benign forms of oesophageal obstruction or dysfunction must be kept in mind and such patients kept under observation. Gastric cancer is prone to occur in developed countries among the poorer people (Doll, 1956), and cancer of the stomach rate is falling in the United States, this being linked to the increasing prosperity. There seem, however, to be factors associated with civilization, and primitive people with few exceptions have little gastric carcinoma, although primary cancer of the liver is common. People who may develop gastric cancer are those who have pernicious anaemia, and such are advised to have periodic and regular medical examinations; patients with chronic atrophic gastritis, those with achlorhydria, and those who have been treated for a gastric ulcer should be kept under observation.

Those patients with congenital abnormalities of the small bowel should be watched, while those with Meckel's diverticulum or benign tumours should have them removed.

Bladder screening by cytological examination is already being employed in industry to detect early tumours in exposed persons, and it has been stated that if circumcision was carried out routinely at birth cancer of the penis would be completely eliminated.

In cancer of the body of the uterus the diagnosis of adenomatous hyperplasia must be made before malignant changes occurred. Any abnormal bleeding must be investigated, and a full diagnostic curettage is best. Women menstruating after 50 years should be suspect, any intra-uterine contraceptive devices should be removed at the menopause, and long-continued oestrogen administration for simple conditions should be avoided.

Screening for Other Conditions

There may be usefulness in developing screening procedure for hospital admissions. Gibson and Pritchard (1965) recommend that the following tests be applied routinely to every elderly patient admitted to hospital—analysis and culture of urine, estimation of haemoglobin, serum urea and electrolytes, blood sedimentation rate, nasal swab, the Wassermann, Kahn, and V.D.R.L. tests, faecal occult blood, E.C.G., chest X-ray, an assessment of the temperature, pulse, and respiration rates.

Where the Medical Officer of Health possesses adequate staff the means for preventive clinical and psycho-social assessments of older people should be provided and integrated in the work of the area geriatric consultant. Such a service has a relationship with patients which is personal and sustaining and may coexist with screening procedures available for mass numbers. Advisory health clinics (Anderson and Cowan, 1963) preferably derive their patients through the general practitioners. The medical examination includes routine estimation of body weight and haemoglobin, urine analysis, electrocardiography, X-ray of chest, and rectal examination. The physical diseases likely to be encountered at such a clinic are hypertension with symptoms, osteo-arthritis, anaemia, chronic bronchitis, fibrositis, previous coronary artery thrombosis, intermittent claudication, neoplasm, angina pectoris, and diabetes mellitus (Anderson, 1960).

It is a misfortune for the elderly that Gillis (1962) is constrained to write that in the course of years of contact with people in varied branches of the medical profession he has been struck by their feelings of inadequacy and need for instruction and concrete help in handling the human situations under discussion. To evaluate successfully the psycho-social problems of the aged the worker should possess a knowledge of the mechanics of human behaviour.

An advisory health clinic is not an isolated entity. It provides physiotherapy and chiropody, directs health visitors on health education, has immediate availability of the domiciliary services of the local authority, and liaises closely with voluntary effort.

Andrews and his colleagues (1971) described an integrated service based on a health centre where general practitioner, health visitor, social worker, and physician in geriatric medicine work together to plan comprehensive medical and psychosocial care of older people in the community.

Cardiovascular Diseases

The number of deaths attributed to coronary heart disease and hypertension has increased enormously in recent years in the western world. Many methods have been advocated for the early detection of these conditions, such as routine electrocardiography, serum cholesterol estimation, blood pressure estimation, etc.

Routine screening by electrocardiography will reveal cases of asymptomatic ischaemic disease, while the major risk factors (family history, blood pressure, serum cholesterol, cigarette smoking, lack of physical activity) can also be identified. However, the value of detection of untreatable disease is very doubtful, and there is as yet no evidence that alteration of the risk factors reduces the actual risk to the individual. There is, however, some support for the view that detection and treatment of moderate hypertension in middle age reduces the chances of stroke. Cochrane (1967) noted a considerable observer difference in the interpretation of E.C.G.s judged to show healed infarcts.

Glaucoma

In a survey of a random sample of the population in Oxford, 1·5 per cent. of persons over the age of 45 years had 'preglaucoma', Luntz et al. (1963); they stress the importance of routine measurement of the intra-ocular pressure, using a Schiotz tonometer in individuals over the age of 45 years. Cochrane (1967) suggests that screeners should concentrate on the relatives of known cases, as there is evidence that they form a high-risk group.

Diabetes

The prevalence of diabetes in 'western' communities is on the increase for two reasons:

1. The greater number of older persons in the community, the disease being eight times as common over the age of 50 years.

2. The discovery of insulin; whereas before this discovery people often died from the disease at a comparatively early age, now they remain alive to a ripe old age. It has been estimated that in the United States 2 per cent. of persons over the age of 40 years suffer from this disease and that there are probably about 1 million persons having the disease who are not aware of it.

The diagnosis of diabetes mellitus has special difficulties in the elderly, and there are now many reports of the results of mass screening surveys for this illness. These have used urine tests and blood tests, usually after a glucose load. The latter are undoubtedly preferable and have been made possible by automated methods for the measurement of blood sugar. There is now fair agreement that tape or stick methods (Dextrostix, etc.) are too inaccurate for this purpose. In the Bedford survey, where glucose-tolerance tests were done on a random sample of the population, a striking deterioration in the tests was noted with age. Over the age of 70 years nearly half the population had abnormal glucose tolerance, and similar findings have been confirmed in all surveys of the elderly population. In elderly people the discovery of glycosuria is an indication for blood-sugar determination. If the random blood sugar is over 200 mg. per cent. the patient has diabetes. If between 100 and 200 mg. per cent. a glucose tolerance test should be done. This test should be carried out after the patient has had a normal amount of carbohydrate in the diet for at least one week. If the test reveals a fasting blood sugar of over 120 mg./100 ml. and the highest blood-sugar level recorded more than 180 mg./100 ml. the likelihood is that the blood-sugar level will not return to the fasting level in 2 hours and that such a patient has diabetes. Some of the patients discovered in random sampling have undoubtedly diabetes by any definition, and their general health is improved by treatment, but when these are subtracted there are many whose abnormality is difficult to classify precisely. It is as yet uncertain what becomes of these people if they are left untreated or whether they benefit in any way from treatment; the answer to this will await adequate follow-up of the patients surveyed.

Keen and his associates (1965) concluded that symptomless impairment of glucose tolerance may be one of the important accompaniments of atherosclerotic disease in the general population, although confirmation of its causal role must await further evidence. It has also been stated that since the two major hazards of diabetes mellitus, namely ketosis and intercurrent infection, can now be controlled effectively, it is the vascular complications of the disease that give doctors the most concern. In our present state of knowledge symptomless diabetics should be detected, and those with symptoms and those without symptoms be treated actively.

Anaemia

There is no evidence that anaemia is ever due to the ageing process, but if figures are taken for hospital admission to geriatric units anaemia among the elderly is fairly common in hospital practice, reflecting as it does a strong pathological basis. Surveys of anaemia in the population have shown that under the age of 65 years, 3 per cent. of men and 14 per cent. of women have haemoglobin levels of under 12·5 g./100 ml. and 12 g./100 ml. respectively (Kilpatrick and Hardisty, 1961) and over that age 20 per cent. of both sexes (Jacobs et al., 1965). Parsons and his colleagues (1965) found anaemia in 10·8 per cent. of men and 15·7 per cent. of women aged over 65. Anaemia of the iron-deficiency type is common, and Bedford and Wollner (1958) concluded from a careful study of 156 patients that whatever other factors may be concerned, intestinal bleeding plays an important part in the pathogenesis of anaemia in old people. Women who have had menorrhagia before the menopause have difficulty in making up their iron supplies, and they remain anaemic even into old age, while partial gastrectomy in both sexes is a cause of anaemia worth bearing in mind.

It is fundamentally important that a proper diagnosis is made in the cases of anaemia detected and that iron is given only to those with hypochromic blood films and/or reduced mean corpuscular haemoglobin concentration (M.C.H.C.). In this way early cases of pernicious anaemia will not be missed. The need for well-organized follow-up is as great as in the cases of hyperglycaemia. Blood diseases in the elderly have been fully described by Thomas and Powell (1971).

Williamson (1966) found an average of 3·9 disabilities unknown to the family doctor in a survey of people over 65 years in three general practices in Edinburgh, and the unreported illnesses were predominantly those associated with locomotor difficulty, including foot troubles, incontinence, anaemia, and dementia. Present trends indicate that public demand will stimulate the further provision of schemes for early detection of disease. It seems essential that the person instituting and in prime control of such projects should be the family doctor. In his hands should rest at least a first-tier scheme. He may require specialist assistance in selective groups of older people, whom he may refer to consultative health centres for a second-tier type of survey [see CHAPTER 50].

MEDICAL AND PARAMEDICAL SERVICES FOR THE ELDERLY

In the past provision for the medical needs of the elderly has often been met in a rather haphazard fashion. Today there is a growing awareness of the need to plan such services on a more scientific and rational basis.

Surveys have been carried out in a number of places to assess the existing demand and future need for hospital and domiciliary services in relation to living conditions. From a review of existing schemes in various parts of the world, two main principles arise:

1. Care for the elderly is no longer considered a principle of charity; it is one of social justice.
2. The elderly have the right to choose how they will live, and it is important therefore to ensure that all the necessary services are available for their needs.

The organization of services for the elderly varies in different countries; thus in eastern Europe voluntary and private agencies are non-existent; in the United States, Switzerland, and the Netherlands they greatly influence public health programmes, while they play a minor role in Scandinavia. In the United Kingdom voluntary bodies still have an important role to play in complementing the welfare services provided by the State.

Medical and welfare services for the elderly should form an integral part of the general health and welfare services, and it is essential that there should be integration and co-operation at all levels and between the various branches of the services, e.g. between health and welfare services and between public and voluntary bodies. In Spain the General Directorate of Health has a special section on geriatrics and geroculture, while in the Netherlands public health service there is a special medical inspector for rehabilitation and care of the aged. In Great Britain and France there are special medical and social officers at Ministry level who deal with the problems of the elderly. In the United Kingdom at Regional level there are geriatric advisory committees, while in many cities there are liaison committees. At some hospitals there is frequent consultation between members of the branches of the service, e.g. at Leeds and Sheffield monthly conferences are held by the geriatric physicians. These various groups have representatives from hospitals, local health authorities, social work departments, and voluntary organizations.

It would appear that the best way to provide medical care for the elderly is by means of a comprehensive geriatric service, which includes domiciliary and hospital services providing for prevention, diagnosis, treatment, rehabilitation, and continuing care; mental health services should be included as an integral part. It is, and must always be, the endeavour of our social services to keep the old person fit and happy for as long as possible in the community [FIG. 95]. In order to accomplish this we must know how and where old people are living, so that ascertainment of disability is essential. Prevention of further disability and early detection of disease can be attempted, supervision of the old person at risk can be undertaken, and the older individual can be kept in the community. It is only when this can no longer be done that the patient is assessed in his own home prior to admission to hospital, and this is the routine in many geriatric units, where diagnosis, therapy, and follow-up can be instituted. The methodology of geriatric medicine is concerned with keeping the older person fit in the community, bearing in mind constantly the three aspects of his illness—physical, mental, and social, and the principle that an old person is ill, not because he is old but because he has a disease process. This concept, however, has

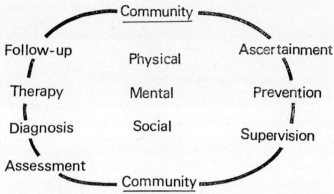

FIG. 95. The methodology of geriatric medicine.

not won universal acceptance, e.g. there are still many doctors who have not accepted the idea of organized medical services for the elderly.

DOMICILIARY SERVICES

In the United Kingdom the responsibility for providing these lies with the Local Health and Social Work Departments, and is augmented by various local voluntary services. Many local authorities, in addition to the normal domiciliary services provide a night-sitter service, a laundry service for the bed-ridden and incontinent with the loan of linen and blankets, a staff of bathing attendants, chiropody, and 'meals on wheels' services. In some areas voluntary organizations have organized such things as libraries, entertainments, friendly visiting, and shopping, hair-cutting, washing, and mending facilities which are not normally provided by local authorities. Domiciliary services should, wherever possible, include the following: advisory health clinics (as at Rutherglen in Scotland), home medical, dental, and nursing care, including the services of specialists; social work and special counselling services; physiotherapy; remedial exercises and graded physical activity; occupational therapy; chiropody; sheltered and home employment; the provision of appliances such as spectacles, hearing aids, nursing aids, and gadgets for the disabled; home help, health visiting, and night care service; supplementary meals, home laundry, and bath services; structural alterations to the homes of elderly people to enable them to live there although disabled; recreational and social activities, such as clubs and free transport facilities. Lunch clubs, all-day clubs and centres provide the opportunity of ensuring an adequate nutrition of older people by giving a midday meal, of laying on keep-fit exercises which can be supervised by physiotherapists, and of offering companionship and a change of environment to people who may live alone. Some authorities provide heating apparatus, furniture, bedding, food, and fuel for those in need. An immensely wide range of services can be provided by whole-hearted co-operation between the local authorities and the many excellent voluntary organizations. The modern trend in the United Kingdom is to extend domiciliary care and to encourage elderly people to remain in their own homes. This means not only a much happier life for them but that any existing relatives should be provided promptly with help to enable them to continue caring for their own elderly people. The Church can provide useful advice and help on spiritual and other matters.

HOSPITAL SERVICES

It is common experience in all acute medical wards that an increasing proportion of patients are to be found in the older age groups. In the United Kingdom, for example, in some general hospitals over 50 per cent. of patients are over 60 years of age. Nevertheless, there are special problems of the elderly which are best dealt with in a specialized unit known as a geriatric unit, which should have all the facilities to be found in a general hospital. This unit should be an integral part of a teaching or district general hospital just as any other specialist medical unit. It can be defined as a relatively high-cost unit, with a high proportion of medical and nursing staff giving active care for a short period of time, with special emphasis on diagnosis and rehabilitation and with adequate accommodation, equipment, and staff for physical medicine, remedial exercises, occupational therapy, diversional therapy, and recreation. The services of a chiropodist should be available. There should be attached to the unit a range of lower-cost units for different types of patients; units for further rehabilitation and continuing treatment and long-term nursing. Co-operation is essential with the authorities providing residential accommodation so that an adequate flow-through of patients is ensured. This accommodation should be able to take physically frail and mentally infirm elderly people. The numbers of beds in these supporting units must be sufficient to prevent a hold-up in the geriatric unit, so that the beds in the geriatric hospital wards have a turnover of the same order as a general medical unit. Ward design of the geriatric unit in the teaching or general hospital is important, and there are certain general principles; it is essential to have two day-spaces, one for those beginning their rehabilitation, who may have anti-social habits and who require constant observation; the second day-space can be more remote from the nursing station, and is for those who have advanced farther along the lines of rehabilitation and do not require such close observation. Day-spaces should always have adjacent lavatory facilities, as this will cut down the incontinent rate of the patients. In these geriatric units space for rehabilitation and day-space for sitting or watching television must be adequate. Day hospitals have been found useful in some countries to enable the patients to stay in their own surroundings while attending the hospital for investigation and treatment and to relieve overworked relatives. Some day hospitals have a few beds and are used as day-wards for special investigation and therapy. Day hospitals should be associated with day centres provided by the social work departments or voluntary agencies to ensure that there is an outlet for patients attending the day hospital. If this is not done the same group of patients will continue to attend the day hospital for many months when there is really no element of hospital treatment or therapy required. Some older people may well need the continued support and supervision provided by the day centre. Transport is of fundamental importance in the provision of such amenities.

A good example of a day-hospital scheme is that which has been set up by Dr. L. Z. Cosin at Oxford. In the morning the patients are collected from home, and in the evenings they are brought back again. Brocklehurst (1970) reviewed day hospital techniques confirming that the day hospital has an essential role in any comprehensive geriatric service.

The geriatric unit in the hospital makes the endeavour to enable old people to live independent lives for as long as possible by early accurate diagnosis and treatment of their disabilities and at the same time to arrange for them whatever practical support the community has to offer. When the disabilities of the elderly cause too much strain on relatives relief should be provided by attendance at day hospitals, day centres, or by admission to hospital or residential home for short or longer periods. At Leeds there is a day occupational centre for handicapped patients closely allied with the hospital follow-up clinic. This has saved a considerable number of hospital beds. An out-patient service is useful for the more ambulant patients, but in any case a transport service is essential. A team of social workers is necessary to ensure the optimal use of domiciliary and hospital services. The functions of a geriatric hospital service are as follows:

1. To accept new elderly patients whether labelled acute or chronic, and to arrange transfer from other wards in the hospital of patients who no longer need the services provided in these specialist units.

2. To provide facilities for the investigation and treatment of geriatric patients.

3. To provide, in partnership with the psychiatrist, a service for the mentally ill elderly for investigation and treatment with an outlet to continuing treatment hospital beds.

4. To afford earlier rehabilitation of the elderly by more adequate and prolonged use of physiotherapy and occupational therapy.

5. To discharge all rehabilitated patients from its wards, and to resettle them in their own homes.

6. To arrange the prompt transfer to continuing treatment hospital beds all irremediable patients.

7. To assess and periodically to review the suitability of all patients in continuing treatment hospital beds, so as to ensure no patient shall be regarded as irremediable while still capable of further improvement.

8. To arrange the co-ordination of medical and social work for the elderly.

9. To provide, on request, for general practitioners under the domiciliary health service special advice about their elderly patients at home or in consultative clinics.

10. To afford facilities for expert advice on the medical aspects of welfare or housing schemes for the aged.

11. In selected departments to provide teaching in the geriatric aspects of medicine, nursing, and physiotherapy.

12. To encourage research in geriatrics and gerontology.

The term long-stay hospital has been changed to continuing treatment unit to indicate that in such places there is physiotherapy, speech therapy, occupational therapy, chiropody, and constant skilled nursing attention. The physician must never be blinded by the diagnosis and, for this reason only, discontinue his efforts to improve the physical, mental, and social health of his patient.

There is a definite place for the full-time geriatric physician (geriatrician), who will co-ordinate all the various branches and who will devote himself whole time to the special needs of the elderly. General physicians are sometimes more interested in the problems of acute disease, and have in the past tended to be rather apathetic about the care of the chronic sick and the elderly. Moreover, they are not always sufficiently experienced in the clinical problems of the elderly, for example, familiar diseases present themselves in a different way, and the special therapeutic problems are not always known. Often elderly patients are sent to hospital for purely social reasons, occupying a high-cost bed, which could be prevented by the provision of lower-cost domiciliary services. For this reason many physicians practising geriatric medicine visit routinely all patients for whom the family doctor has requested hospital admission.

Every call for help or any kind of social service by the elderly should be accompanied by a medico-social assessment, possibly performed jointly by the family doctor and a social worker. It is essential to make sure that the elderly are not provided with social support when in fact what they require is a correct diagnosis and appropriate therapy. In some cases the physician practising geriatric medicine can give advice on the care of a patient at home by carrying out domiciliary visits, and in some areas assessment before admission to hospital is done by the hospital geriatric physician who visits the patient's own home or who may see the elderly person at a health centre and be given a report on the social circumstances by a health visitor or social worker.

Large numbers of old people live in conditions of such isolation that they may become bedridden before their plight is noticed. A register of special cases requiring frequent visiting will help to prevent this from happening. The problem of ascertainment remains the most important one at present in geriatric medicine and in some areas routine visiting of those 70 years and over by a health visitor is being started.

Surveys in the United Kingdom show that where there is a full geriatric service of the type described here, with comprehensive local authority services and good housing, a ratio of 1·2 beds per 1,000 population will give an adequate hospital service. An efficient geriatric service should relieve the need for any more hospital beds than this. Cosin (1952) has in fact been able to reduce the number of beds. Where there are bad housing conditions or inadequate domiciliary services, then a ratio of 2 beds per 1,000 of the population may be necessary. It is better to express the ratio as beds per 1,000 of elderly persons, in which 15–17 beds per 1,000 aged 65 years and over are reasonable figures. These figures do not include beds in psychogeriatric units or mental hospitals which may be required by elderly people. In addition, an accurate estimate of hospital beds required by the elderly sick depends on local housing for the elderly, the number of places available in protected housing or special hostels, the provision of domiciliary services, and the number of general medical and psychiatric beds available for older people in the area.

Training. The problems of geriatrics are not taught adequately either to medical students or in postgraduate courses, and there is much to be said for the setting up of specialist gerontological centres for the study of the problems of ageing, e.g. as at Kiev, Paris, and Glasgow, and to stimulate teaching in all branches of geriatrics. The World Health Organization has sponsored international courses in geriatrics for physicians in Glasgow (1964, 1967), in Kiev (1965), and in Paris (1966). (See Isaacs, 1964; Hobson and Akhmetely, 1963; and Anderson, 1970.)

AN AREA GERIATRIC SERVICE

A description of an area geriatric service based on a local teaching or district hospital and providing for the needs of a population of approximately 200,000 is outlined (Anderson, 1971). For this defined area and population two physicians in geriatric medicine (with supporting medical staff) are stationed at the hospital. These physicians pay routine visits to the health centres in the hospital area. The geriatric assessment unit is situated in the hospital and is supported by:

1. Continuing treatment hospital beds in two situations, near the hospital and also in smaller groups near the places from which the patients come.
2. Specially constructed homes for the physically frail and also for the mentally infirm provided by the social work department of the local authority.
3. Small nests of protected (warden-supervised) housing where elderly people can live with constant 24-hour cover in case of illness or accident [FIG. 96].

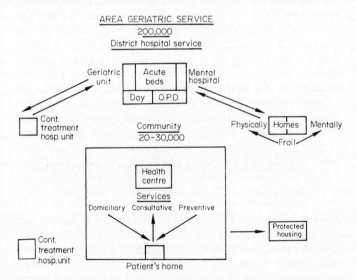

FIG. 96. Area geriatric service. [Anderson, W. F. (1971) *Practical Management of the Elderly*, 2nd ed., Blackwell, Oxford.]

The older people attend their own general practitioner who works at a health centre where the local services for the elderly are co-ordinated. The ascertainment of elderly people by routine home visiting, e.g. of the 70s and over, is carried out by health visitors based on this centre; the domiciliary services, e.g. home (district) nurse, home helps, voluntary services, meals on wheels, are organized from the health centre; chiropody, physiotherapy and occupational therapy can be

provided, and information regarding all the facilities for older people is available there. The old persons, or their relatives, should only have to come to one place to obtain help of any kind. To this health centre the physician in geriatric medicine from the hospital comes routinely to advise on the preventive measures, e.g. the routine visiting of the elderly, and to run an

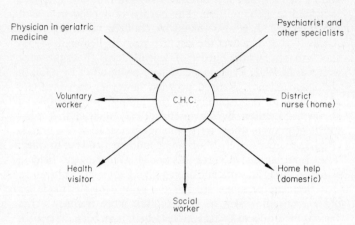

FIG. 97. Community health centre. [Anderson, W. F. (1971) *Practical Management of the Elderly*, 2nd ed., Blackwell, Oxford.]

out-patient clinic for older people. The general practitioners are supported by the health team [FIG. 97] and play an active part in the prevention and treatment of disease in the elderly.

This area geriatric service linked with voluntary workers at day centres, lunch clubs, and hobbies and crafts centres can give comprehensive care to the elderly ensuring that all old people 'at risk' in an area are known about and visited regularly.

In a recent random sample of 800 people 65 years and over (Caird, 1972) where major diability and dependence were estimated, 48 per cent. of the disabled had organic brain disease and 22 per cent. functional psychiatric disorder. Of the dependent people, 93 per cent. had organic brain disease of whom 78 per cent. were demented.

There is no doubt that services for the mentally disordered elderly must be rationalized and expanded. Specially trained home helps, special homes for the mentally infirm, small specialized psychogeriatric units and planned co-operation between psychiatrist and physician in geriatric medicine have been suggested (*Services for the Elderly with Mental Disorder*, 1970).

ECONOMIC AND SOCIAL IMPLICATIONS OF AN AGEING POPULATION

There have been three stages in economic development affecting the care of the elderly:

1. The agricultural stage, in which the aged are cared for and continued to work within the framework of the family. This is the traditional pattern in most parts of the world today.
2. The industrial stage, in which the industrial worker has to save to keep himself in his old age; this is rarely possible,

and has caused most economically developed countries to adopt the third stage.

3. The social stage, in which the aged are taken care of under social insurance or pension schemes.

The increasing number of old persons causes greater demands for pensions. In the United Kingdom, for example, the cost of retirement pensions was about £500 million per annum in 1960, and it is estimated that by 1980 this will have increased to £800 million. The burden of dependency, as it has been called, is also shared by children under 15 years. An analysis of data over the last fifty years by Benjamin (1952) shows that in fact the burden of dependency is about the same as it was in 1901, a rise in pensioners being offset by a fall in child dependency. Retired persons, however, do contribute something to the running of the family; for example, a survey in London by Townsend (1957) showed that two-thirds of grandmothers were looking after at least one grandchild, in many cases enabling young mothers to go out to work. The International Centre of Social Gerontology held a seminar (1971) on work and ageing giving some present trends.

Retirement pensions are not the only demands made by old persons, however, as they require more frequently the various medical and social services which have been described.

Statistics compiled by the Metropolitan Life Insurance Company, New York, 1953–55, show that the average number of days of disability illness in males was 3·2 in the age group 25–44 years, but 27·0 in the age group 60–64 years, while the average number of days in hospital for men rose from 0·7 in

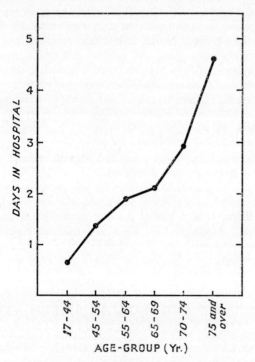

FIG. 98. Days in hospital by age, 1953–55.

those under 45 years to 4·6 for 75 years and over [FIGS. 98 and 99]. In these circumstances the employment and retirement of elderly persons becomes an important question. In an agricultural community old people are traditionally cared for by

the family; in industrial communities there is a tendency for the family to split up, with the result that more old people are living alone, particularly widows (females living longer than males). Even so, in many cities married children live quite

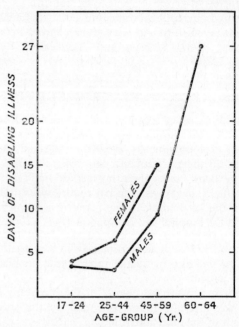

FIG. 99. Annual number of days of disabling illness by age-groups.

close, in the same or next street, and continue to provide care and attention for their old folk. The introduction of comprehensive social-insurance schemes has been blamed for diminution in family responsibility for the care of the elderly; in England, in the cities, approximately 25 per cent. of people over the age of 65 years live alone, and the same percentage have no relatives to help them in time of trouble or difficulty, while at present about two-thirds of all hospital beds in the country occupied by those over 65 years are occupied by the single, widowed, and divorced, and in relation to their numbers this group makes double the demand on hospital beds.

OCCUPATION AND RETIREMENT

The normal retirement age varies in different countries from 50 to 70 years according to sex and type of employment. In Australia, Belgium, Denmark, and the United Kingdom it is 65 years for men and 60 years for women. In the U.S.S.R. 60 years for men and 55 years for women. In Canada, Ireland, and Norway the normal retirement age for men is 70 years, in Argentina it is 55 years of age; in India university staff retire at 55 years. In certain countries, e.g. Belgium, France, and the U.S.S.R., pensionable age varies with the nature of the employment. Thus locomotive drivers and coal-miners retire at an earlier age. The age of retirement for politicians, clergymen, and judges is often over 80 years, while some craftsmen never retire. There are over 6 million retired persons in the United Kingdom today, and over 1,000 people are retiring every day. The ageing of population has brought an increasing need for the employment of older workers from the point of view of the national economy, but there may be other reasons why this is necessary; it has often been said that retirement is bad for old people, although there is little real evidence for this statement; recently retired old people often deteriorate, but that may be due to the fact that ill health may have caused the retirement.

A great deal of research work is being carried out on the physical and psychological capabilities of men in relation to work and the change which takes place with age. The results show that there is little decrease in efficiency with moderately hard physical work up to the age of 70 years, provided the conditions do not become too arduous and provided speed is not an essential factor. This is borne out by a study in Birmingham (Brown *et al.*, 1958) which showed that 75 per cent. of men aged 69 years were still capable of whole time work for which their experience and training suited them. In fact, Logan (1970) pointed out that three-quarters of men over 70 in Britain could do full time work in their previous job if society would let them. Heron and Chown (1967) stated that compulsory retirement provided a striking example of the way in which an arbitrary choice made in one era of social and medical history can become fixed despite later changes. They reviewed the many aspects of compulsory retirement and concluded that the use of a profile in terms of 'functional ages' might be helpful in matching people to suitable work and would be a more rational approach than is represented by the rigid application of limits based solely on chronological age. Evidence from a number of sources indicates that about 20 per cent. of men by the age of 65 years need to change their job if they are to have a chance of permanent employment: there are exceptions for heavy jobs like coal-mining, for example. Where age affects performance, usually some trivial factor is causing it. Future promise in industry is to change the lay-out of tools rather than attempting to find new jobs, because this leads to a wastage of old skills. The evidence lends no support to the idea of a fixed age for retirement from employment, rather there should be an opportunity for older people to continue in work or to change to some job which is best suited for their capabilities. There are certain physical conditions, however, which would disqualify a person from continuing work, for example, severe angina, a previous stroke, or failure of vision. In view of the wide variations in the capabilities of older people, it might be desirable to have some means of discrimination by psychological and other tests. Those with the best educational and cultural background show the least change with age, and diminution in the powers of critical reasoning may be more than compensated by the knowledge and wisdom gained as a result of experience. There is a great need for more refined tests which will measure the intellectual capacity in the aged. The present tests do not measure many of the higher mental abilities and tend to discriminate against the elderly, particularly where speed is a factor. They take no account of difficulties due to physical disabilities, for example, deafness, tinnitus, defects of vision, tremor, weakness, or the fact that tests become more threatening and fearful to the individual as age increases. Thus psychological tests may underestimate the real capacities of old people. It is essential that some form of health supervision should be available to elderly workers, and there should be special counselling programmes and a definite employment policy on the part of employers, employees, and the Ministry of Labour. Special

schemes have been set up in many of the large firms in Britain, France, and the United States to provide suitable alternative employment for older workers. The ideal arrangements would seem to be to place older workers in jobs which form an integral part of work in the factory, rather than to segregate them. Older workers also have a greater need for adequate lighting, and are often sensitive to such things as cold, damp, draughts, and noise. A little relaxation in the hour of starting and finishing may help them to avoid the difficulties of the 'rush hour'. In any case, older workers must have freedom of choice about their future employment. Some of the heavy industries are unable to employ their elderly and disabled at all, in which case it may be necessary to find sheltered or part-time employment, including home employment.

In one London borough a group of old people receive payment for such activities as labelling articles for sale, covering coat hangers, packing small articles. The work is not arduous, they can do it in their own time, and it requires a minimum of training. They are given free transport to the workplace. At Bicêtre near Paris about 1,000 old people are employed in printing for the *Assistance Publique*, while at Basle many old men from one institution help with the staffing of a nearby hospital. In Canada, General Motors has a series of classes to train older people to undertake new jobs; retirement is referred to as 'change of occupation'.

Much work has been done recently on the employment of older workers. A seminar was held at Heidelberg in 1965 with the basic purpose of codifying all existing material in the problem of employment of older workers. A re-employment bureau opened in Glasgow in 1967 has found over 1280 part-time paid jobs for retired people who desire such employment. Discrimination against older workers, which is still a common practice, can be overcome effectively only if the training of older workers and job redesign are applied simultaneously and consistently.

It may be that in the future increasing use of automation will mean that men will have to work shorter hours or retire at an earlier age; certainly when there is unemployment the elderly are the first to be laid off. Unfortunately, one of the chief causes of retirement, apart from ill health, is the criticism of old people by younger workers. The trade unions have been particularly critical, and in the past have not been in favour of employing older people because of the argument that they would keep younger people out of a job or block the promotion line. This attitude is now changing, as many younger workers realize that they, too, will some day grow old.

The proper use of leisure is an important means of promoting health in all ages. Many old people have developed useful hobbies and pastimes of their own, but unfortunately there are still many who have never been able to do this. There should be for them organized programmes which will include creative, cultural, educational, and recreational activities, such as organized holidays, short travels, and Darby and Joan Clubs. The Hudson Community Center, New York, trains elderly persons in games, hobbies, and trades, where in the words of the director, 'they are re-created through recreation'. Preparation for retirement is very important, and since 1959 the Glasgow Retirement Council has been running day-release courses one day per week, for seven weeks, for older employees within five years of their probable retirement and whose employers are willing to release them without loss of earnings. This council also provides hobbies and crafts centre for those who have retired to allow them to make furnishings for their homes or toys for their grandchildren. The formation of retired employees' associations is also encouraged, and this type of organization, means that those who formerly worked together remain as friends after retirement, meeting regularly in the works canteen and being helped by the personnel officer of the interested firm. These associations ensure that any member who is sick, lonely, or in trouble of any kind is visited by one of his former colleagues and by the personnel officer of the sponsoring firm. Such associations contribute greatly to the morale of the retired employee.

HOUSING

Proper accommodation is of primary importance for the health and well-being of old people. It is generally agreed that old people are healthier and happier in their own home surroundings, although some prefer to be in small residential homes or hotels. For this reason the provision of adequate domiciliary medical services is essential. In addition, there should be a range of residential accommodation available for those who are too infirm to look after themselves. The present policy is to provide nests of good housing for older people mixed with the general community, to supply a small number of these with specialized equipment as for the disabled of any age, and to discourage fit older individuals from entering residential accommodation. The slightly frail elderly person should be cared for in some form of protected housing, where she is given a room, or rooms, of her own, with her own furnishings, and in such accommodation a younger person can supervise six to ten such older frail people. In such protected housing added security is given if the warden or caretaker has an efficient intercommunication system which operates in each of the tenant's rooms. If the physical condition of the older person will not allow this, then residential accommodation of frail ambulant type should be provided for those who require help in dressing or assistance in going to the toilet. A modern development has been homes for the mentally frail, where older people who have been completely assessed by the physician practising geriatric medicine and the psychiatrist, and who have irremediable but mild mental deterioration, can be cared for. Such people if collected together can be supervised in specialized accommodation by a minimum of nursing staff. Homes of this type relieve pressure on both geriatric and psychogeriatric beds. Comprehensive and accurate assessment of the patient is essential before admission to welfare accommodation of this type. The correct categorization of the older person can ensure proper placement and greatly enhance her prospects of happiness. Some welfare authorities have solved the problem by 'boarding out' old people in the same way that young children deprived of their parents may be boarded out. The special needs of the elderly are dealt with in more detail in CHAPTER 5.

CONCLUSION

In western Europe the emphasis in public health is now shifting from child health to the problems of old people, due to the remarkable achievements of medicine during the past twenty to thirty years. The doctor and nurse now need to spend more and more of their time dealing with the elderly.

While it is true that we are not yet able to do very much in preventing the process of ageing, nevertheless we can make great contributions to the mental and physical well-being of the elderly by early detection of illness and by controlling what once were regarded as hopeless and progressive infirmities.

The methods of control are by health education, early detection of disease and disability, and by active physical and mental rehabilitation. This requires the provision of a whole range of medical and social services. Teaching of all nurses and medical students should include instruction in the practice of geriatric medicine.

In the care of the elderly the distinction between preventive, social, and curative medicine is especially artificial; they are inextricably bound up in what should be comprehensive medicine. The family doctor should be the central figure in the care of the elderly, and he should have available a wide variety of personnel and services so essential for the multidisciplinary approach to these problems. At all times there should be recognition of the primary importance of services designed to help people remain in their own homes.

The features of life most dreaded by old people are insecurity and loneliness; legislation aided by taxation can solve the former, but the prime responsibility for the latter lies with the family. The Welfare State can never absolve the individual from his moral responsibility to look after 'his ain folk'.

In these days we have given up the idea of rejuvenation; rather should we aim at enabling all persons to reach an old age which is worth living. This is what Aristotle called eugeria, which he defined as 'slowness in the oncome of old age, with freedom from pain'.

It is only since the end of the Second World War that these ideas have gained acceptance even in western Europe, but they are still not sufficiently understood in many parts of the world. It is certain that public health administration and the content of medical curricula will have to be drastically revised in many countries to cope with the changing scene.

REFERENCES AND FURTHER READING

A comprehensive bibliography is contained in the following:

Shock, N. W. (1951, 1957, 1963) *A Classified Bibliography of Gerontology and Geriatrics*, Stanford. This has been kept up to date by appendixes in the *Journal of Gerontology*.

General Works Covering a Variety of Topics on Geriatrics and Gerontology

Agate, John (1970) *The Practice of Geriatrics*, London.
Anderson, W. F. (1967, 1968, 1969/70, 1970/71, 1971/72, 1972/73) Geriatric medicine, in *Medical Progress*, British Encyclopaedia of Medical Practice, London.
Anderson, W. F. (1971) *Practical Management of the Elderly*, Oxford.
Anderson, W. F., and Isaacs, B. (1964) *Current Achievements in Geriatrics*, London.
Bourlière, François (1969) *Progrès en Gérontologie*, Paris.
Brocklehurst, J. C., ed. (1973) *Textbook of Geriatric Medicine and Gerontology*, London.

Gerontology and Geriatrics Year-Book (1970–71) *Ageing of a Cell*, Frolkis, V. V., Kiev.

Gerontology and Geriatrics Year-Book (1971) *Atherosclerosis of Cerebral Vessels and Ageing*, ed. Mankovsky, Kiev.

Hansen, P. From., ed. (1964) *Age with a Future*, Proceedings of the Sixth International Congress of Gerontology, Copenhagen, 1963, Copenhagen.

Hazell, Kenneth (1973) *Social and Medical Problems of the Elderly*, 3rd ed., London.

Hobson, W., ed. (1956) *Modern Trends in Geriatrics*, London.

Proceedings Eighth International Congress of Gerontology (1969) Vols 1 and 2. Abstracts of Symposia and Lectures. Federation of American Societies for Experimental Biology, Washington.

Rossman, Isadore, ed. (1971) *Clinical Geriatrics*, Philadelphia.

Shock, N. W. (1957) *Trends in Gerontology*, 2nd ed., Stanford.

Shock, N. W., ed. (1966) *Perspectives in Experimental Gerontology*, Illinois.

Shock, N. W. (1968) The physiology of ageing, in *Surgery of the Aged and Debilitated Patient*, ed. Powers, J. H., Philadelphia.

Stieglitz, Edward J., ed. (1954) *Geriatric Medicine*, 3rd ed., Philadelphia.

Biological Aspects of Ageing

Birren, J. E., Butler, R. N., Greenhouse, S. W., Sokoloff, L., and Yarrow, M. R. (1963) *Human Aging*, Public Health Service Publication No. 986, Washington.

Bourlière, F. (1970) The assessment of biological age in man, *Wld Hlth Org. Publ. Hlth Pap.*, No. 37.

Brožek, J., and Simonson, E. (1962) Russian research on ageing, *Geriatrics*, **17**, 464.

Burnett, F. M. (1970) An immunological approach to ageing, *Lancet*, **ii**, 358.

Comfort, A. (1956) *The Biology of Senescence*, New York.

Comfort, A. (1969) Test-battery to measure ageing rate in man *Lancet*, **ii**, 1411.

Court-Brown, W. M. (1967) *Human Population Cytogenetics*, Amsterdam.

Cowdry, E. V. (1952) *Cowdry's Problems of Ageing: Biological and Medical Aspects*, 3rd ed., ed. Lansing, A. I., Baltimore.

Goldman, R. (1971) Decline in organ function with ageing, in *Clinical Geriatrics*, ed. Rossman, Isadore, Philadelphia.

Hollingsworth, J. W., Hashizume, A., and Jablon, S. (1965) Correlation between tests of ageing in Hiroshima subjects —An attempt to define 'physiologic ageing', *Yale J. Biol. Med.*, **38**, 11.

Jarvik, L. F., Falek, A., Kallmann, F. J., and Lorge, I. (1960) Survival trends in a senescent twin population, *Amer. J. hum. Genet.*, **12**, 170.

Korenchevsky, V. (1961) *Physiological and Pathological Ageing*, Basel.

Pearl, R. (1931) Studies on human longevity, IV. The Inheritance of Longevity. Preliminary Report, *Hum. Biol.*, **3**, 245.

Shock, Nathan W., ed. (1962) *Ageing Around the World. Biological Aspects of Ageing*, New York.

Strehler, B. L. (1971) Ageing at the cellular level, in *Clinical Geriatrics*, ed. Rossman, Isadore, Philadelphia.

Waldorf, R. L. (1969) *The Immunologic Theory of Ageing*, Copenhagen.

Welford, A. T. (1964) The study of ageing, *Brit. med. Bull.*, **20**, 65.

Yapp, W. B., and Bourne, G. H., eds. (1957) *The Biology of Ageing*, London.

Demographic Aspects

Benjamin, R. (1952) in *The Biology of Ageing*, ed. Yapp, W. B., and Bourne, G. H., p. 55, London.

Geill, T. (1963) *Life Span and Expectation of Life of Elderly People under Different Conditions and Cultures*, Working Paper Euro 245/3 for the WHO Seminar on the Health Protection of the Elderly, WHO Regional Office for Europe, Copenhagen.

Organization for European Economic Co-operation (O.E.C.D.) (1956) *Demographic Trends in Western Europe, 1951–71*, Paris.

Royal Commission on Population, *Report (1949)*, London, H.M.S.O.

United Nations (1964) *Demographic Year Book 1963*, New York.

Economic and Social Aspects

Brockington, F., and Lempert, S. M. (1966) *The Social Needs of the Over Eighties*, Manchester.

National Council of Social Service (1954) *Over Seventy: Report on an Investigation into the Social and Economic Circumstances of One Hundred People over Seventy Years of Age*, London.

Old Age (1968) Number 26, Office of Health Economics, London.

Report of the Committee on the Economic and Financial Problems of the Provision of Old Age (1954) London, H.M.S.O.

Report of the Committee of Enquiry into the Cost of the National Health Service (1956) London, H.M.S.O.

United Nations (1956) Department of Economic and Social Affairs, Population Studies No. 26, *The Aging of Populations and its Economic and Social Implications*, New York.

Valaoras, Vasilios, G. (1950) in *The Social and Biological Challenge of our Aging Population*, New York.

Surveys of the Health and Social Conditions of Old People

Australia

Hutchinson, B. (1954) *Old People in a Modern Australian Community*, Melbourne.

Barrow-in-Furness

Edge, J. R., and Nelson, I. D. M. (1964) Survey of arrangements for the elderly in Barrow-in-Furness, *Med. Care*, **2**, 7.

Birmingham

Brown, R. G., McKeown, T., and Whitfield, A. G. W. (1958) Observations on the medical condition of men in the seventh decade, *Brit. med. J.*, **1**, 555.

Denmark

Lund, E. (1963) Gerontology and geriatrics in Denmark, *Nord. med.*, **70**, 885.

Eire

The Care of the Aged (1968) Report of an Inter-departmental Committee, Dublin.

Finland

Jalavisto, E. (1963) Gerontology and geriatrics in Finland, *Nord. med.*, **70**, 887.

Great Britain

Miller, H. C. (1963) *The Ageing Countryman*, London.

Townsend, P. (1959) Social Surveys of Old Age in Great Britain 1945–1958, *Wld Hlth Org. Bull.*, **21**, 583.

Townsend, P. (1962) *The Last Refuge. A Survey of Residential Institutions and Homes for the Aged in England and Wales*, London.

London

Townsend, P. (1957) *The Family Life of Old People*, London.

Netherlands

Zonneveld, R. J. van (1957) *Health Problems of the Aged*, Essen.

Zonneveld, R. J. van (1962) A national health examination survey of the elderly in the Netherlands, *Geront. clin. (Basel)*, **4**, 198.

New Zealand

Elderly Person Accommodation Needs in New Zealand (1962) Department of Health Special Report Series No. 10, Wellington.

Northern Ireland

Adams, G. F., and Cheeseman, E. A. (1951) *Old People in Northern Ireland*, Belfast.

Norway

Gaustad, V. (1963) Gerontology and geriatrics in Norway, *Nord. med.*, **70**, 888.

Strom, A. (1956) An investigation of the living conditions and health of 1389 persons aged 70 years or more in Norway, *J. Geront.*, **11**, 178.

Scotland

Richardson, I. M. (1964) *Age and Need. A Study of Older People in North-East Scotland*, Edinburgh.

Sheffield

Hobson, W., and Pemberton, J. (1955) *The Health of the Elderly at Home*, London.

Singapore

Davies, T. A. L., and Mills, Rosemary (1956) 'Honour thy Father and thy Mother'. A study of the medico-social needs of old people living in Singapore, *Lancet*, **i**, 835.

Sweden

Eckerstrom, S. (1963) Gerontology and geriatrics in Sweden, *Nord med.*, **70**, 892.

Wolverhampton

Sheldon, J. H. (1948) *The Social Medicine of Old Age*, London.

United States

Bond, F. A., Baber, R. E., Vieg, J. A., Perry, L. B., Scoff, A. H., and Lee, L. J., Jr. (1954) *Our Needy Aged. A California Study of a National Problem*, New York.

The Services Available for the Elderly

Adams, G. F., and McIlwraith, P. L. (1963) *Geriatric Nursing. A Study of the Work of Geriatric Ward Staff*, London.

Adams, G. F. (1969) *Review of Geriatric Services in Northern Ireland Hospitals*, Belfast.

Boucher, C. A. (1962) Services for old people, *Physiotherapy*, **48**, 86.

Brocklehurst, J. C. (1970) *The Geriatric Day Hospital*, London.

Chebotarev, D. F. (1963) Medical Attention for Elderly and Old People in the U.S.S.R. Working Paper Euro 245/13 for WHO Seminar on the Health Protection of the Elderly, WHO Regional Office for Europe, Copenhagen.

European Office of the Technical Assistance Administration, UN (1956) *Report of European Seminar on Social Services for the Aged, Liege, 1955*, Geneva.

Exton-Smith, A. N., Norton, Doreen, and MacLaren, Rhoda (1962) *An Investigation of Geriatric Nursing Problems in Hospital*, London.

Farndale, James (1961) *The Day Hospital Movement in Great Britain*, Oxford.

Fry, J. (1957) Care of the elderly in general practice: A socio-medical reassessment, *Brit. med. J.*, **2**, 666.

Goldberg, E. M. (1970) *Helping the Aged*, London.

Gordon, C., Thomson, J. G., and Emerson, A. R. (1957) Domiciliary services for over sixties, *Med. Offr*, **98**, 19.

Royal College of Physicians of Edinburgh (1963) Publication No. 22, *The Care of the Elderly in Scotland*, Edinburgh.

Royal College of Physicians of Edinburgh (1970) Publication No. 37, *The Care of the Elderly in Scotland: A Follow-Up Report*, Edinburgh.

Services for the Elderly with Mental Disorder (1970) Edinburgh, H.M.S.O.

Shenfield, Barbara E. (1957) *Social Policies for Old Age*, London.

Thomson, A. P., Lowe, C. R., and McKeown, T. (1951) *The Care of the Ageing and Chronic Sick*, Edinburgh.

Wright, Catherine, H., and Roberts, L. (1958) The place of the Home Help Service in the care of the aged, *Lancet*, **i**, 254.

Physical and Mental Capacity

Adams, G. F. (1967) Problems in the treatment of hemiplegia, *Geront. clin. (Basel)*, **9**, 285.

Anand, M. P. (1964) Accidents in the home, in *Current Achievements in Geriatrics*, ed. Anderson, W. F., and Isaacs, B., London.

Anderson, I., Campbell, A. E. R., Dunn, A., and Runciman, J. B. M. (1966) Osteomalacia in elderly women, *Scot. med. J.*, **11**, 429.

Anderson, W. F., and Cowan, N. R. (1959a) The influences of adiposity and varicose veins on arterial pressure in older women, *Clin. Sci.*, **18**, 125.

Anderson, W. F., and Cowan, N. R. (1959b) Arterial pressure in healthy older people, *Clin. Sci.*, **18**, 103.

Belbin, R. M. (1953) Difficulties of older people in industry, *Occup. Psychol.*, **27**, 177.

Brožek, J., Keys, A., and Taylor, H. L. (1966) *Longitudinal Research: The Minnesota Study*. Abstracts of papers presented at the 7th International Congress of Gerontology, p. 38, Vienna.

Busse, E. W. (1966) *The Effect of Aging upon the Central Nervous System*. Abstracts of Papers Presented at the 7th International Congress of Gerontology, p. 40, Vienna.

Caird, F. (1972) Personal communication.

Caird, F., Pirie, A., and Ramsell, T. G. (1969) *Diabetes and the Eye*, Oxford.

Chebotarev, D. F., and Sachuk, N. (1964) Sociomedical examination of longevous people in the U.S.S.R., *J. Geront.*, **19**, 435.

Gatter, R. A., and McCarty, D. J. Jr. (1967) Polymyalgia rheumatica: A rheumatic disease of the elderly, *Geriatrics*, **22**, 3.

Grannis, G. F. (1970) Demographic perturbations secondary to cigarette smoking, *J. Geront.*, **25**, No. 1, 55.

Gsell, O. R. (1967) Longitudinal gerontological research over 10 years (Basle Studies 1955–1965), *Geront. clin. (Basel)*, **9**, 67.

Hamilton, J. B., and Mestlet, C. E. (1969) Mortality and survival: Comparison of eunuchs with intact men and women in a mentally disturbed population, *J. Geront.*, **24**, No. 4, 395.

Haranghy, L. (1965) *Gerontological Studies on Hungarian Centenarians*, Budapest.

Harrison, M. J. G., and Bevan, A. T. (1967) Early symptoms of temporal arteritis, *Lancet*, **ii**, 638.

Hobson, W. (1955) The effects of ageing on mental and physical capacity, *Practitioner*, **174**, 527.

Hughes, G. (1969) Changes in taste sensitivity with advancing age, *Geront. clin. (Basel)*, **11**, 225.

Kay, D. W. K., and Walk, A., eds. (1971) *Recent Developments in Psychogeriatrics. A Symposium*, Royal Medico-Psychological Association, London.

McKeown, F. (1965) *Pathology of the Aged*, London.

Macmillan, A. L., Corbett, J. L., Johnson, R. H., Crompton Smith, A., Spalding, J. M. K., and Wollner, L. (1967) Temperature regulation in survivors of accidental hypothermia of the elderly, *Lancet*, **ii**, 165.

Newman, J. L. (1969) *The Prevention of Incontinence.* 8th International Congress of Gerontology. Proceedings, **2**, 75. Federation of American Societies for Experimental Biology, Washington.

Pathy, M. S. (1967) Clinical presentation of myocardial infarcts in the elderly, *Brit. Heart J.*, **29**, 190.

Pomerance, A. (1965a) Pathology of the heart with and without cardiac failure in the aged, *Brit. Heart J.*, **27**, 697.

Pomerance, A. (1965b) Senile cardiac amyloidosis, *Brit. Heart J.*, **27**, 711.

Welford, A. T. (1958) *Ageing and Human Skill,* London.

Wollner, L. (1967) Accidental hypothermia and temperature regulation in the elderly, *Geront. clin. (Basel)*, **9**, 347.

Employment of the Elderly

Amulree, Lord (1955) The health problems of old workers, *Wld Hlth Org. Bull.*, **13**, 575.

Anderson, W. F., and Cowan, N. R. (1956) Work and retirement: Influences on the health of older men, *Lancet*, **ii**, 1344.

Blythe Brooke, C. O. S. (1955) Sheltered workshop in a London Borough in old age, in *The Modern World*, ed. Tunbridge, R. E., p. 593, Edinburgh.

Clark, F. Le Gros (1956) *The Employment Problems of Elderly Men*, London.

Heron, A., and Chown, Sheila (1967) *Age and Function*, London.

Hobson, W. (1956) Employment, retirement and health, in *Modern Trends in Geriatrics*, ed. Hobson, W., p. 391, London.

International Centre of Social Gerontology (1971) *Work and Ageing*, 2nd International Course in Social Gerontology, Paris.

International Labour Office (1955) *The Age of Retirement*, European Regional Conference, Geneva.

Logan, R. F. (1970) The aged in Britain, *Interdisc. Top. Geront.*, **5**, 83.

National Advisory Committee on the Employment of Older Men and Women (1955) Second Report, London, H.M.S.O.

Nutrition

Andrews, J., Brook, M., and Allen, M. A. (1966) Influence of abode and season on the vitamin C status of the elderly, *Geront. clin. (Basel)*, **8**, 257.

Batata, M., Spray, G. H., Bolton, F. G., Higgins, G., and Wollner, L. (1967) Blood and bone marrow changes in elderly patients with special reference to folic acid, vitamin B_{12}, iron and ascorbic acid, *Brit. med. J.*, **2**, 667.

Exton-Smith, A. N., and Stanton, B. R. (1965) *Report of an Investigation into the Dietary of Elderly Women Living Alone*, King Edward's Hospital Fund, London.

Girdwood, R. H. (1969) Nutritional folate deficiency in the United Kingdom, *Scot. med. J.*, **14**, 296.

Griffiths, L. L., Brocklehurst, J. C., Scott, D. L., Marks, J., and Blackley, J. (1967) Thiamine and ascorbic acid levels in the elderly, *Geront. clin. (Basel)*, **9**, 1.

Hartiala, K. (1963) Study of Nutritional Requirements of the Elderly. Working Paper Euro 245/4 for WHO Seminar on the Health Protection of the Elderly, WHO Regional Office, for Europe, Copenhagen.

Hobson, W., and Pemberton, J. (1955) Diet, nutrition, and budgets, in *The Health of the Elderly at Home*, p. 93 London.

Kataria, M. S., Rao, D. B., and Curtis, R. C. (1965) Vitamin C levels in the elderly, *Geront. clin. (Basel)*, **7**, 189.

McGandy, R. B., Barrows, C. H. Jr., Spanias, A. Meredith, A., Stone, J. L., and Norris, A. N. (1966) Nutrient intakes and energy expenditure in men of different ages, *J. Geront.*, **21**, 581.

Milne, J. S., Lonergan, M. E., Williamson, J., Moore, F. M. L., McMaster, R., and Percy, N. (1971) Leucocyte

ascorbic acid levels and vitamin C intake in older people, *Brit. med. J.*, **4**, 383.

Sinclair, H. M. (1956) Nutritional problems of the elderly, in *Modern Trends in Geriatrics*, ed. Hobson, W., p. 303, London.

Stanton, B. R., and Exton-Smith, A. N. (1970) *A Longitudinal Study of the Dietary of Elderly Women*, London.

Watkin, D. M. (1968) Nutritional problems in the elderly in the United States, in *Vitamins in the Elderly. Symposium*, eds Exton-Smith, A. N., and Scott, D. L., London.

Williams, J. A., Hall, G. S., Thompson, A. G., and Cooke, W. T. (1969) Neurological disease after partial gastrectomy, *Brit. med. J.*, **3**, 210.

World Health Organization Regional Office for Europe (1965) *Studies on Nutritional Programmes for the Elderly*, Copenhagen.

Geriatric Rehabilitation

Cosin, L. Z. (1952) Statistical analysis of geriatric rehabilitation, *J. Geront.*, **7**, 570.

Porsman, V. (1955) Statistical results of rehabilitation in 'The Old Peoples Town' in Copenhagen, in *Old Age in the Modern World*, ed. Tunbridge, R. E., p. 571, London.

Warren, H. W. (1946) Care of the chronic aged sick, *Lancet*, **i**, 841.

World Health Organization (1964) Rehabilitation of patients with cardiovascular diseases, *Wld Hlth Org. techn. Rep. Ser.*, No. 270.

Preventive Aspects

American Medical Association, Council on Medical Services (1955) *Survey of the Study of Multiple Screening*, Chicago.

Anderson, W. F., and Cowan, N. R. (1955) A consultative health centre for older people. The Rutherglen Experiment, *Lancet*, **ii**, 239.

Anderson, W. F. (1960) An approach to preventive geriatric medicine, *Geront. clin. (Basel)*, **2**, 55.

Anderson, W. F., and Cowan, N. R. (1963) Preventive geriatric medicine, *Med. Wld*, **99**, 553.

Andrews, G. R., Cowan, N. R., and Anderson, W. F. (1971) The practice of geriatric medicine in the community, in *Problems and Progress in Medical Care*, Fifth Series, ed. McLachlan, G., London.

Bedford, P. D., and Wollner, L. (1958) Occult intestinal bleeding as a cause of anaemia in elderly people, *Lancet*, **i**, 1144.

Boucher, C. A. (1966) *Accidents in the Elderly in England and Wales*, Abstracts of Papers Presented at the 7th International Congress of Gerontology, p. 226, Vienna.

Breslow, L. (1954) Aging and community health programs, *Amer. J. Geront.*, **9**, 224.

Breslow, L., and Roberts, D. W. (1955) Symposium: Screening for asymptomatic disease, *J. chron. Dis.*, **2**, 363.

Cochrane, A. L. (1967) A medical scientist's view of screening, *Publ. Hlth (London)*, **81**, 267.

College of General Practitioners. Report of a Working Party (1962) A diabetic survey, *Brit. med. J.*, **1**, 1497.

Day, E. (1967) Value of regular medical examinations, in *Prevention of Cancer*, ed. Raven, R. W., and Roe, F. C., London.

Dean, G. (1966) Lung cancer and bronchitis in Northern Ireland, 1960–2, *Brit. med. J.*, **1**, 1506.

Doll, R. (1956) *Gastroenterologia (Basel)*, **86**, 320.

Doll, R., and Hill, A. B. (1964) Mortality in relation to smoking. Ten years of observation of British doctors, *Brit. med. J.*, **1**, 1399 and 1460.

Dunn, J. E. Jr. (1958) Preliminary findings of Memphis–Shelby County uterine cancer study and their interpretation, *Amer. J. publ. Hlth*, **48**, 861.

Durning, J. V. G. A., Taylor, F., and Morris, J. N. (1963) Annual symposium on the preventive aspects of degenerative diseases, *Publ. Hlth (Lond.)*, **77**, 227, 231 and 237.

Fishman, W. H., Bonner, C. D., and Homburger, F. (1956) Serum 'prostatic' acid phosphatase and cancer of the prostate, *New Engl. J. Med.*, **255**, 925.

Gibson, I. I. J. M., and Pritchard, J. G. (1965) Screen investigation in the elderly, *Geront. clin. (Basel)*, **7**, 330.

Gillis, L. (1962) *Human Behaviour in Illness*, London.

Guiss, L. W. (1955) Mass roentgenographic screening as lung-cancer control measure, *Cancer (Philad.)*, 8, 219.

Hitchcock, C. R., and Aust, J. B. (1954) Cancer detection: Report from Cancer Detection Centre, University of Minnesota, *Minn. Med.*, 37, 243.

Hollis, F. (1966) *Casework: A Psychosocial Therapy*, Random House, New York.

Hubbard, J. P., ed. (1957) *The Early Detection and Prevention of Disease*, New York.

Jacobs, A., Kilpatrick, G. S., and Withey, J. L. (1965) Anaemia in adults: Prevalence and prevention, *Postgrad. med. J.*, **41**, 418.

Keen, H., Rose, G., Pyke, D. A., Boyns, D., Chlouverakis, C., and Misty, S. (1965) Blood sugar and arterial disease, *Lancet*, **ii,** 505.

Kilpatrick, G. S., and Hardisty, R. M. (1961) The prevalence of anaemia in the community, *Brit. med. J.*, **1**, 778.

Luntz, Maurice, H., Sevel, David, and Lloyd, J. P. F. (1963) Incidence of unsuspected chronic glaucoma in a population sample at Oxford, *Brit. med. J.*, **2**, 1237.

McKeown, T. (1961) Priorities in preventive medicine, *New Engl. J. Med.*, **264**, 594.

Mills, G. A., and Campbell, A. J. M. (1964) Diabetes in the elderly as part of a selective diabetic survey, *Med Offr*, **111**, 315.

Mullan, H. (1961) The personality of those who care for the aging, *Gerontologist*, **1**, 42.

O'Donnell, W. E., Day, E., and Venet, L. (1962) *Early Detection and Diagnosis of Cancer*, St. Louis, Mo.

Parsons, P. L., Withey, J. L., and Kilpatrick, G. S. (1965) The prevalence of anaemia in the elderly, *Practitioner*, **195**, 656.

Post, F. (1965) *The Clinical Psychiatry of Later Life*, Oxford.

Post, F. (1966) The recognition and treatment of emotional disorders, in *Medicine in Old Age*, ed. Agate, J. N., London.

Raven, R. W. (1971) Malignant disease, in *Medical Progress*, ed. Sir John Richardson, London.

Rechtschaffen, A. (1959) Psychotherapy with geriatric patients: A review of the literature, *J. Geront.*, **14**, 73.

Roth, M. (1964) Prophylaxis and early diagnosis and treatment of mental illness in later life, in *Current Achievements in Geriatrics*, ed. Anderson, W. F., and Isaacs, B., London.

Roth, M. (1966) Some problems of geriatrics common to medicine and psychiatry, in *Medicine in Old Age*, ed. Agate, J. N., London.

Rudd, T. (1960) Security in old age: Its philosophical basis, *J. Amer. Geriat. Soc.*, **8**, 431.

Shulman, R. (1967) Psychiatric aspects of pernicious anaemia: A prospective controlled investigation, *Brit. med. J.*, **3**, 266.

Smoking and Health Now (1971) A Report of the Royal College of Physicians, London.

Sorsby, A. (1966) *The Incidence of Blindness in England and Wales 1955–62*, London, H.M.S.O.

Strachan, R. W., and Henderson, J. G. (1965) Psychiatric syndromes due to avitaminosis B_{12} with normal blood and marrow, *Quart. J. Med.*, **34**, 303.

Strachan, R. W., and Henderson, J. G. (1967) Dementia and folate deficiency, *Quart. J. Med.*, **36**, 189.

Straker, M. (1964) Problems in the management of aged psychiatric out-patients: Survey of 100 cases, *J. Amer. Geriat. Soc.*, **12**, 473.

Thomas, J. H., and Powell, D. E. B. (1971) *Blood Disorders in the Elderly*, Bristol.

Wilkerson, H. L. C. (1949) Diabetes control in the public health program, *N.Y. St. J. Med.*, **49**, 2945.

Williamson, J. (1966) *Ageing in Modern Society*, Paper presented to Royal Society of Health, Edinburgh, 9th Nov.

Wilson, J. M. G., and Jungner, G. (1968) Principles and Practice of Screening for Disease, *Wld Hlth Org. Publ. Hlth Pap.*, No. 34.

Wood, C. H., and Meadows, Susan H. (1963) Experimental clinic for preventing chronic bronchitis, *Brit. med. J.*, **2**, 1088.

Reports of the World Health Organization on Old Age

World Health Organization Expert Committee on Mental Health (1959) Sixth Report, Mental Health Problems of Ageing and the Aged, *Wld Hlth Org. techn. Rep. Ser.*, No. 171.

World Health Organization Regional Office for Europe (1959) *The Public Health Aspects of the Aging of the Population, Report of an Advisory Group Convened by the Regional Office for Europe of WHO at Oslo, 28 July–2 August 1958*, Copenhagen.

World Health Organization Regional Office for Europe (1963) *Report of Seminar on the Health Protection of the Elderly and the Aged and the Prevention of Premature Ageing, held at Kiev, 14–22 May 1963*, Copenhagen.

World Health Organization Regional Office for Europe (1970) Working Group on Education and Training in Long-Term Care, including Geriatrics. Held at Florence 10–13 November 1970 (Euro 5301), Copenhagen.

World Health Organization (1974) The planning and organization of geriatric services. Report of a WHO Expert Committee, *Wld Hlth Org. techn. Rep. Ser.*, No. 548.

Training

Anderson, W. F. (1970) Geriatrics—A Speciality?, *Interdisc. Top. Geront.*, **5**, 44.

Hobson, W., and Akhmetely, M. (1963) The Training of Professional and Auxiliary Staff in Gerontology and Geriatrics, Working Paper Euro 245/16 for the WHO Seminar on the Health Protection of the Elderly, WHO Regional Office for Europe, Copenhagen.

Isaacs, Bernard (1964) The training of a geriatric physician, *Lancet*, **i,** 1339.

40

SOCIO-MEDICAL PROBLEMS OF NOMAD PEOPLES[1]

SIXTEN S. R. HARALDSON

DEFINITIONS

Traditionally a country's population is divided into urban and rural. Conditions and problems of these two groups of people are basically different and therefore need a different approach in community planning, including health and other social services.

There is, however, in most countries an extreme group of rural population, which is usually not sufficiently considered and often neglected in development plans. This group could be called 'scattered populations'. They have special characteristics, and special knowledge and consideration is needed by authorities dealing with their problems. It seems to be necessary, not to say urgent, to separate this population from the traditional one, the urban and the rural, in order to make sure that they are not left aside, but offered a reasonable share of adequate development.

Scattered peoples may be sedentary, static people living in small hamlets or villages spread over wide areas and separated by great distances, or they may be mobile. Scattered populations exist all over the world.

The mobile people can be subdivided into people in seasonal movements or 'pendlers', common in industrial areas of developing countries, or they may be refugees, or real nomads. Refugees are scattered in small groups outside their home country or concentrated in refugee camps or new settlement land offered to them. Refugees as a whole have many problems related to those of nomadic peoples, but their health problems may be acute and resembling catastrophic medicine. Contrary to other scattered people, refugees have not voluntarily chosen mobile life outside their native country but have rather been forced to it.

The American College Dictionary defines nomad as 'one of a race or tribe without fixed abode, but moving from place to place according to the state of the pasturage or food supply'. Pure nomads are people with no permanent dwelling, regular migration and consequently no agricultural activities. Semi-nomadic could be defined as migrating people with one permanent dwelling, where the family stays part of the year, or part of the family during the whole year—usually wife and children. This way of living may permit some gardening and small-scale agriculture. In principle, however, systematic and profitable agriculture puts an end to nomadism.

'Transhumance', finally, is a life model where pastoral people share the year between two fixed camps in order to utilize seasonal variations in rainfall and grazing. One place usually is situated in a mountainous area and the other in a lake or river district. Hence, there is a floating scale of migration models, often passed through in the development of nomadic people today to a settled and sedentary life. With a strict definition of a nomad, very few people in the world today could be classified as full nomads.

To make the picture complete, it should be mentioned that there are also migrating populations with no socially accepted reasons for their nomadism, which rightly could be called vagabondism. Some 'caravaners' in the United States and the United Kingdom and 'woonwagen bewoners' in the Netherlands, as well as 10,000 'tinkers' in Ireland, and some Gipsies could be counted in this group which, because of its unstable life, is difficult to reach with social services as well as development programmes. Traditionally Gipsies are regarded as a pariah group, who some thousand years ago left India, and reached the Donau region in Europe 600 years ago. From this place they invaded other countries in Europe in waves, primarily as a nomadic population. Today about two million Gipsies are spread all over Europe, few of whom are still migrating and practising their old craft as tinsmiths.

Real nomads may be subdivided into one more 'primitive' group—hunters-fishers and collectors, and one with pastoral peoples. The latter group, making up the majority of nomads today, has domesticated animals, usually cows, camels, sheep, goats, and reindeer. For transportation they often use horses and donkeys. The animals are held for provision of meat, milk, and sometimes blood and for utilization of their hides and hair for clothing, tents, and professional equipment.

Originally and basically, nomads have a primitive, pagan religion, often with animism as a dominating ingredient. Nowadays, the majority of nomads in Africa and South-West Asia are Moslems, while those of Central Asia are confessors of Buddhism. However, the nomads' religion is from a ceremonial point of view mostly uncomplicated and less rigid. It is practical and tolerant. Women among the African Mohammedans seldom wear the veil. There is also a tendency to mix elements from different faiths with characteristics of primitive religion.

CHARACTERISTICS OF SPARSELY POPULATED AREAS AND NOMAD POPULATIONS

The decisive characteristics of sparsely populated areas is their low average population density and long distances between the units themselves, and to central and densely populated districts. Usually the density is in the range of 1–5 per sq. km.

[1] Few medical studies of general interest have been made on nomadic peoples, and only occasionally public health research. That which is discussed in this chapter is mainly based on impressions from numerous study visits by the author to a large number of the world's nomadic tribes, fifteen years as a district medical officer among the Lapps of Scandinavia, WHO planning work in various regions of Asia and Africa, catastrophe relief work with the League of Red Cross Societies, and finally work as the director for the Ethiopian Nutrition Institute in Addis Ababa.

When the density is below one, the region should be called and dealt with as an empty area. Nomads mostly occupy remote and isolated areas along frontiers and with sparse road communication. In some cases air communication is well developed (Australia, Kenya).

Due to their isolation and ecological situation, nomads have developed extreme cultural and social patterns and mostly a complete self-sufficient household economy. They have made themselves, voluntarily and by force of circumstances independent of the outside world, their own countrymen and governments. This means that they are sometimes not even under control by the authorities.

Nomads principally do not accept borderlines, which *de facto* were drawn after their arrival and often divided their feeding grounds and tribe into two or more parts. Many of the straight frontiers made by rulers and foreigners are regularly crossed by migrating nomads. The ecological situation has not sufficiently been considered. The whole migratory land of a tribe, whether it is located in one or several countries, is often regarded as their tribal land and their loyalty to any of the governments concerned may be practically none.

The consequence of a nomadic livelihood is a strictly utilitarian, cultural, and professional set-up of equipment and tools, streamlined and simplified, tested for generations and proved to be indispensable—a 'portable culture' in which the personal belongings are few and often can be carried in one hand.

Individual ownership is secondary. Nomads have mostly developed a system of collective ownership in the tribe or clan. The nomad is the present care-taker of the tribe's inherited richness of cattle. He may take out as an income as much food and hides from the herd as is needed for his family's subsistence. He wants to hand over the herd to the next generation if possible in an improved condition and a numerically larger size.

The extended family group, the clan, has often been experienced by nomads to be the adequate basic group for herding and migration. In this group an agile system of leadership develops and a social system, offering complete cradle-to-grave security for all members, independent of their talents or age. These strong bonds and the advantages of them must be understood when nomads hesitate to accept new alternatives and systems offered from outside.

A consequence of the mobile life is a self-supporting economy, a pre-monetary economy with barter, gifts and co-operation rather than selling and buying.

Naturally such groups maintain what from other points of view may be regarded as conservative patterns and attitudes, extreme cultural and social manners and settings with goals and values which may be hard to understand, and constitute obstacles to development inaugurated from outside.

The individual small population unit whether sedentary or mobile, may be separated by desert sand, by impenetrable jungle or rough mountains, by snow and ice or by open ocean. It all brings about the same situation of isolation with low accessibility from the outside and for the people from services such as health, education, and communication facilities.

Thus, any investment on services or other development measures in the area will be non-profitable compared with the same investment in any more densely populated place. This is one of the reasons for neglect of nomads in development programmes. Unfortunately, pastoral and arid areas are largely located in developing countries with poor economy, and the output–input relationship has to be considered thoroughly in any investment.

To this is added the fact that the areas concerned are geographically difficult to reach and the people's political loyalty and respect for frontiers may not keep up to the expectations of the government. Sometimes nomads avoid contacts with the outside, as they suspect hostility and negative effects—they have often been the losers in confrontations. Their loyalty is primarily directed to their own tribe and clan.

Nomads are rather international and do not think much of citizenship. They often have trading of all kinds over the borderlines, which may be classified as smuggling by the authorities, but as the justice of the wilderness by nomads. This results in a striving to avoid confrontation with any authority.

The total situation presents to the nomad a unique position of complete independence, a value which he is aware of and appreciates more than anything else.

THE ORIGIN OF NOMADISM

Reasons for nomadism are several and differ in different parts of the world. Generally speaking, the leading causative factor for a certain area being inhabited by nomads is a low average annual precipitation. It can also be unfavourably distributed over the year. As a rough yardstick, an annual rainfall below 25 cm., being the lower limit for growing of cereals, does not permit gardening or agriculture and below 50–70 cm. agriculture is mostly unprofitable. Extreme winds, temperatures and altitudes may add factors against cultivation of the soil. In the Arctic, the permafrost and too short vegetation period have the same effect, and the precipitation—usually small—may fall entirely as snow.

If people insist on staying in these areas, they are forced to lead a life of hunting, fishing, collecting, or with breeding of domesticated animals as their livelihood. Wide areas must be covered for collecting food or finding enough game, or for grazing, and the people are forced to become nomadic. Generally, searching for water is the number one reason given by nomads for migration, and as number two grazing is mentioned. Both of course go together, as water is a prerequisite for grazing. Primarily the domesticated animals are migrating, and the owner follows his herd and has to become a nomad. There is no such thing as 'nomad blood' or 'travel fever' involved. It is, in most cases, a pure ecological question.

Apart from the eternal searching for water and feeding grounds, there are among some nomads other incentives and motives for seasonal migration and choice of migratory routes: intertribal frictions, seasonal marketing and trading with neighbours, avoiding mosquitoes, flies, and diseases, such as malaria and sleeping sickness. There may also be religious and other ritual forces (Aborigines in Australia), and finally legislation regarding borderlines and disposition of certain grounds may regulate the movements of nomadic people (Lappland, Iran).

In many cases, the land and the nomadic life have been chosen voluntarily by tribes (Afghanistan, Masailand), although the actual area occupied would permit other forms of subsistence such as agriculture. In other cases (Bushmen, Danakil) they have been forced by warfare and frictions to retire to an inhospitable barren area, claimed by nobody else, and practising a nomadic life as the only way of livelihood under the local ecological circumstances. Once adapted to the environment and its resources, the tribe defends its arid area against new intruders and hostile neighbours.

If culture is defined as a human dignified life optimally utilizing available natural resources, a high cultural level may develop, yet they may be primitive in the sense that they cannot or write—arts which, in pastoral life, are considered unimportant talents. The nomad's spiritual, moral, and ethical life may be second to none. In some places (Somali, Afghanistan) the nomadic sector of the population is regarded as superior and graded as the upper social class, both economically and socially. 'The fittest people can migrate, while less capable people have to stay settled.'

THE DIMENSION OF NOMADISM

Scattered populations still occupy a considerable part of the world's total land area. Permafrost covers about 20 per cent. of it already, and this tundra area is inhabited by a sparse population of sedentary and nomadic tribes. In the rest of the world, regions with nomadic populations are mostly arid or semi-arid deserts of sand and stone with a sparse vegetation of grass and shrubs. In total, one third of the earth's land surface is arid and primarily not cultivable land. Much of this situation is man-made and of increasing dimensions.

In some countries, most of the land is unsuitable for agriculture and thus empty or inhabited by nomadic pastoralists, e.g. Somali (about 90 per cent.), Kenya (60), Ethiopia (54), Egypt (96·5), Jordan (86), Syria (65), and Iraq (40). Sahara has an area of 7·5 million sq. km. and a population of about 2·5 million. Although it is difficult to estimate, and largely a matter of definition how many nomads the world accommodates today, an estimate of over one hundred million would not be unrealistic.

In the New World, the Americas, there have—on the whole—only been small groups of nomads in a few places (Nunamiut, Navaho). The problem of nomadism is mainly one of Asia and Africa. In the north of Asian Russia, we find some arctic nomadic groups with reindeer husbandry (Samoyed, Chuckchi, Tungus, Koryak), but otherwise most nomads are found in hot or subtropical regions.

Europe has only small and vanishing groups of real nomads. In the north of Scandinavia, there are about 35,000 Lapps, of whom today only 2,000 could be registered as semi-nomads. However, many more are still living from reindeer breeding. Small groups of sheep-herders on the Balkan Peninsula are nomadic, and as a curiosity about two million Gipsies spread over Europe should be mentioned, of whom today only a very small fraction are mobile.

Africa has three main regions occupied by nomads, the Sahelian region, the Kalahari desert in South Africa, and a belt over Central Africa from Senegal in the West to Ethiopia and East Africa in the East. The original population of Africa is supposed to be the Bushmen, today numbering about 25,000 of whom 5,000 are considered as pure Bushmen, bands migrating as hunters and collectors in a desert area larger than France.

In Somali about 70 per cent. of the total population are nomadic pastoralists, in Kenya, Mali, and Ethiopia about 10 per cent. The total number of African nomads would be about 20–30 millions.

Corresponding figures for Asia could be estimated to be two or three times higher. In all countries in the Middle East there are nomadic peoples, from Turkey to Afghanistan (Kotshi). The Kurds are successively becoming sedentary. Iran, Afghanistan, and the Arabian Peninsula are still to a large extent occupied by nomads. In the desert of Negev in Israel you find a sample collection of all stages between the most old-fashioned Bedouin life as at the time of Abraham, to a settled life in town with industrial work. However, artificial irrigation of this land will in a few year's time convert it to a fertile agricultural area. Tibetans and other Mongolian tribes make up a large portion of the world's total number of nomads (Uzbek, Kazah, Kirghiz, Sart, Tadzjik, Badawin, Turkmen).

When the Europeans entered Australia in 1788 there were some 300,000 Aborigines. Through injudicious treatment by the newcomers their number was rapidly reduced. By 1960 there were 122,000, of whom 44,000 were full-blooded Aborigines living in reserves or spread as small nomadic groups in the interior of Australia. Lately the Federal Government has allocated great resources for help to the Aborigines, training camps for making the assimilation less painful, flying doctor service, etc. The anxious desire to repair the errors of the past can be understood from the switching of the name Native Protection Board to the Welfare Board.

The number of workers in Africa and Asia, moving seasonally between their tribal land and industrial areas, away from their families, is not known, but the figure is likely to be high and constitutes a major social and health problem.

The world has (1971) about 20 million refugees, in many cases former nomads and now living as farmers in new settlement areas, in refugee camps or scattered in small units in foreign lands.

The number of pure nomads in the world is rapidly shrinking, and in some cases the 'half-life' period may be as short as a generation. From a stage of semi-nomadism many are switching over to a sedentary life.

REASONS FOR DEALING WITH NOMAD PEOPLES

Some formulations in the Universal Declaration of Human Rights by the United Nations in 1948 would be a challenge to humanitarian considerations and assistance to all people in need of it, independent of being settled or nomadic. This declaration has been followed up by several national declarations. President Kenyatta of Kenya in his book (1965) on African Socialism pleads for social justice and equal opportunities to all population groups, independent of geographical location, race, and profitableness of investments. As we all know, there are many obstacles to this utopian attitude.

Gaining of political loyalty and solidarity from people in borderline areas has sometimes been the foremost incentive in some African countries to deal with nomads. However, this important motive has also in many places been surprisingly neglected, resulting in perpetual warfare, characteristic of many borderline areas, both in Asia and in Africa. By offering some benefits, the government may secure co-operation from remote groups, benefits which otherwise may be provided by a rival neighbour government.

The fact that nomads often occupy vast land areas, is in itself a strong motive for including them in planning and sharing of the Government's budget cake. In some cases nomadism may be the only way in which one can squeeze a livelihood out of a certain region by exploiting its only potentiality, the grass.

Disturbances of the ecological balance by overgrazing, resulting in erosion of the soil and a dead landscape, will in the future be another reason for authorities to interest themselves in nomads. The rapid growth of both human and cattle population, which has been observed, e.g. in Turkana and in Masailand in Kenya, has seriously upset the natural balance and threatened the future of the two tribes. In most cases, however, nomads have reached an ecological equilibrium with nature instead of exploiting it.

Lately, national and international public health considerations have become leading incentives for a growing interest in pastoral areas and their inhabitants. A health control or eradication programme may be regarded as successful, but if reservoirs of infection are left in nomadic groups not covered by the programme, they may jeopardize the project by serving as foci for flaring up of an epidemic, e.g. malaria or smallpox, making enormous investments wasted. Nomads may also carry a disease to a neighbouring country across the frontier, where the disease may have been eradicated.

Thus, pure self-defence and instinct for self-preservation have become a major force in the engagement for nomadic peoples. The WHO malaria control programme in places such as Somali put the spotlight on this situation and called for special design of programmes for pastoral areas and nomadic people—for 'travelling human vectors'.

The explanation of the fact that many pastoral areas in the world still are neglected in development work, is primarily the limitation of funds, the necessity of careful consideration of the profitableness of any investment, and the accessibility ratio of health service units constructed. Secondly, the lack of knowledge and information, sometimes underestimation and prejudices, are obstacles to occupation with extreme groups of countrymen. The lack of understanding of other cultures, their goals, values, and expectations may finally be a complete hindrance for co-operation. Health, happiness, and material standards of living may to them mean something totally different, compared with settled or urbanized people.

HEALTH PROBLEMS AMONG NOMADS

The harsh way of life has usually left the nomad with a high tolerance threshold for suffering, and he feels a reduced need for health services. He is well adapted to nature and an extreme climate, and he has a slow, swinging gait which is energy-saving and does not overheat him. A fair degree of harmonious co-existence with flies and disease has also been evolved.

It is widespread and popular to classify minorities or people living in a different way from our own as having a lower social and cultural status. This attitude often includes statements suggesting that the concerned group is slowly dying out or

vanishing, that it is weak and degenerated and ridden by diseases such as veneral diseases, leprosy, and malnutrition.

Usually the actual situation is the contrary, especially when it concerns nomadic peoples, who are growing with the same ratio as their settled countrymen. There is no reason to believe that the fertility rate is different in nomadic populations compared with sedentary. Through assimilation with surrounding ethnic or cultural populations it may look as though certain tribes are dying out, but mostly it is just a change of profession and place of residence. The fact that a primitive tribe of hunters, the Navaho Indians, during some hundreds of years have been able to migrate 2,400 km. from the Arctic taiga of Canada to the hot desert of Arizona and in 100 years has increased its population ten times, shows how wrong it is to consider some cultures as weak or vanishing.

As a whole, efficient birth control is unknown among nomads. Thus the birth rate is high. Studies of Lapps noted a higher

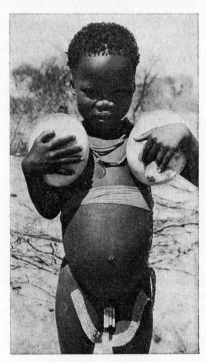

FIG. 100. Water 'buckets', Kalahari Bushman.

birth rate for Lapp women than for their settled neighbours. This in spite of a suggested higher abortion rate among the Lapps. The converted proportions between newborn girls and boys have been explained through a higher abortion ratio, which is known to hit the male foetus more than the female. The Lapps give birth to 2–4 per cent. more girls than boys, while the common figure in the world is 2–5 per cent. more newborn boys.

In the past all nomad Lapp babies were born in the camps, while today almost 100 per cent. of the deliveries are institutional. Helicopter transports are widely used for this purpose. This has considerably contributed to a reduced infant mortality among the Lapps. From 1940 to 1956 the infant mortality for all Sweden changed from 42 to 15.9 per thousand, and in the same period among the Lapps from 67 to 17.6 per thousand. Only in few other nomad populations in the world similar services have been offered and therefore the infant mortality could be expected to be high. Shaffer estimated (in 1960) the infant mortality in the Kenya pastoral areas at 250 per thousand, and the average life expectancy was estimated to be the same as for the rest of Kenya, or 35 to 40 years. Only 30 years ago the average life expectancy of newborn Lapp babies was about the same as in Sweden in general 200 years ago, or around 35–40 years. For Greenland Eskimos in 1959 the average life expectancy was 32 years.

Due to a more hazardous life, infant and child mortality as well as accidental deaths in hunting and herding tend to be high among nomads. This is, on the other hand, compensated by better general health, due to better nutrition and to a healthy life near nature. The nomadic life demands a certain physical condition. Weak people have to stay settled.

In 83 adult Kalahari Bushmen, living as nomad hunter-gatherers, studies by Hansen *et al.* showed that some medical conditions were not seen—obesity, heart disease, cirrhosis, hypertonia, varicose veins, rheumatoid arthritis. Hunting accidents were common. Comparable studies of nomad Masai give about the same picture of a surprisingly healthy population.

In a survey 1962/63 of 406 Masai 35 (or 8·6 per cent.) were found to have serological evidence of syphilis, indicating that this disease was not as serious a problem in this population as had been suggested. The prevalence was lower than for the native population of Nairobi.

Exact information is seldom available as neither demographic figures nor health statistics exist in pastoral areas, and are often insufficient in the country as a whole. Studies have revealed that nomadic tribes, such as the Masai and the Somali have the best nutritional status of all native groups in Central Africa. As most nomads have domesticated animals, there is plenty of milk and meat, and in some cases blood is regularly taken from the cattle for drinking (Masai).

The nomad's diet is usually very uniform. Reindeer meat may be eaten 4–5 times a day by the Lapps from ages below one year. Somalis drink camel milk several times a day. Both meat and camel milk have high contents of calories (fat) and protein, and the daily protein requirement is covered many times over. Milk makes up to 90–95 per cent. of the calories in the Masai diet, with cows' meat and blood consumed at intervals. Fish and wild animal meat are taboo.

Characteristics of many pastoral and nomad peoples, are hungry seasons with semi-starvation towards the end of the dry season. It has been reported that Bushmen killed babies born at the beginning of the dry season as the chance for the baby to survive was regarded as small. During these seasons the protein intake may be critical, although most nomad peoples' diet is fairly well balanced in specific nutrients. Hunters and collectors (Bushmen, Australian Aborigines) cover their calorie and protein need by a rich variety of game, larvae, insects, ants, eggs, etc. The Bushmen get meat from game, mainly antelopes, brought down by primitive hunting with bows and arrows. Poison for hunting is prepared from herbs and snakes.

Everything including the roasted hide and the bone marrow is consumed. The bulk of their calorie need over the year, however, is covered by vegetables, fruits, and roots. They have a choice of 85 different species of edible plants. They know

exactly where, when, and how they grow, what is edible and what is poisonous, a knowledge gained through generations of life in a desert. It has been observed that people who are suddenly forced to live as gatherers (Tirma) have a scanty knowledge about nature and cannot survive on a collecting economy. Any switching between the three basic models of livelihood, gathering–herding–farming is hazardous for the first generations as there are no inherited funds of experience to build on.

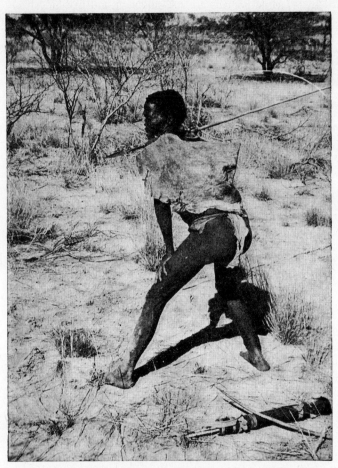

FIG. 101. Hunting Bushman in the Kalahari desert (Botswana).

The high intake of milk and meat and consequently protein by pastoral peoples is accompanied by a simultaneous high intake of animal fat and saturated fatty acids. Fatty acids have been suggested by modern research as an essential factor in development of cardiovascular diseases and heart infarction. Among nomads, however, other causative factors in this pathology are absent, as they have plenty of physical exercise, no over-consumption of calories and presumably no mental stress. Studies of some tribes (Masai, Somali) have confirmed a very low prevalence of cardiovascular diseases and deaths in degenerative diseases as a whole.

The most noteworthy biochemical findings reported by teams studying the Kalahari Bushmen (Hansen, etc.) were very low serum cholesterol values. Mean level in 83 adults studied was between 100 and 121 mg. per 100 ml. This was looked upon as a consequence of low calorie intake and walking long distances, often carrying heavy loads. The percentage of linoleic acid in their serum triglycerides plus cholesterol esters was not unusually high. A clinical survey (in 1964 by Mann *et al.*) of 400 Masai showed almost no evidence of chronic cardiovascular diseases. An American team (Taylor *et al.*, 1967) studied 24 Masai and found again very low serum cholesterol values, which they suggested as being a consequence of a 'built-in' immunity, a metabolic mechanism for neutralization and suppression of the great amount of cholesterol known to be absorbed.

In principle nomads are self-sufficient and live only from what nature provides. This means that carbohydrates, flour, and sugar are minor, if any, portions of the diet. Until monetary economy and systematic trading were introduced dental caries was unknown in many nomadic peoples. Their teeth were also, thanks to their special diet, given sufficient exercise. However, periodontal diseases are common in some groups.

Bread, if used by nomads, is often prepared in a simple way with flour, salt, and water as the only ingredients. This unfermented and unsweetened bread, baked over the open fire is tough and tooth-friendly, and together with dried meat a perfect travel food, resembling the 'pemmican' of the Red Indians.

Indigenous beer is brewed by many nomads and mostly they smoke some substitute for tobacco. Masai seldom smoke, but make beer from wild honey.

Malnutrition has been largely unknown among nomads. The Turkana nomads in Kenya did not know kwashiorkor until the drought catastrophe in their region in 1960. It was then rather a general starvation than lack of any particular ingredient such as protein in the food. Studies of children of nomad Bushmen revealed no case of kwashiorkor, and marasmus only as secondary, e.g. to malaria infection. Dental caries and otitis media were rare, and little or no evidence of mineral or vitamin deficiency was found.

Concerning the intake of vitamins and minerals in other tribes little is known, but it is generally accepted that a high meat consumption reduces the requirements of B-vitamins and that C-vitamin needs are covered by consumption of plants and berries. 'Juobmo' among the Lapps, made from a green plant (*Rumex Acetosa*) has been analysed and found to have high C-vitamin content, which is also known from cloud-berries, consumed by the Lapps.

Increasingly the world's nomads are becoming omnivorous. With a monetary or mixed economy, products such as rice, corn, millet, and sugar have crossed the cultural barrier and found their way to the nomad world.

Nomads' breast-feeding patterns are interesting contributions to the general discussion of the successively decreasing breast-feeding in industrialized countries. When there is no alternative, no substitute for breast-feeding, this is carried out in full scale and often for 1 or 2 years. Studies among the Lapps recorded breast-feeding exceeding 6 months in 70 per cent., while the corresponding figure for neighbouring urbanized population was 20 per cent.

Studies of physical capacity with test bicycles (Masai) showed a very good standard, and in some cases the highest oxygen intake ever recorded in men—Olympic competitors included—was found. Due to ecological and climatic factors certain diseases tend to be prevalent among nomads. Trachoma is favoured by hot, dry and dusty climate—which also may

make the place suitable only for a nomadic cattle herding economy. It has been observed in Kenya that nomads generally develop milder forms of trachoma than the neighbouring population. This is believed to be a consequence of their nutritional status.

Bilharziasis and hookworm do not thrive in this climate and are therefore minor problems in nomad populations. Trypanosomiasis, both human and cattle (Nagana), is in some areas a serious obstacle for pastoralism, which in some places (Tirma in Ethiopia) has forced nomads to settle down and initiate farming. Malaria and tuberculosis are other scourges, which nomads share with settled people. Due to handling of hides

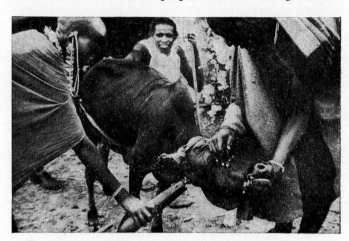

Fig. 102. Masai letting blood from a cow for drinking (Kenya.)

anthrax is more prevalent in some areas with nomad pastoralists (Kenya). Accidents, such as burns and scalds, cold injuries, drowning, animal bites, etc. are common among people living in nature. Accidents also substantially form the mortality pattern of some primitive peoples (Eskimo, Lapps).

Although latrines and 'soap-and-water' cleanliness are abhorrent to the traditional nomad, the general impression is that they have more feeling for personal hygiene than settled people. Furthermore, their mobile life favours hygiene, as they move away from dirt and rubbish, and nature cleans it up until they return to the same place next year. Both heat and cold are favourable factors in this cleaning. Portable dwellings are also convenient to keep clean, while there is a tendency among nomads who become settled to develop a slum situation as soon as they move into a house. It seems as if at least one generation of experience is needed until people know how to live in a house.

In some nomadic tribes pits and caves (Jate in Afghanistan) or *ad hoc* constructed shelters (Australian Aborigines, Turkana, Bushmen) are used, and no dwelling is transported during migration.

Due to their living close to domesticated animals some zoonoses have been prevalent among nomads, but are today decreasing, e.g. hydatid cysts (Echinococcus) which are spread from the reindeer via the watch dogs to human beings, where cysts may develop in lungs, liver, or brain (Lapps, Eskimos).

Cultural and social patterns in many African tribes claim ritual operations, often carried out as ceremonies at the age of puberty, e.g. circumcision, extraction of front teeth and uvulectomy, perforation of ears, nose, and lips, clan-branding tattoo with dye or scarification. Circumcision, and in some cases also infibulation (Somali) on girls are mostly extensive operations, by which labia majora and minora as well as clitoris are removed with primitive instruments and without anaesthesia. There is a certain mortality in all these operations, but there seems to be little lasting disability of the female circumcisions from the gynaecological and obstetrical point of view.

Due to extreme cultural patterns and their need of integrity for their land, nomadic people often develop isolates with a high rate of inbreeding. Nine per cent. of all marriages were found to be cousin marriages in a Lapp population in Norway. Corresponding figure for all Norway is 0·5 per cent. One

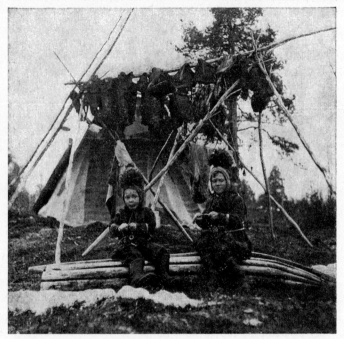

FIG. 103. Lapp camp.

could expect a high incidence of genetic, physical, and mental disorders, congenital malformations, etc. caused by this custom.

The incidence of congenital hip joint luxation among Lapps is about fifty times higher than among other Scandinavians which has partly been explained as a genetic effect. The traditional Lappish method of keeping a baby with the stretched legs bound together has been accepted as a trigger factor for an inborn disposition. As a whole geneticists today consider inbreeding as a rather harmless factor, genetically seen. How much of the small stature of primitive people and of many populations in developing countries can blame genetics is a difficult question to answer. In any case, part of the smallness is in many places related to nutritional patterns, which has also been demonstrated, e.g. among the Lapps in Sweden.

The new-born Lapp baby is smaller than the average Swedish. Mellbin compared (in 1940–60) 491 new-born Lapps with 1,008 new-born Swedish babies, and found a statistically significant difference between the two groups. The male Lapp babies had an average weight of 3,470 g., the Swedish 3,600. The Lapp female babies 3,320 and the Swedish 3,490 g. The

difference is further stressed by the fact that Lapp women give birth to more children than do Swedish women, The first baby—representing a proportionally larger group among non-Lappish babies—has a lower average birthweight.

Observations by Almeida of Bushmen in Angola suggest that chronic or seasonal calorie insufficiency may be a major reason why Bushmen do not reach the same adult stature as most other people. A distinct fall-off in growth rate starts after the first year of life, and the adult Bushman has an average height of 150 cm.

Congenital malformations and mental deficiency are surprisingly seldom seen among nomads. It is known from East Africa that traditionally and as a necessity of racial hygiene, defective new-born babies are killed in some tribes—a custom which is likely to be widely spread over the world.

HEALTH SERVICES AMONG SCATTERED AND NOMAD POPULATIONS

For several reasons nomadic people have made themselves independent and self-sufficient in most fields. There has mostly been no other choice, as they have not been offered much of social services from outside. Thus, they have, over generations, developed their own health services, often in charge of persons of their own tribe, who inherited secrets and talents in their medical profession—the medicine man, sorcerer, or witch doctor, nojd (Lapps) shaman (Siberia), laibon (Masai, Nandi, Samburu), herbalist, or holy man.

Certain treatment performed by these highly trusted native doctors has definitely an adequate curative effect on ailments for which they are prescribed, but doses are often maximal and in some cases even lethal. However, the main part of the therapeutic effect—and not to be underestimated—is purely psychological and based on magical practice, and the enormous prestige and confidence which among primitive people are inherent in the medicine man. In the common situation in these societies, when no help from outside can be reached and transport facilities are insufficient, security feeling and safety are linked to him. Amputations, open repositioning of fractures (Masai) and even trepanation of the skull have been carried out by medicine men.

In most countries where nomads exist, the national budget is limited, and therefore sparsely populated areas are neglected. There is a total shortage in these countries of professional as well as auxiliary health personnel and of health service units. In addition there are serious malproportions between different categories of health personnel, e.g. with one nurse for each doctor, whereas one doctor could supervise the work of several nurses and thus much more work could be performed. There is also in many places an unrealistic perfectionism claiming university trained doctors, where the main problems are elementary and could be done by auxiliaries specifically trained for local problems.

With the present trend of development and training capacity, it will take an estimated 230 years in Ethiopia to reach the pastoral areas for which the World Health Organization suggested the minimum standard for Africa of one doctor for 10,000 population. This presumes that one insists on university trained doctors. A compromise with auxiliary doctors (health officers, medical assistants, etc.) specially trained for the urgent local health problems would solve the problem in Ethiopia—as well as in many other developing countries—in a considerably shorter time, and immediately improve the situation; all at a lower cost and avoiding brain drain from the country that always follows professional training.

Finally, there is often a grotesque geographical maldistribution, resulting in an agglomeration of, for example, doctors in the capital and a few other big cities, whereas rural areas have few, if any doctors. In Ethiopia (in 1970) over 50 per cent. of all doctors (about 370) worked in the capital, Addis Ababa, where 3 per cent. of the total population are located. Most of the others were in a few cities, and the rural areas had nothing. The pastoral areas covering over 50 per cent. of the total land area of Ethiopia have practically no health services, and the existing services have an extremely low accessibility rate due to the low population density and vast distances. The doctor/population ratio is ten times higher in Stockholm than in the areas where the Lapps migrate.

In Kenya, where 10 per cent. of the population, or about one million, are nomadic pastoralists, these people occupy over 65 per cent. of the total land area. Of all doctors in Kenya, native and expatriate (together about 900), only 1·4 per cent. serve the 10 per cent. portion which are nomads. Thus, considering only the population figure, their share of doctors is seven times lower than that for the rest of the Kenya population. To this situation comes an average population density twenty times lower in the pastoral areas, which *de facto* should justify a higher doctor/population ratio than in densely populated and urban areas. The result of this distribution is that there are in Kenya, as well as in Ethiopia, wide areas with scattered populations, who have no access whatsoever to any government or other health service from the outside.

A total of 15–20 per cent. of Ethiopians have access to health service units. As the density of population in the pastoral area is fifteen times lower than in the central parts of the country, the accessibility rate is higher in these latter regions than in the 54 per cent. of the land where 8 per cent. of the people live, and the accessibility rate is 2–3 per cent. The service unit/population rate is also lower in the pastoral areas, which adds to the distances.

Traditionally, missions cover districts and needs in remote areas. The native health personnel tend to concentrate in urban areas and are unwilling to leave these. On the provincial level international programmes often offer their assistance.

PLANNING OF HEALTH SERVICES AMONG SCATTERED AND NOMAD POPULATIONS

Most of what has so far been accomplished by national and international development programmes has affected urban areas. Latterly, problems of rural areas in developing countries have attracted increasing attention, resulting in rural projects. For reasons discussed above it is more profitable from an immediate economic point of view to make investments in densely populated areas. This concerns especially health services, where a new unit in a sparsely populated area will be only modestly utilized because of the low population density in the area and consequently long distances and low accessibility rate.

With the limited budgets for development as well as for current expenditures on health available in these countries, it is understandable that rural areas have to a great extent been neglected and seldom have got their fair share of the national budget. This is even more apparent for the extreme rural, the pastoral and sparsely populated areas, where we find the nomads. The accessibility ratio for a health unit may in these areas be 10–100 times lower than in densely populated areas of the country.

In Ethiopia, the capital, Addis Ababa, had (1969) 56 hospital beds for each 10,000 population, while the corresponding figure for the pastoral province of Bale was 0·5 or one hundred times lower. In the pastoral areas of Ethiopia, accommodating 1·5 to 2 million people, the accessibility rate for health services is extremely low. This means that existing units serve only narrow circles of neighbours. Mobile units as well as wheeled transportation facilities, if available, can widen the circles and reduce the number of people outside the range of service units.

Although the output of any investments in sparsely populated districts will usually be meagre in relation to the input, one must not glance too much at profitableness. Humanitarian reasons, social justice, and political considerations call for at least a minimum of assistance to all population groups of a given country, independent of their geographical localization and contribution to the national economy.

Therefore, long-term plans have to cover these areas as well. The primary question which has to be answered before any development steps are initiated is—is it likely that the particular area has sufficient natural resources for securing a reasonable material standard of living? Otherwise prospects for the future are dark. Most people will not in the future accept today's standards. If the standard of living in the future has to be based to a major extent on 'artificial breathing', on assistance from the outside, it is likely that the people concerned will slowly lose their cultural self-confidence and identity.

Thus, planning has to be commenced at an early stage to decide whether a certain area is to remain inhabited or should rather become an empty area through migration of the people to places where there are prerequisites for the standard which the next generation will ask for—food, schools, communications, and health service. However, even emigration should be planned in order to avoid a selective migration of breadwinners, leaving less capable individuals behind in a place which demands full capacity of its inhabitants for their survival.

Anything done by authorities in a particular district may be taken as an indication that further development will take place and will make people stay in the area. If promises are not fulfilled, people are misled. To be realistic in this planning needs a firm hand and a thorough knowledge of people and areas dealt with. Once a decision has been taken that a certain area is likely to be inhabited in the future and to foster its occupants, a modest long-term plan of development must be presented, especially for keeping the adequate chronological order between priorities. The first step to be taken may be a demographic study and collecting of some baseline health statistics.

It can be expected that international donor organizations will become interested in pastoral areas, where certain basic facts are known and the needs can be specified and motivated. In some cases projects for pastoral areas and nomadic populations should focus on populations rather than be bound to a certain country, as a tribe may migrate to two or three countries. Thus a new model of international and even inter-regional programmes would be needed.

Extreme conditions warrant extreme solutions. Designs of health services in urban or densely populated regions can seldom be transferred to pastoral areas, which need their own tailor-made design of service, adapted to its purpose in order to utilize resources in the most economic way. In many of these areas the adequate and realistic solution has been the establishment of a network of many small static units, staffed with a team of multipurposely trained personnel, dedicated to their work and duty station. These units must then be supervised by mobile units, wheeled or winged. Apart from supervising the remote units, mobile teams should assist with their more qualified medical personnel, bring drugs and medical equipment and transport sick people to and from hospitals. The mobile teams—as well as the static ones—could serve departments other than health, to justify the arrangement economically, if needed. A kind of multipurpose mobile service, specially designed for the situation in Kazakhistan (U.S.S.R.), was carried out in the 1920s by the 'red caravans' (kyzylkeruen). They were accompanied by doctors, teachers, and representatives of various social organizations, and camels carried manufactured goods, foodstuffs, medicaments, and even libraries for outlying nomadic camps.

Postgraduate training of professional, and especially auxiliary, personnel specifically for 'pastoral medicine' and for work with mobile units has been discussed in some countries, but not yet carried out. It is important that all personnel involved, whether static or mobile, should be dedicated people and multipurposely trained. The system carried out in some places to deport health personnel to pastoral areas as punishment for misbehaviour may add to the hardship of a population, which may already have much suffering. The grass-root contact of the team and 'kraal-side service' have been regarded as essential.

It may be necessary to favour personnel in remote places by offering higher salaries, longer vacations, free transport, assistance for schooling of children, and making professional literature available. In some cases youngsters taken from the actual tribe for training and returning to their fellow men, has only resulted in 'brain drain'.

An early and inexpensive method for raising the standard of health services, when a certain infrastructure has been established, is to introduce radiotelephones for consultation with hospitals, doctors, and nurses, and for ordering of transportation. Drug kits with detailed prescriptions may be an acceptable alternative in places where no health personnel is stationed.

Apart from small static units and mobile supervisory service, the guiding star should be a reliable transportation system, so that qualified medical service can be reached in emergency situations. This demands radiotelephones first, and secondly often aircraft.

Mobile units have a tendency to start gloriously and soon die out, when the car breaks down or the petrol allowances dry up. In some cases, such as the mobile eye-clinic in Kenya, a team

goes on for many years covering vast areas, where treatment of trachoma and eye operations are badly needed.

For national programmes, such as against smallpox, leprosy, and malaria, a special design of campaign is needed. This has been painfully experienced in malaria control programmes by WHO (Somali). If the area is left aside the whole programme

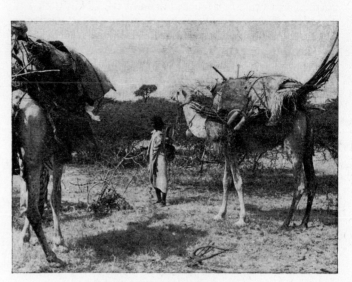

FIG. 104. Migrating Somali nomads.

may be wasted, as the nomads may keep the infection running and act as foci, when the programme has been accomplished and regarded successful. They may even carry the disease over the frontier to the next country, where it may already be eradicated.

To any nation-wide control of disease the minimum requirement is a sparse network of health stations or centres. Optimistically an infrastructure with one unit for 10,000–20,000 population has been suggested. The present utterly sparse infrastructure in nomad areas of the world makes adequate control of a series of diseases still unrealizable.

PRESENT AND FUTURE TRENDS IN PUBLIC HEALTH DEVELOPMENT OF PASTORAL AREAS

Nomad peoples and other scattered populations have so far not received their legitimate share of government and international benefits. In many cases they have been totally self-sufficient and asked for nothing from the outside, while in other cases the ecological situation is—or has become—unfavourable, keeping people on the verge of destitution. There is often only a narrow margin between survival, famine, and death from starvation, as the reserves are small or non-existent in the nomad's economy.

In some cases ecological catastrophes (Turkana, 1960; Sahel, 1973) have put the spotlight on nomadic tribes, and their future has been discussed. Assistance, tending to be everlasting, has been food and establishment of emergency camps or offering of new settlement areas. Any measure of this kind has to be used with the utmost consideration as they are likely to disrupt the traditional economy, produce an acultural and allowance-minded population, not inclined to return to their former livelihood.

Successively international organizations and especially the International Labour Organization (ILO) have been focusing on problems of pastoral groups, and United Nations funds have been earmarked for programmes in this field. The problems of pastoral areas were first touched upon by the UN in 1949, and since 1954 ILO has held a number of sessions, where particular problems of nomads in the Middle East and the Sahelian region have been debated. In 1964 ILO called a technical meeting on Nomadism and Sedentarization, and in 1966 ILO sponsored a study tour and seminar in the Soviet Union on the same subject. Health services for nomadic populations were discussed in the WHO Inter-Regional Seminar on National Health Planning in Addis Ababa in 1965 and in a seminar in Shiraz in 1973.

The interest shown by the United Nations has also been substantiated in its Inter-Agency Working Party on Problems of Rural Development in Africa. In a territory in Cameroon and Chad, containing a semi-nomadic population of over 2·5 million persons, the UN Development Programme has (since 1967) undertaken a survey aiming at control of the Logone River's seasonal floods. This would permit the people to change from flood agriculture and nomadic herding to permanent irrigating farming. Other projects for nomadic populations aim at developing semi-desert areas of Chad and control of syphilis in Niger (WHO). Lately the Awash Valley Development Scheme in Ethiopia has been started, in which the World Bank and bilateral donors are involved.

The main aspect on migrating peoples discussed at conferences and by planning of projects has been sedentarization and assimilation of nomads to the national communion. To some extent social anthropologists have been consulted, whereas socio-medical aspects have not been paid due attention to. The settlement of nomads has often been seen merely as a technical problem, but that is by no means the whole story. Beyond the technical problems loom also the far more serious and intractable human problems which merit equal if not greater care and expertise, and should be taboo for amateur efforts.

The motivation given for sedentarization of nomads has been the fact that people in a static village can be reached by social services, including health, at a reasonable cost. Furthermore, a reasonable utilization of the units can be expected, making the investment profitable from a pure economic point of view. One other motivation has been the improved opportunities to control a population in critical border-line areas if they are settled.

The disadvantage of sedentarization is, that the reason for the area being inhabited mostly by nomads is that no other livelihood could be squeezed out of the region, as the grass may be the only natural resource. The climate may permit no agricultural or ranging activities. The whole local culture may also be closely connected with and centred around nomadism. Thus switching to a settled living may rapidly rub out their cultural distinctive character and their independence, and at the same time disrupt the economy.

Sedentarization may be forced by authorities, offering no alternative, or encouraged by being linked to certain advantages and benefits, or it may be entirely voluntary and spontaneous—the latter way being the most physiological and considerate to their culture. If sedentarization is considered, one has to go the full length of one's tether in long-term planning, and see if a reasonable economy can be offered to the people in static villages. If, for example, cattle nomadism is the only possible livelihood, the family will stay in the village, while the herders have to continue their migrating life with the cattle. Thus milk and meat provided by the animals will be far away and not available to the family. Furthermore, the husband will lead a lonely life without his family and has to arrange his camps and food himself.

In marginal pastoral land sedentarization, and starting of ranging, has been stimulated (Masai) with some success, but the tribal ownership of feeding grounds raises legal obstacles. The subtribe or clan may have an area which they have claimed for generations for grazing, but the individual is not a land owner. Another drawback is that subcultures will develop, conflicting with traditional patterns. Individuals who are co-operative with authorities are sometimes already marginal people in the nomadic society.

As the primary need of a nomad is water, it seems that provision of water supplies would be the key to development of arid areas and for settlement of nomads. Water is needed for drinking by humans and animals—a camel can drink 130 litres at one time—and for irrigation in order to improve grazing, which in turn may limit the migration. In fact, no other single investment seems to have a more striking development effect and be more rewarding than the provision of water, and this concerns both nomadic and settled populations in many developing countries. Health conditions are automatically raised as hygiene improves. Cultivation of the soil may be made possible and a small scale agriculture started.

Housing, if not sufficiently guided when nomads settle down, tends to turn to slums very early. In any case, living in a house claims certain experience and different behaviour. The mobile life permits a rather lax hygiene without being harmful. However, many nomads continue to live in tents, although they have left nomadism and are leading a static life.

Arrangements have sometimes (Lappland) been offered pastoral people for a controlled slaughter, which should result in higher prices of their products. The idea does not necessarily please or tempt as the monetary economy may be unimportant to them, and any organized trading may take away the charm of private family trading. Finally, producing a surplus for sale does not always fit into their traditional system. Switching from intensive to extensive breeding of cattle or reindeer means a cultural change, which may not be wanted. To a Masai, cows have less to do with economy and food than the provision of recognized wealth and 'raison d'être'.

Once an agglomeration of a suitable size—maybe 2,000 people within a limited settlement area—has been established, health services of somewhat higher quality could be offered, e.g. a health centre with a team of auxiliaries. There will then be a reasonable accessibility and utilization rate making the investment economically justified. Radiotelephones can improve the services in an inexpensive way, and transportation facilities be made available. Primary schools may be added to the social services and a dry-season track constructed to the place, making it accessible by wheeled mobile units.

Any interference in foreign cultures is associated with a

great responsibility. Aculturation may result—people cannot change culture as one changes a shirt. Extinction of cultures has occurred, and even during a complete assimilation a loss of valuable cultural inheritance may take place. People do not always know how to make the right choice, to keep the best of their own culture and adopt the best of the new they are entering. A mixture of cultures may be disastrous, as the bad points of each may be adopted. Cultural conversions always imply lost generations.

It is often primarily a question of time and of education of the people, slowly to make them more qualified to choose and to ask for adequate development steps. The programme should be theirs and not ours. In this sensible procedure, sociological and even health guidance from outside is valuable in order to

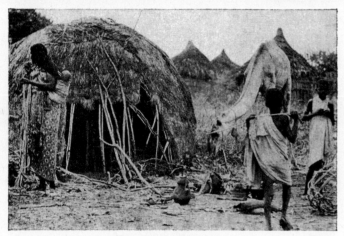

FIG. 105. Somali camp.

introduce modifications in a considerate and painless way, with respect for 'the total man in his total environment'. Standards of living may mean something totally different to them than to the national planner.

In the conventional dichotomy between policies of sedentarization versus *laissez-faire* in the administration of nomads, a careful consideration of modification as an alternative is recommended by the Norwegian anthropologist, Barth, in his paper on 'Nomadism in the mountain and plateau areas of South-West Asia'. Barth stresses that, 'a comparison of nomadic and settled communities in their present form reveals a clear difference in the average standard of living in favour of the nomad camp. Even in spite of recent great advances in public health in the villages of the region, the diet, hygiene, and health of all but the poorest nomad communities is better than that of most villages . . . wholesale assimilation of nomads into the sedentary population can only be achieved through economic and social proletarization: the nomad can find a place near the bottom of sedentary society. . . . The resistance to sedentarization among nomads can be understood simply in terms of self-interest; few men are willing to accept the reduction in standard of living which sedentarization implies. . . .'

Exploration and exploitation of natural resources such as oil, gold, and diamonds (Alaska, Kalahari, etc.) in a pastoral area, naturally turn things upside-down and there will hardly be any cultural considerations in the industrial development of the region.

Equality and complete social justice will always be a chimera as the profitableness of any investment, including health services, will always dominate development programmes. And also, many primitive people are ready to pay the price of limited services for their complete independence. There are advantages and disadvantages in nomadic life too.

Scattered populations other than nomads may have international organizations specially occupied with their problems. For refugees, the smallest member of the United Nations family, the United Nations High Commissioner for Refugees in Geneva, is responsible for the need and rights of the world's refugees, with an annual current budget of about 6 million U.S. $. Through this organization *ad hoc* assistance from donor countries can also be channelled to needy groups. In 1971 about 130 million U.S.$ went this way to the 10 million Pakistan refugees in India. Another organization, United Nations Relief and Works Agency, is responsible for the 1·5 million (1971) Palestine refugees in the Middle East.

Despite attempts—which may not have been the adequate solution at the adequate time—by various governments to settle nomadic people, nomadism continues to flourish and constitutes an accepted and respected way of life for large groups of the world's people. With an increasing communication between populations of the world today, information about conditions and standards of neighbour populations will reach everyone, and if a certain standard asked for does not become available, certain areas are soon likely to become empty, e.g. Turkana, Danakil, and Kalahari semi-deserts in Africa.

On the other hand, the population explosion of the world, which is expected, will in a not too far off future, lead to a global crisis. People will then have to look around the world, and any part of the surface may be considered or reconsidered for human habitation and survival.

Permafrost takes away 20 per cent. of the earth's land surface from this planning, as does the tundra, even with the most limited demands on standards of living, and are deemed to be almost uninhabitable, in spite of the experiences gained by Eskimos and other Arctic peoples. The first areas to be studied are those pastoral and arid areas, which today or in the past, have been occupied by primitive people, nomad collectors, and hunters and pastoralists. Therefore their techniques of survival and art of living may be worth noting, not only for planning the development of the present population, but also for planning of presumptive invaders in the future. It will be necessary to classify all these areas with regard to their climatic conditions and in relation to survival possibilities as hunters, collectors, fishers, small or large-scale farmers, cattle herders, and rangers. The situation should be studied on untouched conditions and be estimated after projected investments in water supply and irrigation.

REFERENCES AND FURTHER READING

Abel-Smith, B. (1967) An international study of health expenditure, *Wld Hlth Org. Publ. Hlth Pap.*, No. 32.

de Almeida, A. (1965) Bushmen and other non-Bantu peoples of Angola, Johannesburg.

Barth, F. (1962) Nomadism in the mountain and plateau areas of South-West Asia. Report of a UNESCO Symposium, The problems of the arid zone, p. 341.

Bhagwati, J. (1966) *U-ländernas ekonomi*, Aldus Universitet, Sweden.

Chang, W. P. (1969) Development of basic health services in Ethiopia, *J. Formosan med. Ass.*, **68**, No. 6.

Chang, W. P. (1970) Health manpower development in an African country—the case of Ethiopia, *J. med. Educ.*, **45**, 29.

Elkin, A. P. (1964) *The Australian Aborigines*, London.

Elliott, K. (1973) Doctor substitutes, *Health and Social Service Journal*, July 1973.

Famine Relief Committee, Government of Kenya (1962) Report on the Flood/Drought Catastrophe 1961/1962.

Fendall, N. R. E. (1963) Health centres: a basis for a rural health service, *J. trop. med. Hyg.*, **66**.

Hansen, J. D. L., and Truswell, A. S. (1968) Serum-lipids in Bushmen, *Lancet*, **ii**, 684.

Hansen, J. D. L., Truswell, A. S., Freeseman, C., and Mac-Hutchon (1969) The children of hunting and gathering Bushmen, *S. Afr. med. J.*, **63**, 1157.

Haraldson, S. (1963) Socio-medical conditions among the Lapps in Northernmost Sweden. Scand. School of P.H., *Svenska Läk.-Tidn.*, **59**, 2829.

Haraldson, S. (1968) Pastoral and nomadic populations in Kenya with special consideration to development of health services, WHO Report to Regional Office for Africa, Brazzaville.

Haraldson, S. (1970) Appraisal of health problems and definition of priorities in health planning, *Ethiop. med. J.*, **8**, 37.

Haraldson, S. (1973) Aspects on development of health services in pastoral areas. In the press.

International Labour Organization (ILO) (1964) Report on technical meeting on problems of nomadism and sedentarization.

International Labour Organization (ILO) (1966) Report on conference in Moscow on nomadism, etc.

Kimble, G. H. T. (1961) *Tropical Africa*. The Twentieth Century Fund.

Mann, G. V., Shaffer, R. D., and Rich, A. (1965) Physical fitness and immunity to heart disease in Masai, *Lancet*, **ii**, 1308.

Mann, G. V., Shaffer, R. D. *et al.* (1966) Survey of serologic evidence of syphilis among the Masai of Tanzania, *Publ. Hlth Rep. (Wash.)*, **81**, No. 6.

Marshall-Thomas, Elizabeth (1969) *The Harmless People* (Bushmen), Harmondsworth.

Mellbin, T. (1962) The children of Swedish Nomad Lapps, *Acta ped. (Uppsala)*, **51**, Suppl. 131.

Ministry of Health, Nairobi (1966) Reports on North-Eastern province.

Shaffer, R. (1965) Health in Turkana (Kenya). Dupl. by the African Medical and Research Foundation (AMRF), Nairobi.

Shaffer, R. (1965) Health in Olkejuad District (Kenya), Dupl. AMRF.

Shaffer, R. (1965) Narok District health survey (Kenya), Dupl. AMRF.

Truswell, A. S., and Hansen, J. D. L. (1968) Medical and nutritional studies of Kung Bushmen in North-West Botswana, *S. Afr. med. J.*, **42**, 1338.

Truswell, A. S., Hansen, J. D. L., Wannenburg, P., and Sellmeyer, E. (1969) Nutritional status of adult Bushmen in the Northern Kalahari, Botswana, *S. Afr. med. J.*, **63**, 1157.

Visser, W. M. (1965) Malaria eradication among the Nomads of Somalia, *Wld Hlth Org. Chron.*, p. 232.

Wehmeyer, A. S., Lee, R. B., and Whiting, M. (1969) The nutrient composition and dietary importance of some vegetable food eaten by the Kung Bushmen, *S. Afr. med. J.*, **63**, 1157.

World Health Organization, *Techn. Rep. Ser.*, No. 123 (1957), No. 162 (1959), No. 205 (1961).

World Health Organization (1965) Report on Inter-regional Seminar on National Health Planning, Addis Ababa, Regional Office for Eastern Mediterranean, Alexandria.

World Health Organization (1973) Report on a Seminar on Health Problems on Nomads, Shiraz/Isafan, Regional Office for Eastern Mediterranean, Alexandria.

41

PLANNING OF HEALTH SERVICES AND THE HEALTH TEAM

J. H. F. BROTHERSTON and G. D. FORWELL

'Let us first be reminded that "health planning" is a relatively new venture . . . what deserves to be named by this term in fact started in the Soviet Union after the Russian revolution as part of the over-all economic and social planning. I am, by the way, old enough still to recall vividly how the whole planning process in the Soviet Union was ridiculed and laughed at in the western world at that time. Now, I think, few countries with any national self-concern refrain from producing "five-year plans" or plans for shorter periods practically in all important fields. As far as health planning is concerned, most countries, however, only started it after the Second World War.'

Evang, 1965

Introduction

The World Health Organization definition of health is 'a state of complete physical, mental and social well-being and and not merely the absence of disease or infirmity'. In keeping with this is the comprehensive definition of public health by Winslow (1951), quoted in full in the preface to this book. In this comprehensive sense, public health includes the planning of health services.

The term 'medical care' is now widely used as somehow separate and different from public health, which in consequence is restrictively defined. Abel-Smith (1967) defined the terms of public health, medical care, and health services for his international study of health expenditure. He regards 'public health' as covering services which are primarily of a promotional or preventive character and 'medical care' as intended, apart from obstetrics, to denote only health services which are primarily for diagnosis or treatment. However, he does use the term 'health services' as describing the sum not only of public health and medical care but also related education and research. This definition of health services is applicable to the present chapter. In the planning of health services it is now a distortion to think of the medical care organization as other than a vital and integral part of the total health system. In keeping with this is the definition of medical care used by the WHO Expert Committee on Organization of Medical Care (1959): 'a programme of services that should make available to the individual, and thereby to the community, all facilities of medical and allied sciences necessary to promote and maintain health of mind and body. This programme should take into account the physical, social and family environment, with a view to the prevention of disease, the restoration of health and the alleviation of disability.'

THE CONTEXT OF PLANNING

Health services are only one aspect of the complex matrix of a society. By and large, they take their shape from that society.

The determinants of health services and their planning may be classified as political, historical, cultural, economic, demographic and epidemiological, and scientific and technological.

Political Determinants

The form of government and delivery of health services reflects, in outline and in detail, the political system and tradition of the country. Evang (1960), in a world review of health-service organizations, distinguished four main types of health services, the Western European, the American, the type evolved by the People's Republics, and the type in developing countries. Although Evang's classification is based on the comparison of national health services, it is significant that this approximates to political groupings of nations in the world today. A system of state socialism such as that seen in the People's Republics assumes the provision of health services as a direct responsibility, whereas an American 'free-economy' system will assume provision by private enterprise and arrangement. Similarly, hierarchical administration in the former group is reflected in the structure and staffing of the health service system, just as the tradition of individualism is seen especially in the United States. The extent of consensus seeking before decisions are made and the methods employed also reflect national and local traditions; for example, Evang points to the complexity of health service systems in his Western European type, in which central authority tends to be divided between several government departments, with much decentralization of decisions to local responsibility.

Despite these differences, all forms of government have a vested interest in the health of their people, although very different methods may be adopted, and different levels of priority given, to advance this interest. Even government systems which assume provision through private enterprise will seek, if deemed necessary, to support the provision of health services. In this connexion it is notable how the free-market system in the United States has been modified in the decade since Evang made his classification.

Historical Determinants

Like other facets of government and administration, normally the strongest influence in shaping the future of a service is its past. This is true, even when apparently drastic organizational changes are made: in Britain the form of the National Health Service introduced in 1948 was shaped largely by historical determinants. Commonly the earliest interest of government in health services was through quarantine arrangements to prevent the introduction of infection from other countries. Eventually, the impact of industrialization and urban growth, for example, in the eighteenth and nineteenth centuries in Europe and North America, led to government intervention to control epidemic disease among overcrowded populations through sanitary measures. Usually government interest in personal health promotive services for children and mothers formed a next stage of development. Although government measures to provide custodial and medical care for selected groups, e.g. armed forces, mariners, paupers, may be of long-standing, active intervention to provide or support such services for larger populations is comparatively recent, coinciding with the evolution of medicine and surgery as effective therapeutic disciplines. The pressure for government intervention mounts steadily with the increasing effectiveness, cost, and complexity of medical care.

Certain of the common characteristics of health services which are historically determined persist, although they may be recognized to be unhelpful anachronisms in modern times: the tendency in developed countries for the administration and delivery of preventive services to be separate from curative responsibilities derives from historical development rather than from the inherent needs of their existing health situation.

Cultural Determinants

The cultural determinants of health care systems are complex and ramifying, the ethos of Western medicine is itself shaped by its Greco-Christian origins. The extent to which health personnel and services are sought after for support by individuals and communities is influenced not only by their technical capacity but also by the extent, availability, and acceptability of other types of support. Thus a society in which traditional religion still plays a strong part in individual and social life will be less likely than a more secular society to seek assistance from its health services for problems of unhappiness, social maladjustment, and even mental illness. The extent to which illness itself, the *sickness role*, is acceptable in society will vary from one culture to another. Thus behaviour syndromes, which in one society will be acceptable as sickness, and elicit medical care and supporting financial benefits, might in another society be stigmatized as delinquent or irresponsible behaviour, and accordingly evoke condemnation and even punishment. Public understanding, types, and levels of education, both formal and informal, are clearly of great importance, Contemporary pseudo-scientific philosophy, especially as regards mental health, may lead to demands on medical science and medical care which cannot be realized. Health services, as an easily recognized and esteemed source of help, may be approached with problems of social need or social maladjustment. In this situation there is a danger of medicine making unwarranted claims to solve problems for which it has no answer. The more useful alternative is for the medical services to develop close links with social and counselling services and transmit these problems to whichever of these services is appropriate.

The public demand for medical care is growing and showing evidence of acceleration with increasing confidence in modern medicine, advancing levels of education, and rising standards of life, with diminished tolerance of pain and disability. The level of amenity to be provided is also, especially in privately funded health services, in part determined by rising standards of comfort. In the past, 'need' for health services, in the sense of the pool of ill health in the community, has often been seen as the sole and absolute determinant of what has to be provided. Today not only is there scepticism of the capacity to measure need in that ultimate sense but also whether the concept of need itself is helpful. In addition, there is a growing awareness of the importance of public expectations as a major factor in determining the pressure of demand on health services. Although pockets and strata of relative ignorance and resistance manifestly still exist, the problems today, in both developed and developing countries, are more those of meeting demand than of persuading people to use services. There is the beneficial tendency for previous attitudes of fatalism towards disease to become erased, although such attitudes are still prevalent, especially in the older age groups. This is a very recent change, and this world-wide interest in, and demand for, health care is perhaps the most significant phenomenon of our times for the health planner. Even so, there remain pockets of relative resistance. Generally speaking, the elderly are more cautious in their demands relative to their needs; there are problems where fear and mistrust still create resistance, notably as regards mental illness and cancer. However, in general, the trend is for resistance to lessen, and thus for the pressure of demand to increase.

Much of the change in public attitudes is the consequence of the considerable improvement which has taken place in the quite recent past in average standards of living and education, at least in developed countries. Long-term economic forecasts assume a steadily rising gross national product, with rising income levels in real terms, and increasing expenditure on education and other social services. This affects health services in many ways, some obvious and direct, and others more subtle. Social differences are narrowed, and the relationship between doctor and patients is bound to be influenced by this. While doctors sometimes complain that their status has changed, it is in fact the status of the patients which has altered (Platt, 1963).

Education, propaganda, and publicity take different forms in different countries. The tendency as yet is for emphasis to be placed largely on what the health service has to offer to the exclusion of consideration of the active role which the individual himself can play in determining his own health, or in making intelligent and responsible use of services. Within any country it tends to be the better educated and more intelligent who exploit the services more effectively to their advantage. Even where the provision of services is totally free from economic barriers or restraints, the more ignorant, who are often also those in greatest need, may tend to make least effective use of services.

In Britain mortality and other personal statistics are available classified by socio-economic state ('social class'); persons are classified into five groups by the level of skill and social status of the occupation of the head of their household. The classification broadly correlates with education and income. The overall mortality experience for males shows an upward gradient from the professional occupational group to the unskilled group, but there is a number of important causes of death in which the mortality is greatest in the professional and managerial groups, notably ischaemic heart disease. A high standard of living brings with it its own mortality risks. As one would expect, trends in serious morbidity follow the same curve as those for mortality; in general, one adverse for the less-privileged social groups. When a group of general practitioners in England examined all their male patients aged 60–69 the proportion of men with disease detected increased in social class order from two out of three in professional occupations to six out of seven in unskilled occupations, and the proportion with disability from one in seven to two in three (Brown *et al.*, 1958). The proportion of men with disease who were in some degree disabled was one in four in professional occupations and three in four in unskilled occupations. The prevalence of six of the eight most common diseases (bronchitis, coronary disease, hypertension, peptic ulcer, defective hearing, and defective vision) was related in similar fashion to socio-economic status. Although there was no uniform gradient with social class, in seventy-six general medical practices in England and Wales standardized patient consulting ratios were higher in unskilled than professional males aged 15–64 years (Logan, 1960). In Scotland hospital admission rates, duration of hospital stay, and bed usage showed an upward trend from professional to unskilled group in both men and married women; the interclass differences were less for the married women than for the men (Carstairs and Patterson, 1966).

The extent to which services are developed towards seeking patients differs between countries. Since most health services still operate largely on an 'on-demand' basis, it is the individual himself who initiates action from the service. Although it is axiomatic that the patient himself is potentially one of the most important agencies for the early detection of serious disease, deliberate public education towards the recognition of personal signs and symptoms for subsequent professional investigation is still controversial. There is a need for a study of the preventive value of many proposed screening techniques; for example, the value of self-examination of the breast in the early diagnosis of breast cancer has never been adequately assessed (Wilson and Jungner, 1968).

There is a tendency for public expectations as regards health services to be too readily satisfied. There is evidence that in every country which has a health service which is well known to its population this service is popular and rated highly, irrespective of its organization or system of financing. However, it is probable in the future that there will be a tendency for public attitudes to become more discriminating, sophisticated, and demanding. Health care systems tend to develop insensitivity or resentment towards public criticism. This attitude fails to take account of the fact that public interest must ultimately be the main source of support for improvement and progress in health services. Accordingly, there is a need to educate professional as well as public opinion in this field, and

the aim should be to take the public into a partnership of understanding.

As a generalization, it may be concluded that partnership with the consumer, the public, is one of the least studied, and in the long run most important, responsibilities of the health planner. In the ultimate analysis it is the public's interest as client, as tax-payer, and discerning user and critic which will determine levels of support and quality of health services.

Economic Determinants

The importance of economic factors in the planning of health services is manifest. They influence directly the levels of provision, and indirectly the scale and types of problem with which the service must deal. The scale of operation is largely a function of the economic strength of the country; so much so that the convention has developed of quoting levels of expenditure in terms of the percentage of gross national product allocated. These calculations are subject to considerable error, but they show a good deal of variation as between nations of approximately similar economic strength. There is also great variation in the sources of expenditure incurred by different systems; varying from the simplest kind of arrangements, where virtually all expenditure is directly from governments, to complex mixes of expenditure by private individuals, charitable foundations, industry, private and public, insurance, and local and central taxation.

When compared with *per capita* daily national income the cost, for example, of a day in a general hospital varies widely between countries. In this relative sense, Abel-Smith (1967) found that general hospital care was far more expensive in low-income than in high-income countries; in a low-income country, where a day in a general hospital cost ten times the average daily national income, 4 per cent. of the national income would be required to provide four hospital beds per thousand of the population. On the other hand, health services were more expensive in absolute terms in high-income than in low-income countries, because in high-income countries the price of direct labour tends to be high compared with the price of goods, and the possibilities of automation and mechanization in health services are relatively more limited than in most other industries.

Mounting costs of health care are the most obvious contemporary pressure on the health planner. This is as much a reflection of provision extending to meet the demand as of the increasing technical potential and complexity of modern medicine. In consequence, the costs of health services in most countries are increasing at a higher rate than the rise of national income. Abel-Smith (1967) has shown that in high-income countries there was a secular trend between 1953 and 1961 for expenditure on health services to increase as a proportion of gross national product. In general, the rate of increase was such that an additional 1 per cent. or more of gross national product was absorbed in health expenditure in a decade; if this trend continues, before the end of the present century there will be countries in which more than 10 per cent. of the gross national product is devoted to health services. In all the countries studied by Abel-Smith an increasing proportion of total health expenditure was being devoted to hospitals. Planning to achieve a more rational and effective use of medical institutions, notably hospitals, is becoming an urgent matter; the same is true of the many types of medical and paramedical personnel, engaged on health service work. The medical profession has demonstrated relatively little interest in these and other administrative aspects of health services (Evang, 1967).

Improvement in material conditions increases disproportionately to other types of consumption, the demand for all kinds of service, including health services; the same influences which increase the demand for all categories of health personnel, simultaneously tend to diminish their working hours (Biörck, 1965). General demand in the labour market for skilled people tends to accelerate the rise of wages and salaries of health service personnel. Mounting costs create their own pressures in health systems which manifest in different ways. In systems which have been largely privately financed there is a shift towards increasing government support. There are pressures towards rationalization; but, generally speaking, health services do not readily respond to market pressures.

The elements of the calculations which determine the proportion of national expenditure which goes on health services are usually difficult to discern. Much the biggest element in most systems is simply a historical determinant, the carry forward of past expenditure with gradual addition and subtraction of services. In government-supported services national economic planning will increasingly tend to lead to deliberate decisions to allocate national resources in a planned fashion between different services. Clearly many different factors influence the decision how much to allocate to health services compared with, for example, to education or roads. Expenditure aimed to raise standards of living in terms of nutrition, housing, and education may in the long run influence the national health as much as, or more than, direct expenditure on health services. In general, those responsible for health services are in difficulties as compared with other services in demonstrating an economic return for expenditure incurred. Many calculations have been made in many places over many years to demonstrate the economic value of health and health services, but the fact remains that the propositions are difficult to demonstrate in any conclusive way, except in rare and limited circumstances. In fact, in recent years supporters of a specious neo-Malthusian analysis have asserted that health services have an adverse effect on national well-being in some developing countries by increasing population pressures on resources through instituting death control without any corresponding control of births.

Demographic and Epidemiological Determinants

Age. In the developed countries, especially during the last fifty years, the expectation of life at birth has risen sharply till it has now reached 70 years. However, during this period, the further expectation of life for a man aged 65 has not altered significantly. At all ages the expectation of life has been consistently slightly greater for females than for males; during the last thirty years there has been an accelerating trend for the mortality experience of the sexes to diverge after middle age, so that a woman aged 65 can now expect to live several years longer than her male contemporary. In Britain today there are two women aged over 80 years for every one man.

In the young population the health service emphasis moves progressively from the hazards of birth, to congenital and other malformation, to services for the early detection of disability, and to the acute illness of infancy and young childhood. In adolescence and young adult life importance centres on physical injury and emotional disorders, perhaps attended by drug addition or self-poisoning. Education in turn for parenthood and infant welfare is associated with the provision of obstetric services. The working and middle-age period is where services for early diagnosis of chronic degenerative disease are most required, together with emphasis on the morbidity and disability which cause absence from work or family duties.

The characteristic difference between the age structure of developing and developed countries is the proportion of the elderly in the latter. This elderly population inevitably carries a mass of disease processes with consequent physical and mental disabilities which, at least quantitatively, dominate the other calls on health service resources. The prevalence of chronic disease and disability increases rapidly and progressively after middle age. The proportion of persons in Baltimore, who were found to have no chronic diseases ranged from 71 per cent. for those under 15 years of age to only 5 per cent. for persons aged 65 and over (Commission on Chronic Illness, 1957a). This trend was paralleled by the prevalence of limitations on the activities of daily life. While 30 per cent. of those 65 years of age and over had some limitation of activity, only a little over 1 per cent. of persons under age 55 had any limitations. Ciocco and Lawrence (1958) found that in Hagerstown, Maryland, of every 1,000 persons who were well at 45 years of age, about 100 needed medical attention during the next five years because of the onset of some chronic illness or major impairment. Some of these needed medical care from time to time, a smaller number needed also constant treatment or care of some kind until death occurred. Of those who were well at 60 years of age, almost 25 per cent. acquired a chronic illness within five years, for which, in many cases, continuing medical care was necessary.

The increased use of health services with age has been illustrated by Engel (1965) in terms of 'consumer units'. Where the average use by the entire population of all types of health service was one unit, the 0–9 age group used an average of 0·4 units, and the 80 years and over group, 2·4 units. Although the use of services by the intermediate decades ranked with increasing age in regular ascending order, this did not begin to rise rapidly till the 50–59 age group [TABLE 116].

Illness and disability in old age arises from conventional physical and mental diseases. Wilson *et al.* (1962) found an average of six disease processes in patients, mainly over 70 years old, admitted to a hospital medical geriatric unit. With the notable exception of arterial hypertension, which was significantly related to disorders of heart and brain, these multiple disorders were not usually the varied manifestation of one disease but rather an expression of several apparently independent processes.

In addition, difficulties arise because the chronic and normally multiple nature of the pathological processes is productive of long-term disability, which creates a special responsibility for long-term supervision. This disability is commonly both physical and mental, and frequently linked to requirements for social care and supervision, when the normal domestic arrangements fail through incapacity, overload, or bereavement. This complex of social, physical, and mental problems of ageing creates a spectrum of need to be met by health services and society through the provision of housing, income, and domestic help, substitute homes and long-term hospital beds. At any point on the spectrum medical care may be required. The nature of these medical needs is not specific to the elderly, but their problems are more unstable, are more commonly multiple, and apt to diminish independence, sometimes permanently. Although the great majority of the elderly are self-maintaining or maintain themselves with the assistance of relatives or friends (Townsend and Wedderburn, 1965), the total medical care need of the elderly is so great that it may create problems of overload throughout the entire system. An appropriate range of provision, both social and medical, must be provided to match this load, its spectrum of need, and the speed with which the individual may move from independence to dependence, and back again.

TABLE 116

Number of Medical-care Consumption Units per Individual at Different Ages (Engel, 1965)

| Age | An individual at the stated age corresponds to the number of consumption units given below | | | | |
	Care in general, tuberculosis, and isolation hospitals	Long-term care for somatic diseases	Mental care	Ambulatory care	All forms of care (in round figures)
0–9	0·63	0·00	0·00	0·35	0·4
10–19	0·47	0·02	0·01	0·27	0·5
20–29	0·78	0·02	0·27	0·53	0·5
30–39	0·82	0·03	0·49	0·73	0·6
40–49	0·90	0·09	0·90	0·83	0·8
50–59	1·29	0·21	1·30	1·24	1·2
60–69	1·74	0·69	1·87	1·68	1·6
70–79	2·00	2·09	2·15	2·07	2·0
80–	1·37	6·85	3·01	2·30	2·4

Family Structure. Age and family structure of the population have to be taken into account by the health planner, not only nationally but also locally, since significant differences may exist between different communities. Localities from which much emigration has taken place tend to have higher than average proportions of elderly, as do suburban and health-resort communities popular for retirement. New communities, such as housing estates, dormitory areas, and planned new towns, have disproportionately large populations of children. The age structure of such communities may present special challenges for the planner, because the health service requirements shift as the child population grows up. The family ties, and the strength of the kinship and neighbourhood social structure, vary greatly between communities of different types, and is of significance to the planner. The extent to which mothers of young children can call upon the traditional support of the grandmother and other relatives materially affects the need for supporting services to assist when the family is in trouble from illness or other reasons. The isolation of the young mother from traditional support in new communities may increase her vulnerability and need for support from health and social services (Martin *et al.*, 1957). Paediatric hospital policies of planned admission of mother and baby may be more easy to implement in communities where relatives and neigh-

bours are at hand to look after older children. Similar differences will exist with any service which includes large elements of community care. For example, in planned community care of mental illness it is dangerous to make assumptions based on the experience of other localities without careful assessment of the social strengths and weaknesses of the community for which the service is planned.

These social background factors are, perhaps, most clearly seen in services for the care of the aged. Traditional communities, with kinship and neighbourhood ties strong and intact, can support heavy problems of care within the family. In other situations where the elderly have been left behind, or have moved from their families, for example, in the decaying centres of cities or in retirement resorts, health and social services may have to substitute for almost every element of domestic need in situations of waning independence (Nuffield Foundation, 1947).

Admission to hospital and use of other health services, especially by the mentally ill and the elderly, is closely related to family structure. Abel-Smith and Titmuss (1956) compared hospital in-patients with the total population on the night of a population census; in the hospital population there was an excess of single and unmarried persons, and, indeed, more than two-thirds of those over 65 years of age in hospital on census night were single, widowed, or divorced.

Townsend and Wedderburn (1965) compared the family structure of the less than 5 per cent. of persons aged 65 and over in Britain living in hospitals and other institutions with the remainder living at home. Far more of the old people in institutions were unmarried, more lacked children, more lacked brothers and sisters, and more of those who had children had only one, and had sons rather than daughters. Persons who had relatives but found themselves in institutions were persons who had more often led their lives in seclusion from their relatives. In summary, in family structure and propinquity the elderly institutional population differed sharply from the rest of the elderly population. Similarly, those who received health and welfare services at home differed in family structure and propinquity from the rest of the elderly population at home. For example, 39 per cent. lived alone, compared with 22 per cent.; 30 per cent. were unmarried or childless, compared with 22 per cent.; 41 per cent. did not have any relatives living within 10 minutes' journey of their houses, compared with 31 per cent. There was little evidence of health and welfare services being 'misused' or 'undermining family responsibilities'. Those who benefited from the services were mainly infirm or incapacitated persons who lacked a family or had none within reach. The survey suggests that the family does in fact play a positive role for many old people, with a considerable body of data to support this suggestion. For example, there were over four times as many bedfast or otherwise severely incapacitated old people living at home as in all types of institutions; most of them were living with members of their families, and were cared for by them. Townsend and Wedderburn also provided evidence that in illness and infirmity the role of the family dwarfed that of the social services. Of those who were ill in bed at some time in the course of a year, 77 per cent. relied on a spouse, children, or other relatives for help with housework, 80 per cent. for help with shopping, and 82 per cent. for help with meals, compared with 5, 2, and 1 per cent. who relied on the public social services. An interesting point shown by the survey was that some services, such as home nursing and chiropody, were required by persons whether or not they could rely on the resources of the family, simply because the family is not equipped to provide such skilled professional services. This suggests that the respective roles of the family and of domiciliary services in meeting the needs of the aged should increasingly be thought of as complementing each other rather than as alternatives. The domiciliary services perform two main positive functions: they furnish expert professional help which the family cannot supply, and they furnish unskilled or semi-skilled help for persons who do not have families, and whose families living in the household or near by are not always able or available for help. In all health-care systems it is manifestly an appropriate priority to develop the capacity of the domiciliary services to keep the maximum number of individuals fit and active, and to prolong their independence to the utmost.

Scientific and Technological Determinants

Scientific and technological factors are increasingly significant determinants of health services for two reasons: the degree of involvement of scientific techniques in medicine is growing, and so also is the rate of change of these techniques. One inevitable consequence of this trend is for increasing institutionalization of medical care; another is for staff specialization, because skill in the application of practical techniques requires concentration of training and experience.

In some ways the relatively abrupt change consequent on the introduction of science and technology into medicine resembled the Industrial Revolution: the doctor's place of work is moving from the patient's home to the hospital or other health service institution. This institutional setting permits the concentration of skills and equipment; it affords access to complex and sophisticated health teams and elaborate investigative and treatment facilities. However, a potential contrary trend also exists, in that the power of the individual doctor to treat patients outside hospital has been vastly increased, especially in the last thirty years, by the scientific development of potent drugs. Scientific changes have also the indirect effect of creating a public attitude that quality of care is appropriately associated with an ambience of science. The public attitude may be ambivalent and combine a predilection for an aura of science with a desire for personal care and for privacy. The net balance in the two-way results of scientific development is in the direction of increasing resources being required to exploit the new possibilities. The rate of scientific advance in medicine is escalating, bringing in train new opportunities as challenges for the planner and new competing demands for support. Together with all the other pressures for increased services, there arises a situation for the planner demanding the greatest economy, flexibility, and ease of redeployment in the use of resources.

OBJECTIVES OF HEALTH SERVICES

The general objectives of health services are frequently expressed as health promotion, and the prevention and treatment of disease. Treatment services are sometimes referred to as curative services, although cure is possible in a relatively small proportion of the cases of established chronic disease which occupy so much of the attention of services in developed countries; for the majority of such patients mitigation, or even only palliation, is all that is possible. Inseparable from treatment services is the need for rehabilitation to begin simultaneously with treatment.

Promotion of Health

The improvement in health which has taken place in developed countries over the last 200 years was the result of a rising standard of living till a century ago, when preventive medicine became a potent factor, followed by treatment of the individual in the twentieth century. In developed countries the most important health-promotive factors are normally not the direct concern of health services. However, any or all of these factors, notably nutrition, housing, education, and conditions of work, may become of direct concern to health services, at any rate for particular categories or age groups, for example, mothers and children. Where infection and malnutrition are the principal causes of ill health, disease and death (as in many developing countries today, but as in the past in the developed countries), material progress and rising standards of living are strongly positive influences in improving general levels of health. However, today the tide of material progress is no longer wholly favourable to health in the developed countries. Indeed, their endemic plagues of cardiovascular disease and cancer are partly caused by the habits of a prosperous society.

One promotive activity of relevance to all health services is health education. In many health systems this is an activity to which insufficient effort and resources are devoted. Most current health-education activities are comparatively simple and unsophisticated, and achieve their greatest successes in situations where relatively simple lessons have to be taught. The greatest immediate gains obtainable from health promotion in developed countries will have to come from persuading populations to modify or abandon cherished habits of excess and self-indulgence. Progress towards more sophisticated techniques of health education capable of making some impact in such situations must come from fundamental research on human behaviour, attitudes, and motivations.

Prevention

Preventive measures ('primary prevention') have never required any justification, as prevention is a self-evident basic general objective of health services. However, a more recent motivation to develop services for prevention has been the recognition that the mounting costs of treatment, and public demand for it, make the very credibility of treatment services depend on the maximum effort being expended on prevention.

Apart from health-promotive factors such as nutrition, environmental control has been the most effective type of health care activity in producing the improved standards of health in the developed countries. It is commonly and incorrectly believed that all the important environmental hazards are today adequately recognized and controlled. We are in fact contending with familiar hazards spread by new or newly recognized means, and are only now recognizing fully the significance of many environmental hazards, for example, atmospheric pollution and radiation. In addition, man is continually creating new artificial hazards; for example, the control of food additives sets a problem of increasing extent and complexity.

Communicable disease control is related to environmental control, at least in so far as the latter is concerned with importation of infection and prevention of its spread. In epidemic control, as in other aspects of communicable disease control, there is an obvious need for a unified attack by epidemiological and treatment services. Hospital infection, where exogenous, is an increasingly important facet of communicable disease control. Primary prevention by immunization is practicable in an increasing range of diseases. The public response has sometimes been poor, and this is a potentially fruitful field for health education. In addition, it is important to provide the immunization services in a fashion convenient for the public, and economical in the use of health service staff. Such a service for the management of a vaccination and immunization scheme, including follow-up, was developed by Galloway (1963) using electronic data processing.

For most populations of the world the first priority is to control infections, in a social context which is adverse in many respects, especially in respect of widespread sub-nutrition. In general, in such situations the established techniques and 'know-how' of public health and preventive and curative medicine have the answers to the prevailing problems. The obstacles to progress lie in the fields of economic development and control of population expansion. A heavy problem for many developing countries is how to find the huge capital resources needed to establish basic environmental controls, such as providing plentiful and safe water supplies and efficient methods of sewage disposal. In situations of rapid urbanization such needs, along with the squalor created by multiplication of miserable shanty-type houses, may escalate to truly daunting proportions. Yet no effective health service can be envisaged without a plan for provision of such essentials.

Primary prevention of other than communicable disease is limited by lack of knowledge of aetiology. In a few instances, where the disease is a response to a known hazard, this hazard can be controlled, for example, by eliminating contact with a toxic industrial substance. If prevention of the common degenerative diseases is to be achieved the sphere of preventive medicine must move from the environment to the individual; this exposes the artificiality of the traditional distinction between prevention and treatment in the care of the individual where diseases are caused or aggravated by personal habits. Progress is dependent on our ability to persuade individuals to alter their own adverse behaviour. Changed individual habits of eating, drinking, smoking, and physical exertion may be as difficult to achieve as termination of drug taking or abuse of alcohol. The condemned behaviour may be cherished and, unlike the provision of a clean, chlorinated, fluoridated water supply, personal effort and inconvenience is required.

Treatment

Two main factors affect the potential of treatment services, the scientific possibilities and the pattern of disease. In considering the pattern of disease, the priorities depend on the state of socio-economic development of the country and the age structure of its population.

The developed countries are confronting problems of de-generative disease for which modern medicine has still little to offer in the way of cure; the possibilities of prevention ('primary prevention') are equally limited or fraught with great difficulty. A range of health services is required to deal with this pattern of disease so that individual patients may receive treatment appropriate for the stage reached in the disease process. Increasing interest is shown in the development of schemes for early detection of disease, so-called 'screening' and pre-symptomatic diagnosis. This development is a much more difficult exercise than is often realized. Certain criteria require to be satisfied (Commission on Chronic Illness, 1957b), notably that the detection procedure proposed is valid, reliable, acceptable, and by yield and cost deserves priority over more conventional medical measures. Also there is a presumptive undertaking that treatment is possible and will be made available to those who require it.

The World Health Organization recently commissioned a publication on the principles and practice of screening for disease (Wilson and Jungner, 1968). This provides an excellent summary of current progress, including the following principles as guides to public health services in planning schemes for early disease detection:

1. The condition sought should be an important health problem.

2. There should be an accepted treatment for patients with recognized disease.

3. Facilities for diagnosis and treatment should be available.

4. There should be a recognizable latent or early symptomatic stage.

5. There should be a suitable test or examination.

6. The test should be acceptable to the population.

7. The natural history of the condition, including development from latent to declared disease, should be adequately understood.

8. There should be an agreed policy on whom to treat as patients.

9. The cost of case-finding (including diagnosis and treatment of patients diagnosed) should be economically balanced in relation to possible expenditure on medical care as a whole.

10. Case finding should be a continuing process and not a 'once and for all' project.

Following early diagnosis, ease of patient access from first point of recognition to point of definitive diagnosis and treatment is very important. Obstacles to this may lie primarily with health service and social organization or with the patient. It is incumbent on the health service to ensure that the patient, probably rendered anxious by being called for medical attention, does not require to join a waiting-list or suffer from communication delays within or between health services. As regards patient obstacles, fears of costs of major or long-term illness itself can largely be circumvented only where there exists an adequate social-security system or private insurance; fear of loss of employment, at least in the private sector, is more difficult to overcome, although here again the social-security system or private insurance can be a compensating factor. A further frequent obstacle to rapid follow-up and treatment is the presence of domestic responsibilities, for example, that of a mother for young children or of an adult for the care of an elderly relative.

Rehabilitation

In the interests of both patient and health service, efforts are required to ensure maximum long-term benefit from therapeutic effort expended, even where complete cure is not possible. There is, however, widespread failure to realize the importance of after-care and rehabilitation. It is axiomatic that the rehabilitative process should begin as soon as the diagnosis has been reached; this axiom is commonly preached, but rarely practised. The series of 'Hospital and Community' studies supported by the Nuffield Provincial Hospitals Trust has convincingly shown the consequences of failure to give attention to after-care and rehabilitation. Ferguson and MacPhail (1954) studied the subsequent histories of 705 men discharged from the acute medical wards of four hospitals in Scotland. Within the five years immediately preceding the admission on which the study was based, one-third of these patients had already had one or more spells of inpatient treatment, or outpatient hospital care, for the condition responsible for their recent hospital admission, or for one closely related. Ten per cent. died within three months of leaving hospital, 5 per cent. had been readmitted, and a further 10 per cent. seen in their own homes three months after discharge had clearly deteriorated. By two years after discharge 25 per cent. of the original 705 men were known to have died, many after further spells of hospital treatment; 30 per cent. of the survivors had worked for less than one of the two years since leaving hospital. In the further study carried out by the same authors (Ferguson and MacPhail, 1962) a similar type of follow-up was used, except that help, usually of a social nature, was sought for the patients. The outcome was as disappointing as in the initial study, although evidence is presented that the development of efficient rehabilitation and after-care services, together with an intensified approach to the resettlement in work of disabled men, would lead to better results. Previous studies elsewhere in Britain showed an equally depressing picture and similar need for development of rehabilitation services (Brown and Carling, 1945; Beck et al., 1947; Pemberton and Smith, 1949).

DELIVERY OF HEALTH SERVICES

Front-line and Domiciliary Care

In all health care systems there is a particular service or range of services, which is normally the point of first contact by the patient. There is great variety between countries in the staffing of this front-line. Where there is a doctor in the front-line, he tends to be a general practitioner. In most developed countries similar problems for the front-line doctor have been demonstrated, and recruitment to general practice is becoming difficult. The reasons given are everywhere practically identical: loss of status in relation to specialists and medical institutions, heavy work load, irregular working hours, bureaucratization of practice with too much paper work, professional isolation and therefore reduced possibility for postgraduate training, and, on the whole, professional frustration (Evang, 1967). Nevertheless, in the foreseeable future the early recognition of disease will still depend predominantly on the front-line health service. The problem as regards early diagnosis by this service

is how to enable the staff to remain alert to the early signs of serious disease among the large volume of minor illness.

The supporters of a front-line service provided by general practitioners acting as personal physicians advance many reasons, in addition to early detection of disease, why such a system is desirable: the individual's need for a personal, informal, well-known point of contact with the health care system; the paradoxical necessity in a medical world of increasing specialization and sub-specialization that there should be someone to construe the system in the best interests of the patient; the increasing emphasis which must be given to continuity of care as degenerative disease processes become proportionately more significant; the insights of social and psychological medicine into the importance of cultural and emotional pressures; and the new knowledge reinforcing the old wisdom that there are no diseases, only sick people.

It is interesting to note the increasing awareness, in countries where general practice has dwindled or disappeared, of a serious gap which has opened up as a result in their patient-care services. Many individuals and committees have concluded that general practice is an essential speciality in medicine and that it requires urgent study. The WHO Expert Committee on Professional and Technical Education of Medical and Auxiliary Personnel (1963) recommended research into the different forms which family practice can assume not only in various countries but also in different situations in the same country, for example, urban and rural areas.

In most systems the relatively large share of medical care carried out by the domiciliary services in comparison with the hospitals makes essential close integration with at least the support services of the hospital. Moreover, there is a very considerable overlapping of problems dealt with at home and in hospital.

At first sight it appears incontrovertible that it is cheaper to keep a patient at home than to send him to hospital. However, Jones (1964) has pointed out, at least as regards mental health services, the question of cost is not so simple, because concentration of services is more efficient than dispersal in the use of staff resources. For the sake of efficiency, children are concentrated in schools and students in universities, workers in factories and scientists in laboratories. Accordingly, Jones believes a major dispersal of mental health facilities in Britain would lead to a drop in standards of care unless more money and more workers were provided than would be necessary in a service concentrated largely on the mental hospital.

Ambulatory care may be given by general practitioners or specialists. At present in many countries ambulatory care is given at premises used by only one or two doctors and often relatively close to the homes of the patients. The centre for ambulatory care by doctors at front-line contact level should be capable of accommodating a group of doctors and ancillary workers, should be well equipped with facilities for investigation and treatment, and should be reasonably accessible to the homes of patients who use it; the first two attributes eliminate most doctors' homes or other consulting premises, and the third, in some areas, rules out any hospital site. Hence there is, at least in these areas, a role for a health centre for ambulatory care between home and hospital (McKeown, 1965). The location of centres for ambulatory care on hospital sites, if reasonably accessible to the homes of patients, would allow all doctors to share the use of the comprehensive investigative and therapeutic facilities of a well-equipped hospital.

Second-line and Hospital Care

The second-line health team is normally the locus of specialized skills, and is institutionally based. The dominant medical in-patient institution is the hospital. 'The hospital is an integral part of a social and medical organization, the function of which is to provide for the population complete health care, both curative and preventive, and whose out-patient services reach out to the family in its home environment; the hospital is also a centre for the training of health workers and for bio-social research' (WHO Expert Committee on Organization of Medical Care, 1957). This definition illustrates how the concept of hospital functions has developed from custodial care to include curative care, education of a range of types of hospital staff, medical research, and preventive medicine (Lentz, 1957). In terms of scientific and technical progress in medicine, subsequent to its development from its custodial function, the hospital has become highly productive, and is in turn greatly strengthened by the fact that it is the mother house of the main health professions. This educational role has been one of the main reasons the hospital has been able to adapt so successfully to change and innovation, so as to become the prototype for the medical profession of the environment of professional stimulus. Professional interaction, continuous exposure of clinical work to the view of senior and junior colleagues, the old tradition of teaching, and the new tradition of research have all made it an institution of professional stimulus and refreshment (Evang, 1960).

Evang (1951) has pointed out that the hospital must be built on the various forms of medical activity already in existence; no hospital pattern can be the best for all countries and at all times. Hospitals are so closely interwoven with the social and cultural structure of a given society, the status of medicine, the habits of doctors, dentists, nurses, and the population that the pattern will vary from country to country, and inside each country. For example, urban and rural conditions call for different types of hospital (Evang, 1951).

Hospital admission often takes place for a combination of reasons, but logically, each patient admitted should need the specialized resources of the particular hospital to which he is admitted. In practice, many patients whose needs do not include technical hospital services are admitted to hospital. Crombie and Cross (1959) estimated that at least 12·5 per cent. and perhaps 43 per cent. of the patients of all ages admitted to the medical beds of a large acute general hospital in England required only hotel care, in that they 'had no diagnostic, therapeutic or nursing requirements at hospital level'. The proportions of adult in-patients requiring hotel care only in similar studies carried out by Forsyth and Logan (1960) were one-quarter for males and two-fifths for females. However, Mackintosh et al. (1961), in an assessment of patients in the same medical wards as those used by Crombie and Cross (1959) but using different criteria, estimated that while 13 per cent. of the patients did not need hospital care on strictly medical grounds, in only 4 per cent. of patients might admission have been prevented by augmented domiciliary medical and social services; these proportions were considerably higher in chronic and mental hospitals, so that it is in these hospitals that im-

provements in domiciliary medical and social care can be expected to make their greatest impact on the pattern of hospital admissions.

While, in general, hospital admission in the developed countries depends on the severity of the illness and not on the possibility of a cure (Candau, 1965), Crombie and Cross (1961, 1963) have provided evidence that, in Britain, the domiciliary services care for two-thirds of the patients with serious medical illness, and an even higher proportion among the elderly. This situation calls for strong supporting services for home care.

Like industrial enterprises, and for similar reasons, general hospitals are tending to become larger. In 1961, 14 per cent. of all hospitals in England and Wales were of less than 100 beds; it has been estimated that by 1975 this proportion will have fallen to 8 per cent. (Cowan, 1963).

Industrial health services play a role in the delivery of health services the significance of which varies greatly with the country's pattern of health services. In industrialized areas it is practicable to deliver a range of ambulatory services to workers. Wilson and Jungner (1968) point out that industrial health services offer advantages in the early detection of disease, in that it is possible to ensure the regular attendance of a relatively large population and that continuity of attendance is usually of a higher order. In some countries this route of delivery of health services is extended to dependants of workers, frequently as part of a paternalistic system of family support.

Relationships between Front- and Second-line

It is difficult to make valid international comparisons of front- and second-line care. There are very significant differences between countries in the relative medical responsibilities of general practitioners and specialists. For example, Stevens (1966) has pointed out that in Britain, taking doctors at the height of their careers, seven out of ten doctors are in general practice, whereas in the United States the balance is reversed; there more than six out of ten doctors are in full-time specialist practice, and many of the remaining four are specialists in a part-time capacity. She found hospital 'service' specialties such as pathology and radiology account for comparable proportions of medical man-power in both countries. The major difference, and where it might reasonably be supposed that general practice in Britain has made its greatest impact, was in paediatrics, obstetrics, general medicine, and general surgery. The proportion of doctors in these four specialties in Britain was 12 per cent.; in the United States it was 38 per cent.

Furthermore, there are rapid changes taking place in front-line as well as second-line care. It has been recognized that, associated with the diversity of skills required in front-line care, is the necessity for larger groupings and more sophisticated facilities. These changes are necessary in addition to counter the dangers of individualism and isolation. As medicine advances more rapidly so does professional isolation become more of a handicap; isolation carries the further hazard that work remains hidden from view (Evang, 1960). Exposure to criticism and comment of the professional group is one of the most active incentives to professional self-improvement.

Assuming the existence of front- and second-line health services, there are three extremes of relationships between them: complete fusion, total separation, and linkage. These relationships can also be expressed in the form: 'closed' and 'open' front-line and 'closed' and 'open' second-line.

In many countries doctors are now engaged almost exclusively on either hospital or domiciliary work. This arrangement has two types of disadvantage, of which the first is that it restricts the logical development of services: for example, the care of the mentally ill and the aged sick cannot be divided simply into institutional and domiciliary classes; they require a complex pattern of care which cuts across these traditional boundaries. The second disadvantage of separation is that doctors outside of hospital tend to lose touch with the technical advances of medicine, whereas those inside, seeing only selected patients, may lose contact with reality (McKeown, 1961).

The medical staff of hospitals may be derived by two extremes: the closed hospital with fixed staff of hospital doctors, frequently geographical full-time in the hospital; and the open hospital with a staff largely composed of doctors practising outside the hospital, who can send their patients into hospital and treat them there. In practice, population density and other factors may bring about a system which is intermediate between these open and closed extremes.

Evang (1951) gives a summary of the arguments in favour of each system. Major points in favour of the open hospital are: (1) The patient will tend to prefer to be treated in hospital by the doctor who has arranged for his admission there. (2) This doctor will be familiar with the patient's family and his social and working environment, all factors which are of importance in deciding on his care in hospital and also on how soon the patient can safely be sent home. (3) From the medical point of view there is no overlap of doctors or misunderstandings. (4) The average doctor benefits from the stimulus of contact with the hospitals as a medical centre.

In favour of closed hospitals are: (1) The health team within the hospital becomes more integrated, so that the hospital functions are carried out in a more planned way, with consequent gains in efficiency and security for all staff and patients. (2) An emergency occurring while a patient is in hospital is dealt with by a doctor who is familiar with him. (3) Progress in scientific medicine and teaching within the hospital is facilitated.

PLANNING

In the technical discussions on health planning at the Eighteenth World Health Assembly attention was drawn to the following requisites for planning, and necessary data.

1. An understanding of the government's interest, aims, and assessment of objectives, in national socio-economic development, and of its policy in respect of health planning as one of its integral parts.

2. Enabling legislation for planning and subsequent implementation.

3. An organization for overall socio-economic planning and a health planning organization.

4. Arrangements for co-ordination between all planning organizations and between these organizations and the government departments concerned.

Necessary data

1. Demographic data—national, regional, or provincial and for local districts.

2. Vital and health statistics (crude and infant mortality rates, deaths by causes, morbidity, data, hospital admissions, etc.).

3. An inventory of public and private health service institutions, including training institutions, and a complete statement by categories of health service manpower, whether employed officially or practising independently.

4. National economic background. Information regarding the present national economic background and general manpower position.

5. A statement of the financial allocations to the health services.

Some authorities, however, regard the above data as too restricted in scope and would request the addition of the following:

(i) hospital morbidity and mortality data;

(ii) the results of mass screening investigations into the prevalence of certain specified or asymptomatic diseases and the physical fitness of certain vulnerable groups, data as to the growth of urbanization, and information as to the extent of nomadism.

The usefulness of surveys under certain conditions was stressed, and also the need for research into suitable forms of methodology for the intended planning process. Because of their selective character a warning was given about the reliability of hospital statistics, particularly in developing countries. Finally, the need on occasions to undertake planning with only the minimum of data was emphasized. Such data should not be regarded as final. Upon simple and even primitive data it was possible by patience and persistence to build over the years statistical systems for the periodic review and correction of operating plans, and to assist in forward planning (WHO Expert Committee on Hospital Administration, 1968).

There is no single optimal level for planning of all health services. The level appropriate for a particular service depends on the resultant of two main factors: it is desirable for planning to be carried out at as near as possible to the population to be served; the more specialized the particular health service, the larger the population served and, accordingly, normally the larger the population unit for planning.

Health service planning requires the interaction of planning personnel of a range of disciplines, some of which are not represented among the staff responsible for patient care. It is difficult to recruit, build up, and use economically and effectively the skills of this interdisciplinary planning team except by the formation of planning units which provide for relatively large populations.

Critical sizes of population for planning depend on such factors as population density and geography. However, for developed countries the following approximate population and functional levels may be considered to be appropriate: (1) Central (for 5 million population and upwards). General planning policies of a strategic nature should be executed at this level and also the planning of very highly specialized services. (2) Regional (for 1 million population and upwards). This population is likely to be focused on a medical centre with teaching responsibilities for undergraduate and postgraduate medical students. The planning of specialized services, for example, neurosurgery, would appropriately be carried out at this level. (3) Area (for 250,000 population). The focus of this size of population is likely to be the district hospital and its constellation of associated facilities. Planning at this level would tend to be more tactical than strategic in nature. (4) Neighbourhood (for 50,000 population). The size of population served from this level is crucially related to population density and geography, and may be as low as 5,000. This is front-line unit level, and only tactical planning is appropriate.

The valuable Report of the WHO Expert Committee on Hospital Administration (1968) discusses the allocation of planning responsibilities to three different levels.

At *central level* the principal responsibility is seen as that of policy-making, for example, the determination of the overall plan. There is also a wide range of other responsibilities, including the co-ordination of plans at all levels and with national planning authorities, social services, universities, and public works departments; cost analysis and budget planning; acquisition of adequate funds from fiscal and legislative authorities; establishment of standards for services, personnel, architecture, and equipment; conduct of research in hospital planning and design; advising regional and local authorities; selection of leadership personnel for regional and local levels, and support of training of personnel at all levels (principally by establishment of programmes for training of specialists).

At *regional level* responsibilities will vary greatly, depending on the social organization of the country; from co-ordinated planning to policy-making, supervision, and co-ordination; all the way to direct operational management. A principal factor will usually be the translation of centrally established standards into detailed regional requirements, taking into account the regional situation (e.g. forecasts of size and other characteristics of the population and the social geography of the regions). Detailed regional planning may include the division of the region into areas and ensuring suitable plans for each area.

At *area and local level* lies usually the responsibility for providing service and initiating new developments. A vital responsibility is the co-ordination of all health services and ensuring effective co-operation with other social services and local bodies (WHO Expert Committee on Hospital Administration, 1968).

The area planning organization should be designed to achieve an integrated system of related services, not a series of separate services, front-line and second-line, curative and preventive. It is out of the national total of such constellations that the universe of health service provision is arranged. The essential constellation consists of: (1) the district hospital service, whether this is a single institution or a group of smaller hospitals; in other words, the inpatient services acute and long-term, for physical and mental disease; plus second-line consulting, diagnostic, and reference facilities; (2) the front-line services for preventive and curative care in health centres, polyclinics, group practices, and the consulting rooms of individual general practitioners; and (3) the planning and administrative headquarters for the area. Emphasis should be on the relationships between the components, not on their separateness. By this means it is possible to see more clearly the partnership of

front- and second-line, and to plan for appropriate association between them. The concept allows alignment of the hospital, no longer an enclave, as the power-house helping to turn the wheels of the area health system; and as the mother house to which all members of front- and second-line can come to share the stimulus of work in this atmosphere of the scientific team, and for planned continuous education in its postgraduate medical centre, which is, at once, the library, postgraduate education school, and social meeting-place of the area service.

Neighbourhood teams which constitute vital components of the constellation may be easy to form where all personnel are together in one clinic or health centre; or their members may be scattered and isolated as individual doctors, public health nurses, social workers, etc. In either event the need is to motivate the workers in the system to see and understand their relationship to each other in clearer and more explicit terms. It is also appropriate to clarify the interdependence of front- and second-lines, and to identify and integrate the working groups of front- and second-line personnel who are involved in such problems as care of the elderly and the mentally ill, and provision of obstetric and child-health services.

There are many possible variants of a planning and administrative structure for health services. Each derives from the historical and political background of its country and has its own advantages and disadvantages; there is no one blue-print for health services administration. It is possible, however, to delineate some elements which have significance for planning and administration in all health systems.

Health services require some method of strategy formation and long-term planning. They develop quantitative and qualitative standards of provision. They should have a system of research and intelligence to inform them about the on-going system, to evaluate its effectiveness, and to assess the extent to which the requirements of the population served are met. They need capacity for experimentation and the promotion of development and innovation. They should be able to call upon a variety of expertise for many purposes. They need an efficient system for the day-to-day administration of local services. With this has to be coupled an arrangement of the local services which can easily and effectively exploit the developing opportunities of modern medicine. Since administration is ineffective without the partnership of the key health service personnel and health service teams, there is required also a clinical organization which encourages effective leadership and understanding of the needs of the system, as well as continuous self-evaluation of standards of work.

Strategy Formation and Long-term Planning

Various activities are involved. Forecasting trends of demand, and medical development, assessment of resources; and assessment of priorities. Forecasts are required of the direction and pace of developments in medicine and the resources required for their implementation.

Long-term planning is fraught with difficulties, not least of which is the danger of over-planning into the future, on assumptions which in a few years time are obsolete. The pace of change is such in the scientific and social development of health services that detailed long-term planning may seriously restrict future capacity to respond to new opportunities. The volume of work involved in preparing a long-term plan may turn it into a kind of sacred cow; something which it is difficult to criticize and even more difficult to change. There is also a tendency for plans to act as 'a sleeping pillow', a substitute for action. 'Long-term planning involving also estimates for capital investment and running costs and forming part of the total economic planning of the country or region may also easily be used as a "trap". The health authorities are stuck with the figures they have suggested and may have the greatest difficulty in breaking through this barrier regardless of whether inflation, scientific and technical development or other factors have obviously made the original figures obsolete. One method of counteracting the inflexibility of the process is to build in from the start opportunities for revisions at short intervals' (Evang, 1965).

Long-term planning should therefore be concerned to create a system capable of flexible response. This applies both to accommodation and staffing; the existence of hospitals for tuberculosis in relatively inaccessible locations militated against their subsequent use for other types of health service when the demand in developed countries for in-patient accommodation for tuberculosis patients was reduced. Apart from buildings, the adaptation of senior specialist health service staff to a new specialty from, for example, tuberculosis raises difficult, and occasionally insoluble, problems.

Administrative arrangements which create artificial barriers in the health system are also a source of inflexibility. Thus separate administrative and financial responsibilities for curative and preventive medicine, and for front-line and second-line care, may inhibit the exploitation of new possibilities for integrated care.

Flexible response to patients' needs is another characteristic of good planning. The range of health services available should be such that they present a continuous gradation of support in response to individual patient need. Patients should not be fitted into a Procrustean bed of services. As the patient's needs change, he should be able to move freely and quickly from one combination of services to another. This freedom of movement may be restricted by financial or administrative barriers; it is facilitated where the health services are under one financial and administrative control. Gradation and diversity of service is as important in the care of mental illness as of physical disease. Recent developments in Britain illustrate ways in which this can be attempted. A gradation of mental health services has been developed between completely institutional and domiciliary care: hostel, day hospital, diversional therapy, industrial training, night care for patients who work in the community, and supportive services for patients living in their own homes (Jones, 1966).

The long time scale of the chronic disease process makes continuity of care and supervision an important goal. This is helped where the patient has a personal doctor who can make arrangements for the individual's changing needs, based on his knowledge of his patient's problems and environment, and of the services available to meet them.

The assessment of priorities is a difficult exercise. For the most part it is conducted by a series of informed guesses, value judgements and percentage additions to or subtractions from past effort. The process may be refined by good information from research and intelligence activities into the effectiveness of on-going services. The techniques of cost–benefit analysis

may in future bring greater clarity to the planners' judgements. Economists are showing increasing interest in the health field and 'one of the major roles of the economist, which has even been defined as *the* role is to give advice on "the allocation of scarce resources between competing uses". The economist's business is to try to work out beforehand the prospective yields on alternative uses of resources, and to rank them accordingly in an order of priority' (Foster, 1968).

Techniques analogous to those of 'Planning, Programming, and Budgeting' used by the Rand Corporation in long term plans for defence in the United States might eventually bring new insights to the health planner, although health service objectives are intangible indeed compared with the hardware needs of a defence system. However devised, it is certain that the health service planner greatly needs some grid of appropriate objectives to set against the efforts of his service to give him a more systematic means of judging the relative short-falls and excesses in its expenditures on different fields. Perhaps such a grid may most appropriately be devised from within the stated objectives of the system itself, to test how far priorities allocated in terms of actual resources match the objectives outlined in policy reports and statements of intent.

One systematic approach to the evaluation of health service programmes has been proposed by Deniston *et al.* (1968), who distinguish four categories of evaluative questions: (1) appropriateness: the importance of the specific problems selected for programming and the relative priority accorded to each; (2) adequacy: how much of the entire problem the programme is directed towards overcoming; (3) effectiveness: the extent to which pre-established objectives are attained; (4) efficiency: the cost in resources of attaining objectives.

Although international, or even interregional, comparisons of health services are difficult to interpret, it is manifest that there are wide ranges in the scale of provision of particular types of health services. This diversity will be illustrated with reference to one particular form of provision. Much published work on the subject has dealt with the ratio of the hospital beds to the population served. There is a voluminous literature which seeks to advocate precise formulae to predict demand for hospital beds, but it is now apparent that no precise ratio exists which is valid when applied to different health service contexts; Anderson (1964) has satirized this search for the 'Holy Grail' of hospital use.

A plan must be related to the needs of the population and community for which it is intended. The WHO Expert Committee on the Organization of Medical Care (1957) cited the following relevant factors to be considered in hospital planning: (1) the age distribution of the population; (2) the general standard of living, special habits, local housing conditions, and transport facilities; (3) the population density, urban areas requiring more beds per thousand inhabitants than rural areas; (4) the incidence of disease and injuries; (5) the standard of development of medical care provided outside the hospital by private practitioners and health centres; (6) the system adopted by a country to finance its hospitals; government legislation or social security schemes.

Estimates of need and measurements of demand are largely conditioned by the availability of existing services. The most readily available practical estimate of demand during a given year for any individual hospital or area is provided by the amount of use during the previous year. Many methods of predicting demand depend on the application of this principle, with varying degrees of sophistication. However, none of these methods does other than recognize that hospitals, like dinosaurs, appear to rely mainly on the momentum of their habits and conditioned reflexes (Logan, 1964).

Feldstein (1963) makes the economist's point that to think about the provision of one particular facet of a health service in terms of need is misleading. Since there are not enough doctors, hospital beds, and other resources, a decision to give more to one service is a decision to deny resources to another. To find the optimal use of resources the relative benefits and cost of alternative programmes have to be weighed. Accordingly, it is more appropriate to strive after optimal allocation rather than meeting needs. Health care programmes should be planned not so much to attempt to meet all existing needs and demands but rather so as to find the optimal use of available resources; thus it is not enough to show that maintaining the existing hospital bed/population ratio will meet future demands for hospital care. It is necessary also to show that resources used to maintain this ratio cannot be better used in other ways (Feldstein, 1964). We have to think of balanced systems of care, both institutional and community services, rather than planning in terms of isolated facets such as hospital beds.

Research and Intelligence

To carry out planning functions, including evaluation, an effective research organization is required. Since health service requirements are continually changing, planning must be a continuous process, subject to revision in the light of experience. Accordingly, evaluation is desirable during all stages of planning, implementation, and application.

Medical research has long been recognized to be an essential activity, but it is only within the last generation that there has been significant development of 'operational research' in health services 'the application of scientific methods of investigation to the sort of problems that confront executive and administrative authorities' (Bailey, 1959); relevant techniques include analysis of routine statistics, patient-care evaluation, work study, and systems analysis.

It is a characteristic of *ad hoc* operational-research studies, especially work study and systems analysis, that they require a multi-disciplinary approach with co-ordination of a range of skills. Projects are normally so closely related to patient care that members of the health professions are required in the team. There is the need for statistical advice, preferably from statisticians experienced in health service problems.

During its early development operational research as a whole tended to show two main deficiencies: the organizational and support relationships between hospital departments received emphasis, at the expense of studies of the effectiveness of patient care (Flagle *et al.*, 1960); there was a failure to link with other types of health service studies. The essential interrelationships of effectiveness in dealing with sickness or its prevention and efficiency in administration are now more clearly recognized. Attempts are being made to design studies so that they fit into a wider study of the service as a whole (Cottrell, 1966). As Kerr White (1968) says, 'No longer is it adequate to deal *only* with the input side of the equation, the costs of providing care; it is now necessary to deal *also* with the output

side, in terms of values—human values, received. . . . Nor is it adequate to have an "activity" budget in which we talk about the *number* of patients admitted to hospitals, the *number* of visits made to doctors, and the *number* of visits made by nurses. What is needed is a "performance" budget. To what extent are health activities reflected as achievements measured against defined objectives.'

All health services require the capacity to experiment, and to promote development and innovation. Experimentation may be the logical and necessary extension of research and intelligence. Operational research is limited in its capacity to assist by its curtailment within the existing methods and assumptions of the system examined. For many purposes, and not least the search for more economical use of resources, health service planners may require to launch bold experiments into new methods of deploying health care and using health service personnel. Although many experiments have been made in the history of health care systems, too few have been adequately evaluated.

It is necessary to encourage generation, acceptance, and implementation of new ideas, processes, and services. This requirement flows from the increasing rate of technological change in medicine. Innovation is as much a matter of the spirit and the climate of opinion of a service and its key personnel as it is of central planning and the allocation of resources to specific ends. One of the functions of the planning team is to stimulate health service personnel to research and innovate, rather than regarding this as a monopoly of planners and professional medical care and operational research workers. Apart from other benefits, the involvement of larger parts of the health services in the search process also increases the chances of acceptance and implementation peripherally of new ideas. It follows from this that the planning exercise should be conceived of as a collaboration between the health services staff and the planning team.

The Planning Team

Methods of staffing and organizing central, regional, and local health departments will vary widely with time and place, but whatever system of organization prevails, the importance of quality of recruitment and training of key staff is paramount. The prestige allocated to health service administration as a career differs in different systems. In a good many systems the qualities and skills required are insufficiently recognized; whereas clinical work commands high prestige and remuneration, administration and planning may be regarded only as necessary chores of a less-demanding nature. The risks of such a value-system are not to the *amour propre* of the planners but to the whole balance, priority system, and *élan* of the service. As health services become increasingly complex and integrated systems of applied scientific and social technology, the significance and contribution of planning and administration increases. The need increases also to make explicit the specialized professional skills required for health service administration, so that the quality of training for the important tasks involved may be raised. Different professional skills will be required to make up the large administrative and planning teams of modern health services; financial, legal, architectural, as well as from the social and health sciences and professions. While valuable insights into health service problems are to be gained from experience of other fields, including industry, emphasis must be laid on the importance of expertise in the special requirements of a health service.

The medical administrator has a role of special responsibility and leadership in health service planning. His recruitment, education, and career structure are matters of great significance for the well-being of the system. No amount of training will compensate for poor-quality recruits. Capacity to interest and attract high-quality candidates will depend on many things, not least the attitudes towards community medicine inculcated during basic medical education. Candidates should be able to see in front of them the possession of professional expertise comparable with other medical specialities, and a career structure which compares favourably in prestige and financial terms with other branches of medicine.

Professional training should now be seen as a planned high-level experience of combined academic education and apprenticeship comparable in depth and duration to other specialties. The cutting-edge disciplines of the medical administrator are quantitative and derive from scientific training and field practice in statistics, epidemiology, and operational research. Important insights also come from social and administrative sciences. The practical success of a medical administrator stems not only from his skills in community medicine but also from his capacity to motivate and change the social system which constitutes a health service (Evang, 1966; WHO Working Group, 1967; General Medical Council, 1967; Royal Commission on Medical Education, 1968).

It is necessary in health service administration and planning teams to recognize the need for continuing education and stimulation for staff, including the most senior. Excellent library arrangements, inservice discussion and seminars, opportunities for travel and study leave are at least as necessary in this as in other health professional fields. It is desirable in dealing with long-term planning that capacity should also exist for individuals or groups to be taken out of day-to-day administrative commitments for intensive attack on the most difficult problems.

In addition to its own range of skills, the planning organization needs access to outside expertise and up-to-date information not only in the medical field but also in a wide range of natural and social sciences and professional and technical skills. To ensure the availability of this expertise requires, as a minimum, free access to advice from any health service personnel and the capacity to seek and pay for advice from outside the health services, for example, from university economists or other social scientists. In complex health systems such sources of expertise should no longer be left to the hazard of random availability. In some countries, and notably the Peoples' Republics, there is an impressive constellation of institutes related to Central Health Departments. Such institutes have responsibilities in given fields for research, teaching, and policy formation and direction.

The Clinical Team

Health service administration is almost unique in the relationships involved between the administrative and planning team and the key clinical workers in the system. Specifically the medical profession inevitably play a dominating role in determining the direction of work and the use of resources. It is undesirable that the key professional personnel should be subordinate to the administrative hierarchy in any fashion which impairs clinical decisions. Initiative and responsibility are key characteristics of good clinical work, and these are encouraged by freedom of professional judgement. At the same time under the impact of scientific and technical change clinical work is changing rapidly, from situations of individual activity, towards the build-up of bigger and more complex teams. The stereotype of the *prima donna* and his individual clinical *tour de force* is obsolete. The need now is for team leadership within the peer group and for systems of clinical organization which embody these new requirements; for the clinical division with its chairman rather than the individualist or small unit.

There are a variety of reasons why this change is desirable. The complexity and highly specialized nature of modern medicine makes the individual clinical conscience no longer adequate as sole monitor and judge of practice. It is only by organized comparison of experience and peer-group criticism that the individual can effectively judge his performance. Medical audit and patient-care evaluation are necessary activities which require clinical organization in larger groups. Patient-care evaluation is to be regarded as educational and promotive, rather than investigative or punitive in intent; professional review of professional activities is properly viewed as a bulwark of autonomous but responsible professionalism, rather than a negation of it (Donabedian, 1968).

A truly effective partnership between administrative and clinical organization is more difficult to achieve where clinical work is arranged only on an individual or small-group basis. The tendency in such situations is for the most vocal and prestigious clinicians to gain the ear of the administrator, who is thus deprived of more widely based clinical advice. A more structured clinical organization will give the medical administrator greater opportunities for effective partnership with his clinical colleagues; for example, in exercises to determine priorities, to discuss the use of resources, and to create the data necessary for systematic medical audit and patient-care evaluation. Clinical organization of the divisional type may also be the necessary device to group together front- and second-line clinicians concerned with the same area services.

A further point of significance relates to use of resources. Clinicians as leaders of the health teams are the major determiners of how health service resources are used. It is difficult to clarify the alternatives in use of resources effectively when the decisions are fragmented among many individuals. For example, the use of expensive acute beds is determined largely by hospital clinicians. Redeployment of use is inflexible, if beds are allocated in many small packages. Moreover, clinical policies for duration of stay in a hospital bed are easier to discuss and change in the larger clinical group rather than with a series of individuals. Should the ordinary case or appendectomy stay in a surgical hospital bed six days or sixteen? This is not an isolated and academic question. Upon this answer may depend the capacity of a surgical service (as opposed to an individual surgeon) to overtake queues of patients in the community who are waiting for operations for hernia repair and other non-urgent but important surgical procedures.

It is now fashionable to talk about the managerial responsibilities of the clinician. Certainly in an increasingly complex clinical world there are many things for the clinical leader to learn about the place of his service within the whole context of health care and the health system. This is a process which can be assisted by planned opportunities for learning. These should start during basic medical education, and recur in appropriate terms through professional training; with special opportunities for staff-college-type experiences for the fully trained clinician and leaders of divisional organizations (Advisory Committee for Management Efficiency, 1966; Joint Working Parties, 1967a, 1967b) [see also CHAPTER 3].

MANPOWER AND THE HEALTH TEAM

Health service personnel can be categorized and counted in different ways. In broad terms a distinction should be made between total employees engaged in the 'health service industry' and the 'health occupations'. Our concern and our discussion here is mainly with the health occupations which have a specific and special content of work concerned with health. Pennel (1966) gives a list of thirty-five categories and over 300 sub-categories of health occupations listed by the United States Employment Service. We cannot, however, neglect categories of less-specific kind, such as cooks and clerical workers. As the health service grows, so do specialities in such occupations begin to develop.

Rapid increase in the numbers of health service personnel has been a striking feature of the scene in many countries during the last generation. For example, the health service industry as defined by the United States Bureau of the Census came third of all industries in the United States in the size of work force employed in 1960. The work force had expanded by 54 per cent. during the decade 1950–60, and only seven out of seventy-one major industries had expanded at a greater rate. Most estimates of future requirement predict further steady increases. Therefore, manpower needs tend to be viewed in many health systems as the major contemporary issue for solution, and potentially as a narrowing bottleneck in the forward planning of service.

Anne Somers (1966) recites some of the social and economic pressures already discussed in this chapter which will produce an effect of steady enlargement of demand for health services and personnel: for example, the overall increase in population; increase in the proportion of the population over the age of 65; rising socio-economic status of lower-income groups; increasing proportion of women in the population; steady increase in urbanization and industrialization; the rise in educational levels, and in income levels, both individual and national.

Manpower Planning

An increasing preoccupation is how best to make forward estimates and plans for manpower. A good deal of current discussion on this subject is concerned to criticize existing and traditional methods without yet reaching very clear conclusions on what to substitute. Economists criticize the use of population ratios, e.g. the number of doctors or nurses or dentists needed per 10,000 population, as being based simply on extensions of value judgements. Hiestand (1966) points out 'the term shortage tends to be used in one way by non-economists and in a distinctly different way by economists. Non-economists use the term to describe a discrepancy between the situa-

tion which they view as necessary or desirable, and the situation which does in fact exist; i.e. "shortage" often has meaning primarily in relation to the norms and value systems of those in the leadership of particular professions.' Economists point out that in a market economy the community indicates its own judgement on what is desirable within the limits of the total resources available to it. In a sense this is true also where priorities are allocated by government policies rather than the market. For the economist the word 'shortage' in this context has a different meaning. It indicates some discrepancy between the actual level of manpower supply and that which is possible within the limits of the existing effective demand. This may be due to a lag in supply keeping up with a rapidly expanding demand, or to artificial restrictions on the flow of manpower, e.g. where there are monopolist professional tendencies (Hiestand, 1966).

However, estimates of manpower shortage based on 'needs' do have their uses, provided that the limitations of the method are kept in mind. They are most useful when devoted to comparatively narrow and specific fields of study: e.g. an analysis of the requirement for dentists based on known community incidences of dental disease, and well-studied estimates of the work which a dental team can accomplish in a given time.

Baker (1966), from the Johns Hopkins University Division of International Health, has outlined a framework for manpower planning which has been used in a number of developing countries. He discusses the method under four headings. (1) Supply analysis: measuring the current supply of all types of health workers in some detail. (2) Projection of supply: projecting the supply of health workers forward to target dates ten and twenty years in the future with anticipated new graduates, and estimated subtractions for death, emigration, retirement, and change of profession. (3) Demand analysis: evaluating the effective economic demand for health service from both the public and private sector. (4) Projection of demand: projecting the effective economic demand forward to the ten- and twenty-year target dates. Will supply match demand? Here comparison is made of the projected supply with the projected demand, and necessary recommendations are made to effect a balance. Baker says that a most important concept in this kind of planning is 'start from where you are'. It does no good to propose grandiose schemes for the complete redesign of manpower structures and training. It is essential to bear in mind in all man-power planning the long time-lags between formulating plans and increased production of personnel. Especially where educational processes are involved which necessitate increased numbers of teachers, the process is bound to be slow.

Specialization and Diversification

The process of enlargement of total health service manpower has been one not only of increasing numbers but also of change in the nature and mix of the groups concerned. There has been a marked trend towards the development of specialization, best recognized within the medical profession itself, but also taking place by the development and expansion of other existing professional, sub-professional, and auxiliary categories, and by a tendency to evolve totally new categories of personnel to meet new tasks. There has also been a greatly increased diversification or widening of the range of types of workers involved. Within the trend of increase of numbers for all categories of personnel, there has been a relatively greater increase in the supporting grades relative to the older-established leadership professions of medical practitioner and registered nurse.

In traditional consideration of manpower needs there tends to be an almost complete preoccupation with a few old-established professions, notably medical practitioners and registered nurses. This is understandable, but is no longer sufficient. As Hiestand (1966) says, they are the key groups 'indeed in a way unparalleled in any other industry, the physician controls and influences his field and all who venture near it. For many functions no direct substitute for the physician exists. This has a great impact on the manpower problems of the health service industry. However, other personnel groups may substitute directly and indirectly for physicians and nurses. . . .' He, and other contemporary students of health service manpower problems, call attention to the need for much more study of the many other categories of workers involved in providing a modern health care system. Hiestand asks the question, in relation to the contemporary proliferation of many supporting grades of personnel, whether this is a temporary response to shortage or a more fundamental change in the technology of producing medical services akin to the shift in industry from hand-craft to mass methods. He points out that the problems of management, work organization, selection, training, and placement take on entirely new meanings as the work force becomes increasingly differentiated in function and skill level. Kissick (1968), pursuing the same point, quotes an analysis carried out in the United States into changes in utilization of health man-power during the period 1940–60. Health occupations were grouped into three levels of job content: high, medium, and low. Comparing employment at each level over the period, it was found that the largest percentage increases took place in those occupations with low job content, and the smallest increases in the occupations with high job content.

The move towards increasing specialization in the health field has been much more publicized than the movement of increasing diversification; this is especially true in relation to the medical profession. Rosemary Stevens (1966) has given an excellent account of the combination of scientific and other factors which has led to the existing pattern of specialization in Britain. Although, in general, the number of specialties is increasing, since specialization is a dynamic process, specialties may also diminish in appropriateness. For example, with changes in disease prevalence in developed countries, chest medicine and infectious diseases are tending to become absorbed into general medicine and paediatrics. Specialties based on a technology may disappear entirely; this could occur to radiotherapy should a new form of effective treatment for cancer be introduced. Not all specialties emerge because of increase in volume and complexity of scientific knowledge and technological advance in relation to medicine. The types and degree of specialization of medical practice is related in part to the health service structure. In Britain geriatric medicine has emerged as a specialty in consequence of social as well as demographic change.

Inextricably bound up with the use of the most sophisticated techniques is their application by a congeries of specialists. Although specialization of health services and the health team is advantageous, and indeed inevitable, it may be associated with rigidity. Specialization may impair flexibility of health services by making adaptation to scientific, technological, or social change sometimes less easy. Scientific advance does not necessarily fit into the boundaries of existing specialties, and effort may be wasted because of boundary disputes and vested interest. A price paid for the enhanced skill of the specialist is some loss of the flexibility of the natural scientist. Another price paid is the need to man every specialty with leaders and their replacements (Rutstein, 1965). Brockington (1964) has pointed out that since in developed countries much of the existing work for the doctor concerns chronic physical and mental disease, for which home care under a general practitioner is most appropriate, specialization is of more limited significance for man's total needs for medical care than might be imagined.

Hiestand (1966), in his discussion of the trend to specialization, points out once again the different viewpoint of the economist from that of the traditional health service planner. In his view as an economist the increasing degree of specialization of health manpower, either within a health occupation or in the form of new health occupations, is the direct result of improvements in utilization practices. Specialization is usually said to flow from increased scientific knowledge, which forces a practitioner to limit himself to a smaller and smaller part of the whole. For the economist, however, specialization is a function of the scale of the enterprise or market. As the population becomes more concentrated, and as transportation improves for both patients and doctors; as more patients are concentrated in hospitals, increasing numbers of medical practitioners can occupy themselves fully while restricting their type of patients. With a limited practice in this way, they gain increased skill and productivity through deeper explorations into particular diseases and techniques. Specialization, in fact, is the source of increased knowledge, not the result. More importantly, it leads to higher quality and an increased supply of services, since the specialist can usually handle a given problem better and in less time than a less skilled practitioner (Hiestand, 1966).

Manpower Utilization

Kissick (1967a) has discussed in an interesting way the new insights provided for health manpower planners by examination of the processes which have resulted in rapid increase in numbers, diversification of personnel, and further trends towards specialization. Adopting the language of economics, he says that up to now manpower has been considered as an output, e.g. a new doctor is considered as a product of an education programme. In discussing shortages the focus has been on the number graduating each year and the number of graduates required to fill projected needs. This approach, although necessary, has tended to take attention off the fact that health services are moving away from independent and isolated personal performance into methods of functioning which call for integrated and institutionalized planning; we are increasingly moving towards a fabric of interrelated health care services into which individual components must be fitted with appropriate attention to the relationships with other parts of the system.

Kissick goes on to say that institutionalization of health

services has brought about the concept of manpower as one of a series of *inputs* into the health care system, the other inputs being facilities (including equipment and supplies) and bio-medical knowledge. Organization and finance become the mechanisms translating these resources into health services for the consumer. The level and type of *output* from the system depends on the way in which the *inputs* are organized (Kissick, 1967*a*).

It is necessary to think in future more clearly about manpower as a whole, the relationship of different kinds of personnel, and the ways in which they can divide out the tasks to be done, as well as the implications for manpower planning of the forecasts in regard to the other *inputs*. To illustrate the relatedness of one aspect of manpower to other aspects, Klarman (1951) proposed studying existing utilization of manpower, and making estimates under alternative policy assumptions. For example, if intravenous fluids are administered only by medical practitioners one set of manpower requirements results; whereas if they are administered by nurses another set of requirements emerges; a third possibility with yet another set of requirements is where intravenous administration is by specially trained technologists.

A major implication of this altered view of manpower's place in the scheme of things is to shift attention from total enlargement of manpower categories towards improved utilization and increased productivity of the man-power force. To achieve this goal of more effective utilization we need much more accurate data than usually exists on the current use of manpower; we also require research and experimentation into alternative uses, with exploration of possible models of health systems which would utilize and organize manpower in very different ways and yield greater outputs than our present arrangements. Such research and experimentation will require built-in measurements to test for the risks to the patient from redeployments of tasks; and assessments of the quality of service provided as well as its quantity. Detailed study of health services is required 'followed by subdivision of specific functions into component tasks'. This will allow individuals possessing only a limited range of skills and competence to be drawn into the manpower pool to perform the tasks identified as being within their capabilities (Kissick, 1967*b*).

An interesting example of use of auxiliary personnel and downward transfer of functions is quoted by Kissick (1968) from a study of dentists in the United States. In the study it was found that productivity per dentist (as measured by income) was increased with each additional chair-side assistant employed. Furthermore, the addition of a second chair-side assistant increased productivity more than the first, and the employment of a third assistant increased productivity more than the second.

These trends of thought on manpower have major implications for special aspects of health service planning; e.g. education of personnel; preparation and arrangements for leadership and team-work; communications and staff relationships; professional and public attitudes; and expenditure.

Training Programmes

In the field of education a new look is required to increase our capacity to make the best use of a wide variety of sources of recruitment and ranges of talent. In contrast to other fields of endeavour, many health services give little or no opportunity for movement of personnel either upwards to higher grades of work or laterally into related fields of work. Professional and sub-professional restrictions on licensing place serious obstacles to this kind of movement. Presumably real possibilities of promotion to higher grades of work would enhance the attractiveness of lower grades to recruits, as well as permitting the best use of talent revealed in simpler work situations. As well as financial support for additional training, to be attractive such a policy would necessitate real educational concessions in the way of time and work credit for previous experience.

Increased lateral mobility is also desirable so that an individual can move easily from one category of work to another closely related in skill content. This is one means of reducing the inflexibility in use of manpower which comes from creating many sub-categories of skills; it may also produce desirable economies in use of scarce teaching resources in the educational plan. Such a policy implies bringing together similar categories of trainees into common training programmes which develop generic or core-courses applicable to the needs of all the students, with specialized courses for special requirements. This kind of educational rationalization is especially necessary in those countries which have devised a wide variety of professions and sub-professions, each with its own training programme designed *ad hoc* to meet a particular need as it arose in the course of health services development. Another solution has been arrived at in the Peoples' Republics, where the tendency has been to use the older professions, e.g. medicine and nursing, as the basic training on to which most new categories of requirement, e.g. physiotherapy, speech therapy, and similar skills, could be grafted.

Teamwork and Communications

The move from the idiosyncratic individualist beloved of medical mythology towards teamwork requires new concepts of the individual's role and understanding of the roles of others. The health service worker today is almost invariably a member of a complex team, whether this be manifest, as in the hospital, or hidden from view, as with the individual general practitioner, who nevertheless is virtually helpless in most advanced health services today, without the aid of whole congeries of other medical men, nurses, social workers, etc., in other parts of the system. The skill of teamwork, like any other skill, has to be learnt, and the process of learning can be accelerated or stultified by the apprenticeship and learning process. The effectiveness of the team can also be enhanced or damaged according to the amount of care taken to develop team work. There is an increasing tendency to create manifest team situations, e.g. in health centres and polyclinics for front-line care. But there is still insufficient attention in research and education to the study of the implications of such situations for those who must work in them.

Communication is a vital element in the health system, and its importance increases with the complexity of the system. The importance in a therapeutic community of satisfactory working relationships between the health-profession types might have been presumed, but experimental evidence has been provided by the studies of Revans (1964*a*, 1964*b*, 1966*a*, 1966*b*). Revans defines the concept of the hospital as a therapeutic community as 'an institution in which the governing element not only knows what is actually going on but is also itself capable of learning from this knowledge, as well as teaching its subordinates'.

Revans (1964a) ranked fifteen acute general hospitals by the following five criteria:

1. Charge nurses' opinions of senior staff, medical and nursing.
2. Charge nurses' attitudes towards student nurses.
3. Length of service of qualified nursing staff.
4. Average length of patient-stay in general medical wards.
5. Average length of patient-stay in general surgical wards.

He found that hospitals which ranked high or low in any one of these five characteristics tended also to rank high or low in the other four. Experimental evidence is thus provided in favour of the opinion, commonly held on empirical grounds, that the communications between the various staff groups have a considerable bearing on patient care in the hospital.

Revans (1964b) compares these findings to the feedback loop used in engineering, where a machine is controlled by a device which monitors its performance, slowing the machine down should it run too fast, speeding it up should it run too slowly. He regards learning as a feedback process also, in that it consists essentially of seeing the effects of one's own behaviour; on this analogy, unless one receives intelligible responses to, or clarifying information about, what one is trying to do, it is impossible to learn. It is significant that Revans (1966b) concludes from his own studies and those of others, notably Georgopoulos and Mann (1962), that while external research workers do have an effective contribution to make in raising standards of hospital organization and control, senior hospital staff themselves are the persons best fitted to pursue research into the operational problems of hospital management.

Professional and Public Attitudes

Professional attitudes and assumptions are severely tested by change. In the progress of health services there is a tendency for social institutions and organizations to lag behind scientific and technical developments, and we must remember that professions are social institutions and in some ways conservative. Evang (1967) has contrasted the medical profession's acceptance of scientific progress with its unwillingness to see that new conditions demand new settings. There may be difficulties in changing the boundaries of professional franchise embodied in statutes dealing with licensure—where the legislation was enacted to cover the needs of a situation substantially different from, and simpler than, the present complex field of health work. There may be legal and other difficulties in sharing tasks which have traditionally been regarded as those of the doctor or registered nurse.

Sometimes the question of professional ethics is introduced; the ethical issue may be real, but more often there is a confusion between ethics and traditional professional *mores*. There is an understandable psychology of indispensability bred by professional education, which may lead a profession to cling on to tasks well within the capacity of sub-professions with much shorter and less expensive training. Kissick (1968) points to the fact that in some situations there may be 'economic vested interests that are supposed to be the hallmark of guilds rather than professions. In such situations the forces of logic and rationality may be no match for tradition and vested interest.'

In general, it can be said that the greatest spur and the greatest hope for innovation and change comes when there is an urgent sense of 'shortage' of personnel in significant categories. In many countries it is almost only in such circumstances that there is any possibility of acceptance by the professions concerned of a cool and rational examination of traditional work distributions and responsibilities.

Public resistance to change may be as conservative and irrational as that of the most hide-bound professional. Therefore, there may go along with any programme for change the need for a plan for public discussion and education. Silver (1963) notes in relation to the social needs of patients that the patient may desire to consult with a doctor, and only a doctor, when the problem involved could in fact be handled better by a professional social worker. Public attitudes and expectations may also be inherently irreconcilable: for example, where the wish is for a family doctor round every corner, and at the same time for a clinical ambience of chromium plate and all the trappings of modern technology.

Mechanization

A well-established process in other fields of endeavour, in situations of skilled labour shortage, is substitution by other types of personnel, by machine, by pre-packaging, by automation, etc. To give an economist's view on this Kissick (1967b) quotes Professor Eli Ginzberg, who discusses the problems of what he calls 'capital poor institutions' in the United States, e.g. universities and hospitals. 'Partly because we have so many non-profit institutions which tend to be capital poor, productivity tends to be low. . . . The kind of supporting personnel that even broken down business organisations would have on the payroll, to economise the use of the more expensive personnel, are scarce in non-profit institutions. Being capital poor, these institutions squeeze their dollars and try to make them go as far as they can. From a productivity point of view I think you have a substantial under-investment in capital, with corresponding under-utilisation of personnel which on balance gives you a bad result.' A policy of pennywise, and pound-foolish.

Progress in this direction is difficult in health services, where so much of the work in support of sick and handicapped people demands face-to-face contact for psychological reasons, as well as clinical requirements. Despite the difficulties, a certain amount has been done to capitalize health systems, and certainly much more is necessary. Examples of labour-saving developments can be cited to show the possibilities of still further development. Disposable supplies—syringes, needles, transfusion sets, and gloves—are one example. Pre-package formulae, pharmaceuticals, and intravenous solutions illustrate a similar trend. So also do the simplified versions of laboratory tests, e.g. the 'Clinitest' substituted for Benedict's solution, in the examination of sugar in urine. The potential of automated laboratories, computer analysis of electrocardiograms, and similar developments are suggested by the Kaiser Permanente multiphasic screening project in California. Approximately 40,000 individuals are screened annually with a battery of twenty automated and semi-automated tests, including a self-administered health history questionnaire. Approximately 2½ hours are required to complete the automated survey, and it is conducted by nurses, technicians, and other supporting health personnel. Conventional methods would require 2 days, and four or five times the existing 42 dollars cost per head (Kissick, 1968).

Incentives and Continuing Education

The subject of the health team and manpower can scarcely be discussed without some brief mention of incentives and the process of professional stimulus and refreshment. The issues in relation to incentives are complex and varied. Only a few points will be mentioned here. The simple issue of financial rewards is as important in this field as in any other. In many countries the problems of recruitment are increased because there is an unrealistic hang-over of low wage-rates from days gone by, when work in medical institutions was regarded as a charitable activity. This concept tends to perpetuate wages which are low by comparison with other fields and the rewards of comparable levels of skill and responsibility elsewhere. The situation is not improved by the extent to which the field of nursing has been kept in a low wage bracket because of the predominance of female labour. For example, there is little reality from an economist's point of view in complaints about shortage of nurses in situations where the salary rates are demonstrably well below the earnings of equivalent occupations in the same economy.

The importance of promotion prospects has already been mentioned. Clearly the incentives to enter, and once in, to study and learn, are very different where the prospects of advancement are good as compared with situations where these are limited or non-existent.

A special question to be asked relates to the extent to which the skills taught and the expectations created for the future are fulfilled in the actual work situations to which the student goes after he is trained. This question is particularly relevant with the highest levels of skilled professional training. The morale of the skilled professional person is much related to his circumstances of work. If the educational process creates expectations of work opportunities which the later service situations cannot fulfil, then morale may be low and work may suffer. Such conditions may exist, for example, in certain circumstances of general practice where the highly trained practitioner may be largely spending his time in solving comparatively limited problems, and where he may have few

resources with which to investigate his more complex problems; an analogous situation may arise with the registered nurse trained to special interest in direct patient care, who is put into a role of administrator with little or no patient contact.

Incentives may be social as well as directly financial or related to the work situation. One of the great problems in many health services is how to persuade key personnel to work in rural areas. Here processes of recruitment and education may be in conflict with the needs of the system. It may be intended that many of the students should choose careers in rural situations, yet the educational process may be one of acclimatization to urban life, with resultant lack of interest in working outside towns. Sometimes too little attempt is made to provide for the general social and cultural needs of the individual who does go to the rural area. It may be that many of the students are intended for practice outside hospitals as doctors or nurses, etc., yet the educational process may condition them to expect conditions and facilities which can be provided only in hospitals. It may be intended that students should be as much concerned about the health of communities as they are about individual patients, about prevention and health promotion as well as cure, yet if the main interest of learning and the prestige situations of later life appear to centre on therapeutic medicine in hospital, student interest and ambitions are likely to remain fixed at that level.

There is increasing awareness in health systems of the need to provide a process of postgraduate and continuing education for all categories of health occupations. The need was first perceived in relation to medical practitioners and registered nurses, but increasingly the principle is being applied to other categories. Such a process, to be effective, needs a serious effort of organization and expenditure, perhaps most clearly demonstrated in the health services of the U.S.S.R.

The scientific and technical changes in the health sciences are so rapid that the content of required knowledge is continually changing. In such circumstances it is necessary for the health services and their agencies to provide opportunities for stimulus to keep up-to-date through planned refresher courses, opportunities for reading and attending scientific and professional meetings, and continuous programmes of in-service discussion and stimulation. A system of postgraduate and continuous education becomes an essential ingredient of the health service itself. Medicine has indeed become a life-time study for practitioners and planners alike (see World Health Organization, 1970).

REFERENCES

Abel-Smith, B. (1967) An international study of health expenditure, and its relevance for health planning, *Wld Hlth Org. Publ. Hlth Pap.*, No. 32.

Abel-Smith, B., and Titmuss, R. N. (1956) The hospital population, in *The Cost of the National Health Service in England and Wales*, Appendix H, Cambridge.

Advisory Committee for Management Efficiency (1966) *Management Functions of Hospital Doctors*, London.

Anderson, O. W. (1964) Research in hospital use and expenditures, *J. chron. Dis.*, **17**, 727.

Bailey, N. T. J. (1959) Operational research, in *Medical Surveys and Clinical Trials*, ed. Witts, L. J., p. 148, London.

Baker, T. D. (1966) Dynamics of health manpower planning, *Med. Care*, **4**, 205.

Beck, I. F., Gardner, F. V., and Witts, L. V. (1947) Social service for a medical ward, *Brit. J. soc. Med.*, **1**, 197.

Biörck, G. (1965) The next ten years in medicine: attempt at an analysis of factors determining medical and social development, *Brit. med. J.*, **2**, 7.

Brockington, C. F. (1964) A community health service, in *Trends in the National Health Service*, ed. Farndale, J., p. 101, London.

Brown, M., and Carling, F. C. (1945) A social study of hospital treatment, *Brit. med. J.*, **1**, 478.

Brown, R. G., McKeown, T., and Whitfield, A. G. W. (1958) Observations of the medical conditions of men in the seventh decade, *Brit. med. J.*, **1**, 555.

Candau, M. G. (1965) Hospital organisation in developing countries, *Wld Hospitals*, **1**, 439.

Carstairs, V., and Patterson, P. E. (1966) Distribution of hospital patients by social class, *Hlth Bull. (Edinb.)*, **24**, 59.

Ciocco, A., and Lawrence, P. S. (1958) Illness among older people in Hagerstown, Maryland, *Publ. Hlth Serv. Publs. (Wash.)*, No. 170.

Commission on Chronic Illness (1957a) *Chronic Illness in a Large City; The Baltimore Study, Chronic Illness in the United States*, Volume IV, Cambridge, Mass.

Commission on Chronic Illness (1957b) *Prevention of Chronic Illness; Chronic Illness in the United States*, Volume I, p. 48, Cambridge, Mass.

Cottrell, J. D. (1966) The consumption of medical care and the evaluation of efficiency, *Med. Care*, **4**, 214.

Cowan, P. (1963) The size of hospitals, *Med. Care*, **1**, 1.

Crombie, D. L., and Cross, K. W. (1959) Serious illness in hospital and at home, *Med. Press*, **242**, 316.

Crombie, D. L., and Cross, K. W. (1961) The care of seriously ill patients in hospital and general practice, *J. roy. Coll. gen. Practit.*, **4**, 270.

Crombie, D. L., and Cross, K. W. (1963) The relationship of hospital and domiciliary care, *Med. Care*, **1**, 245.

Deniston, O. L., Rosenstock, I. M., and Getting, V. A. (1968) Evaluation of program effectiveness, *Publ. Hlth Rep. (Wash.)*, **83**, 323.

Department of Health and Social Security (1972) National Health Service Reorganization, England Cmnd 5055, H.M.S.O., London.

Donabedian, A. (1968) Promoting quality through evaluating the process of patient care, *Med. Care*, **6**, 181.

Engel, A. (1965) Health planning in a changing society, *Wld Hospitals*, **1**, 255.

Evang, K. (1951) Trends in the development of hospital functions and administration, in *Public Health Lectures*, Medical Teaching Mission to Israel, p. 36, Boston, Mass.

Evang, K. (1960) *Health Service, Society and Medicine*, Heath Clark Lectures, 1958, London.

Evang, K. (1965) *Health Planning*, World Health Organization, Eighteenth World Health Assembly, 30 April 1965.

Evang, K. (1966) The position of the medically trained person in the administration of health services, *Amer. J. publ. Hlth*, **56**, 1722.

Evang, K. (1967) Political, national and traditional limitations to health control, in *Health of Mankind*, ed. Wolstenholme, G., and O'Connor, M., p. 196, London.

Feldstein, M. S. (1963) Operational research and efficiency in the health service, *Lancet*, **i**, 491.

Feldstein, M. S. (1964) Hospital planning and the demand for care, *Bull. Oxf. Univ. Inst. Statist.*, **27**, 361.

Feldstein, M. S., Piot, M. A., and Sundaresan, T. K. (1973) Resource allocation model for public health planning; a case study of tuberculosis control, *Bull. Wld Hlth Org.*, **48**, Suppl.

Ferguson, T., and MacPhail, A. N. (1954) *Hospital and Community*, London.

Ferguson, T., and MacPhail, A. N. (1962) The Glasgow study, in *Further Studies in Hospital and Community*, ed. Ferguson, T., London.

Flagle, C. D., Huggins, W. H., and Roy, R. H. (1960) *Operations Research and System Engineering*, Baltimore.

Forsyth, G., and Logan, R. F. L. (1960) *The Demand for Medical Care*, London.

Foster, C. D. (1968) Cost benefit analysis in research, in *Decision Making in National Science Policy*, ed. De Reuck et al., p. 61, London.

Galloway, T. McL. (1963) Management of vaccination and immunization procedures by electronic computers, *Med. Offr*, **109**, 232.

General Medical Council (1967) *Recommendations as to Diplomas in Public Health and Similar Qualifications*, London.

Georgopoulos, B. S., and Mann, F. C. (1962) *The Community General Hospital*, New York.

Goodwin, C. S. (1972) Medical information systems, *Lancet*, **ii**, 871.

Hietand, D. L. (1966) Research into manpower for health services, *Milbank mem. Fd Quart.*, **44**, 146.

Hilleboe, H. E., Barkhuis, Anne, and Thomas, W. C. (1972) Approaches to public health planning, *Wld Hlth Org. Publ. Hlth Pap.*, No. 46.

I.E.A. (1973) Uses of epidemiology in planning health services, *Proc. 6th International Scientific Meeting*, Belgrade.

Joint Working Party (1967a) *Organisation of Medical Work in Hospitals, First Report*, Ministry of Health, London.

Joint Working Party (1967b) *Organisation of Medical Work in the Hospital Service in Scotland, First Report*, Scottish Home and Health Department, Edinburgh.

Jones, Kathleen (1964) Revolution and reform in the mental health services, in *Trends in the National Health Service*, ed. Farndale, J., p. 202, London.

Jones, Kathleen (1966) British experience in community care, in *International Trends in Mental Health*, ed. David, H. P., p. 87, New York.

Kissick, W. L. (1967a) Forecasting health manpower needs; the 'numbers game' is obsolete, *Hospitals*, **41**, 16 September, p. 47.

Kissick, W. L. (1967b) How imagination and innovation can bridge manpower gaps, *Hospitals*, **41**, 1 October, p. 76.

Kissick, W. L. (1968) Effective utilisation: the critical factor in health manpower, *Amer. J. publ. Hlth*, **58**, 23.

Klarman, H. E. (1951) Requirements for physicians, *Amer. Econ. Rev.*, **41**, 633.

Klein, R. (1972) National Health Service reorganization. The politics of the second best, *Lancet*, **ii**, 418.

Lentz, Edith M. (1957) Hospital administration—one of a species, *Adm. Sci. Quart.*, **1**, 444.

Logan, R. F. L. (1964) Studies in the spectrum of medical care, in *Problems and Progress in Medical Care*, ed. McLachlan, G., p. 3, London.

Logan, W. P. D. (1960) *Morbidity Statistics from General Practice, Vol. II (Occupation)*, General Register Office, Studies on Medical and Population Subjects, No. 14, London.

McKeown, T. (1961) Limitations of medical care attributable to medical education, *Lancet*, **ii**, 1.

McKeown, T. (1965) Medical education and medical care: an examination of traditional concepts and suggestions for change, in *Hospitals, Doctors and the Public Interest*, ed. Knowles, J. II., p. 154, Cambridge, Mass.

Mackintosh, J. M., McKeown, T., and Garratt, F. N. (1961) An examination of the need for hospital admission, *Lancet*, **i**, 815.

Martin, F. M., Brotherston, J. H. F., and Chave, S. P. W. (1957) Incidence of neurosis in a new housing estate, *Brit. J. prev. soc. Med.*, **11**, 196.

Nuffield Foundation (1947) *Old People*, Report of a survey committee on the problems of ageing and the care of old people, London.

Pan American Health Organization (P.A.H.O.) (1973) *Ten-year Health Plan for the Americas*, Washington.

Pemberton, J., and Smith, J. C. (1949) The return to work of elderly male hospital in-patients, *Brit. med. J.*, **2**, 306.

Pennel, M. Y. (1966) Identification of health occupations, *Employ. Serv. Rev.*, **3**, 55.

Platt, R. (1963) *Doctor and Patient: Ethics, Morale, Government*, The Rock Carling Fellowship, Nuffield Provincial Hospital Trust, London.

Popov, G. A. (1971) Principles of health planning in the U.S.S.R., *Wld Hlth Org. Publ. Hlth Pap.*, No. 43.

Report of a Steering Committee (1972) *Management Arrangements for the Reorganized National Health Service*, H.M.S.O., London.

Revans, R. W. (1964a) *Standards for Morale, Cause and Effects in Hospitals*, Nuffield Provincial Hospitals Trust, London.

Revans, R. W. (1964b) The morale and effectiveness of general hospitals, in *Problems and Progress in Medical Care*, ed. McLachlan, G., for Nuffield Provincial Hospitals Trust, p. 55, London.

Revans, R. W. (1966a) Hospital attitudes and communications, in *Operational Research and the Social Sciences*, ed. Lawrence, J. R., p. 601, London.

Revans, R. W. (1966b) Research into hospital management and organisation, *Milbank mem. Fd Quart.*, **44**, 207.

Royal Commission on Medical Education (1968) *Report*, 1965–68, London.

Rudoe, N. (1973) Health planning in national development, *Wld Hlth Org. Chron.*, **27**, 6.

Rutstein, D. D. (1965) At the turn of the next century, in *Hospitals, Doctors and the Public Interest*, ed. Knowles, J. H., p. 293, Cambridge, Mass.

Silver, G. A. (1963) *Family Medical Care*, Cambridge, Mass.

Somers, A. R. (1966) Some basic determinants of medical care and health policy: an overview of trends and issues, *Hlth Serv. Res.*, **1**, 193.

Stevens, Rosemary (1966) *Medical Practice in Modern England; The Impact of Specialisation and State Medicine*, London.

Townsend, P., and Wedderburn, D. (1965) *The Aged in the Welfare State*, Occasional Papers on Social Administration No. 14, London.

White, K. L. (1968) Research in medical care and health services systems, *Med. Care*, **6**, 95.

Wilson, J. M. G., and Jungner, G. (1968) Principles and practice of screening for disease, *Wld Hlth Org. Publ. Hlth Pap.*, No. 34.

Wilson, L. A., Lawson, I. R., and Brass, W. (1962) Multiple disorders in the elderly, a clinical and statistical study, *Lancet*, **ii**, 841.

Winslow, C. E. A. (1951) The cost of sickness and price of health, *Wld Hlth Org. Monogr. Ser.*, No. 7.

World Health Organization (European Region) Working Group (1967) Report on the Evaluation of Courses in Hospital and Medical Services Administration, Copenhagen.

World Health Organization Expert Committee on Organization of Medical Care (1957) First Report, Role of Hospitals in Programmes of Community Health Protection, *Wld Hlth Org. techn. Rep. Ser.*, No. 122.

World Health Organization Expert Committee on Organization of Medical Care (1959) Second Report, Role of Hospitals in Ambulatory and Medical Care, *Wld Hlth Org. techn. Rep. Ser.*, No. 176.

World Health Organization Expert Committee on Professional and Technical Education of Medical and Auxiliary Personnel (1963) Eleventh Report, Training of the Physician for Family Practice, *Wld Hlth Org. techn. Rep. Ser.*, No. 257.

World Health Organization Expert Committee on Hospital Administration (1968) *Wld Hlth Org. techn. Rep. Ser.*, No. 395.

World Health Organization (1970) Training in national health planning. Report of a WHO expert committee, *Wld Hlth Org. techn. Rep. Ser.*, No. 456.

World Health Organization (1971) Planning and programming for nursing services, *Wld Hlth Org. Publ. Hlth Pap.*, No. 44.

World Health Organization (1973) Interrelationships between health programmes and socio-economic development, *Publ. Hlth Pap.*, No. 49.

World Health Organization Regional Office for Europe (1973) *Report of a Working Group on Health Planning in National Development, Stockholm 1972* (Euro 4104), Copenhagen.

World Health Organization (1974a) The work of WHO in 1973, *Wld Hlth Org. Off. Rec.*, No. 213, 95–102.

World Health Organization (1974b) Modern management methods and the organization of health services, *Wld Hlth Org. Publ. Hlth Pap.*, No. 55.

42

ECONOMIC ASPECTS OF HEALTH PLANNING

A. P. RUDERMAN

Introduction: Varieties of Economic Doctrine

A discussion of the economic aspects of health planning must begin by explaining why some economists are concerned with the subject while others consider planning of any kind to be a bad thing.

One of the most popular English-language textbooks on the subject defines economics as '. . . the study of how men and society *choose*, with or without the use of money, to employ scarce productive resources to produce various commodities over time and distribute them for consumption, now and in the future, among various people and groups in society'. The choices often have to be made under political pressure, and this is not only the pressure of their constituents on the decision-makers but the pressure of the decision-makers on their economic advisers. Because of this, and in the absence of accurate statistical information and strict scientific tests of hypotheses of cause and effect, a variety of doctrines have come into being to justify the recommendations that economists inevitably seem called on to make.

The main stream of classic Anglo-American economics has firm roots in eighteenth-century moral philosophy (the doctrine of leaving things to work themselves out: *laissez faire, laissez aller*), and in the business experience and crude statistics of Victorian England. It starts from the belief that the interplay of supply, demand, and prices under conditions of perfect competition in free markets will ensure that optimum choices are made. It assumes that organized human activity exists in order to satisfy wants, that greater wants reflect themselves in a willingness to pay higher prices, and that such prices elicit greater supplies of the wanted goods and services. The role of government in this system is to maintain public order and insure the least possible impediment to the working of the prices system.

Popular contemporary offspring of this doctrine has shown considerable mathematical and statistical sophistication in demonstrating the imperfections of the market-place and of the price mechanism. The adherents of this modified doctrine believe that the management of economic life by socially responsible governments—using instruments such as tax policy and control of the rate of interest to influence factors such as the amount of investment and the distribution of income—will assure that market forces lead in fact to the best possible choices.

While it is by no means inappropriate to classify Karl Marx himself as an Eminent Victorian, contemporary Marxist–Leninist doctrine—despite some concessions to the role of the price system and the profit motive—places its main reliance on refined and computerized comprehensive planning of economic life as a whole to ensure that socially desirable choices are made.

Applied economists of all doctrinal schools, concerned as they are with the solution of concrete workaday problems, share a common ground of statistical method and scientific inference. There is an encouraging tendency to escape the emotional polarization of economic thought into Capitalist and Communist schools, and to classify economic systems rather by the preponderance of 'market' or 'command' elements in their structure.[1]

Health planners, whether they turn to economists for general policy recommendations for the solution of specific problems or for allocations of funds, should recognize that economics is by no means monolithic. The attitude of individual economists towards health planning, their specific recommendations, and their willingness to see money spent on the provision of health services, depend in some measure on the doctrines which they profess. Adherence to any given school of economic thought is influenced by academic training, by work experience, and by the prevailing doctrinal climate, but is seldom wholly predictable.

Applying Economics to the Study of Health Planning

Some general non-specific relationship between health and economic activity, typified by the 'vicious circle of poverty and disease', has long been recognized. Serious attempts to apply economics as a formal discipline in the planning of health services, however, have only acquired momentum in the past decade.

One of the reasons for slow progress was that market-oriented economists, whether of the *laissez-faire* or money-management school, encountered conceptual difficulties in applying theories that derived from the assumption that prices reflect wants and lead in turn to the satisfaction of wants. It was found, when the first descriptive statistics were compiled, that many health services were not particularly responsive to price, and were often devoted to the satisfaction of needs rather than wants in any case. Some authority had decided that a given set of health programmes was 'good for people' in some instances and had gone about the task without reference to people's desires. It also became clear that simple demand–price–supply relationships could not obtain in the case of hospitals, or of prescription drugs, where a third-party, the referring or prescribing physician, was interposed between buyer and seller.

This particular set of difficulties was not encountered in command economies, and the dilemma of the market economist

---

[1] While it is hoped that the terms 'market' and 'command' are self-explanatory it may be helpful to think of them as alternative ways of allocating resources—letting free-market prices bring about the allocation in the former case, and issuing direct administrative orders in the latter.

was whether to abandon the study of health services because they did not follow market rules or to abandon market rules in order to analyse health services realistically. While this is still a dilemma in some cases, many economists have come to view the provision of health services as a 'command area' in market economies, even though the income of doctors and nurses may affect their supply, or the price of drugs affect their utilization. Once this position is adopted, it follows that the comprehensive planning of health services by administrative agencies of government is necessary and desirable even in societies where the allocation of resources to the production of bicycles or of laundry services is determined by free market forces. Health is considered to be an inherent right of all persons, as expressed in the Constitution of the World Health Organization, rather than a commodity to be bought and sold according to market rules. This may be taken as a majority view of health economists in the late 1960s.

The practical problem is to apply the tools of economic analysis to health planning. The goal is to provide the responsible authorities with rational bases for deciding how best to employ the scarce resources of the health sector in order to satisfy present and predicted service requirements of the population at the least cost, as well as to measure the costs and returns from health activities that are initiated on other than economic grounds.[1]

The problem is usually broken down into two areas of study that require different technical approaches—the macro-economic and the micro-economic. Macro-economics is concerned with providing health planners with criteria for allocating resources in the aggregate. It is concerned with relative shares—with the share of national income that should be devoted to health rather than to other activities, and with the human resources that should be devoted to health from the pool of all available man-power. Macroplanning at this level compares the relative return to society from investment in health services, from investment in education or other parts of the social infrastructure, and from investment in directly productive activities such as farming and manufacturing. Once decisions have been reached at this level, the allocation of money and man-power to different classes of health activity, and the calculation of relative returns within the health sector, can be based on similar aggregative statistics and analysis.

The micro-economics of health concentrates on the individual service or service unit, be it a network of health centres or an individual hospital. It is concerned with determining operating efficiency, the optimum combination of human and material resources, and the optimum scale of operations for full utilization and least cost. It involves considerations of managerial rather than social accounting. Finally, it provides health planners with local data on costs and output that can be summed at the regional and national levels to provide the raw material of macroplanning.

How Much Money for the Health Sector?

The criteria for allocating resources to health in the aggregate are important to health planners not so much as a basis for their own decisions but because they guide national authorities at the highest level in deciding what share of total national resources shall be devoted to the health sector. The basic national decisions may be made for a variety of political or economic reasons. Whatever the criteria, health services are often considered as a dependent sector of activity, expected to do the best possible job with the resources provided, but by no means provided with all the resources desired when higher priority is conceded to other 'social infrastructure' areas such as education, or to directly productive activity, because of the higher returns anticipated.

A certain consistency has been observed in the share of national resources usually spent for health. Some illustrative figures for fourteen countries are shown in TABLE 117.

TABLE 117

Percentage of Gross National Product Going for Health, and Health Share of General Government Budgets, Circa 1961

Country	Total current expenditure on health services as per cent. of gross national product	General government expenditure on health services as per cent. of total general government expenditure
Australia	4·9	25·8
Canada	5·5	17·1
Ceylon	3·7	14·9
Chile	5·6	16·4
Rhodesia and Nyasaland	4·1	13·2
Finland	4·3	18·8
France	4·2	25·4
Israel	5·9	9·0
Netherlands	4·5	18·7
Sweden	4·9	21·0
Tanganyika	2·5	11·8
United Kingdom	4·0	19·8
United States	5·5	7·0
Yugoslavia	4·4	21·3

Source: B. Abel-Smith (1967) An International Study of Health Expenditures, *Wld Hlth Org. Publ. Hlth Pap.*, No. 32.

Despite their limited coverage, they serve to demonstrate the rather narrow range of variation in the share of gross national product devoted to health in rich and poor, large and small countries. Some slight change in the percentages is introduced when a roughly similar measure such as national income is used instead of gross national product as a basis for comparison, and a large element of potential error is introduced in countries where a significant portion of medical care is provided privately. In general, however, it would appear that many countries devoted about 5 per cent. of gross national product to health care, although the percentage of government expenditure going for governmental health services varies over an extremely wide range.

It is conceptually and administratively important, although statistically quite difficult, to distinguish clearly between expenditures on current account (payroll, drugs, supplies, and other recurring costs) and capital expenditures (buildings and grounds, durable equipment, and other non-recurring or seldom-recurring items). While not all countries have yet adopted the practice, the establishment of separate current and capital budgets makes it possible to separate the long-term considerations involved in planning capital investment

---

[1] Scarcity can be relative as well as absolute, and even the best-endowed countries fall short of being able to provide all the health services that could conceivably be desired. Hence the need to economize.

(hospitals, roads, factories, etc.) from the short-term budgetary forecasts of the cost of routine day-to-day operations.

In some countries, unfortunately, current and capital items are so mixed in accounting practice that it is not certain how many of the latter have been included in statistics of current expenditure. To the extent that the statistics of gross national product or national income follow the Standard National Accounts system of the United Nations, the data cannot be compared directly with figures for countries like those of Eastern Europe that use the conceptually different Material Balance System. In data referring to any single year it is also important to recognize that the signing of the contract for a single major building, particularly in a small country, can introduce a decided shift in the ratio of health to total capital expenditure for that year.

Despite their manifest inaccuracy, the 'fact' that countries devote 5 per cent. of gross national product to health, and the companion notion that 10 per cent. of government expenditure goes for government health services, have been quoted so often and so widely that in some countries they have taken on a magical quality and have been interpreted as indicating the share of national resources that *should* be spent on health. So far as can be determined, however, the share of national resources spent on health seems to be the result of historical accident more than any other single factor. Even in the U.S.S.R., where considerable effort has been devoted to systematic health planning for more than fifty years, the share of national resources devoted to health appears to be limited by a 'law of proportional growth' so that the health sector cannot grow more rapidly than the economy as a whole. In contrast to the detailed studies that have led to the establishment of standard ratios of health man-power and hospital beds to population with provision for adjustment in special cases, the relative share of the health sector as a whole—so far as the author has been able to determine—seems to have a historical rather than an empirical basis.

Quite simply, there is no objective means of ascertaining what the relative share of resources for health should be. There is no known method of comparing the returns from expenditure on health, education, agriculture, manufacturing, etc., since the only common unit available to measure returns on a single scale is money. Many ingenious efforts have been made to guess at the money value of health activity, but even if it were possible to assign money values to improved health or longer life, it is not always possible to identify the direct contribution of health services. Multiple causation must be taken into account, and such elements as higher incomes, more food, better housing, and higher levels of education are known to be positively correlated with lower infant mortality, higher life expectancy at birth, and other available health indices.

In the absence of objectively verifiable rules for determining the share of resources that should be spent on health the economist is forced to concede second place, after historical accident, to political pressure. It was noted above that health services are often oriented to satisfying needs rather than wants, and that wants, in the form of market demand working through the price mechanism, seem to have little direct influence on the supply of health services. In the absence of market mechanism, however, wants can influence the supply of health services through their political expression in terms of votes or of organized public opinion. Decisions as to public spending on health are often taken in response to such political pressure.

Interestingly, the political expression of wants makes it more than ever important to maintain the economic distinction between current and capital expenditures—perhaps because political decisions are often characterized by such short-run considerations as the tenure of an individual or a party in office, and their 'economic time horizon' is seldom extended beyond the period of forseeable political power. This probably explains why it is common experience, in countries with a wide variety of economic and political structure, that it is easier to get administrative or parliamentary (or the dictator's) approval for investment in buildings and equipment than to obtain added staff to man them; easier to get increased staff than to get improved wages and working conditions for existing staff. To many Chiefs of State a hospital is a more satisfactory monument than a memorial garden or arch of triumph. Certainly, some of the unutilized and underutilized capacity in some of the less-developed countries results from the fact that politicians, faced with uncertain tenure, have erected hospitals and health centres without devoting sufficient thought to the man-power, supplies and equipment, and operating budgets that the new construction makes necessary.

When it is possible to surmount political pressure and attempt to draw up objectively justifiable investment plans the administrator is faced, as in the case of determining priorities for current expenditure, with vague and unsatisfactory criteria. Construction may be determined by the mere availability of funds or credit, or by crude empirical formulae that equate a given number of beds with some other number of out-patient services in an attempt to set overall service targets rather than construction targets *per se*.

Finally, it should be understood that, in the absence of a precise formula for determining relative shares, the allocation of health funds involves a range rather than a precise figure. The lower limit to this range is the politically irreducible minimum, below which considerable difficulty could be anticipated by any government. In practice, this lower limit usually represents the contemporary level of service or expenditure per head of population, and can be expected to increase over time as population and prices rise. The upper limit is the maximum amount that scientific argument and personal and political suasion can induce national authorities to concede. Economic and technical considerations are therefore more useful in determining allocations within the range thus established than in setting the upper and lower limits. The criteria for determining allocations of funds within the general range set by higher national authority on a largely political basis are discussed below.

Setting Priorities within the Health Sector

The area of free choice in deciding how money should be distributed among health programmes is bounded by two major constraints. The upper limit to total expenditure is the sum of the money made available to the health sector by higher authority and the funds collectable from the public through insurance and prepayment contribution or the payment of fees in partial or total reimbursement for services provided. The lower limit is the politically irreducible minimum below which further reductions in expenditure would meet powerful opposition from public opinion or legislative action.

Within these limits, other constraints operate to reduce freedom of choice within the health sector. Certain activities (for example, the sort of organized effort to achieve total coverage that is found in malaria programmes) are essentially indivisible. Others, such as house connexions for drinking water, lend themselves to the imposition of a charge on the individual or the household. Funds for some general promotional activities such as health education may be assigned to school budgets, or water and sewer construction to public works budgets, and are thus beyond the decision-making authority of the health services. Above all, popular demand for medical care (in the sense of curative services) usually means that three-fourths or more of all health expenditure, the portion commonly devoted to medical care, becomes part of the politically irreducible minimum.[1] There are, indeed, possibilities for affecting the delivery of medical care services and influencing both quantity and quality through efficient planning, but this does not effect the constraint on expenditure as a whole. This leaves only expenditure on a limited number of community-wide preventive and promotional activities in the full discretionary power of health planners, although it is often possible to influence medical care services to some degree, above all where the system of financing is such as to make the public aware of costs as well as benefits.

Within the health authorities' area of discretion, it is common experience for available resources to fall far short of satisfying all identifiable needs. This in turn imposes the need for establishing priorities.

The basic considerations in establishing priorities can be expressed in the vocabulary of mathematics in the simple relationship:

$$P = f(M, I, V, C)$$

P stands for relative priority, and f means that the priority is a function of (bears an identifiable but unspecified relation to) each of the other variables. M stands for the magnitude of the disease or other condition under attack, commonly measured by statistics of mortality and morbidity, alone or in combination. I represents the relative impact or importance of the disease; in the present state of health economics it cannot be measured with precision, and is usually given an arbitrary numerical value based on the relative incidence among children, the aged, and those of working age, or some similar factors. V is the vulnerability of the disease to attack by known and available means, and, like importance, cannot be measured with precision, so that arbitrary rating scales must be used. C is the cost of the proposed activity; it can be measured with a fair degree of accuracy, as can morbidity and mortality under favourable conditions.

No formula, of course, is a substitute for common sense. In Latin America the same variables have been widely used in the less flexible relationship:

$$P = \frac{M \times I \times V}{C}$$

This avoids the need to seek out and measure the technical coefficients that relate M, I, and V in the formula proposed

earlier. Yet while it simplifies the arithmetic, the multiplicative formula embodies implicit equal weighting of the factors, regardless of the units in which they are measured. TABLE 118 shows an experimental calculation based on data for the state of Aragua, Venezuela, in 1960.

TABLE 118

Priority Calculation for Premature Birth and Pulmonary Tuberculosis, Aragua, Venezuela, 1960

Cause of death	Magnitude (M)	Importance (I)	Vulnerability (V)	Relative priority $(M \times I \times V)$
Premature birth	8·5	1·00	0·33	2·80
Pulmonary tuberculosis	2·8	0·68	0·66	1·25

Source: Pan American Health Organization (1963) *Health Planning: Problems of Concept and Method*, Table 3, Washington.

The above table illustrates both the advantages and the difficulties of the basic formula. In this example M was based solely on the fact that premature birth represented 8·5 per cent. of deaths from all causes recorded in the year, and pulmonary tuberculosis 2·8 per cent. The importance factor of 1 was assigned to premature birth, because all deaths occurred in the first year of life, and 0·86 to pulmonary tuberculosis because the recorded deaths occurred in the 15–49, 50–69, and 70+ age groups. The vulnerability rating was arbitrary, and reflects the fact that expert consensus in Venezuela was that more could be done to avoid deaths from tuberculosis than to prevent deaths occasioned by premature birth. It could, of course, be argued convincingly that deaths in the working years should be assigned a higher, rather than a lower importance, compared with deaths at birth, for economic reasons. This would reverse the I values assigned in the table.

It might also be argued that the premature infants who do not die cannot be said to have a disease, while adding morbidity to mortality for tuberculosis would show a more serious problem in terms of incapacity for work and the possibility of communicating the disease to other persons. If basing the calculation of M on morbidity and mortality had the effect of doubling M, the final product would be 3·5 and the order of priority of tuberculosis and prematurity would be reversed. Finally, the more flexible formulation $P = f(M, I, V)$ permits a variety of possible relationships to be explored, not necessarily multiplying $M \times I \times V$ but using an additive relationship $(M + I + V)$ if this were to seem more realistic, or applying weighting co-efficients to the terms of the expression. Using sums instead of products, the combined relationship would be 9·83 for prematurity and 4·14 for tuberculosis; giving a double weight to the element of vulnerability would yield 0·924 and 0·825 respectively. Clearly, the choice of formula and the method of expressing the relative importance of the elements in the calculation have a substantial effect on the resulting priority.[2]

[2] Another formula suggested for setting priorities by the Indian Health Service of the U.S. Public Health Service is:

$$M \times D \times P + \left(\frac{274A}{N}\right) + \left(\frac{91B}{N}\right) + \left(\frac{274C}{N}\right)$$

Here (with apologies for the authors' assigning different meanings to M and P than are used elsewhere in this chapter) M stands for the ratio of the

[1] Health administrators occasionally encounter a strong politician who is able to cut back health services; in such a case the irreducible minimum is the level below which even a strong political position is threatened.

From the economic point of view, of course, cost is as important as all the remaining elements of the comparison. Calculating cost means obtaining agreement on the part of the health authorities for a standard procedure or group of procedures for each condition (prenatal visits, sputum examinations, standard therapy, etc.), which can then be assigned a money value on the basis of the man-power, materials, and buildings and equipment used. The final priority for operating plans of a health service would then depend on the interrelationship between M, I, and V, and on the relative cost of avoiding the death of a premature infant and preventing the occurrence of a case (or death because of) tuberculosis.

Even for the limited portion of the health budget over which some strict rule of priority might be imposed, a difficulty arises because the statistics usually relate to individual *diseases* while the priority must in practice be assigned to identifiable *activities* in the health service budget. It is of little help to decide that tuberculosis is more or less important than premature birth unless the expenditures for the tuberculosis programme and the expenditure for maternal and child health are separate budget items, unless personnel can be assigned to one or the other task, unless, in other words, the priority calculation can be followed by the indicated administrative action.

It should be observed that the use of any 'objective' formula or system to determine allocations of funds within the health sector may run into conflict with either political or economic demand for medical care, with historical or traditional priorities, and with vested interests in health services. Without a strong political commitment on the part of national authorities to support the priority-setting system, and without considerable education and promotional effort within the health services themselves, the rational allocation of funds may end up as nothing but wishful thinking.

Criteria that Consider Health as the Dependent Variable

Up to this point, the allocation of funds within the health sector has been discussed in terms of the possibilities for rational decision on the part of the health authorities when they set priorities for that portion of health expenditure over which they can be said to have discretionary power. It should also be recognized, however, that even within this area there may be occasions when considerations other than M, I, V, and C will over-ride the calculated priority for a given activity. A country may be faced with the need to meet critical development targets in another sector, to economize on foreign exchange because of a balance-of-payments problem, or simply

to adjust to the fact of poverty by adopting systems and classes of health service consonant with national ability to pay rather than with 'ideal' patterns observed in richer or more advanced countries. Under these circumstances the health authorities may well be called on to abandon their planned priorities for the sake of other national goals.

This may happen so subtly that conscious decision remains subliminal. A case in point is the use of social-security or social-insurance mechanisms to provide health services in poor and underdeveloped countries. Such a trend has in fact been clearly observable since the Second World War. It usually means that in the first instance health services are made available to employed wage earners and salary earners in the major cities, spreading only slowly thereafter to cover family dependants and workers in small towns and rural areas. In an era of urbanization and industrialization this means concentrating health services not in the area of greatest need (morbidity and mortality may well be higher from all causes among underemployed peasants in rural areas) but in the area considered to be of greatest importance for the future economic development of the country. If it were possible to identify the importance for national development of individual health programmes this factor could be rated on a numerical scale and introduced in the I term of the priority formula. Without this possibility, it becomes a matter for political or administrative decision.

The decision can also be made consciously and directly. In Peru, for example, the national health plan presented to the Congress in 1965 recognized the overriding national priority given to development of the Amazonian region by making specific allocations for new construction of health centres in the plan period to be concentrated in that region. The development importance of the projected Andean highway was recognized by the Ministry of Health in special health provisions recommended for road workers (and eventually colonists) in the high mountains. In Buenaventura, Colombia, an important port on the Pacific coast, the most active and best-financed health centre observed by the author was not part of the Departmental network of the Cauca Valley (the administrative district in which Buenaventura is located) but was a dependency of the national government, operated by the port authorities for the benefit of the dockers and their families.

Economic development involves more than the growth of urban industry and trade, however. There are countries which rely heavily on agriculture to feed the domestic population, provide export earnings, and accumulate a surplus for investment in non-agricultural development projects. The colonial plantation health services that grew up in the early twentieth century constituted tacit recognition of the need for a healthy, stable, and productive agricultural labour force. In the postcolonial era many of the newly self-governing countries of the world are attempting to create rural health service networks with similar aims (and the satisfaction of increasingly vocal demand) in mind.

The allocation of resources to health services on the basis of other than health considerations does, of course, run counter to the commonly accepted views of universality (the right of all persons to health care) and of the importance of maintaining the highest possible quality standards. But when the money does not stretch to cover the need arguments of equity are

---

deaths from a disease observed per 100,000 population in the group being planned for (in this case, Indians) to the deaths per 100,000 of the population as a whole or some other rate which is chosen as a target. D is the crude death rate per 100,000 in the group being planned for. P represents years of life expectancy lost because of death from the disease in the group being planned for. A is the number of in-patient days of care, B the number of out-patient visits, and C the number of days of restricted activity, used by the disease in the population being planned for. N is the actual population for which services are being planned. The figure 274 represents 100,000 divided by 365 (reducing hospitalization and restricted activity rates to a daily instead of a yearly basis) and 91 is simply one-third of 274, a weighting factor that seemed appropriate to the planners in the case of out-patient visits. Formulae of this type require more sophisticated basic statistical information than M, I, and V as defined in this chapter, but by means of this they can give more weight to the demand for treatment caused by ill health and to the factor of disability. As might be expected from a service designed for a small minority in an affluent country, cost is not a term in the formula.

countered by the scarcity of resources. Allocating equal funds to all areas and all classes of the population would often mean inadequate health services for all instead of adequate services for a select (hopefully, productive) few.

Human Resources for Health

The decision as to what numbers and what classes of professional, sub-professional, and unskilled man-power should be devoted to health must clearly be based on the decisions determining national health policy, the relative priority of different activities, the allocation of funds for capital investment in health service facilities and the current budgets for their operation, of the relative cost of capital and labour, the various ways in which they can be combined, and the choice among available technologies for combining them. The optimum staffing pattern for the planned health services, however, may be more of an ideal than a feasible design, because human resources in many fields are often scarce.

Health services often plan on the basis of existing numbers of physicians, nurses, medical technicians, etc., making appropriate allowance for attrition owing to death, retirement, and migration to other fields of work or other places. The provision of *additional* health man-power as distinct from the maintenance of existing strength, however, is inseparably linked with the educational system as a whole. Medical schools, for example, are in competition for the output of the limited pool of secondary-school graduates with schools training basic scientists, engineers, business managers, public administrators, agriculturists, and a variety of other professionals. There are cases where students enter the health professions because of family tradition, idealism, social prestige, or some other non-economic motivation, but countries that confer greater status or greater financial rewards on factory managers, soldiers, or politicians may find difficulty in attracting sufficient high-calibre candidates to the health professions.

The problem is, of course, most severe in the less developed and poorer countries. In Jamaica, for example, less than 10 per cent. of individuals in the 15–19 age group were reported as enrolled in secondary schools in the 1960s. This provides a far smaller pool of candidates for higher education than was available in the United Kingdom or the United States, where more than 80 per cent. of the same cohort received secondary education.

Under favourable circumstances, when the health professions exert adequate attraction for young people making career decisions, the principal problem in planning is to take into account the intricate network of time lags of varying length, as well as the relative costs involved in training individuals for the different professions. Starting with the cohort of children entering elementary school at the age of 5, 6, or 7, there is a lag of at least ten years before any are available for recruitment to the least skilled general services or apprenticeship or technical training for jobs of higher skill. As much as twenty years may elapse between entry into the school system and the completion of medical education.

The least skilled occupations have the highest substitutability, in that within broad limits almost any sweeper or kitchen helper or watchman can be substituted for any other. On the other hand, individuals in these occupations seldom have the professional's motivation to work in health services.

Except in the rare (and undesirable) situations where forced labour exists, attracting and keeping unskilled and semi-skilled labour in health institutions depends more on wages and conditions of work than on the service goals of the institutions. Even at higher levels of skill (electricians, book-keepers, junior management staff) health services are in competition with other sectors of the economy (industry, commerce) that employ persons of equivalent skills and sometimes offer more attractive long-run career prospects. Against this, the health administrator is reduced to the argument of job security, since health services are the least likely of activities to be terminated when economic conditions are bad.

As was noted in the discussion of the allocation of funds, there are situations where man-power as well as money allocations respond to national priorities rather than the objectives of the health sector as such. In many developing countries the highest priority among social services is in fact given to basic education, and it is considered important to train far more schoolmasters before training any more physicians. Indeed, the students trained by the new schoolmasters may well serve to expand the pool for later recruitment into the health professions.

The relative cost of training professionals in different fields must also be taken into account. It is possible, for example, to train philosophers with a minimum of capital investment—the main requirements being a supply of able teachers, some reading matter and writing materials, and some 'grove of Academe' where teachers and students can meet. In the health professions, as in other branches of natural science and technology, a far higher investment in laboratories and teaching aids is required, and classes in many subjects must be small so as to provide direct experience for each student. In Canada the different financial requirements were reflected in the formula used for financing by the Ontario Department of University Affairs, which paid universities about $1,500 per annum for Arts undergraduates in 1970, compared with some $7,500 for Medicine.

In the search for criteria to govern the allocation of human resources to health in the aggregate, the planner encounters many constraints imposed by the wage structure, by the organization of the labour market, by the attitudes of different types of health worker towards one another, by the educational system, and by the determination of general national priorities at the highest level. The technical design of an ideal staffing pattern for the planned health services may be relatively straightforward, but the scarcity of trained human resources to satisfy all the demands of complex modern society leads to a great, and sometimes growing, gap between the desirable and the feasible.

The Use of Man-power within the Health Sector

Whatever the external constraints, it might be imagined that the decision as to priority ratings for programmes within the health sector determines once and for all the priority ratings for the allocation of man-power to the programmes. This is not so because labour and capital are substitutable to a certain extent, because some categories of labour may be substituted for others, and because health programmes differ from one another in their capital and labour requirements.

An example of the substitutability between labour and

capital is provided by the use of the jet injector in mass small-pox vaccination programmes. A single operator trained in the use of this rather costly piece of equipment can vaccinate as many persons in an hour as several vaccinators using conventional scarification technique can vaccinate in a day, albeit with far cheaper instruments. The jet injector, then, is a substitute for the additional vaccinators. This example also serves to underscore the importance of utilization; if only a few persons have to be vaccinated, or if the year's work load can conveniently be spread over many working days, vaccination with the jet injector may prove more costly than the manual technique. Other things being equal, if sustained high numbers of persons are to be vaccinated, and the jet injector can be used for many hours each day and many days in the year, the cost per vaccination will be lower by this method.

The decision whether to substitute capital for labour will depend in each case on the volume of service to be provided and the relative cost of capital and labour. In the less-developed countries, where workloads are uneven, unskilled labour is cheap and plentiful, and capital equipment is imported, scarce, and expensive, it may well prove economical (and have the political advantage of helping to provide employment) to refrain from the introduction of labour-saving capital equipment even when the volume of service would justify such substitution in an advanced country where wages were higher and capital costs lower.

Similar considerations underlie the basic decision whether to emphasize in-patient or out-patient care in planning a general system of personal health services. Elaborate hospitals with modern diagnostic and treatment aids are expensive to build and require a variety of skilled professionals to provide a full range of services. An equal number of people could be cared for in lower-cost health centres by preponderantly semi-skilled and auxiliary personnel. In this case the choice of system and the kind of capital investment undertaken can be said to pre-determine to some extent the kinds of man-power needed, and a 'reverse feedback' would be to take the cost of the different kinds of man-power into account in planning the kinds of facilities to be constructed. It is also clear that the alternative systems of health service may take care of equal *numbers* of people, but not necessarily the *same* people. One individual may die of uraemia when there is no hospital where a prosta-tectomy can be performed, while at the same time the life of another may be saved at low cost by a simple rehydration of an infant with diarrhoea, performed in a local health unit. When neither funds nor man-power are available to serve the entire population, the decisions of health planners determine in a very real way who will live and who will die.

The problem of substituting some categories of man-power for others has been studied in a wide variety of settings. Countries experiencing man-power shortages (and shortage relative to demand exists even in affluent societies) have commonly seen a planned or spontaneous devolution of functions from the physician to the trained nurse and from the trained nurse to the nursing auxiliary or dresser. A variety of intermediate professional categories—the feldscher in the U.S.S.R., the assistant doctor in Fiji, the public health nurse with responsibilities that approach the general practice of medicine in certain remote areas of the United States—have been established. An even more important development has been the growing awareness of the possibilities of ensuring better utilization of physician time in professional tasks by using various combinations of professional and supporting personnel as a team. To the economist this is a somewhat tardy rediscovery of the eighteenth-century doctrine that economies and efficiency arise from the appropriate division and specialization of labour, but it is no less fruitful for being delayed.

Finally, it should be noted that the divergencies between money and man-power requirements of health programmes arise because of the varying requirements of the programmes themselves. Perhaps the problems of man-power substitution and combination have been studied too much in the context of medical care, with a resultant lack of emphasis on the differences between kinds of health programmes. When the whole spectrum of health activity is studied it is apparent that medical care of the sick makes the greatest demands on skilled professional man-power, while mass preventive and promotional activities rely far more heavily on sub-professional or non-medical skills.

It is a commonplace in advanced countries that the greatest demand for hospital beds, for individual attention by physicians, and for skilled nursing care, exists in the relatively small, if growing, group of individuals suffering from the chronic and degenerative diseases associated with advanced age. In the less-developed and poorer countries, in contrast, most deaths occur at earlier ages and are attributable to the general group of infectious and parasitic diseases. The so-called 'vertical' or 'penetration' campaigns against such diseases as smallpox, yellow fever, and malaria rely heavily on unskilled labour—drivers, spraymen, warehousemen, plus vaccinators and microscopists with specific limited skills. Far smaller numbers of physicians, nurses, or for that matter, parasitologists and entomologists, are employed.

Environmental sanitation activities—whether for the provision of potable water or for excreta or refuse disposal—principally involve digging, drilling, earth-moving, and pipe laying. These activities call for far more unskilled labourers than foremen or supervising engineers. At least in the early stages of health-programme development, unskilled labour in preventive, promotional, and environmental programmes may contribute more to overall health in terms of death and illness avoided than physicians and nurses contribute by treating those already sick. In such cases high money allocations may well be associated with low demand for professional medical man-power.

In brief, the problem of man-power in health planning is to obtain the highest output of services for a given cost by selecting the most appropriate combinations of capital and labour, the optimum 'mix' of personnel skills, types of capital, and health technology, and the 'mix' of programmes that best reconciles man-power availability in the different categories with the targets set for the health services.

Estimating the Total Return on Investment in Health

While the amounts of money and the human resources assigned to health services may have been determined in part by a variety of political and other non-economic criteria, the basic *economic* criterion for decision-makers is the return on investment in health or health services.

Investment usually denotes spending on capital goods such as hospitals or factory equipment, but current expenditures on health can also be viewed as an investment in the health of the population, or indirectly as an investment in the goods and services which are expected to be produced by individuals in better health.

From the point of view of statistical measurement, the distinction between investing in *health* or in health *services* is important. An investment in health must measure its return in indices of health. In the absence of such indices, the negative aspect, reduction in morbidity and mortality, is commonly used. While this may indeed reduce health to its measurable reciprocal, the problem of determining the return on the investment is complicated by the multiple causation mentioned earlier, which makes it impossible to attribute improvements in health (or reductions in morbidity and mortality) to the sole agency of the health professions. It is quite clear and unambiguous, however, to set a target of service; service units such as bed-days of hospitalization, physician-hours of consultation, nurse-hours of patient care, or vaccinator time, can be calculated relatively easily, and the return on investment in health services can be measured in terms of the units of service provided.

The pioneering work of Dublin and Lotka, *The Money Value of a Man*, dates back to the 1920s, and subsequent students of the return on investment in health have pursued the problem with increasing statistical virtuosity. The common method of such studies is to use statistics of morbidity and mortality as the basis for calculating the wages foregone (including, at times, an imputed wage for housewife services) because of avoidable illness or death. These earnings are then viewed as the positive return on investment in programmes to prevent or cure the diseases causing absenteeism, disability, and death. Many studies also calculate the cost of treatment of the diseases, and add this to the estimated return on health investment on the basis that prevention or early treatment means subsequent medical-care costs forgone.

There are a number of criticisms of this approach. It has been argued that the existence of unemployment as a variable and unpredictable future quantity makes it impossible to obtain a valid present estimate of future wages lost. It is also evident that the calculations must be made for individual diseases, since the data on death and disability are available on this basis, with combined results depending on the aggregation of a large number of individual estimates which may introduce new errors.

Some attempts have also been made to calculate the value of the goods and services produced by investment in health, in the sense of production losses avoided by prevention or treatment of disease in the labour force. These studies have usually been very limited in nature, for it is only in exceptional circumstances that a clear and direct relationship between disease and economic activity can be established. Malaria has been a favourite subject for such studies, since successful malaria programmes are usually marked by a rapid and dramatic decrease in the incidence of the disease that can often be correlated successfully with statistics of agricultural production in single-crop cultivation, such as sugar cane, which depends heavily on manual labour with clear-cut seasonal requirements. The resulting estimates of economic loss from disease, however crude,

have the advantage of being directly comparable in money terms with the anticipated return from alternative uses of the funds proposed to be invested in health. Comparisons of the alternative return on investment (known to economists as 'opportunity cost') provide a key measure of the economic desirability of different activities.

In contrast to the rough but economically important estimates of return to health investment when the target is either health or the gains in production attributable to health, the statistically more feasible and accurate calculation of returns in units of service, when the target is set in service terms, cannot be used for economic comparisons of the yield on investment. In addition, some classes of investment in health itself do not provide a calculable economic return: medical care of the aged, for example, responds to a moral rather than an economic imperative. As noted earlier, much of the demand for medical care services is related to the chronic and degenerative diseases of old age. In such cases a true 'cure' can hardly be said to exist and, as in the case of cancer, is often arbitrarily defined as survival for a given number of years. Palliation is the more likely product of medical care of many older people, and complete cure, or rehabilitation in the sense of a return to productive economic life, is rare. In other cases, such as vaccination against smallpox in a country where the disease is not known to exist, the money value of protection against the possible importation of the disease cannot be calculated even if the persons protected are employed workers with known rates of pay.

From the viewpoint of the health planner, it is important to find measures to reconcile the moral imperative to prevent and treat disease in cases where there is no apparent economic return, with the estimated yield from investment in those areas of health activity where income forgone because of illness and death, and the cost of treatment avoided by preventive activities, can in fact be calculated. Neither economic nor moral criteria alone will suffice, and the reconciliation of the two is usually a matter of political compromise at the decision-making level.

Applications of Cost–Benefit Analysis in Health Planning

Since estimates of the economic return on investment in health are commonly related to individual diseases, the problem of aggregating the results into some measure of the return on investment in 'total health' runs the risk of compounding errors. When the yield on investment in health (assuming that it can be estimated) is to be compared with the alternative yield from investing the same money in schools, roads, or factories it is virtually impossible to arrive at a satisfactory calculation of 'opportunity cost' because the outputs of the different activities are not commensurable (e.g. lives saved, graduates from secondary schools, miles of road, pairs of shoes). Even when the outputs are all expressed in money terms, there are cases where an 'educated guess' must be used when market prices are not available, and there is no assurance that the available market-price quotations for different goods and services reflect the value of the relative contribution of each activity to society; it is more likely that they reflect what consumers are disposed to pay at a given time and place. In addition, any major health planning decision may alter prices, wage levels, and other elements entering into the original calculation if its impact is sufficiently great on the economy as a whole.

Within the health sector the problem of common measures of output is somewhat more manageable, even if some difficulty remains in comparing death deferred by organ transplant with sickness or death avoided by vaccination, health restored by chemotherapy of tuberculosis, or pain and anxiety relieved by active therapy in terminal cancer. Many planning decisions, however, involve deciding among alternative ways to reach the *same* goal. Should X-rays or examination of sputum be made standard in tuberculosis case-finding? Should chemotherapy or house spraying with insecticide be the method of choice in a given malaria situation? In such comparisons the benefits are clearly measurable in common units, and the decision will relate to the output (benefit) of the proposed methods and their relative cost. A useful technique in such cases is that known as cost–benefit analysis.

Cost–benefit analysis was first applied to estimates of the utility of public works about the middle of the nineteenth century, and is still quite popular in that field. More recently it has been extended to other areas of economic activity, including the planning of health services at the project level. The distinguishing characteristic of cost–benefit analysis is not the comparison of costs and benefits at a given moment but rather the present comparison of a stream of anticipated future benefits and costs. To take the most common example encountered in practice, when a water or sewer system is installed in a community it is anticipated that the short-run investment of capital will bring about long-run returns over succeeding years. Yet before one investment project is chosen above another it is necessary to anticipate those returns and compute the present value of the expected future benefit to compare with the present cost of the proposed investment and the present value of future operating costs.

This is done by means of the compound-interest formula, which permits economists to calculate the 'discounted present value' of future benefits and costs at any given rate of interest. In the conventional business calculation the future value of a sum of money P invested at interest rate r for a period of t years is $P(1 + r)^t$.[1] This means that the present value of future benefits is, other things being equal, inversely related to the rate of interest. Common sense bears this out, for when the rate of interest is low (i.e. when capital is cheap) an investment promising given benefits is more attractive than when the rate of interest is high (i.e. when it costs more to obtain the capital that promises the same benefits).

It happens in practice that the interest rate does act as a principal determining factor when the attractiveness is measured by the relation between present costs and future benefits. Just as an individual may hesitate to purchase a house when mortgage interest rates are high, so a community may hesitate to undertake the construction of a water system or a hospital or other major public works under similar circumstances.

The question of the choice of interest rate for cost–benefit

calculations is of particular interest to economists because it has not been solved satisfactorily and is still a matter of debate. At any given time several rates of interest may be quoted in capital markets—the rates of interest on local authority and national government bonds will seldom be the same; higher rates will be charged for consumer credit or high-risk loans than for other credit. Exactly as in the case of goods and services, it is not certain to what degree the market price of money (the rate of interest) reflects a social valuation of the future return from present investment, and to what degree a given rate of interest mainly reflects businessmen's and bankers' short-term expectations of the relative profitability of different kinds of investment and lending.

In terms of the priority-setting formula $P = f(M, I, V, C)$ cost–benefit analysis can be viewed as the examination of the C and V terms (perhaps, ideally, of all four terms) over time, with emphasis on the calculation of a present value for future reduction in M (evidently dependent on V) that can be compared with the investment term C. As in the priority formula, the numerical results must be subject to the same cautious interpretation, and the same reservations must be made with respect to the adequacy of the statistical indicators to provide a precise reflection of social valuations.

Finally, it should be noted that some future benefits of health services cannot be given a present value, since they cannot be identified until they occur. The long-run benefits accruing from a healthier population (ranging from higher potential productiveness to intangibles such as a more satisfying life) are mainly a matter of conjecture at present, and the effect of certain non-specific inputs, such as health education of the public, is also hard to put in numerical terms.

Budgeting and Cost-effectiveness Analysis

While the principal use of cost–benefit analysis is in long-run investment planning, the related concept of cost-effectiveness is often used in planning current activities. The emphasis in both long-run and general health planning is on the yield from investment in health; in short-run operational planning, particularly at the level of the local project or service unit, the general priorities and programme choices are taken as given, and the focus is on efficient fulfilling of planned tasks. Cost-effectiveness analysis is simply a way of making budget decisions with the goal of maximizing the delivery of service and minimizing cost by making the best choice among alternative ways of reaching planned targets.

Since one of the basic economic decisions in planning health programmes is the choice among alternatives, models can be constructed to facilitate analysis by relating inputs with each other and with outputs. Some possibilities are illustrated in FIGURE 106A.

The cost model calculates the cost of an alternative by applying cost–estimating equations to specified resources and their rates of use. The specifications stem from the design of a particular system to deliver the services in question. The relationship among quantities of resources, their use, and the organization of the delivery system can be termed an organization-and-systems model. A third possible model is concerned with the relationship between a delivery system and its output of services—this is the effectiveness model. Finally, when the cost model is related to the effectiveness model, the

---

[1] In numerical terms, \$100 invested at present at 6 per cent. interest compounded annually will be worth $100(1·06)^{10}$ after 10 years, or \$179. If it is *anticipated* that \$179 will result at 6 per cent. interest after 10 years, then the present value of that future benefit is held to be \$100. It is also clear from the formula that, in order to have \$179 at a higher rate of interest such as 10 per cent. at the end of 10 years, a smaller initial investment is required, and at a lower rate of interest a higher initial investment is required.

well-known cost–effectiveness model results. Programme choices are commonly based on cost–effectiveness criteria.

The budget is an essential instrument at the project or operating level because it provides a two-way flow of information for planning purposes. The budget request or submission from the project or service unit to the next higher authority (be it a local governing body or the next unit in a bureaucratic chain of command) embodies the ideas of the operating unit

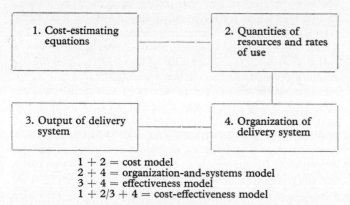

1 + 2 = cost model
2 + 4 = organization-and-systems model
3 + 4 = effectiveness model
1 + 2/3 + 4 = cost-effectiveness model

FIG. 106A. Possible models for programme planning.

as to how it conceives its tasks and how it plans to go about them. The budget submission may be technically justified in every detail, or experience with the reviewing authority may lead to deliberate over-estimates (in the hope that anticipated cuts will leave adequate resources for operation) or under-estimates (based on a realistic assessment of the limited resources likely to be provided). The process of budget review and approval involves evaluation of the submission, and also serves to communicate the constraints on funding and human resources at the next higher level and the priority decisions made at that level for the allocation of funds and man-power to operating units.

Simplistic as it may sound, experience in a number of countries has shown that it is possible to plan activities that are not realized for lack of budgetary provision, as well as to maintain activities that are not included in current plans or are scheduled by the planners for de-emphasis or termination, simply because a concurrent change from previous budgetary allocations is not made by the financial authorities.

Aside from its use as an instrument of financial accountability and control, the budget ideally should be the monetary expression of the activities embodied in the health services plan. The difficulties in achieving this goal are administrative rather than economic in nature. For example, common sense indicates that the budget should refer to the same time period as the plan. In point of fact, however, budgets are usually established on a yearly basis, and seldom more than one or two years ahead, while plans may be drawn up to cover five- or ten-year periods. Clearly, a ten-year plan should involve at least a gross estimate of the ten-year operating and investment budget, while if the annual budget is the real operating instrument of the health service, then the plan of activities must also have a yearly component corresponding to the budget year.

There is also some conflict between the budget as the first step in an accounting process whose basic goal is the control

over disbursement of funds and the budget viewed as the grant of money that enables a series of planned programme activities to be undertaken. From the viewpoint of accounting control, the budget clearly has to be broken down into items that are classified in the same way as expenditures—wages and salaries, drugs, medical supplies, office supplies, etc.—even though any of these categories of expenditure may be shared among a number of different planned activities. The salary of the director of a health service, for example, it attributable in part to direction of each activity the service undertakes.

The conventional budget for control of disbursement is referred to as a 'line item budget' because each line in the budget relates to an item of expenditure, while budgets where the line items are regrouped so as to show expenditures for different planned activities are commonly referred to as 'programme budgets', 'activity budgets', or (when the emphasis is on evaluation) 'performance budgets'. The planning–programming–budgeting system (abbreviated to PPB or PPBS in different English-speaking countries) is perhaps the most popular new approach. It was made general at the Federal level in the United States in 1965 after successful experience in programming military activities, was subsequently adopted in Canada, and by 1971 had been adopted for a number of government activities in the United Kingdom as well. In brief, the PPB system combines the setting of planned priorities with the budgeting of the activities designed to achieve the plan targets. The basic criterion for choice among operating programmes is a cost–effectiveness comparison [see FIG. 106A].

In contradistinction to the cost–benefit technique of estimating the discounted present value of future streams of costs and benefits, cost–effectiveness models typically involve a shorter-term comparison. Classic cost–benefit analysis is usually limited to projects with long-term aspects and a major investment component, but the cost–effectiveness approach is capable of wider application. The technique has been applied to road accidents, heart disease, cancer, and stroke in the United States, but these efforts have emphasized benefits (reduction of treatment cost and of losses in earnings) rather than programme effectiveness. The principal impediment to measuring the effectiveness of health programmes in economic terms remains the difficulty of arriving at medical consensus on the effect of such programmes on health.

Operational Research and Operations Research

Budget and cost-effectiveness studies differ from the health planning techniques discussed earlier in their applications to local operating units and in their emphasis on managerial efficiency once priority decisions and major sectoral allocations of resources have taken place at higher levels. To conclude the discussion of economic aspects of health planning, mention must be made of two general classes of research that can be applied at the project or operating unit level to improve managerial efficiency. While the term 'operational research' is sometimes used for the general descriptive and analytic study of operations, in the United Kingdom it has the more specific meaning of the mathematical analysis of activities. In North America the mathematical field of study is known as 'operations research'.

One of the important goals of operational research is the study of efficient utilization of resources, and in this connexion health services can borrow from the economic analysis of the individual business firm the important distinction between fixed and variable cost. Fixed costs are those which, up to the limit of capacity, do not change with the volume of service provided, while variable costs change with the volume of activity. An illustration of different kinds of cost is given for a hypothetical X-ray unit in FIGURE 106B.

The costs are assumed to be of three kinds. The cost of the floor space and equipment is $100,000, charged off at $50 per day over an expected working life of 2,000 days. This is fixed cost in the day under consideration. The cost of X-ray film and electricity is assumed to be $1 per exposure. This is

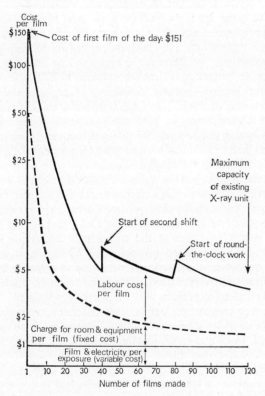

FIG. 106B. Fixed, variable, and total costs per film in a hypothetical X-ray unit.

variable cost. The payroll is assumed to be $100 per shift. This is a fixed cost per shift, but three variations can occur, since the X-ray unit may be operated for one shift, for two shifts, or around the clock. It is assumed that forty films can be made per shift. The base line of FIGURE 75 shows the $1 cost which is constant for any number of exposures. The broken line shows the room and equipment charge, which is $50 per exposure if only one film is made, and falls continuously to $0·42 per exposure when the service is fully operated around the clock and 120 films are made. The uppermost line shows the total cost per exposure, falling within each shift, rising when the second and third shifts are underutilized, and reaching a minimum at full round-the-clock operation. At this point further expansion of service is not possible without the introduction of a second X-ray unit. If the expansion of the floor space and addition of a second machine enable the same or a slightly increased number of technicians to handle the volume of service lower costs will result from full use of the expanded

unit, and these are referred to as economies of scale. The choice of scale of operations follows the same minimum-cost criterion as does the determination of the most economic operating point within the original unit.

The higher the proportion of fixed to variable costs, the greater will be the economies that can be realized from full utilization. Obviously, the cost of leaving a thousand-bed hospital half empty would be greater than the cost incurred by the same degree of underutilization of a rural health post staffed by a single nurse. In either case, however, full utilization is not necessarily within the power of the service unit to achieve. Careful study of anticipated demand for service is essential in determining the size of the unit that can achieve full utilization, and the ideal point is seldom reached. Experience has shown that the introduction of new health facilities stimulates demand because of their education and demonstration effect. Add to this the unpredictable future course of population size, structure, and causes of sickness and death, and it is clear that frequent reappraisals of demand and readjustments of service plans may be required. Nevertheless, the closer the scale and organization of services approach the optimum (whether by good planning, efficient management, or sheer luck), the greater will be the economies realized.

There is, however, an upper limit to utilization. In the case of physician services, quality may possibly be unimpaired, as the average time spent per patient is reduced from 1 hour to 20 minutes as demand increases. But if utilization is so great that the physician cannot spend more than 5 minutes per patient—as has occurred in some instances—even the lower cost per patient attended will not justify the resulting dilution in quality of service. A growing number of countries are studying indices of quality as concern with the cost of medical care increases, and there is every hope that practicable indices will be developed to aid health planners in the future.

Operations research also holds the promise for more efficient planning as mathematical techniques of decision-making are refined and the growing availability of computers makes it possible to achieve rapid solutions of realistic models with large numbers of variables.

Many of the techniques once known only to professional mathematicians and statisticians were introduced into general postgraduate instruction in administration and the social sciences in recent decades, and by the 1970s were becoming more common in undergraduate work as well. While it is impossible to cover the entire field here, some highlights can be pointed out.

Bayesian probability. Conventional statistical studies, when they involve the likelihood of an event occurring, are based on what is commonly termed Neyman–Pearson probability. It is assumed that past events have no influence on future events— that the probability of an event occurring is not affected by whether or not it has occurred before. A growing number of statisticians are finding use for methods based on Bayes' Theorem which enable them to calculate prior probability (i.e. of an event occurring for the first time) and posterior probability (i.e. of an event occurring *again*). This has numerous applications in the field of health—one has only to think of the difference between the risk of an accident in the abstract and the risk of an accident-prone individual!

Simulation. Health service planning is growing increasingly sophisticated through the application of simulation techniques to enable the planner to forecast the likely occurrence of events that tend to occur at random. Examples would be forecasting the optimum staff and facilities for a hospital emergency or maternity service where the arrival of patients can be simulated on a random basis. Incidentally, the reader is urged to remember that, when random processes are at work, the term *stochastic process* is commonly used in the technical literature.

Simulation methods include the Monte Carlo method (in which conceivably the planner could use a roulette table if one were available!) and various mathematical functions that can be used to generate random series under different assumptions and limitations. This type of simulation has also proved important for the analysis of waiting lists in terms of queueing theory.

Considerable use has been made in health planning in the United States of the *Markoff process* which simplifies computation by assuming that only one past state (the immediately preceding state) affects the probability of a subsequent change of state. This provides a handy analytic framework when a population can be classified into discrete states of health care (e.g. out of the system, out-patient care, acute hospital, chronic care, etc.) and the probabilities of moving from one state into another provide a guide to the services that will be needed in the future.

Linear programming is probably the most widely applied method of mathematical problem-solving. Essentially, it is the study of how to juggle a number of (often interrelated) variables simultaneously in the search for an optimum solution. While the sets of simultaneous relationships may look bewildering to the casual reader, particularly since they are usually set out in an algebraic language known as matrix notation, reference to any good introductory algebra textbook and working out a few of the basic matrix exercises should make the mathematics quite comprehensible even to a reader who would hesitate to perform the calculations himself.

Finally, the importance of *multiple regression* and *multiple correlation* should be recognized. Much of the econometric research in health is devoted to the search for cause-and-effect relationships. For example, is a change in the demand for hospital beds related to (or caused by) changes in one or more of the patterns of morbidity, supply of doctors, supply of nurses, supply of patients, personal or national income, ratio of medical specialists to general practitioners, or some other variables? The techniques used to answer this question are an extension of the simple two-variable correlation and regression analysis that is part of every basic course in elementary statistics.

Because of the number of variables, and the interactions among them, the mathematics can get rather involved, but most of the literature in this field can be successfully 'followed with the finger' once the reader has got the knack of simultaneous equations and matrix notation as noted above, and once the jargon of endogenous (dependent) and exogenous (independent, predetermined) variables is understood.

Modern mathematics has run through a number of alphabets in the search for ever more symbols for its condensed speech, and the decision-making aids of the Programme Evaluation Review Technique (PERT) and deceptively simple-looking diagrams used in Critical Path analysis (for the scheduling of operations) are merely the shorthand representation of an underlying body of complex algebra. Descriptive and common-sense operational research can, and probably should, be undertaken by health authorities at all levels of planning, but the mathematics of operations research often require the services of specialized consultants. Once the mathematical operations have been performed, however, operations research loses much of its mystery—it is still concerned with problems like determining the optimum location of an institution with respect to its service area, the optimum size and organization for given anticipated levels of demand, or the flow of staff, supplies, and patients within a building.

Conclusion

The basic function of economics is to point out how to economize—how to get the greatest output per unit of input. This essentially managerial function at the local project or operating level requires the modern tools of operational and operations research. At higher levels the process of economizing involves comparing returns from alternative projects within the health sector, and deciding the relative priorities of health and other activities. For the health planner, economics is primarily a supporting service—providing grounds for decision at each level, and searching for data to point up the complex relationships and issues that sometimes arise. While it is far easier for most health planners to master the principles of economics (or at least the basic vocabulary) than it is to master the mathematics required for operations research, it is often helpful to consult specialists in both fields as part of the decision-making process. The following annotated list is provided as a guide to further reading for students and practitioners of public health who wish to familiarize themselves with economics, and for health planners in need of reference material on the subject.

FURTHER READING

General Economics

The 'most popular' textbook is P. W. Samuelson, *Economics*, New York, various editions. The quotation defining economics appears on p. 5 of the Canadian edition of the same title by P. W. Samuelson and A. Scott (Toronto, 1966).

For those with a historical bent, the Victorian textbook that has influenced many economists still alive and working is Alfred Marshall's *Principles of Economics*, London, various editions from 1890 to 1920 and reprintings to 1930.

A succinct statement of the liberal position that can be found in many health libraries is the speech by Barbara Ward 'Development: The Irreversible Revolution' published in *Manpower for the World's Health*, Association of American Medical Colleges, 1966. The book also provides useful reference material on the general problem of health man-power, and is available in soft covers as a Supplement to the September 1966 issue of the *Journal of Medical Education*.

While Karl Marx' *Capital* is available in English, much contemporary Marxist–Leninist literature has not been translated. A representative selection of modern Soviet economic thought is found in N. M. Oznobina, ed., *Ocherki po sovremmenoy i zarubezhnoy ekonomike*, Vol. I, State Plan Publishing House, Moscow, 1960. An extremely condensed summary in English is given in the review of this book by A. P. Ruderman on pp. 217–18 of the *American Economic Review*, March 1962.

The liberal German position that gave rise to the felicitous terms 'market economy' and 'command economy' is Walter Eucken's. The terms as found in his *Grundlagen der National-ökonomie*, 5th revised edition, Godesberg, 1947, are *Verkehrswirtschaft* and *Zentralgeleitete Wirtschaft*. An English translation by T. W. Hutchison was published as *The Foundations of Economics: History and Theory in the Analysis of Economic Reality*, London, 1950.

Other general texts are Cooper, R. A. (1971) *Statistical Models of Economic Relationships*, London, H.M.S.O., and Wonnacott, R. J. and Wonnacott, T. H. (1970) *Econometrics*, London.

Health Economics

A succinct summary of the 'vicious circle' approach with commentary by a specialist in economic development is the exchange between C. E. A. Winslow and Gunnar Myrdal at the Fifth World Health Assembly, reported in the *Chronicle* of the World Health Organization, August 1952.

The celebrated pioneer attempt of Selma Mushkin, 'Toward a definition of health economics', is to be found in *Public Health Reports*, September 1958.

A comprehensive review of the earlier literature, with emphasis on the market orientation, is provided by H. Klarman in *The Economics of Health*, Columbia University Press, 1965.

The issues that concern health economics in a command economy are outlined in articles by Abel-Smith, B. (1967) An international study of health expenditure and its relevance for health planning, *Wld Hlth Org. Publ. Hlth Pap.*, No. 32. Abel-Smith, B. (1973) Cost effectiveness and cost benefit in cholera control, *Wld Hlth Org. Chron.*, **27**, 407.

Some of the relationships between health services and economic planning are outlined in A. P. Ruderman, 'The epidemiologist's place in planning economic development', *Public Health Reports*, July 1966.

Some examples of modern econometrics will be found in *Empirical Studies in Health Economics*, edited by H. Klarman, Johns Hopkins University Press, 1970. An article that sets out much of the mathematical technique and verbal jargon in lucid English for the benefit of the non-mathematical reader is 'An aggregate planning model of the health care sector' by M. S. Feldstein in *Medical Care*, November–December 1967.

For an account of cost benefit analysis in the planning of Immunization Programmes, see Cvejetanović, B. (1973) Immunization programmes, *Wld Hlth Org. Chron.*, **27**, 66.

Other useful works include Black, H. D. (1973) Economics and medicos, *Med. J. Aust.*, **2**, 101. Helt, E. M. (1973) Economic determinism: a model of the political economy of medical care, *Int. J. Hlth Serv.*, **3**, 475. Malenbaum, W. (1973) Health and economic expansion in poor countries, *Int. J. Hlth Serv.*, **3**, 161. See also World Health Organization, Regional Office for Europe (1971) Report of a seminar on Health Operations Research, Copenhagen. Walsh, H. G. and Williams, Alan (1969) *Current Issues in Cost-Benefit Analysis*, London, H.M.S.O. Wright,

W. M. (1972) Economic impact on schistosomiasis, *Bull. Wld Hlth Org.*, **47**, 559. Young, K. (1973) Value for money in the health services, *Brit. med. J.*, **1**, 165. World Health Organization (1974) Modern management methods and the organization of health services, *Wld Hlth Org. Pap.*, No. 55.

Health Planning

A general review of health planning is provided in *World Health Organization Technical Report Series*, No. 350, *National Health Planning in Developing Countries*, 1967.

The Latin American position is outlined in *Health Planning: Problems of Concept and Method*, Pan American Health Organization, Washington, 1965.

The priority formula suggested for planning purposes in the U.S. Indian Service is taken from Michael, Spatafore, and Williams, 'A basic information system for health planning', *Public Health Reports*, January 1968.

The Soviet position is described by Popov, G. A. (1971) Principles of health planning in the U.S.S.R., *Wld Hlth Org. Pap.*, No. 43.

An interesting outline of mathematical considerations in elementary terms is given by H. A. Thomas, Jr., in 'The animal farm: a mathematical model for the discussion of social standards for control of the environment', *Quarterly Journal of Economics*, February 1963.

A comprehensive review of cost–benefit analysis, with a substantial section devoted to health, is 'Cost–benefit analysis: a survey', by A. R. Prest and R. Turvey, *Economic Journal*, December 1965.

A lucid introduction to the PPB system, with worked-out examples, is *Planning Programming Budgeting Guide*, revised edition, Government of Canada Treasury Board, Ottawa, September 1969.

Operations Research and Basic Mathematics

An excellent elementary introduction to operations research is Eric Duckworth, *A Guide to Operational Research*, second edition, London, 1964, despite the fact that Duckworth says 'operational' where this writer would have said 'operations'.

A simple discussion of many relevant mathematical techniques is found in F. P. Fowler and E. W. Sandberg, *Basic Mathematics for Administration*, New York, 1962. Almost any standard algebra will also prove helpful, and the author would like to thank his son William for pointing out that the basic mathematics is thoroughly covered in Coleman, del Grande, Duff, Egsgard, and Kirby, *Algebra 13*, Toronto, 1966, a standard Ontario high-school text.

For what can be done with Markoff processes, see V. Navarro, R. Parker, and K. L. White, 'A stochastic and deterministic model of medical care utilization', *Health Services Research*, Winter, 1970.

Many of the basic methods and principles of operations research are described in simple though not always non-mathematical language by Tor Dahl in 'Operations research on health care in Chile: An experiment', *International Journal of Health Services*, August 1971.

43

SYSTEMS OF MEDICAL CARE

Some International Comparisons

R. F. BRIDGMAN

It is agreed, among a growing number of health planners, that the concept of medical care covers the whole range of activities from personal preventive health measures to physical rehabilitation, with traditional curative medicine also included as an integral part.

Although this concept widely prevails, yet many countries still do not, in practice, accept this wide definition. At the end of the last century the dualist system was adopted for technical, administrative, and traditional reasons in technologically advanced countries. Curative medical institutions existed for centuries and retained their autonomy whatever their status, public or private. Hygiene and prevention developed independently, and, because they were designed for the community, became the responsibility of the public authorities.

Despite the fact that nowadays practitioners and hospitals play a greater role than previously in the early recognition of pathological disorders among individuals, this dualist system has prevailed in the health organization of most of the western countries. In socialist countries curative medicine and personal health care are now closely integrated. Here one comes across the first cleavage which sometimes makes comparison between the two main systems of medical care difficult.

However, an analysis which restricted itself to a single comparison between western and eastern countries would completely miss the divergences between the different cultural patterns.

Moreover, the developing countries deserve full consideration. This large group, sometimes called the Third World, is, in itself, very heterogeneous. A common factor such as economic underdevelopment and its corollary, a low income *per capita*, hides, in fact, profound social and cultural differences. For our purpose, one may distinguish, on the one hand, between those who some centuries ago were on virgin soil on which the pattern of Western cultures were stamped and, on the other, those who were able to remain relatively independent, at least culturally, because they achieved a high level of development in arts, literature, philosophy, and science before the nineteenth century. They all adopted Western technology because it was based on scientific grounds. However, the first group passively received a superstructure which could not fully develop. In the vacuum between the main Westernized urban centres, the archaic network of rural witches, healers, and medicine men remained, intermingled with mobile health teams and missionary institutions, which resulted in an extremely complicated situation.

The second group, often called the 'Peoples of the Book', had a long tradition of public administration, a network of social services, and a large number of learned physicians practising traditional pre-scientific medicine derived from Graeco-Arabic, Ayurvedic, or Chinese written sources which compared favourably with Western medicine up to the eighteenth century.

In order to take into consideration the different patterns of medical care and to clarify this *exposé*, it is proposed to divide the whole spectrum of medical-care services into two groups, i.e. ambulatory and domiciliary care, on the one hand, and in-patient hospital care, on the other.

In each of the two groups organizational problems are raised, i.e. structure, legislation, administration and management, planning, financing, and staffing. We shall briefly review the situation prevailing for each of these groups in:

1. Countries of western continental Europe (Scandinavia excluded) and Latin America.
2. Northern American countries.
3. Scandinavia and British countries (including Australia, New Zealand, South Africa, and Canada).
4. Socialist countries.
5. Developing countries whose patterns were introduced by Western powers.
6. Developing countries where genuine historical and cultural patterns are still in force.

AMBULATORY AND DOMICILIARY PERSONAL MEDICAL CARE

The corresponding services endeavour to meet the needs of the great majority of patients. In the United States the number of medical consultations *per capita* per year is approximately 4, ranging from 2·8 for the age group 5–14 years, to 7·3 for people over 75. The difference between urban and rural populations is approximately 20 per cent. In Sweden the number of home visits, plus consultations at a physician's surgery, is about 2 *per capita* per year, to which should be added 1 visit to a hospital out-patient department.

In the U.S.S.R. each urban citizen has 9·8 yearly contacts with doctors, while in rural areas this average varies between 5·6 and 9. However, these numbers include all contacts for both curative and preventive cases, and the latter are particularly numerous in the case of children and in vulnerable groups, such as women and industrial workers. Moreover, care given by feldshers or medical assistants is not included in the statistics related to rural populations. In towns feldshers do not participate in curative medicine. In Yugoslavia the number of contacts per head per year varies between 5 in rural areas to more than 12 in towns, but, here also, most of the preventive personal contacts are included. In France, in 1962, the number of annual contacts for curative measures was 3·70 *per capita* in the Centre de Recherche et de Documentation sur la Consommation survey, including X-ray examinations. In the preliminary study undertaken by the International Collaborative Study of Medical Care Utilization team in Great Britain, the United States, and Yugoslavia the number of contacts was between 5·2 and 6·0 for the three countries, regardless of large differences in doctor/population ratio and standards of living.

These numbers are all-inclusive. However, if one considers the number of cases or that of 'first contacts' the total is obviously much lower. In the U.S.S.R. 1·1 first consultations *per capita* per year are registered, in Sweden 0·38.

If one compares these rates with hospital in-patient rates there are, in the U.S.S.R., 19·5 per cent. patients consulting for the first time in the year, who are admitted to hospital, thus the hospital admission rate is 0·2 *per capita* per year. There are therefore 45 times more patients treated ambulatorily and at home than those admitted to hospitals. In the United States, where the hospital admission rate is 0·14, the ratio is 28 to 1, and in France, 46 to 1. Therefore the medical profession devotes most of its activity to ambulatory and home care expressed in working hours.

However, in financial terms this proportion is completely different because of the very high cost of hospital care. Running expenses of hospital care, ambulatory care, collective health, and teaching and research are summarized from the recent study by Abel-Smith (1967).

TABLE 119

Countries	Cost of personal health cure		Public health services, per cent.	Teaching and research, per cent.
	Hospital, per cent.	Home and ambulatory, per cent.		
Austria . .	43·7	52·9	2·07	1·5
Canada . .	42·7	54·5	1·0	1·8
Czechoslovakia	47·75	43·6	2·4	6·3
Ceylon . .	50·0	43·9	4·5	1·7
Finland. .	59·9	35·9	2·5	1·7
France★ .	40·93	55·8	1·7	1·6
Israel . .	45·71	50·0	1·6	2·7
Poland . .	39·92	53·2	2·8	4·1
Sweden. .	52·9	42·4	1·2	3·5
U.K. . .	51·79	44·3	1·9	2·1
U.S.A. . .	38·26	56·9	0·3	4·6
Yugoslavia .	43·28	49·9	3·9	3·0

★ Amortization included.

The total of ambulatory medical services expenditure is approximately equal to 50 per cent. of total health expenditure. It should be noted that pharmaceutical expenses are included both in hospital and ambulatory care costs.

The structure of the medical profession varies widely throughout the world. In the Western world its ethics and its special position within the socio-economic infrastructure is often the cause of discussion about which the public and politicians are often fully aware. However, while fighting for principles which, from their own point of view, protect the quality of the service rendered, professional bodies must adapt themselves to scientific and social evolution. In countries where private doctors do not participate in hospital and health centre work they tend to organize their work through the

group-practice concept and to make up physician and specialist teams. The border line between private liberal practice and institutional practice is therefore somewhat blurred.

European Countries, Continental Western Countries (Excluding Scandinavia), and Latin America

The medical profession has retained its liberal character inherited from the past. This is laid down in a charter composed of four principles:

Confidentiality
Freedom of prescription
Freedom of choice for the patient and the doctor
Direct payment of fee per service

However, it is clear that such principles must be adjusted, since the constitution adopted by the people affirms their right to health protection and promotion. The public authorities who have to implement the constitution have the power to intervene in problems of organization of medical care. Actually, for the past fifty years, the direct relationship between doctor and patient has been distorted either for technical reasons (referral to specialist or institutions), or for financial considerations (social security), or for control (statistics, norms, and technical requirements). Professional unions are studying these problems thoroughly with the institutions concerned and look forward to the organization of group practices as a solution.

In France, Belgium, and Switzerland the physician receives his fees direct from the patient. The patient is partially reimbursed by the social security fund to which he is affiliated. A constant tension exists between the medical profession, social-security organizations, and patients as far as the amount deductible and the ceiling value of the fees are concerned.

In Federal Germany, for practically the entire population, in Italy and in Spain, for insured persons and their dependants, health insurance funds pay the whole or part of the medical fees to the physician. Pharmacists and some private nursing homes have already accepted this system in France.

In western continental Europe the medical profession is bound to accept closer co-operation with public health institutions because of progress in medicine which improves more and more with the use of specialized equipment and skilled personnel attached to hospitals. As a corollary, most of the specialists attached to hospitals are fully employed. This is realized in France, where teaching and hospital centres and many other important hospitals already have full-time staff.

In these countries the number and distribution of doctors and their training arouse passionate discussions. The number of population per physician varies from 560 in Austria to 1,400 in Finland, demonstrating that the correlation between the number of physicians and the level of health is somewhat confused.

Generally speaking, the dualist pattern of health organization, curative and preventive medicine being run separately, prevails in western continental Europe. Preventive measures and public hygiene are the responsibility of local governments (communes or counties and county boroughs). Maternal and child health and tuberculosis programmes are carried out by salaried personnel, but the medical profession treat their patients, and it is very difficult to know what is the total amount of maternal and child health work done. Morbidity statistics are poor. Specialization complicates the problem. For instance, the number of population contacts with doctors is well known through the social-security-scheme registration, but the actual number of cases and the morbidity pattern remain largely obscure.

Even the number of registered specialists gives no clue to differential morbidity, because, if one considers heart diseases, the proportion of cases treated by cardiologists as compared to those examined by general practitioners cannot be ascertained.

In any case, social-security schemes play a considerable role in making medical care available to all salaried personnel, wage-earners, and their dependants, i.e. 70–95 per cent. of the population. No doubt they have contributed to the improvement in the health situation.

However, the health situation is not what it should be considering the number of medical and allied professions and their qualifications, the importance of their equipment and the scope of social and welfare services. The infant mortality rate, the slow decrease in tuberculosis, the number of mental disorders, and the average life expectancy have not been adequately expressed in terms of economics; the output of health measures is not for the best and needs improving. Efforts should be made to increase the efficiency of the health system.

Latin American countries present a special case. Medical care services followed closely on the conquest by the Spanish and Portuguese. Since the sixteenth century they so completely absorbed the socio-cultural pattern of their conquerors that they should be studied with the Latin European countries, even if they are often classified among the developing countries on the sole basis of their low economic level. In this subcontinent there are nearly a hundred medical schools, and most of the countries are developing social-security schemes which considerably assist the development of medical care services. Of course, the problems are many, and two of the most important are the co-ordination between social-security schemes and health services and the obsolescence of hospital administration. Chile is the most organized from that point of view.

In Latin America there were, in 1960, about 5·5 doctors for 10,000 people and in four countries the rate was less than 3. However, 10 per cent. were private practitioners, while among the 90 per cent. who were theoretically engaged in public health work only a quarter were actually employed full time. As a whole, 65 per cent. of the registered doctors divided their time, often very irregularly, between public functions and more remunerative activities (Roemer, 1963).

North American Countries

In the United States and Canada (at least in some provinces) free enterprise is a dogma and the medical profession accepts no encroachment from public authorities on its liberal character. Hence the suspicion, commonly held in America, that European medicine is largely 'socialized', which is only partly true. This opinion is explainable if one considers that the technical, financial, and administrative 'screens' we referred to above are mainly in the hands of private organizations in America. The most sophisticated specialized services are in private hospitals. Most of the best laboratories are in private universities. Health insurance companies are private. The ab-

sence of governmental control is not an obstacle in a streamlined organization of medical care because of the strength of private bodies, such as the American Medical Association, the American College of Surgeons, the American College of Physicians, and the American Hospital Association. Such bodies are, in fact, invested by the government with powers of control in ethical problems, in technical requirements for equipment and staffing (Joint Accreditation Committee), and quality of medical care (medical audit systems). Such powers are exercised without weakness or complacency.

The medical profession participates very widely in hospital and community centre activities, and it is the rule that the great majority of doctors, in a given town, are on the private hospital panel. A striking factor is the increasing proportion of specialists which involves 85 per cent. of all registered physicians. The traditional family doctor is on his way out, and this is a major concern which leads to the contemplation of specialization in general practice or family medical care as well. In accordance with this trend, all doctors would become specialists. As far as ambulatory care is concerned, physicians have organized themselves into group practices, sometimes in conjunction with other professional groups (Health Insurance Plan of Greater New York). The vast extension of private life insurance companies has facilitated the multiplication of periodic 'check-ups'. The cost of these check-ups is such that it rates second or third in the scale of household health expenditure, and this represents an increase of income for medical and allied professions. From that point of view the active approach of the liberal medical profession has been a great contribution in prevention of complications and disabling diseases.

However, some shadows still remain on the horizon. The more depressed social classes do not receive such comprehensive medical care as the majority of the population. The numerous health insurance schemes cover approximately three-quarters of the population, but this coverage sometimes remains very incomplete. Most of the contracts offer satisfactory reimbursement of cost for acute diseases only. In 1961 only 32 per cent. of ambulatory and home medical care expenditure was reimbursed by health insurance schemes, as opposed to 63 per cent. for hospital care. It is now time that there should be free medical assistance schemes for the poor in practically all states. Moreover, certain low-income groups are considered as 'medically indigent' and are eligible for a few home-care programmes. However, the statistical returns are clear. The consumption of medical-care services by low-income groups is largely inferior to that of the middle- and high-income groups.

TABLE 120

Income per household	Medical expenditure per household 1957/58 (subscriptions to health insurance included)
Less than $2,000 .	165
$2,000–3,499 . .	226
$3,500–4,999 . .	287
$5,000–7,499 . .	336
More than $7,500 .	411
Average . .	294 (of which $58 for health insurance subscription)

The same facts are observed for the coloured group as shown below:

Number of Contacts per capita per Year

Race	Age groups					
	0–4	5–14	15–24	25–44	45–64	65 and over
White .	6·6	3·9	4·7	5·0	5·5	6·9
Coloured	3·8	1·9	2·9	4·1	4·6	4·7

(Adapted from United States Public Health Service (1962) Health Economic Series, No. 1.)

However, the average duration of stay in hospital and the length of disability in low-income groups have increased, showing that, here, cases are often more serious than in high-income groups.

The high infantile morbidity and mortality rates of these groups distort the national average, which is still too high compared with other nations of the world, considering the potential of the American medical-care system.

The federal government spares no effort to wipe out these shadows on the social picture. Grants are given to community hospitals and to group practices. Technical requirements are issued, and finally Medicare, an ambitious programme, was voted to offer appropriate medical care to people of 65 years and over, through considerable grants in aid and direct reimbursement to institutions. Of more restricted scope, the medical assistance programme for the Indians was a considerable success.

British and Scandinavian Countries

These countries have adopted a very well-organized system of medical care. In Great Britain, under the National Health Service, all residents benefit from free medical care given by members of the medical and allied professions paid by the state in accordance with the size of their practice. This is the fee *per capita* system which has extended a practice introduced long ago for the benefit of low-income groups. Depending both on the actual government and the economic situation of the country, fees may or may not be charged on medical prescriptions. Administrative problems of the medical profession are dealt with by locally constituted Executive Committees representing both consumer and professional interests. The British Medical Association is one of the representative bodies which discusses the problems of organization with the Ministry of Health.

However, the National Health Service Act missed the opportunity of integrating the different components of the health sector. The service is made up of three branches, medical practice, hospitals, and public health. The machinery is different for the three branches, in that they are largely independent of one another. Co-ordination theoretically dependent on the Ministry of Health is, in fact, loose because of the decentralization of power to regional or local authorities. It is to be regretted that general practitioners remain apart from hospitals and health services. However, it is planned to offer premises within health centres to practitioners and to extend this field of activity, but this project has only been partially implemented, mainly in new towns.

The most noteworthy fact is the total separation of the state health budget coming from general taxation and of the cash benefits for loss of salary, invalidity, and old-age pensions and family allowances which all derive from national insurance. The latter is also a governmental agency, but its budget comes from the value of stamps purchased by salaried workers, wage earners, and voluntary subscribers.

In 1962 the Porritt report recommended changes in the National Health Service to bring about better integration of the three branches of the service: (1) hospitals; (2) general practice; (3) public health. In 1972 the British Government published a White Paper on reorganization of the service and a Steering Committee was set up to discuss management arrangements for the reorganized National Health Service. It listed six key features:

1. Health services should be integrated locally within areas on a district basis.
2. Clinicians should participate actively in management, particularly at operational level (seen as essential in a patient-orientated approach to health care).
3. To achieve integration multi-disciplinary management teams at each level are suggested.
4. Responsibilities must be clearly allocated and defined.
5. Decentralization of decision making is to be balanced against a need for national and regional strategic direction.
6. The arrangements should be flexible.

The new service will come into being on 1 April 1974. Area Health Authorities will be set up under the new Local Government Authorities and will develop a fully integrated service. Important elements will be the Area team of officers, the district management teams, and health care planning teams. The District Community Physician will be responsible for liaison between the various components and for preventive aspects.

Each district will have a Community Health Council which will represent consumer interests (consumerism). Much remains to be done before the final details of this plan are worked out, but it represents a bold effort to initiate change and it will be watched with interest by health planners the world over.

It is not surprising that the economists are worried about the rapid increase in the state health budget and plan to transfer financial responsibility for welfare measures and care for the elderly and mentally deficient to local authorities. Comparable systems exist in Australia, New Zealand, and some provinces in Canada.

Scandinavian countries also adopted comparable schemes, in so far as the majority of medical expenditure is covered by governmental agencies, but they established an economically sound compromise between Great Britain and western continental Europe. The majority of medical-care expenditure is covered partly by social-security funds, partly by the state, and partly by county and county borough authorities. Therefore the financial burden of medical care does not weigh exclusively on salaries, but is partly borne by general and local taxation. This avoids the production cost of goods increasing too heavily on account of the social-security budget, as in the Common

Market countries, where the whole social-security budget reaches 17–18 per cent. of the gross national product.

In Sweden domiciliary and ambulatory care are given by government-employed physicians, private practitioners, and salaried hospital doctors who are authorized to practise outside their hospital. Of a total of 7,631 active doctors in 1962, about 1,200 were private practitioners and specialists, most of them located in big cities. The latter tended to organize group practice teams. Most of the others were hospital doctors, the remainder being health officers. Provincial social-security funds reimburse 75 per cent. of a ceiling fee which is accepted by government-paid doctors but not by private physicians. In 1962 Swedish health insurance funds paid 1,262 million crowns, 189 million of which were for home and ambulatory medical care, 83 million for hospitals, 122 million for drugs, and 40 million for car mileage compensation. The rest was for cash benefits. Every citizen received 24·6 crowns per year from the funds for medical care, 15·9 for drugs, and only 10·8 for hospital care, which shows that a nominal share of hospital cost is borne by social security, local authorities devoting 80–90 per cent. of collected taxes in support of health care. Teaching-hospital costs are mainly borne by the central government, which also supports higher education.

In remote areas, especially in the sparsely populated northern districts, medical care is given by medical officers of health, who use small hospitals.

The number of nurses is considerable. In 1962 there were 38,660 qualified nurses, plus 37,200 auxiliaries, certainly relieving doctors from many minor medical-care activities.

Such a scheme is very efficient if one considers the low morbidity and mortality rates. Even if these low rates can be partly explained by high living standards, it is still obvious that considering the results, the health services are far from the most expensive in the world.

Finally, it should be noted that in Norway medical prescriptions must conform to a list of less than 2,000 specialities, and this restriction does not apparently affect the population's health.

Socialist Countries

Eastern European countries achieved a considerable effort to implement a medical-care programme based on the following principles. One can observe slight differences between these countries, but the U.S.S.R. is taken here as an example.

Free Care. Medical care is provided free of charge either for home and ambulatory treatment or for hospital care for everybody. However, drugs are charged for practically at production cost, except for persons receiving preventive care and those who, suffering from chronic ailments, are put on the 'dispensarization' list (see below).

Veterans and other groups pay only a fraction of the cost of the drugs.

Availability for All. Medical services are available to all, but freedom of choice is restricted to the medical team attached to the polyclinic serving the community to which the patient belongs. Medical-care organization is on a territorial basis. Each community (uchastok) of about 4,000 people has:

One specialist in internal diseases for 2,000 inhabitants
One paediatrician for 750–1,000 children

One stomatologist
One occupational doctor for every 2,000 industrial workers
One surgeon and one gynaecologist deal with several Uchastoks

This medical team is an integral part of the polyclinic staff, which serves 25,000–50,000 persons. The polyclinic may either be geographically isolated, or attached to a nearby district hospital (rayon) serving 50,000–120,000 inhabitants. At the top of the pyramid is the regional hospital (oblast) for approximately 2 million people, with specialists. Medical practitioners perform domiciliary work, consult at the polyclinic, and follow-up their patients if they need admission.

Quality of Medical Care. Physicians are encouraged to follow refresher courses every three years and to undergo post-graduate training. They can become 'half-specialists' and later 'full-specialists'. The latter may have teaching responsibilities. In no case does a doctor remain isolated for a long time, because he is a member of a team and passes through the different levels of out-patient and hospital facilities. In addition, the sanitary and epidemiological centres (sanepid) permanently control the health status of communities through about 150 health indices.

Also, in an effort to improve the quality of medical care, health authorities concentrate diagnostic and therapeutic measures in larger institutions where the staff is more numerous and more specialized. Uchastoks are now reallocated on the basis of 10,000 people, and small hospitals are converted into larger 150–300 bed institutions.

Priority in Prevention. Soviet doctors divide their time between care to patients, preventive work, and health education of the public. However, a special scheme should be briefly described, this is the 'dispensarization' referred to above.

Dispensarization means periodical examinations and treatment of vulnerable persons. As far as children, pregnant mothers, and industrial workers are concerned, nothing, in principle, is very different from that practised elsewhere. However, this scheme applies to individuals suffering from chronic or long-term disorders, such as diabetes, hypertension, rheumatism, glaucoma, peptic and duodenal ulcers, asthma, anaemias, without considering tuberculosis, cancer, and mental diseases, which are treated by specialized services. When such a disease is diagnosed the patient is summoned at intervals fixed by the doctors and receives drugs free of charge. He can be admitted to hospital for a while, as a preventive measure, to protect him against a temporary hazard such as an influenza outbreak.

In this connexion the feldsher's principal responsibility is to arrange for patients to keep the appointments for consultations.

Continuous Health Education of the Public. The population's understanding of health problems is continuously enhanced through a continuous health-education programme. All practitioners participate in giving lectures and demonstrations in schools, factories, sports clubs, governmental offices, etc. The Red Cross and Red Crescent Societies, and a host of volunteers, participate in this propaganda for health promotion.

Specialization. In order to reach all the communities in so vast a territory, it has been necessary to train a considerable number of medical doctors, feldshers, nurses, auxiliaries, sanitarians, pharmacists, dental prosthetists, laboratory and X-ray technicians. At the beginning of 1966, for the whole Union there were 23·9 physicians and 73·0 paramedical personnel for each 10,000 population. In 1967 they reached the ratio of one health technician per 100 inhabitants. This huge army of more than 2 million technicians can reconcile the tendency to specialization with quality of medical care because each patient is examined by a team as soon as he develops something a little more serious than a simple cold.

At the end of his medical studies the young doctor is already orientated in one of the main branches of medical services: therapy (meaning general medicine and surgery for adults), paediatrics, and hygiene. After postgraduate training he may become a 'first-step' or 'wide' specialist in surgery, for instance, of disorders of the gastro-intestinal tract. If he passes higher-grade examinations he then becomes a 'first-class' or 'narrow' specialist in one of the seventy-three recognized specialized disciplines. However, this vertical split up of overall medicine is complemented with a horizontal division according to the age group of the patients. At present the division is between children up to 15 years of age and adults, but it is contemplated to divide the latter into adolescent, adult, and elderly.

Private medicine is not forbidden. Moreover, health authorities organize paying polyclinics where patients can consult the doctor of their choice and pay 2–3 roubles. Doctors in these paying polyclinics are, in the main, professors or retired hospital consultants. The patients mainly come from rural areas where specialists are scarce. Others wish to confirm a diagnosis established at their own polyclinic.

This very strongly structured system has some drawbacks. Each family has its uchastok doctor, but he often changes or is absent due to a refresher course or is away on hospital duty. Children are cared for by different doctors, and the traditional image of the family doctor is somewhat blurred. It is inevitable that the concept of continuity of care is not compatible with the splitting-up of medical practice into numerous specialized disciplines. However, is this not true also of other developed countries where the proportion of general practitioners is continuously decreasing?

Developing Countries where Western Influence Was Overwhelming

Here we have in mind population groups with no written language of their own, living in territories colonized by Europeans during the nineteenth and twentieth centuries. This group of countries comprises approximately Africa south of the Sahara, and some Asiatic and Pacific areas virtually untouched by Chinese, Indian, or Islamic civilizations.

European medical systems were applied both by the army and religious missions. With the advent of medical teams accompanying soldiers and missionary priests, smallpox and trypanosomiasis receded. Medical care was given when mobile teams passed through villages. However, while, on the one hand, plantation and mine workers received basic medical care to protect their working capacity, on the other, European doctors settled in new settlements inhabited by Europeans and influential autochtons. Training of national technical personnel was very slow, often restricted to lower levels of knowledge, leading only to titles of assistant or auxiliary.

During the social troubles following independence most European doctors left, and the resultant disorganization of medical-care services was often dramatic. In many cases European doctors returned as part of bilateral aid, but never in the same quantities as previously.

Considerable effort was made by WHO and some developed countries to train national doctors. This is not the place to study all the difficulties encountered, but we are still very far from an acceptable situation. For instance, in 1961 Tanganyika had 180 private practitioners for 10 million population, but 150 of these were settled in five main cities totalling 200,000 inhabitants (Titmuss et al., 1964).

It is difficult to ascertain the actual situation, because the number of government-employed doctors is generally greater than that of private practitioners. The former are also engaged in part-time private practice for the benefit of the wealthy. This paradoxical situation will exist as long as official salaries are low. The picture remains very bleak indeed, and progress, if any, will be slower than in other socio-economic sectors if original methods are not vigorously applied.

These methods could be as follows:

1. Recruitment of medical students depends on the number of pupils passing secondary education examinations and on the appeal of medical studies. An extensive education for boys and girls is a prerequisite, but is not sufficient. The medical profession should be made attractive through remunerative and stable careers. Hospital-based functions should be offered on a wide basis.

2. Needs of rural and poor urban populations are such that the training of a large number of medical assistants is necessary. They must not be left on their own, but should be part of a well-structured system.

3. Medical training should be adapted to the functions that physicians are required to fulfil, and a thorough revision of the present curriculum of medical schools is necessary.

Equivalence in diplomas is only possible for the most advanced medical students.

4. Cost of adequate medical care—attractive salaries—cannot be wholly borne by state budgets. Social security schemes controlled by the state have to be established as soon as economy in cash is sufficiently developed through adequate salary scales for a significant proportion of the population.

Developing Countries where Original Historical and Cultural Backgrounds Still Operate

Those countries where Chinese, Indian, and Islamic civilizations flourished may apparently look similar to the previous ones in terms of crude statistical data, in regard to relative numbers of physicians, of hospital beds, and of financial resources for health. However, school attendance is now much higher and the young are eager to attain high levels of education. Due to the prestige attached to learning, recruitment of future leaders is easier as economic conditions improve.

TABLE 121, extracted from the *World Directory of Medical Schools* (1963), is self-explanatory:

TABLE 121

	Population in millions	Number of medical schools	Population per medical school in in millions	Number of medical graduates per year	Medical graduates per medical school per year	Medical graduates per million population
Africa, excluding United Arab Republic and South Africa	212·180	8	26·4	79	10	0·37
Asia, plus United Arab Republic . .	983·712	179	5·5	10,900	61	11·1

Moreover, in addition to doctors trained in modern scientific medicine there are a large number of local 'traditional doctors' who already contribute to relieving patients from painful symptoms at very low cost and who could participate in public health programmes as auxiliaries if properly trained.

It can therefore be forecast that, in Asiatic and North African countries, the economic take-off will be followed by a very rapid increase of medical and paramedical manpower. This manpower will be integrated within an administrative framework already accepted by the population of these countries, because the concept of medical services is an integral part of the legacy of their ancient civilizations.

IN-PATIENT HOSPITAL CARE

For centuries hospitals and allied institutions played an essential role in admitting patients and injured persons who could not be treated at home or ambulatorily. Moreover, hospitals were used to solve many social problems raised by children, the elderly, victims of catastrophes, or social troubles. They also served to isolate contagious patients. Finally, some countries were convinced that 100 per cent. of deliveries should occur in hospitals. One knows that Finland and the Netherlands do not accept this latter criterion without any consequence to their infantile and maternal mortality rate.

Moreover, the hospital of today extends its action in two directions. On the one hand, it is used for case finding of early cases of disease, and on the other, it has developed its rehabilitation services.

It was stressed that the overall cost of hospital care was comparable to that of home and ambulatory care. However, if one adds to the cost of in-patient care the increasing costs of out-patient departments, rehabilitation services, geriatrics, and psychiatry, organized within the hospital service, it is unavoidable that the proportion of the health budget governed by the hospital organization absorbs the majority of health expenditures.

Nowadays, the average cost of one patient-day in a general hospital is from four to five times the average income *per capita* per day (Abel-Smith, 1963).

The construction cost of a hospital bed is approximately three to four times the cost of running that bed during the period of one year. The maintenance and the keeping up to date of hospital premises and equipment is costly. The number of personnel and their qualifications have both increased, making their salaries up to more than 60 per cent. of the hospital budget. In many countries the national-health budget cannot afford to pay the whole cost of hospital services. These costs are totally or partly transferred to social security at the risk of achieving two competing medical-care organizations,

one run by governmental authorities, the other under social-security administration.

It was repeatedly stressed that prevention should be given absolute priority in order to release the pressure on curative services. However, facts did not confirm this view. The reasons are many. First, demands for medical care, including hospital care, are very elastic and depend more on perception of disease and availability of services than on morbidity. Therefore it is in countries such as the United States, in Europe, and the U.S.S.R. where preventive services have attained their full development that demand for hospital care is higher. Admission rates between 150 and 200 per 1,000 population per year are commonly observed. Each inhabitant spends an average of 1·5 to 2 days in hospital per year.

Secondly, the ageing population entails an accelerating demand for hospital care. Thirdly, fully developed hospital care, including rehabilitation, obviously has a favourable economic output in avoiding invalidity, shortening disablement periods, saving man-power working days, and avoiding deaths of children, adolescents, and adults in their productive age.

Let us now scrutinize the salient factors governing hospital care organization in the above-mentioned groups of countries.

Continental Western European Countries Excluding Scandinavia and Latin America

Despite important differences between the countries, the general pattern of hospital administration was influenced by the French Revolution of 1789, which brought in reforms, enforced through the Napoleonic era, all through western continental Europe. Most of the general hospitals are public, but they are administered by local authorities with a participation by local governments. However, most of the specialized hospitals for tuberculosis, psychiatry, and cancer are run by governmental authorities at intermediate level: *Département* in France, *Provincia* in Italy, *Land* in Germany, *Canton* in Switzerland.

Hospitals enjoy administrative and financial autonomy in so far as the local authorities are themselves autonomous.

In these countries social-security schemes are non-governmental organizations, but they must share the major part of hospital expenditure in paying for each insured person requiring hospital admission. Therefore the budgetary unit is an average all-inclusive cost per patient-day excluding medical fees. The state budget does not support the hospital except for the small amount requested for treatment of the poor (public assistance). In some countries, especially Spain and Italy, the social-security schemes have built and run their own hospitals restricted to insured salaried persons and their dependants.

Construction costs are usually shared by the state, local

authorities, and sometimes social security. Loans and amortization are included in the calculation of the cost per patient-day. As the duties and rights of a hospital are defined by many acts and decrees, hospital administration is highly complex and is usually implemented by qualified lay administrators. However, this autonomy, strongly defended by hospital associations, is encroached upon by governmental control. Budgeting, staffing, auditing, and technical requirements are closely screened by governmental agencies which scrutinize individual hospital administration in great detail, but the principle of local autonomy remains, and there are no regional hospital authorities.

Parallel to the network of public hospitals, a variable proportion of private hospitals exists. Some are voluntary and, as such, are submitted to practically the same rules as public hospitals. They are important in Belgium, the Netherlands, and Italy, where most of them are administered by the Church. Others are profit-making. They can survive only if they are authorized to admit socially insured patients, i.e. to accept a certain degree of control on their finance, staffing, and equipment. However, private profit-making hospitals play a large role in public health planning because they tend to select patients who could be treated at relatively low cost, leaving the complicated expensive cases to public hospitals, at which the average cost per patient day and the length of stay increase with the flow of severe cases and elderly patients.

France tried to control the rapid increase of hospital beds in private hospitals by determining a ceiling for the total bed complement for each district. This ceiling was calculated by hospital utilization statistical studies.

The liberal character of the medical profession, the fee per service system, and the lack of participation of general practitioners in hospital work explain the relatively low hospital utilization rate, which varies between 80 and 110 admissions per 1,000 population a year.

However, the average length of stay being rather long due to social care, the number of hospital beds is on the mean. The following table gives some data concerning exclusively general hospitals for so-called acute cases:

TABLE 122

Countries	Number of hospital admissions per 1,000 per year	Average length of stay in days	Number of general hospital beds per 1,000 population (acute cases)
Belgium .	86	13	4·48
Fed. Germany	110	21	7·2
Netherlands .	79·6	20	4·65
Portugal .	from 29·5 to 42·25	from 14·08 to 24·64	from 1·97 to 3·00
Switzerland .	—	about 16	6·8
Greece . .	—	17	3·7
Spain . .	16	—	2·44
France . .	56·5	19·3	5·95

(Adapted from *King Edward's Hospital Fund for London*, 1962, 1964, 1966.)

In Latin American countries the situation is much the same as it was some decades ago in Latin European countries. There are, of course, wide differences, for example, between Columbia and Bolivia. Chile is an exception, since it has a national health service and a highly developed hospital administration.

Northern American Countries

The American hospital network is very complex. Regarding general hospitals for acute cases (short-term hospitals) private organization is more significant. The federal, state, and local governments take initiative either in depressed areas or for special groups like veterans, Indians, or for special research institutes.

Conversely, most of the special hospitals for mental diseases, tuberculosis, and, depending on the cases, chronic diseases are publicly owned.

The attention of the world is often drawn to American private hospitals as the most glamorous medical care and teaching institutions. This is amply justified by the quality of medical care maintained at a very high level by the joint Accreditation Committee and other professional bodies. However, the private character and spirit of competition lead to over-equipping the wealthiest regions and to multiplying the most expensive equipment, which explains why the crude cost per patient-day (exclusive of many factors, such as the doctor's fees) is exceedingly high.

The use of computers in hospital administration and the steady increase of operating costs make regional co-ordination feasible and desirable. An increasing number of hospitals and medical schools are studying how to create regional hospital services for which administrative, financial, and technical patterns could be organized without encroaching on individualism.

American hospitals are different from European hospitals in three main ways. The average duration of stay is short = 6 days, the cost per day is high = $100, and the hospital admission rate is considerable = 140–150 per 1,000 population per year. These differences are explained by the fact that the open-staff system is very common. This means that the great majority of doctors practising in a given town have free access to the private hospital of that town and admit their patients for minor illnesses and check-ups.

In addition to the general hospitals there are a great number of private nursing homes classified as skilled and unskilled according to their staffing and equipment, which deal with convalescent, long-term care, and chronic sick. Therefore the average American hospitalized patient is very different from his European brother, and this should be taken into consideration when attempting to compare hospital statistics on both sides of the Atlantic.

Britain (England, Wales, Scotland and Northern Ireland)

Whatever the differences between these countries, the hospital systems have in common the fact that they are planned at central governmental level, but administered at decentralized levels, which is either the region, or the county.

In 1962 the Porritt report recommended changes in the NHS to bring about better integration of the three branches of the service: (a) Hospitals; (b) General practice; (c) Public Health. In 1972 the British Government published a White Paper on reorganization of the service and a Steering Committee was set up to discuss management arrangements for the reorganized NHS. It listed six key features.

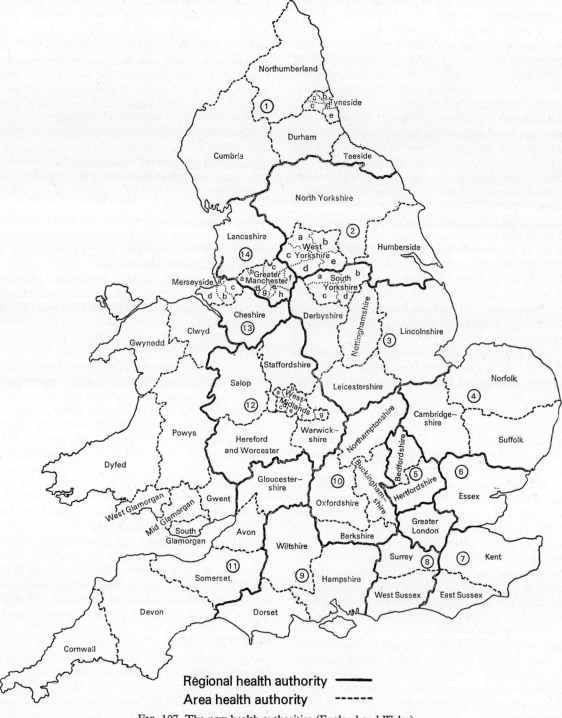

FIG. 107. The new health authorities (England and Wales).

1. Health services should be integrated locally within areas on a district basis.

2. Clinicians should participate actively in management, particularly at operational level (seen as essential in a patient-orientated approach to health care).

3. To achieve integration multi-disciplinary management teams at each level are suggested.

4. Responsibilities must be clearly allocated and defined.

5. Decentralization of decision making is to be balanced against a need for national and regional strategic direction.

6. The arrangements should be flexible.

Radical changes have been made in the National Health Service from 1st April 1974 under new management throughout England, Wales, Scotland and N. Ireland.

Hospitals, family doctors and community health facilities are reorganized into one giant machine. With a £3,000 million annual budget and 850,000 staff, it will be one of the largest civilian enterprises in the world.

The changes mean that the health service, brought in by Aneurin Bevan in 1948, formally ceases to exist.

Regional hospital boards, executive health councils and local authority departments with health responsibilities will disappear. So too will medical officers of health, some of whom will now become 'community physicians'.

Under the three-part structure of the past 26 years, local executive councils were responsible for general practice and the dental, ophthalmic and pharmaceutical services. Hospital management committees ran hospitals and specialist services, and local authorities handled health centres, ambulances, mother and child care and a wide range of other preventive and caring services.

This system will be replaced by a single health service. But GPs and dentists will retain much of their present independence, working as contractors to the new administration— closely linked with it but not under its direct authority.

England will be divided into 14 regions, of which the largest will be the West Midlands, with 5,119,000 people, and the smallest East Anglia, with 1,681,000 [see FIGURE 107]. Scotland, Wales and Northern Ireland will be administered separately, though similarly.

The 14 English regions will be divided into 90 areas, the lowest level with statutory authority. These areas will mostly have the same geographical boundaries as the new local authority metropolitan districts and non-metropolitan counties.

The areas will be further sub-divided into 205 districts, each with about 250,000 people. Their boundaries are not being rigidly defined, so the populations they service will be, as far as possible, existing 'natural' communities.

It is expected that re-organization will cut overlapping and duplication of services, improve inter-departmental co-ordination, and streamline management. If this happens, care for the 500,000 chronically sick, disabled and mentally ill in hospitals and the 1,500,000 similarly affected people who live outside institutions, should be radically improved.

One feature is that an ombudsman will act as a health service watchdog. Community Health councils will also represent the public (consumerism). These 18 to 30 member councils are one of the more controversial features of the reorganizations. The idea is that they will be an 'effective voice' of local people and will have the right to visit hospitals and make representations to higher authorities in published reports. But at least half of the community council members must be nominated by local authorities, and several more by the area health authority. Only about one third will be nominated by voluntary bodies.

Details of the way in which the reorganized Health Service will work start at the top with the Department of Health and Social Security. This will be responsible for central strategic planning. The free family planning for all and monitoring of the entire Health Service were also introduced on 1st April, 1974.

At the next level of responsibility are the 14 regional health authorities (RHA). They will see to regional planning and general supervision of health services.

Although their number is the same as the now defunct regional hospital boards, their function is different. They will take in the family doctor service, previously run by the executive councils, and community health and welfare services. They will be accountable to the Secretary of State for their own activities and those of the area health authorities under them. They will distribute money to the authorities and will be responsible for new hospitals; they will also run special services, like blood transfusion, and must ensure proper support for medical and dental teaching and research.

The 90 area health authorities (AHA) the next tier down will co-ordinate action with the new local authorities. They will have 'operational control' of hospitals, GP services, community health and area planning. Each area, employing thousands of professional and other staff, will have responsibility for up to one million people.

The health districts will be in charge of the day-to-day running of the services. Each district will contain a district general hospital or several hospitals and each will have a district management committee.

Other innovations include health-care planning teams to review the needs of the old, disabled and mentally ill. See Reorganization of the NHS (1972, 1973 and 1974) for detailed accounts.

Scandinavian Countries

In Sweden the central office for planning and administration is the National Board of Health, which supervises the general health and pharmaceutical services and is intended to exercise control over treatment of the sick in both public and private hospitals. Within the National Board of Health hospital bureaux deal with matters concerning general hospitals.

The Board is also a kind of administrative tribunal, and its disciplinary committee deals with notifications regarding maltreatment and professional misconduct.

The Central Board of Hospital Planning supervises plans for the construction of hospitals. Such control is obligatory despite the fact that the hospitals are built by the counties and county boroughs and are owned and financed by them.

The State operates mental hospitals, but the transfer of ownership of the hospitals to the counties was to take effect in 1967. The state also operates three famous university hospitals: Karolinska and Serafimer in Stockholm and Akademiska in Uppsala, but a large part of their expenses are paid by the counties and county boroughs which use the hospitals for their local population.

The cost of hospitals and other health services amounts to 80–86 per cent. of the counties' total gross expenditure. Of course, the county councils have the right to impose rates, which are based on the same principles as the communal tax (local rates). On an average the county council's rates take about 5 per cent. of the taxpayer's income.

The counties and county boroughs are not bound to fulfil their obligations to provide hospital accommodation by running the hospitals themselves. But there are not many hospitals owned by other than the legally responsible authorities. The few private hospitals often receive considerable financial support from the public authorities.

The administration of public hospitals is the task of the County Health Board to be elected by the county council and the county borough council. The daily management is conducted by the medical superintendent and the hospital secretary.

There is a strong trend towards the organization of regional hospital co-ordination, and the county and county borough councils have agreed to co-operate in maintaining regional hospitals in seven regions. These hospitals retain their status as county or county borough hospitals, but are encouraged to make specialized facilities available to the whole region. In five regions university hospitals have been made regional hospitals. An average region has a population of 1 million, the northernmost and smallest has only 700,000.

Socialist Countries (U.S.S.R.)

The most salient point is the integration of hospitals within the general health service. On the one hand, this reconciles the great importance of the hospital service, the large number of beds, and their vast utilization rate and, on the other, the apparent simplicity of hospital administration. The increase in the number of beds was regular from 4·02 per 1,000 population in 1940 to 9·60 in 1965. The number of admissions per 1,000 per year also shows an increase, but it is interesting to point out that the utilization rate by rural population was about 50 per cent. of that of the urban population in 1950, but is now approximately equal. This shows that the ideal target of 'availability to all' is nearly reached.

TABLE 123

Hospital Admission rate per 1,000 population per year

	Admission rate				
	1950	1955	1958	1964	1965
Urban population	150	161	190	203	201
Rural population .	77	114	144	180	189

A large network of hospitals was developed. Four types are described: (1) small local hospitals; (2) central general hospitals (rayon) in urban settlements; (3) central general hospitals (rayon) in rural settlements; and (4) regional hospitals (oblast), most of these being teaching hospitals.

The trend now is to suppress some of the smallest rural units, to increase the bed complement of local hospitals to 150–300 beds, to increase the rayon hospital to 700–800 beds, and also to develop regional centres.

Ambulatory-care facilities, already centred in polyclinics, were integrated within general hospitals, creating 'unified hospitals'. This decision was taken in May 1947. By 1951, 99 per cent. of general hospitals and 75 per cent. of children's hospitals were 'unified', meaning that polyclinics were attached to them. Moreover, 75 per cent. of the independent polyclinics were integrated in unified hospitals.

There are general hospitals with specialized departments for a large range of medical disciplines, but in very large cities specialized hospitals and institutes have been created for paediatrics, maternity, infectious diseases, cancer, tuberculosis, traumatology, etc.

In 1965 the total number of beds was 2,255,500, the number of institutions was 26,303, and that of out-patient departments and polyclinics, 36,696. To this network of institutions run by the Ministry of Health must be added some hospitals organized by factories and collective farms, homes for the elderly and chronic sick run by the welfare authorities, and a large number of rest and convalescent homes with medical facilities, called 'sanatoriums', organized by Workers Unions and social security in climatic resorts such as the Crimea and Georgia.

Strictly speaking, specialized hospital administration has practically disappeared, because hospitals have merely become branches of the health system. In most cases the district (rayon) medical officer of health acts as director of the hospital at the same time. There are no administrative boards, but health committees, at different levels, deal with health matters, including hospitals.

To develop a scheme in such wide territory it was necessary to play quantity against sophistication. Therefore lavish hospitals do not exist in the U.S.S.R. Research on functional planning and a vast use of standardized building components enabled fast and cheap construction. At present a 1,000-bed hospital is erected in a period of eighteen months. Internal comfort is not neglected, and hospital wards have a maximum capacity of six beds with a large number of three- to four-bed rooms. Colour, sound, decoration, and greenery are considered important from a psychosomatic point of view. Equipment is also standardized, and technical apparatus is mass-produced under the control of a new Ministry of Medical Supplies. Practical and sturdy operating tables, lamps, anaesthesia machines, and microscopes can be found everywhere. Architectural plans are drawn up in a central institute, the Guiprozdrav, attached to the Ministry of Health in Moscow, with a complement of more than 400 architects. The location of hospitals is decided upon by town planning committees at which the health authorities are present. The hospital budget is calculated in advance, on a yearly basis, based on norms concerning the expected number of admissions, of patient-days, of surgical operations, of laboratory and X-ray procedures, etc.

Adjustments can be made during the fiscal year. The hospital budget is integrated within the health budget, is submitted to the regional health committee, then to the Republican Ministry of Health and Soviet, and finally to the federal authorities and to the Supreme Soviet Assembly. After final approval allotments are made along the same lines in reversed order. Staffing is abundant, as most of the physicians are attached to the 'unified' hospital and work alternately for domiciliary care, in the polyclinic and wards.

There seems to be no concern about the very high level of hospital admission rate, because in-patient care is considered as a means of improving community health, and thus productivity. A proportion of the patients admitted to hospital were summoned because they suffered from chronic conditions and the physicians thought that a stay in a hospital would prevent further complications. Therefore health authorities consider that the bed complement is not yet sufficient, and contemplate reaching an overall bed population ratio of 13 beds per 1,000 population, including mental and tuberculosis hospitals but not welfare and elderly homes. Efforts were made in Republics which are still under the federal average, but the deviation from the mean never exceeded 20 per cent.

A similar trend is observed in other socialist countries of Eastern Europe. Efforts in hospital construction in Poland,

Czechoslovakia, Eastern Germany, Rumania, and Bulgaria are noteworthy.

Having reached an already satisfactory level of hospital facilities, the tendency is to study in depth new methods for planning hospital services based on utilization surveys and to embark on studies of economics of medical care.

Important results can be expected because of the availability of standardized data.

Developing Countries where Western Influence Was Overwhelming

Patterns of hospital organization which were alien to their own civilization were imposed on these countries. The hospital network was developed without the participation of the people. Many hospitals were built by the army of the ruling power, and were actually run by military doctors under the supervision of the Commissariat.

An important sector was also covered by religious missions, but in many cases the efforts of the churches were directed towards assistance to the chronic sick, lepers, the blind, and welfare cases.

In some countries a considerable effort was made, such as in Zaire, where the number of beds per 1,000 population equalled nearly 4.

It is also worth mentioning the creation of private hospitals for thousands of workers engaged in large enterprises like mines, rubber, fruit, or tea plantation estates, etc.

However, co-ordination of these efforts was poor and even non-existent. International economic crises entailing the interruption of ore extraction or rubber collection resulted in thousands of workers suddenly becoming ineligible for treatment in the local hospital of the firm concerned.

With independence, most of the foreign staff left these countries. The new central administration had very little practical control over the institutions and was deprived of any real legal power. The lack of an efficient administrative framework was strongly felt.

However, where severance from the former ruling power was not too drastic, hospitals continued to receive assistance through bilateral and sometimes multilateral channels. But as a rule the health systems of these countries became more dualist than ever because public health administration was run by the new ministry of health, while hospital administration was cut off from the central competent authorities. Moreover, maintenance problems were insuperable, and nowadays most of these hospitals, poorly staffed, badly equipped, and invaded by a host of chronic sick, absorb an undue amount of the ministry of health budget and give very little service to curable patients belonging to a productive age group.

Planning medical care services is, in most countries, a very urgent matter because unplanned existing institutions drain so much money that, in fact, a decreasing proportion is allocated year after year to preventive services.

The situation is likely to be more serious than it looks at first sight because of the expansion of private or semi-private firms specialized in hospital construction which offer lavish models at very high cost. These hospitals cannot be staffed and operated properly after completion, because they would absorb almost the entire ministry of health's budget, without mentioning the difficulty of maintaining sophisticated installations.

Integration of health services, development of administrative and legislative frameworks, control of construction, selection of patients at basic health-service level, step-by-step development of simple health-insurance schemes strictly controlled by the government are necessary to improve hospital care in these countries.

Developing Countries where Original Historical and Cultural Backgrounds Are Still Operating

As stated above, brilliant civilizations flourished in these countries, which favoured the development of hospitals. For centuries Islamic hospitals had nothing to envy in those of the medieval Christian world. Therefore, if the equipment of these hospitals had to be adapted to the scientific medicine of the twentieth century the concept itself was familiar to the people. Even if the hospitals of today appear inadequate according to western standards, they have their roots in the people, history, and administration.

In these countries hospital administration was in most cases highly centralized. The traditional Turkish administrations favoured concentration of powers. Moreover, in Islamic countries hospitals derived their income from mortmain estates owned by religious authorities (Waqf, Habous). Nowadays, these estates are nationalized and the central government could, in most cases, take over the hospital network without any legal difficulty.

This situation is not without drawbacks. The lack of norms and standards, the insufficiency of financial resources, and the over-concentration of powers make hospital budgeting very difficult. Too often the only criterion for organizing the budget is the amount of money available rather than well-assessed needs.

Here again, a refined legislative framework seems necessary to avoid abuses and to promote planning machinery.

In many of these countries social-security schemes started functioning for the benefit of the salaried workers. Unfortunately, when these schemes are not controlled at governmental level they show a tendency to build up a network of services available only to eligible subscribers and focused on curative medicine.

Such a situation is very detrimental to the harmonious development of health services, and leads to a dual system of curative care in a constant imbalance because, due to economic development and industrialization, the proportion of salaried workers and wage earners progressively increases. The problems of dependants and unemployment make the development of independent medical-care systems within social security even more critical.

Means of co-ordinating social security and health plans must be implemented, as well as participation of social-security schemes in personal preventive care.

CONCLUSION

Medical-care services are often considered a burden to modern societies by economists and planners. If well organized they can contribute to economic development and welfare. Whatever the priority given to preventive services, it is a recognized fact that any population well protected against preventable diseases will still require a very large amount of medical care. The glamour of medical progress, the perception of disease, the increase of degenerative diseases, and the ageing of populations inevitably make the consumption of medical care an important sector of the nation's expenditure.

The ultimate would be for governments to create more efficient planning of their medical-care services. This aim can be achieved through better co-ordination with preventive services and a deeper knowledge of the underlying factors governing medical-care organization.

Many of these factors remain insufficiently known, and it is necessary to explore, on the one hand, the different existing patterns of hospital legislation and administration in order to offer reasonable models to developing countries which have to build up an administrative network. On the other hand, demographic, social, and economic factors influencing consumption of medical care and hospital utilization have to be assessed and weighted.

A certain number of research projects are taking place in developed countries on the utilization of medical-care services. In a few years it is expected that we shall know more about the factors influencing consumption of medical and planning methods.

REFERENCES AND FURTHER READING

Abel-Smith, B. (1963) Paying for health services: a study of the costs and sources of finance in six countries, *Wld Hlth Org. Publ. Hlth Pap.*, No. 17.

Abel-Smith, B. (1967) An international study of health expenditure and its relevance for health planning, *Wld Hlth Org. Publ. Hlth Pap.*, No. 32.

Ahmed, Paul I. (1967) Patterns of health insurance coverage for American families, *Inquiry*, **4**, No. 4, 59–68.

Albinsson, Gillis (1965) *Public Health Services in Sweden*, Swedish Hospital Association, Halmstad.

Babson, J. H. (1972) *Health Care Delivery Systems: A Multi-national Survey*, London.

Bravo, Alfredo Leonardo (1961) *Servicio Nacional de Salud. Doctrina y Política.* Sección Educación para la salud, Santiago, Chile.

Bridgman, R. F. (1963) *L'hôpital et la cité*, Paris.

Bridgman, R. F., and Roemer, M. I. (1973) Health legislation and hospital systems, *Wld Hlth Org. Publ. Hlth Pap.*, No. 50.

Department of Health and Social Security (1972) *White Paper on the National Health Service Reorganization*, England Cmnd 5055, London, H.M.S.O.

Dodge, J. S., ed. (1970) *The Organization and Evaluation of Medical Care*, Dunedin.

Doll, R. C. (1973) Nuffield lecture: Monitoring the NHS, *Proc. roy. Soc. Med.*, **66**, 729.

Fenall, N. R. E. (1972) *Auxiliaries in Health Care Programmes in Developing Countries*, London.

Forsyth, G. (1973) *Doctors and State Medicine*, 2nd ed., London.

Godber, G. E. (1970) *Medical Care: The Changing Needs and Patterns*, London.

Ferrer, H. P., ed. (1972) *The Health Services: Administration, Research and Management*, London.

King Edward's Hospital Fund for London (1962) *The Hospital Services of Western Europe.* Report of the Western European Conference, London.

International Hospital Federation, and King Edward's Hospital Fund for London (1964) *The Hospital Services of Western Europe.* Report of the Second Western European Conference, London.

International Hospital Federation, and King Edward's Hospital Fund for London (1966) *The Hospital Services of Europe.* Report of the Third European Conference, London.

Lerner, Monroe, and Fitzgerald, Sandra W. (1965) A comparative study of three major forms of health care coverage: a review, *Inquiry*, **2**, 1, 37–60.

Logan, R. F. L., Klein, R. E., and Ashley, J. S. A. (1971) Effective management of health, *Brit. med. J.*, **2**, 519.

Mizrahi, Andrée, and Mizrahi, Arié (1964) Un modèle des dépenses médicales appliqué aux données d'une enquête, *Consommation*, No. 1.

Péquignot, H., Rösch, G., Magdelaine, M., and Rempp, J. M. (1962) La consommation médicale des Français, *Rev. Hyg. Méd. soc.*, **10**, 6, 451–83.

Reorganization of the NHS (1972) A series of 6 papers, *Roy. Soc. Hlth J.*, **92**, 12.

Reorganization of the NHS (1973) 3 papers in *Health Trends*, **5**, 22, 42, 72.

Reorganization of the NHS (1974) 2 papers in *Health Trends*, **6**, 2, 7.

Report of a Steering Committee (1972) *Management Arrangements for the Reorganized National Health Service*, London, H.M.S.O. (The Grey Book).

Report of the technical discussions at the 26th World Health assembly (1973) *Organization, Structure and Functioning of Health Services and Modern Methods of Administrative Management*, Geneva.

Roemer, Milton I. (1962) Highlights of soviet health services, *Milbank mem. Fd Quart.*, **15**, 4, 373–406.

Roemer, Milton I. (1963) Medical care in integrated health programmes of Latin America, *Med. Care*, **1**, 182–90.

Roemer, Milton I. (1963) *Medical Care in Latin America*, Pan American Union, Washington.

Titmuss, R. M., Abel-Smith, B., Macdonald, G., Williams, A. W., and Wood, C. H. (1964) *The Health Services of Tanganyika; A Report to the Government*, p. 13, London.

United States Department of Health, Education, and Welfare (1962) *Medical Care Financing and Utilization. Source Book of Data Through 1961*, VIII, Washington, U.S. Government Printing Office.

United States Department of Health, Education, and Welfare Social Security Administration. Division of Research and Statistics (1964) *Social Security Programs throughout the World, 1964*, XXV, Washington, U.S. Government Printing Office.

United States National Academy of Sciences. National Research Council Division of Medical Sciences (1966) *Public Health Problems in 14 French-speaking Countries in Africa and Madagascar. A Survey of Resources and Needs*, xix, Washington, NAS–NSC, 1966, 2 vols.

U.S.S.R. Ministry of Health (1967) *The System of Public Health Services in the U.S.S.R.*, Ministry of Health, Moscow.

White, Kerr L. (1967) Medical care research and health services systems, *J. med. Educ.*, **42**, No. 8, 729–41.

Wofnider, R. C. (1972) Health centres: problems and possibilities, *Community Med.*, **128**, 175.

World Health Organization (1963) *World Directory of Medical Schools*, 3rd ed., Geneva.

World Health Organization (1967) *World Health Statistics Annual 1963*, Vol. III, Health personnel and hospital establishments, Geneva.

World Health Organization (1971) Report of a joint ILO/WHO committee on personal health care and social security, *Wld Hlth Org. techn. Rep. Ser.*, No. 480.

World Health Organization (1974a) Modern management methods and the organization of the health services, *Wld Hlth Org. Publ. Hlth Pap.*, No. 55.

World Health Organization (1974*b*) Health services in the People's Republic of China, *Wld Hlth Org. Chron.*, **28**, 117.

World Health Organization (1974*c*) The work of WHO in 1973, *Wld Hlth Org. Off. Rec.*, No. 213, 96–102.

World Health Organization (1974*d*) The training and status of the physician in China, *Wld Hlth Org. Chron.*, **28**, 268.

World Health Organization, American Regional Office (1966) *Administración de servicios de atención médica. Nuevos elementos para la formulación de una política continental*, Publicación Científica No. 129, Washington.

World Health Organization, American Regional Office. Study Group on Coordination of Medical Care in Latin America (1965) *Relationship between Social Security Medical Programs and those of Ministries and other Official Health Agencies*, Washington, 16 pp.

World Health Organization Regional Office for Europe (1971) *The Role of the Primary Physician in Health Services*, Copenhagen.

World Health Organization Regional Office for Europe. Reports of a series of meetings on the organization of health care, Copenhagen.

(1973) *Health Planning and Organization of Medical Care* (Euro 4102).

(1974) *Chronic Diseases* (Euro 4102).

(1974) *Working Group on Trends in the Development of Primary Medical Care, Moscow 1973* (Euro 4309).

(1974) *Symposium on the Role of Social Insurance Institutions in Preventive Medicine, Nancy 1973* (Euro 4305).

(1974) *Working Group on Psychiatry in General Practice, Lysubu 1973* (Euro 54281).

(1974) *Working Group on the Public Health Aspects of Tourism, Torremolinos 1973* (Euro 4005).

(1974) *Working Group on the Health Aspects of Labour Migration, Algiers 1973* (Euro 4003(2)).

(1974) *Seminar on the Health Aspects of Urban Development, Stuttgart 1973* (Euro 4108).

(1974) *Symposium on the Functions of Central Institutes of Public Health and Hygiene, Moscow 1973* (Euro 4001(2).

(1974) *Health Services in Europe*, 2nd ed. (Euro Monograph).

44

THE CONTROL OF INFECTION IN HOSPITAL

R. F. BRIDGMAN

The potential danger for human beings of becoming infected during a stay in hospital is due to the continuous flow of various species of organisms carried by patients, by all personnel who come in contact with them, and disseminated by fomites, air, body surfaces, linen, and contacts during medical examinations and nursing care.

HISTORY

Up to the last decades of the nineteenth century the situation was tragic. All wounds were infected, epidemics of puerperal fever spread among delivered mothers, killing at their peak 70 per cent. of them. As a rule, the hospital mortality rate reached 25 per cent. and was due to infection in the great majority of cases. Those who survived suffered their whole life from the sequelae of osteomyelitis and abscesses which were developing during their stay in hospital. Special infections such as gangrene and diphtheritic infection of wounds, were seen only in hospital wards.

It is worth recalling that this dreadful situation could have been greatly alleviated if the practice of Guy de Chauliac had been accepted as valid. Guy de Chauliac was a surgeon in Montpellier during the thirteenth century and who used to wash recent wounds with warm wine. Wounds remained 'dry' and healed quickly. A considerable academic dispute stormed throughout European universities. Finally the supporters of the 'humid' wounds won, dragging their arguments from Galen, Arab, and Jewish theoretical writers rather than from practical experience. Thus infection was intentionally developed by putting dirty dilapidated cloths (swabs) on the wounds. Doctors were satisfied with an abundant production of pus, they even considered as a favourable event the coming of blue pus (caused by *Pseudomonas pyocyanea*) which acted indeed like an antibiotic against streptococci and staphylococci but was in itself a deadly agent.

A comparable attitude prevailed during the controversy which arose from Semmelweiss' practice of frequent hand washing he imposed on himself and on his personnel in his maternity department in Vienna.

Theoreticians thought that the permanency of high infection risks within hospital walls was due to the concentration of 'putrid miasmas' mixed with air. This theory lead to diluting the miasmas into the greatest possible volume of air. Ceilings were built 6–8 metres high, cross ventilation was established through large chimneys and, finally, wards were separately built according to the pavilion type which began with the Portsmouth hospital (1762). The idea spread through the Western world. For large hospitals, the pavilion system was also adopted but communications were made shorter according to the recommendations of the French Academy of Sciences (1788). Most hospitals built between 1800 and 1920 were planned accordingly, adopting a lay-out which was essentially designed to reduce hospital infection.

The results of this profound change in hospital architecture were partially favourable until Lister and Pasteur established the germ theory of disease on undisputable grounds. Two techniques developed which are still the basis of most hospital procedures; *antisepsis*, i.e. the destruction of germs by disinfection process, and *asepsis*, i.e. the production of germ-free material and products. After one or two decades the dissemination of antiseptic and aseptic techniques, together with the isolation of infected patients brought spectacular results enabling the development of safe surgery and the practice of injections which was a revolution in pharmacology.

However, some dark spots remained, children's hospitals or paediatric wards kept a high cross-infection rate. It was not infrequent that a child admitted for a certain disease, caught most of the communicable diseases during his stay in hospital against which he was not immunized. In adult departments infectious complications were frequent among surgical patients, urology cases, and in medical wards. The situation could not be compared with that of previous times because the majority of hospital-acquired infection did not endanger life but entailed important prolongation of stay. Socio-economic considerations were brought to the fore. The development of sickness insurance schemes covering a large part of hospital expenditure on the one hand and the rocketing cost of hospital cases on the other, focused attention on length of stay in hospital of patients.

Then came the antibiotic era. In a few years most infectious diseases could be treated successfully and the period of contagion was reduced to a minimum. Added to the use of new or improved sera and vaccines, the antibiotic techniques triggered a sudden fall in communicable disease rates. Infectious diseases hospitals nearly emptied in developed countries. Spectacular improvements were made in the treatment of burns, wounds, sores, abscesses, etc. Sources of hospital infection seemed to have disappeared.

But two factors, one of a psychological nature, the other biological, made this progress a sort of Pyrrhic victory. It is openly recognized by doctors and nurses that the extensive use of antibiotics entailed a disinterest towards the cumbersome antiseptic and aseptic techniques. Why spend so much time and energy on the tedious rites of germ control when their growth could be stopped with antibiotics? Operating techniques became less strict and personal discipline more careless. The practical teaching was inadequate and nurses used faulty dressing techniques. The cleaning was done by domestic staff outside the supervision of ward sisters. There was a rapid turn-over of patients and staff, hospitals became overcrowded thus increasing the risks of cross-infection.

On the other hand, organisms seemed to adapt. Some species changed, probably through the mutation process; resistant strains appeared in a few years. These new strains had not to compete against other species which were more vulnerable and it appeared that use and abuse of antibiotics had produced a selection of a few highly pathogenic strains which were free to develop.

PRESENT SITUATION

It is difficult to know the exact proportion of patients who are suffering from infectious complications coming from the hospital environment. Some post-operative infections develop from the patient's own body. Some lung congestive failures generate in the patient's own upper respiratory tract. Some infectious diseases are brought in the hospital during their incubation period. Moreover, doctors, specially surgeons, do not like to divulge the infection rate in their department, but some do and truth may be discovered through a few objective statistics and also through nurses' experience. The American Hospital Association disclosed that over 13 per cent. of the patients in a large community hospital had developed infections while in hospital. About the same rate, 13·5 per cent., was reported from the Boston City Hospital. The actual rate might be higher if one thinks about the short duration of stay in American hospitals. According to the United States Public Health Service publications, infection from *Salmonella derby* totalled nearly 1,200 cases in 40 institutions of 25 States plus the district of Columbia.

It has been estimated that about one million extra patient days in hospital result from the 1,500,000 operations performed in Britain each year because of post-operative sepsis. Thompson discovered that in many maternity units, over 90 per cent. of the infants carry pathogenic staphylococci in the nose and in the umbilicus when they leave hospital and a high proportion have infective lesions and 'sticky eyes'. Some surgical wards have a wound infection rate as high as 80 per cent. among cold surgery cases. Many of these complications are minor and are barely notified to the surgeon by the nurse who is used to seeing small abscesses of the abdominal wall, urinary infections, and small pulmonary infarcts. In the United States, registered post-operative wound infection rates vary from 1 to 20 per cent. with a mean of 5–10 per cent. Many statistics have been published in developed and developing countries (see bibliography).

The situation seems to have deteriorated to such an extent that most American hospitals have organized Infection Control Committees. The American Hospital Association considering the medico–legal responsibilities of hospitals, recommends organizing committees which should establish a surveillance and reporting programme and a personnel situation programme as well as regulations for hospital visitors. The Infection Control Committee should appoint a bacteriologist, a paediatrician, a surgeon, an internist, a nurse, a hospital administrator, and the local health officer. The personnel should be instructed to report not only on the patient infectious cases but also on their own history of infections. Follow-up of patients should be done to discover infections developed after hospital discharge.

The situation, albeit fully acknowledged by specialized health agencies, has not yet been given enough attention by doctors and nurses. The latter will be ill-informed compared with other technicians who are considering very seriously the contamination problem in their own fields of activity. Considerable progress has been made on the pollution control of closed volumes by gaseous products, dust, and micro-organisms. This concerns the pharmaceutical industry (especially for the preparation of antibiotics, laboratory media, vaccines, sera, and aseptic solutions), the electronic industry (transistors, integrated circuits), spacecraft assembly plants, computer functions, deep sea exploration, etc. In all these various fields the absence of any particles whose size is equal or greater than 0·001 ml. is an absolute prerequisite (bacteria usually measure 2–5 microns). As any failure of the control automatically entails a higher percentage of faulty units to be discarded, which means an economic loss, technicians are eager to improve their methods. The Association for the Prevention and Study of Contamination, organized in 1971 in Paris, was the 2nd International Congress for technicians interested in these problems.

Animal farms devoted to research and production of living cells have also had to study thoroughly cross-infection problems. It is strange to think that in these farms, different species of monkeys, especially prone to bacterial and viral infections, benefit from a better environment than patients in hospitals.

CAUSATIVE AGENTS

All pathogenic micro-organisms are able to spread from one patient to another, but most of those which are sensitive to antibiotics are prevented from doing so by the 'antibiotic umbrella'. In practice, a few strains are responsible for the majority of severe hospital infection cases.

Staphylococcus aureus is found everywhere and may cause many kinds of infection. A United States Public Health Service study was conducted on 1,456 mothers and infants delivered in fifteen community hospitals of a major city within one month. Staphylococci were the cause of 20 per cent. of cases of infant pyoderma, 45 per cent. of those of maternal mastitis, 100 per cent. of those of infant mastitis, and occasioned 75 per cent. of neonatal deaths. In another study, the incidence of staphylococcal infection varied from 0·5 to 5 per cent. of all patients admitted to hospital. The distribution according to clinical services was the following: 50 per cent. among surgical patients, 25 per cent. among medical patients, 25 per cent. among others. *Staphylococcus aureus* may start large epidemics in nurseries with 50 per cent. mortality, disorganizing the whole department for several days.

Gram negative bacteria make up a large group which is highly resistant to antibiotics. They are responsible of 20–50 per cent. of hospital-acquired infections.

The main species are:

Escherichia with 11 types of *E. coli*.

Salmonella and especially *Salmonella derby* which is introduced by contaminated eggs and *Salmonella typhimurium*, usually carried by rodents. Pseudomonas and especially *Ps. aeruginosa* and *Ps. pyocyanea*, both antibiotic resistant. It is also a threat in heart operations.

Achromobacter, Moraxella, Mima, Flavobacterium, Proteus,

Perfringens, are also present in hospital infected patients and can be found in wounds, urine, blood, or spinal fluid with the possibility of severe consequences.

Futhermore, there are active types of infection which are specifically iatrogenic in the sense that they are brought to the patient either by surgical instruments or catgut, or by blood or plasma used for transfusion. These are tetanus and viral hepatitis. Spores of *Clostridium tetani* can be found anywhere and are especially resistant to heat and disinfectants. Hence the danger of epidemics of post-operative tetanus which requires a complete revision of the sterilization process and the careful testing of catgut. Blood and plasma transfusion entail the serious danger of communicating viral hepatitis. Moreover, faulty sterilization of ordinary infectious material is at the origin of outbreaks of hepatitis in hospital from time to time. Unlike tetanus which originates always in the operating block, viral hepatitis is feared at the time of most nursing procedures: it was sometimes called the 'syringe and needle disease'. The use of disposable injection material is a definite improvement. Nevertheless, bacteriological control of disposables can be done only on samples and nobody could state that 100 per cent. of syringes are germ free.

WAYS AND MEANS OF TRANSMISSION

In a general hospital, most of the species above mentioned may be found practically anywhere, but in order to combat a commonly observed attitude it is necessary to proceed systematically.

Patients

Patients carry the main stream of infection continuously entering hospital. Some are infectious patients. They cannot help disseminating bacteria and viruses coming from their saliva, their sputum, their faeces, or simply in using utensils or linen. They require strict isolation techniques. Other patients are carriers and are admitted for quite a different disease. This often happens in paediatric departments where children may be admitted for a fracture of the limb while they are incubating measles or mumps. Hence the usefulness of cubicle isolation (the lazareth) before entrance to the ward. Others become infected while in hospital but they in turn spread their infection to others, being both victims and active agents. Hence the necessity of dividing paediatric departments by partitions, creating individual cubicles for infants up to 12 or 15 months.

Personnel

All sorts of personnel are equally responsible for spreading hospital infection. Physicians, nurses, and auxiliary staff may be infected themselves and disseminate influenza, for example. They may be carriers of streptococci, staphylococci, diphtheria, or salmonella *inter alia* and periodic swabs taken from nose and throat demonstrate this fact. They may be passive transmitters of organisms from patient to patient through their hands, shoes, or dress. It is important to stress the responsibility of medical students who often neglect the antiseptic techniques painfully taught to nurses and, due to their faulty behaviour they spoil the morale and the discipline of the latter. In teaching hospitals, a large number of infections come from the carelessness of the students and their bad influence on the nursing personnel.

Visitors

They are considered in every hospital as a supplementary source of infection which is thought highly undesirable. It is true that visitors may bring bacteria and viruses into the hospital, especially during influenza epidemics. It is fully justified to provide special accommodation and routes for them in maternity and paediatric departments, but they should not be considered as scapegoats. Actually a nurse or a doctor, coming to the hospital during the morning rush hours is, bacteriologically speaking, like a visitor. The main difference, indeed important, is that they wear uniforms and sometimes change their shoes before starting to work. It is likely that streets and houses harbour much fewer pathogenic micro-organisms than hospitals. This might explain the following fact: During the 1870–71 Franco–Prussian war, slaughterhouses were used as emergency military hospitals. The post-operative infection rate was unexpectedly very low despite the incredible dirtiness and smell of the premises. It should be pointed out that dirtiness and pathogenic danger are not the same thing.

Air

There have been many disputes on the role of air versus surface as the source of infection. After the errors of the pre-Pastorian era when airborne miasmas were held responsible for all infections, surface-borne infection became a point of dogma. In fact, both ways of transmission play a role. Air itself is of course harmless but atmospheric whirling currents sustain and disseminate in all directions dust particles and droplets which may harbour dangerous organisms. It was demonstrated by Trillat that microscopic particles of fat, proteins, and carbohydrates are dissolved in floating droplets and produce an acceptable media in which bacteria can remain alive and multiply. Natural cross ventilation is certainly effective in diluting the particles, but artificial ventilation and air conditioning create problems. Filters, humidifiers, and ducts are ideal places for bacterial growth as they produce the same phenomenom as do Trillat droplets. As a consequence of neglect and lack of surveillance, an air conditioner becomes an important source of pathogenic micro-organisms which are continuously disseminated in all the artificially ventilated rooms.

In a hospital the internal air is moved horizontally along the corridors and vertically through vertical shafts, staircases, chutes, and lifts. Some governmental health agencies are rightly forbidding the building of chutes for soiled linen and garbage in hospitals. It is good practice to group the lifts in the centre of the building because a lift and its shaft is comparable to a gigantic double action pump which is dangerously leaking at each floor spreading a part of its contents through the doors. It should be remembered that the walls and shafts of chutes cannot be cleaned. An outbreak of smallpox in a German hospital was proved to be air-borne (Wehrle *et al.*, 1970).

Surfaces

All surfaces are contaminated with dust and bacteria. This is easily demonstrated in placing Petri dishes at different places. Floors are, of course, highly contaminated by shoes and wheels, but they can be washed quite often. Walls are not generally highly contaminated but cracks and spaces between ceramic tiles can harbour bacteria. Acoustic ceilings might be more dangerous because dust may fall from their holes and they are never washed. Some floors are much more contaminated than others. One must think of the dressing and septic rooms, porters, toilets, soiled linen and utility cabinets, and last but not least the floor under operating tables. From these static surfaces bacteria are carried everywhere by mobile surfaces which are essentially shoe soles, trolley wheels, brooms, and cleaning material.

Insects

It is not easy to get rid of insects such as flies and cockroaches. Ticks were responsible for a severe epidemic in an American hospital. The role of chutes cannot be overestimated because their walls are permanently stained with dirt directly coming from the patients' soiled linen. Crowds of cockroaches and ticks may feed on these excreta and wander through the wards and service rooms, being attracted by humidity and smell.

Dangerous Areas

Areas where soiled linen and utensils are permanently brought in are more contaminated than others. The laundry, the reception counter and the scrubbing-up of the Central Supply department, housekeeping spaces, toilets, sinks, septic operating rooms, infectious wards, the urology department, the intensive care unit, are the main areas of hospital contamination.

VICTIMS

Each individual staying in a hospital is proven to be a victim of hospital infection but some are much more vulnerable than others. Infants and elderly are especially endangered. Not so long ago, the admission of children was feared because it was well known that a young child could successfully catch a sequence of diseases while in hospital. The elderly suffer from more insidious forms of infection such as congestion of the lungs, sores, parotitis, urinary infection, from which they often die. Patients with tracheotomy, cystostomy, or a mere bladder catheter left over 72 hours, require special care, but the most vulnerable patients are prematures, burned and aplastics accompanying leukaemia and organ transplantations. The latter requires an intensive exposition to ionizing radiations in order to suppress any immune reaction. Therefore, such a patient, if exposed to a mild infectious source, may be killed in a few days. For such cases, special rooms and equipment and highly trained personnel are an absolute necessity.

THE FIGHT AGAINST HOSPITAL INFECTION

Nowadays the different facets of the hospital infection problem are well identified. The building of large industrial plants which require a dustless environment demonstrated that it is technically possible to manage a large volume in which there is not one particle whose size is greater than one micron and where hundreds of people are working. Filters, laminar ventilation inlets and outlets, and dustless garments exist. The application of these strict techniques is difficult in hospital but it is already a common practice in special centres for allergic and aplastic, premature and burned patients. Nobody would seriously recommend such techniques to an entire hospital, however it is possible to lead the fight against the intolerable scourge of hospital infection without spending too much money and imposing sophisticated techniques on the personnel.

The fight should be directed on two fronts:

1. A continuous action for which the personnel is mainly responsible. This essentially requires an attitude of mind and permanent good will.
2. A favourable environment for which the role of the architect and the engineer is essential; they must show competence and humility because it is necessary to know the best solutions and also to abandon any individualistic idea of perfectionism.

Personnel Action

The most important permanent action is to be directed to individuals such as patients, staff, and visitors. Patients should be kept clean, but specially if they are bedridden, frequent bacteriological controls should be made on axillae, groin, and perineal skin, nose and throat, urine, and surgical wounds. The shaving of hair should be encouraged on explaining its importance. Pyjamas must be autoclaved and telephone receivers thoroughly cleaned. The cleansing of the room must insist on bed areas, wash-basins, and toilets. The personnel should be periodically checked. Specific immunization must be carried out. Swabs should be taken from nose and pharynx. Any infectious episode of the skin, the upper respiratory tract, or the alimentary tract must be notified. The crucial role the personnel has to play requires constant training and strict supervision.

Posters in waiting halls and corridors should explain to visitors that they have to follow the regulations enacted in order to protect their relatives and themselves.

It is useless to insist on the perfect sterilization of instruments, dressings, linen and utensils used by physicians and nurses. Any reliance on the use of antibiotics as an excuse for neglectful techniques should be discouraged. The cleaning of anaesthesic apparatus and accessories is often poorly done. Masks, valves, and intratracheal tubes should be thoroughly sterilized and changed for each patient. Utensils and linen are often neglected when they are related only to the surface of the patient's body. This is a dangerous illusion as a contaminated oxygen tent may be as harmful as a soiled catheter. Inhalation therapy instruments and incubators for prematures require careful disinfection. The role of auxiliary personnel is often underestimated. It is frequently observed that domestic staff are carrying dirty buckets and are spilling large drops of soiled water in a sterile department. The most humble tools such as brooms, buckets, crockery, and towels may be dangerous. An abundance of soap and detergent is not a guarantee of sterility, as contrary to what many people think, they are very poor disinfectants in themselves.

It is rare that food and water be the source of hospital infection except during outbreaks of food poisoning which are not specific to hospitals.

Cleaning of premises goes without saying but special

attention should be paid to toilets, bathrooms, service rooms, lifts, and laundry.

STERILIZATION FACTORS

Moist and dry heat are the classical forms of sterilization. Ethylene oxide is used for medical instruments which would be damaged by heat, but for the cleansing of fomites and surfaces, chemicals are used. The main are alcohol, chlorine, phenols (hexachlorophane), cresols, formalin, etc. An exagerated reliance is often put on soap and detergents which are not real disinfectants. In lowering the surface tension of liquids, they enable mechanical action to remove dirt and bacteria, but it should be remembered that cleansing with a detergent is in fact an exchange of a soiled surface condition for a clean surface plus a soiled detergent. Therefore wet brooms, sweepers, and buckets still harbour living organisms and care should be taken during their removal.

Infected departments, cubicles, and rooms must be disinfected. The most reliable disinfectant is still formaldehyde gas. The use of glycol (triethylene or propylene) and betapropiolactone vapour is still in an experimental stage.

ARCHITECTURAL REQUIREMENTS

The fight against infection is made considerably easier if hospital architecture follows precise rules. The lay-out of operating blocks is dictated by the definition of sterile and contaminated areas and by the avoidance of 'routes' crossing. Therefore there is a classical arrangement for the operating rooms and their annexes (nurses station, substerilization, scrub-up, anaesthesia, and recovery) which should be insisted upon. Four main routes should never cross: those followed by patients, surgeons, theatre nurses, and instruments. Any deviation from the basic layout is detrimental to the maintenance of contamination at an acceptably low level. The creativity spirit of architects may lead to disasters. There should be no more freedom or laxity in hospital architecture than in industrial plants or laboratory construction.

Special planning is also well established for maternity wards, paediatric departments, infection rooms, and intensive care units. The principles of these standard plans are dictated by the necessity of avoiding contacts between patients and between themselves and visitors. Hence small nurseries between two mothers' bedrooms, peripheral corridors, cubicles for the newborn, oxygen for the prematures, and the intensive care unit. Chutes should be abolished, dumb waiters and lifts should be grouped and always open on neutral spaces such as lobbies and surface areas.

Within the nursing unit, the location of service rooms should be seriously considered. The double corridor or racetrack design may raise the level of hospital infection in creating overcrowding of circulation spaces. The recent trend of providing toilets for each patient's room or common to two adjacent rooms is a definite improvement. The reader may find more details in specialized books and periodicals on hospital architecture.

The selection of floor coverings and wall finishes is very important. Floor coverings must be noiseless, shock resistant, nice looking, and also withstand repeated cleaning. Plastic or asphalt tiles are generally considered as good materials. However, no material can exist for a long time to repeated scrubbing with chlorine. This sometimes gives a shabby outlook to floors which are bacteriologically clean. Wall paints should be washable. Finally, the choice of appropriate design for washbasins, sinks, toilets, faucets, and all other sanitary equipment should be dictated by the facility they offer to be decontaminated in all their parts. Dust traps should be eliminated or designed in such a way that they can be easily cleaned. Attention should be given to the proper location of central services and industrial plants which are always a primary source of infection, pollution, and noise.

THE ROLE OF THE ENGINEER

The engineer has a growing role to play in a modern hospital. One of his major activities should be directed towards infection control. The importance of checking the airconditioning system has been pointed out. This involves a periodical inspection of filters, of all air handling units, air conditioner cooling coils and drip pans, refrigerators, etc. Together with the hospital bacteriologist the hospital engineer should check all washing facilities and especially the blade handle faucets of surgical hand-washing facilities. The central supply of sterile water has proved to be a source of danger because algae and micro-organisms can climb up along the pipes, making the so-called sterile water highly contaminated compared with the general water supply to which chlorine is routinely added and whose quality is regularly checked and controlled.

An important point to be discussed is the connexion between the hospital sewage system and the urban network. Before the antibiotic era, hospital effluents were highly dangerous. The large use of antibiotics seemed to alleviate the risk because they pass in the patient's urine and flow also from the rinsing of syringes. The antibiotic concentration in hospital effluents ran high and it was thought that treatment of refuse by an effective disposal plant was no more necessary. However, in recent years, strains, particularly of staphylococci have developed resistance against antibiotics. It is thus safer to provide for a disposal plant. Finally, a central incinerator should be available in which all infected soiled material is destroyed, including laboratory animal carcasses.

CONCLUSION

Infection is a constant threat to all human beings staying or working in a hospital, as far as the most vulnerable of them are concerned, infection would mean death. For a significant proportion of patients it entails more risks and a prolongation of stay. For the country it means an economic loss. The fight against infection should never stop and should not be confused with the search for cleanliness. Cleanliness is not synonymous with sterility.

Therefore auxiliary personnel should be educated in order to think in terms of infection fighting rather than of furniture polishing. Nurses should constantly bear in mind that they themselves and their patients can be sources of infection. Doctors and medical students should strictly follow hand-washing and gown-changing disciplines and not encourage faulty techniques in nursing and auxiliary personnel by their carelessness.

All personnel should notify their own infective episodes. An infection control committee should be established in order to collect statistics, to recommend measures, and to organize the personnel education programme. Architects should respect circulation patterns which have been painstakingly drawn up in order to avoid crossing of sterile and septic routes. Perhaps the most useful team is made up of the hospital bacteriologist and engineer. They must trace the origin of any infection which seems to spread and to take adequate measures to suppress it. The closest co-operation with doctors and head nurses is obviously essential.

It may be a dream to hope bringing an entire hospital to the dust-free condition of an antibiotic plant or a transistor factory, but no effort should be spared to protect patients against lethal danger and increased risk.

SELECTED BIBLIOGRAPHY FOR FURTHER READING

American Hospital Association (1970) *Infection Control in the Hospital*, Chicago.

Baine, W. B. (1973) Institutional Salmonellosis, *J. infect. Dis.*, **128**, 357.

Bhatia, C. K. (1971) Hospital-acquired infections, *New Engl. J. Med.*, **284**, 338.

Baylet, R., et Dauchy, S. (1966) Infections et surinfections dans quelques services hospitaliers dakarois, *Rev. Hyg.*, *Méd. soc.*, **14**, 1, 53.

Charter, D. (1971) Housekeeper is key member of infection control team, *Can. Hosp.*, **48**, 44.

Clamageran, A. (1966) L'infirmière face aux problémes d'infection et de surinfection en milieu hospitalier. Remédes préconisés, *Rev. Hyg. Méd. soc.*, **14**, 1, 41.

Colbeck, J. C. (1962) Control of infections in hospitals, American Hospital Association, *Hospital Monograph Series*, No. 12, Chicago.

Davidson, A. L. et al. (1971) Ward design in relation to post-operative wound infection, *Brit. med. J.*, **1**, 72.

Environmental aspects of the hospital (1966) Vol. 1, *Infection Control*, Washington, U.S.P.H.S., **7**, 67.

Feingold, D. S. (1970) Hospital-acquired infection, *New Engl. J. Med.*, **283**, 1384.

Greene, V. W. (1969, 1970) Microbiological contamination control in hospitals, *Hospitals*, several articles.

Journal of Hospital Research (1968) **6**, No. 1, pp. 9, 15, 25.

Le Riche, William Harding, et al. (1966) *The Control of Infection in Hospitals*, Toronto.

Litsky, B. Y. (1966) Results of bacteriological surveys highlight problem areas in hospitals, *Hospital Mgmt*, **101**, 3, 82.

Llewelyn-Davies, R., and Macaulay, H. M. C. (1966) Hospital planning and administration, *Wld Hlth Org. Monogr. Ser.*, No. 54.

Mochii, E. (1970) The pattern of hospital-acquired infection in the teaching hospitals of East and West Africa, *E. Afr. med. J.*, **47**, 639.

Premières journées internationales de perfectionement en Hygiène hospitalière (1970) (Rouen, 13–17 mai 1968). *Rev. Hyg. Méd. soc.*, **18**, 181.

Report (1963) of a conference held in London 19.6.1963 at the Royal Society of Health, *Prevention of hospital infection. The personal factor*, London.

Report (1966) du 44e Congrés d'Hygiène, Médecine du Travail et Médecine légale, 1966. La Prévention de l'infection et de la surinfection dans les services hospitaliers, *Arch. belges Méd. soc.*, **24**, I. 2.

Sen, R. (1966) Reducing hospital infection, *J. Hyg. (Camb.)*, **64**, 501.

Smylie, H. G., et al. (1971) Ward design in relation to post-operative wound infection, *Brit. med. J.*, **1**, 67.

Top, F. H. (1970) The hospital environment—a crossroads for infection, *Arch environm. Hlth*, **21**, 678.

United States Department of Health, Education, and Welfare. Public Health Service. (1970) *Isolation Techniques for Use in Hospitals*, PHS Publication No. 2054, Washington.

Vic-Dupont, J. F., et al. (1966) Documentation de la clinique des maladies infectieuses de l'Hôpital Claude-Bernard sur les surinfections hospitalières, *Rev. Hyg. Méd. soc.*, **14**, 29.

Wehrle, P. F., et al. (1970) An air-borne outbreak of smallpox in a German hospital and its significance with respect to other recent outbreaks in Europe, *Bull. Wld Hlth Org.*, **43**, 669.

Williams, Robert, Evan Owen, et al. (1966) *Hospital Infection, Causes and Prevention*, 2nd ed., London.

World Health Organization Regional Office for Europe (1973) *Report of a study on the influence of functional changes in hospital design and operation, Copenhagen 1972* (Euro 4307), Copenhagen.

45

USE OF COMPUTERS IN PUBLIC HEALTH

CHARLES D. FLAGLE

INTRODUCTION

A chapter on computers in public health written at this time is likely to be more interesting in its speculative aspects than its factual reporting of the state of practice. The excitement is in the potential impact of computing technology on public health; the highest priorities are in the development of working prototype systems that offer new—or perhaps the fruition of old—concepts in the processes of medical care and organization of services for enhancement of the health of the public.

In most cases the essence of innovation through computer technology is in the speed and volume of communications and transactions, which are by one or more orders of magnitude greater than human capacity. In the area of scientific research this has permitted enormously complex calculations that might have required many man-years of manual effort to be done in minutes. In the area of administration it is less the complexity of calculation than the speed of manipulation of information that is of interest. Our hope is to reduce time delays in processing and analysing data to provide broader data bases and lucid interpretations so that decisions may be made under less uncertainty.

The beneficiary of computers in public health may be the clinician who has available to him, prior to seeing a patient, the print-out of results of a multitest laboratory (here the prototypes do exist) or he may be the public health planner, enabled to forecast future needs by means of simulations of population growth and morbidity accompanied by trends in man-power and facilities. Or he may be the operator of a referral centre constantly apprised through a network of computer terminals of the state of need and the state of resources to meet those needs. Examples and trends in computer applications may be drawn from the health field (World Health Organization, 1968; Collen, 1966; Caceras, 1966), but in the last two instances, having to do with planning and administration, one must look outside the health field for ideas of possibilities.

The public health administrator, concerned over potentials of computer technology for his field, would do well to examine the experiences to date in other ventures, particularly business and industrial administration. He might begin by reading the collection of papers presented at a recent conference on computers, edited by Myers (1968), who observes in his introduction: 'In 1955 there were only 10 or 15 computers installed, worth about $30 million. By 1965, the total had reached nearly 31,000, worth $78 billion. Projections to 1970 indicate that there will be 60,000 computers in use by that time, to be valued at $18 billion. Therefore, within a few years no business firm will be unaffected by computers, especially with the spread of computer utilities selling services and programs to smaller firms.'

He might have added health services to his list of those affected, although it is significant to note that health services are not among the illustrations of managerial users subsequently discussed by Myers. This is not to say that the computer industry and health services are not aware of each other's existence. The use of computers in biomedical research is long established. Some notion of the scope and complexity—as well as some implications of long-term usefulness in administration —may be gained from Ledley (1965). By way of introduction his third chapter gives a description of the working of computing equipment and some definitions of terms.

Ledley is concerned primarily with the computer as a tool of research, an extension of the analytical capability of the statistician and applied mathematician. Much impetus for development of computing equipment and programming languages has come from this motivation. A little later comes the notion of the computer as business machine, an extension of the paperwork capabilities of the corporation treasurer and accountant. To meet requirements of this type one needs machines and a computer language such as COBOL, adapted to simple operations on large masses of data and relatively easy to use over a wide range of equipment.

A discussion of the programming requirements for which FORTRAN, ALGOL, and COBOL have been developed is given by Bailey (1967).

The differing requirements of research computation and business office procedures have led in some cases to two separate and incompatible computer systems within the same organization. Typically in both systems the flow of work into the machine is controlled administratively by the computer centre, operating as a service organization processing batches of data according to programmes prepared by or for it. The user of the service is not involved with equipment, but transports or phones his data to the centre, receiving print-out results a matter of hours or days later.

It remained for the field of education (Kemeny and Kurtz, 1968) to provide impetus for development of another concept of computer use, now rapidly developing and known as 'time sharing'. Under this type of system remote terminals, such as teletype or cathode-ray tubes, may be used to transmit instructions and data directly to a large computer. Since the speed of processing is much greater than the rate any one individual can communicate into the terminal, it is possible for a number of users, of the order of 30–50, to share the same central computer system simultaneously. This development has had enormous effects on users and their methods of working. Costs have been lowered by an order of magnitude to $5.00–$8.00 per hour. Further, the user, receiving responses to his data inputs in a matter of seconds, is immediately aware of errors in his programme or inputs and can 'debug' without delay, unlike batch processing systems, in which he may have to wait for several days only to learn of the flaw. Another aspect of time sharing that has implications for diffusion of computer usage is the ability to share programmes. The owner of one terminal may introduce into the central computer memory a programme he has devised, identified by a unique code name. Once done this same programme may be called up for use on any other terminal sharing the same central processor.

The importance of time sharing to health administrators is discussed by White (1968). We shall say more about the administrative possibilities of all this in a later section on 'on line, real time computers', but first we should look at the information flow aspects of public health and the present state of the art of computer usage in the field.

CURRENT COMPUTER USE IN PUBLIC HEALTH

In the foregoing the evolution of computer use has been described in three phases:

1. A tool for basic research involving complex mathematical analysis—solution of differential equations, statistical analysis.

2. Routine, tabulation, and computation—for business, accounting, and reporting.

3. On line, real time administrative aid with remote terminal devices.

By and large public health usage is in the second phase with a few research projects in the third. Some traditional aspects of public health are intensively involved in information processing, e.g. vital statistics, licensing and certification, and clinic operations. The recent assignment to state health departments in the United States of responsibility for some administrative aspects of Medicaid and comprehensive health-planning legislation has given impetus to computer development to handle the burden of claims processing and analyses of health-services utilization. In the State of California there have been some remarkable advances in development of a computer centre within the Division of Research of the Department of Public Health.[1] Apart from the progressive character of the Department and recent pressures towards administrative data processing for participation in Federal programmes, attention on potentials and requirements for data systems was focused by a series of studies on applications of aerospace industry techniques to public problems carried out in 1965. One study of requirements for a state-wide, inter-agency data system concluded that agencies should develop their own computer centres, guided by a set of compatibility rules that would permit, through a central switching unit, each agency to have access to data banks and programmes of other agencies.

Thus encouraged, the Department of Public Health expanded its existing capabilities, acquired a computer, and established relations for subcontracting to commercial computer services. With an annual budget of approximately a million dollars, the centre is organized into four major line sections: an Operations Section (including keypunch units and

computer and tabulating machine operators), a Control Section, a Programming Section, and an Applications Development Section. The last-named section is intended to be the centre's mechanism for growth into new services, exploitation of new computer and management techniques, and performance of cost/benefit studies. The scope of data-processing requirements for various programmes within the Department[2] are listed below in order of the intensity services:

1. Health Facilities and Services
   (a) Health facilities planning and construction
      (i) Compilation and analysis of health facility utilization data
      (ii) Storage and analyses of audited construction costs
   (b) Licensing and certification
      Lists and tabulations of facilities, their size, location function, and inspection data
   (c) Licensing and certification of clinical laboratories
      (i) Listing of laboratories and directors
      (ii) Statistical tabulations of laboratory data

2. Vital Statistics Registration
   (a) Keypunching and verification of vital records
   (b) Data reduction, analysis, and reporting on birth, death, marriage, and divorce
   (c) Retrieval of data for individual or agency use

3. General Service to other Agencies
   Data processing service and support to special projects and to other State, Federal, and Local Agencies

4. Planning and Support
   (a) Computational services to research
      Health surveillance data
   (b) Health man-power data bank
   (c) Statistical reports to local health agencies

5. Chronic Diseases
   (a) Mortality experience reporting on categories linear or demographic basis
   (b) Tumour registry
      (i) Updating of case files
      (ii) Assist in evaluations
      (iii) Report preparation

6. Air Sanitation
   (a) Data processing for Bureau of Air Sanitation
   (b) Analysis and reporting for studies

The programmes above account for about 90 per cent. of the Data Center's budget. The remainder is accounted for by the following programmes: Crippled Children Services; Radiological Health; Communicable Diseases; Occupational Health; Food and Drug; Mental Retardation; Maternal and Child Health; Water Sanitation; Vector Control.

[1] The author is indebted to Dr. Robert Dyar, Director of Research, Dr. Louis Saylor, Director of the Department of Public Health, and to Mr. Stephen Gibbens, Chief of the Data Processing Center, for opportunities to follow the development of this Center and for descriptions of its current status.

[2] Source: State of California, Department of Public Health, Short and Long Term Data Processing Plan.

In addition to data-processing activities in the health-department programmes described above, activities which tend to extend the hand of the traditional public health functions—in effect to add the equivalent of more clerks to the system—some programmes are under development which can add a new dimension to the administrative process. In its delegated responsibility for monitoring claims payments under Title XIX programme the Department has become involved in a large volume of transactions. Each of the transactions involves matters of patient eligibility, recording medical decisions and prescriptions ordered, updating of records, and payment for services. The process calls for rapid file search and communications; it poses a new set of problems for computer technology and simultaneously opens the door to new possibilities in health services and administration.

The timing of demands on the computer centre becomes the prerogative of a host of users, the physicians, pharmacists, fiscal intermediaries. Data retrieval and computation are needed as part of an ongoing process in the real world—hence computing equipment, its terminals, and its data banks must be 'on-line' operating in real time.

In the health field such systems are in experimental stages. At the time of writing only preliminary reports are available (see Derry, 1968). We have as yet no prototype to emulate but a number of innovative experiments where implications for the future must be pondered [see also CHAPTER 3].

EXTENSION OF COMPUTER USE TO MANAGEMENT DECISIONS

To this point we have spoken of computer use as a substitute or aid for human calculation, accounting, or filing. The assumption has been one of replacement of a machine for human labour, without basically affecting the nature or purpose of the work. New technologies are often conceived in that way, sometimes blinding us to their ultimate potential. Marshall McLuhan has exemplified our tendency to freeze our vision by verbally tagging new technology to the past; hence the steam engine in use became an 'iron horse' and the internal-combustion engine yielded simply a 'horseless carriage'. We are perhaps doing the same thing when we designate our early effort in computer application as automated data processing—computerized patient histories. The very terms bind us to administrative systems that have taken their form in part from the technological limitations of the past. So let us accept good naturedly some of the jargon and the acronyms of the computer scientists. At first glance they may seem meaningless, but the reader is invited to give them meaning in his own field. As noted earlier, the great fascination is with time sharing and on-line, real-time, control systems. Carroll (1967) has defined the terms clearly: 'The following is advanced as a working definition of an on-line, real-time system. Remotely located transaction-origination stations are connected directly ("on-line") to the central processor; and transactions are processed immediately upon origination in ("real-time"), subject only to delays resulting from the processing of the transaction itself and from queuing behind transactions of earlier origination or otherwise higher priority. To fulfill the requirement of "real-time", these delays must be negligible in the context of the particular application. Often, there is maintained a backlog of lower priority "background" programs which occupy the central processor when it is otherwise idle, that is, until a real-time transaction requires processing and interrupts the background operation. It is this background compatibility that makes on-line, real-time systems an extension of rather than a substitute for conventional "batch"-oriented processing.

'One popular application of these systems is in providing remote inquiry of a central status file. Real-time inquiry is the simplest form of management employment. Frequently, but not always, the file is updated in real-time as well. Operations, or more generally, process control, is a more advanced application. If the transactions report changes in the state of the environment, the system is an on-line, real-time control system. The purpose is to obtain control directions before the states have changed materially, so the effect is response to events "while they are happening".'

Two industrial examples of the use of such systems are noteworthy. One is the airlines SABRE system (Parker, 1965) of reservation of seating space. The current state of available space on a future flight may be queried from a terminal, and if a booking is then made the available seats are reduced by one upon instructions from the same terminal. The operator of the terminal has first searched a data base (reservation status) department constantly up to date in the face of transactions from many geographically dispersed terminals. He has, by deciding to book a space, caused the central processor to perform an elementary computation, leaving the data base current after his own transaction.

Substitute for 'airline seat' the term 'clinic appointment' or 'hospital bed'. These are the simplest analogies, but substantially more difficult computations may be brought to bear. The author has a programme for screening asthma using data of Collen et al. (1964). Here the data bank contains a record of confirming diagnosis for hundreds of patients identified by their 'yes' or 'no' answers to a set of six questions. The input to the programme is the pattern of 'yes' or 'no' answer of a new patient. The first step in the programme is a search and print-out of the accumulated data for that pattern, the number of confirmed positives and negatives having the particular pattern and the total number of confirmed positive and negative asthmatics in the data bank. The next step in the programme is to compute the likelihood ratio, the ratio of the percentage of confirmed positives with the given answer pattern, to the percentage of confirmed negatives with the pattern. A high likelihood ratio indicates that further action should be taken for the patient at hand—how high the action threshold is a policy decision that could be aided by further computations taking into account the prevalence of asthma and some economic measures of following costs and benefits (see Flagle, 1968). The outcome of the present case furnishes new data to the data base and gives weight to calculations for the next case having the same pattern of answers to the programme questions.

A second commercial application is the Westinghouse Telecomputer System. Through a dedicated world-wide network connecting company offices and warehouses, the existing stocks of any company product may be located and orders filled from the most convenient store. A transaction, say for an electric motor, corrects stock levels at the shipping warehouse and may check to see if this level has fallen below a threshold for replenishment. In effect, the company has pooled its inventories and has taken advantage of the statistical law of large numbers to reduce total reserve stocks required. Substitute for 'electric motor' the medical supplies of a clinic or hospital—or within a region the 'inventory' of medical and nursing skills.

Somewhere in the SABRE and the Telecomputer developments are the makings of a communication and control system for public health—or better the beginnings, for as management systems go both the industrial examples given are, for all their electronic complexity, the implementation of simple notions. In both cases the system waits for arrival of a potential customer who states his need. The data bank searched is the record of available resources to meet the need. The computation involved thereafter is only the adjustment of recorded inventory levels resulting from the transaction, if one takes place. It is the wide dispersion of points of inquiry or the source of supply that dictates the need for the communication and computing network. The inertness of the inventory of electric motors or future airline seats diminishes the pressure of immediate inventory adjustment—the dynamics of the system are mainly related to rapid completion of a paper transaction. Here is where some basic problems of public health administration exceed the demands of industrial administration.

Our resource inventory is one of costly human skills or complex facilities whose idleness carries a high opportunity cost. Our demands arise from accident or illness of people or the development of hazards to their health or safety. Where need exists it must often be sought out, a process of active surveillance rather than a passive waiting for demand to appear. One might press the comparison further, but to do so would only strengthen an already obvious conclusion: advanced computer systems in use in industrial application are not adequate for the requirements of a sophisticated management system in public health. The difficult fact to be faced is that a great amount of system development work—measured in millions of dollars and many man-years of specialized skills—will be required to exploit the potentials of computer and communications technology for planning and administering of health services. A further imperative of technology—here the word imperative is used in the sense of Galbraith in *The New Industrial State* (1967), a book very relevant to our considerations here—is the need for highly formalized planning. In this case the planning of computer hardware and programmes must be accompanied by or preceded by a formalization of administrative and planning procedures themselves. This is administrative research and development, it may be aided by the computer-system analyst, but it remains the ultimate responsibility of the public health administrator.

At this stage of the simultaneous development of computer technology and evolution of public health administration it is possible to set forth some goals for which we can jointly strive.

GOALS OF COMPUTER USE IN PUBLIC HEALTH

Having reviewed some of the characteristics, capabilities, and problems of computers and their applications to public health, we might now ask 'What should be the substance and organization of a programme for further development and exploitation of this technology for the benefit of health?' We can begin to formulate such a programme by setting forth some of the purposes and procedures of public health

administration, examining the role of information in the administrative and planning processes.

The mission of public health to protect and promote the health of the population conjures up the vision of a large-scale cybernetic system of sensing, communication, and control. In the short term it envisions observation mechanisms for constantly sensing health needs and for maintaining cognizance of resources, their capacities, capabilities, and state of utilization. Given such observations, and a set of norms of performance for the system, the next step in the cybernetic process would be to detect error signals, that is to say, departures from norms. In a well-developed system then error signals would lead directly to a course of action to correct the error. Following such action the original observation mechanisms are brought back into play to detect effects of the action on error. The cybernetic process is nicely exemplified by the speed-control governor on an engine or by the maintenance of homeostasis in the human body. It is less obvious, but nevertheless real, in the day-to-day administrative processes of assigning personnel to tasks, maintaining inventories, and scheduling patients into clinic services. For such a system to function it is essential not only that resources be adequate to demand but also that all the processes of observation, communication, and control be effective. To be effective means that relevant and complete observations are made, that correct inferences are drawn about required action, and that action is ordered within the time frame of the requirements.

The description of an administrative system so far has concerned short-term operations, in economist's terms the allocation of existing resources. The role of computers in such a process is to aid or to enable the processing of observations and the simplification of routine decisions. Such a role is evident in the examples of data-processing functions in California, previously noted. Ideally, the short-term operations should be routinized to free the administrator from short-term decisions for concentration on the difficult problems of intermediate range decisions—the planning and creation of new resources for changing or unmet needs.

The role of the computer in the planning process is less obvious then in short-term operations, but once again the cybernetic system serves as a model to show the functions of observation, communication, analysis, and control. In planning the term 'norms' is replaced by 'goals', or by some projected set of future needs. The error signal becomes the gap between future needs and present resources—or the projection of future resources. Then comes the process of weighing alternative strategies for actions during the intervening period in order to create a set of resources to meet projected needs.

The computer has two major roles to play in the planning process described so far. First is the data-processing role in collection, analysis, and projection of health needs and resource capabilities. Second is the process of simulation or gaming, in which the outcomes of alternative strategies may be played out in condensed time, thus giving the planner some insight into the influence of the variables he can control. Through a set of computer routines described by Balintfy *et al.* (1966) it is possible to simulate, in repeated trials, the behaviour of complex systems in time, where a sequence of events in hours or years of real time may be run through in minutes or seconds. The bulk of applications of simulation and gaming is to be found in military or business contexts where competition is the hallmark of the process. A few examples of experimental simulations in the health field are reported, notably Thompson and Fetter (1963) in their model of hospital maternity services, and Flagle (1966) in a model of flow of individuals in a population represented as a set of age-sex cohorts, through a set of health services in response to cohort-specific utilization characteristics. The model has several uses; first, for a given population, to gain insight into the statistical variations in occupancy of various services and facilities, such as intensive-care units, out-patients clinics, and extended-care facilities. In another application for long-term planning the same model can be used to simulate future demands, given some projections of fertility and mortality. Another potential use of simulation is as a vehicle for training. As in the case of war games or business games, the player may intervene as the simulation progresses and make decisions about allocation of resources or courses of action. He can then in a short time see the results of his choices.

With this picture of a public health system, aided in its communication, control, planning, and to some extent training processes by computers and sophisticated information-processing programmes, it is possible to state some specific activities for which system development should be pushed:

1. Surveillance and forecast of population health need simultaneously with surveillance of resources capacities and utilization. This leads for the short term to systems of patient referral and co-ordination of case management. In the long term it provides the bases for planning by pointing up unmet needs.

2. Construction of patient data bases. One primary use is for retrieval of an individual record for care of that individual.

A record is, detaching the individual's identity from his record, the basis for development of statistics for diagnosis and programme evaluation.

3. Automation of established administrative routines and development of new management systems.

At the time of writing there are many more efforts under way to exploit computer technology for public health than have been reported yet in the literature. The efforts are often local and sporadic. We are speaking of system development rather than research, and there has been relatively little funding of development in the health field—in contrast to a large investment in basic research. Yet development is a costly business; technological development of a prototype system usually costs ten to twenty times as much as the research whose new knowledge makes the development possible. We have seen so far in all fields, including health, that computer development and applications take longer and cost more than original estimates, and ultimately involve a heavy commitment on the part of management in terms of its own intellect and time. Where computer use is intended for an administrative or planning process it cannot be brought into being if the system it is intended to assist either does not exist or has not formalized its own procedures.

To sum up, computer technology has great promise for public health administration and planning. But the fulfillment of the promise is not something to be delivered to us by the computer specialist alone. A complex of skills, and organizational mechanisms—what Galbraith calls in industry the 'technostructure'—is required. If progress is to be sure, the public health administrator must not be far from the centre of effort.

REFERENCES AND FURTHER READING

Bailey, N. T. J. (1967) *The Mathematical Approach to Biology and Medicine*, New York.

Balintfy, J. L. *et al.* (1966) *Computer Simulation Techniques*, New York.

British Medical Journal leading article (1973) What future for computers? *Brit. med. J.*, **2**, 570.

Buckley, J. D. (1973) A computer based medical records system, *Methods Inf. Med.*, **12**, 137.

Caceras, C. A. (1966) Automatic analysis of the electrocardiogram as a service to the community and to the practising physician, in *Proceedings on Automated Data Processing in Hospitals*, ed. Dessau, E., Copenhagen.

Carroll, D. C. (1967) Implication of on-line, real-time systems in management decision-making, in *The Impact of Computers on Management*, ed. Myers, E., pp. 140–67, Cambridge, Mass.

Cheek, Robert C. (1967) TOPS—The Westinghouse Teletype Order Processing and Inventory Control System. Presented at the Business Equipment Manufacturers Association Conference, 1967.

Collen, M. F. (1966) Periodic health examinations using an automated multi-test laboratory, *J. Amer. med. Ass.*, **195**, 830.

Collen, M. F. *et al.* (1964) Automated multiphasic screening and diagnosis, *Amer. J. publ. Hlth*, **54**, 744.

Crystal, R. (1968) Developing a central file of facilities for long term care in the United States, *Publ. Hlth Rep. (Wash.)*, **83**, No. 5.

Derry, J. R. (1968) An information system for health facilities planning, *J. Amer. publ. Hlth Ass.*, **58**, 8.

Eden, M. *et al.* (1973) Feasibility of computer screening of blood films for the detection of malaria parasites, *Bull. Wld Hlth Org.*, **48**, 211.

Feldstein, M. S., Piot, M. A., and Sundaresan, J. K. (1973) Resource allocation model for public health planning: a case study for tuberculosis control, *Bull. Wld Hlth Org.*, **48**, Suppl.

Flagle, C. D. (1966) Simulation techniques applicable to public health administration, in *Proceedings of the Simulation in Business and Public Health First Annual Conference of American Statistical Association*, New York Area Chapter and Public Health Association of New York City.

Flagle, C. D. (1968) A decision theoretical comparison of three procedures of screening for a single disease, in *Proceedings of the Fifth Berkeley Symposium on Mathematical, Statistics and Probability*, Berkeley, Cal.

Galbraith, J. K. (1967) *The New Industrial State*, New York.

Garwin, R. L. (1968) Impact of information handling systems on quality and access to medical care, *Publ. Hlth Rep. (Wash.)*, **13**, No. 5.

Goodwin, C. S. (1972) Medical information systems, *Lancet*, **ii**, 871.

Hearn, Catherine R., and Bishop, J. M. (1970) Computer model simulating medical care in hospital, *Brit. med. J.*, **1**, 396.

Kemeny, J. G., and Kurtz, T. E. (1968) Dartmouth time sharing, *Science*, **162**, 3850.

Ledley, R. S. (1965) *Use of Computers in Biology and Medicine*, New York.

Myers, E. (1968) *The Impact of Computers on Management*, Cambridge, Mass.

Ockenden, J. M., and Bodenham, J. K. E. (1970) *Focus on Medical Computer Development*, London.

Parker, R. W. (1965) The SABRE system, *Datamation*, **11**, No. 10.

Smiley, J. R., *et al.* (1973) The use of computers in assisting school health programmes in Ontario, *Can. J. Publ. Hlth*, **64**, 141.

Smith, C. (1972) Computer programme to estimate recurrence risks for multifactorial familial disease, *Brit. med. J.*, **1**, 495.

Thompson, J. D., *et al.* (1963) Computer simulation of the activity in a maternity suite, in *Actes de la 3ème Conférence Internationale de Recherche Opérationnelle, Oslo 1963*, Paris.

Ulmara, K. (1971) Epidemiological model of typhoid fever, *Bull. Wld Hlth Org.*, **45**, 53.

Whitby, L. G., and Lutz, W. (1971) *Principles and Practice of Medical Computing*, Edinburgh.

White, D. (1968) in World Health Organization Regional Office for Europe (1968) Seminar on the Public Health Uses of Computers, London, 17–21 June 1968 (Mimeographed. Original: English).

World Health Organization (1974) The work of WHO in 1973, *Wld Hlth Org. Off. Rec.*, No. 213, 133.

World Health Organization Regional Office for Europe (1974) *Report of a European Conference on Medical Computing* (CSO1(2)), Copenhagen.

Since its inception in 1972, MEDLARS (medical literature analysis and retrieval) has provided a computer based service for the retrieval of bibliographies on the huge store of information in the computer data base. During 1974, the MEDLINE system was developed; it resembles a computerized airline reservations system. It has a number of terminals situated at remote sites, and by operating the teleprinter keyboard, the searcher can receive an instant list of bibliographical references. This is operated by WHO from tapes received from the U.S. National Library of Medicine. These are also used for the compilation of the Index medicus (see also p. 668).

46

EVALUATION AS A TOOL IN HEALTH PLANNING AND MANAGEMENT

MICHAEL D. WARREN

'The three main concerns confronting us are with health services; with health conditions; and with the concept of health itself; in all three we face important tasks of revaluation.'

Sir Geoffrey Vickers, 1958

Introduction

This chapter is focused on operational and service problems; it is concerned with the process of evaluation from the point of view of an administrator responsible for the management of a health service. To maintain and improve existing services and at the same time develop new programmes within his limited resources is the perpetual quandary of such administrators in every area of the world. There are reasons and some evidence to suggest that the application of even the simplest principles of evaluation (as outlined below) to the management of current health services or programmes would show how efficiency and effectiveness could be increased and resources re-deployed.

An essential part of good management is that every person in the service or organization knows: (1) to whom he is responsible; (2) for whom he is responsible; and (3) for what he is responsible. If each person is set quantifiable objectives that he is expected to achieve within a stated period of time then that person will know exactly what it is he has to contribute to the service, and furthermore, will know the progress he is making. Managers, their staff, and the field workers must go beyond subjective assessments of believing they are doing a worthwhile job, to objective assessments of the results of their work. For such assessments it is necessary to concentrate on measurable results and not vague generalities. The emphasis, therefore, in evaluation is on measurement; but this is not to state that all that is important in health planning is measurable. Immeasurable and profound components are the exercise of judgement and realistic sensitivity to the feelings of others. Statistics cannot replace judgement, nor can judgement replace statistics [see also CHAPTER 3].

Definitions

There are no internationally accepted definitions of some of the terms used in describing components of health planning and evaluation, so it is necessary to state the sense in which the terms are used here. In doing this an attempt has been made to avoid jargon, and what is perhaps a worse fault, attributing an idiosyncratic and peculiar meaning to words in everyday use.

Health planning is the systematic process of defining the health problems of a community, of ascertaining needs, of estimating the availability and supply of resources and of identifying and assessing the relevant social interactions in order to suggest alternative plans for deploying services to meet needs, and to forecast the probable achievements, benefits, costs, drawbacks, and repercussions of each alternative. Health planning must be related to a community which may be the world population, a nation, or the population of an administrative area (e.g. a municipality), or a factory or school, and to a specified period of time. Health planning may encompass all the health problems of the community or concentrate on a single problem. Health planning is the diagnosis of and the prescribing for community health problems; as in clinical medicine, diagnosis before prescription is a sound maxim.

Management is the process of planning, organizing, directing, motivating, controlling and evaluating a department, service, or programme. It is a specific kind of work with its own technology and expertise, although most of management technology has grown out of other disciplines, especially economics, accountancy, statistics, operational research, and the social and behavioural sciences (Stewart, 1968; Gatherer and Warren, 1971).

Evaluation is an essential part of health planning and management, for it enables each to be based on an analysis of data and of measured experience. Evaluation relates results to objectives; it is the process of relating the achievements of a service or programme to the results predicted in the plan. It, therefore, measures the effectiveness and efficiency of a service or programme (Suchman, 1967; Donabedian, 1969; Cochrane, 1972).

Operational research is a term that has been used in a variety of ways. It is defined by the Operational Research Society as 'the application of the methods of science to complex problems arising in the direction and management of large systems of men, machines, materials and money in industry, business, government, and defence. The distinctive approach is to develop a scientific model of the system, incorporating measurements of factors such as chance and risk, with which to predict and compare the outcomes of alternative decisions, strategies or controls. The purpose is to help management determine its policy and actions scientifically.' In health services research, however, some authors have used the term in a broader way; for example, Morris (1967) defines operational research as 'the systematic study of health services with a view to their improvement'.

A plan is a detailed scheme for accomplishing a purpose drawn up before the programme is started. Ideally, in health planning, alternative plans for accomplishing the same purpose should be considered. A plan should contain all the details set out under the definition of 'health planning' above.

A programme is the *accepted* plan of operational activity. It is made up of a number of activities and may involve several related specific objectives.

A service is a term used with two quite distinct meanings. First, it can be used, as it has so far in this chapter, to describe groups of personnel employed and the facilities and equipment used by an organization or department for some over-all, common objective (e.g. health service, nursing service, rehabilitation service, etc.). Such a service may contribute to a number of programmes: or, a programme of a health department might include the creation of such a service. Secondly, service can be used to describe the performance of a duty or function to a community, patient, or client.

Objectives are the results that it is intended will be achieved within a finite period of time by a specified activity, service, or programme (or any part of a programme). Objectives can be both general and specific, the latter often being components of the former (see below). Some writers equate 'aims' with general objectives and 'targets' with specific objectives; some use the word 'goals' instead of objectives (Hilleboe and Schaefer, 1967).

The Planning and Management Cycle

The cycle of health planning and management is shown in FIGURE 108. The community, to which all effective planning

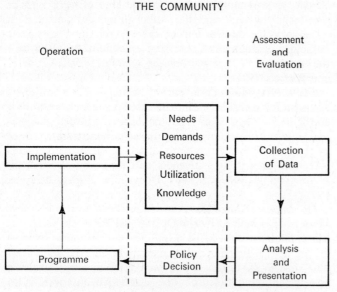

FIG. 108. The planning and management cycle.

and management must refer, has known and unknown needs and will be making demands for health services, but will only have limited resources and knowledge. The first step is the ascertainment of all relevant data; these may be already available or they may have to be specially collected. The data must then be analysed and presented to the policy-making authority. Sometimes this will be the health service ad-

ministrator, but sometimes the policy-making authority will be a board or committee of the central or local government, or of a private organization in the community. Once a policy decision has been taken (and this involves a plan being selected and adopted as the programme), the programme must be implemented. This is usually done by the development of a service to the community, but it may be the alteration of a current service, the withdrawing of a service, or further research within the community. Whatever way the programme is to be implemented, its purpose is either to meet needs and demands, to re-allocate resources or to gain new data about the community. It is therefore necessary to repeat or extend the process of measurement in order to see if change has come about. The cycle then starts again with the evaluation of the new or altered service. The basis of good management is the conscious following of each step in the cycle.

THE PROCESS OF EVALUATION

A systematic procedure should be followed in evaluating health services and programmes. The basic steps of this procedure are set out in FIGURE 109. Although it will not always be possible, and sometimes not even necessary, to obtain all the data discussed below, each stage of the procedure must always be considered whatever the programme and however elusive the data may be. The theoretical concept of evaluation is relatively simple; the practical application can be very difficult. Too often these difficulties have been used as excuses for not starting, but the right approach is to begin; for once begun, experience, techniques, and data grow rapidly. It is better to start even if only with the evaluation of a few aspects of some activities of a programme, than never to have started at all.

1. Statement of objectives

2. Definition of Measurements and Standards

    (*a*) Health Status and Needs of the Community
    (*b*) Coverage and Utilization of Present Services
    (*c*) Resources
    (*d*) Activities and Attitudes of Staff and Clients
    (*e*) Standards of Practice (Process)
    (*f*) Impact, Effectiveness and Output
    (*g*) Costs and Efficiency

3. Collection of Data

4. Collation and Analysis of Data

5. Presentation of Results and Recommendations

FIG. 109. Basic steps in evaluation.

STATEMENT OF OBJECTIVES

The objectives of the programme must be clearly and specifically formulated. Two levels of objectives are distinguished. The first are the general objectives (or aims) which may or may not be measurable, and the second are the specific or component objectives which are measurable. The objectives should set out the health problem that the programme is trying to control or ameliorate and what the programme is trying to achieve.

The general objective of a health service may be to provide for a fixed expenditure the highest quality of health care and protection to a defined community by means of medical-care and public health activities. The general objective of medical-care activities might be to relieve symptoms, cure diseases, increase comfort of the ill, and shorten invalidity; and of public health activities to remove or control all adverse biological, physical, social, and psychological factors in the environment. The general objectives of medical education can be stated as the development of knowledge, skills, and attitudes necessary for the care of people in sickness and in health; such care to include the prevention and treatment of all illness and the after-care and rehabilitation of all patients in the community as well as in the hospital. A health centre may be defined as an institution providing health services to a defined community; its general objectives could include the provision of preventive and promotive health care for individuals, families, special groups, and for the community as a whole, medical care of the sick both at the health centre itself and at the patient's home and rehabilitation and after-care services in close association with the community's welfare, education, and employment services.

These statements of general objectives indicate where investigation might be directed but are not sufficiently specific for the purpose of evaluation. General objectives must be refined into a consistent series of specific objectives which can then be subjected to measurement and incorporated into a coherent system of management control (often referred to as 'management by objectives'). General objectives set out the main intentions but not the details of the 'who', 'where', 'to what extent', 'how', 'at what cost', and 'why' of the programme. These details are referred to as the specific or component objectives of the programme. They are defined in *measurable* terms of the target population and area (answers 'who?', and 'where?'), stated periods of time (answers 'when?'), tangible accomplishments (answers 'to what extent?'), activities (answers 'how?'), resources to be used (answers 'at what cost?') and expected effects upon the health status of the population (answers 'why?'). These components, with examples and references, are discussed below.

DEFINITION OF MEASUREMENT AND STANDARDS

Health Status and Needs of the Community

There is no single index of the health status of a community. The data to be studied must include the age, sex, and mobility of the population, the birth, fertility, mortality, morbidity, and disability statistics, the rates of utilization of services, figures relating to environmental and social factors, the public's knowledge of health and sickness, and attitudes to prevention and treatment and the results of surveys undertaken to measure need (United States Department of Health, Education, and Welfare, 1969; World Health Organization, 1969, 1971; Shonfield and Shaw, 1972; Warren, 1973). Although in some localities there is a paucity of such data, in many places there is an abundance. Unfortunately the data are frequently collected by a number of agencies and presented in such a diversity of forms that a coherent picture of the more important aspects of the health status and needs of the community cannot be adduced. There is need to evaluate the present collection of data in many countries and localities.

The need for medical care must be distinguished from the demand for care and from the use (or utilization) of services. Those in need of a service may perceive and acknowledge this need themselves (perceived need) or they may be defined as in need by health, medical, or nursing professionals who believe that members of the community will benefit from their advice, preventive measures, or specific therapies (these are professionally defined needs). Those in need of a service are all those people who could benefit from the service; this group must be distinguished from those who demand a service and from those who obtain it. People who need a service do not always demand it, for reasons such as not having perceived the need (e.g. a woman with a symptomless carcinoma-in-situ of the cervix of the uterus), unavailability or cost of the service, pride, apathy, or a fear or dislike of the service. People who demand a service do not always need it and may not obtain it; they may have misunderstood the scope of the service or made the wrong diagnosis of their need. So, those who utilize a service do not necessarily represent all who need and all who demand the service. In regard to medical-care services in the developed countries, it is more or less true to state that the more acute and serious the condition and the more amenable it is to treatment, the more likely it becomes that all needs are expressed correctly as demands. Conversely, the more chronic the condition and the less effective the treatment, the less likely is this to be so. Therefore, to assess the magnitude and quality of the individual's and the community's problems relating to the chronic diseases, a special survey is necessary.

To evaluate a health programme on the basis of studies of need is a simple and obvious idea. But, in the same way that defining specific objectives proves difficult in practice, so does the relating of data from studies of need to service resources and activities. First, there is considerable variation in the treatments given for many conditions; this variation is sometimes attributable to the ineffectiveness of the treatments (Cochrane, 1972). Secondly, there is uncertainty whether treatment is desirable at all in some circumstances, especially in the case of borderline abnormalities and symptomless, nonprogressive minor conditions often found in large numbers in surveys (McKeown, 1968). Thirdly, the natural histories of many overt conditions are still unknown so that the effects of intervention are unproven and may, for ethical reasons, be difficult to evaluate. Nevertheless, without base-line data evaluation cannot begin.

Coverage and Utilization of Present Services

The coverage of a health service refers to the number of people eligible for that service; the utilization of the service refers to the number of people using the service. The completeness of coverage is the proportion of the whole population in need of the benefits of the service who are eligible for the particular service under examination. All members of the population may be eligible for the service (as is the case with many of the benefits of the British National Health Service) or various eligibility requirements may be imposed. Eligibility may be defined in terms of diagnostic categories (e.g. all pregnant women may be eligible for the pre-natal and maternity services; all patients with tuberculosis may be eligible for certain services), disabilities and handicaps (e.g. the blind, the limbless, the house-bound), age (e.g. all children under 5 years; all old people over 75 years), socio-economic factors (e.g. all people with an income below a defined limit; people living within defined administrative boundaries) or by contribution requirements to a national, private, or charitable insurance-type scheme. There may be a combination of two or more restrictions. Even in countries with widely available national health services there may be additional benefits available only to certain eligible groups. Surveys are usually necessary to measure the coverage of a service in order to measure the total number of persons in need so that the proportion of those eligible can be calculated. The coverage of a hospital service may be expressed in terms of the population in its geographical catchment area, but this may vary for different specialties within the single hospital. Where alternative hospitals or specialists might be used, it will be necessary to make special calculation of the catchment areas of hospitals concerned (see, for example, Barr, 1957; Forsyth and Logan, 1960; Airth and Newell, 1962). Not everyone eligible for a service will necessarily use the service, therefore it is necessary to measure the utilization of each service. Figures of utilization are often available in annual and other reports of services but are of only limited use in evaluation if the coverage and needs are not known.

A simple example to illustrate these points is an immunization programme for young children. In England all children are eligible for vaccination against, *inter alia*, diphtheria, pertussis, and poliomyelitis; it is recommended that each child should be protected by the age of 2 years. The coverage of this part of the programme is therefore 100 per cent. of all children under the age of 2 years; the utilization figure will be that proportion of children under the age of 2 years who have been fully protected; nationally this figure is between 75 and 80 per cent. Another example refers to a survey of the handicapped (Harris, 1971). This survey found that only one in five of the very severely handicapped were registered with the local authorities and only one in ten of the severely handicapped. Utilization (in terms of registration) was, therefore, found to be 20 per cent. and 10 per cent. respectively. Other studies of utilization and coverage of health services include the pioneering examination of general practice in England and Wales (Logan and Cushion, 1958), studies of the services for the mentally subnormal (Kushlick, 1967), and a detailed collection of utilization data in Exeter (Ashford and Pearson, 1970). The British hospital service has collected and published utilization data based on a 10 per cent. sample of patients (Ashley, 1972); it is now collecting more complete data about every patient (Rowe and Brewer, 1972). The extensive international studies under the direction of Kerr White (White *et al.*, 1967; White *et al.*, 1974), have shown the value of utilization data and developed sound validated methods of collecting such data.

Case registers have been used for some time as an administrative and epidemiological tool in various fields of public health. Originally these registers were used extensively in programmes for the control of tuberculosis. Recently, registers of psychiatric patients, physically handicapped persons and of patients with coronary heart disease have been developed. Registers can provide useful data about utilization provided

they are kept up to date. Case registers can collate information from all health and social services agencies, be based on a defined population and be cumulative over time. If this is done, then the number and kinds of individuals in contact with the existing services can be defined and a basis will be provided for the collection of further information, e.g. about the needs of the patients and their relations and the extent to which the services are meeting these needs (Wing and Hailey, 1972).

Resources

The next area of meaurement to be considered is that of the resources either being used or available for use in a programme. Resources reflect the capacity to give a service and resources used are a major component of the cost of a programme. Resources form the input that is consumed or utilized to produce the effect or output. Resources include money, materials, and manpower. Good resources do not ensure good service and even the full utilization of adequate resources does not prove that the quality of the service rendered was high. For such deductions to be drawn the resources utilized must be related to the standards of practice and the effects produced by the programme.

In the same way that a review of the health status of a community may reveal obvious deficiencies in the present services and programmes, so also may a detailed review of available resources. A model, for the use of this type of measurement in evaluation, is the report of the survey of casualty departments in hospitals in England and Wales (Nuffield Provincial Hospitals Trust, 1960). A number of desiderata for 'good' casualty departments were agreed in discussion with accident and orthopaedic specialists. Each desideratum was quantified into degrees of presence or absence. In this way each feature was scored and a chart showing the capacity for service of each department examined was drawn up. Some examples of the scoring of the desiderata will help to explain the method. One such item was 'consultant cover'. On the assumption that consultant cover was desirable, a full score of 10 was given if a consultant was in charge of the department and attended on a full-time basis. If the consultant attended frequently then 8 or 9 points were given, and the score dropped proportionately down to 3 if the consultant attended for one session a week only, to 2 if he paid only social visits to the department, to 1 if he never visited but was nevertheless nominally in charge, and to 0 if there was no consultant even nominally in charge of the department. Rehabilitation facilities formed another of the 17 features that were examined and scored. Ten points were given if there was a first class physiotherapy department, including gymnasium and pool, and an active occupational therapy department including some industrial work and a daily living activities unit. The mid-point on the scale was given for good physiotherapy, but diversional occupational therapy only; and no marks were given where there were no rehabilitation facilities at all. After scoring each of the features decided upon, the results were presented in the form of a bar-diagram representing the score obtained by each hospital under each of the headings. Those hospitals with grossly inadequate resources were easily identified.

To meet the needs of some groups of people a diversity of services is required; services which may be supplied by different agencies in the spectrum of health and social services.

Under certain conditions, it should be possible in principle to specify an ideal distribution of resources related to the objectives of, the needs for, and demands made on each service. However, we are a long way from such ideal conditions; the present distribution of resources between the different sectors is demonstrably uneven in England (Warren, 1964; Davies, 1968) and in many other countries. In examining the resources of one service (or part of a service) regard must be had to the resources of possible substitute services—especially when the objectives of the services have not been precisely defined. For example, to what extent do the resources of vocational rehabilitation services supply benefits in place of the medical rehabilitation services, and vice versa? To what extent do nursing homes supplement hospital provision? Or institutional care replace community care? In these situations measurements of resources and of costs and benefits must be extended beyond the programme under scrutiny if evaluation is to be achieved.

Activities and Attitudes of Staff and Clients

Activities. Traditional measures of a service are the number of items of work (activities) and of patients attended (utilization) by the staff and the facilities (resources) of the service. Hospitals are graded by the number of beds they contain, by their percentage bed occupancy, turnover per bed per year, number of in-patients admitted or discharged, number of out-patients seen, number of X-rays taken, number of pathological specimens examined, etc. Similarly the activities of public health services are measured by the number of mothers and children attending clinics, the number of visits made by health visitors, home nurses, public health inspectors, the number of people on various registers, the number of vaccinations given, etc. Such measurements are an essential part of the process of evaluation, although the desired effect cannot be assumed always to have occurred because the effort has been expended. For example, it is unreasonable to assume that the display of a large number of health education posters can be equated with acquirement of knowledge and change of attitude and behaviour on the part of those who see the posters. On the other hand the giving of a number of vaccinations may reasonably be assumed to have induced immunity on those vaccinated provided the vaccines contained potent antigens.

The study of activities can be greatly extended by the use of the techniques of *work study*. The term 'work study' embraces method study and work measurement. Method study is 'the systematic recording and critical examination of existing and proposed ways of doing work, as a means of developing and applying easier and more effective methods and reducing costs' (British Standard Definition). Work measurement is 'the application of techniques designed to establish the time for a qualified worker to carry out a specified job at a defined level of performance. A qualified worker is one who is accepted as having the necessary physical attributes, who possesses the required intelligence and education, and has acquired the necessary skill and knowledge to carry out the work in hand to satisfactory standards of safety, quantity, and quality' (British Standard Definition).

Another approach of value in the study of activities is that called *organization and methods* (O and M). O and M is primarily concerned with administrative structure and procedures. Normally O and M systematically reviews every component part of a unit under study, examining in detail its purpose and the way in which it functions, in order to discover how it can be made to function in the most efficient and the most economical way. An O and M review of organization covers such matters as the division of work, the delegation of authority, the line of authority, the span of control of individual officers, functional organization, co-ordination, centralization, and decentralization. The procedure followed is essentially similar to that of evaluation; indeed it is an evaluation of the administration. Full details of these techniques are given in publications by the International Labour Office (1967) and the United Kingdom, H.M. Treasury (1965). It must be emphasized, again, that these methods measure only the activities and not their outcome or effectiveness. Where work study is to be carried out in medical departments, full account must be taken of the medical purpose of the activity and the special relationship between doctor and patient and nurse and patient.

All the activities of staff and patients relevant to the programme should be examined. The activities will include visits, examinations, tests, advice, counselling, prescribing, inspecting, travelling, law enforcement, and clerical activities. A number of such studies have been carried out of the content of the work of general practitioners (for review see Royal College of General Practitioners, 1970; Warren, 1971), of health visitors (Marris, 1971) and of domiciliary nursing services (Allen, King, and Abbott, 1970). These latter studies have shown that when the health visitor is based within a group general practice and concentrates her work on the patients within the practice, there is an increase in the time she spends in discussion with the doctors, a decrease in time spent in clerical work and in travelling. She sees more older patients than a colleague working independently. Studies have been carried out on the work of home nurses which have been shown the disproportionate amount of her time spent in non-nursing activities (Hockey, 1966). Comparable investigations of social workers have shown that time spent in contact with clients and others directly concerned with their problems accounted for only 30 per cent. of all working time and that travelling accounted for just over 15 per cent. of the time worked (Goldberg, 1971).

Measurements of activity have been used in the management of a service. Following an activity study of the work of the home help serice in South Shields (Leitch, 1967), the number of forms, records, and registers was reduced from 27 to 13, and the design of the remaining forms was improved. The work load for each client was devised so that the home help could spend one period of up to 3 hours per week on general household tasks and only a half-hour or so on the other days per person. A year after the start of the survey, it was calculated that the saving in hours of the home helps was in the region of 30 per cent. A study of health visiting and home nursing in Bolton (Gallagher et al., 1970) established 'target times' for a number of items of service using the method of self-recording. These items were then used in the allocation of work with a resultant increase in time spent in direct contact with patients on home visits from 17 per cent. to 26 per cent. and a reduction in travelling time from 15 per cent. to 12 per cent., and on clerical work from 20 per cent. to 14 per cent.

Activity analyses can be used as indicators of the severity of patients' conditions. Barr (1963) has designed a 'nursing dependency score' which reflects by use of a scoring system the intensity of nursing care required by a patient. A patient with a high score, and therefore needing much nursing care, would be considered to have a more severe condition than a patient with a similar diagnosis but lower nursing dependency score. The activities of the patient, particularly those of self-care, have been used to measure the severity of handicap. Townsend (1962) developed a measure based on mobility, personal care, home-care, communication, and bladder and bowel control. This was subsequently modified (Shanas *et al.*, 1968) into an index of incapacity based on the ability of the person to perform those minimal tasks which make him independent of others for personal care. The index required an answer to six questions: (1) Can you go out of doors? (2) Can you walk up and down stairs? (3) Can you get about the house? (4) Can you wash and bath yourself? (5) Can you dress yourself and put on your shoes? (6) Can you cut your own toe-nails? A more elaborate system, but also based on activity, was used by Harris (1971) in her survey of the impaired and handicapped in Great Britain to define 'very severe handicap', 'severe handicap', 'handicap', and 'impairment'.

Activity analyses can be extended to measuring variables in the management of residential institutions. Townsend (1962) observed the daily activities of the residents in old people's homes and Morris (1968) studied the residents in hospitals for the mentally subnormal. King, Raynes, and Tizard (1971) measured four areas of staff–child relationships in institutions for handicapped children. The four areas were the rigidity of the routine, 'block' treatment, depersonalization and social distance which were then grouped together in a 30-item child management scale. The studies clearly distinguished child-oriented management from institutionally oriented management.

The appropriateness of the observed activity and use of resources should be related to the task performed. Studies of home nursing services (e.g. Hockey, 1966; Gallagher *et al.*, 1970) have shown that a significant amount of the work carried out by a fully trained, state-registered nurse could be done by a practically trained state-enrolled nurse and some of the work by a nursing aid. Studies which have examined the medical and nursing needs of patients in acute and long-stay hospitals have revealed the inappropriate placement of up to 20 per cent. of patients (e.g. Forsyth and Logan, 1960; Meredith *et al.*, 1968; Butler and Pearson, 1970). The matching of patients' needs to the resources and activities is the basis of 'progressive patient care' whereby seriously ill patients in need of concentrated and almost continuous nursing and medical care are looked after in specially equipped and staffed intensive care units and at the other extreme patients capable of their own self-care are located in pre-discharge wards or even hostels attached to the hospital.

Attitudes. An aspect that is frequently ignored in measuring activity and utilization of services is the attitude of the person concerned. Organizational, economic and scientific considerations can lead too easily to a rigid system that cannot or will not allow for the idiosyncrasies of human personality or the fears and aspirations of professional groups, patients, and clients. Extensive surveys have been carried out into some of these problems and a number of techniques developed. Revans (1964) studied the attitudes of nurses in hospitals. He pointed out that the methods most frequently used in studying the attitudes of employees are either questions framed to produce unambiguous replies put either by an interviewer or by means of written questionnaires, or non-directive interviews in which the interviewer records the opinions and feelings of each employee. Revans used the latter method and showed, among other findings, that there is a significant relationship between the ward-sisters' opinions of the senior staff, their attitudes towards student nurses, and the stability of qualified nursing staff on the wards and the mean length of stay of general medical and general surgical patients. Jefferys (1965) interviewed members of the health and social welfare staff of a county council in England. Thirty-five of the 46 health visitors stated they were glad they had come into health visiting and, on the whole, found their work satisfying and absorbing. However, in three important ways, clearly related to each other, health visitors' dissatisfactions significantly exceeded those expressed by any other group of workers interviewed. The first was their inability to use in practice all the techniques and knowledge acquired during training, the second was that their job was not clearly enough defined and thirdly that some of the tasks they were asked to do they felt were valueless.

Cartwright (1967) interviewed general practitioners and their patients, using standard question forms. She found that the patients were generally satisfied with the medical service they obtained but that some doctors expressed dissatisfactions similar to those of the health visitors in Jefferys' survey. The most obvious flaw, she concluded, in the organization of the general practitioner service (in England and Wales) is the uncertainty about the doctor's role. This lack of job definition bedevils the relationship between general practice and hospital, hinders effective collaboration with the local community services, and adversely affects the relationship between doctors and patients. In an earlier study Cartwright (1964), again using a structured questionnaire, interviewed 739 patients in 12 randomly selected districts in England and Wales who had been in hospital during the preceeding 6 months. Most patients were grateful for the way the nurses had looked after them; altogether two-thirds of the patients described some disadvantage of being in a ward with other patients, and a rather similar proportion described some advantage. The disadvantages were lack of privacy, illnesses of other patients, habits and behaviour of a minority of other patients, and discussions about illnesses which were upsetting. The advantages were enjoyable discussions with other patients and discussions about illness which were helpful. Only 8 per cent. of all patients wanted a room of their own; the majority said they preferred the size of ward they were in. A major finding was that over half the patients described some difficulty in getting information about their illness while they were in hospital.

Surveys of patients' opinions tend to produce results expressing satisfaction with the service. People seem to like what they know. As the public become more informed about health services and more vocal, it is probable that patients' opinions will be more critical. Despite present limitations, surveys of the opinions of staff, patients, and the public should form a part of a complete evaluation of service.

Standards of Practice

The 'quality' of medical care is often referred to, but this factor can have a number of dimensions. In one sense the quality of a medical service can be equated with the results of a total evaluation; at another extreme, to a patient, quality may mean degrees of kindness and attentiveness, and may be confused with plausibility and ingratiation from physicians and nurses. Quality is an important aspect of evaluation, but it is not a unitary concept that can be assessed by the measurement of a single comprehensive criterion.

One aspect that can be measured and has been used in a number of studies is the extent to which an activity or service matches a pre-determined code or standard of practice. For example, if it is agreed that pre-natal care should include a haemoglobin estimation, taking and recording the blood pressure at each visit, and rhesus typing, then it is possible to measure the percentage of pregnant women not having these items of care and so express numerically the short-fall in the accepted standard of practice. Butler and Bonham (1963) found that 4·7 per cent. of women attending for pre-natal care at hospital had no haemoglobin test, 1·6 per cent. did not always have their blood pressure recorded and 0·7 per cent. failed to have a rhesus test. For women attending local health authority clinics the figures were 35·2, 18·6, and 4·8 per cent. respectively.

Two methods are used in setting the 'standards of practice'. The first is to base the standards on studies of actual practice, the content of this having been ascertained by previous surveys. The second approach is to base the standards on the judgement of an expert group. The standards defined must be explicit, complete, reliable, and repeatable by different observers or recorders. The standards should also be acceptable to the professional groups concerned in the survey, whose co-operation and advice should be sought from the beginning. If the professional groups have helped to define the standards, then the standards are more likely to be acceptable to them. The investigator should act as convenor and chairman of the 'standard-setting group' and encourage the setting of high standards by asking, for example, doctors and nurses what they would want to have done for themselves or their relatives in the situations to be evaluated.

These techniques of defining standards of practice have been extended and developed by the Commission on Professional and Hospital Activities at Ann Arbor, Michigan, United States, into a monitoring system of quality control called Professional Activity Studies (PAS) and Medical Audit Plan (MAP). The basis of the Professional Activity Study is a case abstract which is completed by the medical records officer from the patient's clinical notes. The abstract includes the identification code, personal data of the patient, dates of admission and discharge, diagnoses, operations performed, clinical investigations, and details of treatment. The abstract sheets are forwarded for central processing and analysis by computer and the information is returned to the participating hospitals. The essential feature of the medical audit is the comparison of accepted standards of medical care against the content of the care actually provided. The information received by the hospital is presented in a form which draws attention to departures from accepted standards. Limited possibilities for review of some aspects of clinical work have arisen with the development of Hospital Activity Analysis in Great Britain (Heasman and Carstairs, 1971; Rowe and Brewer, 1972).

Impact, Effectiveness, and Output

The resources available, the activities and the maintenance of standards of practice all relate to the process of care and the structures and staff that surround and form the process. The objective of these processes is to improve the health status of individuals and of the community. In achieving this there may also be unwanted repercussions of the programme that must be taken into account in evaluation. For example, the specific impact of a malaria control programme might be a marked fall in the number of clinical cases of malaria seen. The secondary effects might include an increase in morbidity from other causes among those previously liable to malaria, a rise in the population and socio-economic effects varying from increased productivity to increased unemployment.

Since health services seek to improve the health status of populations, it is logical to evaluate their work by using the same indices that were used in the planning of the programme. Perinatal mortality rates, infant mortality rates, maternal mortality rates, case fatality rates, standardized death rates, morbidity rates, invalidity and disability rates can all be used. An obvious example is the measurement of the impact of an immunization programme by the subsequent incidence of the target disease. A pre-symptomatic screening programme should be measured not only in terms of activities, but also in terms of a reduction in mortality or disability among those screened and found to have the precursors or early stages of the target disease. Generally accepted objectives of medical-care services are the prevention of death, disease, disability, discomfort, and dissatisfaction (the five Ds). This alliterative list can be extended to include reduction in the time elapsing between onset of symptoms and receipt of care; prevention of complications and improvement in social (and occupational) functioning. These 'end' results present complex problems of measurement. The incidence of death and the incidence and prevalence of disease can be measured with more and more accuracy as definitions become nationally and internationally accepted. Some disabilities (e.g. blindness, deafness, mental subnormality, and anatomical defects and deficiencies) can be ascertained and measured, but others (e.g. personality defects, and disabilities due to chronic fluctuating medical conditions such as chronic bronchitis, cardiac failure, or senility) pose considerable problems in measurement and resort is usually had to measures of social functioning (Garrad and Bennett, 1971). Discomfort and dissatisfaction are subjective phenomena and therefore difficult to measure.

In recent years a number of consultants in hospitals have investigated the results of earlier discharge of their patients. The average length of stay of maternity patients admitted to hospital after delivery in England and Wales was 8 days in 1966. In Bradford, a total of 9,718 babies and their mothers were discharged from hospital, between 1959 and 1965, within 72 hours (3 days) of birth (Arthurton and Bamford, 1967; Craig and Muirhead, 1967). During that period the perinatal mortality rate declined. The mortality, morbidity, and breast-feeding experiences of the babies discharged within 3 days were compared with those of babies born at home. The differences between the two groups were not significant, except that mothers confined in hospital began to breast feed their babies and continued breast feeding more often than did women delivered at home. Maternal mortality rates could not be used in the evaluation as there were no maternal deaths. To gauge the obstetric effects, the incidence of readmission of mothers discharged within 3 days was compared with the admissions to hospitals of patients confined in their own homes. No significant differences between these groups were observed. Theoretically, this study should have used a method of random allocation of mothers admitted to a short-stay or long-stay group and then compared the results in each group.

Morris *et al*. (1968) have described a controlled trial of early discharge from hospital after hernia repair operations. They compared a number of factors relating to the recovery of a group of patients discharged the day after an operation for the repair of an inguinal hernia and another group discharged 6 days after operation. The names of all the patients entering the trial were arranged in chronological order of their being put on the waiting-list and were then allocated alternately to long or short stay. The two groups were found to be of similar composition. The effects of the long and short periods of stay in hospital were considered in relation to the development of post-operative complications, duration of convalescence, recurrence of hernia, and the repercussions in terms of the workload for general practitioners. The post-operative progress of patients in both groups was similar, but, not unexpectedly, the short-stay patients required some additional domiciliary care. In terms of achievement, the programme to introduce a shorter length of stay for patients after an operation for repair of hernia increased the availability of hospital beds, reduced the hospital costs per patient treated without affecting the post-operative recovery of the patient, but at a cost of a slight increase in expenditure on domiciliary services.

Other measures of outcome (in this example of case fatality rates) have been used in the study of hospital services. In 1957, attention was drawn to the higher case-fatality rates for patients with common surgical conditions treated in regional-board hospitals compared to those for patients with similar conditions treated in teaching hospitals in England and Wales (Lee *et al*., 1957). Subsequently, hyperplasia of the prostate was used as a 'marker' condition (see below) for a detailed study of factors contributing to the differences in case-fatality rates (Ashley *et al*., 1971). It was found that 78 per cent. of the admission of patients with hyperplasia of the prostate admitted to two of the regional-board hospitals were unplanned, the operation rate on these men was generally low and case fatality among them was 14 per cent. In contrast, only 22 per cent. of the admissions to the two teaching hospitals were unplanned, nearly every case was operated on, and the case fatality was 4·3 per cent. Men admitted urgently and especially those not operated on were older than the rest and mostly in acute retention, and many had cardiovascular and other disease. Thus the two regional board hospitals with proportionately less resources than the teaching hospitals were carrying more than their share of the most difficult cases.

Costs and Efficiency

Estimating the economic benefits and costs of a programme is a task for the economist. Problems of health economics and the costing of social services are discussed in another chapter; they have been reviewed historically by Fein (1971) and in deatil by Klarman (1965), Abel-Smith (1967), Feldstein (1967), and in a series of papers edited by Hauser (1972).

Expenditures for medical care to diagnose and treat a disease or injury are not the total costs of that disease, they are only the direct ones. There are also indirect costs such as loss of output of the individual with the disease and social costs involved in the care of a disabled person. Direct costs can be reduced by not providing services, but indirect costs would continue; indeed, it is usually assumed that the indirect costs would rise in the absence of medical services. In a cost–benefit analysis the comparison is between the costs of the actual programme on the one hand and the estimated reduction in costs (both direct and indirect) on the other hand. The costing of the services, losses and benefits is in practice very difficult. The loss of production and earnings through death, sickness, and incapacity can be computed from the age of the patient, duration of illness, and the expected earnings and productivity. Disability and injury can be priced in accordance with social security benefits and the awards made by law courts in compensation cases. Great difficulties arise where multiple diseases are present or the person is over retirement age. A programme may only be concerned with one disease and the economic effect of coping with this on the general condition of a patient may be problematical.

Some of these problems are simplified where direct comparisons are made between the expenditures of alternative programmes that produce the same degree of health improvement (cost–effective studies), as in the examples of early discharges from hospital that have already been quoted. But hospitals are concerned with many diseases and many patients. Measures of hospital costs per day per patient can be related to a variety of hospital and patient characteristics, e.g. hospital size, levels of activity, and the diagnoses, ages, and sexes of the patients treated. In a study of acute-care hospitals in Ontario, Evans (1971) found that the mix of diagnoses accounted for 80 per cent. of the variance in cost per case between the hospitals and about 50 per cent. of the variance in cost per day; diagnoses are, of course, related to the age and sex of the patient. As has already been discussed, different programmes are likely to have different outputs. Therefore, if the interest lies in the comparison of programmes, a common denominator for the different outputs must be used; a common way must be found of comparing the value of a life saved with a patient in whom the onset of disability has been postponed or with an elderly handicapped patient who has been enabled to die peacefully and with dignity. If only measurable outputs are measured and costed, then programmes that have such measurable impacts may be over-valued by administrators, because other, equally socially desirable, programmes cannot be shown to have measurable benefit (Logan *et al*., 1971). Peterson *et al*. (1967) reviewed the published data on health, expenditure, staffing, and the use of services by patients in England and Wales, the United States, and Sweden and concluded that insufficient facts were available for decisions on the best use of necessarily inadequate resources to be made. Details for the input of the health services (expenditure, numbers of beds, staff, buildings) were readily available, but morbidity rates, patient-demand rates and measures of outcome were too deficient for comparison and for the true effect of the different systems for providing medical care to be understood.

Interrelationships of Measurements

Evaluation is the measurement of the features discussed in the preceding pages and the *relating* of the results to each other and to previously defined objectives and standards. Each feature (health status, coverage, utilization, resources, activities, attitudes, process, impact, and costs) overlaps with and is effected by the others; all are interrelated in complex ways. Although the examples that have been quoted have been selected to illustrate a particular feature, many of the studies (as already indicated) have examined a number of features of various programmes. Research work is under way to understand the interrelationships of the features and to construct mathematical models which describe these.

COLLECTION OF THE DATA

The discussion, so far, has been about the data that should be collected for evaluation. This section discusses briefly some aspects of the methodology of the collection of the data. The main points to be decided are:

1. How should the data be collected?
2. When should the data be collected?
3. From whom should the data be collected?
4. By whom should the data be collected?

If routinely collected statistics on mortality, morbidity, disability, and the utilization of services reflect the health status of the community, they should serve to measure the effect of programmes to improve health. Being collected routinely, the data are available for evaluation more cheaply than data obtained from special studies; routine data should therefore be fully exploited before undertaking such studies. However, even in developed countries, where mortality statistics are reasonably complete and accurate, the data are of limited use for the evaluation of specific programmes; and the use of morbidity data is hampered by the fact that such data is often incomplete and inaccurate (Peterson *et al.*, 1967). In less developed countries reliable data are not usually available. As statistical services become more concerned with current health problems, the data provided from this source will be more useful for evaluating health programmes and for planning (Bodenham and Wellman, 1972). An outstanding advance in this respect can be expected from the development of automated record linkage (Acheson, 1967). It is axiomatic that all new programmes should have a system of data collection for evaluation built in as an integral part of the programme.

Principle Survey Techniques

Meanwhile, surveys have to be carried out in order to establish the basic facts about a community's problems and its current programmes. This is not to suggest that surveys will one day cease to be necessary, for special surveys will always be required to identify new problems and investigate changing aspects of old problems. A health survey utilizes one or more of four principal approaches, depending upon its purpose and the local circumstances. The four approaches are:

1. Use of existing or specially designed records of the activities of hospitals, clinics, family doctors, social security services, and occupational health services, etc.

2. Collection of data by postal questionnaires addressed to the administrator of a service, a field worker, a patient, a client, or a member of the public. A response rate of over 70 per cent. should be obtained; the skill in the use of this method lies in the phrasing of the questions and the design of the questionnaire (see Moser and Kalton, 1971).

3. Special interrogation of individuals carried out by trained interviewers either using structured questionnaires or in open interviews and discussions. This technique, with examples, is discussed under 'Attitudes' above. It is not, of course, limited to the investigation of attitudes; it can be used very helpfully to inquire about health and illness, as it was in the United Kingdom Government Social Survey to collect data about perceived morbidity (Logan and Brooke, 1957) and is currently used in the United States in the U.S. National Health Survey. The technique, combined with the respondent completing a structured questionnaire is used in many national and local censuses (see Moser and Kalton, 1971).

4. Special health examinations of individuals to determine the prevalance of morbidity in general, of a selected disease or of any abnormal state in the population in the area under investigation.

Time of Surveys

There are two distinct decisions to be taken about the time of surveys and investigations. The first relates to the possible effects that the seasons of the year might have on the result both from the point of view of disease prevalence and of probable activities of staff. Obviously either during an epidemic or the usual holiday period would be bad times for a survey unless its objective was to investigate some aspect of those actual occurrences. The second decision relates to the evaluation procedure. Should evaluation be continuous or episodic? Should all programmes be continuously evaluated or should programmes be specially selected for evaluation from time to time? Both methods should be used. Data should be continuously collected and considered by the director of the programme. In addition a deeper analysis of progress should be carried out at predetermined intervals during the execution of the programme, and a full evaluation of results and side-effects should be done when the programme reaches the conclusion of some particularly important phase or stage.

Use of Samples

Data have to be collected from a large number of sources and people. Wherever possible, samples of the population at risk should be used, because of the economy achieved. The techniques of this are common to epidemiology and need not be repeated in this chapter. There is now considerable knowledge about the practical and theoretical aspects of sampling so that in many instances it is possible to select a sample that will give results that are representative of the whole population. Special techniques are used to select a sample of people from a population or a sample from records; the same meticulous approach should be used in the evaluation and quality control of environmental hygiene programmes by methodically sampling specimens of food, water, and air for examination and analysis (World Health Organization, 1966).

'Marker' Conditions and Situations

Another method of limiting data collection is to concentrate on a 'marker' condition or situation which while not representative of other conditions is considered to be illustrative of the factors likely to be involved. Mention has already been made of the study of patients with hyperplasia of the prostate (Ashley *et al.*, 1971) to examine the effects of differences in case-mix and treatments in two types of hospital service, using case-fatality rates as a measure of outcome. In England and Wales there has been for many years a system of detailed and confidential inquiries carried out on every maternal death—maternal deaths, being relatively infrequent (in 1970 there were only 109), are used as 'markers' or indicators of possible breakdown in the maternity services. The report on these inquiries relating to the 3 years 1964–66 (Department of Health and Social Security, 1969) showed that in 579 of the deaths directly due to pregnancy and childbirth there were considered to be avoidable factors in 45 per cent. Somewhat similar inquiries have been carried out into post-neonatal deaths (Department of Health and Social Security, 1970). The technique has been applied to a study of tuberculosis mortality (British Thoracic and Tuberculosis Association, 1971); 884 deaths were fully investigated; avoidable factors responsible for or contributing to death were identified in 211 of the 263 cases in which death was due to active tuberculosis. In 106 cases the patient was responsible for delay in diagnosis or failure of treatment; the most clearly defined factors were old age, mental disorder, and alcoholism. In 149 medical care was unsatisfactory—19 in general practice, 92 at a chest clinic and 39 in hospital. Another study (Warren *et al.*, 1967) looked at problems of emergency admissions to hospitals in London, and found that there was greater difficulty in admitting older patients and patients suffering from abortions, strokes, heart failure, and terminal cancer. Although 62 per cent. of the patients who were not admitted to hospital at once got into hospital within a few days, the investigators found that the help of the community services was only sought in 33 per cent. of all patients not immediately admitted. All these studies while focusing on special groups of patients or categories of outcome were able to contribute to the understanding of more general health service problems.

Use of Controls

The use of 'controls' in evaluation is essential in certain circumstances. Surveys (such as those described in the preceding paragraph) collect facts about situations, services, programmes, and the community; and surveys are an essential feature in the observation of any innovation. An innovation is introduced because it is believed that it will be beneficial; a preliminary trial of the innovation is then organized and the results measured and observed. If these results suggest that the innovation is beneficial, then to prove that the improvement was due to the innovation, a more extensive survey with proper controls must be carried out.

A survey establishes the base-lines of the current situations and is an essential prerequisite of health planning and evaluation. As part of the evaluation of an innovation or experiment, survey methods will be used to collect data from the index programme (that is the innovation or experimental situation) and the control situation. To answer the question, 'Would the objectives have been equally well achieved in the absence of the new programme?' a control situation must be measured. The model for evaluation of experimental services is that of the therapeutic trial using random allocation of patients into 'treated' and 'untreated' groups (see World Health Organization, 1968, and Cochrane, 1972). Ideal control groups for an evaluation procedure can be established only if the programme to be evaluated is applied to individuals rather than to the community at large. To divide a group of people with similar needs receiving the old service or no service randomly into two groups, one continuing as before and the other to receive the new service is the goal. However, it is not always attainable in the deployment of health services, particularly in the provision of community health services such as the provision of a health centre, the abatement of air pollution or the addition of sodium fluoride to drinking water. Here a 'treated' community is compared with an 'untreated' community. The idea that one community acts as a control to the other is only as good as the initial matching of the communities, and since people select the neighbourhood or community in which they live, selective factors may be involved that will bias the results. The New York Hospital—Cornell Project, 1960–65 (Goodrich *et al.*, 1970) was an experiment in the organization of welfare medical care services. Participants were selected at random from welfare patients in New York City. One group was offered integrated medical care of all kinds by the New York Hospital: the controls were left untouched to continue to use the piece-meal services then available in the district of New York. The two groups were observed systematically for 2 years. Equality of need and background was ensured by the random selection; and evaluation of the two systems of care was based on the patients' use of services, the cost of care provided, and various measures of the activities, processes, and attitudes. The results support the hypothesis that integrated care is better than unintegrated care, though it may not be cheaper. Another ambitious effort to use randomized controls in the evaluation of a service is the study by Goldberg (1970) of the help given by a social service department to their aged clients.

Collectors of Data and Evaluators

The final question about the collection of data to be discussed refers to the people who should collect the data and carry out the evaluation. Alternatives are the field workers of the programme, a special group or unit within the department responsible for the programme or a special group or unit from outside the department such as from a regional headquarters, from a university, or independent research unit. Evaluation is more profitable, because implementation is more likely if the field workers are involved and convinced of its help and relevance. Large organizations should be able to support their own evaluation and operational research units and smaller organizations may make joint arrangements between each other or with a larger organization. The universities and central government departments should initiate some of the necessary research, develop methodology and train personnel in evaluation and operational research. All grades of professional staff need, at the very least, to be aware of the procedures of evaluation; the clinical staff within a health service should be encouraged to undertake operational research in the same way as they are encouraged, at present, to undertake clinical research. In addition health-services research units (a combination of operational, epidemiological, and applied research and development units) are needed as an integral part of the health services organization.

COLLATION AND ANALYSIS OF DATA

Having defined and collected the data, the final steps are to collate and analyse it and to present the results with suitable recommendations for further action. Collation is the checking of completeness and sequence and the bringing together of the facts for comparison. Much of this should be done during the collection of the data. The amount of computing and analysis required will depend on the problem and the complexity of the programme; it will vary from simple tabulations, standardizations, percentages, and tests of significance to complex analyses of multiple variants, and the construction of mathematical, or simulation models. These models may then be used to calculate yardsticks for the programme, and so re-define the specific objectives (Luck *et al.*, 1971). The physical handling of the data may be by card-sorting using manual methods or a counter sorter or by electronic data processing machines. The choice will depend upon the amount of material, the complexity of the analysis and associated calculations, and the probable repetitiveness of the process (see Holland, 1970).

PRESENTATION OF RESULTS AND RECOMMENDATIONS

The form of presentation of results of evaluation must vary depending on the reader for whom it is intended. A report written for members of the department concerned will emphasize different things to one written for publication in a scientific journal. More than one report may be necessary. But whoever the readers are intended to be, the report should be as brief as possible; the results must be stated simply, emphasizing their practical implications and with a sensitivity to, and understanding of, the problems of the field workers. Clear, practical recommendations should be made. The report should be prepared as soon as possible after the completion of the evaluation, so that its results refer to the current situation and not to history.

The contents of the report should follow the usual pattern. There is first an introduction setting out the purpose of the evaluation and stating clearly for whom the results are intended and by whom the survey was carried out. Reference is made to any previous surveys relating to the service or programme. The next section describes the methods used, particularly the sampling procedure and the data collected. Then the results are presented. Illustrations should be used to enable the readers to grasp information clearly and quickly. Many of the results can be presented in tables which may be included in the body of the report or be collected together in an appendix; in either case, attention should be drawn in the text to the tables and the conclusions to be drawn from them should be stated. Figures given in the tables should not be repeated in the text except for the purposes of comment and comparison. The text should not be decorated in rococo style with calculations and statistical symbols and formulae. The next section

contains the discussion; it should comment on the accuracy and completeness of the results and whether they can be considered representative of the programme or service as a whole and whether they apply regionally as well as locally. Finally, the implications of the findings and recommendations for change and further action form a concluding section. Without such recommendations the whole process of evaluation becomes an intellectual exercise of interest to a few, but of no immediate value to the programme or service. The summary should state briefly the purpose, method, main results, and recommendations; it should not merely be a statement that these are to be found in the report. The summary is best placed at the beginning of the report; considerable thought must be given in writing the summary, because it will be the only part of the report read by many readers.

COMMON DIFFICULTIES IN EVALUATION

Evaluation is so obviously necessary; much of the procedure is straightforward; and it is within the capacity of a medical administrator to carry out some evaluation of his programmes with his own resources. Why then has evaluation not been widely and routinely applied in the planning and management of health services? There are a number of reasons, some of which are discussed below.

The demands for health services exceed the provision so that any or all expansion of services seems beneficial. The health services have therefore grown in response to social and emotional pressures and many administrators have adopted opportunistic approaches. Where there was a demand and money available, there a service would develop. Sometimes this would result in the creation of a new and independent organization to meet the new demand. This piecemeal development of health services has been the bane of economic and planned progress, and has frustrated and hindered evaluation.

A second reason for slow progress in evaluating health services is the lack of expertise. Evaluation requires the involvement of specialists from a number of academic disciplines such as social medicine, statistics, sociology, social psychology, economics, social administration, and computer science. Such people are scarce. The techniques and terminology of evaluation are often strange to the clinical staff in the health services; many of the techniques have been developed in the fields of industry and commerce and carry such forbidding titles as marketing research, consumer survey, management audit, network analysis, cost-benefit analysis, and management by objectives.

Many doctors and nurses feel that economists, management consultants, and evaluators view medicine as a marketable commodity, whereas they see the practice of medicine as a humanitarian vocation. They, therefore, distrust evaluation of their work.

Some of the objections to evaluation that are voiced by staff, although sometimes rationalizations of their opposition, often reflect methodological difficulties. Thus the objections that the effects of the programme are long-range and cannot be measured in the immediate future; that the effects are general rather than specific; that the effects are small and subtle and cannot be measured by the crude standards suggested; or that the process of evaluation will itself change the quality of the programme are all valid to a degree. There is another problem —the pressure of the day-to-day work. This can make demands to analyse and record activities seem to be an unnecessary additional burden.

To overcome the resistance of staff, careful attention must be given to the process of introducing evaluation and an attempt made to harness their co-operation and gain their enthusiasm. With an established programme a small start may be indicated. Commence with partial evaluation of minor problems and parts of a programme; and then as experience is gained and staff interest and confidence are built up, more complete evaluation can be introduced. The co-operation and confidence of the staff can be achieved by seeking their advice. Most field-workers already have to complete a number of forms about their work. A useful starting point is to convene a conference of field-workers on the need for and design of the forms and records they use. The purpose of these documents can be discussed, as well as the use that is made of the information and the greater use that could be made if somewhat different data were collected. The next step is to discuss the possibility of using the data for evaluation. At this stage the planning of evaluation and the setting of criteria and standards can be jointly discussed. After the evaluation, and before the report is finalized and circulated, further joint discussions between the evaluators and the field-workers should be held. In these discussions, value judgements of 'good' and 'bad' should be avoided; to fall short of one's own standards *may* be bad, but there may be peculiar circumstances to account for the short-fall. The objective of evaluation is not to condemn or praise, but to state the facts (e.g. these standards were not maintained to this extent because those resources were not available; the objectives of this programme were not achieved because the means suggested were found inappropriate to the problems actually encountered; or, the objectives of this programme were achieved at so much less cost in money and staff than in another programme). Throughout, the evaluators must have genuine joint discussions with all the staff. The objectives of the joint discussions are to gain the co-operation and advice of the staff, to help them receive and interpret the results with understanding so that they will be able to modify their own actions in the most useful way and without emotional strife.

ENVOI

Much has been said about the importance of evaluation; it applies equally to the process of evaluation. Population surveying and the medical examination of large numbers of people are expensive. Evaluators must state their objectives and relate their costs to their results. They cannot be exempt from the application of their own logic and methods.

REFERENCES AND FURTHER READING

Abel-Smith, B. (1967) An International Study of Health Expenditure, *Wld Hlth Org. Publ. Hlth Pap.*, No. 32, Geneva.

Acheson, E. D. (1967) *Medical Record Linkage*, London.

Airth, A. D., and Newell, D. J. (1962) *The Demand for Hospital Beds*, Newcastle-upon-Tyne, University of Durham.

Alderson, M. R. (1973) Towards a health information system, *Hlth Soc. Serv. J.*, **83**, 1524.

Allen, W. H., King, V. M., and Abbott, G. M. (1970) Domiciliary nursing services in Hertfordshire, *Med. Offr*, **124**, 217.

Arthurton, M. W., and Bamford, F. N. (1967) Paediatric aspects of the early discharge of maternity patients, *Brit. med. J.*, **3**, 517.

Ashford, J. R., and Pearson, N. G. (1970) Who uses the health services and why?, *J. roy statist. Soc.*, Series A, **133**, Pt. 3, 295.

Ashley, J. S. A. (1972) Present state of statistics from hospital in-patient data and their uses, *Brit. J. prev. soc. Med.*, **26**, 135.

Ashley, J. S. A., Howlett, A., and Morris, J. N. (1971) Case fatality of hyperplasia of the prostate in two teaching and three regional-board hospitals, *Lancet*, **ii**, 1308.

Asvall, J. E. (1973) Evaluation of public health programmes in WHO European Region, *Wld Hlth Org. Chron.*, **27**, 3.

Barr, A. (1957) The population served by a hospital group, *Lancet*, **ii**, 1105.

Barr, A. (1963) *Measurement of Nursing Care*, Oxford Regional Hospital Board Report No. 85, Oxford.

Bodenham, K. E., and Wellman, F. (1972) *Foundations for Health Service Management*, London.

British Thoracic and Tuberculosis Association (1971) A survey of tuberculosis mortality in England and Wales in 1968, *Tubercle (Lond.)*, **52**, 1.

Brooke, Eileen M. (1974) The current and future use of registers in health information systems, *Wld Hlth Org. Offset pub. Ser.' No. 7.

Butler, J. R., and Pearson, M. (1970) *Who Goes Home?*, Occasional Papers on Social Administration No. 34, London.

Butler, R. N., and Bonham, D. C. (1963) *Perinatal Mortality*, Edinburgh.

Cartwright, A. (1964) *Human Relations and Hospital Care*, London.

Cartwright, A. (1967) *Patients and Their Doctors*, London.

Cochrane, A. L. (1972) *Effectiveness and Efficiency*, London.

Craig, G. A., and Muirhead, J. M. B. (1967) Obstetric aspects of the early discharge of maternity patients, *Brit. med. J.*, **3**, 520.

Davies, B. P. (1968) *Social Needs and Resources in Local Services*, London.

Department of Health and Social Security (1969) *Report on Confidential Enquiries into Maternal Deaths in England and Wales 1964–66*, London, H.M.S.O.

Department of Health and Social Security (1970) *Confidential Enquiry into Postneonatal Deaths, 1964–66*, London, H.M.S.O.

Dodge, J. S. (1970) ed., *The organization and evaluation of medical care*, Dunedin.

Donabedian, A. (1969) *A Guide to Medical Care Administration*, Vol. II, *Medical Care Appraisal*, New York, American Public Health Association.

Evans, R. G. (1971) Behavioural cost functions for hospitals, *Canad. J. Econ.*, IV, 198.

Fein, R. (1971) On measuring economic benefits of health programmes, in *Medical History and Medical Care*, London.

Feldstein, M. S. (1967) *Economic Analysis for Health Service Efficiency; Econometric Studies of the British Health Service*, Amsterdam.

Forsyth, G., and Logan, R. F. L. (1960) *The Demand for Medical Care*, London.

Gallagher, E., Howe, J. E., Richardson, E. M., and Ross, A. I. (1970) A study of health visiting and district nursing in Bolton, *Med. Offr*, **123**, 161.

Garrad, J., and Bennett, A. E. (1971) A validated interview schedule for use in population surveys in chronic disease and disability, *Brit. J. prev. soc. Med.*, **25**, 97.

Gatherer, A., and Warren, M. D. (1971) *Management and the Health Services*, Oxford.

Goldberg, E. M. (1970) *Helping the Aged*, London.

Goldberg, E. M. (1971) Research in social work, in *Portfolio for Health: Problems and Progress in Medical Care*, Sixth Series, London.

Goodrich, C. H., Olendzki, M. C., and Reader, G. G. (1970) *Welfare Medical Care: An Experiment*, Cambridge, Mass.

Grundy, F., and Rinke, W. A. (1973) Health practice research and formalized managerial methods, *Wld Hlth Org. publ. Hlth. Pap.*, No. 51.

Harris, A. I. (1971) *Handicapped and Impaired in Great Britain*, (SS 418), London, H.M.S.O.

Hartley, R., O'Flynn, W. R., Rake, M., and Wooster, M. (1968) Experiment in progressive patient care, *Brit. med. J.*, **3**, 794.

Hauser, M. A. (1972) *The Economics of Medical Care*, London.

Heasman, M. A., and Carstairs, V. (1971) Inpatient management: Variations in some aspects of practice in Scotland, *Brit. med. J.*, **1**, 495.

Hilleboe, H. E., and Schaefer, M. (1967) *Papers and Bibliography on Community Health Planning*, Albany, New York, Graduate School of Public Affairs, State University of New York.

Hockey, L. (1966) *Feeling the Pulse. A Survey of District Nursing in Six Areas*, London, Q.I.D.N.

Holland, W. W. (1970) *Data Handling in Epidemiology*, London.

International Labour Office (1967) *Introduction to Work Study*, Geneva.

Jefferys, M. (1965) *An Anatomy of Social Welfare Services*, London.

King, R. D., Raynes, N. V., and Tizard, J. (1971) *Patterns of Residential Care. Sociological Studies in Institutions for Handicapped Children*, London.

Klarman, H. E. (1965) *The Economics of Health*, New York.

Kushlick, A. (1967) A method of evaluating the effectiveness of a community health service, *Social and Economic Administration*, **1**, No. 4, p. 29.

Lee, J. A. H., Morrison, S. L., and Morris, J. N. (1957) Fatality from three common surgical conditions in teaching and non-teaching hospitals, *Lancet*, **ii**, 785.

Leitch, I. D. (1968) Value for money in health and welfare. A local study of the Home Help Service, *Roy. Soc. Hlth J.*, **88**, 159.

Logan, R. F. L., Klein, R. E., and Ashley, J. S. A. (1971) Effective management of health, *Brit. med. J.*, **2**, 519.

Logan, W. P. D., and Brooke, E. M. (1957) *The Survey of Sickness 1943 to 1952*, Studies on Medical and Population Subjects No. 12, London, H.M.S.O.

Logan, W. P. D., and Cushion, A. A. (1958) *Morbidity Statistics from General Practice*, General Register Office, London, H.M.S.O.

Luck, G. M., Luckman, J., Smith, B. W., and Stringer, J. (1971) *Patients, Hospitals, and Operational Research*, London, Tavistock Publications.

McKeown, T. (1968) Validation of screening procedures, in *Screening in Medical Care*, London.

McLachlan, G., ed. (1973) *The Future—and Present Indicatives*, London.

Marris, T. (1971) *The Work of Health Visitors in London*, Research Report No. 12, London, Greater London Council.

Meredith, J. S., Anderson, M. A., Price, A. C., and Leithead, J. (1968) *Hostels in Hospitals? The Analysis of Beds in Hospitals by Patient Dependency*, London.

Morris, D., Ward, A. W. M., and Handyside, A. J. (1968) Early discharge after hernia repair, *Lancet*, **i**, 681.

Morris, J. N. (1967) *Uses of Epidemiology*, Edinburgh.

Morris, P. (1969) *Put Away. A Sociological Study of Institutions for the Mentally Retarded*, London.

Moser, C. A., and Kalton, G. (1971) *Survey Methods in Social Investigation*, London.

Nuffield Provincial Hospitals Trust (1960) *Casualty Services and their Setting*, London.

Peterson, O. L., Burgess, A. M., Berfenstam, R., Smedby, B., Logan, R. F. L., and Pearson, R. J. C. (1967) What is value for money in medical care? Experiences in England and Wales, Sweden and the U.S.A., *Lancet*, **i**, 771.

Revans, R. W. (1964) *Standards for Morale. Cause and Effect in Hospitals*, London.

Rowe, R. G., and Brewer, W. (1972) *Hospital Activity Analysis*, London.

Royal College of General Practitioners (1973) *Reports from General Practice* 16 (3rd edn). *Present State and Future Needs*, London, R.C.G.P.

Shanas, E., Townsend, P., Wedderburn, D., Friis, H., Milhof, P., and Stehouwer, J. (1968) *Old People in Three Industrial Societies*, London.

Shonfield, A., and Shaw, S. (1972) *Social Indicators and Social Policy*, London, Social Science Research Council.

Stewart, R. (1968) *The Reality of Management*, London.

Suchman, E. A. (1967) *Evaluative Research*, New York, Russell Sage Foundation.

Townsend, P. (1962) *Last Refuge. A Survey of Residential Institutions and Homes for the Aged in England and Wales*, London.

United Kingdom, H.M. Treasury, Management Services Division (1965) *The Practice of O and M*, London, H.M.S.O

United States Department of Health, Education and Welfare (1969) *Towards A Social Report*, Washington.

Vickers, G. (1968) What sets the goals of public health?, *Lancet*, **i**, 559.

Warren, M. D. (1964) Demands and needs for in-patient care for elderly people, *Med. Care*, **2**, 113.

Warren, M. D. (1971) The National Health Service and the planning of general practitioner services in England and Wales, *Acta socio-medica, Scandinavica*, **1**, 1.

Warren, M. D. (1973) *Problems and Opportunities in the New Towns*, London.

Warren, M. D., Cooper, J., and Warren, J. L. (1967) Problems of emergency admissions to London hospitals, *Brit. J. prev. soc. Med.*, **21**, 141.

Wing, J. K., and Hailey, A. M. (1972) *Evaluating a Community Psychiatric Service*, London.

White, K. L., Andjelkovic, D., Pearson, R. J. C., Marboy, H. J., Ross, A., and Sagen, O. K. (1967) International comparisons of medical care utilization, *New Engl. J. Med.*, **277**, 516.

White, K. L., et al. (1974) *The World Health Organization International Collaborative Study on Medical Care Utilization*, in press.

World Health Organization, Expert Committee on Health Statistics (1966) Sampling Methods in Morbidity Surveys and Public Health Investigations, *Wld Hlth Org. techn. Rep. Ser.*, No. 336. Geneva.

World Health Organization (1968) Principles for the Clinical Evaluation of Drugs, *Wld Hlth Org. techn. Rep. Ser.*, No. 403, Geneva.

World Health Organization, Expert Committee on Health Statistics (1969) Statistics of Health Services and of their Activities, *Wld Hlth Org. techn. Rep. Ser.*, No. 429, Geneva.

World Health Organization (1971) Statistical Indicators for the Planning and Evaluation of Public Health Programmes, *Wld Hlth Org. techn. Rep. Ser.*, No. 472, Geneva.

World Health Organization (1974) Modern management methods and the organization of the health services, *Wld Hlth Org. publ. Hlth Pap.*, No. 55.

World Health Organization Regional Office for Europe (1973) *Report of a Working Group on the Evaluation of Public Health Programmes, Burgos 1972* (Euro 4004), Copenhagen.

World Health Organization Regional Office for Europe (1974) *Report of a Conference on Health Information Systems, Copenhagen 1973* (Euro 4914), Copenhagen.

Yates, J. M. (1973) Monitoring in the hospital service, *Hosp. Hlth Serv. Rev.*, **69**, 322.

47

SOCIAL SCIENCE AND PUBLIC HEALTH

M. W. SUSSER

Students of society can rarely make planned experiments; in lieu of experiment they use the natural contrasts between societies and opportune changes within them. But they do not ignore measurement, although they must often rely on verbal communication and direct observation of behaviour. Physicians should well understand the importance and validity of these methods (even though they are beset with large margins of error) for they resemble those of medicine; the clinician uses direct observation, and the epidemiologist measures and compares groups.

Doctors can hardly avoid learning empirically, in day-to-day practice, a good deal about the social aspects of their work. Such knowledge, however, is comparable to that which a priest might have about the prevalence of disease in his parish; it is usually not ordered and interpreted in a theoretical framework. Despite this deficiency, doctors often feel that they do command special competence in questions of behaviour. This feeling may take on the flavour of authority, for medical education in the past has not been prone to emphasize what the physician did not know. It could be argued that one task of medical education has been to breed confidence in the physician's own judgements, and through this confidence to promote his authority and ability to act; for the practice of medicine is beset with uncertainties in diagnosis, in treatment, and in prognosis which hinder decision.

In the times when medicine had little scientific basis, personal authority was the more necessary to the doctor, and such authority may still have value in inducing compliance in patients. In recent times, advances in organic medicine have enabled doctors to abandon some of this personal authority and to practise scientific humility, because they could rely on the growing authority of scientific knowledge. The substitution of scientific for personal authority has not been easy; as late as the end of the nineteenth century Samuel Gee, whose surname is the eponym for coeliac disease, is said to have advised his students not to bother with physiology.

The substitution of science for authority is even more difficult when judgements must refer to the psyche and to society. The objective study of society requires the examination of value systems. To do this the social scientist, in his scientific role, must stand outside society. But each of us is a product of society, of its mode of rearing children, of its moral beliefs, and of its assumptions about people and society. Each of us knows right from wrong according to the special values that obtain in our own culture. The social scientist must detach himself from these built-in attitudes and modes of thought; this is to stand outside himself.

The social sciences are in their infancy. Their productivity is much less than that of the physical sciences, for the study of society is among the most difficult of scientific endeavours. At each level of observation in the study of human beings, through the molecular, the cellular, the organic, the individual, and the social, the number of uncontrolled variables is successively multiplied. As with the whole of medicine, proved facts are relatively few, and must be linked by hypothetical constructions. But we learn from social science to adopt a position of scientific detachment towards society; to analyse, classify, and generalize observations in terms of social groups; and to measure and define the objective, if intangible, regularities of social relationships.

One can treat social science in medicine under four heads:

1. Social factors in health and disease.
2. Patients as social beings.
3. Health professionals in relation to patients.
4. Systems of medical care.

Henry Sigerist, writing about the history of medicine, summed up these social relations of medicine:

'In every medical action there are always two parties involved, the physician and the patient, or in a broader sense, the medical corps and society. Medicine is nothing else than the manifold relations between these two groups. The history of medicine, therefore, cannot limit itself to the history of the science, institutions and character of medicine, but must include the history of the patient in society, that of the physician, and the history of the relationship between physician and patient.'

SOCIAL FACTORS IN HEALTH AND DISEASE

Social Science in Epidemiology

Epidemiology is the study of the distribution and determinants of health and disease in populations, and part of its province is the study of the related social factors. Indeed, every epidemiological variable is in some sense a sociological variable. But these variables also have social meaning, and their distribution in populations implies a particular configuration of statuses in society; each of these statuses carries its own set of obligations and duties and social relations. The factors affecting the distribution of disease in populations may be biological or environmental, and both have social implications. The populations to whom the biological dimension refers are not mere aggregates of discrete individuals. They comprise, as groups of people with some order of relationships between them, the elements of society. The environment which contains the populations is equally a facet of society in its physical and biological as well as its social components; civilization, however primitive, is natural environment modified by human groups.

Epidemiologists have tended in the past to interpret such basic attributes as sex and age and marital status in biological terms. But these variables also have social meaning, and their distribution in a population implies a particular configuration of statuses in society; each of these statuses carries its own set of obligations and duties and social relations. Each marital status, for instance, has implicit in it distinctive expectations of support for the individual should he fall ill. We may, therefore, predict that an individual's marital status will affect his decision to seek help from a medical agency, or to enter a medical institution. Such decisions give rise to unrepresentative populations which distort the view of disease obtained by any one agency, whether it is general practice, or a hospital, or a public health department. The forces which determine whether an individual or a group breaks through the surface of anonymity to recognized morbidity are thus not only pathological but psychological and social. They need to be interpreted in terms of psychology and sociology.

The influence of such demographic factors as the age and sex structure of the population appears in the different courses of individual and family life cycles in different social classes. In this century women of the lower social classes have borne more illigitimate babies, have had more pre-nuptial conceptions, married younger, had larger families, and in sum have been more fertile. Although their youth has given them some advantage in child-bearing, all these other factors concentrated in the lower social classes act against efficient reproduction. High fertility with close spacing is not only wearing to maternal health, but also leads to high foetal and child death rates, and in infancy their children have high mortality rates. Moreover, after the neonatal period young mothers lose more infants than older mothers, and the incidence of infections is greater among their children. Illegitimacy in young mothers, too, is associated with high infant mortality. It is evident that physical, economic, social, and cultural factors combine to produce the distinctive life cycles on which rest the gradients in morbidity and mortality between the social classes. Variations in health hinge on the whole pattern of living. Since these patterns are changing, so is the incidence and prevalence of disease.

Sociological Concepts

Many doctors are agreed that social factors are important in disease. Nor is it any longer a question whether they need to be equipped to handle the notions relating to these factors or whether an empirical, amateur approach is sufficient. Sociological notions tend to be many-sided and unamenable to simple, finite definitions. One example with wide currency is the concept of social class. The phenomenon it describes is real enough, but even sociologists disagree about its fundamental nature. For the 1911 British Census, Stevenson, chief statistical medical officer to the General Register Office, devised a method of measuring social class by arranging all occupations within a hierarchy of five classes. His classification, somewhat modified, has come to be regularly used in national statistics and in medical research. If it is to be used with confidence, however, some understanding of the assumptions and the criteria which divide the classes is needed. Yet half a century after the classification was introduced it is not clear how far

these are arbitrary, or theoretical, or empirical, and anomalies of classification ensue.

In trying to devise a unilineal scale of social class which is valid for the nation, the Registrar General faces an impossible task. Each occupational group has a very wide span, so that pedagogues can include vice-chancellors of universities as well as kindergarten teachers. Specific occupations may embrace an equally wide range of social classes; a farmer may be a duke or a tenant, and a company director may direct anything from a small local business to the Bank of England.

Individuals have multiple social roles which cannot be described by a single index such as occupation. Over a period of time they may have multiple occupations as well, and their mobility between occupations will tend to be in different directions at different ages, upward before retirement and downward after. This effect of age on occupational mobility varies with occupational category; for instance, downward mobility after retirement occurs less often among entrepreneurs and the self-employed. Difficulties are increased by the technical problems of recording. In one national survey 12 per cent. of the information recorded by health visitors had later to be reclassified.

More fundamental problems of classification are caused by the inescapable subjective elements that enter into the ranking of occupations. A blurring of the social gradations recognized by an observer tends to accompany increased geographical or social distance, and the Registrar General is not immune to this. Thus his scale discriminates fairly well at the upper end of the social spectrum, for instance between the learned and the other professions, but poorly at the lower end. Half the population falls into Social Class III, which includes such large and divergent occupations as colliers and clerks. The pitfalls of subjective judgements are multiplied by the relative rigidity of any scale which has to be applied to the constant flux over time of an expanding industrial economy. The content and structure of occupations change, and so does their social prestige, and the elements of skill and training necessary to them as new methods of production are introduced.

Anomalies also reside in the classification itself. Any method of stratifying society aims to reflect its real structure. But Britain is not a social pyramid divided into five horizontal layers, which is the model the classification suggests. The lines of cleavage are vertical as well as horizontal. Moreover, social groups are not static; the movement of individuals between social groups, and the movement of whole social groups, obscures the pattern. We can hardly hope to understand the distribution of schizophrenia, or mental subnormality, or coronary heart disease, or bronchitis, unless we can grasp both the cleavages in society and the constant reshuffling of social and genetic attributes that accompanies social mobility.

Social mobility thus complicates the distribution of populations within a class system, and epidemiological studies are beginning to take account of this. Allowance must be made for it in framing genetic and environmental hypotheses, both of which have often treated the social classes as stable populations with fixed characteristics. Individuals may be selected for mobility by genetic and social traits through education and occupation, or through marriage, and so alter the distribution of the traits between the classes. Moreover, vertical social mobility may bring with it special stresses, similar in kind to those ascribed to the lateral movement of migration. To handle such material we need the most rigorous methods that social science can offer; studies of social factors in health and disease which do not use them neglect a vital dimension.

PATIENTS AS SOCIAL BEINGS

Patients are social beings, and much of their response to disease and their behaviour with doctors is socially determined.

Many doctors have come to accept that what causes a particular individual to present as a sick person should in part be interpreted in psychological terms. Whether a patient's symptoms rise above the threshold of complaint depends on the way in which he perceives illness and in which he is moved to act about it. Perception and motivation, however, are determined by the particular social context in which the individual lives and in which he performs his social roles. During growth he learns the behaviour expected in the roles appropriate to each new stage of development, and what he learns becomes an integral part of his personality. All behaviour is to some extent a reflection of social roles, and of the duties and expectations implicit in them.

It follows that to be sick is a social phenomenon. The sick person, as Sigerist long ago pointed out, has a special position, a social role with implicit rules and privileges. Sickness is not synonymous with disease although it includes it. Disease can be defined as a state of physiological or psychic dysfunction which affects the individual organism, whereas sickness is a state of social dysfunction which affects the individual's relations with others.

The conditions in which sick privileges are conferred therefore vary between societies, between cultures, and between particular social situations. The typical sick role is temporary; society expects that most patients will get well. This appears most clearly in simple societies, where all sickness is temporary, in the sense that there are no permanent bedridden sick. In the Mambwe tribe in Central Africa, for instance, 'natural' sickness is considered to make a man ill for only 2 or 3 days. If he continues to feel sick after this time, he suspects that someone is using sorcery against him, and calls in the witch-doctor. If the witch-doctor confirms that sorcery is the agency at work, the patient pays him to turn the sorcery away and to provide a cure. In the outcome the patient either recovers within a short period, or else he dies, for the environmental conditions are too harsh to favour protracted crises. The majority of the Mambwe, like millions of other tribal Africans, suffer constantly from chronic illnesses such as malaria, treponemal infections, tuberculosis, and malnutrition. But such chronic complaints are so commonplace that they do not qualify a sufferer to be treated as 'sick', and he must carry out his social obligations and duties. In Uganda, the symptoms and the diagnosis of peptic ulcer are rarely encountered among Africans, but at necropsy the scars of peptic ulcers are no less common than in Britain. In primitive conditions, there is no place for the bedfast patient, for neither the economy, the technology, nor the culture of tribal societies is advanced enough to support non-productive individuals for any length of time. Chronic sick roles appear only under civilized conditions, where there is an economy to support unproductive patients, a technology to cure or aid them, and a system of values that insists that they should be cared for.

Chronic sick roles are of two kinds, the bedridden and the ambulant, and each has its own problems. The bedridden and dependent invalid in Britain has long had a recognized role in the past: a person on his feet and at work was usually considered healthy. Lepers provide an apparent long-standing exception, but although they have been recognized as sick persons ever since Biblical times, most societies could not provide them with a positive social role and tended to exclude them altogether from normal social life.

The distinction between the ambulant and the bedridden is no longer clear-cut. This came prominently to public notice at the time of the Boer War, when the British forces rejected a large number of young recruits on medical grounds. It was evident that many apparently healthy people were, in fact, in need of medical care and attention. (Public alarm at the state of the nation's health led to the appointment of the Inter-Departmental Committee on Physical Deterioration, which reported in 1904. Its findings helped to hasten the introduction of the School Health Service in 1908, which was intended to check the extent of the health problem by regular inspection of schoolchildren.)

Standards of health have been raised since then, and the expectation of life increased. A large and increasing number of people now survive to suffer from such chronic disorders as hypertension, coronary disease, heart failure, diabetes, and rheumatoid arthritis. They are kept on their feet and at work by continuous medical treatment. Such persons do not fit the stereotyped sick role, and their families often experience difficulty in according them the necessary relief from normal obligations warranted by their condition, for they appear to be neither ill nor well, and their condition is not temporary, but permanent.

The chronic sick role offers a prolonged escape from everyday responsibilities, and for this reason some patients may prefer this role, despite the disadvantages of disablement and unemployment that follow. In such a case, the patient's preference is influenced by his family situation as well as his personality, and in any given illness the threshold of disordered function which produces disablement and unemployment varies accordingly. Variations in the threshold are bound up with the social norms and values which define malingering, hypochondria, and neurosis, for these norms and values determine whether certain forms of behaviour are tolerated or rejected. Many persons recognized and persecuted as witches in Britain in the past, as in Ghana today, would be diagnosed in contemporary Britain as suffering from depression.

Family norms and values, and their material resources, govern the initial interpretation of the nature of the individual's problem, the recognition of his illness, and his participation in treatment. The chance of a diabetic child surviving, for instance, may virtually depend on these factors; certain families may be unable to appreciate the full importance of the physician's instruction, or to equate them with their own view of the illness, or else their material and social resources may be inadequate to sustain the exacting regime of diet and medication.

The relationship of the patient with the doctor is only one aspect of his total situation and derives from it, and an adequate assessment of the patient requires analysis of his social context. Social science enables the doctor to make the analysis systematic; this should be as much a part of medical history-taking as systematic inquiry about symptoms. The analysis would examine the structure and content of the patient's relations in the home, in the wider community, and in his occupation, and consider the relevance of these various associations in the clinical setting. The structure of the relationships is determined by the status of the interacting individuals—in terms of age and sex and social position—and by the ramification of formal and informal ties between them. The content of the relationships depends not only on the personality of those who interact, but on the nature of their ties, and on the expectations and sanctions attached to them by the culture. Interaction is mediated by what is right and proper in the appropriate system of values.

Communication

Analysis of this kind places the health professional in a better position to comprehend the problems of patients. It may also help him to communicate more effectively with them by supplementing intuition with intellectual appraisal. Effective communication in the face-to-face situation between doctors and patients is fundamental to diagnosis and treatment. Much evidence shows how frequently communication by doctors does not produce the hoped-for result in their patients.

In an Israeli study patients were asked, before seeing the doctor and again afterwards, whether they considered they had a dangerous or a minor illness; the doctors were asked to make a similar rating. Forty per cent. of those patients rated by the doctor as having minor illness had thought, before seeing him, that their condition was serious. After seeing the doctor, 1 in 10 of the 40 per cent. no longer thought their condition serious, but the original number was exactly restored by others who had come to think their illness serious. In the patients' perception of their illnesses there had been hardly any shift which could be attributed to the consultation. Although the doctors had succeeded in communicating instructions to these patients, they had not succeeded in communicating either reassurance or information about illness.

The practice of medicine always involves communication between at least two people, patient and doctor, and sometimes more, as between a medical officer of health and the community. The need for exact interpretation exists not only in the privacy of the consulting-room, but also in the health educator's lecture in the maternity clinic.

All doctors have been harassed at one time or another by the apparent illogicality of some patients, who appear to hold ignorant and mistaken beliefs concerning the nature of their troubles. But consideration of the patients' beliefs in terms of their social background may show that the 'illogicality' is relative. Failure to communicate or to understand may result from a clash in cultural values.

When a doctor in Britain makes the diagnosis of influenza in a young adult patient, both patient and doctor understand that the patient will need only symptomatic treatment, and that the patient will be obliged to stay away from work for only a few days. The patient will also assume without being told that his life is not in danger. This common understanding does not apply to every similar situation. People who do not share the same cultural background may attach divergent meanings to the same words, and, as a result, fail to communicate their exact intentions to one another.

Should a doctor make a diagnosis not of influenza but of tuberculosis, then a very different situation often arises. The doctor will understand that the patient has a serious and possibly long-lasting disease, although nowadays, in an early case, he will expect to achieve a cure within a few months by appropriate treatment. He no longer fears later complications, nor subsequently imposes restrictions of the patient's habits other than those of moderate living. But the patient may view the matter quite otherwise. To him, tuberculosis may conjure up 'galloping consumption'; he may regard it as a sentence of death; he may sometimes consider it a curse on his family, a punishment for some obscure family sin.

In public health the main emphasis of the problems of communication has shifted with time. The upsurge of public health in the nineteenth century was aimed at control of the elements of the physical environment which were known or thought to be important to health. The great tasks were to purify water and food supplies, dispose effectively of sewage, improve housing, control working conditions. All these sources of ill health could be attacked physically given the necessary legislative power and administrative resources. The work of public health was therefore dependent on political and administrative change. In these circumstances communication by the public health official was directed chiefly to the organs of central and local government; thereafter the task called for energetic local administration.

This form of endeavour, however does not deal effectively with many of the problems which preventive medicine now takes into its demesne, for it has since recognized the contribution to preventable disease of personal behaviour in everyday life.

Child welfare and maternity clinics were set up to attack 'ignorance' and to eradicate practices harmful to health. 'Health education' became an important part of the work of public health. But habits that affect health in childbearing and midwifery, in nutrition and in daily living, are not merely the negative result of ignorance among people who know no better. They are often an integral part of a way of life, customs which for the people concerned have positive value and explicit and implicit symbolic significance.

Health education aims at changing the behaviour of individuals and groups in a direction favourable to health. It cannot achieve this by exhortation in the face of values, beliefs, and social relationships that the educators have failed to appreciate. This is not a problem confined to one type of society. In such matters as cigarette smoking in industrial societies the need to alter personal and group behaviour has become a public health problem no less crucial than, say, infant feeding in non-industrial societies.

HEALTH PROFESSIONALS IN RELATION TO PATIENTS

The Professional's Social Situation

The doctor is the professional of the two parties involved in the transaction of medicine, but he, too, is a social being; his social situation influences the transaction. The ideal type or model of the doctor's relationship with the patient takes no account of this; as Talcott Parsons has put it, his position is one of 'affective neutrality'. The doctor tries always, according to the medical ethic, to give priority to the patients' interests and needs, but at the same time he must remain emotionally detached from him. Theoretically the doctor elicits the necessary information about the patient, collates it, and makes his judgements and decisions on dispassionate rational grounds.

A major revision of this computer-like model of the doctor's role took place when psychoanalysts began consciously to use the doctor's relationship with the patient for therapeutic purposes. They first recognized and analysed the nature of the patient's emotional involvement with the doctor. However, all relationships are reciprocal, and they were soon led to recognize the doctor's involvement with the patient.

These psychological insights had to be revised in their turn when sociological studies began. Since the primary aim of the doctor is to serve the best interests of his patients, the medical ethic must forbid discrimination against them according to colour, class, or creed. The doctor in the bygone charity hospital was probably firm in the belief that he was trying to do as much for his patients in the hospital as for those in his consulting-rooms. But what he consciously believed was unlikely to be the same as what he unconsciously did.

A study of psychotherapy in New Haven provides a notable example of such unconscious social bias. In each of the psychiatric agencies, the treatment given was related to the social class of the patient in its type, frequency, and duration. Among private psychiatrists, for instance, the average time for the therapeutic session declined from the higher social classes to the lower. Clearly psychotherapy is not all a matter of psychodynamics. The gulf of class and culture between the doctor and his patients affected his ability or readiness to treat them.

The ideal position of 'affective neutrality' on the part of the doctor helps him to avoid making moral judgements about the behaviour of individual patients. His proper response is to judge the problem for which the patient seeks help on clinical grounds; if it is a question of behaviour he seeks its cause and helps the patient to modify it. The same position holds for the public health professional who is called upon to make judgements about groups in the community. Such judgements may hinder communication and understanding if they become morally loaded by values derived from the culture of the public health worker; he needs to take account of the variability of norms of human behaviour between social groups.

The Professional's Work Situation

Many other factors influence the health professionals' relations with patients and communities and the quality of their performance. To take one example, a study of the Health Insurance Plan in New York suggests that the situations in which doctors work, and the groups to whom they refer to approve their behaviour, exert a marked effect on their relations with patients. The general practitioner, who stands close to the community and is subject to many pressures from it through his practice, tends to be sensitive to the personal aspects of care. In contrast, the hospital physician is under little pressure from the surrounding community or from patients, and he tends to be sensitive to pressures from professional colleagues. While such pressures are likely to maintain

the doctor's technical competence, they do not promote attention to the personal needs of patients. In line with this we have found that the mistakes of hospital practice often seem to arise from failures of communication, and the mistakes of general practice from technical failures.

The reference groups of the health officer will include the representatives of his community on local government to whom he is responsible and the organs of public opinion such as the Press. He must be sensitive to pressures from such sources if, as his work requires, he is to influence them and not alienate them; for the possibilities of action in medical and health problems will inevitably be affected by them.

The work situation is immediate to the professional's behaviour. The professional personality which reacts to the situation is founded on more remote factors, and to search them out one must examine his profession as a whole, its political and economic interests, its organization, and its values. At the heart of its values lies the system of professional education. Professional education is more than a means of teaching the skills necessary to the practice of a health profession. It is a chief channel through which the values of the profession are transmitted and their continuity ensured.

In the process of professional education the doctor, for example, gradually acquires a concept of his proper functions, of the sphere of his competence, of his obligations and duties and of the nature of his relations with patients. The role concept generated by present-day medical education is predominantly that of the hospital doctor, technically competent, concerned with the patient as a case and an object of scientific study, and intent on treating and hopeful of curing the seriously ill. This role concept is not appropriate to all doctors, for instance, the general practitioner. Like his colleagues in hospital he is trained to act by scientific and professional criteria and to deal with serious acute disease. But he must frequently give greater weight to the wishes and the circumstances of his patient and of those close to him than to scientific criteria, and he must often deal with minor complaints or psychological disturbances which do not threaten life.

In a different way the professional role concept is inappropriate to the work of the doctor in preventive medicine. The health officer does not contribute to the treatment of serious acute disease, and much of the time he does not deal with individual patients. If he seeks to practise personal preventive medicine through such techniques as mass screening he finds himself reversing the traditional relationship of patient and doctor. Instead of the patient seeking the doctor's help, the doctor solicits the patients attendance. In some circumstances the health officer may even find himself exercising legal power to compel the compliance of an individual with his instructions. Compulsion is at variance with the voluntary nature of the traditional professional relationship between doctor and patient. The conflict between the traditional role concept and the actual role of a doctor may thus give rise to strains which affect his mode of work and his choice of career.

SYSTEMS OF HEALTH AND MEDICAL CARE

The 'efficiency engineer', whose job was to eliminate inefficiency in organizations 'scientifically', was discredited among industrial sociologists by the crudeness of his schemes. Medical care likewise does not respond to the simplicities of rational planning, and requires an appreciation of its social dynamics. Systems of health care can be considered in terms of their external relations with the larger society, and in terms of their internal relations—that is, in terms of the structure and content of relations within particular health organizations.

External Relations of Health and Medical Systems

The actual functions of medicine in society extend beyond its avowed functions. In industrial societies its avowed function is at the organic level, to cure and prevent disease. But it is quite evident that medicine has an additional function at the personal level. This is to reassure and to allay anxiety in individuals, whether healthy or diseased, who turn to the doctor to alleviate their distress. Work at the personal rather than the organic level is the standby of the traditional doctor of pre-scientific societies; his credits in this field balance his debits with organic disease.

In all societies medicine has a third function, at the social level, by which it helps to absorb the social strains of sickness. I have noted above that sickness can be seen as a form of social dysfunction in which the individual's relations with others deviate from the norm. This sick role is regularized by his relationships with the doctor. Hence the heavy commitment of doctors in all modern societies to duties of certification, whether for absence from work or school, or for deaths, or for a multitude of other matters. Society uses the doctor to legitimize departures from such expected behaviour as continuing to work, or continuing to live. It has used him, too, to legitimize the custody of deviants such as the psychopath and the mentally ill, and to legitimize the support of dependent or disabled persons—for instance, the severely subnormal and the victims of industrial accidents.

The balance between medical functions at the organic, the personal, and the social level varies between societies and social groups. In New York, for example, psychotherapy appears to have served functions different from those in Manchester or in Moscow. In a survey of the prevalence of mental illness in Manhattan 23·6 per cent. of the population were considered to be functionally impaired by mental disorder. Only 5 per cent. of this staggering proportion were in treatment at the time, but an equal number of persons not evidently impaired were also in treatment. One explanation for this anomaly is that treatment was related less to the 'organic' level of severe psychiatric disorder than to personal or social needs. Such variations emphasize that in all societies doctors share some or all of their functions with other agents and institutions whose part in absorbing the strains of sickness must be recognized. The distribution of the functions of medicine can only be comprehended in relation to other purveyors of care.

Public health exemplifies those social functions of medicine which are most explicitly avowed. Although in the past public health has been concerned chiefly with the prevention of disease at the organic level, its object has been to influence the health of the community as a whole. Indeed, it has been necessary to the practice of preventive medicine that the representative organs of society assume formal responsibility to health. Moreover, most factors which cause disease and are preventable reside in the environment, whether physical or biological or social; by the nature of its task, public health has been obliged to take account of the social relations of disease and sickness. Modern public health has, therefore, added to its concern for the physical and natural environment those problems of social disability and resettlement which arise in the course of medical care. These problems, and the related problems of social deviance, are illuminated by the methods of social science.

Internal Relations of Health and Medical Systems

The formal structure of an institution and the quality of communication within it is likely to influence the effectiveness of its officers, including doctors and other health professionals, and the services they provide. Studies of the internal working of health and medical organizations are one aspect of the general study of organizations. They warn us of the ravelled nature of the problems of organization, and of the difficulties to be expected in such apparently simple matters as achieving co-ordinated care for patients, for example in Britain, between the three branches of the National Health Service. In any attempt at co-ordination the forces within each organization must be recognized and coped with. Each organization has a life of its own, and the forces which generate this life may be quite divorced from the ostensible purpose of serving the client. Some of these forces are concerned with the maintenance of the power, the prestige, and the stability of the organization and its various sectors.

Stable persisting organizations develop distinctive cultures and beliefs about their functions. An organization tends to see its work in terms of its own culture, and any medical agency's outlook is inevitably centred in its own functions. This centripetal view is limited by the world of the institution in which the medical transaction takes place. The patient in a hospital bed has extremely restricted roles and a narrow range of explicit needs. Consequently some of his needs—for instance, for resettlement in normal social roles—may not be recognized or they may not be thought quite proper to the sphere of the hospital doctor.

In contrast the view of a public health department, which may recognize social needs, may yet be restricted in respect of technical needs. A characteristic constraint on the function of public health departments is their typical bureaucratic structure (using the description in a technical and not a pejorative sense). A public health department will usually have such a structure, that is to say, it is arranged in a hierarchy of offices, each with a well-defined sphere of competence, and a chain of command that rises through them and ends with the medical officer of health. Bureaucratic organization is rational and to that extent efficient and predictable. Rules may help to eliminate the personal vagaries of officials, but they also tend to produce impersonal formal relationships. Hence the impersonal judgements which are the foundation of 'red tape' can become a danger in public health work.

The various settings in which doctors work and the values they acquire in these settings cause them to act by differing criteria and priorities. Because of the limits set on experience and perception by professional training and institutions, it cannot be assumed that health professionals have common ends, even though they share their patients. Public health will be frustrated in its attempts to live up to its ethical ideals, and will fail to give its best service, until it can recognize the hidden social forces that intervene between intention and action.

This chapter is based in part on Susser, M. W. (1964) *Lancet*, **ii**, 425; and Susser, M. W., and Watson, W. (1971) *Sociology in Medicine*, 2nd ed., London.

FURTHER READING

Freeman, H. E., Levine, S., and Reeder, L. G., eds. (1963) *Handbook of Medical Sociology*, London.

Freidson, E. (1963) *The Hospital in Modern Society*, London.

Freidson, E. (1970) *Professional Dominance: The Social Structure of Medical Care*, New York.

Levine, S., and Scotch, N., eds. (1970) *Social Stress*, Chicago.

Mechanic, D. (1968) *Medical Sociology: A Selective View*, New York.

Moser, C. A., and Kalton, G. (1971) *Survey Methods in Social Investigation*, London.

Paul, B. D., ed. (1955) *Health Culture and Community*, New York.

Prins, H. A., and Whyte, Marion B. H. (1972) *Social Work and Medical Practice*, Oxford

Scott, W. R., and Volkart, E. H. (1966) *Medical Care: Readings in the Sociology of Medical Institutions*, New York.

Suchman, Edward A. (1963) *Sociology and the Field of Public Health*, New York.

Susser, M. W., and Watson, W. (1971) *Sociology in Medicine*, 2nd ed., London.

48

THE SOCIAL SERVICES AND THE HEALTH OF THE COMMUNITY

HARDY WICKWAR

INTRODUCTION

The term 'social services' came into use in Britain early in this century in order to distinguish government outlay on direct services to its own citizens from spending for 'defence services'. The corresponding broad term in North America has been 'social programs' and in France 'programmes d'action sociale'.

Within this broad classification, it has become customary, however, to use the term 'social services' also in a more restricted sense, for those services which cannot be classed conveniently as health, housing, or education. The corresponding restricted term in North America is 'welfare programs' and in France 'prévoyance sociale'. Since the other social services, in the broad sense, are covered in other chapters in this volume, it is with the social services in this narrower sense that this chapter is concerned.

The principal reason for government action in the social field is that the ordinary working of the economy does not produce all the services consumers need. Government has therefore been called upon to provide not only educational and health services but also other social services. In other words, social 'need' has been translated into effective 'demand' only through government action.

During the past 150 years, all these public social services have become well-established institutions in all countries. They are now part of the social milieu in which we grow up and live our lives. Since public health is concerned with the relationship between human beings and their environment, it has to take account of institutional as well as physical aspects of the human environment.

This is reflected in the definition of health goals on which the world's governments agreed when they set up the World Health Organization: 'a state of complete physical, mental, and social well-being, and not merely the absence of disease or infirmity'.

Social services other than health, housing, and education help people meet some of their most pressing needs under certain specially disadvantageous circumstances which would otherwise prevent their functioning. These circumstances and these needs are mainly of two kinds. Persons or families may not have enough earnings and savings to be able to live as they expect to do: their own slender resources may then be supplemented by guaranteeing them a certain income in partial replacement of what they have lost or in addition to what they have. (These income guarantees are known in French, as 'prestations sociales'.) Or persons may need special help in order to look after themselves or cope with their environment, because of youth or handicap or age: what they can do for themselves and what their family can do for them may then be supplemented by providing them with personal attention, care,

or protection. (These social welfare services are called in French 'services de protection sociale'.) These are the two principal categories under which social services will be analysed in the next two sections of this chapter.

Both kinds of social service in these narrow senses differ from health, housing, and education in requiring a different mix of human services and physical facilities. Whereas modern health care is inconceivable without hospitals or education without schools, these other social services require comparatively little investment in buildings for use by their beneficiaries. Instead they depend mainly on efficient organization of income-guarantee services and good staffing of social welfare services; and good services may even diminish the need for investing scarce capital in expensive institutions.

The two kinds of social service may also differ from one another in the ways in which they are organized. The income-guarantee services may tend to be administered by the national government or its local agents as impersonally as possible. The social welfare care and adaptation services may tend, on the other hand, to be administered by the local community with as much personal attention as possible. This distinction has become especially clearcut in Britain.

Both kinds of public social service are highly developed in all the 'developed' countries of the temperate zone. Neither kind is much developed in the 'developing' countries of the tropical and arid zones. This difference is part of the general difference in their patterns of living. In tropical and arid countries, the majority of the population get their living directly from the soil and tend to live and work together in some kind of kinship group. Their basic needs both for subsistence and for care are therefore met within their kinship group, except when they are stricken by some disaster, whether natural as with earthquake or flood, or man-made as with civil or international war. In the temperate countries since the industrial revolution, on the other hand, the majority of the population have moved off the land into urban settlements; instead of growing their own food, they have become employed for wages or salaries, so that, whenever they cease to be employed, their livelihood is threatened; and, instead of living in extended families or clans, they have come to live in 'conjugal' or 'nuclear' families, which may leave many persons without any relatives able to care for them. The less developed and the more rural the society, the greater the probability of the need for subsistence and care being met spontaneously and on a small scale. The more developed and the more urban the society, the greater the extent to which large-scale government action has been required to help people meet these needs.

We are here particularly concerned with the pattern of income-guarantee and social welfare services that has taken shape in all developed countries during the twentieth century. This pattern did not emerge full-blown, however, during the lifetime of persons still living, but was preceded in early modern times by a transitional form of public social service. This was the system of 'poor relief' which emerged in most European countries about 1600, under which each government held each local parish responsible for the subsistence and care of its local poor. Under the name of 'Elizabethan poor-law', this system spread from England to the English colonies overseas. It is only since about 1900 that this system has everywhere been broken up into the specialized services discussed in this chapter.

INCOME-GUARANTEE SERVICES

If people are to be healthy, they have to have access to food, clothing, housing, and other basic necessities. Experience has shown that the increase in life expectancy in developed countries has been closely linked to the rise in the level of living among the mass of the population. Public health is therefore concerned not only with removing specific health obstacles that may stand in the way of people living normal lives, but also with all other policies and programmes that can help people meet their vital needs.

Consumption Levels

In order to pay for their basic necessities, people who live in a money economy need an income. The usual way to get an income is to earn it by working. Since the Great Depression of the 1930s, governments have therefore adopted 'full employment' policies. That is to say, they have committed themselves to using their fiscal, monetary, and other powers in such a way as to lessen the probability of unemployment exceeding a certain agreed percentage (e.g. 2·5) of the economically active population.

If a full employment policy fails to keep unemployment below the agreed level, a government may feel that it ought to act as 'employer of last resort' and create temporary public jobs.

If there are certain areas within a country which fail to reach the general level of employment, a government may feel that it ought to adopt a special policy in the hope of turning these depressed or backward regions into 'development areas'. If the country has a general development plan, it may aim at the equal development of all the country's regions.

If people are to meet their basic needs by working, mere employment is not enough: they need a living wage. Some workers may be in a good bargaining position, because they have scarce skills for which employers compete or because they benefit from collective bargaining between organized labour and organized management. Others, however, may be at a great disadvantage in bargaining, especially if they are unskilled or unorganized. On their behalf, minimum wages are therefore set, either by a special procedure to meet the different circumstances of each particular industry, as in the United Kingdom, or by uniform nationwide legislation, as in France and the United States. There are, however, many different principles on which a minimum wage may be based. It may aim at enabling an individual worker to subsist, or it may aim at enabling him to reproduce his kind, that is to say, at support-ing a family of four. It may aim at basic necessities or at a few amenities.

Risk-pooling and Income-transfer

There are certain contingencies, however, under which all persons risk being unable to earn their livings: they may be too aged or handicapped to obtain employment; they may be dependent spouses or children who have lost their breadwinner; or there may be no employment for them to take. There is also a contingency in which every minimum wage becomes less than a living wage: the family may have more children than it can afford to raise; most wage-earners who assume parental responsibilities are financially worse off than those who do not; and even a government which wishes to prevent large families has to consider the health and welfare of children brought into the world by an act for which they were not responsible.

In the modern world there are risks that everyone runs. An African kinship community may be able to assure the subsistence of its members, whatever happens to them as individuals; and a self-employed farm family working its own land may usually manage to get by, even when for a while it has less hands to work or more mouths to feed. In a rural economy where people get their subsistence in kind from their family labour, the land and its produce have been their 'income security'. With the triumph of a money economy and the breaking of the link between land and people, only a declining minority retain this kind of landed security on which to fall back, and only a still smaller minority enjoy enough of a family fortune to substitute for it. Artificial substitutes have therefore been devised, in four methods of risk-pooling which amount to income-transfer from the more fortunate to the less fortunate under a system of social solidarity organized on a national instead of a kinship scale.

Some of these forms of risk-pooling are called 'universal' because the risks they cover are considered universal in developed countries. Others are called 'selective' because they make benefits available only to certain especially 'vulnerable' segments of the population.

Under a universal system, the need in any individual case is 'presumed' rather than actually proved; and, by not inquiring into the 'means and needs' of each individual applicant, the cost of administration is kept down to between 1 and 3 per cent. of the benefits paid. Under the selective method, on the other hand, administrative overheads amount to 9 or 10 per cent. of cost.

Under a universal system, if any government feels that it is unfair for a person to accept an income-transfer payment who has a sufficient fortune to put him above real risk, it can counteract this situation simply and cheaply through its income-tax system if it so desires.

After a country has crossed a certain threshold of development, income guarantees become a legal right to which all are entitled. When introduced into developing countries, on the other hand, they cover only the minority who have left the land and are fortunate enough to have found paid urban employment.

Universal Pensions

The simplest way of operating a universal income-guarantee system is for the government to give a statutory right to a flat-rate pension to every citizen who is too old or too young to work, and then finance this out of the general taxes. This is what the British and Australian governments do when they pay children's allowances, or the Canadian and New Zealand governments when they pay pensions to all persons over a certain age. A similar result is reached, but in kind rather than in cash, when health care, schooling, and school milk are made available free to all. The merit of this approach has been its administrative simplicity, and its assurance of a 'floor' beneath everyone's level of living. Its political weakness has been that it depends entirely on parliamentary budget appropriations.

Social Insurance

A second method of risk-sharing has been social insurance. In all developed countries in the nineteenth century there arose mutual aid associations under various names—friendly societies, fraternal orders, and craft unions—through which their working members could insure against some at least of the risks of loss of earnings. Governments then converted this voluntary system into compulsory social insurance, obliging workers and employers to pay certain rates of compulsory 'contributions' (premiums), and obliging the insurance funds to pay certain 'benefits' in certain contingencies. This system, initiated in Bismarck's Germany, spread to Britain in 1911. Its merit was the political one of linking benefits to contributions, thus creating a feeling that participants had a right to 'covenanted' benefits, and doing this outside the country's regular budget. Its defects were that it did not cover the whole population impartially and that its administrative overheads were high.

Universal Social Security

Experience with these earlier methods led on to the idea of a comprehensive system that would guarantee most citizens against most risks. To this the American term 'social security' was applied. The first country to enact such legislation was New Zealand (1938); but the spirit of solidarity that arose in West European countries during the Second World War facilitated its rapid adoption among developed countries, especially after the publication in Britain of the Beveridge Report (1942).

The contingencies covered first by social insurance and later by social security have to be defined. Old age, retirement, or superannuation permits of several definitions; for example, a national social security system may say that one can become entitled to a pension either when one retires or when one reaches an advanced age. A degree of invalidity such that one cannot work may be equated with premature retirement. Loss of a family breadwinner may necessitate benefits for surviving children, while leaving room for different definitions of the benefit rights of widows. These contingencies call for continuing payments. For unemployment, on the other hand, provision has been made for only a limited term; but the limits have been frequently redefined; and if the unemployment lasts indefinitely it can shade off into redundancy and premature retirement.

With regard to one set of risks an important innovation is being made. All countries have developed work injuries compensation and rehabilitation to cover accidents and diseases due to occupational risks regardless of whether anyone is at fault. New Zealand has now extended this to cover all the risks of modern life, in the home and on the highway as well as at work.

In most of these contingencies, social security guarantees a 'substitute' income when the regular earned income is lost or seriously diminished. In one other contingency a 'compensatory' income has been provided, as when France pioneered with family allowances in respect of each child and also of the mother who stays home to look after it, in order to reduce morbidity and mortality among children, and to increase the chances of persons who assume parental responsibilities being not too much worse off materially than those who do not.

In each of these contingencies, detailed provisions differ greatly from country to country and from year to year, and may be found in standard reference works: here it is more appropriate to review issues and principles.

Guarantee against loss or inadequacy of income in all these contingencies is of two-way importance to public health: one way because people's physical and mental health depends on their being able to obtain the material necessities of life; and, the other way, because effective public health services can lessen the frequency of income being lost through chronic invalidity, premature bereavement and acute illness, or of income proving inadequate through parents' having more children than they can afford to raise.

In fixing the amount of social security benefit, governments hesitated initially between two principles. Britain began with the idea of a 'flat rate' to enable all beneficiaries to reach a 'subsistence minimum' indispensable to physical health, whereas the United States began with a scale of benefits graduated to correspond to different income levels and presumed conducive to mental health. Most national systems have now reached a compromise between these two principles —they aim both at 'minimum adequacy' and at being 'income related'.

Social security has provided a reliable income floor, and by pooling risks has enabled 'high risk' as well as 'low risk' persons to insure against income loss. In insuring most of the population against total loss of income, it has guaranteed them only part of the earnings they have lost. It has nevertheless provided a foundation on which a family can build, by private savings, work-connected insurance, and pension schemes and other 'fringe benefits' negotiated between organized labour and organized management; in a few countries these collective-bargaining pension schemes have been subjected to public regulation in order to ensure the rights of participants.

Owing to the large-scale development first of social insurance and then of social security, a new system of remuneration has now emerged. Only part of a person's earnings becomes his individual 'take-home pay': the other part goes into a 'social income' pool from which he and others will be entitled to draw in time of need. This latter portion varies from one worker to another according to a country's laws, but reaches between one-tenth and one-third of the wage bill.

There is no absolute necessity for financing most income-guarantee out of premiums levied on the wage bill, and saying that some of this constitutes the employee's and some the employer's 'contribution' to the premium. This method has been more followed than any other, however, because risk-pooling through autonomous funds rather than annual parliamentary appropriations originated in workers' mutual aid funds, developed under social insurance, has been promoted by the International Labour Organization, is flexible, and above all has been found politically convenient. For all of these reasons, the dominant current approach towards a universal income guarantee is through contributory social security rather than non-contributory pensions and allowances. Its method of financing has been slightly modified in communist countries by charging 'pensions' entirely to state and co-operative business enterprises as part of their cost of production instead of deducting a contribution from workers' wages.

Selective Social Assistance

Although the main responsibility for providing substitute or supplementary income has been placed on universal public pension and social security systems, these alone have proved inadequate to enable some people to meet all their basic needs. In every country there are persons who have not met all the statutory conditions and therefore do not qualify, or there are needs which have not been provided against, or, above all, the social security benefits or universal pensions have not by themselves been sufficient to meet all the basic needs of every recipient. In particular, nationwide standards may need adjusting to local differences in housing costs. Every government providing national pensions or social security benefits has therefore 'supplemented' this universal system with a 'selective' system of social assistance on behalf of the minority who remain exceptionally needy. This social aid to needy persons has been financed from general taxation, and the allowances granted to each individual applicant have varied according to his means and needs. These payments have come to be known as 'supplementary benefits' in Britain, 'public assistance or supplementary security income' in the United States, 'aide sociale' in France, and 'social assistance' internationally.

Since the systems of universal and selective transfer payments are complementary, it is obvious that, the more adequate the universal minimum, the smaller the role of social assistance as a method of compensating for loss or insufficiency of income. Conversely the expansion of social assistance in some countries suggests that a lag may have occurred in carrying out the original intention of making universal public pensions and social security adequate to meet basic needs.

Assistance allowances (supplementary benefits) can also be used to supplement wages, where the minimum wage is aimed only at the support of one or two children. In many parts of the United States, wage supplementation through 'general assistance' has been widely practised. Canada decided in 1970 that it could combat poverty more effectively by this means than by universal children's allowances. Britain has also abandoned its former policy of regarding persons in full-time employment as ineligible for social assistance, by introducing selective 'family wage supplements' rather than increasing universal children's allowances. And the United States national government has considered financing this form of assistance to the 'working poor' as a way of guaranteeing a minimum income related to family size.

If social assistance payments (supplementary benefits) are to be calculated fairly as between one applicant and another, there has to be a scale relating payments to differences in means and needs. The construction of this scale opens up a wide range of policy options. What needs shall be met? A government can draw up a list of what it thinks is needed for physical and mental health, including food, housing, clothing, furnishings, utilities, memberships, and recreation, and can then decide how many of these needs it can afford to meet out of annual budget appropriations and to what extent. The result is that, in some countries and at some dates, assistance projects suffice for little more than subsistence and shelter, whereas in others they aim at some selected level of 'human needs' or 'decency'. The scale selected may or may not be in line with the funds available: in countries where it is based on a comparatively modest poverty line, it may be actually followed, as in the United Kingdom, whereas, where it aims higher, it may be customary to pay only some fraction of what it entitles the recipient to, as in much of the United States. And what resources shall be taken into consideration? To a large extent this boils down into a question of 'Whose resources?' and this is answered by accepting as the norm the two-generation nuclear family that has become common in all developed countries. It is thus presumed that marriage partners have assumed responsibility for one another and parents for their children, but that the normal course for children to follow is to hive off and renew this cycle. Thus the traditional responsibility of children for parents and grandparents, including that of teen-agers living in the same household, has everywhere tended to be limited, abolished, or not enforced, while the former responsibility of collaterals has almost everywhere disappeared. In a mobile society, it has even become difficult to enforce the responsibility of an absent male parent. In most countries it is also assumed that if an applicant for assistance owns more than a limited amount of property or savings, this must be counted in some way as part of his income.

Assistance allowances may be granted to any who can prove that their means and needs justify them. This has become the British policy. On the other hand, they may be available only to categories of persons presumed to be exceptionally unlikely to be able to fend for themselves. This is Australian and French policy, and is the practice in many parts of the United States, where national funds have hitherto been provided for assistance to only certain specified 'categories' of applicant: the aged, the blind, the permanently and totally disabled, and families with dependent children.

In a money economy, in which most people get their living from their earnings, it is natural to pay social benefits and assistance allowances in money. In some countries, however, there are some survivals or revivals of assistance in kind instead of in cash. For example, the United States Department of Agriculture has sought ways of disposing of surplus farm products while at the same time supporting high food prices; it therefore sells 'food stamps' for a lower price than their face value, to families below a certain poverty line.

All assistance systems differ from social insurance and social security in that the applicant is expected to be in actual rather than presumed need. Arrangements are therefore made to check the veracity of his statements; and administrative costs tend consequently to be high. If income-guarantee payments were made only to persons in provable need, they would presumably be lower, although their administration would cost more. This has not seemed like a good reason for transferring responsibilities from social security to social assistance; but it has served to prevent any recent expansion of universal non-contributory pensions or allowances or their introduction into the United States, or even the retention of non-contributory pensions for children in Canada or old people in Britain; and it has been used to justify family supplements for large low-income families in these three countries.

SOCIAL WELFARE SERVICES

The income-guarantee services, along with the health and education services, enable many families and individuals to look after themselves without much further aid. Many, however, are also helped towards adaptation and survival by other social services.

Community Participation

Certain of these social welfare services are available to all, and can help everybody reach a higher level of health and well-being than would otherwise be possible. These tend to be services associated with groups, to which individuals or families belong who have something in common, and which can operate only with their members' active participation. Community centres, neighbourhood associations, leisure-time clubs of many kinds, and some vacation centres, are typical examples in all European countries. French Canadians have created a network of credit co-operatives (caisses populaires, credit unions) to encourage saving and keep down the cost of borrowing among members of the same parish or workplace. The Soviet Union puts great emphasis on 'people's organizations' of all kinds. India and its neighbours use village 'panchayats' even for settling disputes. The idea that civic associations are an essential part of the organized social milieu, and that they open up opportunities for individual self-realization and for habits of working together, has been greatly promoted in Britain by the National Council of Social Service.

In a developing and rural country, community development is a policy aimed at helping village communities invest their surplus labour in endowing themselves by their own efforts with such modern communal facilities as schools, health posts, water-supply, bath-houses, and markets. In a developed and urban country, on the other hand, where specialized institutions have developed for economic activity and for building educational and health facilities, community participation tends to focus on 'social' action, and particularly on consumer needs, family needs, and leisure-time activities.

Social Adjustment

Most social welfare services, however, have been aimed at helping individuals and families in situations in which they would not otherwise be able to adapt to a modern social environment. Even where such services are open to all, they may in fact focus on the exceptional problems of selected disadvantaged or vulnerable minorities who might lose rather than gain by economic and social development if special measures were not taken on their behalf.

In a primitive village, there are few such problems. The child and its family do not have to cope with the transition from home to school; nor does the adolescent have to cope with the transition from school to work. The grown person does not have to move from one employer to another, perhaps with a painful gap between jobs; nor is there an age at which no one will employ him any more. If he becomes physically or mentally unable to fend for himself, he is surrounded with relatives able to help him out. Nor is it only the primitive village that makes it easy and natural for the individual and his social milieu to fit in together at every passing phase in his life-cycle. Much the same has usually been true also of more developed rural societies, from the freeholding peasants of some European countries to the freeholding farmers of North America.

With the passing of these settings, abrupt transitions and life crises have grown greatly in importance. Instead of the individual functioning all his life within one set of closely interlocking groups—household, extended family, and kinship neighbourhood—he has to move abruptly from one group to another: from home to school, from school to workplace, from one working group to another, and from work to the comparative isolation of the home, with a risk that he may end his days alone and lonely or confined to an institution.

To help people cope with the complexities and transitions of modern life, social welfare services have been evolved by various kinds of organizations. Some might be called 'horizontal' associations: the community groups already mentioned, friendly societies, fraternal orders or mutual aid groups, trade unions and churches have all taken some responsibility for helping their members face life's vicissitudes. Others might be called 'vertical': voluntary agencies have been founded by charitable or philanthropic patrons, to help some exceptionally handicapped clientele, or to provide a special service such as marriage counselling today. Many attempts at improved 'charity organization' have been made in the past 100 years, and two of these are currently important: local Citizens' Advice Bureaux in Britain have provided information and referral to persons who would not otherwise know to what agency they could go; and social agencies that function in the same town have tended to federate together in a community social service or health and welfare council. In some countries, they also federate to make joint appeals to the public for contributions. Governments usually encourage voluntary social agencies by grants-in-aid, tax privileges, or contracts of service. Many helping services, however, have been provided by public bodies themselves, and especially by local government, as for example, when accommodation is provided for persons who are temporarily homeless.

The overriding aim of all such social welfare services has been to help individuals be as self-supporting as is practical. To the greatest possible extent, they have helped them earn their livings. When this has not been possible, they have helped them fend for themselves at home. And when even this has seemed impractical, social welfare services have taken full responsibility for the individual in the last resort.

Preparation for Self-support

The first important set of social welfare services concern the growing-up process and are intended to help children grow into self-supporting adults. They relate particularly to passage from early childhood through schooling to school-leaving.

Early childhood development is no longer left entirely to the accident of such care and affection as may be given by a mother and the relatives and neighbours who help mind the child, but is becoming the object of organized services. Under modern conditions, it is felt that it may be possible to increase the chances of a child having a fair chance in life, by supplementing what its home can give, and making sure that it gets the care and attention that it needs, that it has contact with interesting things and learns to cope with them, that it learns to talk intelligibly and has something to talk about, and that it begins to learn to get on with its peers. A health service may provide day nurseries, or an education service nursery schools, or a social welfare service day-care centres: but, whichever takes primary responsibility in a particular country, the co-operation of all these services is helpful. Public support for such centres was originally regarded as something exceptional—they were for poor working mothers—and, in some European countries, there was a statutory obligation on employers to provide them for the young children of their women employees. Gradually, however, they have come to be regarded as a universally available community social service, open to use by any mother who feels that they can usefully supplement the all-important early upbringing she gives her child. As a matter of social policy, such centres are regarded as especially important wherever a particular effort seems necessary to help bring about a drastic change in people's attitudes; they have therefore been greatly encouraged in some developing countries as a key to their modernization, in the United States to give a 'headstart' to children whose families have seemed locked in to poverty, and in Britain with a special government grant in aid of children of immigrants.

For more than 100 years, it has been accepted that the school should share with the home the responsibility of educating all children. The government of every developed country sees to it that schooling shall be universal and compulsory and that it shall be available free. The content and method of school education are being continually modified to meet changing conditions. Among other things, they may be enlisted to help meet pressing social problems; United States schools, for example, played a big part in helping immigrant families integrate into a new country, and now face their biggest challenge in trying to integrate the children of non-white field hands from the South into the urban life of the North; and a similar role is now expected of British schools in immigrant neighbourhoods. Of recent years, it has become normal for schools in most countries to contribute formally to sex education, much as they have always been expected to contribute in one way or another to various aspects of health education; and in the United States, they are now expected to help combat drug abuse. Although formal education is the essence of schooling, there has also been a considerable accretion of other social services around the school. It may be so built that it can serve as a neighbourhood or community centre for use by all age-groups. It may try to spot defects in a child's health that would affect its ability to learn, and then make sure that it gets treatment. School milk and meals may be a form of children's allowance in kind where they are available to all and, in some circumstances, a school breakfast may be needed to ensure the attentiveness of the child who is not adequately fed at home, besides contributing to a balanced diet; not least, a special service is required to make sure that

every child that is enrolled will really be able to attend—that it has the shoes or clothes it needs, or that the family can cope with its problems in some better way than keeping a child home from school.

A major critical turning-point comes with the adolescent's passage from school to work. In many countries, unemployment is much more frequent among teen-agers than among older age-groups, because there is a considerable lag in the time it takes many of them to find a job that fits their capacities or ambitions. Special services have therefore been developed to ease this transition, as for example, counselling both from the side of the school and from that of a youth employment service. Some observers suspect that youth opportunity may offer a key to the lessening of lawbreaking among adolescents.

Restoration of Self-support

Another important group of services is to persons of working age, for the purpose of helping them fulfil their normal responsibilities as parents and workers.

For persons who have become handicapped, it is often not enough that they recover from their heart attack, stroke, tuberculosis, or other disabling illness, or that their glandular, mental, or nervous disorder has been brought under control, or that a physical impairment to their sense perception or locomotion has been corrected by an artificial appliance. They may need 'social' and 'vocational' as well as 'physical' rehabilitation if they are again to find employment. The need for this service has grown with the incidence of work injuries and traffic accidents, as well as the increasing possibility of treating what would formerly have been irremediable conditions. Even so, vocational rehabilitation alone may not be enough: Britain and some other countries have therefore required employers to reserve a percentage of their jobs for handicapped persons; and, for persons who can work but are physically or mentally unable to earn a full day's pay by a full day's work, many countries have subsidized 'sheltered workshops', sometimes under the name of 'training centres'. It is assumed that it is better for most persons' mental health for them to feel they are contributing to their keep by being productively occupied. Moreover, in developed economies, there is sometimes a shortage of labour; and it seems uneconomic for a person on whom health and other services have been expended, not to make some contribution in return. Other civilizations have looked on this problem differently; and in some developing countries, it has been considered better for a blind or otherwise crippled person to keep alive the spirit of individual charity by begging for alms.

Other handicaps requiring special remedial measures are essentially economic or social. For persons who have lost their jobs but have not found others before their unemployment insurance runs out, retraining schemes and aid for removal to a locality where work is available have been developed by many governments; and continued public aid is often made conditional on participation in such retraining, although its effectiveness depends on the availability of jobs of the kind for which the person is retrained.

A difficult problem of social handicap is posed by the release of ex-offenders after long-term imprisonment. Rehabilitation implies readaptation. They may need 'aftercare' to help them find a place again in self-supporting free society. This service thus becomes a 'secondary prevention' procedure: a way of lessening the chances of their repeating their offence. Their counsellors in prison therefore try to put them in touch with a voluntary aftercare and resettlement agency in their community.

Maintenance of Self-care

Another group of social welfare services are for helping individuals and couples care for themselves even when there is little likelihood of their again earning their living. This is particularly the case with people who are irreversibly handicapped by injury, disease, or age. They may be totally incapacitated so far as employment is concerned, but may still be able to shop, to look after themselves, and to keep house, to some extent at least. It may be more satisfying to their mental health, as well as more economic, to help them fend for themselves in their own homes, than to care for them in congregate institutions. If this policy is adopted, several services may be required to help make it possible. Housing that is specially convenient for people with physical handicaps is often provided. Podiatry may help them get around. 'Home help' (domestic service) and 'meals on wheels' may be needed to help them tide over periods when they are less well than usual. A geriatric service has to aim, not only at treating their infirmities, but also at helping them function on their own.

Care, Custody, and Guardianship

A final group of social welfare services deals with persons who for one reason or another cannot look after themselves or cannot be looked after satisfactorily by their families. For some this is temporary; for others it is permanent. The needs of socially incompetent persons have always stimulated much private philanthropy; but, in order that the needs of all such persons may be met, government has had to actively exercise its role of ultimate guardian, to the point where some persons are formally adjudged 'wards of the state' and committed to the care of a 'fit person', which in Britain may often be a local government authority.

This happens frequently with children who do not have homes capable of bringing them up satisfactorily. In many cases, another home has to be found for them. In North European and North American countries, it has become usual for the local authority to board them out with a foster family which it supervises. In Mediterranean countries, both Christian and Muslim, it remains more usual for them to be placed in orphanages. Since it was shown that neglect, malnutrition, disease, and death were more common in congregate institutions than in family households, there has been a trend away from large institutions towards cottage homes with their own house-parents and with children of all ages and both sexes attending ordinary schools, in the belief that it is better for their mental and social as well as physical health to grow up in a group resembling a natural family.

A special instance of this problem is the child who is formally adjudged to be in need of care, protection, or control. He may be found neglected, unmanageable, or delinquent; and, if delinquent, his behaviour may have been illegal only when committed by a minor, or may have been illegal when committed by a person of any age. In North European and North American countries and in Japan, an effort has been made to treat as many such children as possible in their own homes; in some countries the juvenile courts are helped by considerable staffs of probation officers; and in some Scandinavian countries, the child welfare boards have appointed co-guardians for as many as one child in ten. To supplement or replace the home, and yet still stay with this principle of 'treatment in the community', some localities have provided probation hostels or leisure-time attendance centres. For the minority whom it is judged better to send away, all countries have special boarding schools ('approved schools' in Britain); but here again the trend is towards staffing these corrective schools generously, making them as much like ordinary homes as is practical, keeping the child there for as short a time as can be arranged, and helping him back into the community, unless he is adjudged incurably dangerous. To help it decide what is best for a child, a juvenile court in some countries can send him to a temporary hostel ('remand home' in Britain), where he can be observed while his social situation is being investigated.

There is a small minority of adults who do not submit to prolonged treatment voluntarily, but who must be treated for the protection of the public as well as of themselves. They may, for example, be spreading tuberculosis or syphilis, or may be dependent on illegally distributed drugs, or may suffer from a dangerous mental disorder. Most governments arrange for their civil commitment for compulsory detention and treatment, for a long or indeterminate time, often until they are adjudged cured. In some countries, including Britain, the possibility of effective treatment has induced most persons with these kinds of sicknesses to seek treatment voluntarily; but in some countries, the judicial and custodial approach remains more frequent; and it has everywhere to be retained as a measure that can be resorted to at last resort.

For offenders, 'treatment in freedom' has become in English-speaking and Northern European countries as common as imprisonment. Their freedom is limited by a Court instead of being suspended. This is done in a number of ways: their sentence may be suspended or they may be bound over on their own recognizance or placed on unsupervised probation, conditional on good behaviour; or they may be placed under supervised probation, and bound by certain specified restrictions on their activities, aimed at freeing them from the influence of their former comrades. Hostels may form a useful adjunct to such treatment, especially for young adults; or the conditions imposed may include the making good of damage done or participation in some form of service to the community.

A person who has been found guilty by a Court may be sentenced to prison if no other sentence seems more appropriate. It then becomes necessary to so organize prisons as to increase rather than decrease the probability of their inmates complying with the law after their release; and this requires a work discipline and a regime of justice within each prison, and the maintenance of links with family and potential employers outside. Thus viewed, a prison is not merely a place of custody for persons whose freedom has been judicially suspended, but is also an occasion for 'secondary prevention' of crime. A modern penal service keeps such deprivation of freedom to the indispensable minimum. Insofar as brief suspension of freedom is believed to have an educative value, it tries such devices as weekend imprisonment. Insofar as long-term imprisonment is considered an unavoidable necessity, it tries to place the prisoner in the institution most appropriate to his own personality, and to prepare him for his return to freedom by special readaptation services and halfway houses. Countries vary greatly in the extent to which they house their populations in prisons: 30 per 100,000 in Denmark and the Netherlands, 70 in Britain, France, and Sweden, 100 in Canada, 180 in the United States, and 400 in South Africa. Congregate residential institutions for lawbreakers are dangerous social medicine, to be used with great care: a corrective school or penal institution may be 'criminogenic', just as a psychiatric hospital may generate secondary psychoses.

Lastly, there is a small minority of persons whose conditions may be adjudged irreversible and who may need constant care and attention, though not necessarily medical treatment or hospital facilities. Some may be severely subnormal. Many may be becoming senile. Special kinds of well-staffed residential accommodations are provided for them in most European countries; British local authorities, for example, have of recent years tried to move away from the nineteenth century 'infirmaries' to homelike 'homes' receiving not more than 35 persons. All governments have also established procedures for granting to others certain powers of guardianship over socially incompetent persons and their affairs.

Relations between Social Welfare and Income Guarantee Services

This chapter has assumed that income-transfer and social welfare services are usually distinct and separate social functions, which may even be organized by different levels, national and local, of government. There are, however, some situations in which they come together.

Under a universal payment system, a beneficiary receives what he is entitled to, with no strings attached: he does not have to receive services along with the public income payment. An exception is that on behalf of a small minority of orphans and of old-age pensioners adjudged incapable of managing their own affairs, a guardian has to be appointed to receive the pension on their behalf. Offering services to income-recipients but leaving them free to use them or not is another matter. French social insurance and family allowance funds are even obliged by statute to devote part of their outgo to 'collective benefits', and French family allowance funds in particular have made many services available to their contributors.

Under a selective income-transfer system, the situation may be different. In particular, it has been unusual to extend social assistance payments to an adult who is adjudged employable, without asking for evidence that he is truly seeking work, and, after a certain time, without requiring him to attend training courses even if this means a temporary absence from home. Some countries have gone much further than this. Thus in nineteenth-century Germany, the city of Elberfeld started a system under which every family receiving public assistance had to accept supervision for the purpose of helping all its members become self-supporting. Hence, the German use of the term 'welfare' for a system of assistance-payments-cum-services. This same principle has been adopted in North American 'public welfare', often more in theory than in practice; but, where successfully applied, it has usually meant

putting the assistance recipient into effective contact with educational, employment, or health services; for example, in New York City between 1968 and 1970, public provision of family planning counselling to women receiving 'aid to families with dependent children' reduced their birth rate from 20 per cent. to 10 per cent.

Moreover, one of the uses of a selective income-transfer system is to enable a person to meet the expense of exceptional needs, such as the hiring of a helper, or a particular kind of equipment needed to help him function, or, above all, long-term care.

SOCIAL DEVELOPMENT POLICY
Practical Inputs

Social policy is much broader than the social services. It covers the whole range of advantages and disadvantages that are meted out by government to one or other segment of the population. This often happens as an aspect of what is thought of primarily as economic or fiscal policy, with only secondary attention to its social consequences. For example, a government's agricultural policy may help make food dear or cheap; if food prices are low, families with low incomes may be better able to afford good food, and the publicly supported income floor may also be kept low; on the other hand, if food prices are high, low-income families may be less able to afford good food, and more public income-support services may be required. Again, the detailed structuring of the tax system may make it easier or more difficult for poor people to get along without support from social services; if taxes fall directly or indirectly on necessities such as food and housing and if income taxes are levied on low incomes, the chances are that the fiscal levies will be compensated for by increased public income transfer-payments.

When setting policy, there is often a balance of advantage and disadvantage that has to be weighed. It may happen that a policy that aims at economic or political benefits may result in social costs. In all such cases, there tends to be a certain pressure to balance the economic or political action of government with an expansion of social services, so as to keep the social costs down to a tolerable level.

Even social policy itself may result in unexpected social costs which then have to be counteracted by a further development of social services. For example, the right to compensation for work injuries may make employers less willing to employ categories of persons whom they regard as accident-prone, such as young, old, and handicapped persons, unless special measures are taken to induce them to do so. Again, the right to retire with a pension at a certain age may be customarily interpreted as an obligation to retire. Or, the level at which a minimum wage is fixed may have important consequences; if it is fixed at a low level, there may be pressure for public supplementation; but if it is fixed at a less low level, it may induce employers to dispense with unskilled labour, thus increasing pressure for a public substitute income. In short, every intervention of government in economics and social processes may bring with it a chain of unintended and unanticipated consequences which are met with further state interventions. It therefore becomes important to constantly evaluate the actual working and effects of every policy in order to take steps for correcting those social consequences that are not really desired. Social policy is thus not merely the introduction of new models of social service intended to provide a basic solution to a social problem; instead it requires continual adaptation and adjustment.

Inputs of Principle

The policy that is adopted may also be influenced partly by different people's different ideas of social justice. For example, we have already looked at the principles of universalism and of selectivity—the former aimed at meeting presumed needs on a basis of equal treatment for all, without distinction, and the latter at meeting only the proved poverty of the most disadvantaged minority.

Other principles may have to do with people's ideas of the kind of society they wish to see develop. Thus, some may emphasize the service of the state to the individual, a point of view that has come to dominate income-support services in English-speaking countries, whereas others may emphasize the role of civic groups other than the state, including voluntary agencies and local government bodies, a viewpoint that has tended on the contrary to affect the provision of social welfare services, particularly in Britain. With these two contrasting emphases come two others: on the one hand a preference for a service that operates as impersonally and automatically as possible, which is what we have tried to achieve in some methods of income-support, and on the other hand, a preference for a human and personal quality, such as may be sought after in social welfare services.

Scientific Inputs

Social service policy, however, does not derive only from the problems created by previous policies or from the ideas and ideals of those who have the power to mould it. Its planning is also affected by certain scientific approaches. Of these one of the most important is the conception of a 'poverty line'. This originated in Britain nearly 100 years ago in the great study of *London life and labour* financed by Charles Booth of Liverpool; but it was put on to a scientific basis when it was linked with growing knowledge of nutrition—first calories and then minerals and vitamins—by Seebohm Rowntree at York and (Lord) Boyd-Orr in Scotland. Thanks to this knowledge, incomplete though it still is, we have acquired a yardstick for estimating minimum food needs for the average person to subsist and to function. This has at least given a rough notion of a 'floor' beneath which society should not allow any member to fall except by his own choice. In affluent developed countries, this has become the starting-point for all income-support measures. In poor developing countries, it has provided the basis for calculating what proportion of the population is undernourished, and for planning to raise agricultural production to the point at which there should be enough food to meet minimum human needs. It will be noted that, in developed countries, with highly productive economies, social policy may be expressed in terms of equitable distribution of social resources, whereas, in some developing countries, the previous question may have to be posed, of how to raise production to the level needed for meeting minimum nutritional needs. Nutritional needs are not, of course, the only factor that goes into evaluation of a poverty line; they are, however, a quantitatively calculable factor, as well as being basic. Nor does the meeting of average nutritional needs exclude the need for meeting the nutritional deficiencies of non-average persons, e.g. by 'welfare foods' distributed to persons who show symptoms of under- or malnutrition.

Another important scientific approach is provided by demography. It is only since we learned to measure life expectancy at the end of the eighteenth century that first private life insurance and then social insurance have become possible. Demographic projections also give us some indication of the size of the age groups that are likely to need the various social services in the course of the next decade or so; and it is only by knowing ahead the order of magnitude of a problem that we can plan to meet it. Trends in population structure result from the decisions of millions of individuals. They constitute a natural process which has to be taken into account in many respects when formulating social policy. For example, the kind of non-working population that has to be supported by people in their working years may vary greatly between a developed country or community with a heavy proportion of aged persons and a developing country or community with a heavy proportion of persons of or below school age. Population policy is still in its infancy: thus far, it has aimed only at helping individuals make their own decisions by way of family planning; and it is not yet clear what additional public measures, if any, could be devised for increasing the probability of world population stabilizing itself, if it is decided that this is desirable.

Organization and Management

The effectiveness of a social service policy depends to some extent on how it is administered: the choice of organization to carry it out, the way it is financed, and the selection of personnel to staff it.

We have already seen two organizational trends at work, the one towards the centralizing of all income-support services in national government departments, and the other towards devolving responsibility for social welfare services on to local government and voluntary agencies. In both cases, the problem arises of how to make sure that people actually get the service to which they have a legal right.

In the case of all income-guarantee services, efforts have been made to narrow the range of administrative discretion. It is at its narrowest in universal pensions and allowances, which are almost automatic. It is slightly less narrow in social security, where more qualifying conditions have to be met. It is at its broadest in social assistance (supplementary benefits), where room is left for a little flexibility. Nevertheless, provision is everywhere made for dissatisfied applicants to appeal to a specially constituted administrative tribunal.

In the case of social welfare services, on the other hand, there may be room for a wide range of discretion, and special efforts may therefore be needed to increase the probability of the client getting the services that will help him most. The professional training of social welfare workers may help; so may central government inspection of the local authority or voluntary agency; and the political answerability of the local authority to its constituents may also count for something, especially if the beneficiaries among them are organized. In social welfare services, as in health and education, there can be no absolute certainty that professional discretion will be correctly exercised; but everything possible has to be done to lessen the chances of error.

People not only have a right to schooling, but also have an obligation to go to school or to send their children there; and local education authorities enforce this obligation. With some public social welfare services, it is different; they offer rights or opportunities, which persons who are entitled are free to use or not to use. A special effort may therefore be needed to increase the likelihood of people applying for the services to which they are legally entitled. This may require search-and-enroll campaigns or be one of the roles of a citizens' advice and referral service or of a person who works with a family as social worker or public health nurse.

Social services, in general, have become a major charge on the budget in every country. Hence, a tendency to finance as much of them as possible outside the regular budget. The principal way in which this is done is through autonomous social insurance or social security funds fed mainly from employers' and employees' contributions. This strategy is followed to a different extent in different countries. For example, in France it is used for financing family allowances, health care costs, and many social welfare services as well as guaranteed incomes and therefore takes one-third of earnings, while in Britain it takes one-tenth. The chief objection to this method of financing is that workers' 'contributions' to these funds are less 'progressive' than income tax; that is to say, the burden falls more heavily proportionately to income on the poor than on the well-to-do. For this reason, most European governments make their social insurance 'tripartite', by having government contribute alongside workers and management; and all make some use of non-contributory allowances or pensions. Some of the financial responsibility for social welfare services is similarly devolved on to local authorities which can levy rates or to voluntary agencies which try to collect funds from their supporters, with the central budget meeting only part of the cost through a grant-in-aid.

The administration of public social services requires also an adequate personnel. Insofar as income-support services are kept strictly to that function, what they need primarily is machinery for applying the law correctly. In the case of the social welfare services, however, many persons with different kinds of specialized professional or auxiliary training are needed: employment advisers, social and vocational rehabilitation technicians, home teachers of the blind, home economists, home helps, school attendance officers, house parents, probation officers, and professional social workers, among others. The problem has naturally arisen of how to lessen the chance of the same family being contacted by a number of different health and welfare workers; for this reason, the French have evolved an assistante sociale who is to some extent social worker and to some extent public health nurse, in the hope that she will normally co-ordinate all the health and welfare services provided to a family.

This suggests the advisability of planning all the various services to people in such a way that they work together. If all the different kinds of health and welfare workers have different employers, teamwork is hard to enforce, but has nevertheless to be sought after. The problem is how to make all services as available as possible to the persons who need them. This challenges the city planner and the municipal authority to develop a multi-service centre in every community and neighbourhood, so that people may know where to go for the help they need and may move easily from one service to another. The services on which this chapter has focused have to radiate out from physical facilities; and the planning that is required relates not only to national policy and services to people, but also to the localities in which people live and function with the help of these health and welfare services.

REFERENCES

Family Welfare Association (annual) *Guide to the Social Services*, London.

George, V. N. (1968) *Social Security*, London.

Hall, M. P. (1969) *Social Services of Modern England*, London.

Kuenstler, P. (1961) *Community Organization in Great Britain*, London.

Marsh, D. C. (1964) *The Future of the Welfare State*, London.

National Council of Social Service (annual) *Public Social Services:*
(1963) *Councils of Social Service*, London.
(1966) *Voluntary Social Services*, London.
(1968) *The Elderly*, London.

United Kingdom Central Statistical Office (annual) *Social Trends:*
(1942) *Social Insurance and Allied Services* (Beveridge), London, H.M.S.O.
(1966) *Health and Welfare: the Development of Community Care*, London, H.M.S.O.

(1966) *The Sentence of the Court: a Handbook for the Courts on the Treatment of Offenders*, London, H.M.S.O.
(1968) *Government Social Survey: Social Welfare for the Elderly*, London, H.M.S.O.
(1968) *Local Authority and Allied Personal Social Services*, London, H.M.S.O.

United Nations (annual) *International Review of Social Development:*
(annual) *International Review of Criminal Policy*, New York.
(1969) *Report on the World Social Situation*, New York.
(1967–69) *Organization and Administration of Social Welfare Programmes: a Series of Country Studies*, New York.

Wilensky, H. L., and Lebeaux, C. N. (1968) *Industrial Society and Social Welfare*, New York.

Wilmott, P. (1967) *Consumer's Guide to British Social Services*, London.

World Health Organization (1963) *The Care of Well Children in Day-Care Centres and Institutions*, Geneva.

FURTHER READING

Branton, M. (1967) *Race Relations*, London.

Feldstein, I. (1969) *Later Life*, London.

Heywood, J. S. (1965) *Children in Care*, London.

International Labour Review (periodical) articles:
(1967) *Minimum Living Standards*, Geneva.
(1969) *Reflections on Fifty Years of Social Security*, Geneva.

Jones, R. H. (1971) *The Doctor and the Social Services*, London.

King, J. (1964) *The Probation Service*, London.

Kowley, T. H. (1965) *Social Security in Australia*, Sydney.

Morris, N. (1970) *The Honest Politician's Guide to Crime Control*, Chicago.

Moser, C. A., and Kalton, G. (1971) *Survey methods in social investigation*, London.

P.E.P. *Broadsheets*, London.

Newman, T. S. (latest edition) *Guide to British Social Insurance*, London.

New Zealand Royal Commission (1967) *Compensation for Personal Injury*, Wellington.

Prins, H. A., and Whyte, Marion B. H. (1972) *Social Work and Medical Practice*, Oxford.

Rodgers, B. (1968) *Comparative Social Administration*, London.

Steiner, G. (1971) *The State of Welfare*, Washington.

Susser, M. W., and Watson, W. (1971) *Sociology in Medicine*, 2nd ed., London.

Titmuss, R. M. (1963) *Essays on the Welfare State*, London.

Titmuss, R. M. (1968) *Commitment to Welfare*, London.

Townsend, P. (1965) *The Aged in the Welfare State*, London.

Townsend, P. (1968) *Old People in Three Industrial Societies*, London.

Wickwar, W. H. and M. (1949) *The Social Services: an Historical Survey*, London.

Wootton, B. (1959) *Social Science and Social Pathology*, London.

World Health Organization Regional Office for Europe (1974) *Report of a Working Group on the Role of the Social Worker in Psychiatric Services, Nice 1972* (Euro 5438I), Copenhagen.

49

HEALTH EDUCATION IN BEHAVIOURAL MEDICINE

JOHN BURTON and LEO BARIĆ

It is easier to destroy our villages than to change our customs.
Bosnian proverb.

Human behaviour plays a dominant role in the aetiology and epidemiology of many of the diseases of greatest importance in contemporary society. Likewise, in the promotion of health and the prevention of disease the effectiveness of modern public health measures is ultimately dependent on the health consciousness of legislators and citizens and the preparedness of every man to help himself by making the best use of available knowledge and health services.

In the eternal triangle of host, agent, and environment it is the two latter elements which have attracted most scientific attention in the past. The difficulty of modifying human behaviour may be responsible for a certain apathy on the part of health workers regarding the host, and an over-emphasis on dealing with health problems in ways which involve his behaviour as little as possible. Though this approach has been strikingly successful where general environmental improvement was required and in diminishing the prevalence of many infectious diseases, we are now left with an assortment of conditions for which an attack on the agent or the environment is either impracticable or has proved ineffective. The conditions in which human behaviour plays this primary role in aetiology are now sufficiently numerous and distinct to merit a separate grouping in the classification system. We propose, therefore, to call them behavioural diseases.[1] Included in the grouping are such conditions as the venereal diseases, schisostomiasis, some forms of cancer, heart disease, malnutrition, diabetes, chronic bronchitis, and neurosis; infectious diseases for which immunization is available and effective; drug dependency, alcoholism, obesity; some industrial dermatites and many forms of accident at work, on the roads, or at home.

By using this classification of diseases we give value and importance to the intellectual, emotional, and social factors which constitute the major impediment to their prevention and treatment and which should be uppermost in our minds when conducting services or planning research. By considering them as behavioural diseases, we cut across traditional boundaries and put ourselves in a position to perceive hitherto unrecognized connexions between them and other medico-social problems. In the case of lung cancer, for instance, we do not yet know the ultimate cause of the neoplastic changes, but we do know that the recognition of the behavioural factor of smoking cigarettes has led to the most fruitful approach to controlling this disease. Gonorrhoea and syphilis are classical examples of behavioural disease. Though the infections are caused by different organisms, the behavioural element is constant. The differences in incubation periods, however, lead to different levels of success when health education is applied to their prevention (Glass *et al.*, 1968).

Under the banner of behaviour we include both voluntary and involuntary acts, habits, customs, learned responses, and conditioned reflexes, all of which are of interest to the physician and health educator.

If we accept the concept that host behaviour is primary in the causation of a disease and the agent and the environment are secondary it is logical that health workers should ensure that their diagnoses, therapy, prophylaxis, and research reflect this order of priority.

In a book on public health it is appropriate to concentrate on the behaviour of groups. However, in attempting to make any diagnosis of the behavioural diseases or render any service on a community basis, we must bear in mind that many public health services are rendered on an individual basis, many group reactions are dependent on the leadership of individuals, and that health behaviour is an expression of the culture as a whole, of which health workers are a part.

HEALTH WORKERS IN THEIR CULTURAL SETTING

To most men and women the way of life of their community is its most precious possession. To outsiders who have their own habits and assumptions this way of life often appears incongruous and misguided.

The doctor and health worker is very often an outsider for the community in which he works, because of his education, his income, or his habits of scientific thought, as well as the frequency with which he practises in places and among social classes which are not his own. One of the prescribed duties of the Medical Officer for Environmental Health in England is to know his area, and health educators likewise, in their training, are exhorted to study every aspect of the lives of the people whom they serve. The effectiveness of the clinician and public health worker and the prestige of their subject and profession, even in cultures which accept scientific medicine, depend to as great an extent on their understanding and participation in the life of the community in which they work as on their technical ability. This is hard to accept for those who have undergone a

---

[1] Behavioural disease may be defined as any pathological condition in which human behaviour plays a leading aetiological role or the treatment and prevention of which depends mainly on changes in the behaviour of individuals or groups.

modern medical training with its technological emphasis, but to those numerous experienced practitioners, like Pickles (1939) working in a remote rural area of his own country, or to others working in cultures quite foreign to their own, the value of a deeper and more systematic understanding of the nature of their patients' way of life becomes apparent. Knowing your area in this sense is not simply a matter of vital statistics and local economics and geography but an understanding and curiosity about the customs and beliefs, family relations and social roles, and the patterns of communication of the people and the ceaseless changes and developments which are afoot among them. It means understanding how disease appears to them, how they rationalize tragedies, and what problems people will encounter in making any changes in their accustomed practices. This does not mean that every health worker must be fully trained in the social sciences. Sensibility and good manners will take him far, but a grasp of the way of thinking and methods of the social scientists can speed up and make more interesting and enjoyable the inevitable process of learning by experience.

Dealing, as they do, with matters of life and death, practitioners of medicine hold a very ambivalent position in society. They are endowed with semi-magical powers and regarded with love and distrust, fear and hope, to an extent far greater than any other profession. The way their patients expect them to behave professionally and morally is often very strictly codified. This inevitably gives them great power and authority, but tends to isolate them from ordinary people. In discussing the role of health personnel in the United States, Foster (1956) observes that: 'Experience shows that when health personnel, doctors, nurses, health educators and sanitarians work with people of their own general social and economic background, they accomplish more. In part this is because they are able to communicate more effectively. . . .' Communication difficulties mean much more than simple language differences—they stem from very different premises on which the outlook and understanding of people of diverse backgrounds are based.

After considering some of the material reasons for the continuing lag in the health statistics of social groups IV and V in England, Jefferys (1957) goes on to say: 'There are, however, other factors which may not be so readily discernible, but which may have contributed to the lag of the lowest social classes behind the others so far as health is concerned. These factors are facets of the relative positions which unskilled workers, doctors and educationists occupy in the social structure and of different ideas, expectations and customs of different groups in the community. An understanding of them may make the work of those concerned with the health and welfare of unskilled workers and their families more effective.'

By virtue of a long process of pre-conditioning or learning, the doctor acquires a way of thinking, a set of attitudes, and a scale of values and preferences which are quite different from those of the lowest ranks of society. The social distance between general practitioner and patient in the therapeutic relationship or between infant welfare doctor and mother in the educative relationship can lead to misunderstandings which, in their turn, mitigate against a successful outcome of the relationship. Some doctors are intuitively aware of the complications of social distance for the patient and are able to bridge it successfully, others learn in the hard school of experience; but some do not appear to realize either how wide the distance is that separates them from their patients or how by their own actions they can help to narrow it.

In Koos' (1954) study of the health of Regionville, a patient is recorded as saying: 'Nobody should blame the doc if he doesn't fix them up right away—or never. But maybe things would be better if the doc understood us and if we always knew what the hell he was driving at.'

The poorer people of Regionville, in spite of the mixture of love and distrust displayed by this observation and the high social esteem in which doctors were held, seem to have preferred the local chiropractor. 'You are important to him' was repeatedly stated, and again: 'It ain't—isn't—our fault if we are poor, and the chiropractor seems to know this better.'

When the qualified doctor practises in a culture which is not his own he is often in much the same position as a witch doctor would be in a teaching hospital in London, if he does not adapt his procedures to the expectations of his clientele.

Marriott (1955), in a study of medicine in India, points out that many of the features which orthodox medicine holds most dear are meaningless and even discouraging to many Indian patients. Such things as questioning and examination merely display the doctor's ignorance, and the presentation of a bill for a consultation relegates him to a low class. But perhaps the most important observation Dr. Marriott makes is that scientific medicine, to succeed in India, must strip itself of its nonscientific elements. 'Western ideas of personal privacy, of individual responsibility, of the dignity of certain techniques and of the democratic nature of interpersonal trust are not intrinsic parts of scientific medical practice but are cultural accretions upon it.' This observation has considerable significance for health education, because many seemingly fundamental concepts, such as individual responsibility, have become woven into the texture of its philosophy.

MEDICINE AS A BEHAVIOURAL SCIENCE

The social sciences have since the days of Herodotus been engaged in studying and comparing the factors in the ways of life of communities which give them their character, and by so doing are enabling others to understand the behaviour of groups as a whole and the pressure this exercises on the individuals within them. It is comparatively recently that interest has begun to centre on the behaviour of people when confronted with problems, such as sickness, and innovations, such as preventive medicine, but as health becomes more and more a feature of social policy, the need for considering social and cultural factors in the aetiology and epidemiology of disease increases.

It may appear to us now that the introduction of scientific medical measures, such as the great sanitary reforms of the last century, which did as much to transform our way of life as the steam engine, came about with comparative ease in an atmosphere uncontaminated by the sort of strife which surrounds measures like the fluoridation of water supplies today. We may feel that even the least-developed areas will accept gladly the obvious benefits which scientific medicine has to offer if they are clearly and thoroughly explained. Suffice it to quote *The Times* leader of the last century which stated: 'We would prefer to take our chance of cholera and the rest than be bullied into health.' However, it was during this period that the idea of an aggressive public health service backed by active education in health was born in those countries which had chosen the scientific modes of thought. It was rapidly seen by such philosophers as Sir John Simon and Florence Nightingale that, for the new discoveries to become effective, great changes were needed in the outlook and behaviour of all classes in society from the legislators on a national and local scale right through to the women who carry the major responsibility for the health of families. As Sir John Simon wrote in 1890: 'Education, in the full sense of the word, is the one far-reaching true reformer: not the mere elementary school business of reading and writing and arithmetic, nor even merely those bits of learning with some super-addition of a bread-winning technical proficiency; but the education which completes for self-help and for social duty, by including wisdom and goodness among its objects. Education in that sense is not something which one man can receive passively from another, as he might receive an inunction or a legacy, but is something which his own nature must actively grow forth to meet. It in truth is a process of fertilisation, a process in which one generation of minds can only awaken the germs of another, a process in which fructification requires time.'

Health education thus became the ideology and one of the main executive techniques of the new era of public health, in the same way that the precepts of the Jewish and Mohammedan and other religions or the humoral teachings of Galen had served the pre-scientific cultures. The main difference, however, between health education and its predecessors is that, being part of scientific medicine, it eschews dogma and aims to bring about necessary change by the conscious and free choice of those concerned. The study of what people choose to do and why they choose it thus becomes a prime factor in the good practice of behavioural medicine. We can do little more in a general article such as this than mention some of the cultural elements that health workers will encounter in developing their educational activities. Some elements are general to all cultures, others are specific to a small group. The quality of the educational work depends to a great extent on the ability of the health workers to understand the uniqueness of the culture in which they are working and tailor-make their plans accordingly.

Authority

All peoples have some system of authority within the state, within the locality, and within the family, and these authorities are related to one another, and to the people they influence, in various ways. Health education is concerned at every level because, to initiate any action or change any custom, it is generally necessary to deal with these authorities and obtain their active support and participation. Without their goodwill and co-operation they are at best neutral, and if ignored will most likely be in active opposition. Though it is not difficult to identify the formal authorities, such as headmen or chiefs, Members of Parliament or councillors, priests, schoolteachers, etc., it may be more difficult to find out who is the main influence within the family; is it the father, the mother, or even the children? Many public health measures are devised on the assumption that all men and women are of equal influence, and the approach is made direct to the individual concerned, for instance, young mothers regarding baby care. Logical as

this seems, it is often found that all power of decision devolves on the grandmother, and to gain co-operation she must, like the formal authorities, be consulted. In many communities it is the father who decides on budgeting, and in some even purchases the food. Apart from its obvious value in general education, it is often proposed that health education is best carried out in schools, because thereby the parents will be influenced by the children. This may be the case in some cultures, but in others it is doubtful, because the views of young children often carry little weight with the older generation, who may even consider their innovations an impertinence.

There is also another class of informal authority in most communities which is often difficult to discover but which may in fact be wielding more influence than all the others when it comes to public health questions. Such a person may be the secretary of a local voluntary organization, the witch doctor or chiropractor, the wife of the local schoolmaster, or some modest private person of intelligence and attractive personality to whom people naturally turn for advice. These informal leaders of opinion are often different for different situations. They may be the health worker's strongest allies or opponents when it comes to getting things done, because they often dominate one of the most influential forces in the population—the 'gossip group'—that small gathering of friends (Steuart, 1957) where things are talked over at leisure and attitudes are formed. There is no set pattern for the power of various types of authority to influence the choices of members of the community. In one the elected representatives or traditional leaders may carry weight, in another little or none. In some communities the religious leaders have great importance, in others very little, but it is worth underlining that assumptions are often made, and acted on regarding the proper authority, without much inquiry and with a negative or disappointing result. For instance, it is assumed that because the members of a town council agree to a measure like fluoridation of town water supplies, the townspeople will therefore accept. In some cases the very fact that the authorities favour a measure renders it suspect, because the authorities have no prestige, are associated with raising taxes or some other unpopular measure. In the case of fluoridation, all sorts of informal leaders spring up to defend the liberty of the subject against officialdom. Such incidents generally occur where the authorities are remote from the people and have taken no trouble to consult them, particularly have taken no trouble to satisfy the informal leaders. Medical personnel and health educators are often part of, or acting on behalf of, government authorities. To them it is of the utmost importance that they should be aware of their double role in society, and the way in which their patients and the public regard them.

Economics

Economic factors of interest to health education permeate every aspect of society. They often decide the material basis and the extent to which proper health services can be established. They influence or may even determine the attitudes and relationships between people, and are deeply involved in the self-interest or motivation of both individuals and groups. The power structure already discussed frequently depends on economic considerations, though it must always be borne in mind that this dependence is rarely complete and is usually indirect. The very dynamic element of business enterprise is moulding social behaviour in such matters as nutrition, budgeting, and social values.

The change from mainly agricultural to largely industrial methods of production has brought, and is bringing, about certain radical changes in the culture of communities by changing the relationships between men and women, parents and children, and men and work. Commerce is introducing new products which can bring about major changes in the family budget in both advanced industrial societies and remote and primitive agricultural groups. Television, transistors and Coca-cola symbolize these universal instruments of change.

Many traditional family patterns, however, remain largely uninfluenced by these changes, and recent studies in Bethnal Green have drawn attention again to the strength of the relationship between daughters and their mothers, even in highly industrialized areas. This maintains a strong maternal influence on ideas about the upbringing of children, the feeding of the family, and other matters of vital interest to health education. Significant social change may take a generation.

Industrialized and non-industrialized communities display important differences in their attitude to man himself. In the former man is looked on primarily as an isolated producer–consumer. It is his obligations to impersonal things like the production process, formal education, or as a consumer that are highly considered. In the latter he is looked on primarily as a member of a family, and his obligations to people in a wide human circle are highly prized. This provides for the family labour on the farm and for considerable social and emotional stability and security. But it is precisely this stability that the reformer sees as his chief enemy. While it remains, new ideas cannot be accepted, and he is tempted to throw the baby of security out with the bath water of conservatism. Industrialized countries are becoming only too aware of the stress and cost in human terms of their way of life, with its tiny family, cramped living space, and impersonal factory-dictated rhythms of life. Those countries that have recently embarked on industrial development are already becoming aware of the cost. But if industrial living poses new problems it also offers new solutions to old ones by forming new groupings, opening minds to new ideas, and providing essential economic resources. This point is briefly mentioned, because mobility of labour and large-scale migrations, industrialization and urbanization are in progress all over the world, such as the West Indian in Britain, the Puerto Ricans in the United States, and the peasants in all those countries embarking on industrialization for the first time. In China and Russia radical changes are occurring in the pattern of rural life with a view to introducing industrial organization to farming. Health services and health education, in applying themselves to the needs of people in settled agricultural, or industrial communities or to the groups in flux, encounter quite different problems in each, and must strive to understand and adapt their approach. In settled agricultural groups the ideas and methods of the urban health educator may be seen as a threat to the whole way of life, as in many cases they may seem to challenge recognized divisions of labour or ways of using the family budget. This is particularly the case in relation to the economic emancipation of that most important group, the employed young women, who are in many cases still more or less subject to a triple pressure, from a male-dominated society, from older women, and from husbands.

To the health educator, experienced in rural affairs, the non-industrialized communities, however, present equally great advantages in that the reservoir of native intelligence and initiative has not been creamed off into the towns, and he may have far more promising material to work with than in the rural areas of industrialized countries.

In considering economic factors one is tempted to speculate on the importance of economic incentives in conditioning people's behaviour about health matters. Poor people are insecure and are quite reasonably unwilling to be the first to change. Until the new methods have demonstrated their value, they will cling to what they know.

The richer groups in most countries have a consistent superiority in infant survival rates over poor groups. They are prepared to invest heavily in the health and education of their children. Boyd Orr showed many years ago that there is a tendency with increasing income to select nutritionally superior diets. Some governments declare that investment in health measures, such as water supplies, immunization, maternal and child health, and accident prevention pays handsome dividends.

Whether health services should be paid for by the client or rendered free of charge on demand varies in importance with the situation. As we have seen in India and some other parts of the world, charging a fee for medical services may demote the whole profession to that of shopkeeping in the eyes of many patients, whereas in the United States the high cost of treatment has a long tradition, and may increase a patient's respect and perseverance or enable a parent to make the sacrifice for the family which proves to him that he has done his best. Free services are held in low esteem. It is the experience of the medical profession in many countries that have adopted free medical services or insurance schemes that the prestige of the family doctor has declined. Though there are many factors which contribute to this, the personal element of payment is certainly one. If 'welfarism' is to succeed it must exact from the patient some equally meaningful and immediate contribution to his own cure. Health education, by expecting people to help themselves and showing them how they can do it, supplies a possible alternative. This is particularly true in preventive services, where the degree to which a community is prepared to invest in its future and make use of health services is one of the sensitive indicators of social maturity.

The Epidemiology of Beliefs and Customs

Epidemiological investigation has not yet expanded to embrace the effects of people's knowledge, attitude, and customs on the incidence of disease, and social anthropologists have until recently conducted their investigations mostly among remote and isolated communities, so that we know much more about the people of New Guinea than about those of New York.

Though epidemiology is extending its sphere of interest towards the social, psychological, and cultural determinants of disease, and some social scientists are reaching out towards epidemiology, there is still a substantial methodological gap between the two. It is probably true to say, however, that the social scientists interested in health matters are still the people most qualified to study in depth the groups selected by the epidemiologist, and until such time as the gap has been bridged the next stages in the investigation of behavioural disease will require the skills of sociologists, psychologists, and cultural anthropologists. The social sciences have demonstrated the importance of certain of their assumptions to all health workers, particularly in their health education function.

Education in health is an innovation in most societies, and often an intervention from outside, and health workers are perforce innovators. If we accept that social scientists have rendered them a service by drawing their attention to the ways in which their clients may regard them and their need to be aware of their own role in the communities they wish to influence (Freedman, 1957), and if we accept that health workers have been accustomed in their medico-social diagnoses to lay most stress on the material factors, such as income, housing, crowding, occupation, etc., then perhaps we can agree to explore jointly some of the other determining factors in human behaviour which have been largely neglected in the conduct of health services.

Values

The Expert Committee on Health Education of the World Health Organization (1954) maintained that the first general purpose of health education was to make health a valued community asset. In the system of values of communities, health has varied considerably. Among upper social classes of the Greek city states and of Rome, health was a highly prized individual and community asset, and much capital and organization were devoted to its promotion in the form of baths, waterworks, sewers, and medical services, and the profession of medicine had prestige. In the European Middle Ages the spiritual life was considered more important; the rigorous and verminous life of pilgrims was admired; the priesthood gained high prestige. The resources of the community were devoted to cathedral building, leaving us a glorious architectural heritage, but the pestilence was treated with a fatalistic incompetence and objective medical studies, such as human dissection, were arrogantly discouraged. But it was from the contradictions of this society that the great innovators, Dante, Leonardo da Vinci, and William Shakespeare, were born, bringing back to philosophy the humility necessary for the objective study of man, of his spiritual aspirations, of his physical nature, and of his psychological motivation. Today health occupies a middling place in the value system of most societies and, as between sickness and health, sickness services are still more valued than health services in many. In spite of all the evidence that such a choice is uneconomical, most peoples continue to invest most of their resources in treatment rather than prevention, and accord greater prestige to the physician and surgeon than to the medical officer of health, the sanitarian, and the public health nurse.

This same aspect of value systems appears in the daily conduct of family life. Entertainment (the cinema and television) are valued by certain age groups and classes more than nutrition, and the bottle of medicine more than a change of habit. Caries-forming feeding habits have a high prestige in England, while not to break with traditional diets is prized in Uganda (Burgess, 1954). In most societies an attachment amounting almost to a religious feeling is associated with traditional dietary habits, and the reformer, unaware of the ultimate consequences of even minor changes, may, if he succeeds, produce more harm than good.

The idea of prevention, that human beings by their own conduct and efforts can improve their state of health is difficult to introduce, because in many social groups there is no standard of comparison, no realization that a better situation could exist, often no appreciation that a disease like trachoma is an abnormal state of affairs, that children need not die in infancy, and that women need not suffer from anaemia and that accidents need not happen.

It is important to remember that the real social gradient in such things as infantile mortality and morbidity continues to exist in the most developed countries and that this gradient most likely exists for preventive services also. Dr. Alison Glover showed that tonsillectomy was performed in 90 per cent. of children in private schools on the Kent coast, but in only 2 per cent. of children in state schools. Circumcision follows a similar pattern. It is hard to imagine that there are any medical reasons for this discrepancy, because generally speaking, the health of children in the top social grades has remained consistently better than that of those in the lower social groups. But it may be an indication of what is happening in other and more important fields. It is noticeable in some countries that conditions which mainly affect the poor have a low prestige, get less treatment, and come low on the list of priorities when preventive and treatment programmes are being planned. It may even be that preoccupation of public health departments with the health problems of the poor affects the status of their personnel in the eyes of the community.

The importance of health and disease also varies greatly in relation to who has them. Much in the same way as the Italian religious pictures of the Quattrocento used a perspective of social status, God being depicted large in the background, the angels smaller, and the donor of the canvas, most likely a rich and important mortal, smallest of all in the foreground, so we link the importance of various health practices with that of the people who carry them out. When poliomyelitis immunization was introduced in England many people waited to see what the Queen would do about her children.

Beliefs

Value systems are built up on traditional beliefs and concepts of disease, and change only when those beliefs are altered by new experience, technical innovations, education, economic trends, or such upheavals as wars and revolutions. Generally this is a slow process of a generation or two.

The Maoris of New Zealand believed (Newell, 1957) that disease was caused mainly by social wrongdoing, which exposed one to attack by a spirit and was a form of punishment which could be put right by exorcism and retribution. Under the impact of western medicine a division was beginning to grow up between those diseases—mainly accidents, infections, and those treatable by surgery and Maori diseases, including all mental illness and medical conditions requiring treatment by drugs. This situation is closely paralleled in recent investigations of tuberculosis in London, and of people's attitudes to cancer in the Manchester area, where a substantial minority considered the diseases to be a punishment for bad living. The essential feature of this type of belief system is that it is moral rather than magical, and constitutes a useful explanation of incomprehensible phenomena, and that, in the case of the Maoris, by taking certain social action the situation can be put right.

The desire to find explanations for the certain kinds of misfortunes frequently assumes magical influences. As Loudon (1957) points out in relation to the Zulus, magic accounts for only part of the aetiology of sickness, and many misfortunes are explained and solutions provided on a purely rational basis. But when the misfortune is out of the ordinary the sufferer begins to ask 'why?' and the answer is often the operation of supernatural forces. Such beliefs are firmly established in European cultures too; for example, the evil eye in Italy. In England a similar ambivalence towards the supernatural is displayed in the following quotation from the *Manchester Guardian*:

'Prayers for rain were offered in churches of all denominations in County Durham, where from 8 a.m. today water will be rationed for the five hundred thousand people supplied by the county water board. Mr C. F. Grey, M.P., joined in the prayers from Easington Lane Independent Methodist Church.

'Mr Grey, who has had no reply to his request to the Air Ministry to send rainmakers to Durham said, "I believe in prayer: we have not just to sit back. If we can get rain by artificial means, so much the better. I shall catch an early train to London and get in touch with the Air Ministry to urge them to act."'

Many individuals in any community reflect one or other of these magic and moral concepts of aetiology which have no particular significance for the culture as a whole, but when these beliefs are held by well-knit groups they are reinforced, and any solution becomes more difficult because as Koos (1954) puts it: 'To do anything about it would have meant denying all the expectations of his group and going counter to social heritage.'

This becomes of the utmost importance to the health educator because, though many are harmless, some of these beliefs are dangerous, and some might be described as lethal, for instance, the notions that cancer is never curable; that tuberculosis is hereditary and not infectious; that 'one for the road' is good for your driving; that children's diseases are best treated in institutions; that female circumcision promotes chastity; that smoking is soothing, stimulating, socially attractive; that certain protein-rich foods are taboo to pregnant and nursing mothers and young babies; that children should be kept in ignorance of sexual matters; that disease is the will of God; and many others which every experienced worker will have come across.

Dangerous as many of these beliefs are, and ineffective as are the customs and behaviours they give rise to, they have an important place in the health culture of many communities and condition behaviour; they may be the most satisfactory way that culture has evolved of rationalizing its desires and its calamities. Much medical folklore is thus carried over into cultures which boast the most advanced scientific tradition. It may help us greatly in understanding why so many people fail to make use of baby welfare clinics in England to know why they welcome or shun them in other parts of the world.

In the same Maori community it was believed that tuberculosis had been introduced by Europeans and was always fatal. It was also held that the disease was in some way caused by the doctor's diagnosis. At a public meeting the chairman of a tribal committee said to Dr. Newell, 'We hate pakeha [western] doctors and we do not want you, although we have nothing against you personally. You come to us and you say you and you have TB; we then go away and die. This is no good. When you come to us and say you and you will not die, then you will be welcome.' In reply Newell mentioned B.C.G. There was an immediate response, and the tribal committee bullied authority until they got the necessary materials and finally learned to read the tests and carry out the inoculations themselves. Newell remarks in conclusion: 'This action suggested quite a number of important ideas. The disease, although a very important one, had a different importance for one as a doctor than it had for the community . . . there were certainly many more pressing problems which could have shown a greater return for far less effort. However, this disease was the most pressing problem to the community as a whole.' We have a parallel in England in the exaggerated importance given to poliomyelitis in the industrialized world.

Medical authorities frequently have different opinions on what is important from that of the community itself, and generally have different views on the causation and treatment of disease. One of the main services that the social sciences can render the health worker is in assisting him to estimate the relative importance to the community of its various problems. They can also help health workers to an objective appreciation of how the disease is perceived by the community, its supposed causes, acceptable methods of handling them; they can throw light on the prestige value of certain diseases like smallpox in some areas of Africa, and gastric ulcer and liver troubles in business circles in Europe and the United States. If the health worker wishes to gain the active co-operation of the population he is well advised to start his activities with those aspects which appear important to the community rather than those which appear important to the health authority.

It would be a pity if health workers were to be deterred from making use of the concepts and methods of the social sciences by making perfection the enemy of the good. There is much that they can do themselves by way of cultivating the necessary objectivity towards their own assumptions, and their own cultural backgrounds. There is no doubt that a thorough understanding of at least one foreign culture can make them a great deal more sensitive to their own. 'Vive la différence.'

Since the word culture embraces the whole way of life of a community, we should not be satisfied with studies of beliefs, however significant they may appear to be. In arriving at a diagnosis it is equally important to observe objectively what people do. Looked at scientifically, people's behaviour may be in advance of their beliefs or far behind.

There are many mothers who continue the excellent practice of breast feeding their babies because they believe it will prevent pregnancy. There are certainly many smokers who fully understand the dangers of their behaviour, but persist for other reasons.

HEALTH EDUCATION IN PRACTICE

For the purpose of this chapter the term health education includes the *state* of health consciousness of individuals or groups which expresses itself in behaviour; a *process* of learning and teaching and a *relationship* between partners—the public patients and health workers—in the business of promoting health, preventing disease, treating and rehabilitating the sick.

Like the practice of medicine, health education is eclectic and draws on a wide variety of health and social sciences, communication techniques, and organizational methods, but like medicine the success of its practice depends mainly on the status, resourcefulness, and empathy of its practitioners.

Since the relationship between client and practitioner is central to the whole activity, we have devoted a section to the consideration of some of the theoretical aspects of status and role definition in this relationship.

Both with individuals and countries the application of health education requires a stage of diagnosis, a stage of decision-making and a stage of treatment. This implies following certain broad rules of procedure which enable practitioners to reach reasonable conclusions about health problems as they affect the individual patient or the social group, about the objectives they should work towards and about the methods most likely to attain these objectives.

The *diagnostic phase* is devoted to identifying the problem, exploring the state of health consciousness and the behaviour patterns of the clients in relation to the problem including the social and psychological setting in which this state exists. The conclusions reached, combined with a knowledge of the resources available, form the basis for *deciding* on realistic objectives and *planning* the steps which will lead to their attainment.

The *treatment phase* is essentially one of choosing among the wide variety of resources available, those which are most appropriate and which are not likely to do harm. All phases are susceptible to evaluation and all phases require a suitable organizational plan and possibly a variety of practitioners, qualified to carry them out.

In the diagnostic phase are included consultation, observation, and surveys, in the decision-making phase synthesis and the definition of objectives in behavioural terms, and in the treatment phase teaching, learning and motivational activities, publicity and environmental manipulation.

The Diagnosis

If we are to educate, we must know as precisely as possible who to educate and who does the educating. Perhaps the most important single item we need to explore is who is at risk? This implies not only their age, sex, race, geographical location, etc., but their social, psychological, and economic characteristics. Do they constitute definable groups? On the side of the educators, we may need to know about the attitudes and competences of school and university teachers. We must find out what is being done about health education in clinics and services and what clinicians consider to be their role in educating patients.

Knowledge in greater depth about the behavioural epidemiology of the disease will put us in a better position to decide whether the educational activities should be extensive or intensive. The tools for such epidemiological work are already well developed but still need to be applied more thoroughly. The information health education requires about patients and educators and on which health workers can base

their questions to themselves and to social scientists may be grouped for practical purposes under three main headings: (1) states of health consciousness; (2) social environment; and (3) patterns of communication.

Health Consciousness. This includes those intellectual and emotional factors which condition people's behaviour about health. This applies as much to the health authorities and the professional workers as to the patients and the public at large. We need to know:

1. *The degree of awareness* of the problem among those professionally concerned, among patients, and among the general public.

2. *The knowledge and beliefs* they have concerning the causation, prevention, and treatment of diseases.

3. *Their attitudes* regarding the significance of diseases and the value they attach to controlling them.

In the attitude studies we should pay particular attention to motivational factors favouring or restricting treatment, rehabilitation, or prevention.

4. Lastly, we should endeavour to find out about *professional and patient behaviour* which increases or diminishes the risk of disease. From the professional workers we wish to know what steps they take to provide patients with some protective education; among patients we need a detailed breakdown of the behaviour which led to the condition and what kinds of precaution, if any, they take.

Such information constitutes the essential base-line data on which the planning, the choosing of objectives, the training of staff, the educational activities, and the evaluation of health education depend. Though studies of this kind may be costly and the information laborious to collect, it is technically possible to make a start using the existing clinical and research methods.

Social Environment. In exploring the social environment of patients, we need to know particularly about the social structure of the milieu from which they come, their family situation, peer groups, and those persons who influence them. We also need to find out about patients affiliated to other social groups, such as work groups, professional and recreational associations, voluntary bodies, and religious organizations. We should also inform ourselves about legal and economic pressures which favour or prejudice the health objective. These may be of particular importance where special groups are concerned. On the health service side we need to study the provisions made by the health authorities with particular reference to their convenience and acceptability to patients.

Communication Patterns. Communication takes place through *personal exchanges*, such as conversations, interviews, and discussions, and through *impersonal means*, such as radio, films, notices, and newspapers. Communication also has recognizable *patterns*, such as the clinical consultation, meetings of groups for recreation, views expressed by an accepted family or social authority, regular reading of chosen publications which may circulate widely after purchase, pamphlets distributed at health centres, the contents of which are retailed to the family or to friends, school lessons which are discussed with parents, film shows followed by discussion, gossip groups, etc.

In order to reach a chosen group of the population, we need

to know the communication patterns used by that group and, if possible, the importance the group attaches to particular modes of communication. In the first place, professional workers must master the language used by the patients and the public in relation to the health problem in question and the style in which the language is used. Secondly, the educator must be proficient in the use of the media through which the individual is most likely to receive this kind of information. Those we most wish to reach are often the most inaccessible. The richer sections of the population are generally those best supplied with sources of information, whether it be the spoken word, the newspaper, or television. The poorer sections may be reached effectively only by a single medium or are not reached at all.

Market research workers are well aware of the problem and have developed fairly precise methods of investigation, but the value of the market-research approach depends on the ability of the health authorities to define the group they wish to reach.

The approach is long term, but this is inevitable in any problem where human behaviour plays a leading role. Though health educators, like general practitioners, are often compelled to act on inadequate evidence, there is a basic minimum below which no professional person will feel ethically justified in taking decisions. Diagnosis must come before treatment.

The Treatment

Health education in the behavioural diseases is presented with three main opportunities: in the primary prevention of risk; in secondary prevention through early treatment, and in tertiary prevention of transmission and recurrence. The defences against behavioural diseases are within the people, and all types of prevention ultimately depend on the decision of individuals. Making a decision depends on *knowledge*, *motivation*, *reinforcement* and *convenience*. The imparting of *knowledge* is mainly a question of organization and technique, and is within the power of health and education authorities to arrange. *Motivation* is a product of an individual's feelings, his personal identification with the problem, and the social pressures to which he is subject. These are only partly and occasionally within the ambit of influence of health and education authorities. *Reinforcement* is generally necessary to refresh knowledge, to strengthen motivation, to counteract doubt, apathy, and conflicting influences. *Convenience*, being mainly a question of making it easy for the individual to use the services, is almost entirely within the competence of health authorities. Thus, it is possible for health and education agencies to provide two of the main elements which enable people to make sensible decisions which may be enough to protect many from risk and to cause others to report early for treatment.

The only practical methods that can be used by health workers to modify the behaviour of individuals or groups involve *compulsion*, *changing the environment*, and *education*.

Compulsion is an ambivalent weapon in the hands of health authorities. It has been widely used, and sometimes successfully, in attempts to control infectious diseases and prevent accidents, but if wrongly used its benefits may be of very short duration, and its scars take long to heal. It is certainly not a method that has much relevance in the majority of health problems, nor one with which health workers should become

identified. *Changing the environment* and *education* are interrelated methods which are widely used by health workers in clinical medicine and which have shown promise in such fields as maternal and child health, nutrition, rehabilitation, the management of diseases such as diabetes, in coronary disease and in sanitation.

SOME EXAMPLES OF HEALTH EDUCATION IN PRACTICE

What part can the health services and the schools play in improving the health consciousness and social situation of the people of their area? Which groups of workers in the health and education field should be contributing and what allies will they need to make their educational work effective? What educational methods are at their disposal and how can they best be adapted for the groups at risk?

Primary Prevention through Health Education

In seeking answers to these questions with regard to primary prevention, health education is only one element, but it is an element which can be applied immediately if the responsible authorities are prepared to undertake the necessary organization. Two examples from the field of venereal disease suffice to illustrate this point.

A good example of a comprehensive programme is described by Donald Campbell (1963), a health education consultant in the State of Ohio. The essential feature of the Ohio programme was the involvement of all the community agencies concerned in long-term planning and the effective inclusion of venereal disease education as part of the classroom work of teachers. The two major co-operating agencies were the department of health and education. The state director of health set up a committee which included classroom teachers, parents, health education consultants, a local health commissioner, and representatives of the medical profession in the State and one or two other interested persons. It was decided to focus attention on the high schools. An inquiry revealed that little venereal disease education was undertaken throughout the school system. Three reasons appeared to account for this: teachers did not feel adequately prepared to introduce the subject in the classroom; there were very few educational aids and materials on venereal disease which were suitable for classroom use; teachers and school administrators doubted whether venereal disease education of secondary school children would be accepted by parents. These three essential aspects were then tackled systematically. Inservice training of teachers was started. By using discussion methods, teachers began to use the technical words without embarrassment. Materials, including brochures and an excellent film, were produced and carefully tested for acceptability on teachers and pupils. Meetings were held with parents at which the intentions of the programme were explained and their support solicited. Contrary to the anxieties expressed by the teachers, parents welcomed the initiative.

Schools were approached and a good response was obtained for introducing the subject into the curriculum as part of health education. Assistance from the health department was often necessary in getting teaching started and building up confidence of the teachers in their ability to handle the subject.

The reception by students was very favourable, and the programme has gradually spread to cover most schools in the State. In this case venereal disease education was recognized as a legitimate part of health education in school and community. Though the focus was on the pupil, the involvement of all the professional and voluntary groups concerned provided a much wider educational coverage.

Programmes of this kind would have to be worked out, taking account of the local cultural setting. This should not be impossible in any area where the urgency of the problem demands it and the will to protect young people exists.

In a report on the incidence of syphilis in the 15–19 years age group in Los Angeles it is stated that a 73 per cent. reduction took place following intensive educational efforts in the schools and clinics between 1962 and 1966. A reduction was also recorded in the 20–27 years age group. No significant change was recorded in the gonorrhoea incidence among these age groups during the period.

This significant finding emphasizes the important point that the short and long incubation periods of gonorrhoea and syphilis must be taken into account when deciding on the emphasis the educational work should have.

The Limitations of Health Education in Primary Prevention

Such a programme of information and discussion can lay the foundation on which enlightened public opinion can grow. It cannot be expected to deal with the behaviour problems of the high-risk groups, such as the children of low intelligence, the neglected, the maladjusted, and the homosexuals. Though we can reasonably hope that information and discussion will help the majority of youngsters, it may not have much effect on the 'problem children', who as Loeb (1960) puts it 'act out their fantasies in promiscuity'. Special diagnostic and preventive action is needed from the school health service in detecting particularly the maladjusted girls and boys whose promiscuity and failed treatment can have such wide social and epidemiological consequences. Their education, social rehabilitation, and psychological treatment merit a high priority in school health work for more reasons than that of preventing venereal disease.

Intermediate between primary and secondary prevention we have health education in relation to high-risk groups, such as women in their middle years, who are more at risk from cancer of the cervix and breast. A fine example of a carefully developed and controlled programme, covering a population of approximately 4 million inhabitants and designed to reduce the delay between recognition of symptoms and seeking professional advice, is described in a series of articles from the Manchester Committee on Cancer (1954–59), which has now continued for more than 20 years. Among many other important findings on cancer consciousness, the detailed preliminary studies and the careful follow-up have demonstrated that in that area the significance of lumps in the breast was well understood by most women, and delay was caused by fear of the diagnosis. The significance of irregular vaginal discharges was not recognized, and delay in seeking advice was mainly due to ignorance of their significance. The emphasis in the health education activities took these psychological factors into account by attempting to reduce anxiety in the former and increase it in the latter. A steady reduction in delay has been recorded since the third year of the programme's existence.

Secondary and Tertiary Prevention

Clearly those most at risk are patients. For many this may be the first occasion on which they come in contact with anyone with sufficient knowledge, sympathy, and time to discuss their problems. In secondary and tertiary prevention therefore the first place to be considered from an educational point of view is the doctor's surgery, health centre, or hospital, and the most important educator the physician or other well-informed person, such as the nurse or health visitor.

If we agree with this proposition several questions arise, however: does the public at large know about the health services? What kind of reputation has the service acquired? What efforts are clinic staff prepared to make during treatment to tackle the educational problem? A large proportion of doctors do not consider that the education of the patient is part of their responsibility, and a large proportion of clinics carry out no serious educational activities.

Since early treatment is one of the most important preventive measures in many conditions, publicity for the health services and education of the public in their proper use is an important but often neglected first step towards prevention. Many new public-relations approaches, such as patients' clubs (Naish, 1954), open days, 'friends of the hospital', and advice by telephone can bring the health service nearer to their public and the potential patient.

In the therapeutic services generally the aim is twofold: securing adequate treatment and preventing recurrences.

The interview with the doctor is undoubtedly the most impressive educational opportunity. Does he have time for conversation? If not, is any other competent person available? Are simple illustrations and persuasive leaflets ready at hand for the doctor to give the patient? Is the doctor willing and able to use the language of the patient and to provoke questions? Has the doctor any facilities for referring patients for group education? The nurse and the social worker can ascertain from the patient by questioning whether he has understood what the doctor has said and can follow up and interpret his doctor's advice. In some cases (Davies, 1948; Dalzell-Ward et al., 1960) group discussions with patients can be arranged so that the educational treatment can be taken to a deeper level and even a group solidarity built up. Such discussions have psychotherapeutic value and may go a long way to meet the social problems of disturbed patients.

SOME THEORETICAL CONSIDERATIONS RELATING TO ROLES, STATUS, AND BEHAVIOUR

The actors in the educational relationship have more or less well-defined roles and statuses. On the one hand there are well people, people 'at risk', the sick, and the convalescent. On the other, there are doctors, nurses, sanitarians, and teachers who use the health education process as part of their professional armamentarium. In addition, there are health educators whose primary concern is the communication process in relation to health.

Whether they are aware of it or not, all these people display a state of health consciousness and behaviour, are involved in the process of learning and teaching about health and maintain relationships with one another which directly or indirectly affect one another's behaviour. They play their parts on a variety of stages, ranging from the intensity and depth of the individual consultation to the simplification and breadth imposed by the television screen.

When planning health education it is necessary to draw the distinction between its informal and formal manifestations as well as between the objectives of such activities in terms of health 'related' and health 'directed' behaviour. We are aware that such distinctions are arbitrary and that it will never be possible to draw a sharp dividing line between them. However, it is useful when building a theory of an activity because it helps in differentiating between what happens and what was intended to happen as well as in allocating the achievement to the relevant actor. Health education is presented here as a system described in a model (Barić, 1972) which differentiates between informal and formal health education on the one hand and between health related and health directed behaviour on the other. It further differentiates between various influences decisive for a certain type of behaviour in terms of either adherence to certain norms or application of certain forms of knowledge, or a combination of both, as well as between different stages in acquiring both norms and knowledge by means of a process generally referred to as socialization.

Informal health education existed always; it is a part of the evolutionary process which involves the transmission from one generation to another of information relevant to the survival and continuation of the human species, based on accumulated empirical knowledge. The process takes many different forms and involves many different actors. It is, therefore, impossible to define precisely the contribution of each one, although we have certain ideas about the importance of each one. We know the importance of the family on the attitudes of the child and the consequences of early experiences on future health-related behaviour.

Formal health education is a planned process initiated and carried out by professionals with the aim of providing knowledge and experience which will favourably influence attitudes and practices related to individual, family, and community health. It is considered to be the action-oriented aspect of preventive medicine and the applied aspect of behavioural sciences in the field of medicine. Its function is to bridge the gap between recommended behaviour for the cure and prevention of disease and the practices of the population under consideration.

Though the aim of health education is to influence behaviour affecting people's health, one cannot in many cases define exactly in advance what kind of behaviour affects a person's state of health. But the attempt should be made to distinguish general behaviour which may affect health, 'health related behaviour', from 'health directed behaviour' which is intentionally carried out with a specific health aim in mind.

Many aspects of *health-related behaviour* are a part of a person's adherence to social norms, are considered as 'normal' forms of behaviour and do not require any conscious effort for their performance. *Health-directed behaviour*, however, requires a certain amount of conscious effort on the part of the actor, initiated by awareness based on knowledge, and

directed towards preservation of health and avoidance or cure of disease.

In our society, health is a defined state, forming a part of our value-system, and illness represents a deviance from this socially defined 'normal' state. Being healthy, therefore, implies a formalized status with an appropriate role attached to it. Since illness is considered to be a deviance from this socially defined norm, society has developed institutionalized ways of dealing with it. This deviant state is defined by the presence of symptoms which imply the presence of illness, or by behaviour which implies an increased health threat, has a defined role attached to it, and is legitimized by a doctor of accepted status. Since these statuses, with appropriate roles, are socially defined, they form a part of 'reality' as perceived by the members of that society. The process of transmission of concepts which make up a person's perception of 'reality' is known as 'socialization'. Under socialization we understand the process of integrating new members into a society. This process can take different forms, such as primary or secondary socialization or

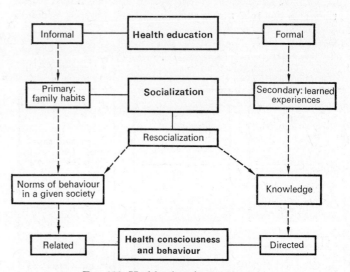

FIG. 110. Health education as a system.

resocialization. Primary socialization takes place in the family or home into which a child is born, and is based on emotional identification of the child with 'significant others' such as its parents on which it models itself. By this process a child learns what is 'normal' in terms of health and illness, how to behave and what to expect from others. Secondary socialization usually takes place in formal settings such as schools, is carried out by persons with a formalized status, is concerned with the transmission of knowledge and is considered to be more or less rational. Through this process a person acquires the accumulated knowledge of his society, such as how to recognize symptoms indicating an illness, what to do about them, where to seek help and how to avoid risks of acquiring them.

If a person does not internalize certain norms during primary socialization, or does not acquire certain knowledge during secondary socialization, or if the existing norms or items of knowledge change, the person will have to reorganize his perception of reality by integrating the new or changed knowledge. This process of readjustment is known as resocialization.

The term 'health education' is composed of two concepts, the first one denoting the concept (health) and the second one the process (education). The contents are a part of our medical knowledge and reflect the value-system of the health professions. The process of education involves socialization for certain future roles, in our case those of a person at risk from a health threat trying to reduce that risk, or of a person who is ill trying to obtain a cure and become healthy again.

Thus, by describing the contents and the processes involved, we are now able to redefine health education as two separate (but often parallel) processes. Informal health education is considered to be concerned with the learning of health norms by an individual, essentially by means of primary socialization, resulting in desirable 'health-related behaviour'. Formal health education is concerned with the acquisition of knowledge about health and disease as a part of secondary socialization resulting in desirable 'health-directed behaviour'.

Professions and Roles in Health Education

We have stressed the importance of informal health education and the role the 'significant others' play on a child's

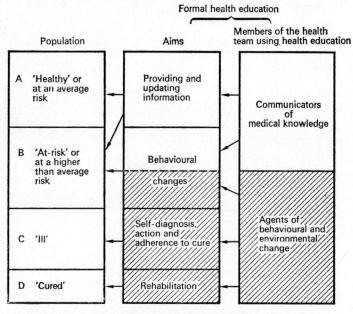

FIG. 111. Formal health education.

integration into a society. It will, therefore, be necessary to find out whom the child considers to be the 'significant other' before we can define the roles of various people who represent the child's immediate social environment. The important point at this stage is to remember that education for health in later life is rarely concerned with innovations alone. It is mostly the case of changing one behaviour to another or resocialization, which means that we are faced with two different processes: one is the process of erasing the existing attitude, habit, or behavioural pattern, and the other is having the innovation adopted by the client.

We are here mainly concerned with formal health education as a part of the health care delivery system. Within formal health education we can distinguish two main interacting factors: the client or client population and the health education

service. The model presented (Barić, 1972) divides each interacting factor into several categories, while the arrows indicate the general direction of the flow of intervention. The shaded area represents the part of the system which in our opinion should be carried out by people with professional standing in medicine, nursing, or sanitation but remains poorly developed. The white area should be the responsibility of those with a professional standing in teaching or communications.

The process of health education is essentially problem-oriented and therefore its function must be defined by the problems existing in the client population. The first part of the model categorizes the population according to its exposure to health threats into (A) the vast majority of people who are at certain risk from a number of diseases but whose level of risk is not above the average for the whole population; they can be defined as 'healthy'. Category (B) denotes the people who are at a higher risk than average risk from certain health threats because of their genetic make-up, behaviour, or environment; they can therefore be recognized as being 'at risk' (Barić, 1969). The category (C) is made up of people who are already ill. The category (D) consists of people who have been ill but are now cured and trying to return to normal life.

From the model it is obvious that different population groups require different services, carried out with different involvement and intensity. The 'healthy' group (people at average risk) require scientifically based information about the health threats to which they can be most commonly exposed so that they may decide upon the necessary action. This, today, is being provided by health educators or 'communicators' through publicity, lectures, publications, and group activities. The 'at risk' group (people at higher than average risk from certain health threats because of their behaviour) need more than information—they need to change their behaviour. At present this group, too, is being catered for partly by the health educators of the 'communicator' type and partly by doctors and nurses acting as communicators. The groups of 'ill' and 'cured' have been left so far largely to the curative services and have hardly been catered for by the health education services as such.

The approach shown in the model emphasizes the need to differentiate between the roles of the various clients on the one hand and to differentiate between statuses and roles of the professional workers within the health team on the other.

For the first group the goal of health education is to reinforce or create social norms related to the desired health behaviour. To do this, health educators must take the role of communicators, bridging the gap between scientific findings and public knowledge about health threats and behaviour related to illness. To fulfil this role, health educators must gain a professional recognition in the field of communications. Their target population will be predominantly in the group of 'healthy' people and their code of ethics must comply with professional standards required in the field of public communications or teaching related to health.

For the second, third, and fourth groups the main goal, that of changing behaviour, requires health educators who can identify and legitimize each individual's 'at risk' role with all its implications. For this an appropriate medical status is required. Doctors and nurses have such a status but may have received no adequate preparation in the art of communication or may have reservations about the extent to which such communication benefits the patient.

Structural analysis based on this model shows that there is room for conflict between the expectations and achievements of the various types of present-day health educators. The work of health educators who provide information for the general public is often judged on a short-term basis according to the amount of behavioural change achieved among special groups of people who are at higher than average risk because of their behaviour. This is most likely unfair to them and further emphasizes that within the framework of a health service a clear understanding of the status and roles of the various members of the health education team is essential if appropriate activities are to be assigned to its members.

THE WORK OF THE HEALTH EDUCATION CONSULTANT

Health education activities within a clinic and in the wider field of public health and education require careful organization and their planning, development, and evaluation will benefit from the advice of an experienced health education consultant. Such a professionally qualified person may also serve the school programme and any out-of-school youth activities that may be going on through youth clubs, the Junior Red Cross, and other voluntary bodies.

The availability of the health education consultant to work in the wider social context and even across departmental frontiers can be a potent force in what Popchristov (1960) in Bulgaria has described so eloquently as building up public opinion and social customs which support a constructive way of life.

Though changes in society are slow, technical progress is rapid. The existence of an enlightened public opinion will be a major element in gaining their acceptance by the public. The investment in staff well qualified in health education will pay a worthwhile dividend in speeding what experience has shown can be a very slow process.

The World Health Organization is actively encouraging governments to establish within their Ministries of Health departments with qualified staff in health education. Their work includes carrying out inquiries, planning, evaluating, and organizing health education in all fields of clinical medicine, public health, and general education in co-operation with other departments and professional groups. If the fruits of scientific discovery are to benefit mankind, modern medicine requires interpreters of the highest skill and integrity.

REFERENCES

Barić, L. (1969) Recognition of the at-risk role, *Int. J. Hlth Educ.*, **12**, 1.

Barić, L. (1972) The behavioural sciences as a basis for health education, in *Behavioural Sciences in Health and Disease*, ed. Barić, L., Geneva.

Barić. L. (1972) The teaching of behavioural sciences and health education at the University of Manchester, *Int. J. Hlth Educ.*, **15**, 1.

Burgess, A. (1954) Letter, *Lancet*, **ii**, 869.

Campbell, D. A. (1963) Strengthening VD education, *Int. J. Hlth Educ.*, **6** (2), 66.

Dalzell-Ward, A. J., Nicol, C. S., and Haworth, M. C. (1960) Group discussions with male VD patients, *Brit. J. vener. Dis.*, **36**, 106.

Davies, M. (1948) Royal Society of Health Report.

Foster, G. M. (1956) Working with people of different cultural backgrounds, *Calif. Hlth*, **13**, 107.

Freedman, M. (1957) Health education and self education, *Hlth Educ. J.*, **15**, 78.

Glass, L. H., Atkisson, L. M., and Rickett, M. S. (1968) What do the educated know about VD, *Int. J. Hlth Educ.*, **11**.

Jefferys, M. (1957) Social class and health promotion, *Hlth Educ. J.*, **15**, 109.

Koos, E. L. (1954) *The Health of Regionville*, New York.

Loeb, M. B. (1960) Future problems of VD control affected by increased teenage population, *Brit. J. vener. Dis.*, **36**, 191.

Los Angeles County Health Dept., Progress Report, Teenage (15–19) VD.

Loudon, J. B. (1957) Social structure and health concepts among the Zulu, *Hlth Educ. J.*, **15**, 90.

Manchester Committee on Cancer:
Aitken-Swan, Jean, and Easson, E. C. (1959) Reactions of cancer patients on being told their diagnosis, *Brit. med. J.*, **1**, 779.

Aitken-Swan, Jean, and Paterson, R. (1955) The cancer patient: delay in seeking advice, *Brit. med. J.*, **1**, 623.

Aitken-Swan, Jean, and Paterson, R. (1959) Assessment of the results of five years of cancer education, *Brit. med. J.*, **1**, 708.

Paterson, R., and Aitken-Swan, Jean (1958) Public opinion on cancer—changes following five years of cancer education, *Lancet*, **ii**, 791.

Paterson, R., Metcalfe Brown, C., and Wakefield, J. (1954) An experiment in cancer education, *Brit. med. J.*, **4**, 1219.

Marriott, McK. (1955) in *Health, Culture and Community*, ed. Paul, B. D., New York.

Naish, F. Charlotte (1954) *Lancet*, **ii**, 1342.

Newell, K. W. (1957) Medical development within a Maori community, *Hlth Educ. J.*, **15**, 83.

*PAHO/WHO Inter-Regional Conference on the Postgraduate Preparation of Health Workers for Health Education (1964) *Wld Hlth Org. techn. Rep. Ser.*, No. 278.

Pickles, W. N. (1939) *Epidemiology in Country Practice*, Bristol.

Popchristov, P. (1960) Incidence of veneral diseases and the campaign against them in Bulgaria, *Brit. J. vener. Dis.*, **36**, 125.

Simon, J. (1890) *English Sanitary Institutions*, London.

Steuart, G. W. (1957) Experiences in the health education of mothers, *Hlth Educ. J.*, **15**, 7, 178, 240.

Steuart, G. W. (1964) School health education: an appraisal of instruction, *Hlth Educ. J.*, **22**, 158.

World Health Organization Expert Committee on Health Education of the Public (1954) First Report, *Wld Hlth Org. techn. Rep. Ser.*, No. 89.

FURTHER READING

Abercrombie, M. L. J. (1960) *The Anatomy of Judgement*, London.

Bibby, C. (1951) *Health Education: A Guide to Principles and Practice*, London.

Burgess, A., and Dean, R. F. A., eds. (1962) *Malnutrition and Food Habits*. Report of an international and interprofessional conference held by Josiah Macy, Jr. Foundation, New York.

Burton, J., ed. (1954) *Group Discussion in Educational, Social and Working Life*, London.

Burton, J., ed. (1955) Visual education, *Hlth Educ. J.*, **13**, No. 1.

Burton, J., ed. (1957) Social anthropology and health education, *Hlth Educ. J.*, **15**, No. 2.

Burton, J., ed. (1958) Preparation for health education, *Hlth Educ. J.*, **16**, No. 2.

(The above three editions of the *Health Education Journal*, edited by J. Burton, were special editions concerned exclusively with one subject.)

Burton, J. (1958) Doctor means teacher, *Int. J. Hlth Educ.*, **1**, 4.

Health Education Journal (1959) The Journal generally, and particularly Vol. 17 giving articles on the history of health education and in relation to the major religions.

Health Education Monographs (1963) Review of research related to health education practice, Suppl. No. 1, New York.

Health Education Monographs (1967–1969) Review of research and studies related to health education. Young, M. A. C., No. 23, What People Know, Believe, and Do About Health; Young, M. A. C., and Simmons, Jeanette, J., No. 24, Psychosocial and Cultural Factors related to Health Education Practice; Young, M. A. C., No. 25, Review of Research and Studies related to Health Education Communication: Methods and Materials; No. 26, Patient Education; No. 27, Program Planning and Evaluation; No. 28, School Health Education. Society of Public Health Educators, New York.

Hobson, W. (1963) The place of health education in the medical curriculum, *Roy. Soc. Hlth J.*, **83**, 36.

International Journal of Health Education, Geneva.

Leavell, H. R., and Clark, E. G. (1958) *Preventive Medicine for the Doctor in his Community*, pp. 13–39, New York.

Mace, D. R., Bannerman, R. H. O., and Burton, J., eds. (1974) The teaching of human sexuality in schools for health professionals, *Wld Hlth Org. publ. Hlth Pap.*, No. 57.

Paul, B. D., ed. (1955) *Health, Culture and Community; Case Studies of Public Reactions to Health Programs*, New York.

Pirrie, D., and Dalzell-Ward, A. J. (1962) *A Textbook of Health Education*, London.

Read, M. (1957) Social and cultural backgrounds for planning public health programmes in Africa, *Wld Hlth Org. Reg. Off.*, Brazzaville.

Read, M. (1966) *Culture, Health, and Disease*, London.

Turner, C. E. (1964) *Community Health Educator's Compendium of Knowledge*, Geneva.

*Turner, C. E. (1966) *Planning for Health Education in Schools*, UNESCO, Paris.

World Federation for Mental Health (1953) *Cultural Patterns and Technical Change*: a manual, ed. Margaret Mead, Paris, UNESCO.

*World Health Organization Expert Committee on School Health Service (1950) *Wld Hlth Org. techn. Rep. Ser.*, No. 30.

*World Health Organization Expert Committee on Health Education of the Public (1954) *Wld Hlth Org. techn. Rep. Ser.*, No. 89.

*World Health Organization Expert Committee on Training of Health Personnel in Health Education of the Public (1958) *Wld Hlth Org. techn. Rep. Ser.*, No. 156.

*World Health Organization (1963) Health Education in the U.S.S.R., *Wld Hlth Org. Publ. Hlth Pap.*, No. 19.

World Health Organization (1969) Report of a WHO Expert Committee on Planning and Evaluation of Health Eduaction Services, *Wld Hlth Org. techn. Rep. Ser.*, No. 40.

*World Health Organization/UNESCO Expert Committee on Teacher Preparation for Health Education (1960) *Wld Hlth Org. techn. Rep. Ser.*, No. 193.

World Health Organization Scientific Group on Research in Health Education (1969). In preparation.

World Health Organization (1971) Report of a study group on health education in health aspects of family planning, *Wld Hlth Org. techn. Rep. Ser.*, No. 483.

World Health Organization (1974a) The work of WHO in 1973, *Wld Hlth Org. Off. Rec.*, No. 213, 114–117.

World Health Organization (1974b) The selection of teaching/learning materials in health sciences education. Report of a WHO Study Group, *Wld Hlth Org. techn. Rep. Ser.*, No. 538.

World Health Organization (1974c) Editorials on WHO activities in health education, *Wld Hlth Org. Chron.*, **28**, 250, 251.

World Health Organization (1974d) WHO programme reviews, *Wld Hlth Org. Offset Publ. Ser.*, No. 8.

World Health Organization Regional Office for Europe (1974) *Report of a Working Group on the Evaluation of Mental Health Education Programmes, Nancy 1973* (Euro 5432 III), Copenhagen.

* Available in English, French, and Spanish.

50

EVALUATION OF SCREENING PROCEDURES

J. CHAMBERLAIN

INTRODUCTION

The detection and treatment of disease at an early stage in its development is an attractive idea to the health professions, which are too often faced with the late stages of chronic disease which they can do little or nothing to alleviate. It seems reasonable to suppose, that if patients were diagnosed earlier, treatment offered then would have a greater chance of success in curing the disease or at least in delaying its progression. Screening of large populations, in order to identify individuals who will later develop overt illnesses, has therefore been increasingly advocated and practised, catalysed by the development of more and more sophisticated diagnostic techniques. This so-called 'prescriptive screening' (McKeown, 1968) can be defined as the presumptive identification of unrecognized disease, or risk of disease, by investigation which does not arise from a patient's request for medical aid. Screening may also be practised for other purposes, of which the major one is the control of communicable diseases by identifying and removing infected individuals from the community. It is also frequently used as a research instrument in epidemiological studies of the prevalence, incidence, and natural history of disease. While many of the principles applicable to prescriptive screening apply also to these other forms, this chapter will be confined to the evaluation of prescriptive screening, with examples drawn from chronic non-communicable diseases prevalent in Western Europe and North America.

The doctor who offers prescriptive screening to people who have not sought his advice is in a rather different ethical position from that in his usual role. Normally, when he is consulted by a patient with a complaint, he must obviously do his best to help that patient within the limits of medical knowledge of the illness, but he cannot be held responsible if the available treatments fail to help. When he offers screening, however, the implication is that he *knows* it will do good; he is, as it were, a missionary persuading people to be screened with the promise that they will have better health as a result. He therefore has an ethical responsibility to be sure that the good resulting from screening far outweighs the harm. It is for this reason that a strict evaluation of screening procedures should always precede their development as a service.

FACTORS INFLUENCING THE EFFECTIVENESS OF SCREENING

In seeking methods for evaluation of screening, one must first explore the various factors which can affect the success of a screening programme. A number of interdependent factors can be identified and are shown in diagrammatic form in FIGURE 112.

By *natural history* is meant the course of the disease from the earliest stage at which an individual may be identified as being at risk through the stage of early, perhaps presymptomatic disease, to overt disease, disability, and death. We need to know what course the disease would follow if not treated in any way, and how effective previous methods of preventing or treating it have been.

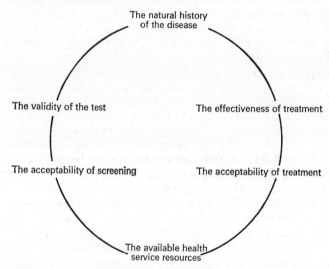

FIG. 112. Factors influencing the effectiveness of a screening programme.

The *effectiveness of early treatment* in altering this natural history is obviously of vital importance in the evaluation of screening. Commonly, reports of screening programmes are given which claim to show value simply by the number of abnormalities found, as though having reached the point of diagnosis there were no further problems. Implicit in this is the assumption that all disease is easily curable, which unfortunately is certainly not true for many chronic diseases which it is possible to detect presymptomatically.

Most methods of treating chronic disease are inconvenient, often lifelong, and not infrequently associated with distressing or even dangerous side-effects and complications. Because of this they may prove *unacceptable* to the people for whom they are prescribed, particularly if these people had no symptoms before being put on treatment. Obviously, even if all other factors affecting the success of screening are satisfactory, it will not succeed in controlling the disease, if there are many 'dropouts' from treatment.

The *efficiency of the screening test* itself is also of great importance in assessing the value of a screening programme. A test which is insufficiently sensitive gives a large number of false-negative results, letting many diseased people slip through the net. On the other hand, a non-specific test, giving a high proportion of false-positives, causes many healthy people to be submitted to the worry, inconvenience, and in some cases even danger of further diagnostic tests.

The provision of screening needs to be organized in a way that is *acceptable* to the people most likely to contract the disease, for otherwise considerable resources will be wasted in screening low-risk people with no prospect of controlling the greater part of the morbidity from the disease. In considering the acceptability of both screening and treatment, behavioural factors such as perception of need are of prime importance and may outweigh all efforts to organize the testing in a way that is both convenient and comfortable. There is a major role for health education in this context.

The last factor shown in FIGURE 112 is the *availability of resources* for the screening programme. Before embarking on screening it is necessary to have resources available not merely for performing the screening test, but also for further diagnostic tests on all who screen positive (in order to sort out the false-positives from the true), and for treating all the people found to have early disease. It is sometimes claimed that the costs of providing a screening and follow-up service will be more than offset by savings in expensive treatment of the 'late' cases averted by screening, but this hypothesis has never really been put to the test. In such an assessment the importance of the disease(s) to be screened for, looked at in terms of both prevalence and severity must be considered. Cochrane and Holland (1971) illustrate this using the extreme example of porphyria variegata—a condition for which screening could well be effective in preventing deaths due to barbiturate sensitivity, but one which is so rare that it would not be worth devoting resources to this end. More often though, the health administrator may be faced with the difficult decision of whether to allocate his inevitably scarce resources to limited control of an important disease by screening of uncertain value, rather than spending them in some other field of medical care. It is therefore essential for him to have information as complete as possible on all the factors influencing screening mentioned above. Each of these will now be examined in detail, with examples from diseases for which screening has been studied, to show how the necessary evidence can be obtained.

NATURAL HISTORY

Many of the diseases for which screening is advocated are chronic, with an insidious development often continuing over many years. Collecting sufficient evidence to give a scientifically accurate description of their natural history is therefore a lengthy undertaking, requiring prospective study of a large population for a long time. This cannot be done retrospectively, for even though possible risk factors can be identified more frequently in people with the overt disease than in control cases, the contribution of these risk factors to the development of the disease can only be found by prospective study; the prevalence of risk factors in a population cohort is measured, and then by repeated examinations of the same cohort the subsequent incidence of the disease in question can be determined and related to the previous findings. Such studies, which identify the aetiology and early warning signs of later disease

are of practical importance in suggesting appropriate stages at which to intervene, either by early treatment or by other preventive measures, such as health education.

Ischaemic Heart Disease

The natural history of *ischaemic heart disease* has been investigated perhaps more fully than any other chronic condition. Several prospective incidence surveys, such as the Framingham study (Kannel *et al.*, 1962) and the London busmen's study (Morris *et al.*, 1966) have been carried out and are continuing. These, and others, have identified the many factors, familial, environmental, behavioural, and physical, which lead to increased risk of ischaemic heart disease. Morris *et al.* suggest that these can be divided into *causes* and *precursors*. The causes include factors such as increasing age, obesity, physical inactivity, smoking (and diet high in animal fat); to this list can perhaps now be added living in a soft water area (Crawford, Gardner, and Morris, 1971) and having a 'Type A' competitive personality (Rosenman *et al.*, 1970). These causes, operating separately or together, lead to the precursors, which include raised blood pressure, raised serum cholesterol, and other lipid changes, and ECG changes. Discriminant function analysis has been used to isolate the risk factors which, independently of the others, are the most accurate predictors of subsequent disease. Both the London busmen and the Framingham studies (Truett, Cornfield, and Kannel, 1967) found that raised blood pressure and raised serum cholesterol were much the most important predictors of subsequent disease, although only one in seven men identified as high risk by these factors developed the disease within five years. Work is continuing in trying to find out how the causes operate (Morris *et al.*, 1973; Carruthers, 1969), but meanwhile several intervention studies have been started in which people identified by screening as being at risk are randomly allocated to treatment (including diet and health education) or control groups. It is unfortunately true that although much has been learnt about the development of this condition, we still do not fully understand the disease process, and, at least until the results of the intervention studies are available, there is no case for mass prescriptive screening for ischaemic heart disease [see CHAPTER 27].

Diabetes

Another chronic disease in which prospective studies are elucidating the natural history is *diabetes mellitus*. The particular problem here lies in determining which people who are found to have a moderately raised blood sugar are eventually going to develop clinical features of diabetes. This is a good example of the borderline problem, very frequently met in screening. In a population, many variables, of which blood sugar is one, are distributed in a unimodal curve, slightly skewed to the 'diseased' side of the population mean. FIGURE 113, using data from the United States National Health Survey (1964) shows the distribution of blood sugar one hour after a loading dose of 50 g. of glucose in a population of middle-aged women. From this the size of the borderline group can be seen; over 15 per cent. of the total population of adults tested had a blood sugar level of 160 mg. or over (an accepted screening level in the United States), although the number of overt diabetics is known from other surveys to be less than 1 per cent.

Cochrane and Elwood (1969) suggest that distributions of this nature may be composed of a large healthy distribution concealing a small separate diseased distribution within the tail,

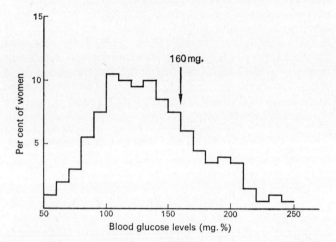

FIG. 113. Distribution of blood glucose levels in women aged 45–54 (United States National Health Survey, 1964).

as shown in FIGURE 114. However, in the absence of further tests to distinguish the healthy from the diseased, a purely arbitrary decision may have to be taken on whom to treat. In the past, in reporting results of many biochemical tests the convention has been to classify as abnormal results which are outside the range of plus or minus two standard deviations from the mean value of the variable for the whole population. This judgement is based on the fact that 5 per cent. of values (2·5 per cent. at either end of the distribution) lie outside this

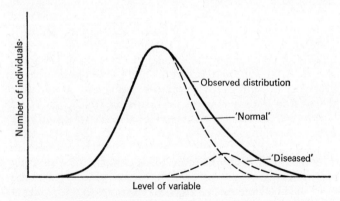

FIG. 114. Model of 'normal' and 'diseased' populations within an observed distribution (Cochrane and Elwood, 1969).

range, if the variable has a statistically normal distribution— i.e. one that is bell-shaped with an equal number of values on either side of the mean. However, as already seen, most physiological variables are skewed so that this calculation does not apply to them (Elveback, Guiller, and Keating, 1970), and in any case is inappropriate as a criterion of disease. The influence of other factors, of which the most obvious is age, also needs to be taken into account in assessing whom to label as diseased; a one-hour blood sugar of 160 mg. in a man of 20 for

example would be taken much more seriously than the same level in a woman of 70.

If the natural history of the disease were known, however, the decision on whom to treat could be based on firm evidence rather than on a value judgement. In the case of diabetes this would entail identifying a cohort of people with moderately raised blood sugar and, without giving them any treatment, following them over several years to determine the subsequent incidence of disease. Provided that the original group was large enough, it would then be possible to define the level of blood sugar which predicted later disease in people of different age-groups. The control group of a randomized controlled trial of treatment of borderline diabetes, such as the Bedford study (Keen, 1966) provides just such a cohort in whom the natural history is being followed. Trials such as this have the added advantage that they not only show which people will develop overt disease, but also indicate which people will benefit from treatment, thus conforming with Cochrane and Elwood's (1969) definition of the cut-off point between 'normal' and diseased—'the level below which treatment does more harm than good'.

Phenylketonuria

Screening has sometimes been introduced as a service without adequate evidence of the natural history of the condition, and hence of the effect which screening and early treatment will have. An example of this is screening for *phenylketonuria*, in which it is assumed that sustained excess phenylalanine in the blood in early life is always associated with subsequent mental retardation, and that dietary treatment to keep the serum phenylalanine level down results in normal intelligence. This assumption is based on the fact that many treated phenylketonuric children have developed with normal intelligence. But the natural history is unknown and it has been suggested that screening may pick up a proportion of children who only have the biochemical abnormality and who would not later develop mental retardation, thus introducing a bias into the reported effects of treatment (Wilson, 1968). Reports of individual cases (Mabry, Denniston, and Coldwell, 1966) have also shown that intelligence may be normal or only slightly impaired in the presence of a high serum phenylalanine level. If this occurred frequently there would be a large number of mentally normal people with raised phenylalanine levels in the general population. In order to investigate this, Levy *et al.* (1970) tested the serum of 250,000 adults for phenylalanine, as part of a serological study for other diseases. They found only three cases of phenylketonuria all of whom were mentally subnormal. Thus, this provides indirect evidence that the postulated natural history of the biochemical abnormality almost always leading to mental defect is very probably correct.

Carcinoma-in-situ of the Uterine Cervix

This is another condition for which screening is widely practised even though its natural history is unknown. Pathologically, there seems to be a continuum from cells showing dysplasia or dyskaryosis through carcinoma-in-situ, to microinvasive, preclinical invasive, and eventually clinically invasive tissue, and it is assumed that the disease process follows this course. However, as Knox (1968) has pointed out, it is impossible ever to follow the natural history of the cellular abnormality, because in order to diagnose the lesion accurately (being sure that there is no area of invasion) it has to be removed completely. The only way of collecting evidence about the proportion of cellular abnormalities which would become invasive would be by comparing the incidence of and mortality from invasive cancer of the cervix in a population in whom cervical cytology screening was practised, with that in a randomly selected control population not offered screening. The opportunity to do such a trial when it would have been ethically acceptable (i.e. when screening was first suggested) was missed, and it is very doubtful now if the natural history of pre-invasive lesions will ever be understood. Attempts have been made to show the effectiveness of cervical cytology by demonstrating a fall in incidence and mortality in populations offered screening, such as that in British Columbia (Fidler, Boyes, and Worth, 1968) but as shown by Ahluwalia and Doll (1968) and by Hammond (1971), so many other factors may contribute to the decline that the value of cytology is still in doubt. As Wilson (1970) has pointed out, the lesson to be learnt from cervical screening is that we should always try to obtain some experimental evidence about the natural history of a condition before providing a screening service for it.

THE EFFECTIVENESS OF TREATMENT

From what has already been said about natural history, it should be clear that the surest way of obtaining evidence about the effectiveness of screening and early treatment in altering the natural history is by a randomized controlled trial. Because of the chronic nature and usually low prevalence of diseases for which screening is suggested, these trials are necessarily long-term and involve large numbers of people. This in part accounts for the fact that, for so many conditions, we still do not know the answer to the question of whether screening can help to control the disease. It is important to appreciate the fact that the effectiveness of treatment can only be properly assessed by looking for positive end-points which really measure the effect of treatment on the patient's life, such as reduced mortality from the disease or a reduced number of major episodes of illness. It cannot be assumed that because a treatment is able to convert an abnormal test result to a normal level, the patient is necessarily any better off for this change—he might indeed have a worse prognosis due to long-term complications of the treatment.

Diabetes

This point is well illustrated in the results of two randomized controlled trials of treatment of *diabetes* in middle-age. One is the Bedford study (Keen, 1966) already mentioned, in which subjects with borderline diabetes identified by screening have been randomly allocated to treatment with tolbutamide or a placebo, and then each group subdivided into diet or no diet categories. The other trial is that run by the University Group Diabetes Program (1971) in the United States, in which subjects presenting at hospital clinics with mature onset diabetes were randomly allocated to treatment with insulin, oral diabetic agents, or placebo. These trials, both very well designed and well executed in their follow-up, give conflicting results as to the long-term value of the oral treatment. After seven years in the Bedford trial, the value of treatment in the study group as a whole is inconclusive, although in subjects classified as low-risk there has been a significant reduction in incidents of cardiovascular disease in the group treated with tolbutamide (Keen and Jarrett, 1970). In the UGDP study, however, after eight years of follow-up, a significantly *increased* mortality was found in the tolbutamide-treated group. Because the subjects in these two trials were not identified in the same way (those in the UGDP study presumably having more symptoms than those identified by screening in the Bedford study) and because there may have been a chance bias towards low-risk subjects in the placebo group in the UGDP study, the two trials are not exactly comparable. However, as Cochrane (1972) has pointed out, the fact that the results of treatment by tolbutamide are in conflict indicates that whatever effect it may have—in either direction—must be small.

Hypertension

A more conclusive result of the effects of early treatment comes from the United States Veteran's Administration (1970) trial of treatment of *hypertension*. This again was a randomized controlled trial in which 523 middle-aged men, who in the course of medical care for some other condition were incidentally found to have diastolic blood pressure levels between 90 and 129 mm. Hg, were randomly allocated to treatment with hydrochlorothiazide, reserpine, and hydralazine, or to a placebo. A favourable effect of treatment was apparent very quickly in the group with diastolic pressure above 115 mm., and the trial was stopped and all put on treatment after an average follow-up of 1·6 years. The remaining group were followed for an average of 3·3 years, after which time those with pressures above 105 mm. were also doing significantly better on treatment than on placebo. TABLE 124, taken from a summary of the study by Freis (1970), shows the results. The complications which were reduced in the treated group were principally cerebrovascular accidents, and no difference was found between treated and placebo groups in the incidence

TABLE 124

Incidence of Major Complications in the Treated and Control Groups in the VA Trial of Treatment of Symptomless Hypertension (Freis, 1970)

Pre-randomization Diastolic BP	CONTROL GROUP			TREATED GROUP		
	Number randomized	Number with complications	Per cent. incidence	Number randomized	Number with complications	Per cent. incidence
115–129	70	27	38·6	73	1	1·4
105–114	110	35	31·8	100	8	8·0
90–104	84	21	25·0	86	14	16·3

of myocardial infarction. This study, however, does give positive evidence that treatment of a symptomless condition can benefit the people concerned, and thus suggests that screening would be valuable. But it cannot be assumed that the same level of effectiveness would necessarily be reached by treating men of different age-groups, or women; similar trials of screening and early treatment of these groups in well populations are now being started which it is hoped will eventually show similar benefit, possibly, in the case of younger men, showing an effect on myocardial infarction as well as cerebrovascular accidents.

Breast Cancer

For some conditions, of which cancer is the most obvious example, a trial in which the control group is left untreated or placebo-treated is impossible for ethical reasons. The effectiveness of screening, however, can still be measured by a randomized controlled trial of screening versus not screening. The Health Insurance Plan of Greater New York has carried out such a trial of screening for *breast cancer* by clinical examination and mammography, and provides an excellent example of the size and complexity of the epidemiological studies needed to evaluate screening (Shapiro, Strax, and Venet, 1971). In this study, 62,000 women between the ages of 40 and 64 registered with a number of group practices were stratified by age and various other factors and then randomly divided into a study group and a control group. The study women were offered screening by clinical examination and mammography annually for four successive years, and their experience of breast cancer is currently being compared with that of the control women, for whom no special provision was made. Fortunately, the Health Insurance Plan, for actuarial purposes, keeps accurate statistics of health service utilization by all its members, and hence it is possible to identify virtually all breast cancers occurring in both groups. The effectiveness of screening is being measured by comparing mortality from breast cancer, and fatality rates in breast cancer cases, in the two groups.

Results are now available for a period covering 5 years from the women's date of entry to the study. During this time there have been 296 histologically confirmed cases of breast cancer in the study group and 284 in the control group. The cancers in the study group can be divided into three groups; 132 of them were detected by screening, 73 presented in women who had refused the invitation to be screened (about one-third of the total group), and 91 occurred between screening examinations. Of the cancers detected at screening, 45 per cent. were found by clinical examination alone, 33 per cent. by mammography alone and only 22 per cent. were positive to both these tests. TABLE 125 shows the number of deaths from breast cancer in both groups after 5 years. From this it can be seen that there is an over-all reduction in mortality in the study group of about one-third, but that this is related to age. In women under 50 there was no difference; in those between 50 and 59 there was a mortality reduction of about two-thirds, statistically significant at the 1 per cent. level; and in those over 60 there was a lesser reduction, which, with these small numbers, was not statistically significant.

The favourable effect of screening suggested by these results is borne out by a comparison of fatality rates in women diagnosed as having breast cancer in the two groups; this also

TABLE 125

Five Year Mortality from Breast Cancer in the HIP Breast Cancer Screening Study (Shapiro, Strax, and Venet, 1971)

Age at death	DEATHS FROM BREAST CANCER	
	Study Group	Control Group
40–49	13	12
50–59	16	34
60–69	11	17
Total	40	63

illustrates the difference between the various subgroups of cancer detection in the study group. TABLE 126 shows how the reduced case-fatality rate in the study group as a whole was apparently entirely due to the cancers detected by screening. Cases detected in women who had refused screening, or which presented between screening examinations, did not differ significantly from those in the control group.

The figures shown in TABLE 126 allow for a 'lead time' of 1 year in cases detected by screening; in other words, the fatality rate 5 years after diagnosis in cases detected by screening is being compared with that 4 years after diagnosis in cases presenting in the other groups. Lead time is defined as the interval between the early diagnosis achieved by screening and

TABLE 126

Five Year Case-fatality Rates in the HIP Breast Cancer Screening Study (Shapiro, Strax, and Venet, 1972)

Population	5-year case fatality rate per cent.
Control group	42·1
Total study group (screened and refused screening)	27·9
Total screened group	25·8
Detection by screening . . .	16·9
Not detected by screening . .	38·7
Refused screening	34·5

Rates for study group cases allow for 1 year average lead time in cancer detection due to screening.

the time when the disease would have been diagnosed if screening had not been performed. It should always be remembered, and if possible, estimated as has been done in this case (Hutchison and Shapiro, 1968), in comparisons of survival following screening with survival following conventional diagnosis, as otherwise the results will inevitably be biased in favour of screening.

A related point which can also lead to bias in favour of screening is the selection of longer duration, presumably slower growing cases by screening. If a disease has a variable preclinical history, a population will, at any given point in time, contain some short-duration and some long-duration preclinical cases. As Feinleib and Zelen (1969) have illustrated in the model shown in FIGURE 115, screening at a single point in time will detect a greater proportion of the longer duration cases; if such cases of long preclinical course are also those of long clinical course—i.e. more benign variants of the disease— then cases detected by screening will contain a disproportionate number of them. There is a suggestion that this is so in the breast cancer screening study in relation to cases detected by mammography alone, which contained a greater proportion of intraductal carcinomas, generally considered to be more benign.

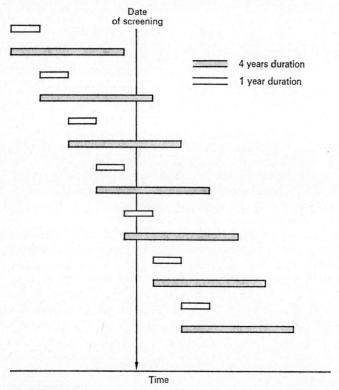

FIG. 115. Selection of longer duration cases by screening (Feinleib and Zelen, 1969).

The possible biases in survival comparisons, however, do not apply to the over-all reduction in mortality shown in TABLE 125, and this can be regarded as firm evidence of benefit. But breast cancer has a long natural history, sometimes recurring 10 or even 15 years after diagnosis, which would make it preferable to have comparisons of mortality over these longer intervals, in order to know whether lives have in fact been saved or merely prolonged.

These two studies—on hypertension and breast cancer—provide what is virtually the *only* positive evidence so far available that prescriptive screening of middle-aged people for non-communicable diseases has a favourable effect on prognosis. Moreover, they both illustrate that the level of effectiveness is certainly not complete, and refute the claims still heard from ill-informed proponents of screening that mortality from certain conditions could be completely averted by early detection. This question of the extent of the effect likely to be achieved in practice is of great interest to the health administrator in his difficult decision as to the resources he is able to allocate to a screening programme, in which the balancing of costs versus effectiveness is an essential ingredient.

THE ACCEPTABILITY OF TREATMENT

One of the factors which makes it unwise to extrapolate the results of the Veterans' Administration study of treatment of symptomless hypertension to a general population, is that the group of men involved were not typical. Before embarking on the trial, a much larger group of symptomless hypertensives was started on a regime of 'treatment' with placebo drugs. The placebos were marked with riboflavine, which can later be detected in the urine, and the men were periodically tested by urine fluoroscopy, and by pill counts. After 3 months, some 50 per cent. of the original group were judged as unsuitable for inclusion in the trial of treatment, because they were not taking the drugs as prescribed (Freis, 1970).

It is well known that this non-acceptance of treatment can be of major proportions in the treatment of chronic disease, particularly where the treatment concerned involves prolonged courses of drugs with unpleasant side-effects. Fox (1962) found that some 50 per cent. of people being treated with oral anti-tuberculous drugs were not taking them.

If non-acceptance occurs in people who have already sought care for symptoms, it is likely to be very much greater among those detected at screening, in whom the result of the screening test causes an abrupt change from being healthy to being labelled as a patient, though not necessarily accompanied by any change in illness behaviour. If the person feels worse on treatment than he did before it is hardly surprising if he ceases to take it as prescribed. The role of a personal doctor or other health professional in educating the patient about his treatment regime can have a major effect, as shown in a recent study by Finnerty, Mattie, and Finnerty (1973). Two hundred and eighty-four hypertensive patients found at screening and subsequently attending a follow-up clinic were randomly allocated to a 'stepped-up care' group with frequent visits and investigations, and close identification with paramedical clinic staff, and to two general medical clinics, in one of which reminder letters to attend for scheduled appointments were sent. After an average of 8 months, 84 per cent. of people in the study group were still being followed compared with 33 per cent. and 26 per cent. in the general medical clinic groups. It is not stated how many of the patients were actually taking the treatment prescribed, but it is noted that the diastolic pressure was controlled in 70 per cent. of patients in the study group compared with less than 10 per cent. in the other groups.

Perception of need and attitudes towards health services in general are determinants of the acceptance of treatment. In a follow-up of elderly people found by screening to have unreported disabilities of hearing, vision, mobility and feet, half of those recommended for treatment had not received it after 6 months (Garraway, 1972). The commonest reason for this was that the person had not taken up the offer of treatment, probably indicating that the attitude which had led her not to report her discomfort in the first place also caused her to turn down the offer of help. A certain stigma still attaches to being a patient, particularly among the elderly who—perhaps rightly —may consider that preserving their independence of health services is worth a certain amount of discomfort.

The attitude of the doctor is also important; in the same study Garraway found that many recommendations (which had been made by specialists at a screening clinic) had not been acted upon because the general practitioner considered that the person would not benefit from treatment. This again underlines the necessity to show, by randomized controlled trials, how effective early detection and treatment is in improving prognosis. If the level of benefit is known, then the general practitioner or other doctor can be taught to base his decision about treatment on factual evidence.

THE EFFICIENCY OF THE SCREENING TEST

The efficiency of the test, in sorting out those people who really have the early disease from those who do not, influences the success of every screening programme. The criteria for judging screening tests have been listed by Cochrane and Holland (1971). Some of these are virtually self-evident, such as that the test should be safe, quick and easy to perform, accurate, and reasonably cheap. The validity of the test and its reproducibility, however, may require further explanation. In defining screening, the United States Commission on Chronic Illness (1957) stressed that screening was really a sorting process and was not intended to be firmly diagnostic. This implies that a proportion of false results can be expected, and that confirmatory diagnosis is always needed.

TABLE 127
Classification of Screening Test Results

Screening test results	TRUE DIAGNOSIS		Total
	Diseased	Not diseased	
Positive . .	a	b	a + b
Negative . .	c	d	c + d
Total .	a + c	b + d	a + b + c + d

a = true-positives   c = false-negatives
b = false-positives   d = true-negatives

Before introducing a new screening test, it should be studied in order to see how efficient it is in diagnosing the disease in question, in terms of the proportion of false results which are given by it in practice. The terms *sensitivity* and *specificity* are commonly used to express the validity of a test in this way. Sensitivity is defined as the proportion of diseased people in the population tested who are detected by the test; if a test has a sensitivity of 90 per cent., 10 per cent. of diseased people screened by it will give false-negative results. Specificity, on the other hand, is the proportion of non-diseased people in the population tested who are classified as non-diseased by the test; a test with a specificity of 90 per cent., will give false-positive results in 10 per cent. of the non-diseased people tested by it, and these people will be wrongly referred for follow-up as a result. TABLE 127, adapted from Thorner and Remein (1961), illustrates that sensitivity is calculated by the true-positives as a proportion of all diseased people in the population tested, while specificity is calculated by the true-negatives as a proportion of all non-diseased people in the population tested.

To find out these indices of a screening test it is necessary to compare the results given by screening a representative population with the true disease status of that population, the latter being determined by the best diagnostic measures available. This is not always easy in practice, since it necessitates a double examination of each individual, by the screening test and by the definitive diagnostic test, and often the latter is inadequate or absent. In such cases, sensitivity and specificity can only be

estimated by confirmation of the presence or absence of disease by later follow-up of the people screened, regardless of whether their screening result was negative or positive.

TABLE 128
*Validity of Ophthalmoscopy as a Screening Test for Glaucoma
(Graham and Hollows, 1966)*

Ophthalmoscopy	GLAUCOMA		Total
	Present	Absent	
+ve	20	65	85
—ve	0	4,129	4,129
Total	20	4,194	4,214

Sensitivity = 100%
Specificity = 99·4%

TABLE 128, showing the validity of ophthalmoscopy as a screening test for glaucoma, is derived from a prevalence study in which a number of different methods were used to determine the true prevalence of glaucoma in a middle-aged population (Graham and Hollows, 1966). As can be seen, ophthalmoscopy (performed by ophthalmologists) proved a very satisfactory test in terms of both sensitivity and specificity. This was in contrast to tonometry, which had a sensitivity of only 50 per cent. In this case, the 'true' presence or absence of glaucoma was determined by the number of cases found by all methods of testing. TABLE 129 (Wilson, 1973) shows another example of a good screening test—the Guthrie bacterial inhibition test for phenylketonuria—but here the 'true' presence or absence of disease could not be obtained directly by confirmatory tests on all babies who screened negative. It is deduced from the

TABLE 129
*Validity of Guthrie test in Screening for Phenylketonuria
(Wilson, 1973)*

Serum Phenylalanine	PHENYLKETONURIA		Total
	Present	Absent	
4 mg. + per 100 ml. .	9	419	428
< 4 mg. per 100 ml.	0	117,016	117,016
Total . .	9	117,435	117,444

Sensitivity = 100%
Specificity = 99·6%

fact that no cases of phenylketonuria, other than those detected at screening, in babies born in the region and time period overed were notified to the phenylketonuria register.

Both these tables illustrate the fact that, in screening for conditions of low prevalence, the specificity is always high because the number of true-negatives (forming the numerator of the specificity calculation) is inevitably very large. Poor specificities are more likely to occur in conditions of high prevalence, as can be seen in TABLE 130, which shows the results of screening questions about financial need administered by nurses to people over the age of 70, compared with a definitive assessment of their need, based on an interview with an expert in the supplementary pensions field (Chamberlain, 1973). This illustrates, as well as any, the dilemma which may face those organizing screening about what to regard as a satisfactory level of sensitivity and specificity. The two-thirds

TABLE 130

Validity of Questionnaire in Screening for Eligibility for Supplementary Pension

Screening Questions	SBC INTERVIEW		
	Entitled	Not entitled	Total
Entitled . .	13	16	29
Not entitled .	7	30	37
Total . .	20	46	66

Sensitivity = 65%
Specificity = 65%

of needy old people found by screening must surely benefit from receiving more money, but what about the one-third who were missed, who because their need had not been detected would presume they were not eligible? Conversely, one-third of those not fulfilling the criteria for supplementary pension, would, as a result of screening, be put through the embarrassment or distress of a detailed financial examination on the assumption that they would receive more money, only to find that they were not eligible.

Deciding on satisfactory levels of sensitivity and specificity in such situations has to be done on an arbitrary basis weighing up the disadvantages of false-negatives against those of false-positives.

It should be noted that sensitivity and specificity have a relationship with each other which varies according to the cut-off point between the normal and diseased populations. Therefore, when the screening test measures a continuous variable such as serum phenylalanine or blood sugar, the sensitivity and specificity can be made to vary according to the screening test level—as sensitivity increases specificity decreases and vice versa. This is illustrated graphically in FIGURE 116; moving the screening test level X to the left would decrease c, the false-negatives, thus improving sensitivity, but would increase b, the false-positives, thus diminishing specificity. Wilson (1973) has shown how the screening level of serum

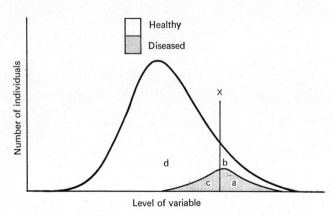

FIG. 116. Relationship between sensitivity and specificity.

phenylalanine in the series shown in TABLE 129 could be raised (i.e. moved to the right in FIGURE 116) from 4 to 6 or even 8 mg., to improve the specificity still without missing any cases. This is shown in TABLE 131. This would have the obvious advantage of relieving a large number of families of the anxiety and inconvenience of further diagnostic tests on the baby. The first positive case in this series occurred at a test level of 8 mg./100 ml., but presumably it is felt that the disadvantage of missing a case is so very much greater than the anxiety engendered by false-positives that the screening level should be set low.

So far, screening tests have been considered from the point of view of the people who are tested, judging their value by the proportion of people who may be misclassified by screening. When looked at from the point of view of the resources required for follow-up, however, a third index—the *diagnostic power* (or predictive value) of the test—is important. This measures how well the test discriminates the disease in question and is calculated by the true-positive results as a proportion of all positive results—$\frac{a}{a+b}$ in TABLE 127. In the examples given it can be seen [TABLE 128] that the diagnostic power of

TABLE 131

Effect of Altering Screening Level of Serum Phenylalanine (Wilson, 1973)

	SCREENING LEVEL OF SERUM PHENYL-ALANINE		
	4 mg.	6 mg.	8 mg.
Number of false-positives	419	28	16
Sensitivity (%) . .	100·0	100·0	100·0
Specificity (%) . .	99·6	99·9	<100
Diagnostic power (%) .	2·1	24·3	36·0

ophthalmoscopy as a test for glaucoma is 20/85 or 23 per cent., that of the Guthrie test [TABLE 129] at a screening level of 4 mg. is 9/428 or 2 per cent., and that of the financial need questions [TABLE 130] is 13/29 or 45 per cent. As with sensitivity and specificity, altering the screening level will alter the diagnostic power; it can be seen from TABLE 131 that if the serum phenylalanine screening level were set at 8 mg., the diagnostic power of a positive test would be increased to 36 per cent. The diagnostic power of a test can also be increased if the prevalence of the condition in the population can be increased. In practice this can be achieved by restricting screening to those previously identified as being at high risk of the disease.

Resource implications of the diagnostic power of the test need to be assessed in the context of the prevalence of positive results to the test and the complexity of the further investigations which will be needed to sort out the false-positives from the true. In the case of phenylketonuria, the prevalence of positive results is low (0·4 per cent. with the screening level at 4 mg.) and the further investigation required is simple, often requiring only a repeat Guthrie test. The fact that the diagnostic power is low is therefore not a major disadvantage. In the case of testing for glaucoma by ophthalmoscopy, however, the prevalence of positive tests is higher, at 2 per cent., and the further diagnosis means referral to ophthalmic outpatients for a full range of specialized tests. This assessment of 2 per cent. of the adult population, presumably repeated at regular intervals, might so swamp the ophthalmic service that treatment facilities for other conditions could be seriously reduced. This, together with the fact that the screening itself in this study was done by specialists and might be much less efficient in non-expert hands, makes this method of screening impractical, quite apart from the fact that the effectiveness and acceptability of therapy for presymptomatic glaucoma remains to be proved (Cochrane, Graham, and Wallace, 1968).

The measures of efficiency of screening tests discussed above compare the results given by a test with the results of more definitive diagnostic procedures. It is also necessary, however, to know whether the test will give consistent results when applied to the same subject at different times or by different observers—in other words to measure the *reproducibility* of the test. This can be done by comparing the results given by testing the same individuals twice, and is usually expressed as the percentage agreement between the two results. Where the prevalence of the condition is low, however, the large number of negative results to both tests almost invariably gives a high reproducibility percentage, but there may still be very poor agreement as to the positive results. For this reason it is advisable to express reproducibility as the proportion of agreement out of all positive results.

Variability in test results in the same individual can arise in three ways. First, there can be variations within the individual, either of a physiological nature or (particularly important in questionnaire testing) of a psychological nature; secondly, there can be variation in the test technique or instrument; thirdly, there can be variation in the observer's interpretation of the test result. Taking cervical cytology as an example, the cell pattern of cervical epithelium may vary within each woman, the method of taking and staining the smear may vary, and the interpretation of the microscopic appearance of the specimen may vary between different observers or within the same observer on different occasions (Yule, 1973).

When the biological variation within an individual is known to be large, as for example in blood pressure readings, it is advisable to use more than one reading as a screening test (Armitage *et al.*, 1966) and, so far as possible, to standardize testing according to variables known to affect the result—e.g. testing blood sugar at a set time after a known loading dose of glucose. Variability of the test technique can, if appropriate, be reduced by mechanical means, for example by regular calibration of instruments against known standards, but a clearly laid-down programme of training and regular testing of screening staff is also of prime importance in this connexion. The same methods of ensuring consistency apply to interpretation of results, and are widely used as 'quality control' measures in laboratories.

ACCEPTABILITY OF SCREENING

A fifth factor affecting the value of every screening programme is its *acceptability* to the people at whom it is aimed. A number of behavioural studies have established the fact that recognition of a current medical need leads an individual to seek care, but people's perception of need and perhaps their belief in what the service has to offer them varies, and has been shown to decline with age and with social class. Consequently preventive health services including screening, where immediate need is not felt, are consistently under-used particularly by those people subject, in general, to higher rates of morbidity (Bloor and Gill, 1972). Because of this under-utilization, various inducements may have to be used in order to persuade a worthwhile proportion of those at risk of getting the disease in question to be tested.

Undoubtedly the highest response rates to screening are achieved in 'captive' populations where the individual has little or no opportunity to refuse. This applies to neonatal screening (virtually all neonates being in contact with health services) and to school examinations, where it is likely that the small proportion remaining unscreened can be attributed more to failure of the organization rather than to refusal of the individual (or parent). Another captive population consists of people attending hospital who are very commonly screened in so far as they are subjected to investigations not related to their presenting complaint; this may vary from simple routine testing of urine on all admissions to the extremely sophisticated techniques of biochemical and haematological profiling. As we shall see later, such profiling raises some problems, but lack of response is certainly not included among them.

With cervical cytology on the other hand, lack of response from those most at risk is a constant finding and may largely account for the failure of cervical screening to influence mortality from carcinoma of the cervix. One possible method of getting more of the high risk group screened would be to take advantage of their attendance at hospital for some other condition, particularly if the latter required a vaginal examination. This could be achieved by undertaking routine testing of all previously unscreened women attending gynaecological and venereal clinics, and those over a certain parity attending antenatal clinics. It is not known to what extent this is already being practised.

The primary-care doctor also has a potentially large influence in persuading people attending him to be screened, either by testing them himself or by referring them to a screening clinic. For this to be effective it is necessary that the doctor himself should be convinced of the possible value of early detection and accept preventive as well as curative medicine as part of his role. This can be accomplished in the long term by education, although in the short term other inducements to the doctor, such as financial incentives to undertake screening, may be necessary. Antenatal care is one example of a form of screening which is accepted by the profession as an integral and necessary part of any health service, and this fact must contribute to a large extent to its high utilization. The involvement of the primary-care doctor in a screening service does not, of course, stop at screening itself for, regardless of who does the testing, he will be involved in the subsequent care of people who screen positive.

Nurses and health visitors in the primary-care team have also proved useful in persuading people to be screened, especially if they are able to do the testing themselves. Response rates of well over 80 per cent. have been obtained by nurses administering questionnaires and simple tests to elderly people in their own homes (Chamberlain, 1973). In a small experiment to try to find ways of screening women in deprived social circumstances for carcinoma-in-situ of the cervix, Osborn and Leyshon (1966) found that district nurses were able to take smears from women at home, and achieved a good response from women all known to belong to 'problem families'; the prevalence of positive or suspicious smears in these women was ten times that in women from the general population attending clinics. Bloor and Gill (1972), in discussing screening of the well child, also emphasize that working-class under-users of services feel more at ease in their own home environment than in impersonal clinic surroundings, and consequently are more likely to accept domiciliary screening. Another method successfully exploiting a personal approach to 'high risk' women is described by Fulghum and Klein (1967). In this study, social workers identified 'opinion leaders' among an indigent population in Florida, and educated these leaders about the value and technique of cervical screening. The leaders then proved very effective in persuading their peers to attend screening clinics.

An approach which has the advantage of testing in the person's home environment but obviates the need for skilled staff is the development of 'do-it-yourself' screening methods which can be delivered to people's homes. The postal self-administered questionnaire is the most obvious of these, but its use so far has been largely restricted to epidemiological surveys and it has seldom been used in a prescriptive screening service. The probable reason for this is that conditions detectable by self-administered questionnaire techniques have not so far been proved to benefit from early treatment, but if intervention studies eventually do show benefit, there could be an increasing place for such questionnaires in detecting unreported angina and other cardiovascular risk factors, and in the early detection of psychiatric disease.

Postal 'do it yourself' tests have also been used in screening for diabetes and for cervical carcinoma-in-situ. In the case of diabetes, paper strips for testing for glycosuria have been mailed to large populations (e.g. nearly one million inhabitants in the city of Munich) in various 'diabetes drives'; however, it has been clearly shown that testing for glycosuria is an insensitive method of diabetes detection compared with blood sugar testing, and there therefore seems little place for it in a screening programme. In the case of screening for carcinoma-in-situ of the cervix, the cytopipette technique, which the woman can use herself to obtain a sample of cells from the posterior fornix of the vagina, has been shown to be nearly as sensitive as the conventional technique (Husain, 1970) and to be more acceptable to women than a clinic attendance (Carruthers et al., in preparation). However, although more acceptable overall, particularly in rural communities, the high risk, older, high parity, low social class women are still largely under-represented among women who will use it.

The use of special mobile screening units is another method of bringing the service to the people who need it. Such units, which can make periodic visits to factories or other places where large numbers of people are employed, and to large supermarkets or shopping areas, have been successfully used in screening for tuberculosis and some other conditions. They have the advantage that people can act immediately on their decision to be screened, usually without having to make appointments, but have the attendant disadvantage that they do not fit easily into the normal health care system, and hence

often have little or no facilities for follow-up of people screening positive.

Inviting people by postal invitation to come to be screened can usually achieve a good response, particularly if the letter comes from the general practitioner or other health professional known personally to them. The principal drawback to this method is the need for a population register which ideally should, at the least, include each individual's age and sex, as well as name and address.

General publicity about the availability of the service is still perhaps the most widely used method of persuading people to be screened, but is also probably the least effective in making symptomless people see the immediate relevance of screening to their own situation. An extreme method of persuasion is to build some punitive element into the system; this is done in some countries for example by withholding social security maternity benefits from women who have not attended for antenatal screening in the first three months of pregnancy. Such measures, however, even if effective in persuading a majority to use the service, are likely to cause harm to the very people who most need help.

From the few sociological studies which have looked in depth at people who do not use preventive services (e.g. Fink, Shapiro, and Lewison, 1968), it is apparent that these non-users are characterized by negative attitudes to curative as well as preventive medicine. Although often reporting more symptoms, they less often seek care. They tend to be less educated, of lower social class, and older than the people who will accept screening. These characteristics, which, with many conditions, also mean they are at high risk, must be taken into account in trying to devise methods of communicating to them the value (if proved) of early detection of disease.

HEALTH SERVICE RESOURCES FOR SCREENING

In considering the resources needed for the introduction of a screening programme, several aspects should be estimated. These include the staff and facilities required for inviting people to be screened, for performing the screening test, for confirmatory diagnosis of those screening positive and for treatment of the confirmed cases. In addition, an efficient recording system will be needed, preferably one which incorporates a method of recalling each individual for repeat screening at an appropriate interval. Staff training and testing must be organized and ideally, some on-going quality control measures should be incorporated to ensure that the standard of the screening test does not deteriorate when widely applied over time.

Because adequate follow-up services are so important it is necessary that the screening organization should fit easily into the whole health care system of the population, in a way which is acceptable to both the people and the health service personnel. Some commercial multiple screening organizations which may well have been very efficient as diagnostic centres, have failed because they were divorced from the normal health service and hence were unable to ensure a follow-up for cases screening positive. Involvement of health service staff in screening as a preventive measure in addition to their normal curative activities is desirable, although not always practicable.

Provision of staff for screening is one of the main resource problems to be overcome. Many screening tests require two categories of staff; first, to perform the test procedure on the individual being screened and, secondly, to interpret it in laboratory, X-ray department, or other technical service. Although medically qualified staff are used in both these capacities, they are expensive, require a long training, and are in very short supply in some specialities. Where a screening examination can be incorporated into a medical examination which the individual is undergoing for other purposes, it is, of course, economical for the doctor to do it, but in general population screening, paramedical workers such as nurses or technicians will often be found more feasible. With suitable training in the test technique there seems no reason why such workers should not be as good as medical staff, but their availability, or rather lack of it, may be a problem. Redeployment of existing staff may be a better proposition than recruitment and training of new staff specially for screening but, of course, such redeployment must be based on firm evidence that the priority to be accorded to the screening service is greater than that of their alternative work.

The development of computer techniques for interpretation of test results is an expanding subject which should eventually reduce the need for staff. It is already widely practised in automated biochemical and haematological testing, and is used to a lesser extent in interpreting questionnaires and other test results. Automated pattern recognition for reading of histological slides or X-rays has so far proved disappointing.

It is probable that automation will also play an increasing part in screening information systems but at present these are still largely manual. The purposes of record systems for preventive as for curative services are to assist in the management of individual patients, to assist in the administration of the service, and to provide data required for evaluation of its effectiveness and efficiency. With regard to individuals, a record of the test result is, of course, essential to further follow-up if the result was abnormal, but may also be of value in subsequent care of the person if it was normal. This implies that some means of linking the screening record with the person's other health record should be possible; at the simplest level this may merely be a notification to the person's general practitioner, at the most automated it may consist of linking by some identification code the screening record to the person's whole health record on magnetic tape or disc. From the administrative viewpoint, the information system should be capable of ensuring that all positive results are acted upon, of recalling individuals for repeat screening after the appropriate interval, and of providing routine information on factors such as numbers of people screened in a given time. Wherever possible, information from the screening record should also be able to be used to evaluate how well the programme is meeting its objective. The factors which require to be measured for this include the proportion of the population who have been screened (a population register is needed for this), the proportion with positive tests, and the proportion of these confirmed as having early disease. Information about the last group should include details of the treatment prescribed, and if possible the patient's acceptance of this. These factors, looked at in association with disease incidence registrations and mortality registrations for the whole population, should enable some assessment of the impact which early detection may have in control of the disease.

In service as distinct from research screening programmes, there are few existing systems which can provide sufficient information in this way. One of the factors conflicting with the establishment of an information system for evaluation is the need to maintain confidentiality of personal medical records; it can be seen that linkage of different records from the same individual is necessary for statistical analysis, and this implies some identification particulars on each separate record, available to a central data-processing unit as well as to the individual's personal doctor.

It can be seen that provision of resources for any early detection programme is likely to be a major item of health service expenditure, and therefore methods of improving the efficiency of screening by increasing the yield of treatable disease per unit cost have been studied.

High-risk Screening

One method of increasing yield is to limit screening to people of known high risk. This has the effect of increasing the prevalence of disease in the screened population, and hence also increasing the diagnostic power of the screening test. Thus, a greater number of cases are identified per unit screening cost. There are, however, both ethical and scientific constraints to selective screening of high risk subjects. Is it ethically justifiable to withhold a valuable early detection service from low risk subjects who still have some chance of developing the disease? The answer to this will, of course, depend on how small their chances of getting it are. Attempts have been made to draw up 'at risk' registers of infants, on the basis of adverse antenatal and perinatal events and to screen only the risk infants for developmental abnormalities. However, the detection rates based on selective screening have been disappointing because of the difficulty of defining a relatively small group of children in whom the majority of handicaps would occur (Oppé, 1967). Nevertheless, Alberman and Goldstein (1970) have shown that differentially devoting resources to screening children at different risks could be more efficient than a uniform allocation of resources to screening all children.

Scientifically, the procedure for identification of high risk subjects should be evaluated in the same way as outlined above for the screening procedure. For example, Bulbrook, Hayward, and Spicer (1971) have shown that measurement of the excretion of androgenic steroid hormones in the urine can identify women at increased risk of breast cancer. Present evidence suggests that this test can identify 30 per cent. of women who will develop 60 per cent. of the breast cancers, but it is possible that if combined with known epidemiological indicators of risk (e.g. a late age at first pregnancy (MacMahon et al., 1970), better prediction could be achieved. But the acceptability, validity, and cost of the prescreening urine test (requiring a 24-hour specimen) has not so far been studied.

Multiple Screening

The combination of screening tests for several conditions into a procedure which can be performed at one clinic attendance is another potential method of improving efficiency in using resources. Such multiple screening is well established in specialized areas such as antenatal care and school examinations.

More recently, it has been developed, particularly in the United States, as a preventive health measure for middle-aged adults. A large effort has gone into the technology of computerized testing and diagnosis, with the result that the term Automated Multiphasic Health Testing, or AMHT, has become common parlance, and the number of AMHT units operating in the United States now runs into hundreds (Thorner, 1971). However, these units are limited to diagnosis and there is as yet very little evidence of the effect which they may have on people's health.

Wherever multiple screening of adults has been practised, it has detected large numbers of abnormalities, often leaving only a minority of people who are classified by the screening as entirely 'normal'. This is particularly true of biochemical screening, where Murphy and Abbey (1967) have pointed out that increasing the number of tests increases the probability of 'abnormal' results occurring by chance. The significance of many abnormalities to the person's health is still obscure, emphasizing again our lack of knowledge of the natural history of disease, and our lack of a clear understanding of what constitutes 'health'. In one study of biochemical profiling of hospital inpatients, Whitehead, Carmalt, and Widdowson (1967) found that in 8 per cent. of patients a new diagnosis could be made as a result of profiling, but a further 36 per cent. of patients had unexpected abnormalities which could not be explained.

The worry and inconvenience to all these people of repeated further tests, and their use of resources, must be counted in the cost of screening. One of the problems in laboratory profiling is that the selection of tests for inclusion in the profile has so far been based on the convenience of their automation to laboratory organization rather than on their value in detection of treatable disease. It is hoped that future work both on laboratory screening and on non-laboratory tests to be included in multiple screening programmes may lead to batteries of tests that have been shown by evaluative studies to be of benefit.

Evaluation of the effectiveness of multiple screening is more complicated than merely summating the effectiveness of early detection of separate diseases included in it. Baseline information about several measures of the individual's health will be obtained, and the availability of this to his doctor may influence long-term management, with possible effects both on prognosis and on use of resources. Consequently, there is a case for conducting trials of multiple screening in its own right, looking at a variety of end-points to measure the total effect which such screening may have over several years. Two reports of controlled trials of multiple screening are available. One, in Sweden (SPRI, 1972), screened about 1,000 people between the ages of 45 and 65 in 1964, and again in 1969; a control group of similar age and sex structure was selected but not screened in 1964, and was examined for the first time in 1969. Comparisons of the two groups showed that, although many of those screened in 1964 were then considered to benefit, after 5 years no statistically significant difference could be demonstrated in the state of health (represented by 20 parameters) of the screened group compared with that of the controls. Another attempt to evaluate multiphasic screening is being undertaken at the Kaiser Permanente Foundation in the United States where a study group of 5,000 people are invited to be screened annually and are being compared with a control group who are screened on request. After 7 years, Ramcharan et al. (1973) reported no clear-cut difference in mortality or hospital utilization between study and control groups, although there was a suggestion (based on results of a self-administered questionnaire) that the study group had a lower rate of absence from work. A third study (Holland, 1970), for which no results are yet available is a randomized controlled trial of multiple screening of people aged 40–64 in London. This will compare approximately 3,000 individuals, screened every 2 years, with 3,000 unscreened controls, measuring mortality, prevalence of disease and disability, perception of health, and occupational functioning, and the demand on financial and health service resources that such a multiphasic screening programme creates.

Thus there is, as yet, insufficient evidence to suggest that multiple screening in middle-age is a valuable method of preventive medicine. Even if looked at in terms of individual conditions, there are really only two—hypertension and breast cancer—for which screening has been proved to be effective. Although there is no wholly convincing evidence that screening for cervical carcinoma-in-situ is effective, it is already widely practised, so that there may be reasonable grounds for offering multiple screening as a service to middle-aged women, with tests limited to those for breast and cervical cancer, and hypertension.

CONCLUSION

Knowledge of the effects of screening for early detection of chronic disease has considerably increased during the past few years. The principles of screening as set out in 1968 by Wilson and Jungner, have since then been subjected to careful scrutiny in relation to several different diseases. The results of this research so far available have confirmed the emphasis which Wilson and Jungner placed on the importance of evaluating screening by measuring its long-term value rather than judging it by the short-term achievement of finding 'positives'. The extent to which it can help to control disease is dependent on very much more than our ability to diagnose. This is not to deny the relevance of accurate diagnosis, and the work which has been done in measuring and trying to improve the validity of tests is obviously of great importance. However, the effects of screening are so dependent on our ability to improve prognosis by treatment that it is to be hoped that future research may concentrate more on studying and developing effective therapies. For most of the major diseases afflicting Western countries, including ischaemic heart disease, mature onset diabetes, and many cancers, we still do not know the extent to which early treatment can alter prognosis.

The success of screening is also very dependent on the attitudes and behaviour of people in relation to health and disease. Too little attention has been paid in the past to providing services, both curative and preventive, in a way which encourages those people in need to use them, and a potentially effective screening and treatment service could fail completely if it is not used by those who need it.

The decision on whether or not to provide a screening service to control one or more diseases can seldom be an easy one for the health administrator. He not only has to devise an efficient method of organization within the existing health care system, but he also has to measure the total cost of this and decide whether the extent of benefit likely to be achieved is greater than that which could be derived from alternative ways of spending his scarce resources. To make this decision rationally requires a scientific evaluation of screening and early treatment, taking into account all the factors which can influence its success.

REFERENCES

Ahluwalia, H. S., and Doll, R. (1968) Mortality from cancer of the cervix uteri in British Columbia and other parts of Canada, *Brit. J. prev. soc. Med.*, **22**, 161.

Alberman, E. D., and Goldstein, H. (1970) The 'at-risk' register: a statistical evaluation, *Brit. J. prev. soc. Med.*, **24**, 129.

Armitage, P., Fox, W., Rose, G. A., and Tinker, C. M. (1966) The variability of measurements of casual blood pressure, *Clin. Sci.*, **30**, 377.

Bloor, M. J., and Gill, D. G. (1972) Screening of the well child, *Community Medicine*, **129**, 135.

Bulbrook R. D., Hayward, J. L., and Spicer, C. C. (1971) Relation between urinary androgen and corticoid excretion and subsequent breast cancer, *Lancet*, **ii**, 395.

Carruthers, M. E. (1969) Aggression and atheroma: a hypothesis, *Lancet*, **ii**, 1170.

Chamberlain, J. (1973) Screening elderly people, *Proc. roy. Soc. Med.*, **66**, 888.

Cochrane, A. L. (1972) in *Effectiveness and Efficiency*, Nuffield Provincial Hospitals Trust, London, p. 55.

Cochrane, A. L., and Elwood, P. C. (1969) Laboratory data and diagnosis, *Lancet*, **i**, 420.

Cochrane, A. L., Graham, P. A., and Wallace, J. (1968) Glaucoma, in *Screening in Medical Care*, Nuffield Provincial Hospitals Trust, London, p. 81.

Cochrane, A. L., and Holland, W. W. (1971) Validation of screening procedures, *Brit. med. Bull.*, **27**, 3.

Crawford, M. D., Gardner, M. J., and Morris, J. N. (1971) Cardiovascular disease and the mineral content of drinking water, *Brit. med. Bull.*, **27**, 21.

Elveback, L. R., Guiller, C. L., and Keating, F. R. (1970) Health, normality and the ghost of Gauss, *J. Amer. med. Ass.*, **211**, 1.

Feinleib, M., and Zelen, M. (1969) Some pitfalls in the evaluation of screening programs, *Arch. environm. Hlth*, **19**, 3, 412.

Fidler, H. K., Boyes, D. A., and Worth, A. J. (1968) Cervical cancer detection in British Columbia, *J. Obstet. Gynaec. Brit. Cwlth*, **75**, 392.

Fink, R., Shapiro, S., and Lewison, J. (1968) The reluctant participant in a breast cancer screening program, *Publ. Hlth Rep. (Wash.)*, **83**, 479.

Finnerty, F. A., Mattie, E. C., and Finnerty, F. A., III (1973) Hypertension in the inner city, *Circulation*, **47**, 73.

Fox, W. (1962) The chemotherapy and epidemiology of tuberculosis, *Lancet*, **ii**, 473.

Freis, E. D. (1970) Value of antihypertensive treatment in mild and moderate hypertension, *Bull. Int. Soc. Card.*, **11**, 4, 6.

Fulghum, J. E., and Kelin, R. J. (1967) *Cancer Detection through Cytology*, Florida Department of Health and Rehabilitative Services, Monograph 11.

Garraway, M. (1972) *Follow-up Study of Elderly People found at Screening to Have Some Disability*, unpublished report for M.Sc. (Social Medicine), University of London.

Graham, P. A., and Hollows, F. C. (1966) A critical review of methods of detecting glaucoma, in *Glaucoma, Proceedings of a Symposium Held at the Royal College of Surgeons of England*, Edinburgh, p. 103.

Hammond, E. C. (1971) *The Early Diagnosis of Uterine Cancer, Symposium on the Early Detection of Cervical Cancer*, British Association for Cancer Research, University of Hull.

Holland, W. W. (1970) *The Value of Surveillance and Multiple Screening, Proceedings of the Eighth International Congress of Gerontology*, **1**.

Husain, O. A. N. (1970) The irrigation smear, *Amer. J. Obstet. Gynec.*, **106**, 1, 138.

Hutchinson, G. B., and Shapiro, S. (1968) Lead time gained by diagnostic screening for breast cancer, *J. nat. Cancer Inst.*, **41**, 665.

Kannel, W. B., Kagan, A., Dawber, T. R., and Revotskie, N. (1962) Epidemiology of coronary heart disease, *Geriatrics*, **17**, 672.

Keen, H. (1966) The presymptomatic diagnosis of diabetes, *Proc. roy. Soc. Med.*, **59**, 1170.

Keen, H., and Jarrett, R. J. (1970) *The Effect of Carbohydrate Tolerance on Plasma Lipids and Atherosclerosis in Man, Proceedings of the Second International Symposium on Atherosclerosis*, New York, p. 435.

Knox, E. G. (1968) Cervical cancer, in *Screening in Medical Care*, Nuffield Provincial Hospitals Trust, London, p. 43.

Levy, H. L., Karolkewicz, V., Houghton, S. A., and MacReady, R. A. (1970) Screening the 'normal' population in Massachusetts for phenylketonuria, *New Engl. J. Med.*, **282**, 1455.

Mabry, C. C., Denniston, J. C., and Coldwell, J. G. (1966) Mental retardation in children of phenylketonuric mothers, *New Engl. J. Med.*, **275**, 1331.

MacMahon, B., Cole, P., Lin, T. M., Lowe, C. R., Mirra, A. P., Ravnihar, B., Salber, E. J., Valaoras, V. G., and Yuasa, S. (1970) Age at first birth and breast cancer risk *Bull. Wld Hlth Org.*, **43**, 209.

McKeown, T. (1968) Validation of screening procedures, in *Screening in Medical Care*, Nuffield Provincial Hospitals Trust, London, p. 1.

Morris, J. N., Chave, S. P. W., Adam, C., Sirey, C., Epstein, L., and Sheehan, D. J. (1973) Vigorous exercise in leisure-time and the incidence of coronary heart disease, *Lancet*, **i**, 333.

Morris, J. N., Kagan, A., Pattison, D. C., Gardner, M. J., and Raffle, P. A. B. (1966) Incidence and prediction of ischaemic heart disease in London busmen, *Lancet*, **ii**, 553.

Murphy, E. A., and Abbey, H. (1967) The normal range—a common misuse, *J. chron. Dis.*, **20**, 79.

Oppé, T. E. (1967) Risk registers for babies, *Develop. Med. Child Neurol.*, **9**, 13.

Osborn, G. R., and Leyshon, V. N. (1966) Domiciliary testing of cervical smears by home nurses, *Lancet*, **i**, 256.

Ramcharan, S., Cutler, J. L., Feldman, R., Sieglaub, A. B., Campbell, B., Friedman, G. D., Dales, L. G., and Collen, M. F. (1973) Disability and chronic disease after seven years of multiphasic health checkups, *Prev. Med.*, **2**, 207.

Rosenman, R. H., Friedman, M., Straus, R., Jenkins, C. D., Zyzanski, S. J., and Wurm, M. (1970) Coronary heart disease in the Western Collaborative Group Study, *J. chron. Dis.*, **23**, 173.

Shapiro, S., Strax, P., and Venet, L. (1971) Role of periodic breast cancer screening in reducing mortality from breast cancer, *J. Amer. med. Ass.*, **215**, 1777.

SPRI (1972) *Follow-up Study of Health Screening in Eskilstuna*, Rapport 9/72, Stockholm.

Thorner, R. M. (1971) The status of activity in automated health testing in the U.S., in *Automated Multiphasic Health Testing*, Engineering Foundation, New York, p. 225.

Thorner, R. M., and Remein, Q. R. (1961) Principles and procedures in the evaluation of screening for disease, *Publ. Hlth Monogr.*, **67** (P.H.S. publication, No. 846).

Truett, J., Cornfield, J., and Kannel, W. (1967) A multivariate analysis of the risk of coronary heart disease in Framingham, *J. chron. Dis.*, **20**, 511.

United States Commission on Chronic Illness (1957) *Chronic Illness in the United States*, Vol. I, Cambridge, Mass.

United States National Health Survey (1964) *Glucose Tolerance of Adults*, National Center for Health Statistics, Series 11, 2, U.S. Department of Health Education and Welfare, Washington, D.C.

United States Veterans Administration Co-operative Study Group on Antihypertensive Agents (1970) Effects of treatment on morbidity in hypertension, *J. Amer. med. Ass.*, **213**, 1143.

University Group Diabetes Program (1971) A study of the effects of hypoglycaemic agents on vascular complications in patients with adult onset diabetes, *Diabetes*, **19**, Suppl. 2.

Whitehead, T. P., Carmalt, M. H. B., and Widdowson, G. M. (1967) *Hospital Admission Profiles, Automation in Analytical Chemistry*, Vol. II, New York, p. 77.

Wilson, J. M. G. (1968) Evaluation of prescriptive screening for phenylketonuria, in *Screening in Medical Care*, Nuffield Provincial Hospitals Trust, London, p. 97.

Wilson, J. M. G., and Jungner, G. (1968) Principles and practice of screening for disease, *Wld Hlth Org. Publ. Hlth Pap.*, No. 34.

Wilson, J. M. G. (1970) Problems in the evaluation of screening for disease, *Ann. Soc. belge Med. trop.*, **50**, 4, 489.

Wilson, J. M. G. (1973) Current trends and problems in health screening, *J. clin. Path.*, **26**, 555.

Yule, R. (1973) The prevention of cancer of the cervix by cytological screening of the population, in *Cancer of the Uterine Cervix*, ed. Easson, E. C., Philadelphia, p. 11.

51

INTERNATIONAL HEALTH ORGANIZATIONS

LEO A. KAPRIO

Introduction

Co-operation in the health field across national borders is continually increasing. Scientific collaboration is now world wide, as no country can afford to isolate itself from the development of research elsewhere. Co-operation in improving the application of scientific research also calls for mutual contact on an international scale. Moreover, many countries need direct assistance from more fortunate ones in setting up a national health organization. Every government, if it is properly to serve its population, must build up its teaching institutions and services; otherwise their peoples will not be able to enjoy in the reasonably near future the major benefits made possible by the medical advances of the past hundred years.

International co-operation over health is not an isolated phenomenon. International action to improve social and economic conditions throughout the world has been approved in principle by the Charter of the United Nations and spelt out in various documents accepted by nations of the world such as the 'Universal Declaration of Human Rights' and in the constitutions of various organizations belonging to the United Nations' family.

Despite the 'cold war', limited 'hot wars', and many political and economic problems, there has, since the Second World War, been a growing concern for the well-being of mankind as a whole. The results of action taken may still be meagre and may have been counteracted by such phenomena as rapid population growth (as such, a sign of the improvement of certain conditions) or by unexpected food shortages. However a growing number of people are coming to realize that all human beings live on the same globe, share the same risks and, hence, cannot afford to live in isolation. Accordingly, we share responsibility for seeing that there is balanced social and economic development in the world as a whole. The prime motivation may be negative—fear of the hydrogen bomb making us opt for peace, or positive—a real sense of unity. But these more philosophical problems are best left to each to analyse for himself.

History of International Co-operation in the Field of Health

International co-operation in the health field goes back to the time when the first industrialized countries sought to keep international trade going despite epidemics such as cholera. Another early impetus derived from humanitarian motives which found expression in attempts to reduce suffering during wars. The International Sanitary Conferences, which sought to reach quarantine agreements, and the International Red Cross, can be singled out as successful examples of international co-operation. They led on gradually to large permanent international agencies such as the World Health Organization (WHO) and the League of Red Cross Societies.

The first International Sanitary Conference was held in Paris in 1851–52. This started a series of international meetings which finally, in 1903, led to an international agreement—the International Sanitary Convention—to control certain epidemic and quarantinable diseases. This was the early predecessor of the modern International Health Regulations now administered by WHO. The International Sanitary Convention needed an organization to deal with its practical application and, in 1907, in Rome, an agreement was signed by twelve countries to set up an International Office of Public Health in Paris known by its French name of l'Office international d'Hygiène publique (OIHP). The main function of OIHP was to disseminate to Member States information of general public health interest, and especially relating to communicable diseases such as cholera, plague, and yellow fever, and the measures taken to combat them. It was also to suggest improvements in the International Sanitary Convention and to publish a monthly bulletin. The OIHP continued its work despite the disruption of the First World War. When the League of Nations was later established the merging of OIHP and a health organization to be established by the League of Nations was discussed. A proposal to this effect was made by the International Health Conference which took place in 1920 in London. However, the OIHP continued its independent work, albeit in close co-operation with the new Health Organization of the League of Nations. The latter, which started work in 1921, developed further the work of combating epidemic diseases, on an international scale, established an Epidemiological Intelligence Service with an Eastern Bureau in Singapore, and set up a special commission to tackle the problem of malaria. In the next few years the League of Nations Health Organization broke new ground through the work of its Cancer Commission and gradually extended its work to the fields of biological standardization, housing physical fitness, typhus, leprosy, medical and public health training, rural hygiene, and unification of the pharmacopoeias. The most outstanding example in leadership by the Health Organization is perhaps to be found in its work on nutrition, later again taken up and expanded by WHO and FAO. With the outbreak of the Second World War international health work came once more almost to a standstill. The remaining staff members of the League of Nations Epidemiological Intelligence Service were transferred from Geneva to the United States to organize an epidemiological intelligence service in the health division of the United Nations Relief and Rehabilitation Administration (UNRRA), which was the new social agency created by the war time allies to take care of social reconstruction in liberated countries in the immediate post-war period. In January 1945 UNRRA also assumed responsibility for OIHP's duties in respect of the international sanitary conventions. Although UNRRA was a temporary organization created to deal with an emergency situation during and after the war, the work of its Health Division provided all indispensable links between intergovernmental health activities before and after the war. It combated epidemics, administered the international sanitary conventions, provided essential medical supplies, and helped the governments of fifteen countries to rebuild and even improve their health services.

Before going on to the establishment of UNRRA's successor —the World Health Organization—mention should be made of the work of a regional body—the Pan American Sanitary Bureau (PASB), which strongly influenced the future structure of WHO. As early as 1902, representatives of the republics of the Americas established the first International Health Bureau with its own Secretariat to deal with common regional health problems in that continent. From 1923 on it was known as the Pan American Sanitary Bureau. Its regional organization, which now co-operates closely with WHO is called Pan American Health Organization (PAHO). PASB, under an agreement signed in 1949, now represents WHO in the Americas.

Turning to non-governmental international health activities, mention must be made of the Rockefeller Foundation and its International Health Board formed in 1913. This agency dealt with international health problems, supported disease eradication, medical education, the development of rural health services, and the establishment of schools of public health all over the world. Its training programme and fellowships created several generations of internationally oriented health experts and greatly influenced developments in the international health field.

The experience of all these international health organizations was available when the United Nations Organization was set up at the San Francisco Conference in 1945, and this conference decided that a special international health organization should be established.

An International Health Conference was convened in June and July 1946 in New York. It approved the Constitution of WHO and decided that its functions should include those of OIHP. At the same time it created a regional organization which could accommodate PASB.

After an interim period WHO officially started its work in 1948. Its official birthday is 7 April—World Health Day— when twenty-six Member States of the United Nations ratified WHO's Constitution. It is now celebrated in practically every country in the world. A special topic is selected each year: 1971, 'A Full Life Despite Diabetes'; 1972, 'Your Heart is Your Health'; and 1973, 'Health Begins at Home'.

INTERNATIONAL HEALTH ACTIVITIES

WHO is now the only international global governmental health agency. It has well-established relations with other United Nations organizations such as UNICEF, FAO, and ILO, and co-operates closely with the League of Red Cross Societies. Before going into its structure and activities it would be useful to note the various auspices under which international health is being conducted at the present moment. The major ones are: governmental, Red Cross, non-governmental organizations, universities and research institutions, foundations, religious orders, and missions, and industry with international interests.

Governments

Governments carry out international health activities on a global scale through WHO. Certain international activities, such as child welfare, are supported by UNICEF, nutrition by FAO, education by UNESCO, and so on, but in close coordination with WHO. On a regional basis, governments are also developing health activities, mainly through WHO's Regional Offices. In the case of the Americas the Pan American Sanitary Bureau is, at one and the same time, the office of the Pan American Health Organization of American States as well as the Regional Office for the Americas of WHO. The Council of Europe has a special Public Health Committee working closely with the WHO Regional Office for Europe. A new Asian medical organization, SEAMHO, the South-East Asia Medical and Health Organization, has been established and works in close co-operation with the Regional Office for the Western Pacific of the World Health Organization. Governments support United Nations' multilateral activities by yearly contributions assessed in principle on a similar basis to a tax, but may, in addition, provide voluntary contributions via the United Nations Development Programme or by donations to UNICEF.

In addition to these multilateral activities, several governments provide through bilateral agreements with friendly countries, support for health activities as part of their broader aid programme, or engage in joint activities with neighbouring countries—co-operation is sometimes militarily or politically directed. The actual financial contributions in bilateral programmes are, in most cases, higher than for multilateral assistance; bilateral assistance is much more geared to medical supplies, vehicles, construction materials, whereas multilateral assistance provides rather for advisory services, fellowships, and meetings.

Of course, one of the examples of interesting, but almost constantly changing, bilateral assistance is that provided by the United States. France and the United Kingdom, too, for example, provide continuous, rather large-scale bilateral assistance with a 'health component' to several territories which were formerly under their political control. The Federal Republic of Germany, the northern countries of Europe, and many others, run a considerable number of growing bilateral assistance programmes with health components. The government of Sweden was one of the first to support family planning on an international scale.

International Red Cross and League of Red Cross Societies

The International Red Cross Committee, established in 1863, and the League of Red Cross Societies, established in 1919, serve specific humanitarian purposes, especially in wartime. The national Red Cross or Red Crescent and Red Lion and Sun Societies in many countries have pioneered health activities, training programmes, and the establishment of health institutions. The League of Red Cross Societies has a permanent health programme and co-operates closely with WHO.

Red Cross activities are of special importance in war- or peace-time crises and, together with the United Nations Office of the High Commissioner for Refugees, the League has played an important role in alleviating suffering at times when political and economic measures have been unable to prevent catastrophes. Since 1972, the UN has had a 'Disaster Relief Co-ordinator' who works in full co-operation with the League of Red Cross Societies. Of course, the charitable work of organizations such as CARE and OXFAM can have a great influence on health conditions in emergency situations.

Non-governmental Organizations

A large number of voluntary organizations of different kinds have been accorded consultative status in the United Nations family. In the health field they are mainly of two types; on the one hand, large international bodies formed by professional associations such as the World Medical Association, the International Council of Nurses, and, on the other, international groups interested in combating specific diseases, such as the International Union Against Tuberculosis, the International Union Against Cancer, the International Society of Cardiology and the International Union for Health Education. The membership of the World Federation of Public Health Associations, which has consultative status with WHO, consists of important national organizations such as the Royal Society of Health and the American Public Health Association. At the end of January 1973, there were 106 non-governmental organizations in official relationship with WHO. (See p. 673)

Universities and Research Institutions

In medical research it is generally accepted that new achievements in medicine should be made internationally available to all other institutions and services interested in applying them for the benefit of the people. Accordingly, there is often close international co-operation between groups of universities having the same research interests. Lately there has been a growing tendency for universities in the developed countries to assist in building up new teaching institutions and research centres in the developing parts of the world. There are, for example, a number of interdepartmental links between British and overseas teaching institutions in the field of medicine, where there has been interchange of teaching staff and the same type of relationship has long existed between American schools of public health and universities and institutions overseas.

In addition to the traditional bilateral co-operation between research institutions, WHO, and the International Agency for Research on Cancer (which is part of WHO and situated in Lyon, France) illustrate the growing tendency to support research on a world-wide scale.

The CIOMS (Council for International Organizations of Medical Sciences) secretariat in Geneva is concerned with scientific contacts at international level and works in close co-operation with, and is supported by, UNESCO and WHO.

Foundations

Reference has already been made to the international health work undertaken by the Rockefeller Foundation. It still makes a large contribution to the development of medical education. However, it is not the only foundation which has been involved

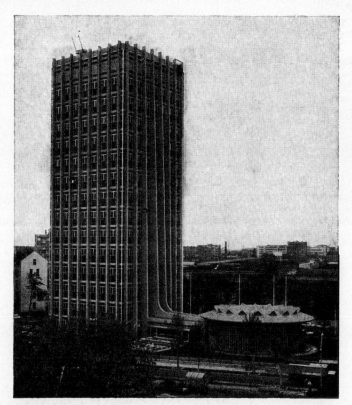

FIG. 117. The new building of the International Agency for Research on Cancer, Lyon, France.

in health work, medical education, and research. The Ford, Kellogg, Milbank, and, in the United Kingdom, the Nuffield Foundations are other examples. The Ford and Rockefeller Foundations support agencies such as the Population Council which has played an important role in research and field work in family planning and population problems at world level. The Milbank Foundation has assisted, in particular, in medical manpower studies.

The Religious Orders and Missions

The religious orders and missions have done work for sick people since their establishment which, in some cases, goes back in history to the time of the Crusades and even earlier. There are similar examples from the other religious movements. However, in the modern world many religious orders and missions continue, especially in developing countries, to give extremely worthwhile services. They provide hospital care or special treatment facilities for diseases such as leprosy. In many cases they are becoming more and more involved in training international health personnel. Similar work, of course, is done by some of the non-governmental organizations described above and for similar human motives to those of the religious orders and missions.

Industry

Several different industries having international interests and subsidiaries in many countries have contributed positively to the development of health services, especially in developing countries, or have strongly supported internationally important research.

The drug industry has often been attacked for its commercial aspects but, at the same time, its internal competition has produced innovations which have helped to solve international health problems. WHO and UNICEF find themselves in the position of having to demand from the industry, for example, new drugs for tropical diseases and new pesticides or, as in the last few years, new birth control methods.

WORLD HEALTH ORGANIZATION

The World Health Organization is today the most important of the international health organizations. It is the only health agency that aims at global coverage and can hope one day to

However, as with the United Nations and other Specialized Agencies, there have been conflicting political opinions among powerful Member States, or groups of them, that have affected the general will to co-operate. Differences as to how WHO should work have also inhibited, up till now, full use of the Organization's potential. Its terms of reference, as spelled out in its Constitution, would allow much more to be done.

The Aims of the Organization

The Constitution of WHO bears remarkable witness to the optimism of public health leaders of a generation ago. Among other things it declares, in conformity with the United Nations Charter, that:

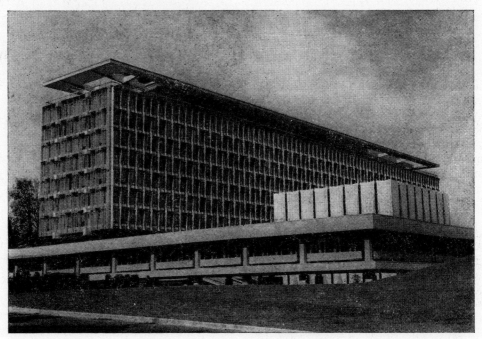

FIG. 118. General view of the World Health Organization headquarters building in Geneva.

count all countries of the world as members. Indeed, its membership is already so extensive and its work so far developed that an analysis of its objectives, function, structure, and activities will, in itself, give an over-all picture of how international health problems are being dealt with in our time.

WHO's Role in International Health

With more than 20 years' experience as an international health organization, WHO has now become the focal point for the intergovernmental co-ordination of health activities on a world scale. Close co-operation is also maintained with non-governmental organizations over a broad field of medical and health problems.

WHO is in a position to follow health trends and the development of health services and conditions throughout the world. Where the Member States have so wished and have given it the means, the organization has also been able to take action in a number of fields. It has even influenced countries in the achievement of permanent improvements in their health conditions by means of technical assistance.

Health is a state of complete physical, mental, and social well-being and not merely the absence of disease or infirmity.

The enjoyment of the highest attainable standard of health is one of the fundamental rights of every human being without distinction of race, religion, political belief, economic, or social condition.

The health of all people is fundamental to the attainment of peace and security and is dependent upon the fullest co-operation of individuals and States.

The achievement of any State in the promotion and protection of health is of value to all.

Unequal development in different countries in the promotion of health and control of disease, especially communicable disease, is a common danger.

Healthy development of the child is of basic importance; the ability to live harmoniously in a changing total environment is essential to such development.

The extension to all peoples of the benefits of medical, psychological, and related knowledge is essential to the fullest attainment of health.

Informed opinion and active co-operation on the part of the

public are of the utmost importance in the improvement of the health of the people.

Governments have a responsibility for the health of their peoples which can be fulfilled only by the provision of adequate health and social measures.

The Constitution then goes on to state: 'The objective of the World Health Organization shall be the attainment by all peoples of the highest possible level of health.'

The principle of 'complete' health quoted above has sometimes been criticized as non-scientific, but it has to be read in the right context. It is a political statement and not an exact scientific biological definition. The functions, some very specific, listed in the next chapter of the Constitution are still valid and show the basic realism of the founders of WHO.

WHO Functions and Programme of Work

The Constitution starts by committing the Organization to 'act as the directing and co-ordinating authority on international health work'.

Several specific functions are then listed which, even now, are still somewhat broader than the Organization can cope with in practice. Nevertheless, this list has served as a guide to the Organization's governing bodies in selecting priorities.

The early World Health Assemblies requested the Organization to attack certain problems as a matter of priority, and soon a special four-year plan—the first of a series of general programmes of work—was hammered out and implemented from 1952 to 1955. The present plan is the Fifth General Programme of Work Covering a Specific Period (1973 to 1977 inclusive). It defines WHO's present functions as a combination in varying proportions of global, interregional, regional, and intercountry activities, and of direct assistance to individual countries for specific programmes aimed at achieving better health for their people through national effort.

An important role of WHO is to consolidate these broad types of basically interrelated activities as complementary aspects of an international health programme. Global activities are interpreted and adapted at regional and country level and thus often have immediate and practical implications for national health programmes; and, similarly, direct assistance to countries for specific programmes contributes to international health programmes. The major programme objectives are:

Strengthening the Health Services of Member States. This concentrates on health planning, implementation of health plans, management of health services and institutions, evaluation of health systems, programmes, and services and development of comprehensive community health services. Within the framework, the Organization's aim is to assist Member States that need such help to achieve complete coverage of the population by permanent health services. In co-operation with the United Nations Children's Fund (UNICEF), family and child health services are given high priority. Family planning services form part of this programme, when requested by governments, and WHO and UNICEF now have funds available from the UNFPA (UN Fund for Population Activities) for this purpose.

Development of Health Manpower. Strengthening of health services implies in large measure strengthening of health manpower and the optimal use of professional and auxiliary personnel.

Training of national health personnel has been the concern of WHO since its inception. In almost all of its varied activities the Organization has found that inevitably governments have requested help to overcome the personnel shortage that has hampered the execution of their health programmes. The training of greater numbers of people for specific types of health work has increasingly become one of WHO's main preoccupations and is strongly emphasized in its Fifth General Programme of Work. The Organization will concentrate its activities in the field of education and training on the following main areas: (1) the adjustment of education schemes, curricula, and teaching methods and media to meet the local requirements, with emphasis on the team approach to the education of health workers; (2) the training of auxiliary personnel; (3) the training of teachers; (4) the provision of continuing education; and (5) educational methodology and technology. Assistance to individual countries as well as the development of intercountry programmes will, accordingly, be along these lines.

Disease Prevention and Control. In the Fifth General Programme of Work this refers both to communicable and non-communicable diseases. WHO exerts a leading role in promoting and co-ordinating epidemiological surveillance at national, regional, and global levels, the principles of surveillance being common to all forms of disease of public health importance, even though details vary with the type of disease.

The surveillance and control of many communicable diseases is made more difficult by the increasing speed and volume of national and international travel and migration. However, specific programmes against malaria, smallpox, cholera, yellow fever, trachoma and other communicable diseases will continue, depending on national and international needs. The malaria eradication programme has already freed a large part of the world population of the scourge of malaria and there is a possibility that, in the near future, the world will be free of smallpox. After eradication, maintenance programmes will continue in the context of national public health programmes with WHO support.

In the field of non-communicable diseases, WHO's attention was drawn early to the problem of widespread cardiovascular diseases, causing premature death and invalidity, and it is expected that work in this field will be intensified. Since 1968, in the European Region a specific long-term programme has been mobilizing both governments and institutions dealing with cardiovascular diseases towards a uniform approach to the prevention, early cure, and rehabilitation of cardiovascular disease.

The International Agency for Research on Cancer has already been mentioned but WHO will continue to develop programmes in cancer control—cancer registers and the evaluation of screening programmes—as well as the development of personnel, for example, for cytology, radiation treatment, etc.

However, other chronic diseases can be assisted on the basis of individual requests from countries—diseases such as diabetes, rheumatoid arthritis, chronic respiratory diseases and renal conditions.

WHO's work in the prevention of accidents, especially traffic accidents, also belongs to this part of the General

Programme of work. Considerable attention has been given to this matter in the European Region where traffic accidents are one of the biggest public health problems.

The prevalence of mental disorders is an important public health problem in both developed and developing countries. Under conditions of social stress, such as may occur in the process of rapid urbanization and industrialization, the incidence may rise, as it does with the ageing of populations. WHO will continue with the international collation and analysis of reliable statistical data, based on comparable criteria, with a view to arriving at a more precise definition of the scope of the

communities, a problem that has become of international concern not only to WHO but also to other United Nations agencies. Close co-operation in this field encouraged the establishment of the UN Environment Secretariat in Nairobi in 1973.

Subjects of General International Health Interest. Implementation of the aims outlined above is usually achieved by direct assistance to, and co-operation with, the Member States. However, WHO's programme of work also includes subjects with legal implications and of general international health interest. Action in this field is based on Article 21 of the

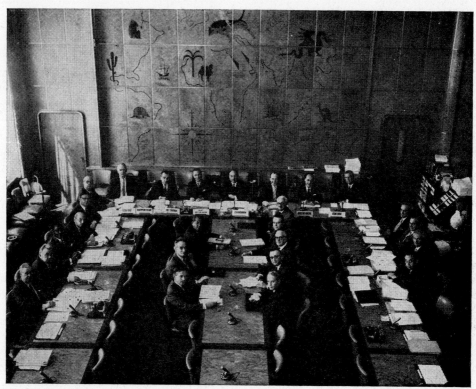

FIG. 119. Top scientists meet in Geneva. The world-wide medical research programme of the World Health Organization being reviewed by nineteen top scientists.

problem. It will continue to assist in the delivery of mental health care through the general health services. In spite of the improved prognosis for most mental patients in recent decades, owing to important advances in treatment and in social attitudes towards them, and in spite of the fact that many can now be successfully and rapidly adjusted to community life, if not cured, the control of mental disorders will depend on further knowledge of their aetiology and long-term evolution. The Organization will therefore concentrate on research in respect of socio-psychological, epidemiological, and biological aspects of mental disorders as an essential part of efforts to reduce the heavy burden on communities.

Promotion of Environmental Health. From the outset, environmental health has held an important place in the Organization's programme. In addition to supporting the improvement of general community sanitation, it has faced special challenges in the need to provide, on the one hand, clean water supplies for developing countries and, on the other, to reduce environmental pollution in industrialized and urban

WHO Constitution. One example is the International Health Regulations (1969) which came into force on 1 January 1971. These now form the basis of the obligatory international reporting system for four infectious diseases—plague, cholera, yellow fever, and smallpox—and recommend continuous national surveillance of paralytic poliomyelitis, louse-borne typhus, louse-borne relapsing fever, malaria, and viral influenza. A second example, concerned with the nomenclature of diseases, is the International Classification of Diseases (1965 revision). WHO inherited from the League of Nations the right to provide standards and has used it mainly for biological and pharmaceutical products. The Twenty-sixth World Health Assembly approved the latest list of international standards for biological substances which include various tuberculins, toxoids, vaccines, serums, antitoxins, antibiotics, hormones, as well as insulin, heparin, vitamin D, and digitalis, to mention but a few.

A series of recommendations on various subjects has been made on the basis of Article 23 of the WHO Constitution.

Research. The World Health Organization is an agency which co-ordinates research in selected fields of medicine and public health that are of international importance. Research in insecticide resistance and on new insecticides presents but one example of the very wide field in which the Organization is acting as a co-ordinating centre. The International Agency for Research on Cancer under the aegis of WHO co-ordinates cancer research on a world-wide scale. Various divisions of WHO Headquarters maintain continuous contact with research workers in their own field and obtain the latest information on research applicable to the national services. WHO also en-

Membership of WHO

Membership of the Organization, under its Constitution, is open to all states. By the end of April 1974 WHO had 140 Member States and 2 Associate Members (territories not responsible for the conduct of their international relations). The universality of WHO—as of the United Nations and its Specialized Agencies—long a controversial subject, is now almost complete as the People's Republic of China, the German Democratic Republic, and the Democratic People's Republic of Korea have now become active members.

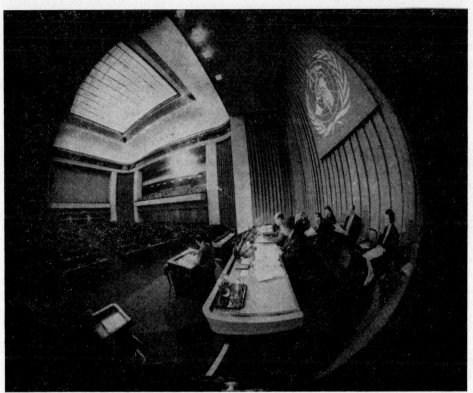

FIG. 120. World Health Organization headquarters. The World Health Assembly seen through the fish-eye lens.

courages multidisciplinary research on an international scale of which a recent, and still expanding, example is research in the field of human reproduction.

Co-ordination. The WHO programme is not without influence on other aspects of socio-economic development, such as labour productivity and population growth. At the same time availability of food, shelter, education, and transport, as well as the income level of the population, has a far-reaching influence on health services. Close co-operation is needed with many other agencies: over child health and welfare with UNICEF; over nutrition with the United Nations Food and Agriculture Organization (FAO); over education with UNESCO; over the use of isotopes and disposal of radioactive wastes with the International Atomic Energy Agency (IAEA); and with the United Nations itself over town planning and population policy, to list only a few important items.

Administrative co-ordination between the United Nations and its family of organizations also calls for constant attention to ensure uniform policies and avoid duplication of effort.

Every member of the Organization contributes to its regular budget and has a vote in its constitutional meetings.

The Structure of the Organization

The work of WHO is carried out by the World Health Assembly, the Executive Board and the Secretariat.

The World Health Assembly is composed of delegates representing Members. It meets in an annual session, usually at Geneva, Switzerland, but occasionally elsewhere, as in 1969 at Boston.

The Assembly determines the Organization's policies, names the Members entitled to designate a person to serve on the Board, and appoints the Director-General. It reviews and approves reports and activities of the Board and Director-General, supervises financial policy, and reviews and approves the budget of the whole Organization. It also has authority to adopt international regulations and make recommendations to Members in any matters within the competence of WHO.

The Executive Board—the executive organ of the Assembly

—consisted in 1973 of twenty-four persons designated by as many Members. However, an amendment to the Constitution in process of ratification would expand the membership to thirty. The Board then meets twice a year to prepare for the Assembly and to advise the Director-General.

The Head of the Secretariat is the Director-General, who is appointed by the Assembly on the nomination of the Board, and is the chief technical and administrative officer. The first Director-General of WHO, from 1948 to 1953, was Dr. Brock Chisholm, the second, from 1953 to 1973, Dr. Marcolino Candau. The World Health Assembly in 1973 appointed Dr. Halfdan Mahler as the third Director-General.

WHO has staff at its headquarters in Geneva, at six Regional Offices and in the field in various countries whose health programmes are supported by WHO projects. The Organization also provides staff and technical guidance for a number of projects financed by the United Nations Development Programme and by UNICEF. WHO representatives co-ordinate WHO assistance in a large number of developing countries, acting as advisers to the ministries of health.

Budget

The regular budget of WHO, based mainly on income from the contributions of Member States, has increased from $5 million in 1949, the first full year of operation, to approximately $115 million, the effective working budget approved for 1975. In 1973, 31·8 per cent. of the funds available for the operating programme were directed to strengthening basic national health services. Ten per cent. went to environmental health and 22·8 per cent. to communicable disease control. Another 12·5 per cent. was earmarked for health manpower development and 4·6 per cent. for non-communicable diseases; the remainder covered world-wide services to be rendered by WHO in the fields of epidemiology, statistics, biology, pharmacology, and toxicology. WHO medical research funds were spent mainly on investigating communicable diseases, with smaller allocations for other fields.

Funds from the United Nations Development Programme and UNICEF for health projects carried out by WHO in developing countries form an important additional source of assistance.

Expert Advisory Panel

To ensure that WHO is kept fully up to date with every aspect of health services throughout the world, a large body of expertise is at the disposal of the Director-General and the Secretariat. Individuals from the Expert Advisory Panel are called to man expert committees and scientific groups which meet in Geneva at the WHO Headquarters and whose reports guide the work of the Organization, even if they are not always necessarily accepted as official policy. The Regional Offices use national administrators and other experts to advise on the development of Regional activities. All this results in a large number of reports which are made available to the Member States.

WHO Publications

Such reports are published in the Technical Reports Series (references to which appear after practically every chapter in this book), the Monograph Series and the Public Health Papers and, at Regional level, in various regional series. In the Americas they are usually on sale but in other Regions they are chiefly available to the governments and institutions concerned. However, WHO Headquarters has a large publication programme including historical documents such as *The First Ten Years of the World Health Organization*, and *The Second Ten Years of the World Health Organization*; handbooks such as *The Medical Research Programme of the World Health Organization*, *Basic Documents*, the *Constitution of the World Health Organization*, *Handbook of Resolutions and Decisions of the World Health Assembly and Executive Board*, and the *Official Records of the World Health Organization*. 1973 saw the beginning of the new *Offset Publications Series*. Periodicals include the *Bulletin of the World Health Organization*, the *WHO Chronicle*, the *International Digest of Health Legislation*, the *World Health Statistics Report*, the *World Health Statistics Annual*, and the *Weekly Epidemiological Record*.

Publications are usually in English and French but are increasingly available in other languages such as Russian and Spanish. The Pan American Sanitary Bureau, WHO's Regional Office for the Americas, publishes mainly in English and Spanish.

The World Health Organization also operates a Medline Centre. Medline is the on-line version of MEDLARS (Medical Literature Analysis and Retrieval System) of the US National Library of Medicine, Bethesda, Maryland (see also p. 602).

WHO International Reference Centres

An international reference centre may be defined as an institution designated by WHO or by competent and specialized international bodies to assist, where needed, in the development and maintenance of high standards of work in specialized fields. The WHO centres provide certain services of international value to practice and research in medicine and public health, with the aim of improving precision, reliability, consistency, and comparability in medical practice and in national and international studies of medical or public health problems.

Together with regional and national reference centres, the international reference centres form an important world-wide network of institutions that facilitate the use of specific standards in materials and practice. They may also develop collaborative research on problems arising from their work and from the material and information they receive.

These centres cover an ever-increasing range of subjects. Responsibility for some of them passed to WHO from the Health Organization of the League of Nations.

Regional reference centres have responsibilities similar to those of international reference centres, but restricted to those they are fitted to accept and limited to a group of geographically related countries. They collaborate closely with the related international reference centres and with national reference centres.

There are also WHO collaborating laboratories, which assist in particular WHO activities related to the work of reference centres, in conjunction either with the Organization or with an international reference centre.

The international reference centres undertake some or all of the following activities: consultation, the collection of material or data, assistance in establishing standards and material at the request of the Organization, the production and distribution of standard materials, the exchange of information, and training. WHO may contribute to the cost of those activities that are additional to the work of the host institution.

It can thus be seen that the work of these centres is an integral part of the technical activities of WHO, and is appropriate to the international breadth of the Organization's responsibilities and interests.

With the valuable help of the centres, WHO strives to establish standard substances, nomenclatures, etc. that will be internationally accepted and used. In all these activities, the assistance of collaborating laboratories in many countries ensures that full use is made of scientists with a wide range of experience.

A complete list is available from the Headquarters of the World Health Organization, WHO, Geneva.

Regional Offices and Field Activities

Typical of WHO is that its Regional Offices deal with technical assistance and direct practical co-operation with Member States; they are also responsible for the supervision of field activities supported by WHO in individual Member States.

There are six Regional Offices, located in Brazzaville, Washington, Alexandria, Copenhagen, Manila, and New Delhi. These are in direct contact with member governments. WHO's programme is first discussed by the six Regional Committees, which review and approve the annual reports of their Regional Directors and recommend the regional budget proposals to be included in the Director-General's budget. A large number of smaller conferences, symposia, training courses, and other training activities, are arranged regionally. Studies of health conditions in Member States are conducted by the Regional Offices and various reports made available.

WHO's large fellowship programme is also mainly a regional responsibility, the Regions for the Americas and Europe receiving the largest number of fellows from other parts of the world. WHO fellowships are mainly for postgraduate students, but a number of undergraduates have been trained from those countries which do not as yet have their own universities.

Under Headquarters' guidance, the Regional Offices are responsible for United Nations Development Programme (Special Fund) projects. These are usually large-scale programmes providing, for example, for big public health institutions, the training of sanitary engineers, occupational health facilities, or water supply and sewage installations.

The Regional Offices establish, with the Resident Representatives of the UNDP and the national authorities, the health sector of the UNDP country programme; an example of the co-ordination of UN assistance to developing countries.

The Organization, in many cases, maintains staff in the developing countries which it assists. Thus, in a number of Asian, African, or Latin American countries, it has a WHO Representative as chief adviser to the Ministry of Health. WHO Representatives are senior medical officers or public health administrators, with more than ten years' experience at senior level in their own countries or in international work. They may have a public health adviser to assist them, as well as a public health nurse/midwife and sanitary inspector to contribute to building up basic rural health services, and a health engineer to deal with water, sewage, and vector control

problems. An epidemiologist, specializing in infectious and tropical diseases, may be appointed to help develop an epidemiological service and a group of nurse educators to teach in a nursing school and help to organize nursing services. A malaria and smallpox eradication team will establish a mobile staff group to support permanent health workers tackling those

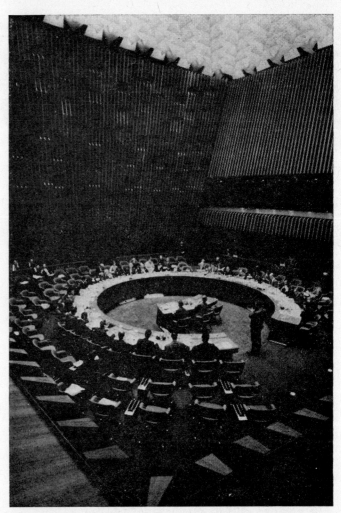

FIG. 121. World Health Organization headquarters building. The 24 members of the Executive Board during its 38th Session, the first to be held in its new headquarters, at their places around the circular table.

two diseases. An expert in maternal and child health may train medical and nursing staff to give proper emphasis to the child population, teach mothers, undertake health education, particularly as regards acceptance of vaccination, promote better nutrition, and introduce new methods of work to national staff.

In more than sixty countries staff groups are working in this way under WHO Representatives, and in others there are many more smaller groups dealing with specific problems that have been neglected in the past. Consultant services are provided for all countries of the world.

Other Important Health Organizations

No review of international health organizations would be complete without mention of the United Nations Children's Fund (UNICEF). It was set up as a post-war emergency

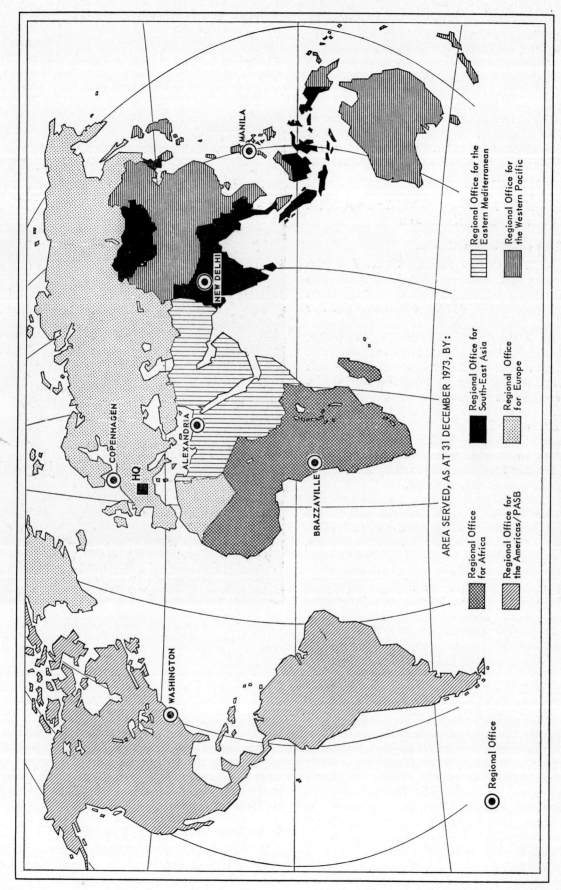

AREA SERVED, AS AT 31 DECEMBER 1973, BY:

Regional Office
for Africa

Regional Office for
the Americas/PASB

Regional Office for
South-East Asia

Regional Office
for Europe

Regional Office for the
Eastern Mediterranean

Regional Office for
the Western Pacific

⊙ Regional Office

Fig. 122. WHO Regional Offices and the areas they serve.

agency, but has continued as a permanent international 'children's bureau', devoting almost half of its budget to health activities, the remainder being spent on educational work and social welfare. UNICEF has paid special attention to nutrition, maternal and child health, and campaigns against communicable disease, including malaria. Equipment, vehicles, drugs, and stipends provided for local training activities have greatly increased the ability of governments to make use of WHO's advisory services.

The Pan American Health Organization is at the same time WHO's American Regional organization, but has its own long history and a large budget in addition to WHO's regular budget. Accordingly it is distinct from other WHO Regional Offices in that it conducts a more varied type of work in the field of publication and research, which would, in other parts of the world, be the responsibility of WHO Headquarters. It recently, 1972, celebrated its seventieth anniversary.

Reference has already been made to the new South East Asia Medical and Health Organization which may play a similar important role in the future.

In Europe, the WHO Regional Office co-operates with the Public Health Committee and other health activities of the Council of Europe. The Council's health section, while it consults WHO regarding important health problems, works in close contact with the Ministries of Health of its own Member States, concentrating on the standardization of health legislation and making recommendations in matters of public health

importance. Its group fellowships have produced interesting reports.

WHO's Influence on the Public Health Movement

The Organization, in 1973, has been in existence for twenty-five years and has clearly established itself as the co-ordinator of international health activities; its almost universal membership guarantees that it will continue to play this role. As the central world health agency responsible, among other things, for international quarantine, epidemiological intelligence, and the classification of diseases, and assistance to Member States, it has had a considerable influence on attitudes to public health throughout the world.

The wider acceptance today of the importance of health planning and of health manpower policies, readiness to analyse the economic aspects of medical care and the increased attention given to health education by central health administrations are certainly due to the continuous contact maintained between all leading health authorities through WHO. It is thanks to WHO's existence that a dialogue can take place between countries with greater economic resources and those with less. Such problems as the flight of talent in medicine and medical and biological research from one country to another, can also be discussed. On the whole, a more preventive and rational approach to disease and health is developing throughout the world and a greater readiness is being shown by health administrators to benefit from the experience of others (Mahler, 1974).

REFERENCES AND FURTHER READING

Abt, G. (1933) *Vingt-cinq ans d'activite de l'Office international d'Hygiène publique, 1909–1933*, Paris.

Berkov, R. (1957) *The World Health Organization. A Study in Decentralized International Administration*, Geneva.

Brockington, Fraser (1967) *World Health*, 2nd ed., London.

Bustamante, Miguel E. (1955) *The Pan American Sanitary Bureau. Half a Century of Health Activities, 1902–1954*, Washington. (PASB Miscellaneous Publ., No. 23.)

Ciba Foundation (1967) *Health of Mankind*, London.

Goodman, N. M. (1971) *International Health Organizations*, 2nd ed., Edinburgh.

Hobson, W. (1963) *World Health and History*, Bristol.

Howard-Jones, N. (1972) Threescore Years and Ten. The Pan American Sanitary Bureau 1902–1972, article in *World Health*, December 1972.

Howard-Jones, N. (1974) The scientific background of the International Sanitary Conferences, 1851–1938. 1, *Wld Hlth Org. Chron.*, **28**, 4, 5, 8, 9, 10 and 11.

International Classification of Diseases—1965 Revision (1967), World Health Organization, Geneva.

International Health Regulation (1969) First Annotated Edition, World Health Organization, Geneva, 1971.

Mahler, H. (1974) An international health conscience, *Wld Hlth Org. Chron.*, **28**, 207.

Pan American Health Organization (1972) *Basic Documents of the Pan American Health Organization*, 10th ed., Washington, D.C.

Reports on the World Health Situation, 1954–68. First (1959), Second (1963), Third (1967), Fourth (1971).

Rockefeller Foundation (1964) *Toward the Well-being of Mankind*, New York.

Roelsgaard, E. (1974) Health regulations and international travel, *Wld Hlth Org. Chron.*, **28**, 265.

World Health Organization (1958) *The First Ten Years*, Geneva.

World Health Organization (1964) *The Medical Research Programme of the World Health Organization 1958–1963*, Report by the Director-General, Geneva.

World Health Organization (1967) *Twenty Years in South-East Asia 1948–1967*, New Delhi.

World Health Organization (1968) *The Second Ten Years; 1958–67*, Geneva.

World Health Organization (1969) *The Medical Research Programme of the World Health Organization 1964–1968*, Report by the Director-General, Geneva.

World Health Organization (1971) Fifth General Programme of Work Covering a Specific Period 1973/1977 inclusive, Offprint from *Official Records of the World Health Organization*, No. 193, Geneva.

World Health Organization (1972a) *Basic Documents*, 23rd ed. Geneva.

World Health Organization (1972b) *Training of Research Workers in the Medical Sciences*, Proceedings of a Round Table Conference organized by CIOMS with the assistance of WHO and UNESCO, Geneva, 10–11 September 1970.

World Health Organization (1974a) The scientific programme of IARC, *Wld Hlth Org. Chron.*, **28**, 269.

World Health Organization (1974b) The work of WHO in 1973, *Wld Hlth Org. Off. Rec.*, No. 213.

World Health Organization (1974c) *World Health Statistics Annual for 1970*, Geneva.

Vol. 1. Vital Statistics and Causes of Death.

Vol. 2. Infectious Diseases: Cases, Deaths and Vaccinations.

Vol. 3. Health Personnel and Hospital Establishments.

(Up-to-date information on WHO's activities can always be obtained from the latest report of the Director-General to the World Health Assembly and the Proposed Programme and Budget Estimates which are published in the Official Records of the World Health Organization, Geneva.)

Nongovernmental Organizations in Official Relations with WHO at 31 December 1973

Biometric Society
Christian Medical Commission
Council for International Organizations of Medical Sciences
Inter-American Association of Sanitary Engineering
International Academy of Legal Medicine and of Social Medicine
International Air Transport Association
International Association for Accident and Traffic Medicine
International Association of Agricultural Medicine
International Association for Child Psychiatry and Allied Professions
International Association of Logopedics and Phoniatrics
International Association of Medical Laboratory Technologists
International Association of Microbiological Societies
International Association for Prevention of Blindness
International Association on Water Pollution Research
International Astronautical Federation
International Brain Research Organization
International Commission on Radiation Units and Measurements
International Commission on Radiological Protection
International Committee of Catholic Nurses
International Committee on Laboratory Animals
International Committee of the Red Cross
International Confederation of Midwives
International Council on Alcohol and Addictions
International Council on Jewish Social and Welfare Services
International Council of Nurses
International Council of Scientific Unions
International Council on Social Welfare
International Council of Societies of Pathology
International Cystic Fibrosis (Mucoviscidosis) Association
International Dental Federation
International Diabetes Federation
International Epidemiological Association
International Ergonomics Association
International Federation of Fertility Societies
International Federation of Gynecology and Obstetrics
International Federation for Housing and Planning
International Federation for Information Processing
International Federation for Medical and Biological Engineering
International Federation of Medical Student Associations
International Federation of Multiple Sclerosis Societies
International Federation of Ophthalmological Societies
International Federation of Pharmaceutical Manufacturers Associations
International Federation of Physical Medicine
International Federation of Sports Medicine
International Federation of Surgical Colleges
International Hospital Federation
International Hydatidological Association
International League of Dermatological Societies
International League against Epilepsy
International League against Rheumatism
International Leprosy Association
International Organization for Standardization
International Organization against Trachoma
International Paediatric Association

International Pharmaceutical Federation
International Planned Parenthood Federation
International Radiation Protection Association
International Society of Biometeorology
International Society of Blood Transfusion
International Society for Burn Injuries
International Society of Cardiology
International Society of Endocrinology
International Society of Hematology
International Society of Orthopaedic Surgery and Traumatology
International Society of Radiographers and Radiological Technicians
International Society of Radiology
International Society for Rehabilitation of the Disabled
International Sociological Association
International Solid Wastes and Public Cleaning Association
International Union of Architects
International Union against Cancer
International Union for Child Welfare
International Union for Conservation of Nature and Natural Resources
International Union for Health Education
International Union of Immunological Societies
International Union of Local Authorities
International Union of Nutritional Sciences
International Union of Pharmacology
International Union of Pure and Applied Chemistry
International Union of School and University Health and Medicine
International Union against Tuberculosis
International Union against the Venereal Diseases and the Treponematoses
International Water Supply Association
Joint Commission on International Aspects of Mental Retardation
League of Red Cross Societies
Medical Women's International Association
Permanent Commission and International Association on Occupational Health
Population Council
Transplantation Society
World Association of Societies of (Anatomic and Clinical) Pathology
World Confederation for Physical Therapy
World Council for the Welfare of the Blind
World Federation of the Deaf
World Federation of Hemophilia
World Federation for Mental Health
World Federation of Neurology
World Federation of Neurosurgical Societies
World Federation of Occupational Therapists
World Federation of Parasitologists
World Federation of Public Health Associations
World Federation of Societies of Anaesthesiologists
World Federation of United Nations Associations
World Medical Association
World Psychiatric Association
World Veterans Federation
World Veterinary Association

Abbreviations Used in Volumes of the **Official Records of the World Health Organization**

ACABQ	Advisory Committee on Administrative and Budgetary Questions
ACAST	Advisory Committee on the Application of Science and Technology to Development
ACC	Administrative Committee on Co-ordination
CIOMS	Council for International Organizations of Medical Sciences
DANIDA	Danish International Development Agency
ECA	Economic Commission for Africa
ECAFE	Economic Commission for Asia and the Far East
ECE	Economic Commission for Europe
ECLA	Economic Commission for Latin America
FAO	Food and Agriculture Organization of the United Nations
IAEA	International Atomic Energy Agency
IARC	International Agency for Research on Cancer
IBRD	International Bank for Reconstruction and Development
ICAO	International Civil Aviation Organization
ILO	International Labour Organization (Office)
IMCO	Inter-Governmental Maritme Consultative Organization
ITU	International Telecommunication Union
OAU	Organization of African Unity
PAHO	Pan American Health Organization
PASB	Pan American Sanitary Bureau
SIDA	Swedish International Development Authority
UNCTAD	United Nations Conference on Trade and Development
UNDP	United Nations Development Programme
UNEP	United Nations Environment Programme
UNESCO	United Nations Educational, Scientific and Cultural Organization
UNESOB	United Nations Economic and Social Office in Beirut
UNFDAC	United Nations Fund for Drug Abuse Control
UNFPA	United Nations Fund for Population Activities
UNHCR	Office of the United Nations High Commissioner for Refugees
UNICEF	United Nations Children's Fund
UNIDO	United Nations Industrial Development Organization
UNITAR	United Nations Institute for Training and Research
UNRWA	United Nations Relief and Works Agency for Palestine Refugees in the Near East
UNSCEAR	United Nations Scientific Committee on the Effects of Atomic Radiation
USAID	United States Agency for International Development
WFP	World Food Programme
WHO	World Health Organization
WMO	World Meteorological Organization

INDEX